Biologic and Systemic Agents in Dermatology

Paul S. Yamauchi

Editor

Biologic and Systemic Agents in Dermatology

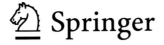 Springer

Editor
Paul S. Yamauchi, M.D., P.h.D.
Division of Dermatology
David Geffen School of Medicine a UCLA
Los Angeles, CA
USA

ISBN 978-3-319-66883-3   ISBN 978-3-319-66884-0   (eBook)
https://doi.org/10.1007/978-3-319-66884-0

Library of Congress Control Number: 2017963299

Printed on acid-free paper

This Springer imprint is published by Springer Nature
The registered company is Springer International Publishing AG
The registered company address is: Gewerbestrasse 11, 6330 Cham, Switzerland

This book is dedicated to my parents Mitsuko and Floyd Yamauchi, my wife Jennifer Yamauchi, and my brother and his wife Raymond Yamauchi and Veronica Partida. Without their love and support, this book would not have been possible.

Preface

The field of medical dermatology has rapidly evolved within the past 15 years. Indeed, these are exciting times in dermatology with the introduction of safer and more effective agents to treat various inflammatory dermatosis. Patient outcomes have improved tremendously due to advances in immunology that have led to the development of more targeted and selective therapies. The goal of this textbook is to provide an overview of the various biologic and systemic agents used to treat various dermatologic conditions such as psoriasis, atopic dermatitis, immunobullous disorders, skin cancers, urticaria, acne, alopecia, and numerous others. In addition, important topics such as pharmacoeconomics, compliance, combination therapy, pharmacovigilance, off-label uses, clinical trial interpretation, health outcomes, and several other subjects are discussed.

This book provides a useful all-in-one resource that encompasses various aspects pertaining to biologic and systemic agents in dermatology. Dermatologists, residents, physician assistants, nurse practitioners, and any health care provider who treats dermatologic conditions can find pertinent information at their fingertips in one setting. In addition, a case report-oriented approach is emphasized in this book. Many chapters have included a practical case report relevant to that topic so that the reader can gain better appreciation of utilizing a particular systemic or biologic agent in clinical practice. In addition, there is a chapter devoted to complex cases and managing adverse events and complications.

The overall intent of this book is for the practitioner to gain a greater comfort level in treating patients with biologic and systemic agents for various dermatologic conditions.

Los Angeles, CA
Paul S. Yamauchi, M.D., P.h.D.

Contents

Contributors

William Abramovits, MD, FAAD Baylor University Medical Center, The University of Texas Southwestern Medical School, Dallas, Texas, USA

Amber Alcaraz, BA Clinical Research, Southern California Dermatology, Inc, Santa Ana, CA, USA

Kyle T. Amber, MD Department of Dermatology, University of California, Irvine, CA, USA

Mina Amin, BS School of Medicine, University of California, Riverside, CA, USA
La Crescenta, CA, USA

April W. Armstrong, MD, MPH Department of Dermatology, University of Southern California, Los Angeles, CA, USA

Patrick Armstrong, MD Division of Dermatology, UCLA Medicine, Los Angeles, CA, USA

John W. Baddley, MD, MSPH Division of Infectious Diseases, Department of Medicine, University of Alabama at Birmingham, Birmingham, AL, USA

Jerry Bagel, MD, MS Psoriasis Treatment Center of Central New Jersey, University of Pisa, Pisa, Italy

Kristyn D. Beck, MD EVMS Dermatology, Norfolk, VA, USA

Brian Berman, MD, PhD Department of Dermatology and Cutaneous Surgery, University of Miami Miller School of Medicine, Miami, FL, USA
Center for Clinical and Cosmetic Research, Aventura, FL, USA

Andrew Blauvelt, MD, MBA Oregon Medical Research Center, Portland, OR, USA

Emily Boes, DO Des Moines University College of Osteopathic Medicine, Des Moines, IA, USA

Jennifer Cather, MD Modern Research Associates, Dallas, TX, USA

J. Christian Cather, MD Modern Research Associates, Dallas, TX, USA

Nancy Cheng, MD Pediatric and Adolescent Dermatology, University of California, San Diego/Rady Children's Hospital, San Diego, CA, USA

Catherine G. Chung, MD The Ohio State Wexner Medical Center, Columbus, OH, USA

Catie Coman, MA Health Advocacy Partners, Portland, OR, USA

Jeffrey J. Crowley, MS, MD, FAAD Bakersfield Dermatology and Skin Cancer Medical Group, Bakersfield, CA, USA

Kavita Darji, BA School of Medicine, Saint Louis University, St. Louis, MO, USA

Sean Dreyer, BA MS4 at David Geffen School of Medicine at UCLA, Los Angeles, CA, USA

Kristina Callis Duffin, MD, MS Department of Dermatology, University of Utah, Salt Lake City, UT, USA

Boni E. Elewski, MD Department of Dermatology, University of Alabama at Birmingham, Birmingham, AL, USA

Steven R. Feldman, MD, PhD Department of Dermatology, Wake Forest School of Medicine, Winston-Salem, NC, USA

Katherine Ferris, MD Departments of Dermatology, University of California, Irvine, CA, USA

Alexandra G. Florek, MD Department of Dermatology, Feinberg School of Medicine, Northwestern University, Chicago, IL, USA

Amit Garg, MD Department of Dermatology, Zucker School of Medicine at Hofstra/Northwell, SVP, Dermatology Service Line, Northwell Health, Lake Success, NY, USA

Joel M. Gelfand, MD, MSCE Department of Dermatology, University of Pennsylvania, Philadelphia, PA, USA

Allan Gibofsky, MD, JD Fordham Law School, New York, NY, USA

Weill Medical College of Cornell University, New York, NY, USA

Hospital for Special Surgery, New York, NY, USA

Carolyn Goh, MD David Geffen School of Medicine at University of California, Los Angeles, CA, USA

David J. Goldberg, MD, JD Icahn School of Medicine at Mt. Sinai, New York, NY, USA

Fordham Law School, New York, NY, USA

Jose A. Gonzalez, BS The Laboratory for Investigative Dermatology, The Rockefeller University, New York, NY, USA

Melinda Gooderham, MD, MSc, FRCPC Skin Centre for Dermatology, Peterborough, ON, Canada

Probity Medical Research, Waterloo, ON, Canada

Queen's University, Kingston, ON, Canada

Kennethk B. Gordon, MD Department of Dermatology, Medical College of Wisconsin, Milwaukee, WI, USA

Sergei A. Grando, MD, PhD., DSc Departments of Dermatology, University of California, Irvine, CA, USA

Biological Chemistry, University of California, Irvine, CA, USA

Institute for Immunology, University of California Irvine, Irvine, CA, USA

Tamar Hajar, MD Oregon Health and Science University, Portland, OR, USA

Peter W. Hashim, MD, MHS Department of Dermatology, Icahn School of Medicine at Mount Sinai, New York, NY, USA

Jason E. Hawkes, MD Department of Dermatology, University of Utah School of Medicine, Salt Lake City, UT, USA

The Laboratory for Investigative Dermatology, The Rockefeller University, New York, NY, USA

Peter W. Heald, MD Yale University School of Medicine, New Milford, CT, USA

Emma Hill, BA Oregon Health and Science University, Portland, OR, USA

Alexander S. Hoy, BS EVMS Dermatology, Norfolk, VA, USA

Amy Huang, MD Department of Dermatology, State University of New York Downstate Medical Center, Brooklyn, NY, USA

Jordan Huber, MD Department of Dermatology, University of Utah School of Medicine, Salt Lake City, UT, USA

A. Jarad Peranteau, MD New York Medical College, New York, NY, USA

Robert E. Kalb, MD Suny At Buffalo School of Medicine, Buffalo, NY, USA

Primal Kaur, MD, MBA Biosimilars Development, Amgen Inc., Thousand Oaks, CA, USA

Andrew Kim, MD Department of Surgery, Division of Dermatology, Dartmouth-Hitchcock, Concord, NH, USA

Alexa B. Kimball, MD, MPH Department of Dermatology, Harvard Medical School, Beth Israel Deaconess Medical Center, Boston, MA, USA

Grace W. Kimmel, MD Department of Dermatology, Icahn School of Medicine at Mount Sinai, New York, NY, USA

John Koo, MD Department of Dermatology, University of California San Francisco, San Francisco, CA, USA

Neil J. Korman, MD, PhD Case Western Reserve University, Cleveland, OH, USA

James G. Krueger, MD The Laboratory for Investigative Dermatology, The Rockefeller University, New York, NY, USA

Gerald G. Krueger, MD Department of Dermatology, University of Utah School of Medicine, Salt Lake City, UT, USA

Gary Lask, MD Dermatology Laser Center, David Geffen School of Medicine at UCLA, Los Angeles, CA, USA

Lauren Bonomo, BA Department of Dermatology, Icahn School of Medicine at Mount Sinai, New York, NY, USA

Mark G. Lebwohl, MD Department of Dermatology, Icahn School of Medicine at Mount Sinai, New York, NY, USA

Katrina Lee, BS School of Medicine, UC Irvine Medical Center, University of California, Irvine, CA, USA

Jacob Levitt, MD Department of Dermatology, Icahn School of Medicine at Mount Sinai, New York, NY, USA

Roger Lo, MD, PhD Division of Dermatology, Department of Medicine, University of California, Los Angeles, Los Angeles, CA, USA

Emily B. Lund, MD Departments of Dermatology and Pediatrics, Feinberg School of Medicine, Northwestern University, Chicago, IL, USA

Raman K. Madan, MD Department of Dermatology, State University of New York Downstate Medical Center, Brooklyn, NY, USA

Andrea D. Maderal, MD Department of Dermatology and Cutaneous Surgery, University of Miami Miller School of Medicine, Miami, FL, USA

Stephanie Martin, MD UCLA/WLA VA Derm Surgery Fellowship Program, Dermatologic Surgery and Mohs Micrographic Surgery, Department of Dermatology, VA Greater Los Angeles Healthcare System, Los Angeles, CA, USA

Julia Mayba, BSc University of Manitoba, Winnipeg, MB, Canada
Skin Centre for Dermatology, Peterborough, ON, Canada

Philip J. Mease, MD Swedish Medical Center, Seattle, WA, USA
University of Washington School of Medicine, Seattle, WA, USA

Alan Menter, MD Baylor University Medical Center, Dallas, TX, USA

Margaretta Midura, BA MSIII, Zucker School of Medicine at Hofstra/Northwell, Hempstead, NY, USA

Mio Nakamura, MD Department of Dermatology, University of California San Francisco, San Francisco, CA, USA

Jared J. Nathan, BS chemistry Biosimilars Development, Amgen Inc., Thousand Oaks, CA, USA

John K. Nia, MD Department of Dermatology, Icahn School of Medicine at Mount Sinai, New York, NY, USA

Mathew N. Nicholas, BMSc Faculty of Medicine, University of Toronto, Toronto, ON, Canada

Daniel J. No, BA School of Medicine, Loma Linda University, Loma Linda, CA, USA

Megan H. Noe, MD, MPH Department of Dermatology, University of Pennsylvania, Philadelphia, PA, USA

Allen S.W. Oak, MD Department of Dermatology, University of Alabama at Birmingham, Birmingham, AL, USA

Martin M. Okun, MD, PhD Fort HealthCare Department of Dermatology, Fort Atkinson, WI, USA

Amy S. Paller, MS, MD Departments of Dermatology and Pediatrics, Feinberg School of Medicine, Northwestern University, Chicago, IL, USA

K.A. Papp, MD, PhD K Papp Clinical Research and Probity Medical Research, Waterloo, ON, Canada

Timothy Patton, DO Department of Dermatology, University of Pittsburgh, Pittsburgh, PA, USA

Gregory Peterson, MD Baylor University Medical Center, Dallas, TX, USA

Brian Poligone, MD, PhD Rochester Skin Lymphoma Medical Group, Fairport, NY, USA

Martina L. Porter, MD Department of Dermatology, Clinical Laboratory for Epidemiology and Applied Research in Skin (CLEARS), Beth Israel Deaconess Medical Center, Boston, MA, USA

Monica Ramchandani, BS, MS pharmacy, PhD pharmaceutical sciences Biosimilars Development, Amgen Inc, Thousand Oaks, CA, USA

Amanda Raymond, MD Department of Dermatology, University of California San Francisco, San Francisco, CA, USA

James Q. Del Rosso, DO, FAOCD, FAAD Touro University Nevada, Henderson, NV, USA
JDR Dermatology Research, LLC, Las Vegas, NV, USA
Private Dermatology Practice, Thomas Dermatology, Las Vegas, NV, USA

Suzanne M. Sachsman, MD Division of Dermatology, David Geffen School of Medicine at UCLA, Los Angeles, CA, USA

Sahil Sekhon, MD Department of Dermatology, University of California San Francisco, San Francisco, CA, USA

Kevin Sharghi, MD Virginia Tech Carilion School of Medicine, Roanoke, VA, USA

Jessica Shiu, MD, PhD Departments of Dermatology, University of California, Irvine, CA, USA

Annika Silfast-Kaiser, BS Texas A&M Health Science Center College of Medicine, Temple, TX, USA

Eric Simpson, MD, MCR Oregon Health and Science University, Portland, OR, USA

Jaclyn Smith, BS Department of Dermatology, Wake Forest School of Medicine, Winston-Salem, NC, USA

Jennifer Soung, MD Clinical Research, Southern California Dermatology, Inc, Santa Ana, CA, USA

Bruce Strober, MD, PhD Department of Dermatology, University of Connecticut Health Center, Farmington, CT, USA

Wynnis L. Tom, MD Pediatric and Adolescent Dermatology, University of California, San Diego/Rady Children's Hospital, San Diego, CA, USA

Stephen K. Tyring, MD, PhD University of Texas Health Science Center at Houston, Houston, TX, USA
Center for Clinical Studies, Houston, TX, USA

Ramya Vangipuram, MD University of Texas Health Science Center at Houston, Houston, TX, USA

Abby S. Van Voorhees, MD EVMS Dermatology, Norfolk, VA, USA

Daniel J. Wallace, MD, FACP, MACR Cedars-Sinai Medical Center, David Geffen School of Medicine Center at UCLA, Beverly Hills, CA, USA

Guy Webster, MD, PhD Department of Dermatology, Sidney Kimmel Medical College of Thomas Jefferson University, Philadelphia, PA, USA

Jeffrey M. Weinberg, MD Department of Dermatology, Icahn School of Medicine at Mount Sinai, New York, NY, USA

Scott Worswick, MD Assistant Professor of Dermatology at UCLA, Los Angeles, CA, USA

Jashin J. Wu, MD Department of Dermatology, Kaiser Permanente Los Angeles Medical Center, Los Angeles, CA, USA

Paul S. Yamauchi, MD, PhD David Geffen School of Medicine at UCLA, Dermatology Institute and Skin Care Center, Santa Monica, CA, USA

Kaitlyn M. Yim, BA Department of Dermatology, University of Southern California, Los Angeles, CA, USA

Melodie Young, RN, ANP-C Modern Research Associates, Dallas, TX, USA

Abby S. Van Voorhees and Jeffrey M. Weinberg

Introduction

This chronicle of psoriasis begins in ancient times when psoriasis, leprosy, and other inflammatory skin disorders were thought to be the same condition. The identification of psoriasis as a distinct entity did not occur until the nineteenth century, when clinical descriptions distinguished it from other cutaneous disorders. Histopathologic descriptions in the 1960s and 1970s shed some light on the pathophysiology of psoriasis, but many aspects of the disease remain unknown to this day. As Bechet expressed, "Psoriasis is an antidote for dermatologists' ego" [1].

Given the lack of understanding of its pathophysiology, early psoriasis therapies were discovered serendipitously. Chance observations by early clinicians of psoriatic improvement in patients prescribed medications for other conditions led to advancements in therapy. As our understanding grew, this serendipity evolved into detailed targeting of specific immunological processes. These newly directed therapies clarified aspects of the pathophysiology and treatment of psoriasis and other immune-mediated diseases.

Ancient History: Lepra, Psora, Psoriasis

The roots of the identification of psoriasis lie in Ancient Greece. The Greeks, who pioneered the field of medicine, divided skin disease into the categories of *psora, lepra*, and *leichen* [2]. *Psora* referred to itch, while *lepra* was derived from the Greek words *lopos* (the epidermis) and *lepo* (to scale)

[3]. Hippocrates (460–377 BC) was one of the first authors to write descriptions of skin disorders. He utilized the word "lopoi" to describe the dry, scaly, disfiguring eruptions of psoriasis, leprosy, and other inflammatory skin disorders [4].

Similar to Hippocrates' works, the Old Testament also lumped together many cutaneous disorders. The biblical term *tsaraat,* or *zaraath,* described a range of skin conditions including leprosy and psoriasis. Lepers were often ostracized because they were considered divinely punished, and cruelty was imposed upon those who suffered from psoriasis and leprosy alike [5, 6].

Many historians credit the Roman thinker Celsus (ca. 25 BC–45 AD) with the first clinical description of papulosquamous diseases [1, 2, 5]. Celsus described impetigines and specified that the second species of impetigo was characterized by red skin covered with scales. This description suggested a type of papulosquamous disease, such as psoriasis [7].

Galen (133–200 AD) first utilized the term psoriasis, but his description was not consistent with the disorder that we now call psoriasis. He described psoriasis as a pruritic, scaly skin disease of the eyelids and scrotum. Although he used the term psoriasis, his description is now believed to most likely represent seborrheic dermatitis [4, 5, 8].

Indiscriminate grouping together of all inflammatory skin diseases led to stigmatization of patients with psoriasis. For centuries, patients with psoriasis received the same cruel handling as lepers. They were required to carry a bell or clapper to announce their approach, and had to wear a special dress. In addition, they could only touch or dine with others considered lepers. In 1313, Phillip the Fair of France ordered that they be burned at the stake [1].

Distinguishing Psoriasis as a Distinct Entity

In 1809, Willan built on Celsus's description of papulosquamous conditions by detailing features of what we now know as psoriasis. However, he described modern psoriasis under the term lepra vulgaris, which perpetuated confusion of

A.S. Van Voorhees, MD
EVMS Dermatology, 721 Fairfax Avenue Suite 200, Norfolk, VA 23507-2007, USA

J.M. Weinberg, MD (✉)
Department of Dermatology, Icahn School of Medicine at Mount Sinai, 1090 Amsterdam Avenue, Suite 11D, New York, NY 10025, USA
e-mail: foresthillsdermatology@gmail.com

© Springer International Publishing AG 2018
P.S. Yamauchi (ed.), *Biologic and Systemic Agents in Dermatology*, https://doi.org/10.1007/978-3-319-66884-0_1

psoriasis and leprosy. Lepra vulgaris was described as enlarging, sharply marginated erythematous plaques with silvery-white scale that occurred most frequently on the knees, and were associated with nail pitting [8, 9].

For decades after Willan's description, some authors favored using the term psoriasis [1, 2, 10–12], while others chose the term lepra [9, 13]. Physicians lacked clarity regarding the word psoriasis and the ability to distinguish psoriasis from diseases with similar cutaneous manifestations.

Finally, Gibert and Hebra matched Willan's description with the term psoriasis, ending much confusion. Psoriasis was now finally acknowledged as a distinct disease, leading to improved perception of psoriatic patients.

In his books, Gibert (1797–1866) used the term psoriasis, recognized secondary syphilis as a contagious entity, and established pityriasis rosea as a clinical syndrome. Gibert's pivotal publications included thorough accounts that made important distinctions between papulosquamous diseases [5, 10, 14]. In 1841, shortly after Gibert's works, Hebra further distinguished the clinical picture of psoriasis from that of leprosy. Only 165 years ago, this differentiation set the stage for psoriatic patient's freedom from extreme persecution [15, 16]. The distinctions made by Gibert and Hebra were essential to accurately diagnosing patients and developing tailored therapies.

Advancements in the Description of Psoriasis

The nineteenth-century identification of psoriasis as a separate entity ushered in a period of increasingly accurate descriptions of the disease. One of Hebra's students, Heinrich Auspitz (1835–1886), noted bleeding points upon removal of scale in patients with psoriasis. We now refer to this as the Auspitz sign [14, 17]. Along with the Auspitz sign, the Koebner reaction is a characteristic feature of psoriasis. In 1876, Koebner described the propensity of psoriatic lesions to arise in areas of prior trauma. Koebner's observation provided insight into the importance of the vascular compartment in the initiation of the psoriatic lesion [18]. Two decades later, in 1898, Munro described microabscesses of psoriasis that are now known as Munro's abscesses [17].

The start of the twentieth century ushered in further descriptions of psoriatic lesions. In 1910, Leo von Zumbusch first described generalized pustular psoriasis, or von Zumbusch disease [19]. Additional descriptions included Woronoff's 1926 description of a pale halo referred to as the "Woronoff ring" encircling a plaque of psoriasis [20]. The portrayals of the Auspitz sign, Koebner phenomenon, Munro's abscesses, pustular psoriasis, and the Woronoff ring allowed physicians to more confidently diagnose patients with psoriasis.

Understanding Pathophysiology

In addition to clinical observations, histopathologic descriptions of psoriatic skin advanced understanding of the roles of epidermal hyperplasia and the immune system in psoriasis. Epidermal hyperplasia in psoriasis was first observed in 1963, when Van Scott noted a significant increase in mitoses of psoriatic epidermis [21]. Three years later, Van Scott and Weinstein noted that psoriatic basal cells rose to the stratum corneum in only 2 days, in contrast to their 12-day transit through normal epidermis [22].

Therapeutic discoveries and histopathologic observations linked the immune system with psoriasis. In 1951, Gubner treated rheumatoid arthritis with the folic acid antagonist aminopterin, and serendipitously noted clearing of the skin in patients with psoriasis [23]. At that time researchers did not understand the mechanism of action of folic acid antagonists in psoriasis treatment, but later understanding revealed that these medications modulated the immune system. Two decades after Gubner's report, Mueller prescribed cyclosporine to prevent rejection in transplant patients, and found improvement of lesions in patients with psoriasis [24]. Reports of psoriatic improvement provided by immunosuppressive drugs implicated the immune system in the pathogenesis of psoriasis. Histopathologic observations, that cellular infiltrates in psoriasis were composed primarily of T cells and macrophages, further highlighted the role of the immune system in psoriasis [25, 26].

In spite of these discoveries, much remains unknown about the pathogenesis of psoriasis and other immune-mediated diseases including arthritis and inflammatory bowel disease. Psoriasis serves as a model for immune-mediated diseases because the response to therapy can be readily seen [27].

History of Treatment of Psoriasis

The history of the treatment of psoriasis is relatively short, and initially treatment discoveries were serendipitous. Early psoriasis therapies included arsenic and ammoniated mercury use in the nineteenth century. In the first half of the twentieth century, anthralin and tar were discovered as effective psoriasis treatments. Corticosteroids were developed in the 1950s. These therapies were followed in the 1970s by use of methotrexate and PUVA on psoriasis. In the 1980s, psoriasis treatment discoveries included narrowband UVB, retinoids, and vitamin D therapies. From the 1990s to the present time, manipulating the immune system to treat psoriasis has been explored first with cyclosporine and more recently with targeted molecules.

Nineteenth Century: Arsenic and Ammoniated Mercury

Throughout history, arsenic has been utilized as both a poison and therapeutic. In 1806, Girdlestone reported on the efficacy of Fowler's solution with 1% arsenic in treating many dermatologic conditions including psoriasis [1, 28]. With similar toxic potential, ammoniated mercury was used as a medication before the twentieth century [16, 29]. In 1876, Duhring recommended mercurial ointments to treat psoriasis [30].

1900–1950s: Anthralin and Tar

In 1876, Squire inadvertently discovered anthralin as a treatment of psoriasis. Squire prescribed Goa powder, which was until then known only to be effective in ringworm, and the patient's psoriasis improved. The active ingredient of Goa powder is chrysarobin, also known as 2-methyl dithranol [31]. During World War I, this treatment was further refined, as a synthetic form of chrysarobin called anthralin, or dithranol, was formed. In 1916, Unna reported the effectiveness of dithranol as an antipsoriatic treatment [32].

The next advancement in psoriasis treatment was coal tar. Hippocrates and other ancient physicians treated dermatologic conditions with pine tar and other types of tar. Coal tar became available when coal gas production developed in the late nineteenth century, and Goeckerman found that coal tar was particularly useful in psoriasis therapy [33, 34]. Many observed that psoriasis improved with summer sun. In 1925, Goeckerman reported an additive benefit of coal tar and UVB radiation in psoriasis treatment [16, 35]. Goeckerman's method remained the mainstay of psoriasis treatment for decades. In 1953, Ingram reported the successful treatment of psoriasis with a combination of Unna and Goeckerman's modalities. He established the first day care center for psoriasis in which patients were treated with a tar bath, then UVB therapy, and lastly 0.42% dithranol in Lassar's paste [36]. This treatment improved the morbidity of psoriasis for many patients, but was time intensive.

1950s: Corticosteroids

In the 1950s, the corticosteroid era began and revolutionized the treatment of many diseases. In 1950 Hench, Kendall, and Reichstein received the Nobel Prize for the development of cortisone [37, 38]. A mere 2 years later, Sulzberg and Witten reported that compound F, or hydrocortisone, was the first moderately successful topical corticosteroid in inflammatory skin diseases including psoriasis [39]. From that time forward, additional topical corticosteroid preparations were developed to treat inflammatory dermatoses such as psoriasis.

1970s: Methotrexate and PUVA

Although methotrexate was first developed in the 1950s, it was not used to treat psoriasis until the 1970s. In 1946, Farber developed aminopterin to treat leukemia [40]. Five years later, Gubner reported that aminopterin used in the treatment of rheumatoid arthritis also cleared psoriasis [23]. In 1958, Edmundsun and Guy introduced methotrexate, a more stable derivative of aminopterin with lower toxicity [41]. Investigators initially believed that folic acid antagonists prevented keratinocyte hyperproliferation, but later the effect on lymphocytes in psoriatic lesions was elucidated. In 1972, the FDA finally approved the use of methotrexate for psoriasis [42].

Also in the 1970s, PUVA therapy was reported to be effective in psoriasis. PUVA, based on the interaction between UV radiation and a photosensitizing chemical, has its own rich history [43]. The concept originated in about 1500 BC when Egyptian healers treated vitiligo with a combination of sunlight and ingestion of plants known as psoralens, including fig and limes [44]. An article published in 1974 reported the efficacy of oral PUVA therapy in a group of patients with psoriasis [43]. Three years later, a multicenter study confirmed that most patients with psoriasis experienced clearing of their skin using oral PUVA [45]. Shortly after the development of oral PUVA, alternative bathwater delivery systems of psoralens were also created to minimize adverse effects associated with oral PUVA [46].

1980s: Narrowband UVB, Retinoids, Vitamin D

Although often therapeutically successful, PUVA therapy carries an increased risk of skin cancer. Therefore, further study of UVB therapy was undertaken. In 1981, Parrish and Jaenicke demonstrated that UVB wavelengths between 300 and 313 nm caused the greatest remission of skin lesions

[47]. Subsequent trials reported that the 311 nm spectrum showed improved clearance of lesions with less erythema [48, 49].

In the 1980s, researchers also established the use of retinoids in psoriasis treatment. Prior to its use in psoriasis, in the 1960s physicians prescribed retinoids for hyperkeratosis and acne. At this time, first-generation and synthetic topical retinoids did not have significant antipsoriatic activity [50, 51]. In the early 1980s, reports demonstrated the efficacy of the second-generation retinoids etretinate and its derivative acitretin, in the treatment of psoriasis [52, 53]. Although etretinate is no longer available in the USA due to its lipophilia and protracted adverse effects, acitretin has a shorter half-life and remains an important therapy in psoriasis [54]. Third-generation acetylenic retinoids developed in the 1980s allowed for the production of a topical retinoid, tazarotene, with demonstrated antipsoriatic efficacy [55].

The next class of drugs developed for psoriasis, vitamin D and its analogs, was also developed by chance observations in the 1980s. In 1985, a patient who received oral vitamin D3 for osteoporosis experienced dramatic improvement of his psoriasis [56]. The active form of vitamin D3 plays a part in the control of intestinal calcium absorption, bone mineralization, keratinocyte differentiation, keratinocyte proliferation, and immune modulation [57, 58]. Despite extensive research, the exact mechanism of action of vitamin D analogs remains unknown. In 1988, a topical form of vitamin D proved useful in the treatment of psoriasis [59].

1990s: Cyclic Immunosuppressive Medications

In 1997, cyclosporine was FDA approved for psoriasis treatment. Cyclosporine was isolated in 1969 from a fungus and was screened for antibiotic properties. In 1976, Borel reported immunosuppressive properties of cyclosporine in animal models [60]. Three years later, cyclosporine A was used experimentally in transplant patients to prevent graft rejection, and psoriatic patients in these trials experienced relief of their lesions [24]. FDA approval was delayed until the 1990s due to concerns about toxicity. Cyclosporine is prescribed for severe psoriasis that is not responsive to other therapies [61].

Biologic Therapies

Although our understanding of the immunological basis of psoriasis had expanded greatly by the turn of the millennium, many details still remain unknown. Understanding of the role of immunology in psoriasis, together with the knowledge of protein engineering techniques, has given us the capability to manufacture specific proteins that can selectively alter the immunological processes in psoriasis. These therapies continue to improve the treatment of psoriasis and shed further light into its pathogenesis.

Beginning in January of 2003, a number of biologic agents were approved by the FDA for the treatment of psoriasis including alefacept, efalizumab, etanercept, and infliximab. Alefacept binds to CD2 to prevent the activation of T lymphocytes in psoriasis [27, 62], while efalizumab binds to CD11 to inhibit T cell activation and migration into the skin [63]. Both of these therapies strengthened the understanding of the role of T lymphocytes in psoriasis. Tumor necrosis factor inhibitors also demonstrated efficacy in the treatment of psoriasis [64]. The efficacy and mechanism of etanercept, infliximab, and adalimumab suggest that psoriasis pathophysiology also involves immunologic mediators in addition to T cells.

Understanding the importance of immunosuppression in the treatment of psoriasis was another example of gains achieved by serendipitous findings.

While heralded in with great promise, the T cell-targeting compounds alefacept [62] and efalizumab [65] have subsequently been removed from the market because of potential side effects and/or lack of efficacy. However the TNF inhibitors—adalimumab [66], etanercept [64], and infliximab [67] and the IL-12/23 compound ustekinumab [68]—have revolutionized the care of patients with psoriasis. Over the past few years, three new drugs in the IL-17 class, secukinumab, ixekizumab, and brodalumab, have been approved for the treatment of psoriatic disease [69]. Three new medications which inhibit IL-23 are in development [69]. With each new class of medication developed, the importance of the immune system in psoriasis has become increasingly apparent.

Additional agents targeting different sites of the inflammatory cascade are currently under development and may further add to both our understanding of psoriasis and our therapeutic armamentarium. The expectation for treatment response has increased to levels unimaginable only 20–30 years ago.

References

1. Bechet PE. Psoriasis, a brief historical review. Arch Derm Syphilol. 1936;33:327–34.
2. Hebra F. On disease of the skin. London: New Sydenham Society; 1868.
3. Fox H. Dermatology of the ancients. JAMA. 1915;65:469.
4. Sutton RL. Sixteenth century physician and his methods mercurialis on diseases of the skin. Kansas City, MO: The Lowell Press; 1986.
5. Pusey WA. The history of dermatology. Springfield, IL: Thomas, Charles C; 1933.
6. Glickman FS. Lepra, psora, psoriasis. J Am Acad Dermatol. 1986;14(5 Pt 1):863–6.
7. Celsus AC. De re medica. London: East Portwine; 1837.

8. Willan R. On cutaneous diseases. Philadelphia: Kimber and Conrad; 1809.

9. Rayer P. Treatises on diseases of the skin. 2nd ed. London: J.B. Bailliere; 1835.

10. Gibert CM. Traite pratique des maladies speciales de la peau. 2nd ed. Paris: Germer-Bailliere; 1840.

11. Wilson E. Diseases of the skin. Philadelphia: Blanchchard and Lea; 1863.

12. Fox T. Skin diseases: their description, pathology, diagnosis, and treatment. New York: William Wood and Co.; 1871.

13. Milton JL. Diseases of the skin. London: Robert Hardwicke; 1872.

14. Crissey JT, Parish LC, Shelley WB. The dermatology and syphilology of the nineteenth century. New York, NY: Praiger; 1981.

15. Hebra F, Kaposi M. Lehrbuch der Hautkrankheiten. Stuttgart: Ferdinanand Euke; 1876.

16. Fry L. Psoriasis. Br J Dermatol. 1988;119(4):445–61.

17. Farber EM. Historical commentary. In: Farber EM, Cox AJ, Nall L, Jacobs PH, editors. Psoriasis: proceedings of the third international symposium, Stanford University, 1981. 3rd ed. New York, NY: Grune and Stratton; 1982. p. 7-7-11.

18. Kobner H. Zur aetiologie ppsoriasis. Vjschr Dermatol. 1876;3:559.

19. von Zumbusch LR. Psoriasis und pustuloses exanthem. Archiv Dermatol Syphiliol. 1910;99:335–46.

20. Woronoff DL. Die peripheren verandergunge der haut um die effloreszenzen der psoriasis vulgaris und syphilis corymbosa. Dermatologischen Wochenschrift. 1926;82:249–57.

21. VanScott EJ, Ekel TM. Kinetics of hyperplasia in psoriasis. Arch Dermatol. 1963;88:373–81.

22. Weinstein GD, Van Scott EJ. Turnover time of human normal and psoriatic epidermis by autoradiographic analysis. J Inves Dermatol. 1966;45:561–7.

23. Gubner R. Effect of aminopterin on epithelial tissues. AMA Arch Derm Syphilol. 1951;64(6):688–99.

24. Mueller W, Herrmann B. Cyclosporin A for psoriasis. N Engl J Med. 1979;301(10):555.

25. Bjerke JR, Krogh HK, Matre R. Characterization of mononuclear cell infiltrates in psoriatic lesions. J Invest Dermatol. 1978;71(5):340–3.

26. Baker BS, Swain AF, Fry L, Valdimarsson H, Epidermal T. Lymphocytes and HLA-DR expression in psoriasis. Br J Dermatol. 1984;110(5):555–64.

27. Schon MP, Boehncke WH. Psoriasis. N Engl J Med. 2005;352(18):1899–912.

28. Girdlestone T. Observations on the effects of dr. fowler's mineral solution in lepra and other diseases. Med Phys J Lond. 1806;15:298–301.

29. Farber EM. History of the treatment of psoriasis. J Am Acad Dermatol. 1992;27(4):640–5.

30. Duhring LA. Atlas of skin diseases. Philadelphia: JB Lippincot & Co.; 1876.

31. Squire B. Treatment of psoriasis by an ointment of chrysophanic acid. Br Med J. 1876;2:819–920.

32. Unna PG. Cignolin als heilmittel der psoriasis. Dermatologische Wochenschrift. 1916;6:116–37. 151-163, 175-183

33. Hjorth N, Norgaard M. Tars. In: Roenigk HH, Maibach HI, editors. Psoriasis. New York, NY: Marcel Dekker; 1991. p. 473–9.

34. Squire B. Atlas of skin diseases. London: J&A Churchill; 1878.

35. Goeckerman WH. The treatment of psoriasis. Northwest Med. 1925;25:229–31.

36. Ingram JT. The approach to psoriasis. Br Med J. 1953;2:591–3.

37. Lundberg IE, Grundtman C, Larsson E, Klareskog L. Corticosteroids—from an idea to clinical use. Best Pract Res Clin Rheumatol. 2004;18(1):7–19.

38. Hench PS, Kendall EC, Slocumb CH, Polley HF. Effects of cortisone acetate and pituitary ACTH on rheumatoid arthritis, rheumatic fever and certain other conditions. Arch Med Interna. 1950;85(4):545–666.

39. Sulzberger MB, Witten VH. The effect of topially applied compound F in selected dermatoses. J Invest Dermatol. 1952;19:101–2.

40. Farber S, Diamond L, Mercer R, Sylvester R, Wolff V. Temporary remissions in acute leukemia in children produced by folic acid antagonist 4-amethopteroylglutamic acid (aminopterin). N Engl J Med. 1946;238:787–93.

41. Edmundson WF, Guy WB. Treatment of psoriasis with folic acid antagonists. AMA Arch Derm. 1958;78(2):200–3.

42. Roenigk HH Jr, Maibach HI, Weinstein GD. Use of methotrexate in psoriasis. Arch Dermatol. 1972;105(3):363–5.

43. Parrish JA, Fitzpatrick TB, Tanenbaum L, Pathak MA. Photochemotherapy of psoriasis with oral methoxsalen and longwave ultraviolet light. N Engl J Med. 1974;291(23):1207–11.

44. Benedetto AV. The psoralens: an historical perspective. Cutis. 1977;20:469–71.

45. Melski JW, Tanenbaum L, Parrish JA, Fitzpatrick TB, Bleich HL. Oral methoxsalen photochemotherapy for the treatment of psoriasis: a cooperative clinical trial. J Invest Dermatol. 1977;68(6):328–35.

46. Fischer T, Alsins J. Treatment of psoriasis with trioxsalen baths and dysprosium lamps. Acta Derm Venereol. 1976;56(5):383–90.

47. Parrish JA, Jaenicke KF. Action spectrum for phototherapy of psoriasis. J Invest Dermatol. 1981;76:359–61.

48. Green C, Ferguson J, Lakshmipathi T, Johnson BE. 311 nm UVB phototherapy—an effective treatment for psoriasis. Br J Dermatol. 1988;119(6):691–6.

49. Picot E, Meunier L, Picot-Debeze MC, Peyron JL, Meynadier J. Treatment of psoriasis with a 311-nm UVB lamp. Br J Dermatol. 1992;127(5):509–12.

50. Wolbach SB, Howe PR. Tissue changes following deprivation of fat-soluble A-vitamin. J Exp Med. 1925;42:753–78.

51. Stuttgen G. Zur lokalbehandlung von keratosen mit vitamin A-saure. Dermatologica. 1962;124:65–80.

52. Tsambaos D, Orfanos CE. Chemotherapy of psoriasis and other skin disorders with oral retinoids. Pharmacol Ther. 1981;14(3):355–74.

53. Ward A, Brogden RN, Heel RC, Speight TM, Avery GS. Isotretinoin. A review of its pharmacological properties and therapeutic efficacy in acne and other skin disorders. Drugs. 1984;28(1):6–37.

54. Ellis CN, Voorhees JJ. Etretinate therapy. J Am Acad Dermatol. 1987;16(2 Pt1):267–91.

55. Weinstein GD. Safety, efficacy and duration of therapeutic effect of tazarotene used in the treatment of plaque psoriasis. Br J Dermatol. 1996;135(Suppl 49):32–6.

56. Morimoto S, Kumahara Y. A patient with psoriasis cured by 1 alpha-hydroxyvitamin D3. Med J Osaka Univ. 1985;35(3-4):51–4.

57. Smith EL, Walworth NC, Holick MF. Effect of 1 alpha, 25-dihydroxyvitamin D3 on the morphologic and biochemical differentiation of cultured human epidermal keratinocytes grown in serum-free conditions. J Invest Dermatol. 1986;86(6):709–14.

58. Kragballe K, Wildfang IL. Calcipotriol (MC 903), a novel vitamin D3 analogue stimulates terminal differentiation and inhibits proliferation of cultured human keratinocytes. Arch Dermatol Res. 1990;282(3):164–7.

59. Kragballe K, Beck HI, Sogaard H. Improvement of psoriasis by a topical vitamin D3 analogue (MC 903) in a double-blind study. Br J Dermatol. 1988;119(2):223–30.

60. Borel JF, Feurer C, Gubler HU, Stahelin H. Biological effects of cyclosporin A: a new antilymphocytic agent. Agents Actions. 1976;6(4):468–75.

61. Griffiths CE, Dubertret L, Ellis CN, Finlay AY, Finzi AF, Ho VC, Johnston A, Katsambas A, Lison AE, Naeyaert JM, Nakagawa H, Paul C, Vanaclocha F. Ciclosporin in psoriasis clinical practice: an international consensus statement. Br J Dermatol. 2004;150(Suppl 67):11–23.

62. Ellis CN, Krueger GG, Alefacept Clinical Study Group. Treatment of chronic plaque psoriasis by selective targeting of memory effector T lymphocytes. N Engl J Med. 2001;345(4):248–55.

63. Kupper TS. Immunologic targets in psoriasis. N Engl J Med. 2003;349(21):1987–90.

64. Leonardi CL, Powers JL, Matheson RT, Goffe BS, Zitnik R, Wang A, Gottlieb AB, Etanercept Psoriasis Study Group. Etanercept as monotherapy in patients with psoriasis. N Engl J Med. 2003;349(21):2014–22.

65. Gordon KB, Papp KA, Hamilton TK, et al. Efalizumab for patients with moderate to severe plaque psoriasis: a randomized controlled trial. JAMA. 2003;290(23):3073–80.

66. Menter A, Tyring SK, Gordon K, et al. Adalimumab therapy for moderate to severe psoriasis: a randomized, controlled phase 3 trial. J Am Acad Dermatol. 2007;58:106–15.

67. Chaudri U, Romano P, Mulcahy LD, et al. Efficacy and safety of infliximab monotherapy for plaque-type psoriasis: a randomized trial. Lancet. 2001;357(9271):1842–7.

68. Krueger GG, Langley RG, Leonardi C, et al. A human interleukin-12/23 monoclonal antibody for the treatment of psoriasis. N Engl J Med. 2007;356:580–92.

69. Dong J, Goldenberg G. New biologics in psoriasis: an update on IL-23 and IL-17 inhibitors. Cutis. 2016;99:123–7.

Kristina Callis Duffin

History of Outcome Measure Development and Methodology

Over the past several decades, numerous outcome measures have been developed for skin disease therapies, but development of most measures did not employ rigorous methodologies for development or validation of the measures. In the field of rheumatology, it was noted in the 1980s that rheumatologists varied considerably in the way they utilized clinical measures to make judgments about the efficacy of treatments [1]. Recognition of the need for a common approach led to the formation of OMERACT (Outcome Measures in Rheumatology, formerly Outcome Measures in Rheumatoid Arthritis Clinical Trials, www.omeract.org) which sought to unite the methodologies around outcome measures of academic and professional organizations such as the World Health Organization, American College of Rheumatology, and the International and European Leagues Against Rheumatism (ILAR and EULAR). Since their first meeting in 1992, OMERACT has led consensus efforts overseeing development and assessment of outcome measures in many rheumatologic diseases, utilizing the methodologies summarized in an ever-evolving road map known as the OMERACT Handbook [2, 3].

The field of dermatology has faced the same challenges. Most instruments used in dermatology have been developed by individuals, organizations, and industry, and often modified at the request of the US Food and Drug Administration (USFDA) to meet trial and regulatory needs. For example, the Psoriasis Area and Severity Index (PASI) and the multitude of physician/investigator global assessments (PGA or IGA) are the most commonly used primary or co-primary

efficacy outcome measures mandated by the USFDA for registered plaque psoriasis RCTs, but the PASI and nearly all of the PGA/IGAs were not subjected to rigorous psychometric evaluation (e.g., not assessed for validity, reliability, and discrimination) before being used.

As a result, many new organizations focused on measurement in skin conditions have been formed and are addressing the need for developing and implementing core outcome sets and gaining consensus. The *Cochrane Skin Group Core Outcome Set Initiative* (CSG-COUSIN) was formed in 2014 and supported by the editors of the Cochrane Skin Group; this group developed a road map with the eczema outcome measure group, *Harmonising Outcome Measures for Eczema* (HOME). The *International Dermatology Outcomes Measures* organization (IDEOM) was founded in 2013 with support and advice from members of OMERACT and has focused initially on psoriasis and hidradenitis suppurativa measures for clinical trials.

Although there is no single accepted methodology, a common pathway has emerged among most outcome measure organizations, which generally follow the OMERACT guidance. First, the scope of the outcome measure core set must be defined, including but not limited to the condition, population, and setting. It is important to establish contextual factors around the condition; for example, the domains and measures used to assess guttate psoriasis may differ from those of chronic plaque psoriasis or palmar-plantar psoriasis. The setting (e.g., clinical trial, longitudinal registry, clinical practice) must be carefully considered as well, as measures utilized in clinical trials may be very different than those used in clinical practice or a longitudinal registry primarily due to issues around cost, feasibility, and training.

Second, a core domain set is developed. Through consensus exercises, which usually involve focus groups, meetings of patients and experts, and Delphi surveys, a set of candidate domains is created. From there, consensus exercises such as Delphi surveys and audience response voting at live

K.C. Duffin, MD, MS
Department of Dermatology, University of Utah,
Salt Lake City, UT, USA
e-mail: Kristina.duffin@hsc.utah.edu

© Springer International Publishing AG 2018
P.S. Yamauchi (ed.), *Biologic and Systemic Agents in Dermatology*, https://doi.org/10.1007/978-3-319-66884-0_2

meetings are conducted to determine a core domain set. A core domain set is defined as "what" should be measured. For example, in atopic eczema, the HOME organization's core domain set includes clinical signs, patient-reported symptoms, long-term control, and quality of life.

Once a core set is defined (what to measure) a core measurement set (*how* to measure) must be defined. Candidate measures within each domain are selected through literature review, and then evaluated for validity, reliability, discrimination, and feasibility. For example, the HOME organization evaluated several potential measures as candidates for patient-reported symptoms of atopic eczema, and ultimately selected the Patient-Oriented Eczema Measure based on good validity and reliability data [4]. For more information, see the most updated version of the OMERACT Handbook at www.omeract.org.

Psoriasis Measures

Psoriasis, primarily generalized plaque type, likely has the largest number of outcome measures of any dermatologic disorder owing to its prevalence, disease characteristics, significant life impact, recent advances in the understanding of its pathogenesis, and related drug development. At least 44 different scoring systems in 171 randomized clinical trials of psoriasis therapies between 1977 and 2000 were described, largely by measuring extent, erythema, scaling, and thickness of the psoriasis lesions [5]. Despite this variety of measures, nearly all phase II and III clinical trials that have resulted in approved therapies used Psoriasis Area and Severity Index (PASI) and/or a physician or investigator global assessment (PGA or IGA) as primary or co-primary endpoints.

Psoriasis Area and Severity Index (PASI)

The most widely used instrument to measure psoriasis disease severity and efficacy of therapeutic agents in the last four decades has been the Psoriasis Area and Severity Index (PASI) [5]. The PASI was developed and first described in a study of etretinate in 1978 [6]. Despite common belief, the PASI did not enjoy immediate adoption as a primary endpoint; 7 years after its initial description in 1978, it had only been used in 3 of 30 published psoriasis studies [7]. However, owing to its sensitivity to change in extensive psoriasis and perhaps other influences, it became the most prevalent scoring system in use [5, 8]. It also has become the framework for many other severity measures used in psoriasis and other diseases, such as the Psoriasis Scalp Severity Index (PSSI), Palmar-Plantar Psoriasis Area and Severity Index (PPPASI), Eczema Severity and Area Index (EASI), the Cutaneous Lupus Area and Severity Index (CLASI), and others (Table 2.1).

Since it has become the gold standard for moderate-severe psoriasis trials, PASI has been subject to critical assessments of its psychometric properties [9]. However, one review of psoriasis measures demonstrated that most instruments developed to overcome PASI's limitations (e.g., the simplified SPASI or linearized LPASI) do not outperform the PASI on its clinimetric properties [10]. As a result, uptake of these measures has not occurred in the clinical trial setting, likely due to the desire to compare efficacy using the original PASI across studies. The European Medicines Agency (EMA) has continued to require PASI as the primary endpoint, and in Europe, PASI is the primary efficacy measure used in clinical practice. As a result, PASI is likely going to remain the gold standard and primary or co-primary endpoint for most plaque psoriasis studies.

To perform PASI, see Fig. 2.1.

Table 2.1 Psoriasis Area and Severity Index

	Erythema 0–4[a]	Induration 0–4[a]	Scaling 0–4[a]	Sum (E + I + S)	Area score[b]	Weighting multiplier	Region score
Head/neck	+	+	+	=	x	x 0.1	=
Upper extremities	+	+	+	=	x	x 0.2	=
Trunk	+	+	+	=	x	x 0.3	=
Lower extremities	+	+	+	=	x	x 0.4	=
[a]Severity score 0 = 4:		[b]Area score 0–6: Determine percentage of region affected		Final PASI score (sum of four region scores)			
0 = None		0 = 0					
1 = Slight or mild		1 = >0–<10%					
2 = Moderate		2 = 10–<30%					
3 = Severe or marked		3 = 30–<50%					
4 = Very severe or very marked		4 = 50–<70%					
		5 = 70–<90%					
		6 = 90–100%					

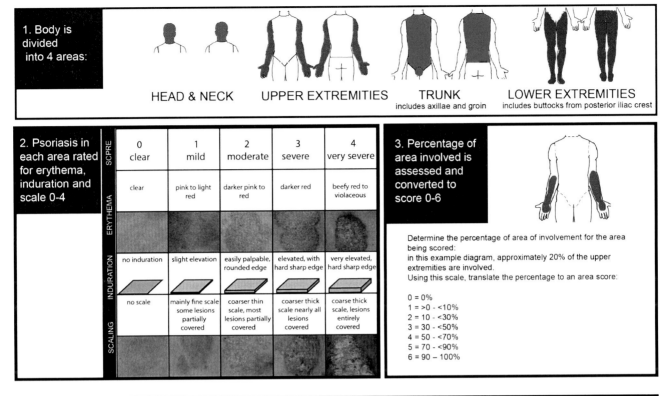

Fig. 2.1 Psoriasis Area and Severity Index. To perform PASI, the assessor rates plaque characteristics and area of involvement in four regions of the body (head and neck, upper extremities, trunk, and lower extremities). When scoring each of the four areas, three plaque characteristics are scored on a scale of 0–4, from clear to very severe: erythema (pinkness or redness), induration (thickness or elevation), and scaling (desquamation). The amount of area involvement is determined for each body area, then assigning a score on a scale of 0–6, where 1 = >0–<10% 2 = 10–<30%, 3 = 30–<50%, 4 = 50–<70%, 5 = 70–<90%, and 6 = 90–100%. (Of note, the original publication described the scale as follows: 1 = 1–9%, 2 = 10–29%, 3 = 30–49%, 4 = 50–69%, 5 = 70–89%, and 6 = 90–100%. This has led to discrepancies in scoring, e.g., what score to assign if the area involved is 9.5%—therefore it is recommended by the author to use the area scores as described in Fig. 2.1.) For each of the four regions, the plaque qualities are summed (E + I + S, maximum of 12), then multiplied by the area score and a weighting multiplier, and the four body area scores are summed for a maximum total of 72. When scoring erythema, most consider residual hypo- or hyperpigmentation to be "clear". (Reproduced with permission from Kristina Callis Duffin)

Psychometric Properties

The PASI has stood the test of time in clinical trials of moderate-to-severe psoriasis as it has been shown to demonstrate good responsiveness to change and reliability. In one small study of 14 trained and experienced evaluators, intra-rater and inter-rater reliability was considered substantial (intraclass coefficient >0.81) [11]. PASI is considered the gold standard, so criterion validity for most measures is assessed against PASI.

PASI Cut Points

Certain PASI cut points and change from baseline are typically used as clinical trial inclusion criteria and endpoints. A PASI score of 10 or 12 is historically and arbitrarily assigned as the usual clinical trial inclusion criterion for moderate-severe psoriasis at screening and/or baseline visits. The PASI 12 is presumably derived from the fact that if every erythema, induration, scale, and area score is scored a 2 ("moderate"), then the PASI score is 12.

The usual co-primary endpoint in a placebo-controlled RCT is the percentage of patients on active therapy who achieve PASI 75 compared to placebo at the primary endpoint (usually 12–16 weeks). PASI 75 is defined as the percentage of patients who achieve *at least* 75% improvement from the baseline PASI score—which means everyone who had 75% *or greater* improvement from their baseline PASI score. The percentage of patients reaching PASI 50, 90, and 100 are typical secondary endpoints; however, with the development of more effiacious therapies, such as the interleukin-17 inhibitors such as secukinumab and ixekizumab, PASI 90 is increasingly being used as a primary endpoint [12].

Although many of the newer therapies are leading to high rates of clearance, it is important not to lose site of the fact that PASI 50 is still a meaningful improvement for patients [13]. Technically, the endpoint PASI 50 includes patients with PASI 50–PASI 74. Patients in this range can have very meaningful improvements: for example, if a patient goes from BSA 49% to 1% but all plaque scores for erythema, induration, and scale stay at 3, they have achieved a PASI 66, which would be included in the PASI 50 category. Carlin et al. also demonstrated that PASI 50 was associated with meaningful changes in quality of life in clinical trials of alefacept and efalizumab [14, 15]. However, as more effective therapies have been developed with higher percentages of patients able to obtain complete clearance, studies have shown that there are statistical differences in the number of patients who obtain a DLQI of 0 or 1 (considered "no impact" on quality of life) going from PASI 90 to PASI 100 [16]. Depending on the study and the therapeutic agent, PASI 75 or PASI 90 may correlate better with the PGA of 0 or 1 (clear/almost clear), which likely is related to the type of PGA used.

Limitations of PASI

The PASI has limitations that have been enumerated in many studies [17, 18]. The PASI score in itself lacks meaning to clinicians. An absolute PASI score could mean extensive area but thin patches, or few plaques that are very thick. It also is not very responsive to change in mild or moderate psoriasis, such as patients with limited BSA involvement. It does not capture the degree of severity of plaques when critical areas such as body folds, face, and genitals are involved. Many feel that it is cumbersome to use, as one must assess 16 data points and then calculate

the final score. It also does not correlate well with patient-reported measures, such as symptom inventories or quality-of-life measures.

Physician/Investigator Global Assessment (PGA or IGA)

In 1998 the US FDA solicited feedback from the Dermatologic and Ophthalmic Drugs Advisory Committee, which recommended that PASI not be used as the sole efficacy endpoint in clinical trials (https://www.fda.gov/ohrms/dockets/ac/cder98t.htm#Dermatologic%20and%20Ophthalmic%20Drugs%20Advisory%20Committee). Following this recommendation, efforts were made by psoriasis opinion leaders and industry to comply with the requirement that the primary efficacy endpoint be a static dichotomous physician global assessment (PGA) or investigator global assessment (IGA). These efforts corresponded closely with phase II and III clinical trials leading to the registration and approval of the first biologics for psoriasis. For the most part, PGA and IGA are synonymous, and therefore will be referred to as PGA for this chapter.

The most important thing to know about "the PGA" is that there is not just one; in fact, there are numerous PGAs that have been developed and used as the primary endpoint in psoriasis clinical trials. The vast majority of the PGA instruments used in psoriasis trials are static, 5-point (0–4), or 6-point (0–5) scales where plaque qualities of erythema, induration (thickness, elevation), and scale (desquamation) are rated from none to very severe. The assessor is generally instructed to consider the totality of the plaques at a single point in time (static assessment) according to descriptions that guide the assessment, and not compared to a past point in time (dynamic assessment). Some score erythema, induration, and scaling separately and then the scores are averaged and rounded to the nearest whole number, whereas for others, the assessor is asked to chose one score based on the anchoring descriptions. The body surface area involvement (BSA) is not included in most versions of the PGA.

Psychometric Properties of PGA

Psychometric properties of some PGAs have been rigorously assessed, although almost none were rigorously developed prior to their use in clinical trials. The five-point, three-item PGA utilized in the tofacitinib phase II and III program (Table 2.2) has been assessed for its reliability and validity, showing that equally weighting erythema, induration, and

Table 2.2 5-point (0–4) static Physician Global Assessment (sPGA) [19]

5-point (0–4) static Physician's Global Assessment (sPGA)

Erythema	Induration	Scale
0 = No evidence of erythema (post-inflammatory hyperpigmentation and/or hypopigmentation may be present)	0 = No evidence of plaque elevation	0 = No evidence of scaling
1 = Light pink	1 = Barely palpable	1 = Occasional fine scale
2 = Light red	2 = Slight, but definite elevation, indistinct edges	2 = Fine scale predominates
3 = Red	3 = Elevated with distinct edges	3 = Coarse scale predominates
4 = Dark, deep red	4 = Marked plaque elevation, hard/sharp borders	4 = Thick, coarse scale predominates
E =	I =	S =

Physician's static global assessment based upon above total average [(I + E + S)/3]:

0 = Clear, except for residual discoloration

1 = Almost clear, majority of lesions have individual scores for [(I + E + S)/3] that average 1

2 = Mild: Majority of lesions have individual scores for [(I + E + S)/3] that average 2

3 = Moderate: Majority of lesions have individual scores for [(I + E + S)/3] that average 3

4 = Severe: Majority of lesions have individual scores for [(I + E + S)/3] that average 4

	[(I + E + S)/3] =	

Table 2.3 5-point (0–4) static physician global assessment (sPGA)—from National Psoriasis Foundation Psoriasis Score, utilized in Amgen etanercept, Janssen ustekinumab, and infliximab programs

6-point (0–5) static Physician's Global Assessment (sPGA)

Erythema	Induration	Scale
0 = No erythema 1 = Faint erythema 2 = Light red coloration 3 = Moderate red coloration 4 = Bright red coloration 5 = Dusky-deep red coloration	0 = No evidence of plaque elevation 1 = Minimal (~0.25 mm) 2 = Mild (~0.50 mm) 3 = Moderate (~0.75 mm) 4 = Marked (~1.0 mm) 5 = Severe (~1.25 mm)	0 = No evidence of scale 1 = Minimal (occasional fine scale over less than 5% of lesions) 2 = Mild (fine scale predominates) 3 = Moderate (coarse scale predominates) 4 = Marked (thick, non-tenacious scale predominates) 5 = Severe (very thick, tenacious scale predominates)
E =	I =	S =

Static Physician Global Assessment: based upon above total average [(I + E + S)/3]:

0 = Clear, except for residual discoloration

1 = Minimal: Majority of lesions have individual scores for [(I + E + S)/3] that average 1

2 = Mild: Majority of lesions have individual scores for [(I + E + S)/3] that average 2

3 = Moderate: Majority of lesions have individual scores for [(I + E + S)/3] that average 3

4 = Severe: Majority of lesions have individual scores for [(I + E + S)/3] that average 4

5 = Very severe: Majority of lesions have individual scores for [(I + E + S)/3] that average 5

	[(I + E + S)/3] =	

Table 2.4 5-point (0–4) static Investigator Global Assessment (sPGA)

5-point (0–4) static Investigator Global Assessment "2011 version"—Novartis

Score		Definition
0	Clear	No signs of psoriasis (post-inflammatory hyperpigmentation may be present)
1	Almost clear	Normal to pink coloration of lesions No thickening No to minimal focal scaling
2	Mild	Pink to light red coloration Just detectable to mild thickening Predominantly fine scaling
3	Moderate	Dull to bright red, clearly distinguishable erythema Clearly distinguishable to moderate thickening Moderate scaling
4	Severe	Bright to deep dark red coloration Severe thickening with hard edges Severe/coarse scaling covering almost all or all lesions

scale is valid [19]. Post hoc studies of prospective RCTs and registries have demonstrated that most PGA measures correlate well with PASI, likely due to the fact that the scales and definitions of erythema, induration, and desquamation are similar for most PGAs and PASI.

Most PGAs in existence have been heavily criticized for the exclusion of BSA as part of their definition. This has primarily been the result of regulatory directives, presumably rationalized by including it as a separate measure. As a result, the product of the PGA and the BSA (PGAxBSA, also called the s-MAPA, discussed below) has been proposed as a measure with better validity. Some PGA instruments, such as the Lattice Scale-PGA (LS-PGA) [20], include BSA but this instrument has not gained favor with the research or regulatory community as it is considered cumbersome. Examples of commonly used PGA measures are provided in Tables 2.2, 2.3, 2.4, and 2.5.

Table 2.5 6-point (0–5) static Physician/Investigator Global Assessment (sPGA)

6-point (0–5) static Physician/Investigator Global Assessment—Amgen, Lilly

Score		Definition
0	Clear	Plaque elevation = 0 (no elevation over normal skin) Scaling = 0 (no scale) Erythema = 0 (no evidence of erythema, hyperpigmentation may be present)
1	Minimal	Plaque elevation = ± (possible but difficult to ascertain whether there is a slight elevation above normal skin) Scaling = ± (surface dryness with some white coloration) Erythema = (faint erythema)
2	Mild	Plaque elevation = slight (slight but definite elevation, typically edges are indistinct or sloped) Scaling = fine (fine scale partially or mostly covering lesions) Erythema = (light red coloration)
3	Moderate	Plaque elevation = moderate (moderate elevation with rough or sloped edges) Scaling = coarser (coarse scale covering most of all the lesions) Erythema = moderate (definite red coloration)
4	Severe	Plaque elevation = marked (marked elevation typically with hard or sharp edges) Scaling = coarse (coarse, non-tenacious scale predominates covering most or all of the lesions) Erythema = severe (very bright red coloration)
5	Very severe	Plaque elevation = very marked (very marked elevation typically with hard sharp edges) Scaling = very coarse (coarse, thick tenacious scale over most of all the lesions; rough surface) Erythema = very severe (extreme red coloration; dusky to deep red coloration)

Target Lesion Assessment and Total Plaque Severity Score (TPSS)

Target lesions are commonly selected and assessed in clinical trials, particularly when the therapeutic agent is topical or serial biopsies are being taken for mechanistic evaluation. Target lesions are typically selected based on size and location and assessed for reduction of size, erythema, induration, and scale. The Total Plaque Severity Score (TPSS) has been used in the Pfizer phase II clinical trial for topical tofacitinib and some validity testing was performed as part of this study. To perform this measure, erythema, induration, and scale are scored 0–4 for selected target lesion (lesion size and location determined by protocol) and summed for a score range of 0–12 [21–23].

PGAxBSA

The product of the PGA and BSA, or PGAxBSA, has risen as a measure of interest in clinical trials and in clinical practice. The notion of using the PGAxBSA as a surrogate for PASI in registries and clinical practice was first published by rheumatologist Jessica Walsh, who, like others, felt that PASI was cumbersome and difficult outside the psoriasis clinical trial venue. It was psychometrically evaluated in the Utah Psoriasis Initiative longitudinal cohort of 226 patients, where it was found to correlate highly with PASI (R^2 of .87) and correlated better with the patient-reported global assessment (PtGA) (R^2 of 0.65 vs. 0.59 with PASI) [18]. Similar results were found in the DCERN cross-sectional study of 1755 patients on systemic or biologic therapies [24]. The PGAxBSA was then used as the primary endpoint in a clinical trial of apremilast for moderate psoriasis (systemic-naïve patients with 5–10% BSA at baseline) where it was shown to correlate fairly well with the PASI but found statistically to be a better measure of effect size [25].

Body Surface Area (BSA)

The body surface area (BSA) in dermatology refers to an estimate of the percentage of the body surface area affected by the condition. It is a commonly used measure of skin disease severity in clinical trials and clinical practice. The acronym "BSA" can be confusing, since fields like oncology use this acronym to mean the total BSA needed to determine doses of chemotherapy. In this context, BSA is calculated using an estimating formula using height and weight, or more precisely with 3D laser technology. For the purposes of this chapter, the BSA will refer to the estimate of the percentage of total body area of disease involvement.

Historically, BSA is calculated by one of the three methods: the "rule of nines," the handprint method, or a general "eyeball it" method commonly used to calculate the PASI. The rule of nines has been used for decades to determine percentage of area involved with a burn. It is performed by dividing the body into regions or multiples of 9% [26]. The Lund and Browder chart is then used to map burns [27].

The second method is the "handprint method," where the patient's handprint is used to estimate 1% BSA (Fig. 2.2) Two studies have assessed the handprint method in adult patients with psoriasis. In the first study, a sample of 50 adults showed that the palmar surface including all five digits was equivalent to about 0.76% in men and 0.70% in women [28]. A similar study found that the whole surface of a man's hand was 0.81% and of a woman's hand 0.67% [29]. In children, the entire child's hand was 0.94% [30]. These studies showed that the palm alone (without digits) was 0.52%. Several authors have noted that referring to BSA with just the "palm" is vague and misleading, as it could mean the full handprint or the just the palm without the fingers (or in some cases, more complex definitions such as the palm to the proximal phalangeal joints of all fingers and the thumb) which all significantly underestimate the BSA. Finlay et al. recommend that the word "handprint," rather than "palm" be used, and that the patient's handprint is a reasonable estimate of BSA 1%, although it is still <1% in adults.

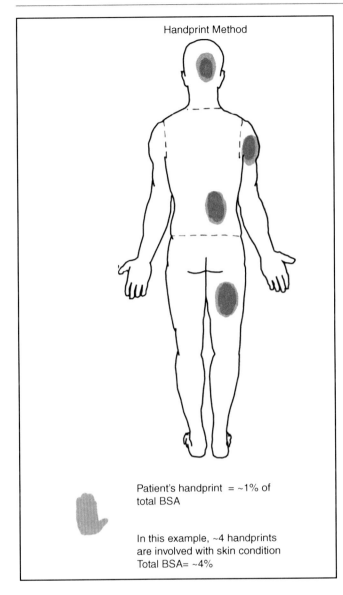

Handprint Method

Patient's handprint = ~1% of total BSA

In this example, ~4 handprints are involved with skin condition
Total BSA= ~4%

Fig. 2.2 The handprint method is typically used to determine body surface area of involvement. First, the patient's hand is used to determine the area of about 1% of their BSA. Second, the assessor determines approximately how many total handprints of the condition are present. It is important to only consider active areas and not to count normal skin between the lesions. ©Kristina Callis Duffin. Reproduced with permission

Psychometric Assessments

Similar to other measures, the BSA has been assessed following its widespread use for validity, reliability, and other clinimetrics, which generally are favorable. Criticisms of the BSA include that it can be overestimated [31]. Pragmatically, in a patient with very high body weight the handprint method will overestimate the true BSA involvement, although one could argue that ten absolute handprints is moderate to severe no matter what percentage of the body it occupies. Like PASI, the BSA correlates weakly with patient-reported measures such as the DLQI [32].

Psoriasis Instruments in Clinical Practice

In the USA, unlike Europe, dermatologists do not routinely utilize PASI or any form of PGA in their practices. The PASI is considered by most to be a research tool and has not had uptake in clinical practice in the same way it has in Europe, where most clinicians do PASI and BSA. In the USA, physicians will commonly document BSA, which is necessary to obtain prior authorization from payers for biologics, as many require documentation of at least 10% BSA or evidence of involvement of critical areas such as face, scalp, palms, soles, or genitals to justify use of these more expensive agents.

There are efforts under way to increase utilization of psoriasis severity measures in clinical practice and to establish treatment targets based on these measures. In 2017, the Medical Board of the National Psoriasis Foundation published a Delphi survey on preferred measures and targets in clinical practice [33]. The most preferred instrument was BSA, primarily chosen because it is the most pragmatic instrument that most US-based clinicians will use, as opposed to PASI or PGA. Utilizing BSA, there was consensus that an "acceptable response" at 3-month BSA should be 3% or less, or 75% improvement from baseline; the target at 6 months should be 1%. Additionally, with quality-based reimbursement measures being instituted, it is likely that there will be uptake in use of instruments like BSA, and possibly PGAxBSA, to demonstrate that the clinician is measuring improvement and at the very least attempting to get a patient to a target BSA or PGA, particularly when treating with systemic agents, phototherapy, or biologics.

The PGAxBSA is being advocated as a tool that is easily performed in clinical practice and in trials, and thus could be a surrogate for PASI. The primary limitations of using the PGAxBSA in trials and practice will be defining which PGA to use in this measure, education of physicians on how to do a PGA, and familiarity with cut points in this score. The PGAxBSA may be better represented as the actual numerical equation rather than its product; much like a blood pressure of 140/90 is a known cut point, a PGAxBSA of 1x1 could be a realistic endpoint in clinical practice.

Scalp Endpoints: Psoriasis of the Scalp Severity Index (PSSI) and PGA of the Scalp

Scalp psoriasis is estimated to be present in 60% of patients with psoriasis, and sometimes is the only manifestation. The PSSI was derived from the PASI to assess plaque psoriasis of the scalp only. It was first used in a trial of topical calcipotriol, and subsequently as the primary endpoint for scalp studies of efalizumab, etanercept, and secukinumab [34–37]. Many studies have utilized it to assess scalp psoriasis as a secondary endpoint in the setting of an RCT for moderate-severe plaque psoriasis.

Table 2.6 PSSI Psoriasis of the Scalp severity Index)

	Erythema 0–4[a]	Induration 0–4[a]	Scaling 0–4[a]	Sum (E + I + S)	Area score 0–6[b]	FINAL PSSI score 0–72
Scalp		+	+	=	x	=

[a]Severity score 0 = 4:	[b]Area score 0–6: Determine percentage of region affected
0 = None	0 = 0
1 = Slight or mild	1 = >0–<10%
2 = Moderate	2 = 10–<30%
3 = Severe or marked	3 = 30–<50%
4 = Very severe or very marked	4 = 50–<70%
	5 = 70–<90%
	6 = 90–100%

To perform the PSSI, investigators are instructed to assess erythema, induration, and scaling in the same way as they are for PASI, but the percent area of involvement and area score assess only psoriasis in the hair-bearing region of the scalp. The final equation is $(E + I + S) \times A_{scalp}$ for total possible PSSI of 0–72 (Table 2.6). Most RCT for psoriasis to date have set the inclusion criterion PSSI score at 12 (where each score = 2, or moderate but the area score must be at least a 3), a global assessment of 3 (moderate), and usually at least 30% of the scalp involved (Table 2.6).

Nail Assessments: NAPSI and mNAPSI

Nail psoriasis is prevalent, affecting about 50% of patients with chronic plaque psoriasis and up to 85% with nail changes in their lifetime. Nails are difficult to assess, due to the lack of specificity of the changes with psoriasis (all of the features such as pitting, onycholysis, splinter hemorrhages, and subungual debris can be seen with many other dermatologic conditions). Additionally, nail changes can happen slowly, as it takes around 6 months for a fingernail to completely regrow, and a year or more for toenails.

The most commonly used investigator-measured nail assessments include the Nail Psoriasis Severity Index (NAPSI) and the modified NAPSI (mNAPSI) [38, 39]. A number of PGAs have been developed as well. A newer composite instrument, the Nail Assessment in Psoriasis and Psoriatic Arthritis (NAPPA), was developed in 2014 [40].

The NAPSI was developed and first published in 2003 as an endpoint for nail psoriasis severity [39]. The NAPSI is performed by first dividing the nail plate into four quadrants with an imaginary horizontal and vertical line. For each quadrant, the nail is evaluated for features of nail matrix psoriasis which include pitting, leukonychia, red spots in the lunula, or crumbling; if any of the features is present in a quadrant, it gets 1 point (maximum nail matrix score for a nail is 4). Next, each quadrant is evaluated for nail bed features which include onycholysis, splinter hemorrhages, subungual hyperkeratosis, or "oil drop"/salmon patch dyschromia; if any nail bed features are present in a quadrant, it gets 1 point (maximum nail bed score for a nail is 4) (Table 2.7).

There is lack of consensus on how many or which nails should be scored when performing NAPSI. Common methods have included scoring all fingernails and toenails (NAPSI total score range 0–160), fingernails only (0–80), and toenails only (0–80), or selecting target nails to conduct the 32-point or 8-point NAPSI. The 8-point NAPSI is performed by selecting the most severely affected nail, which is scored 0–8; the 32-point assesses all 8 features in all 4 quadrants of 1 nail. However, this method has been criticized for lacking responsiveness to change, as no change in score will occur if the nail has 40 pits in all 4 quadrants and goes to 1 pit in all 4 quadrants (score of 4 in each case). A modified "96-point" target nail NAPSI has been proposed as a more responsive target nail NAPSI, where the 8 features of nail bed and nail matrix for the 4 quadrants are scored 0–3 (none-severe) in each quadrant [41]. Most psoriasis studies exclude toenail scoring, as chronic trauma-related nail plate thickening, concomitant onychomycosis, and slow toenail growth can confound the scoring.

The NAPSI was not formally "validated" during its development. An informal assessment of the reproducibility of the NAPSI score was done with 37 dermatologists who were asked to evaluate 8 psoriatic nails and described in the original paper suggesting good interobserver reliability. This was further confirmed by Aktan et al., demonstrating good reliability (ICC 0.781 and 0.649 for total and 32-point nail scores) with 25 patients and 3 dermatologists, with better reliability when scoring nail bed features compared to nail matrix features [42].

Many modifications of the NAPSI have been suggested. Variations on how to calculate the score by giving points for each features (the 32-point target nail score) or rate severity of the bed and matrix features have not been used widely [41]. Leukonychia has been proposed as a nonspecific feature for psoriatic disease, with no statistical difference of this feature in both controls and psoriatic patients in one study [43].

Table 2.7 Nail Psoriasis Severity Index (NAPSI)

1. Divide nail into four virtual quadrants	2. Determine nail matrix and nail bed scores	3. Sum of matrix and bed score = NAPSI score for that nail
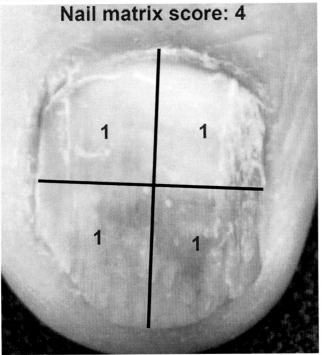	**1. Determine nail matrix score:** Nail matrix psoriasis consists of the following: Pitting, leukonychia, red spots in the lunula, and nail plate crumbling. If **ANY** of these features is present in a quadrant, that quadrant gets 1 matrix point Score for matrix psoriasis: 0 = None 1 = Present in 1 of 4 quadrants 2 = Present in 2 of 4 quadrants 3 = Present in 3 of 4 quadrants 4 = Present in 4 of 4 quadrants	
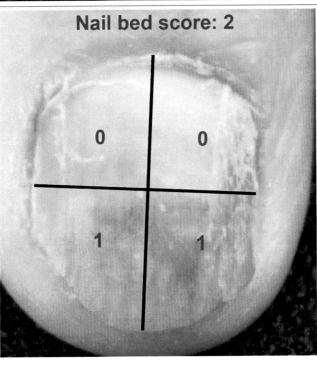	**2. Determine nail bed score:** Nail bed psoriasis consists of the following: Onycholysis, splinter hemorrhages, oil drop (salmon patch) dyschromia, and subungual hyperkeratosis. If **ANY** of these features is present in a quadrant, that quadrant gets 1 point Score for nail bed psoriasis: 0 = None 1 = Present in 1 of 4 quadrants 2 = Present in 2 of 4 quadrants 3 = Present in 3 of 4 quadrants 4 = Present in 4 of 4 quadrants	

Figure legend: The target nail is graded for nail matrix psoriasis and nail bed psoriasis. The sum of these two scores is the total score for that nail. In this example, the nail has pitting and crumbling present in all four quadrants; therefore each quadrant was given a point for presence of matrix psoriasis (matrix score = 4). The two distal quadrants have onycholysis and oil drop dyschromia; therefore the bed score = 2. The total NAPSI score for this nail is 6.

Photograph provided by Kristina Callis Duffin.

Modified NAPSI (mNAPSI)

The modified NAPSI was developed as a validated nail psoriasis measure to overcome some of the deficiencies of NAPSI [38]. Photographs of nails and physician focus sessions resulted in elimination of the quadrant division, adding a four-point scale to better quantify severity of nail pitting, crumbling, and onycholysis, and unweighting features such as splinter hemorrhages, leukonychia, and red spots in the lunula by giving single points if those features are absent or present.

Unlike NAPSI, psychometric properties of the mNAPSI were assessed as part of the instrument development. The inter- and intra-rater reliability was excellent (Spearman's rho 0.85 and 0.9–0.99, respectively) and scores were moderately correlated with various patient- and physician-reported severity measures (Table 2.8).

The Nail Assessment in Psoriasis and Psoriatic Arthritis (NAPPA)

The NAPPA is a newer instrument that was developed and validated through qualitative methods, feasibility testing, and longitudinal validation in six European countries. It includes three components, two of which are patient surveys. The first is a quality of life questionnaire (NAPPA-QoL) which consists of three subscales (nail signs: 6 questions, stigma subscale: 7 questions, and everyday life subscale: 7 questions) each scored 1–5. The second is a two-part patient questionnaire assessing treatment benefits (NAPPA-PBI). This consists of 24 questions, each with an initial stem "so far the treatment has helped me to …" with a response (e.g., … have normal looking nails"), and each is scored 0 (not at all) to 4 (very). The third is a clinical assessment (NAPPA-CLIN). This instrument has not been yet assessed prospectively in a clinical trial of therapeutics.

Palmar-Plantar Psoriasis Area and Severity Index (PPASI or PPPASI)

The assessment of palmar-plantar psoriasis (plaque or pustular variants) has most commonly been done with a palmar-plantar PGA and the PPASI or PPPASI. PPASI and PPPASI were modeled on the PASI as a measure for palmar-plantar psoriasis and palmar-plantar pustular psoriasis. (There is no consensus on the naming convention, but for purposes of this chapter, PPASI will refer to the plaque version, and PPPASI will refer to the pustular version.)

To perform the PPASI, investigators are instructed to assess erythema, induration, and scaling in the same way as they are for PASI, but the four regions assessed are the left palm, right palm, left sole, and right sole. The weighting multipliers are 0.2 for the palms and 0.3 for the soles, so the PPASI score range is 0–72. The PPPASI, used for the palmar-plantar pustular variant, is essentially the same, but severity of the pustules is scored instead of assessing induration (Table 2.9).

Table 2.8 Modified Nail Psoriasis Severity Index (mNAPSI)

Characteristic	Score			
	0	1	2	3
Crumbling (% of nail)	0%	1–25%	26–50%	>50%
Onycholysis and oil spot discoloration (% of nail)	0%	1–10%	11–30%	>30%
Pitting (number)	0	1–10	11–49	50+
Leukonychia	Absent	Present		
Splinter hemorrhages	Absent	Present		
Nail bed hyperkeratosis	Absent	Present		
Red spots in lunula	Absent	Present		
Final mNAPSI score: Sum of 7 components: 0–13				

Table 2.9 Palmar-Plantar Psoriasis or Palmar-Plantar Pustular Psoriasis (PPASI or PPPASI)

	Erythema 0–4[a]	Pustules or induration 0–4[a]	Scaling 0–4[a]	Sum (E + I + S)	Area score 0–6[b]	Weighting multiplier	Region score
R palm	+	+	=	x	x	0.2	=
L palm	+	+	=	x	x	0.2	=
R sole	+	+	=	x	x	0.3	=
L sole	+	+	=	x	x	0.3	=
[a]Severity score 0 = 4:		[b]Area score 0–6: Determine percentage of region (palm or sole) affected		Final PPPASI score (sum of 4 region scores)			
0 = None		0 = 0					
1 = Slight or mild		1 = >0–<10%					
2 = Moderate		2 = 10–<30%					
3 = Severe or marked		3 = 30–<50%					
4 = Very severe or very marked		4 = 50–<70%					
		5 = 70–<90%					
		6 = 90–100%					

Although many trials include the PPASI and PPPASI, these instruments were not assessed for psychometric properties and patients not included in their development. Therefore, the most impactful and symptomatic objective features of palmar-plantar psoriasis (fissuring, erosion, pain, edema) are not assessed. Limitations of the PPASI and PPPASI also include the difficulty in assessing patches of psoriasis as they wrap around to the dorsal aspect of the hand or foot, and it is also not clear how to account for a "switch" in phenotype (e.g., from plaque to pustular) which has been widely described especially with anti-TNF agents.

Patient-Reported Measures in Psoriasis Trials

Over the last 10–15 years, the most commonly utilized patient-reported outcome measures (PROM) have been the Dermatology Life Quality Index (DLQI) and other general quality-of-life measures such as the Short Form-36 (SF-36). However, these measures are not psoriasis specific. Responding to this gap, industry sponsors have followed the US FDA PRO guidance pathway in concordance with the development of three biologics and this has led to several psoriasis-specific symptom inventories and diaries. Three measures have been rigorously developed with qualitative and quantitative methods, and for secukinumab, patient-reported outcomes for the first time were included in the FDA prescribing information label (Table 2.10).

Table 2.10 Patient-reported Psoriasis Symptom Inventories

PSI	Psoriasis Symptom Inventory (Amgen) [70–73]	• 8-item instrument with 24-h and 7-day recall versions • 8 symptoms each assessed for severity on 0–4 scale • Score range 0–32
PSD	Psoriasis Symptom Diary (Novartis) [74, 75]	• 16-item e-diary, performed daily • Each item rated 0–10 (none to as bad as you can imagine) • Assesses symptoms and impact of symptoms on quality of life
PSSD	Psoriasis Symptom and Sign Diary (Janssen)	• 11-item instrument with 24-h and 7-day recall versions • Measures psoriasis symptoms (itch, pain, stinging, burning, skin tightness) and psoriasis signs (skin dryness, cracking, scaling, shedding or flaking, redness and bleeding • 0 (absent) to 10 (worst imaginable) numerical rating scale

Dermatology Life Quality Index (DLQI)

The DLQI was the first dermatology-specific quality-of-life (QoL) instrument and considered the most commonly used non-disease-specific instrument in dermatology studies [44]. A detailed review of its use from 1994 to 2007 described its use in 272 articles, 33 different skin conditions, and dozens of studies [45]. It has been used in 32 countries and is available in 55 languages. There are versions available for use in children's studies (CDLQI) and family members (FDLQI).

The instrument itself is a ten-item questionnaire that assesses skin symptoms, feelings of embarrassment/self-consciousness, impact of skin disease on clothing choice, activities of daily living (work, school, leisure, sports, personal relationships, sexual difficulties), and impact of treatment as a problem over the last 7 days. Each item is rated 0–3 (very much, a lot, a little, not at all). The total score can range from 0 to 30 (Table 2.11).

Its psychometric aspects, including validity, reliability, responsiveness to change, minimal important difference, and others, have been described now in well over 100 studies. Owing to its prevalent use in RCTs for biologics, banding and cut points have been defined. The MCID for DLQI ranges between 3 and 5 depending on the study [46]. A DLQI score of 0–1 means "no impact of skin disease on quality of life"; a DLQI score of ≤5 is considered low impact on QOL. The DLQI of 10 or more is considered moderate and is considered an important cut point, especially in Europe, as it is included in the definition of a threshold for eligibility for systemic or biologic agents [47].

The DLQI has been criticized for its focus on physical limitations and lack of focus on psychological impact. It has been called a "first-generation" instrument, meaning one that was developed with some attention to validity and reliability, but without factor analysis to define item grouping or more modern statistical testing such as item response theory to define dimensionality, response categories, and differential item functioning [48]. Differential item functioning means that responses can be affected by age, gender, diagnoses, or other factors which introduces bias when comparing heterogeneous groups. Other QOL instruments such as SF-36 or SKIN-DEX 29 may function better when comparing groups.

Psoriatic Arthritis Measures

It is estimated that 30% of patients with psoriasis will develop psoriatic arthritis [49]. The musculoskeletal manifestations of psoriatic arthritis include synovitis, dactylitis, enthesitis, and axial features, along with varying degrees of cutaneous involvement. As a result, numerous measures are needed to assess severity of each manifestation, and many composite measures have been developed that combine and weight various musculoskeletal and cutaneous measures. Extensive reviews have covered the instruments now used for assessment of psoriatic arthritis [50]. It is unlikely that most dermatologists will use

Table 2.11 Dermatology Life Quality Index

The aim of this questionnaire is to measure how much your skin problem has affected your life over the last week. Please tick one box for each question

1. Over the last week, how **itchy, sore, painful,** or **stinging** has your skin been?	Very much	☐	
	A lot	☐	
	A little	☐	
	Not at all	☐	
2. Over the last week, how **embarrassed** or **self-conscious** have you been because of your skin?	Very much	☐	
	A lot	☐	
	A little	☐	
	Not at all	☐	
3. Over the last week, how much has your skin interfered with you going **shopping** or looking after your **home** or **garden?**	Very much	☐	
	A lot	☐	
	A little	☐	
	Not at all	☐	Not relevant ☐
4. Over the last week, how much has your skin influenced the **clothes** you wear?	Very much	☐	
	A lot	☐	
	A little	☐	
	Not at all	☐	Not relevant ☐
5. Over the last week, how much has your skin affected any **social** or **leisure** activities?	Very much	☐	
	A lot	☐	
	A little	☐	
	Not at all	☐	Not relevant ☐
6. Over the last week, how much has your skin made it difficult for you to do any **sport**?	Very much	☐	
	A lot	☐	
	A little	☐	
	Not at all	☐	Not relevant ☐
7. Over the last week, has your skin prevented you from **working** or **studying**?	Yes	☐	
	No	☐	Not relevant ☐
If "no," over the last week how much has your skin been a problem at **work** or **studying**?	A lot	☐	
	A little	☐	
	Not at all	☐	
8. Over the last week, how much has your skin created problems with your **partner** or any of your **close friends** or **relatives**?	Very much	☐	
	A lot	☐	
	A little	☐	
	Not at all	☐	Not relevant ☐
9. Over the last week, how much has your skin caused any **sexual difficulties**?	Very much	☐	
	A lot	☐	
	A little	☐	
	Not at all	☐	Not relevant ☐
10. Over the last week, how much of a problem has the **treatment** for your skin been, for example by making your home messy, or by taking up time?	Very much	☐	
	A lot	☐	
	A little	☐	
	Not at all	☐	Not relevant ☐

© Dermatology Life Quality Index. A Y Finlay, G K Khan, April 1992 www.dermatology.org.uk. This must not be copied without the permission of the authors

these measures in practice or in clinical trials, as performance of these assessments requires rheumatologic expertise and training to avoid inter- and intra-rater variability. However, a basic understanding of the ACR score is important in order to understand the efficacy of therapies used commonly for both psoriasis and PsA. Examples of PsA measures including composite measures are listed in Tables 2.12 and 2.13.

American College of Rheumatology (ACR)

The ACR score is a composite measure, originally developed for the assessment of rheumatoid arthritis [51]. The ACR20, which is the typical endpoint, requires at least a 20% improvement in swollen joint count and tender joint count, and 20% improvement in three of five other measures: C-reactive protein level or erythrocyte sedimentation rate, physician global assessment of disease activity (by a visual analog scale or VAS), patient global assessment of disease activity (VAS), patient pain assessment (VAS), and disability, measured by the Health Assessment Questionnaire (HAQ). In most psoriatic arthritis RCTs, the ACR20 is used to define the primary endpoint (e.g., statistically significant difference in the percentage achieving at least 20% improvement in the ACR score from baseline, in patients receiving active therapy vs. placebo). Other typical ACR endpoints are the ACR50 and ACR70 (Table 2.12).

Training for Psoriasis and Psoriatic Arthritis Measures

All clinical trials require evidence of experience and training, particularly industry-sponsored registration trials. The Group for Research Assessment of Psoriasis and Psoriatic Arthritis (GRAPPA) has led efforts to standardize training using online videos for psoriasis and psoriatic arthritis efficacy endpoints [52–56]. The GRAPPA modules include PASI, BSA, several versions of PGA or IGA, PSSI, NAPSI, mNAPSI, PPPASI, TPSS, and several sponsor-specific instruments (Tables 2.1, 2.2, 2.3, 2.4, 2.5, 2.6, 2.7, 2.8, and 2.9). Psoriatic arthritis videos include assessment of peripheral joints for synovitis, enthesitis, dactylitis, and axial disease (most measures in Table 2.12). The majority of the cutaneous psoriasis measures have "certification" testing, where GRAPPA experts have provided consensus scores allowing the user to be scored for how similar their scores are to the expert, and the vendors that host the videos provide certificates of training (ePharmaSolutions, Trifecta ePresentOnline) (for more information, see http://www.grappanetwork.org).

Of the training modules, PASI has been utilized the most by industry. Over 1000 individuals (mostly investigators requiring training) from over 45 countries have viewed the video and completed the 16½-min instructional video and certification portion on performing PASI/BSA assessments. The PASI module was also the subject of an equivalency study comparing PASI assessments performed by

Table 2.12 Psoriatic arthritis measures [50]

Domain	Disease feature measured	Commonly used measures and description
Synovitis: Peripheral joints	Assesses presence of inflammatory features of peripheral arthritis characterized by tenderness ± swelling due to synovitis. May be oligoarticular, monoarticular, asymmetric	68/66 Tender and swollen joint count (TJC, SJC): Assess all 68 joints for tenderness and 66 joints (excludes hip joints) for swelling. Reported as a count Used as a stand-alone 68/66 count and in ACR score Limitations: Time and evaluator dependent [76]
Dactylitis (sausage digit)	Swelling of an entire digit due to synovial inflammation, tenosynovitis, enthesitis, and soft-tissue edema, seen in 16–48% of PsA patients	Leeds Dactylitis Index (LDI): Uses dactylometer to measure circumference of digits and tenderness of digits for an overall score [77]
Enthesitis	Inflammation at sites of tendon, ligament, and joint capsule fiber insertion into bone, present in 35–50% of PsA patients	Leeds (PEST) Enthesitis Index (LEI): Measures six sites for presence/absence of tenderness (bilateral lateral epicondyles, medial femoral condyles, and Achilles tendon insertions) [78]
		Spondyloarthritis Research Consortium of Canada (SPARCC): Measures 16 enthesial sites for presence/absence of tenderness [79]
		Maastricht Ankylosing Spondylitis Enthesis Score (MASES): Measures 13 enthesial sites for presence/absence of tenderness [78]
		Others: Berlin (12 sites), San Francisco (14 sites), 4-point [50]
Spondyloarthritis (axial/spinal and sacroiliac inflammation)	Has overlapping features with ankylosing spondylitis. Occurs in up to 50% of PsA patients Features include spinal joint enthesial inflammation, sacroiliitis, and ankylosis (bridging syndesmophytes)	Chest expansion Schober test Most measures developed in ankylosing spondylitis: Bath Ankylosing Spondylitis Disease Activity (BASDAI) Bath Ankylosing Spondylitis Function (BASFI) Bath Ankylosing Spondylitis Metrology (BASMI) Ankylosing Spondylitis Disease Activity (ASDAS)

Table 2.13 Examples of composite measures used in psoriatic arthritis disease assessment

Examples of composite arthritis measures	
ACR20/50/70 [76]	• 20/50/70% improvement in the TJC and SJC • 20/50/70% improvement in three of five other measures: – C-reactive protein level or erythrocyte sedimentation rate – Physician global assessment of disease activity (VAS) – Patient global assessment of disease activity (VAS) – Patient pain assessment (VAS) – Disability (by HAQ)
Das-28 [80]	• Tender and swollen joint count for 28 joints • Patient's assessment of pain • Patient global assessment • Physician global assessment of disease activity • Patient assessment of physical function • One acute-phase reactant (ESR, CRP)
DAPSA [81]	5-item composite measure, sum of • TJC of 68 joints • SJC of 66 joints • Patient global (by VAS, 1–10 cm) • Pain VAS (1–10 cm) • CRP
CPDAI [82]	Sum of the following five PsA domains: • Peripheral arthritis: TJC of 68 joints + SJC of 66 joints + HAQ • Skin disease: PASI + DLQI • Enthesitis: LEI • Dactylitis count • Axial disease: BASDAI + ankylosing spondylitis QoL (ASQoL)
PASDAS [83]	• Patient GA (by VAS, 1–10 cm) • PGA (by VAS, 1–10 cm) • SF-36 • TJC of 68 joints • SJC of 66 joints • Enthesitis (by LEI) • Tender dactylitis count • CRP

PASI-experienced dermatologists to PASI-naïve physicians and patients pre- and post-viewing the video [57].

Eczema/Atopic Dermatitis

Atopic eczema is a common skin condition that significantly impacts quality of life of patients and their families. A 2007 systemic review revealed that there are numerous outcome measures in existence but little agreement as to which were valid and reliable [58]. The HOME organization, as noted previously, has led the consensus efforts to determining the four core domains ("what" should be measured): clinician-reported signs, patient-reported symptoms, quality of life, and long-term control [4, 59, 60].

Under the clinical signs domain, the EASI and the SCORAD are considered the two best instruments available to measure clinical signs of AD, with general consensus that the EASI is the core outcome instrument for measuring clinician-reported signs in eczema trials [59]. The Patient Oriented Eczema Measure (POEM) has been selected as the core measure for patient-reported symptoms [61]. At this time, there is no consensus on the core measure for quality of life or long-term control.

Eczema Area and Severity Index (EASI)

The Eczema Area and Severity Index (EASI) score was developed by Jon Hanifin MD and modeled after the PASI [62]. Similar to PASI, the body is divided into four areas (head/neck, upper extremities, trunk, and lower extremities), and the percentage of each area involved with AD is determined and translated to an area score 0–6 (exactly how PASI is done). Next, disease characteristics are then scored within each region; however, EASI differs from PASI in that the four disease characteristics are erythema, induration/population/edema, excoriation, and lichenification, and within each region is rated 0–3 (none, mild, moderate, severe) (Table 2.14).

The EASI is considered valid and internally consistent, with adequate intra-observer reliability, intermediate interobserver reliability, and adequate responsiveness [4]. It measures the intensity of lesions in the four areas of the body, unlike SCORAD, which relies on selecting a "representative" area to assess. Interpretability and cut points have been lacking, but recent clinical trials of the biologic dupilumab for moderate-severe atopic dermatitis have set the precedent of defining an EASI score of at least 16 to be considered moderate-severe [63]. A prospective study using IGA to anchor clinical meaning to EASI cut points established the following severity strata: 0 = clear; 0.1–1.0 = almost clear; 1.1–7.0 = mild; 7.1–21.0 = moderate; 21.1–50.0 = severe; and 50.1–72 = very severe [64]. Similar to PASI, criticisms of the EASI in clinical practice include its lack of ease of use, but the interpretability study above also showed that the mean time to administer the EASI is 6 min (±4.5 min), suggesting that it is quite feasible.

SCORe Atopic Dermatitis (SCORAD)

The SCORe Atopic Dermatitis (SCORAD) is a composite score that was developed and published in 1990 by members of the European Task Force on Atopic Dermatitis [65]. To perform the SCORAD, the rule of nines is utilized to determine BSA involvement (total area "A," 0–100%). The intensity score is performed by assessing a "representative area" on a scale of 0–3 for each of six signs: redness, swelling, oozing/crusting, scratch marks, skin thickening (lichenification), and dryness/xerosis (assessed where there is no inflammation). The intensity scores are added together for intensity score "B" (maximum score 18). The patient provides severity of itch and sleeplessness 0–10, which are summed for patient symptom score "C" (maximum score 20). The final score is then calculated: A/5 + 7B/2 + C (Table 2.15).

The SCORAD is considered valid, internally consistent, responsive, and interpretable. It has adequate interobserver reliability, but intra-observer reliability has not been

Table 2.14 Eczema and Area Severity Index

	Redness 0–3[a]	Induration 0–3[a]	Excoriation 0–3[a]	Lichenification 0–3[a]	Sum (R + I + E + L)	Area score[a] 0–6	Weighting multiplier	Region score
Head/neck		+	+	+	=	x	x 0.1	=
Upper extremities		+	+	+	=	x	x 0.2	=
Trunk		+	+	+	=	x	x 0.3	=
Lower extremities		+	+	+	=	x	x 0.4	=
[a]Area score: Determine percentage of region affected with eczema/atopic dermatitis. Refer to PASI area scoring (Table 2.1)					Final EASI score (sum of four region scores)			
0 = 0								
1 = >0–<10%								
2 = 10–<30%								
3 = 30–<50%								
4 = 50–<70%								
5 = 70–<90%								
6 = 90–100%								

Table 2.15 SCORe Atopic Dermatitis (SCORAD)

Investigator scoring portion (A and B)				
Area score (A) perform body surface area using rule of nines	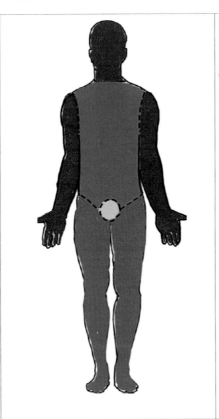		**Maximum per region:** Head and neck 9% Upper limbs 9% each Lower limbs 18% each Genitals 1% Anterior trunk 18% Posterior trunk 18%	
Area score (range 0–100)	A =		0–100	

Intensity score (B): Score each of 6 characteristics 0–3
0 = None
1 = Mild
2 = Moderate
3 = Severe

Redness (erythema)				
0	1	2	3	0–3
Swelling (edema)				
0	1	2	3	0–3
Oozing/crusting				
0	1	2	3	0–3
Scratch marks (excoriation)				
0	1	2	3	0–3
Skin thickening (lichenification)				
0	1	2	3	0–3
Dryness (xerosis)				
0	1	2	3	0–3
Intensity score SUM (maximum score 18)			B =	0–18
Patient scoring portion (C)				

Itch (C_i)

1	2	3	4	5	6	7	8	9	10	C_i=	0–10

Sleeplessness (C_s)

1	2	3	4	5	6	7	8	9	10	C_s=	0–10

Patient itch and sleeplessness score (maximum score 20)	$C_i + C_s$=	0–20
FINAL SCORAD	A/5 + 7B/2 + C =	

adequately assessed. There are no floor or ceiling effects. Criticisms of the SCORAD include the difficulty and the potential drawbacks of identifying an "average representative area" for scoring the intensity of the six clinical signs. It differs from the EASI in that it includes six signs instead of four, but does include the four essential signs as defined by HOME plus oozing/crusting and dryness. The SCORAD gives more weight to intensity than extent, compared to EASI, which weights signs and extent more equally, because the SCORAD includes patient-reported symptoms (therefore is considered multidimensional) and could lead to potential unblinding if a trial had a single-blinded design [65, 66].

IGA (Investigator Global Assessment) in Eczema

Similar to the issues of PGA/IGA in psoriasis, there are numerous global assessments that have been used in atopic eczema trials. A recent review showed that there were over 20 named global assessments, most commonly called Investigator Global Assessment, Physician Global Assessment, and Physician Global Evaluation [67]. The majority included only signs of atopic eczema, with anchoring language including some or all signs such as erythema, population/edema, oozing/weeping, crusting, excoriation, scaling, and lichenification, usually graded 0–4 (none to severe) or 0–5 (none-very severe). The variability and inconsistent/inadequate content that are problematic in psoriasis studies are just as problematic in eczema studies. An example of an atopic eczema IGA is provided in Table 2.16.

Patient Oriented Eczema Measure (POEM)

The Patient Oriented Eczema Measure (POEM) is considered the most validated patient-reported eczema symptom instrument. It was developed and validated in 2004 [68].

Table 2.16 Example investigator global assessment for atopic dermatitis: 5 point (0–4) [84]

5-point (0–4) static Investigator Global Assessment for atopic eczema		
Score		Definition
0	Clear	No inflammatory signs of atopic dermatitis
1	Almost clear	Faint, barely detectable erythema and/or trace residual induration/papulation in limited areas; neither excoriation nor oozing/crusting are present
2	Mild	Light pink erythema and slightly perceptible induration/population; excoriation if present is mild
3	Moderate	Dull red, clearly distinguishable erythema and clearly perceptible induration/population but not extensive; excoriation or oozing/crusting, if present, are mild to moderate
4	Severe	Deep/dark red erythema, and marked and extensive induration/population; excoriation and oozing/crusting are present

The instrument has seven questions that quantify the number of days in the last week that there were symptoms of atopic eczema (itch, bleeding, weeping/oozing, cracking, flaking, dryness, and sleep disturbance). The original validation paper demonstrated that the instrument has good internal consistency, construct validity, responsiveness, and content validity. The test-retest reliability has not been adequately assessed. The minimally clinical important difference is 3.4, and has five bands of severity (clear, mild, moderate, severe, and very severe) [69]. It takes about 2 min to complete, and is free to use and readily available at http://nottingham.ac.uk/research/groups/cebd/resources/poem.aspx (Table 2.17).

Table 2.17 POEM: Patient Oriented Eczema Measure [68, 69])

1. Over the last week, on how many days has your/your child's skin been itchy because of the eczema?				
No days	1–2 days	3–4 days	5–6 days	Every day

2. Over the last week, on how many nights has your/your child's sleep been disturbed because of the eczema?				
No days	1–2 days	3–4 days	5–6 days	Every day

3. Over the last week, on how many days has your/your child's skin been bleeding because of the eczema?				
No days	1–2 days	3–4 days	5–6 days	Every day

4. Over the last week, on how many days has your/your child's skin been weeping or oozing clear fluid because of the eczema?				
No days	1–2 days	3–4 days	5–6 days	Every day

5. Over the last week, on how many days has your/your child's skin been cracked because of the eczema?				
No days	1–2 days	3–4 days	5–6 days	Every day

6. Over the last week, on how many days has your/your child's skin been flaking off because of the eczema?				
No days	1–2 days	3–4 days	5–6 days	Every day

7. Over the last week, on how many days has your/your child's skin felt dry or rough because of the eczema?				
No days	1–2 days	3–4 days	5–6 days	Every day

Scoring:
Each of the 7 questions carries equal weight. For each assign points as follows:
No days = 0
1–2 days = 1
3–4 days = 2
5–6 days = 3
Every day = 4
- If one question is left unanswered this is scored 0 and the scores are summed and expressed as usual out of 28
- If two or more questions are left unanswered the questionnaire is not scored
- If two or more response options are selected, the response option with the highest score should be recorded

Banding:
Bands have been established:
0–2 = Clear or almost clear
3–7 = Mild eczema
8–16 = Moderate eczema
17–24 = Severe eczema
25–28 = Very severe eczema

Permissions:
The POEM scale is copyrighted, but freely available for use and downloaded: www.nottingham.ac.uk/dermatology
The University of Nottingham requests registration of use of the POEM by e-mailing cebd@nottingham.ac.uk with details of how you would like to use the scale, and which countries the scale will be used in

References

1. Kirwan JR, Chaput de Saintonge DM, Joyce CR. Clinical judgment analysis. Q J Med. 1990;76(281):935–49.

2. Boers M, Brooks P, Strand CV, Tugwell P. The OMERACT filter for outcome measures in rheumatology. J Rheumatol. 1998;25(2):198–9.

3. Kirwan JR, Boers M, Tugwell P. Updating the OMERACT filter at OMERACT 11. J Rheumatol. 2014;41(5):975–7.

4. Chalmers JR, Simpson E, Apfelbacher CJ, Thomas KS, von Kobyletzki L, Schmitt J, et al. Report from the fourth international consensus meeting to harmonize core outcome measures for atopic eczema/dermatitis clinical trials (HOME initiative). Br J Dermatol. 2016;175(1):69–79.

5. Naldi L, Svensson A, Diepgen T, Elsner P, Grob JJ, Coenraads PJ, et al. Randomized clinical trials for psoriasis 1977–2000: the EDEN survey. J Invest Dermatol. 2003;120(5):738–41.

6. Fredriksson T, Pettersson U. Severe psoriasis—oral therapy with a new retinoid. Dermatologica. 1978;157(4):238–44.

7. Marks R, Barton SP, Shuttleworth D, Finlay AY. Assessment of disease progress in psoriasis. Arch Dermatol. 1989;125(2):235–40.

8. Manalo IF, Gilbert KE, Wu JJ. An updated survey for the 2007–2013 period of randomized controlled trials for psoriasis: treatment modalities, study designs, comparators, outcome measures and sponsorship. J Eur Acad Dermatol Venereol. 2015;29(10):1945–50.

9. Puzenat E, Bronsard V, Prey S, Gourraud PA, Aractingi S, Bagot M, et al. What are the best outcome measures for assessing plaque psoriasis severity? A systematic review of the literature. J Eur Acad Dermatol Venereol. 2010;24(Suppl 2):10–6.

10. Spuls PI, Lecluse LL, Poulsen ML, Bos JD, Stern RS, Nijsten T. How good are clinical severity and outcome measures for psoriasis?: quantitative evaluation in a systematic review. J Invest Dermatol. 2010;130(4):933–43.

11. Berth-Jones J, Grotzinger K, Rainville C, Pham B, Huang J, Daly S, et al. A study examining inter- and intrarater reliability of three scales for measuring severity of psoriasis: psoriasis area and severity index, physician's global assessment and lattice system physician's global assessment. Br J Dermatol. 2006;155(4):707–13.

12. Thaci D, Blauvelt A, Reich K, Tsai TF, Vanaclocha F, Kingo K, et al. Secukinumab is superior to ustekinumab in clearing skin of subjects with moderate to severe plaque psoriasis: CLEAR, a randomized controlled trial. J Am Acad Dermatol. 2015;73(3):400–9.

13. Carlin CS, Feldman SR, Krueger JG, Menter A, Krueger GG. A 50% reduction in the psoriasis area and severity index (PASI 50) is a clinically significant endpoint in the assessment of psoriasis. J Am Acad Dermatol. 2004;50(6):859–66.

14. Gottlieb AB, Krueger JG, Wittkowski K, Dedrick R, Walicke PA, Garovoy M. Psoriasis as a model for T-cell-mediated disease: immunobiologic and clinical effects of treatment with multiple doses of efalizumab, an anti-CD11a antibody. Arch Dermatol. 2002;138(5):591–600.

15. Krueger GG, Papp KA, Stough DB, Loven KH, Gulliver WP, Ellis CN, et al. A randomized, double-blind, placebo-controlled phase III study evaluating efficacy and tolerability of 2 courses of alefacept in patients with chronic plaque psoriasis. J Am Acad Dermatol. 2002;47(6):821–33.

16. Edson-Heredia E, Banerjee S, Zhu B, Maeda-Chubachi T, Cameron GS, Shen W, et al. A high level of clinical response is associated with improved patient-reported outcomes in psoriasis: analyses from a phase 2 study in patients treated with ixekizumab. J Eur Acad Dermatol Venereol. 2016;30(5):864–5.

17. Robinson A, Kardos M, Kimball AB. Physician global assessment (PGA) and psoriasis area and severity index (PASI): why do both? A systematic analysis of randomized controlled trials of biologic agents for moderate to severe plaque psoriasis. J Am Acad Dermatol. 2012;66(3):369–75.

18. Walsh JA, McFadden M, Woodcock J, Clegg DO, Helliwell P, Dommasch E, et al. Product of the physician global assessment and body surface area: a simple static measure of psoriasis severity in a longitudinal cohort. J Am Acad Dermatol. 2013;69(6):931–7.

19. Cappelleri JC, Bushmakin AG, Harness J, Mamolo C. Psychometric validation of the physician global assessment scale for assessing severity of psoriasis disease activity. Qual Life Res. 2013;22(9):2489–99.

20. Langley RG, Ellis CN. Evaluating psoriasis with psoriasis area and severity index, psoriasis global assessment, and lattice system physician's global assessment. J Am Acad Dermatol. 2004;51(4):563–9.

21. Ports WC, Khan S, Lan S, Lamba M, Bolduc C, Bissonnette R, et al. A randomized phase 2a efficacy and safety trial of the topical Janus kinase inhibitor tofacitinib in the treatment of chronic plaque psoriasis. Br J Dermatol. 2013;169(1):137–45.

22. Boy MG, Wang C, Wilkinson BE, Chow VF, Clucas AT, Krueger JG, et al. Double-blind, placebo-controlled, dose-escalation study to evaluate the pharmacologic effect of CP-690,550 in patients with psoriasis. J Invest Dermatol. 2009;129(9):2299–302.

23. Czarnowicki T, Linkner RV, Suarez-Farinas M, Ingber A, Lebwohl M. An investigator-initiated, double-blind, vehicle-controlled pilot study: assessment for tachyphylaxis to topically occluded halobetasol 0.05% ointment in the treatment of psoriasis. J Am Acad Dermatol. 2014;71(5):954–9. e1

24. Dommasch E, Walsh, J.W., Woodcock, J.A., Shin, D., Callis Duffin, K., Gelfand J. Validity of the simple measure for assessing psoriasis activity (S-MAPA). World Congress of Dermatology, Seoul, Korea: 2011 May 24-29, 2011. Report No.

25. Strober BE, Sobell JM, Duffin KC, Bao Y, Guerin A, Yang H, et al. Sleep quality and other patient-reported outcomes improve after patients with psoriasis with suboptimal response to other systemic therapies are switched to adalimumab: results from PROGRESS, an open-label Phase IIIB trial. Br J Dermatol. 2012;167(6):1374–81.

26. Wallace AB. The exposure treatment of burns. Lancet. 1951;1(6653):501–4.

27. Hettiaratchy S, Papini R. Initial management of a major burn: II—assessment and resuscitation. BMJ. 2004;329(7457):101–3.

28. Long CC, Finlay AY, Averill RW. The rule of hand: 4 hand areas = 2 FTU = 1 g. Arch Dermatol. 1992;128(8):1129–30.

29. Rossiter ND, Chapman P, Haywood IA. How big is a hand? Burns. 1996;22(3):230–1.

30. Nagel TR, Schunk JE. Using the hand to estimate the surface area of a burn in children. Pediatr Emerg Care. 1997;13(4):254–5.

31. Ramsay B, Lawrence CM. Measurement of involved surface area in patients with psoriasis. Br J Dermatol. 1991;124(6):565–70.

32. Ashcroft DM, Wan Po AL, Williams HC, Griffiths CE. Clinical measures of disease severity and outcome in psoriasis: a critical appraisal of their quality. Br J Dermatol. 1999;141(2):185–91.

33. Armstrong AW, Siegel MP, Bagel J, Boh EE, Buell M, Cooper KD, et al. From the medical board of the national psoriasis foundation: treatment targets for plaque psoriasis. J Am Acad Dermatol. 2017;76(2):290–8.

34. Takahashi MD, Chouela EN, Dorantes GL, Roselino AM, Santamaria J, Allevato MA, et al. Efalizumab in the treatment of scalp, palmoplantar and nail psoriasis: results of a 24-week Latin American Study. Arch Drug Inf. 2010;3(1):1–8.

35. Bagel J, Lynde C, Tyring S, Kricorian G, Shi Y, Klekotka P. Moderate to severe plaque psoriasis with scalp involvement: a randomized, double-blind, placebo-controlled study of etanercept. J Am Acad Dermatol. 2012;67(1):86–92.

36. Reich K, Leonardi C, Lebwohl M, Kerdel F, Okubo Y, Romiti R, et al. Sustained response with ixekizumab treatment of moderate-to-severe psoriasis with scalp involvement: results from three phase 3 trials (UNCOVER-1, UNCOVER-2, UNCOVER-3). J Dermatolog Treat. 2017;28(4):282–7.

37. Thaci D, Daiber W, Boehncke WH, Kaufmann R. Calcipotriol solution for the treatment of scalp psoriasis: evaluation of efficacy, safety and acceptance in 3,396 patients. Dermatology. 2001;203(2):153–6.

38. Cassell SE, Bieber JD, Rich P, Tutuncu ZN, Lee SJ, Kalunian KC, et al. The modified nail psoriasis severity index: validation of an

instrument to assess psoriatic nail involvement in patients with psoriatic arthritis. J Rheumatol. 2007;34(1):123–9.

39. Rich P, Scher RK. Nail psoriasis severity index: a useful tool for evaluation of nail psoriasis. J Am Acad Dermatol. 2003;49(2):206–12.

40. Augustin M, Blome C, Costanzo A, Dauden E, Ferrandiz C, Girolomoni G, et al. Nail assessment in psoriasis and psoriatic arthritis (NAPPA): development and validation of a tool for assessment of nail psoriasis outcomes. Br J Dermatol. 2014;170(3):591–8.

41. Parrish CA, Sobera JO, Elewski BE. Modification of the nail psoriasis severity index. J Am Acad Dermatol. 2005;53(4):745–6. author reply 6-7

42. Aktan S, Ilknur T, Akin C, Ozkan S. Interobserver reliability of the nail psoriasis severity index. Clin Exp Dermatol. 2007;32(2):141–4.

43. van der Velden HM, Klaassen KM, van de Kerkhof PC, Pasch MC. Invited reply to "possible reconsideration of the nail psoriasis severity index (NAPSI) score". J Am Acad Dermatol. 2013;69(6):1054.

44. Finlay AY, Khan GK. Dermatology life quality index (DLQI)—a simple practical measure for routine clinical use. Clin Exp Dermatol. 1994;19(3):210–6.

45. Lewis V, Finlay AY. 10 years experience of the dermatology life quality index (DLQI). J Investig Dermatol Symp Proc. 2004;9(2):169–80.

46. Basra MK, Salek MS, Camilleri L, Sturkey R, Finlay AY. Determining the minimal clinically important difference and responsiveness of the dermatology life quality index (DLQI): further data. Dermatology. 2015;230(1):27–33.

47. Mrowietz U, Kragballe K, Reich K, Spuls P, Griffiths CE, Nast A, et al. Definition of treatment goals for moderate to severe psoriasis: a European consensus. Arch Dermatol Res. 2011;303(1):1–10.

48. Nijsten T. Dermatology life quality index: time to move forward. J Invest Dermatol. 2012;132(1):11–3.

49. Mease PJ, Gladman DD, Papp KA, Khraishi MM, Thaci D, Behrens F, et al. Prevalence of rheumatologist-diagnosed psoriatic arthritis in patients with psoriasis in European/North American dermatology clinics. J Am Acad Dermatol. 2013;69(5):729–35.

50. Mease PJ. Measures of psoriatic arthritis: tender and Swollen Joint Assessment, Psoriasis Area and Severity Index (PASI), Nail Psoriasis Severity Index (NAPSI), Modified Nail Psoriasis Severity Index (mNAPSI), Mander/Newcastle Enthesitis Index (MEI), Leeds Enthesitis Index (LEI), Spondyloarthritis Research Consortium of Canada (SPARCC), Maastricht Ankylosing Spondylitis Enthesis Score (MASES), Leeds Dactylitis Index (LDI), Patient Global for Psoriatic Arthritis, Dermatology Life Quality Index (DLQI), Psoriatic Arthritis Quality of Life (PsAQOL), Functional Assessment of Chronic Illness Therapy-Fatigue (FACIT-F), Psoriatic Arthritis Response Criteria (PsARC), Psoriatic Arthritis Joint Activity Index (PsAJAI), Disease Activity in Psoriatic Arthritis (DAPSA), and Composite Psoriatic Disease Activity Index (CPDAI). Arthritis Care Res (Hoboken). 2011;63(Suppl 11):S64–85.

51. Felson DT, Anderson JJ, Boers M, Bombardier C, Furst D, Goldsmith C, et al. American College of Rheumatology. Preliminary definition of improvement in rheumatoid arthritis. Arthritis Rheum. 1995;38(6):727–35.

52. Callis Duffin K, Mease PJ. Psoriasis and psoriatic arthritis video project 2010: a report from the GRAPPA annual meeting. J Rheumatol. 2011;38(3):562–3.

53. Callis Duffin K, Armstrong AW, Mease PJ. Psoriasis and psoriatic arthritis video project: an update from the GRAPPA 2011 annual meeting. J Rheumatol. 2012;39(11):2198–200.

54. Callis Duffin K, Armstrong AW, Mease PJ. Psoriasis and psoriatic arthritis video project: an update from the 2012 GRAPPA annual meeting. J Rheumatol. 2013;40(8):1455–6.

55. Callis Duffin K, Gottlieb AB. Outcome measures for psoriasis severity: a report from the GRAPPA 2012 annual meeting. J Rheumatol. 2013;40(8):1423–4.

56. Mease PJ, Helliwell PS, Boehncke WH, Coates LC, FitzGerald O, Gladman DD, et al. GRAPPA 2015 research and education project reports. J Rheumatol. 2016;43(5):979–85

57. Armstrong AW, Parsi K, Schupp CW, Mease PJ, Duffin KC. Standardizing training for psoriasis measures: effectiveness of an online training video on psoriasis area and severity index assessment by physician and patient raters. JAMA Dermatol. 2013;149(5):577–82.

58. Schmitt J, Langan S, Williams HC, European Dermato-Epidemiology N. What are the best outcome measurements for atopic eczema? A systematic review. J Allergy Clin Immunol. 2007;120(6):1389–98.

59. Chalmers JR, Schmitt J, Apfelbacher C, Dohil M, Eichenfield LF, Simpson EL, et al. Report from the third international consensus meeting to harmonise core outcome measures for atopic eczema/dermatitis clinical trials (HOME). Br J Dermatol. 2014;171(6):1318–25.

60. Schmitt J, Apfelbacher C, Spuls PI, Thomas KS, Simpson EL, Furue M, et al. The harmonizing outcome measures for eczema (HOME) roadmap: a methodological framework to develop core sets of outcome measurements in dermatology. J Invest Dermatol. 2015;135(1):24–30.

61. Spuls PI, Gerbens LAA, Simpson E, Apfelbacher CJ, Chalmers JR, Thomas KS, et al. Patient-oriented eczema measure (POEM), a core instrument to measure symptoms in clinical trials: a harmonising outcome measures for eczema (HOME) statement. Br J Dermatol. 2017;176(4):979–84.

62. Hanifin JM, Thurston M, Omoto M, Cherill R, Tofte SJ, Graeber M. The eczema area and severity index (EASI): assessment of reliability in atopic dermatitis. EASI Evaluator Group. Exp Dermatol. 2001;10(1):11–8.

63. Simpson EL, Bieber T, Guttman-Yassky E, Beck LA, Blauvelt A, Cork MJ, et al. Two phase 3 trials of dupilumab versus placebo in atopic dermatitis. N Engl J Med. 2016;375(24):2335–48.

64. Leshem YA, Hajar T, Hanifin JM, Simpson EL. What the eczema area and severity index score tells us about the severity of atopic dermatitis: an interpretability study. Br J Dermatol. 2015;172(5):1353–7.

65. Consensus Report of the European Task Force on Atopic Dermatitis. Severity scoring of atopic dermatitis: the SCORAD index. Dermatology. 1993;186(1):23–31.

66. Schram ME, Spuls PI, Leeflang MM, Lindeboom R, Bos JD, Schmitt J. EASI, (objective) SCORAD and POEM for atopic eczema: responsiveness and minimal clinically important difference. Allergy. 2012;67(1):99–106.

67. Futamura M, Leshem YA, Thomas KS, Nankervis H, Williams HC, Simpson EL. A systematic review of investigator global assessment (IGA) in atopic dermatitis (AD) trials: many options, no standards. J Am Acad Dermatol. 2016;74(2):288–94.

68. Charman CR, Venn AJ, Williams HC. The patient-oriented eczema measure: development and initial validation of a new tool for measuring atopic eczema severity from the patients' perspective. Arch Dermatol. 2004;140(12):1513–9.

69. Charman CR, Venn AJ, Ravenscroft JC, Williams HC. Translating patient-oriented eczema measure (POEM) scores into clinical practice by suggesting severity strata derived using anchor-based methods. Br J Dermatol. 2013;169(6):1326–32.

70. Bushnell DM, Martin ML, McCarrier K, Gordon K, Chiou CF, Huang X, et al. Validation of the psoriasis symptom inventory (PSI), a patient-reported outcome measure to assess psoriasis symptom severity. J Dermatolog Treat. 2013;24(5):356–60.

71. Bushnell DM, Martin ML, Scanlon M, Chen T, Chau D, Viswanathan HN. Equivalence and measurement properties of an electronic version of the psoriasis symptom inventory. Qual Life Res. 2014;23(3):897–906.

72. Gordon KB, Kimball AB, Chau D, Viswanathan HN, Li J, Revicki DA, et al. Impact of brodalumab treatment on psoriasis symptoms

and health-related quality of life: use of a novel patient-reported outcome measure, the psoriasis symptom inventory. Br J Dermatol. 2014;170(3):705–15.

73. Revicki DA, Jin Y, Wilson HD, Chau D, Viswanathan HN. Reliability and validity of the psoriasis symptom inventory in patients with moderate-to-severe psoriasis. J Dermatolog Treat. 2014;25(1):8–14.

74. Strober B, Sigurgeirsson B, Popp G, Sinclair R, Krell J, Stonkus S, et al. Secukinumab improves patient-reported psoriasis symptoms of itching, pain, and scaling: results of two phase 3, randomized, placebo-controlled clinical trials. Int J Dermatol. 2016;55(4):401–7.

75. Strober BE, Nyirady J, Mallya UG, Guettner A, Papavassilis C, Gottlieb AB, et al. Item-level psychometric properties for a new patient-reported psoriasis symptom diary. Value Health. 2013;16(6):1014–22.

76. van Riel P, van Gestel A, Scott D. EULAR handbook of clinical assessment in rheumatoid arthritis. The Netherlands: Van Zuiden Communications B.V.; 2000.

77. Helliwell PS, Firth J, Ibrahim GH, Melsom RD, Shah I, Turner DE. Development of an assessment tool for dactylitis in patients with psoriatic arthritis. J Rheumatol. 2005;32(9):1745–50.

78. Healy PJ, Helliwell PS. Measuring clinical enthesitis in psoriatic arthritis: assessment of existing measures and development of an instrument specific to psoriatic arthritis. Arthritis Rheum. 2008;59(5):686–91.

79. Maksymowych WP, Mallon C, Morrow S, Shojania K, Olszynski WP, Wong RL, et al. Development and validation of the spondy-loarthritis research consortium of Canada (SPARCC) enthesitis index. Ann Rheum Dis. 2009;68(6):948–53.

80. van Gestel AM, Prevoo ML, van 't Hof MA, van Rijswijk MH, van de Putte LB, van Riel PL. Development and validation of the European league against rheumatism response criteria for rheumatoid arthritis. Comparison with the preliminary American College of Rheumatology and the World Health Organization/International League Against Rheumatism Criteria. Arthritis Rheum. 1996;39(1):34–40.

81. Schoels M, Aletaha D, Funovits J, Kavanaugh A, Baker D, Smolen JS. Application of the DAREA/DAPSA score for assessment of disease activity in psoriatic arthritis. Ann Rheum Dis. 2010;69(8):1441–7.

82. Mumtaz A, Gallagher P, Kirby B, Waxman R, Coates LC, Veale JD, et al. Development of a preliminary composite disease activity index in psoriatic arthritis. Ann Rheum Dis. 2011;70(2):272–7.

83. Helliwell PS, FitzGerald O, Fransen J, Gladman DD, Kreuger GG, Callis-Duffin K, et al. The development of candidate composite disease activity and responder indices for psoriatic arthritis (GRACE project). Ann Rheum Dis. 2013;72(6):986–91.

84. Eichenfield LF, Lucky AW, Boguniewicz M, Langley RG, Cherill R, Marshall K, et al. Safety and efficacy of pimecrolimus (ASM 981) cream 1% in the treatment of mild and moderate atopic dermatitis in children and adolescents. J Am Acad Dermatol. 2002;46(4):495–504.

Interpreting Clinical Trial Data

3

Mina Amin, Daniel J. No, Kavita Darji, and Jashin J. Wu

Introduction

Evidence-based medicine involves the application of clinically relevant research to medical practice [1-3]. The integration of clinical expertise with up-to-date clinical research data is the fundamental basis of optimal patient care. Clinical knowledge ensures that high-quality research is applied to the appropriate patient and is in agreement with the patient's values. Conversely, treating patients based on clinical knowledge without clinical research poses the risk of offering out-of-date care. Thus, the combination of clinical expertise with current evidence significantly improves clinical decision making [1].

The vast amount of clinical trial data available today can make evaluation of clinical research seem overwhelming. However, well-designed, randomized clinical trials convey critical information about the therapeutic options available to patients [4]. Thus, evidence from clinical trials can be directly applied towards patient care [5].

It is imperative that the busy clinician evaluates clinical research carefully and thoroughly. To best interpret clinical trial data, it is important to understand the essential characteristics of experimental trials. The following information is aimed to provide clinicians with the necessary skillset to properly evaluate clinical trials.

M. Amin, BS
School of Medicine, University of California, Riverside, 900 University Ave, Riverside, CA 92507, USA
e-mail: mamin006@medsch.ucr.edu

D.J. No, BA
School of Medicine, Loma Linda University, 11175 Campus St, Loma Linda, CA 92350, USA

K. Darji, BA
School of Medicine, Saint Louis University, 1402 S Grand Blvd, St. Louis, MO 63104, USA

J.J. Wu, MD (✉)
Department of Dermatology, Kaiser Permanente Los Angeles Medical Center, 1515 North Vermont Ave, 5th Floor, Los Angeles, CA 90027, USA
e-mail: jashinwu@gmail.com

Study Designs

An experimental study aims to modify the outcome of a dependent variable in one or more groups of participants. Clinical trials are randomized controlled trials in humans that compare an experimental group with a control group to determine the impact of an intervention. Individual participants are randomly assigned to intervention or control groups. The control group involves an alternate intervention, placebo, or no treatment. With appropriate randomization, minimal differences exist between control and experimental groups at the beginning of the study. Therefore, any differences detected at the completion of study are likely a result of the intervention [6].

Cluster randomization is a method of randomizing groups instead of individuals. Randomization of groups is favorable if the intervention involves a group of participants. For example, a prospective cluster randomized controlled trial evaluated the efficacy of health-related quality of life (HRQoL) intervention for patients on biologic therapy with moderate-to-severe psoriasis. The experimental group received etanercept with an HRQoL assessment and communication while the control group only received etanercept. The locations of the study sites, not the individual participants, were randomly assigned to receive either intervention or control. The locations were separated into four clusters: academic centers, nonacademic centers, sites never exposed to HRQoL assessment and communication, and sites exposed to HRQoL assessment and communication. An advantage of this study is that HRQoL intervention was given in the clinical setting. Additionally, different types of interactions across multiple different locations were compared. A limitation to this study is that participants and dermatologists were not blinded. Additionally, the application of this study to a larger population is challenging because only patients with moderate-to-severe psoriasis receiving etanercept were evaluated [7, 8].

© Springer International Publishing AG 2018
P.S. Yamauchi (ed.), *Biologic and Systemic Agents in Dermatology*, https://doi.org/10.1007/978-3-319-66884-0_3

Study Analysis

Meta-analysis is a statistical procedure that compiles results from multiple distinct but comparable studies. However, the assimilation of data from multiple studies may be challenging when study designs and methods differ. Individual clinical trials are also frequently small, underpowered studies, which creates difficulty applying the derived conclusions to the general population [9]. Clinical trials with small sample sizes may not achieve statistical significance independently, but often become significant when compiled in a meta-analysis [6]. A secondary goal of meta-analysis is to examine factors that may explain the reason for differing results. This is particularly useful when data differs significantly among independent studies. Meta-analysis is also referred to as systematic review based on the qualitative and quantitative characteristics of this analysis. Meta-analysis is considered qualitative because the advantages and disadvantages of study designs are discussed and quantitative because data from different trials is presented [10]. Studies that are flawed or inadequately completed are often omitted. Meta-analyses are becoming increasingly popular as the impact of treatment or intervention can be compared across multiple populations. Despite the fact that many clinical studies are addressing nearly identical questions, their conclusions are often inconsistent with each other [6]. Meta-analysis is a useful technique to resolve these discrepancies to generate one comprehensive conclusion with greater statistical power [6, 9].

Phases of Drug Development

Preclinical research is required before beginning a clinical trial. Chemistry and manufacturing work are used to develop dose and produce a drug candidate to conduct preclinical studies. The goal of preclinical testing is to assess the toxicity, efficacy, and biological activity of an experimental drug. Preclinical testing utilizes in vitro and animal models and typically lasts 2–3 years [11]. This information is used to help predict potential toxic effects in humans.

Clinical trials are often categorized into four distinct phases. Phase I trials are the preliminary trials conducted in "normal" human subjects. The purpose of phase I trials is to evaluate the pharmacokinetics, pharmacodynamics, tolerability, and safety of an experimental drug. Preclinical studies must support human doses. Phase I trials are usually small, involving 5–80 nondiseased participants, and last approximately 6–12 months [11]. Failure can occur due to toxicity or if the pharmacodynamic and pharmacokinetic relationship is not consistent with the hypothesis.

Phase II trials are important in determining if a new drug is clinically effective. Phase II trials also provide important information about dose optimization. Dose ranging helps identify phase 3 dosing. The safety and efficacy of the experimental drug are compared to placebo in patients with the disease. Phase II trials involve 100–500 patient volunteers and last 1–2 years [11]. Failure can occur when the new drug does not show desired efficacy, study design is not feasible, or administration has excessive toxicity.

The primary goal of phase III trials is to compare the safety and efficacy of an experimental drug with existing standard therapy or placebo. Phase III trials are typically larger, involving hundreds to thousands of patient volunteers, and last approximately 2–3 years [11]. They are typically placebo controlled, double blind, and multicenter. Typical reasons for failure include unexpected toxicity, inconclusive efficacy, or lack of financial viability.

Phase IV trials occur after approval of the new drug. The purpose of phase IV trials is postmarketing observation to attain additional information about the risks and benefits of a new drug as mandated by regulatory agencies. Phase IV trials are ongoing to allow for observation of the lasting effects of a new drug along with any delayed side effects [11]. Although an intervention may be beneficial in the short term, long-term side effects may occur and must be monitored [12].

Advantages and Disadvantages of Clinical Trials

A main advantage of clinical trials is the collection of strong evidence to form conclusive results that portray clear cause and effect relationships of an intervention. The comparison of an intervention group with an alternative therapy or placebo in a clinical trial provides an extremely efficient method of observing the impact of an intervention on an outcome. Randomization creates comparable groups that are designed to differ only in respect of the intervention administered. Thus, this design significantly reduces the incidence of bias and confounding factors [13]. Randomized control trials provide valuable information about the efficacy of an experimental drug, along with benefits and risks. The outcomes of clinical trials are of utmost importance as this information ultimately creates the foundation of clinical decision making and public health policies.

Clinical trials are also associated with disadvantages and limitations. For instance, the environment of a clinical trial may be artificial or unrealistic, which can make it difficult to create generalizations to the population of interest. Moreover, randomized clinical trials are more expensive to perform, time consuming, and more complex than uncontrolled observational studies [12].

Ethical problems regarding distribution of treatment must also be considered. Patients receiving a new intervention are at risk of suffering from unknown side effects, whereas participants who do not receive the intervention are at risk of delaying improvement in their disease status. Thus, it is important for participants to fully understand the nature of the trial before agreeing to participate [13]. The recruitment of patients in a clinical trial may also be challenging, especially when examining rare diseases. Moreover, although a trial may convey statistically significant results, these results may quickly lose relevance as new information is constantly released.

P-Values and Confidence Intervals

The *p*-value is a commonly used statistical measurement in experimental research. It represents the probability of acquiring a result equal to or more extreme than the result observed in the study, assuming that the null hypothesis is true [14]. The null hypothesis indicates that there is no difference between the groups of interest. The baseline assumption is that the null hypothesis is true until statistical evidence can prove otherwise. If the calculated *p*-value is below a predetermined limit, such as 0.05, then the null hypothesis is rejected, and the results are considered statistically significant [15]. In contrast, a *p*-value larger than 0.05 would indicate that the null hypothesis is true and there is no statistically significant difference between the groups of interest.

Of note, the *p*-value is often misinterpreted as the probability that the observed results are true. A *p*-value of 0.05, for instance, is often incorrectly assumed to represent a 5% probability that the null hypothesis is true. Under this interpretation, the likelihood that the null hypothesis is false is assumed to be 95%. However, this interpretation is invalid because *p*-values are calculated based on the assumption that the null hypothesis is true. Thus, *p*-values do not provide information on the likelihood that a null hypothesis is true or false [14].

The *p*-value is limited because is it does not consider the strength or direction of an effect [14]. Although very similar in value, a study with a *p*-value of 0.055 is considered insignificant while a *p*-value of 0.045 is considered significant. Similarly, *p*-values of 0.0001 and 0.045 are both considered significant; however, these two results are likely very different [16].

Confidence intervals, on the other hand, contain information about statistical significance, direction, and strength of an effect [15]. Confidence intervals provide a range of values that surround the parameter of interest, such as odds ratio or difference between means. The width of the confidence interval contains information about the accuracy of the measured value of interest. A narrower confidence interval corresponds with increased certainty about the measured value of interest. The width of the confidence interval is influenced by the sample size of the study. Large studies generate more data values, which enhances the certainty about the measured effect and is associated with a narrower confidence interval [15]. A wide confidence interval indicates less certainty about the measured effect and should, therefore, be evaluated carefully as it may suggest an inaccurate result, irrespective of statistical significance [17].

Confidence intervals are also easily misinterpreted. For instance, a confidence interval of 95% does not correspond to a 5% likelihood that the true value is outside of this interval. Instead, it signifies that the confidence interval encloses the true value of interest 95% of the time [14]. Stated differently, a 95% confidence interval indicates with 95% confidence that the parameter of interest exists within the range of values provided. If the value that represents no effect (for instance, a relative risk of one, or the difference between means of zero) is included in the confidence interval, then the results are not considered statistically significant [15].

Survival Analysis

Survival time is the time from a fixed point until the onset of event occurrence. The fixed point may represent the initiation of treatment or enrollment into a trial. The event of interest may refer to death, disease onset, recovery, or relapse. Time is measured as days, months, weeks, or years from the specific set point in time until event occurrence. Survival analysis refers to the set of procedures for analyzing data in which survival time is the variable measured [18].

Analysis can become challenging if the measured event has not occurred by the conclusion of the study or there is a loss to follow-up. Observations are censored if the period of observation was cut off before the event of interest occurred. For example, if a study is completed at 10 months, and the participant is lost to follow-up or the event has not yet occurred by 10 months, then the observations for that participant are censored. [6, 19].

Data depicts time until an event can be graphically represented with Kaplan-Meier survival curves, which are depicted as a stepwise function. If the event measured is death, then the proportion of patients surviving at a particular time point is represented on the vertical axis. The y-value represents the probability of occurrence of the event of interest [6]. The horizontal axis represents the time of event occurrence, and the x-values represent the survival period for a particular interval. At each interval, the probability of event occurrence, or survival probability, is calculated. Censored observations are not included in the calculation. Survival, or no event occurrence, is assumed constant between events and drops in the curve only occur at fixed intervals. Curves that appear close to one another or overlap are less likely to be significantly different. A significant difference can be further assessed using statistical tests such as log-rank test or the Breslow test [18].

The multivariate method of analysis of survival data that is most frequently utilized in medical research is the Cox proportional hazards model [20].

It is a regression model that determines the impact of risk factors on the dependent variable time until event occurrence [20]. The regression equation is

$$h(t) = h_0(t) \times \exp\{b_1 x_1 + b_2 x_2 + \ldots + b_p x_p\}$$

in which $h(t)$ is the probability that an individual will experience the event of interest at time t [20]. Of note, compared to survival probability, which places an emphasis on an event not occurring, the hazard function is interested in event occurrence [21]. The hazard function depends on p covariates (x_0, x_2, ..., x_p). The value of the coefficients (b_1, b_2, ..., b_p) determines the influence of the covariates on hazard. The baseline hazard, h_0, is the hazard if the sum of the covariates equals zero [20].

The hazard ratio compares the ratio of the hazard rate in the treatment group compared to the control group. It refers to the odds that the event will occur in a patient in the treatment group compared to control. If the event of interest is clearance of symptoms, then the hazard ratio would indicate the probability of resolution of symptoms at any point in time in the treatment group compared to the control group. A hazard ratio of two indicates that a patient receiving treatment that has yet to experience resolution of symptoms is twice as likely to have complete resolution at next follow-up compared to the control group. A hazard ratio equal to one implies no difference in the probability of event occurrence in a treatment group compared to a control group [18]. Hazard ratio refers to probability and may be misinterpreted in terms of speed. For instance, a hazard ratio of two does not indicate that resolution of symptoms will occur twice as fast in a patient in the intervention group compared to a patient in the control group [22].

It is important to distinguish hazard ratio from odds ratio. Odds ratio estimates the relationship between an exposure and an outcome. It is the probability that an outcome will occur in an exposed group divided by the probability that an outcome will occur in an unexposed group. Odds ratio is commonly used in case-control studies to determine the effect of exposure to a variable of interest on the likelihood of disease occurrence [23].

An odds ratio equal to one, as with hazard ratio, implies that there is no difference in the probability of event occurrence between the exposed and unexposed groups [18].

An odds ratio greater than one indicates that exposure is associated with a higher probability of event occurrence. On the other hand, an odds ratio less than one implies that exposure is associated with a lower probability of event occurrence [23].

Hazard ratio and odds ratio are both interested in the probability of event occurrence in an exposed group compared to the probability of that same event occurring in an unexposed group. While hazard ratio describes the risk of event occurrence at a particular point in time, odds ratio is a more cumulative measurement of risk that assesses event occurrence without including time as a variable [24].

Missing Data

Subject withdrawal before the end of a longitudinal study is unavoidable. Loss of participants can make an evaluation of safety and efficacy biased, and statistical power may also decrease [25]. Multiple concerns arise when patients withdraw from long-term clinical trials. For instance, patients who comply with treatment often respond better than patients who discontinue treatment. Thus, the remaining subjects at the end of the study may not adequately represent a random subset of the population. Additionally, the possible therapeutic effect of a drug with a prolonged mechanism of action becomes undetected in a patient with early withdrawal. On the other hand, a patient may discontinue treatment due to rapid improvement, yet may subsequently experience undocumented worsening of symptoms [26].

Missing data can be categorized into three groups: missing completely at random (MCAR), missing at random (MAR), and missing not at random (MNAR). In missing completely at random (MCAR), the likelihood of missing data is independent of both observed and unobserved data. The probability of missing data in MCAR is comparable among patients that are receiving different treatments. Lost data or the likelihood of withdrawal due to subject relocation is considered entirely random and irrespective of observed or missing data. MCAR is not a source of bias, yet can result in smaller sample sizes and thus greater standard error, wider confidence intervals, and greater p-values, which may ultimately produce results that are not statistically significant [26–28].

Missing at random (MAR) involves missing data dependent on observed factors only. That is, data is missing independently of unobserved data, but instead may depend on underlying differences among patients. Patients who are older, for example, may have a higher rate of dropout from clinical trials compared to younger patients. In this example, missing data is directly related to the observed outcome of age [26].

In missing not at random (MNAR), missing data is dependent on unobserved factors. For example, patients who experience adverse effects are more likely to drop out compared to patients without adverse effects. Accordingly, patients with disease exacerbation may be more likely to discontinue treatment. Unfortunately, important information about adverse effects or efficacy subsequently remains unreported. In MNAR, the probability of missing data is directly linked to the unmeasured data and can result in a nonrepresentative sample [27].

Methods of Handling Missing Data

Imputation methods create the opportunity to account for missing data in statistical analysis. Imputation methods assign approximated values to missing data. Different methods of imputation are classified based on the type of approximation used. The four strategies of handling missing data are last observation carried forward (LOCF), nonresponder imputation (NRI), as-observed data analysis, and anytime analysis [29]. Imputation allows researchers to obtain a complete data set to conduct statistical analyses [26]. However, each method creates a source of bias that needs to be considered when interpreting long-term clinical trial data.

The last observation carried forward (LOCF) is a frequently used imputation method to evaluate data from lost subjects. LOCF applies the last observed value to all following missed values. Therefore, the last measured value is carried forward until the end of the study [25]. This approach is considered to be less rigorous than other imputation methods and makes the unrealistic assumption that the outcomes of patients do not change after they have dropped out. Thus, response rate may be inappropriately high, as patients marked as responding may have lost response. Additionally, imputation of a single value for missing data can result in lower estimates of standard errors and p-values [30] This limitation is most apparent in long-term studies with many patient dropouts early on, as assigned values are unlikely to reflect true response [29]. A source of bias may also occur if a large number of patients receiving placebo discontinue treatment due to lack of improvement. Under LOCF, responses for these patients, which indicate a lack of improvement, will be continually imputed until completion of the study. Consequently, the estimated difference between the intervention and placebo groups may be inappropriately exaggerated [29]. The use of LOCF should be carefully examined in longitudinal trials evaluating treatment efficacy.

Nonresponder imputation (NRI) is considered to be a more rigorous imputation method. Patients who withdraw from a study are labeled nonresponders and missing data are identified as a nonresponse. A main limitation to this imputation method is that participants who discontinue treatment are classified as nonresponders, regardless of the initial treatment response. For example, a patient may respond well to treatment, yet may need to drop out for reasons that do not pertain to the treatment and all previous data on this participant is omitted. Therefore, valuable information about the effect of intervention on these patients remains undetected. In contrast to LOCF, results are likely underestimated in NRI [29].

As-observed analysis is a method of analysis that utilizes observed data only. Data from withdrawn patients is omitted without substituting values in their place. The advantage to this type of analysis is that data is only depicted from patients who remain in the trial. Thus, important information about patients that discontinue the study is omitted from analysis. The use of the as-observed analysis has the propensity to overestimate response [29].

Anytime analysis is a less rigorous method to analyze data. Data recorded at any point in time after the start of therapy is considered a response. If a trial has a long duration, only the patient's best outcome is recorded. Therefore, efficacy over an extended period of time is likely to be overestimated in this type of analysis [29].

Safety and Efficacy of Apremilast for Plaque Psoriasis

Two randomized, double-blind phase III trials, ESTEEM 1 and ESTEEM 2, evaluated the safety and efficacy of apremilast for moderate-to-severe plaque psoriasis over a 52-week period. In ESTEEM 1, patients received placebo or apremilast 30 mg twice daily for 16 weeks. At week 16, participants in the placebo group were given apremilast 30 mg twice daily. Missing data was handled using LOCF. At the end of the study, 74 patients in the placebo group and 163 in the apremilast group discontinued therapy due to adverse events, lack of efficacy, loss to follow-up, or other reasons. Of note, a clear discrepancy exists in the dropout rate among the placebo and apremilast group. Participants who discontinued after receiving apremilast could have initially responded well to therapy. After dropout, LOCF considers these patients as still responding adequately to treatment, although response may have been lost. A significant improvement in symptoms was reported at week 16 in the apremilast group, achieving a reduction of 75% in Psoriasis Area and Severity Index (PASI-75) in 33.1% of patients compared to PASI 75 response rate of 5.3% in the placebo group. Out of the 73 patients that switched to apremilast from placebo at week 16, PASI-75 was attained among 58.9% of patients at week 52 [31]. Although significant differences were reported, a high withdrawal rate of 41.6% (351/844 participants completed the trial) along with the use of LOCF to account for missing data contribute to an overestimated response.

In ESTEEM 2, participants were given apremilast 30 mg twice daily or placebo. At week 16, placebo patients were given apremilast 30 mg twice daily. Patients with 50% or more reduction in PASI were randomized to resume apremilast or receive placebo at week 32. If symptom improvement was lost, patients were reassigned to receive apremilast. Patients on apremilast therapy attained PASI 75 significantly more often than placebo (28.8% compared to 5.8%) using LOCF at 16-week follow-up. At week 16, patients on apremilast were more likely to attain PASI 50 and PASI 90 compared to placebo (55.5 vs. 19.7%, and 8.8 vs. 1.5%) using LOCF [32]. Of note, the dropout rate in this trial is considerably high (231/413 participants completed the study). It is also important to recognize that the two major reasons for withdrawal were adverse events or loss of efficacy. Patients receiving apremilast may have responded well until an adverse event was noticed, which led to discontinuation of treatment. Although an adverse event was experienced, the recorded positive response to apremilast is carried forward until the end of the study, leading to a misleading interpretation of treatment efficacy. The use of LOCF also implies that in the placebo group, the recorded values for patients that withdrew due to lack of efficacy were carried forward until the end of the study, which may have exaggerated the difference reported between patients receiving apremilast and placebo.

Safety and Efficacy of Secukinumab for Plaque Psoriasis

The NRI imputation method was implemented in a phase 3 randomized, double-blind, placebo-controlled (FEATURE) trial that evaluated the safety and efficacy of secukinumab. Participants received secukinumab 150, 300 mg, or placebo for 12 weeks. Out of 177 subjects, seven patients discontinued therapy due to loss to follow-up, a couple due to adverse effects, and none due to lack of efficacy. The seven patients who discontinued treatment were considered nonresponders. Patients who received secukinumab 300 or 150 mg achieved PASI 75 at 12-week follow-up (75.9% and 69.5% of subjects, respectively). In contrast, none of the patients who received placebo attained PASI 75 [33]. Important information about the participants who discontinued therapy is omitted from analysis. Although NRI is a rigorous method of handling missing data, the low withdrawal rate is reassuring that the results adequately represent the efficacy of secukinumab in plaque psoriasis.

Safety and Efficacy of Ixekizumab for Plaque Psoriasis

Missing data in the phase 3 randomized trials (UNCOVER-2 and UNCOVER-3) that compared ixekizumab to etanercept or placebo was also assessed using NRI. In both trials, subjects were randomized to receive placebo, etanercept, ixekizumab every 2 weeks, or ixekizumab every 4 weeks. In UNCOVER-2, 1224 out of 1161 patients completed the study (95%).

In UNCOVER-3, 1275 out of 1346 patients completed the study (95%). There was no significant difference in withdrawal rates in patients receiving placebo compared to ixekizumab treatment. Lack of efficacy was a major reason for withdrawal in both trials, which was more prevalent in patients receiving placebo versus ixekizumab. In UNCOVER-2, PASI 75 was achieved in patients who received ixekizumab every 2 weeks (89.7%) and 4 weeks (77.5%). Similarly, PASI 75 was achieved in UNCOVER-3 in patients receiving ixekizumab every 2 weeks (87.3%) and 4 weeks (84.2%) [34]. Participants who discontinued treatment were labeled as nonresponders. Many participants may have initially responded appropriately to treatment, yet dropped out for reasons unrelated to the intervention given. That is, the recorded observations for these participants remain unnoticed, leading to an underestimated response [29].

Safety and Efficacy of Secukinumab Compared to Ustekinumab for Plaque Psoriasis

The CLEAR study compared the use of secukinumab to ustekinumab in moderate-to-severe plaque psoriasis. The double-blind trial randomly assigned 676 participants to receive secukinumab or ustekinumab. At week 16, secukinumab was found to be more efficacious than ustekinumab. The amount of patients attaining PASI 100 (44.3% and 28.4%, respectively), PASI 90 (79% and 57.6%, respectively), and PASI 75 (93.1% and 82.7%, respectively) was higher for patients on secukinumab compared to ustekinumab. Out of 676 participants, 651 patients completed treatment. The missing data for 25 participants was handled using NRI. A majority of these participants discontinued treatment due to adverse effect or choice [35]. The rigorous nature of NRI is very appropriately used in this study. The bias towards an underestimated response is beneficial because the reason of discontinuation of treatment was a result of the intervention. Therefore, it is helpful that a stricter method to account for patient dropout was implemented in this trial. We can safely assume that secukinumab was significantly more effective than ustekinumab in treating plaque psoriasis.

Safety and Efficacy of Alefacept for Plaque Psoriasis

Menter et al. evaluated the efficacy of multiple courses of alefacept in patients who did not reach PASI 50 after one 12-week course. Each subsequent course of intravenous alefacept correlated with higher percentages of patients achieving PASI 50, with an improvement from 56% after one course to 74% after five courses of treatment. As-observed analysis was the strategy used to account for missing data.

In this study, it is important to recognize that there was a decline in participants with each treatment course ($N = 521$ in course 1 compared to $N = 39$ in course 5) [29, 36]. It is difficult to assess efficacy with a high subject withdrawal of 92%. Important data from withdrawn patients is omitted in the as-observed analysis and is therefore left undetected. It is assumed that the reported response rate is higher than the actual response rate due to high withdrawal rate and use of as-observed analysis to account for missing data.

Evaluation of Biologic Therapy Comparing Methods of Handling Missing Data

The reported outcome of a study can vary considerably based on the type of method used to handle missing data. An open-label extension of the phase III REVEAL trial assessed the efficacy of adalimumab for moderate-to-severe plaque psoriasis over a 3-year period. After 160 weeks, PASI 75 response rates in patients receiving continuous adalimumab were 76% using LOCF and 88% using as-observed analysis [37]. Evidently, the reported efficacy of adalimumab varies based on the method of analysis applied to account for missing data. As-observed analysis and LOCF both have the propensity to overestimate response. As-observed analysis only includes data that is directly observed, whereas LOCF applies the last recorded response forward until the end of the study. If patients withdraw due to lack of efficacy, then their responses are completely omitted in as-observed analysis. That is, the remaining responses are more reflective of the patients who responded well to treatment, ultimately leading to an overestimated response. LOCF also overestimates response as data from last follow-up is carried forward until the end of the study. However, unlike as-observed analysis, the responses from patients that discontinue are not completely omitted. Thus, as-observed analysis may predict a response greater than the response observed using LOCF.

An open-label study evaluated the efficacy of infliximab over a 3-year period in patients with plaque psoriasis. Out of 131 patients, only 32 patients remained after 3 years. The efficacy of infliximab can be determined by evaluating PASI 75 responses. At 3-year follow up, PASI 75 was 75% using as-observed data, 65.6% using LOCF, and 41.2% using NRI. Thus, the reported efficacy of an intervention can vary drastically based on the method used to handle missing data. Therefore, it is important to carefully review the analysis method used when interpreting long-term clinical data [29, 38].

Conclusion

With the rapid growth in research, the number of clinical trials and studies has steadily increased. The design of clinical trials and data analysis has also become more complex to interpret. It is important for clinicians to be able to interpret clinical trials and ultimately determine if evidence is valid and applicable to clinical practice. The objective of this chapter was to present an overview of the potential sources of bias and uncertainty that occur during study design and approximations of missing data. Identifying sources of error and understanding the limitations of these various methods both help clinicians critically appraise the validity of clinical data. With proper interpretation of clinical trial data, evidence can be effectively applied to medical practice. Evidence from clinical research can thus directly influence clinical decision making, ultimately optimizing patient care.

Conflicts of Interest Ms. Amin, Mr. No, and Ms. Darji report no potential conflicts of interest. Dr. Wu received research funding from AbbVie, Amgen, AstraZeneca, Boehringer Ingelheim, Coherus Biosciences, Dermira, Eli Lilly, Janssen, Merck, Novartis, Pfizer, Regeneron, Sandoz, and Sun Pharmaceutical Industries; he is a consultant for AbbVie, Amgen, Celgene, Dermira, Eli Lilly, Pfizer, Regeneron, Sun Pharmaceutical Industries, and Valeant Pharmaceuticals. All funds go to his employer.

Appendix of Common Biostatistical Terms

- *Adjusted analysis:* A method of analysis that aims to control for baseline patient characteristics, which may otherwise create discrepancies between intervention groups. Also refers to modifications of the *p*-value after multiple testing.
- *Bias:* A misrepresentation of the actual estimated efficacy of an intervention due to flaws in the conduct, design, or analysis of a trial.
- *Blinding (masking):* The act of concealing information from participants, researchers, and healthcare professionals about intervention assignment in order to prevent bias. Clinical trials often implement double-blinding, which blinds participants, healthcare providers, and researchers. Also referred to as masking.
- *Confidence interval:* A statistical measure that provides information about the accuracy of an estimated parameter of interest. The interval consists of a range of values that surround the true value of the parameter of interest with a high degree of confidence, typically 95%. A wide interval suggests less certainty about a measured effect, whereas a narrow interval suggests increased certainty about a measured effect. The units of the confidence interval are the same as the units of the measured parameter of interest.
- *Confounding:* A circumstance in which the observed outcome of an intervention is biased due to extraneous

variables, such as baseline characteristics of participants or alternate simultaneous interventions. A confounding variable must differ among intervention groups and account for the observed outcome.

- External validity: The extent to which the results of a trial can be generalized to other situations and populations. Also referred to as generalizability or applicability.
- *Follow-up:* The practice of recurrent interactions with participants in a trial to administer the allocated intervention, monitor for effects of the intervention, or obtain data values.
- Hazard ratio: A value that explains the probability of event occurrence in the intervention group compared to the control group based on comparison of event rates.
- *Hypothesis:* A statement that offers a proposed explanation for the observed effects of an intervention on an outcome. The null hypothesis implies that there is no difference between the groups of interest and is the baseline assumption until statistical evidence proves otherwise, which produces a *p*-value.
- *Intention-to-treat analysis:* A method of statistical analysis that includes all participants, irrespective of completion of the study, in the analysis. The purpose of this method of analysis is to prevent bias due to subject withdrawal, which could otherwise interfere with the original random allocation of participants.
- *Interaction:* A circumstance in which the effect of one variable is altered by the presence of another variable. Clinical trials evaluate for an interaction by determining if the effect of an intervention differs among subgroups of participants.
- *Interim analysis:* An analysis that evaluates data prior to completion of a trial and oftentimes before the end of recruitment. The trial may be terminated at this point in time, also known as stopping rules, if participants are inadvertently being placed at risk. It is important that the protocol of the clinical trial incorporates the schedule of interim analyses.
- *Internal validity:* The degree to which the design and conduct of the trial reduce the chance of bias.
- *Intervention:* A treatment or healthcare involvement that is under examination in a trial. Outcome measures assess the effect of an intervention.
- *Last observation carried forward*: The last observation carried forward (LOCF) is a method of accounting for missing data from lost subjects by assigning the last observed value to all following missed values.
- *Loss to follow-up:* The inability to complete data collection on certain participants due to loss of contact, most commonly observed in long-term trials.
- *Multiple comparisons:* The practice of conducting multiple analyses on the same set of data. Multiple comparisons increase the likelihood of a type I error, which

attributes an outcome to an intervention when it is more likely due to chance.

- *Number needed to treat (NNT)*: The number of patients who need to receive a particular treatment to prevent one additional bad outcome.
- *Objectives:* A term that refers to the questions that the trial intends to answer. Hypotheses and objectives are related in that testing of the hypotheses also helps answers the objectives.
- *Odds ratio*: The ratio of the odds that an outcome will occur given a specific exposure, compared to the odds that an outcome will occur without exposure.
- *Open trial:* A randomized trial in which both the participants and researches are aware of the intervention administered. In open trials, no one is blinded to the treatment allocation.
- *Outcome measure:* A variable that provides information about the effect of an intervention by comparing the results of the intervention groups. Also referred to as endpoint.
- *P-value*: A measure that represents the probability of observing a result equal to or more extreme than the result observed in the study by chance alone. The *p*-value is calculated based on the notion that the null hypothesis is true, which states that there is no difference between the groups of interest. A lower *p*-value correlates with a greater certainty that the observed difference is attributable to the intervention.
- *Power:* The probability that a trial will appropriately reject the null hypothesis, which indicates that there is no difference between the groups of interest, when it is false. Stated differently, it is the probability that a trial will identify a statistically significant effect of an intervention. It is typically calculated prior to the start of the trial and the sample size is often adjusted to achieve a desired level of power.
- *Protocol deviation:* An unintentional diversion from the initial research protocol. Deviations may occur due to nonadherence to a particular intervention on behalf of a participant or an accidental change to the original protocol on behalf of a researcher.
- *Random allocation; random assignment; randomization:* The purpose of randomization is to evenly allocate participants into separate groups to provide equal opportunity to receive an intervention. In a randomized trial, randomization eliminates the predictability of group assignment and allows researchers to accurately determine the effect of an intervention on an outcome.
- *Recruitment:* The act of acquiring participants into a randomized trial.
- *Relative risk*: A ratio of the probability of event occurrence, or disease incidence, in an exposed group divided by the probability of event occurrence in a nonexposed group. In trials, it often refers to a measure of

the association between an exposure and the risk of developing a disease.

- *Sample size:* The number of subjects in a subset of a population included in a trial. The intended sample size refers to the estimated number of participants included in a trial, often based on calculation of the statistical power before beginning the trial. A large sample size increases the likelihood of exposing a significant effect if one exists. The achieved sample size refers to the number of participants that complete the trial or are included in the analysis.

- *Selection bias:* A bias that occurs when selection of participants for a study or allocation to different intervention groups is not entirely random. Consequently, the different groups vary in baseline characteristics that can impact the observed outcome. Selection bias may also refer to a trial in which the participants inadequately represent the population of interest.

- *Simple randomization:* A method of randomization determined by chance. If only two groups are present, simple randomization is comparable to repeated tosses of a coin. Also referred to as unrestricted randomization.

- *Stratified randomization:* A method of randomization that considers the baseline characteristics of participants, such as demographic information or disease severity, to allow for an adequate balance of these factors across treatment groups.

- *Stopping rule:* A criteria, included in some trials, that specifies the need to prematurely terminate a trial to eliminate placing patients at avoidable risk or if a large effect of an intervention is prematurely observed, deeming further testing unnecessary. A stopping rule is generally established in the original trial protocol and analyzed during interim analyses.

- *Subgroup analysis:* A type of analysis that evaluates the effect of an intervention on a specified outcome within a subset of participants in a trial, often separated by baseline characteristics. Subgroup analysis is often limited by small sample size, which decreases the likelihood of statistical power.

- *Treatment effect:* A measure used to evaluate the effect of an intervention by comparing the difference in outcome between the intervention groups. It is indicated as relative risk, odds ratio, difference in means, or risk difference. Also referred to as effect size.

References

1. Sackett DL, Rosenberg WM, Gray JM, Haynes RB, Richardson WS. Evidence based medicine: what it is and what it isn't. BMJ. 1996;312(7023):71–2.
2. Fletcher RH, Fletcher SW. Evidence-based approach to the medical literature. J Gen Intern Med. 1997;12(s2):5–14.
3. Masic I, Miokovic M, Muhamedagic B. Evidence based medicine-new approaches and challenges. Acta Inform Med. 2008;16(4):219
4. Bigby M, Gadenne AS. Understanding and evaluating clinical trials. J Am Acad Dermatol. 1996;34(4):555–90.
5. Page P. Beyond statistical significance: clinical interpretation of rehabilitation research literature. Int J Sports Phys Ther. 2014;9(5):726.
6. Bonita R, Beaglehole R, Kjellström T. Basic epidemiology. Geneva: World Health Organization; 2006. p. 49–81.
7. Prinsen CA, Spuls PI, Sprangers MA, de Rie MA, Legierse CM, de Korte J. The efficacy of a health-related quality-of-life intervention during 48 weeks of biologic treatment of patients with moderate to severe psoriasis: study protocol for a multicenter randomized controlled trial. Trials. 2012;13(1):1.
8. Prinsen CA, Spuls P, Lindeboom R, Sprangers MA, Rie MA, Korte J. The efficacy of a health-related quality-of-life intervention during 48 weeks of biologic treatment of patients with moderate to severe psoriasis: results of a multicentre randomized controlled trial. Br J Dermatol. 2015;173(4):1091–4.
9. DerSimonian R, Laird N. Meta-analysis in clinical trials. Control Clin Trials. 1986;7(3):177–88.
10. Thompson SG. Meta-analysis of clinical trials. In: Armitage P, Colton T, eds, Encyclopedia of Biostatistics. 2nd edition. Chichester: John Wiley & Sons; 2005. p. 2570–9.
11. Ildstad ST, Evans CH. Small clinical trials: issues and challenges. Washington, DC: National Academy Press; 2001. p. 20–9.
12. Bulpitt CJ. Randomised controlled clinical trials. New York: Kluwer Academic Publishers; 1996. p. 379–85.
13. Stang A. Randomized controlled trials-an indispensible part of clinical research. Dtsch Arztebl Int. 2011;108(39):661–2.
14. Goodman SN. Toward evidence-based medical statistics. 1: The P value fallacy. Ann Intern Med. 1999;130(12):995–1004.
15. du Prel JB, Hommel G, Röhrig B, Blettner M. Confidence interval or p-value. Dtsch Arztebl Int. 2009;106(19):335–9.
16. Raftery S. Confidence intervals. Curr Anaesth Crit Care. 1999;10(4):222–3.
17. Flechner L, Tseng TY. Understanding results: p-values, confidence intervals, and number need to treat. Indian J Urol. 2011;27(4):532.
18. Kleinbaum DG, Klein M. Survival analysis: a self-learning text. New York: Springer; 2006. p. 4–21.
19. Goel M, Khanna P, Kishore J. Understanding survival analysis: Kaplan-Meier estimate. Int J Ayurveda Res. 2010;1(4):274.
20. Bradburn MJ, Clark TG, Love SB, Altman DG. Survival analysis part II: multivariate data analysis–an introduction to concepts and methods. Br J Cancer. 2003;89(3):431–6.
21. Clark TG, Bradburn MJ, Love SB, Altman DG. Survival analysis part I: basic concepts and first analyses. Br J Cancer. 2003;89(2):232–8.
22. Spruance SL, Reid JE, Grace M, Samore M. Hazard ratio in clinical trials. Antimicrob Agents Chemother. 2004;48(8):2787–92.
23. Szumilas M. Explaining odds ratios. J Can Acad Child Adolesc Psychiatry. 2010;19:227.
24. Scott I. Interpreting risks and ratios in therapy trials. Aust Prescr. 2008;31(1):12–6.
25. Saha C, Jones MP. Bias in the last observation carried forward method under informative dropout. J Stat Plan Inference. 2009;139(2):246–55.
26. Myers WR. Handling missing data in clinical trials: an overview. Drug Inf J. 2000;34(2):525–33.
27. Dziura JD, Post LA, Zhao Q, Fu Z, Peduzzi P. Strategies for dealing with missing data in clinical trials: from design to analysis. Yale J Biol Med. 2013;86(3):343–58.
28. Ibrahim JG, Chu H, Chen MH. Missing data in clinical studies: issues and methods. J Clin Oncol. 2012;30(26):3297–303.
29. Langley RG, Reich K. The interpretation of long-term trials of biologic treatments for psoriasis: trial designs and the choices of statis-

tical analyses affect ability to compare outcomes across trials. Br J Dermatol. 2013;169(6):1198–206.

30. Little RJ, D'agostino R, Cohen ML, Dickersin K, Emerson SS, Farrar JT, Frangakis C, Hogan JW, Molenberghs G, Murphy SA, Neaton JD. The prevention and treatment of missing data in clinical trials. N Engl J Med. 2012;367(14):1355–60.

31. Papp K, Reich K, Leonardi CL, Kircik L, Chimenti S, Langley RG, Hu C, Stevens RM, Day RM, Gordon KB, Korman NJ. Apremilast, an oral phosphodiesterase 4 (PDE4) inhibitor, in patients with moderate to severe plaque psoriasis: results of a phase III, randomized, controlled trial (Efficacy and Safety Trial Evaluating the Effects of Apremilast in Psoriasis [ESTEEM] 1). J Am Acad Dermatol. 2015;73(1):37–49.

32. Paul C, Cather J, Gooderham M, Poulin Y, Mrowietz U, Ferrandiz C, Crowley J, Hu C, Stevens RM, Shah K, Day RM. Efficacy and safety of apremilast, an oral phosphodiesterase 4 inhibitor, in patients with moderate-to-severe plaque psoriasis over 52 weeks: a phase III, randomized controlled trial (ESTEEM 2). Br J Dermatol. 2015;173(6):1387–99.

33. Blauvelt A, Prinz JC, Gottlieb AB, Kingo K, Sofen H, Ruer-Mulard M, Singh V, R P, Papavassilis C, Cooper S. Secukinumab administration by pre-filled syringe: efficacy, safety and usability results from a randomized controlled trial in psoriasis (FEATURE). Br J Dermatol. 2015;172(2):484–93.

34. Griffiths CE, Reich K, Lebwohl M, van de Kerkhof P, Paul C, Menter A, Cameron GS, Erickson J, Zhang L, Secrest RJ, Ball S. Comparison of ixekizumab with etanercept or placebo in moderate-to-severe psoriasis (UNCOVER-2 and UNCOVER-3): results from two phase 3 randomised trials. Lancet. 2015;386(9993):541–51.

35. Thaçi D, Blauvelt A, Reich K, Tsai TF, Vanaclocha F, Kingo K, Ziv M, Pinter A, S H, You R, Milutinovic M. Secukinumab is superior to ustekinumab in clearing skin of subjects with moderate to severe plaque psoriasis: CLEAR, a randomized controlled trial. J Am Acad Dermatol. 2015;73(3):400–9.

36. Menter A, Cather JC, Baker D, Farber HF, Lebwohl M, Darif M. The efficacy of multiple courses of alefacept in patients with moderate to severe chronic plaque psoriasis. J Am Acad Dermatol. 2006;54(1):61–3.

37. Gordon K, Papp K, Poulin Y, Gu Y, Rozzo S, Sasso EH. Long-term efficacy and safety of adalimumab in patients with moderate to severe psoriasis treated continuously over 3 years: results from an open-label extension study for patients from REVEAL. J Am Acad Dermatol. 2012;66(2):241–51.

38. Papoutsaki M, Talamonti M, Giunta A, Costanzo A, Ruzzetti M, Teoli M, Chimenti S. The impact of methodological approaches for presenting long-term clinical data on estimates of efficacy in psoriasis illustrated by three-year treatment data on infliximab. Dermatology. 2010;221(Suppl 1):43–7.

Compliance and Persistency

Emily Boes, Jaclyn Smith, and Steven R. Feldman

Abbreviations

EASI	Eczema area severity index
EMR	Electronic medical record
MEMS caps	Medication event monitoring system caps
MI	Motivational interviewing
MPR	Medication possession ratio
VAS	Visual analog scale
Wa	Estimation of medication weight used

Introduction

Skin diseases have an enormous impact on patients' lives; but that does not mean that patients use their treatment well. For the multitude of dermatologic treatments, ranging from topical to injectable medications, poor medication adherence is one of the most common limitations. Biologics have revolutionized the treatment of skin disease due to their greater efficacy and safety compared to topical and oral treatments; however, even biologics are not always used as prescribed. In this chapter we discuss definitions of adherence; how it is measured; how adherence to topical, oral, and biologic medications compare; barriers to adherence; and what can be done to help assure patients' adherence to their treatments.

Adherence, also termed compliance, is the extent to which patients take medications as prescribed [1], or "the level of patient participation achieved once an individual has agreed to the regimen" [2]. Medication adherence is a moving target, a dynamic state that changes with changing attitudes and life circumstances [3].

E. Boes, DO
Des Moines University College of Osteopathic Medicine, Des Moines, IA, USA

J. Smith, BS • S.R. Feldman, MD, PhD (✉)
Department of Dermatology, Wake Forest School of Medicine, 4618 Country Club Rd, Winston-Salem, NC 27106, USA
e-mail: sfeldman@wakehealth.edu

Patient adherence is a complex problem, involving many interconnected variables [4]. Three phases of adherence to medication can be considered: initiation, implementation, and discontinuation. Initiation is when a patient takes the first dose of a medication; it may begin long after a prescription is written, if it occurs at all. Implementation is the extent to which a patient follows the treatment regimen while they are on the medication; between initiation and discontinuation, patients may take their medication very well or very poorly. Discontinuation is when the patient stops taking the medication; it may happen long before the recommended end of the treatment regimen [5]. A term related to adherence is persistence, defined as the time between initiation and discontinuation of medication [5, 6]. This chapter discusses classification of medication adherence, the societal impact of and barriers to adherence, and methods by which to improve adherence to treatment.

Classification of Nonadherence

Nonadherence can be classified in several ways. The concepts of initiation, implementation, and discontinuation help to define classification of different forms of poor adherence. Nonadherence can be classified as either primary or secondary. Primary nonadherence is when a patient does not initiate treatment, a surprisingly common phenomenon among patients with psoriasis. Secondary nonadherence is when the script is filled and treatment is started correctly, but the medication is used poorly (poor implementation) or is discontinued earlier than instructed (poor persistence).

Nonadherence can also be classified as intentional or unintentional [3]. Intentional nonadherence is when a patient makes a conscious decision to not use treatment as prescribed. Unintentional nonadherence is when a patient's intention to use a drug is disrupted by unforeseen barriers such as a misunderstanding or inability to recall the proper directions for medication use (Table 4.1) [7]. Forgetfulness is a frequent cause of unintentional nonadherence.

P.S. Yamauchi (ed.), *Biologic and Systemic Agents in Dermatology*, https://doi.org/10.1007/978-3-319-66884-0_4

Table 4.1 Definitions of nonadherence [data derived from Aslam I, Feldman SR. Practical Strategies to Improve Patient Adherence to Treatment Regimens. South Med J 2015 Jun;108 (6):325–31]

Nonadherence definitions [5]	
Primary nonadherence	No initiation of treatment by the patient
Secondary nonadherence	Prescription filled correctly, but treatment is started incorrectly or cessation of treatment occurs before instructed
Intentional nonadherence	Patient declines consciously to participate in treatment as directed by physician
Unintentional nonadherence	Patient intends to use drug as directed, but unforeseen barriers or patient's misunderstanding or failure to remember directions result in improper use of medications

Measurement of Adherence

Many methods are used to measure medication adherence in a research setting, and as technology continues to progress, so does the accuracy of measurement. Methodology has evolved from self-reported data to objective electronic medication adherence monitoring. Medication Event Monitoring System (MEMS) caps containing microprocessors that record the day and time medication bottles are opened and closed are the gold standard for measuring adherence to treatment [7]. Medications, both oral and topical, can be dispensed into bottles affixed with these caps, and patients can open and close them similar to a standard cap (MEMS caps were also used on injector disposal containers in one study to assess adherence to self-injected biologics) [7]. MEMS caps can record up to 1800 dose events and have a battery life of 18 months. Compared to self-reported medication logs, pill counts, or medication bottle weights, electronic monitoring with MEMS caps is a more precise method of measuring medication adherence; self-reported methodologies commonly overestimate patients' use of medication [6, 8]. For example, psoriasis patients adhered to topical medication 55% of the time as measured by electronic monitors, 90% by patient diary, and 100% by medication weight measures [6, 8].

Collection of self-reported adherence data by way of a medication diary has been used to measure adherence with some success. However, patients may over- and underreport the use of medication [7]. Electronically monitored diaries suggest that most diary entries are completed at a later date than when the medications were taken, creating a significant recall bias [7]. Although self-reported use is less accurate than other methods of measuring adherence, it may be an effective tool to hold patients accountable to adherence to their treatment regimen; a patient group that completed medication diaries in a recent study showed significant improvements in disease severity despite evidence of medication misuse. Although diaries are less than ideal for accurate

measurement of adherence, they may still be an effective method to increase adherence [9]. Pill counts are a means to assess adherence to oral treatment, but many dermatological treatments are topical formulations. Measuring topical medication usage by weight has been used with some success as well. Assessment of adherence based on medication weight used requires knowing the affected body surface area being treated and making assumptions about how much is used per unit surface area [7].

Pharmacy data and prescription refills are other measures of adherence, commonly used when retrospectively assessing adherence from insurance claim information. While useful, inaccuracy can result from assumptions made when using these data to calculate adherence. For example, a prescription filled does not mean a prescription was used or, if it was used, used correctly; a patient may treat a new-onset symptom with antibiotics previously prescribed for a prior infection without consulting their doctor first. Prescription data can be used to calculate days of supply for dispensed prescriptions and the medication possession ratio (MPR = (days of supply)/(number of days between prescription refills)). If the MPR is equal to or greater than one, compliance is assumed; when the MPR is less than one, nonadherence is assumed since there are fewer days of medication supply than number of days between refills.

Other methods of measuring treatment adherence include assessments by a pharmacist or other healthcare providers (i.e., 10–15-min phone calls between physician follow-up visits), pill counts, syrup volume measurements, family member reports, and Internet-based self-reports [10, 11]. From the short history of monitoring medication adherence, it is exciting to see how far these methods have come and evolved.

Clinical Applications of Medication Adherence

In an effort to provide the best quality and most convenient care for busy patients, primary care physicians take on a wide majority of dermatologic complaints without specialty consults. In turn, dermatologists see a filtered patient population [8, 12]. These patients often present with disease that is severe, rare, refractory, and relapsing. Goals of treatment shift from cure to control. To control chronic disease, there is a huge burden on the physician to help their patients take their medications as prescribed. Medication nonadherence is most significant in chronic disease; the longer patients are expected to be on a treatment, the more their adherence drops over time. When 29 psoriasis patients in a clinical trial on single-agent therapy with salicylic acid gel dosed twice daily were observed, medication adherence decreased from 90 to 40% over an 8-week treatment period. If this rate continued to drop at the same rate observed, no one would have been using the medication by 6 months of therapy [13]. Regardless of whether patients know their adherence is being monitored, compliance still drops dramatically over a short time [9].

Systemic medications are commonly promoted to provide greater efficacy and patient adherence to treatment, but despite new ways of treating chronic diseases, adherence is still poor (albeit better than adherence to topicals) [6, 14]. In a healthcare climate that is placing increased emphasis on patient outcomes and patient-centered care, research on the topic of adherence and persistence is pertinent to dermatologists and nonspecialists alike. In a setting where chronic disease without clear-cut curability is addressed on a daily basis, dermatology provides a valid stage to study nonadherence and persistency to treatment. Research related to adherence with dermatologic complaints has implications for all healthcare stakeholders [15].

Other areas of medicine continue to contribute significant research in the area of nonadherence, demonstrating its economic and social impact on our nation. Medication nonadherence is directly linked to approximately 125,000 patient deaths, at least 10% of hospital admissions, and 23% of nursing home admissions per year in the USA. As mentioned above, the cost to the US healthcare system of nonadherence is more than $100 billion annually [1]. 40% of patients admit to not using their medications as directed, and according to one Danish study, 50% of psoriasis prescriptions are never filled [7, 12, 16].

An assumption made when researching adherence is that it directly correlates with greater treatment efficacy and resolution of disease. This is supported by results of studies involving acne patients. Patients with a greater mean percentage reduction of noninflammatory and total lesion counts at baseline, 6-week, and 12-week follow-up appointments had greater adherence to the treatment regimen [10]. Therefore, it is also assumed that poorer adherence leads to worse treatment outcomes. Not only will disease likely progress without treatment, but comorbidity, higher costs, and fatality can also accompany nonadherence to treatment when looking at medication adherence across all medical fields. Nonadherence in all realms of medicine produces shocking statistics that have a significant impact on our nation's healthcare costs annually, in the form of emergency-room visits, hospitalizations, and diagnostic tests [5]. Arguably, a "better understanding of adherence probably will have more impact on patient outcomes than everything else [being studied] " [1].

Reasons for Medication Nonadherence

Common barriers to adherence are plentiful, and vary among different patients. Patients have unique disease presentations, comorbidities, treatment regimens, personalities, and psychosocial and financial stressors that lead to nonadherence. Reasons for nonadherence, like complexity of treatment, apprehension to use of biologics, route of medications, cost of medications, fear of side effects, poor patient-physician relationships, patient motivation, and factors influencing persistence, are discussed in this section.

Complexity of Treatment

Many dermatologic diseases are controlled using combinations of treatments. For example, atopic dermatitis, acne vulgaris, and psoriasis are all conditions for which care commonly involves the concurrent use of multiple drugs for the greatest efficacy and the least likelihood of toxicity [6]. Each medication affects a separate part of a pathologic process, and therefore combination therapy corresponds with greater defense against disease. Also, each drug has significant toxicity (especially systemic medications) and using multiple drugs decreases the dose needed for each individual medication, decreasing the likelihood of side effects without changing treatment outcomes. For example, using biologics in combination with other topical or systemic medications produces an additive effect in the treatment of psoriasis [17–19]. Combination treatment may also be used when monotherapy is not effective. Often, however, monotherapy is not effective because of poor adherence to treatment. Making the regimen even more complicated is not a rational solution to this problem.

Increasing complexity of treatment does not always mean multiple different medications are used; sometimes it means greater frequency of dosing, duration of therapy, or amount of instruction needed for medication application. These can result in poor medication usage leading to poor results, dissatisfaction with treatment, and further poor adherence in a vicious circle. Application of topical medication is inherently complex and time consuming; adherence is better with oral medications and better still with injectables.

Adherence rates of oral systemic medications used in a dermatologic setting correlate closely with frequency of dosing. Adherence to nonbiologic systemic medications used to treat psoriasis decreases when dosing frequency increases. Methotrexate has the greatest adherence and persistence, followed by leflunomide, hydroxychloroquine, and sulfasalazine. Combination therapy has the lowest adherence [6].

Adherence with Biologic Therapy

Biologic medications have been mainstays in treatment of severe and diffuse cases of various conditions. The most commonly prescribed medications for psoriasis are topical corticosteroids [20]. Initial psoriasis treatment uses topical therapies for plaques that are small or few in number, older systemic agents such as methotrexate, phototherapy for plaques that are large or numerous, and biologics for refractory disease. Psoriasis patients are overwhelmingly dissatisfied with treatment, and believe that they are undertreated for their disease [20]. One reason management may fail to meet patient expectations is a disconnect between the physician's and the patient's perception of disease severity, and its affect on patient quality of life [20–22]. Physicians are starting to recognize this disconnect, as more disease-specific systemic therapies are being used [20].

Biologics are associated with better adherence compared to other psoriasis treatments (66 vs. 35%) [17]. An understanding of adherence to biologics and other systemic medications may be obscured by the fact that they are used in a small population of patients with the most severe disease states. Disease severity positively and independently correlates with adherence, as does the use of biologic medications. Adherence and persistence to biologic therapy may be greater in part because of the context in which they are most commonly used [23, 24].

Although the context of use may have some effect on adherence, the efficacy of biologic medications remains superior to other medications (oral and topical) that have been used for psoriasis. Variability in effectiveness of biologic medications is the most common reason for stopping or switching therapy. TNF-alpha inhibitors vary in effectiveness from 40 to 80% after the first year of therapy [19]. Biologics have a greater effect on quality of life and have greater specificity in targeting psoriatic pathogenesis. Three genes known to cause psoriasis are related to the signaling of IL-23, a cytokine that is targeted by the biologic ustekinumab. These genes are related to mutations in TNF-alpha signaling and NF-κB modulation, cytokines, and signaling chemicals that are the targets of adalimumab, infliximab, and etanercept. Biologics prevent disease progression rather than only providing symptomatic relief [25].

Even when biologic and systemic therapies are recognized as viable options, establishing the optimal timing of initiation is not always easy. Scripts involve intimidating prior authorizations and patient fears regarding their use. The mindset of biologic therapy as a last resort should be contested with a "step-down approach" in disease management [2]. A growing body of research is unveiling safety, efficacy, cost benefits, and patient satisfaction which is allowing this change to take place [20, 26]. In one review, overall healthcare costs between the patients' biologic treatment period and pre/post-biologic period were not significantly different in Medicaid patients [17].

Fear of side effects is one barrier that prevents appropriate early use of biologic and other systemic medications. Biologics have fewer drug interactions than other systemic or topical therapies, largely because they target specific cytokines (Fig. 4.1) [17, 27]. Anxiety surrounding the use of psoriasis medications is out of proportion to the prevalence of actual adverse effects [4]. With long-term safety data now available for TNF-alpha inhibitors and 5-year safety data available for ustekinumab, the rate of infections is comparable between nonbiologic medications and certain biologic therapies [26]. The PSOLAR registry data found a decreased risk of serious infections with ustekinumab compared to nonbiologic therapies, a comparable increased risk of serious infections with etanercept and nonbiologic therapies, and a statistically significant increased risk of serious infection with adalimumab and infliximab [28]. It is important to note that diseases that warrant biologic therapy such as psoriasis are independent risk factors for infections. After controlling baseline characteristics, untreated juvenile idiopathic arthritis patients have a hazard ratio of 2.0 for serious infections compared to controls [29]. When treating patients, always consider their disease's baseline infection risk before choosing a medication.

Physicians and other healthcare providers can increase adherence to systemic therapy by educating patients about

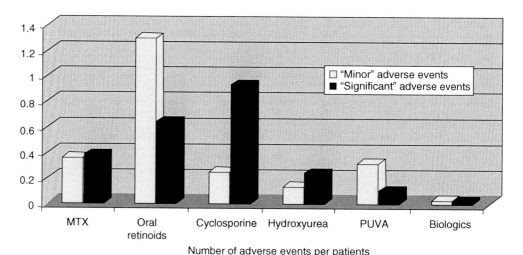

Fig. 4.1 Number of adverse events per patient for commonly used systemic psoriasis medications [18] [permission acquired by Lee-Ann Anderson, Senior Permissions & Licensing Executive, Journals for the Taylor & Francis Group]

the likelihood of side effect development, motivational interviewing and cues to action (Tables 4.2 and 4.3). For example, it is important to give sufficient instructions to patients about the use of their systemic and topical therapy, as well as education regarding side effect profiles of the relevant medications. Motivational interviewing successfully resulted in a positive correlation between increased patient education and greater adherence for osteoporotic patients who received a multidisciplinary patient education program [31]. Another study of seven patients treated with adalimumab showed that patient education can be used as a tool to increase adherence [14].

Another method of decreasing patient fear of medication side effects is by putting into practice the old adage of "start low and go slow." Minimizing drug dosage in systemic therapy may necessitate multimodal therapy for optimal treatment results and limitation of side effects [20]. Though adding more medications may minimize dose and side effects, thus increasing treatment efficacy, it may also confuse patients and lead to lower compliance.

Conversely, more aggressive therapy administered for shorter periods of time may be another approach to avoid adverse effects of medications. This theory supports that short-duration, high-potency pharmacotherapy can be better than lower potency medication administered over a longer period of time, and may be ideal for patients who tend to be nonadherent [9]. Aggressive therapy places the focus on decreasing time of intervention and increasing efficacy, providing an alternative to increase patient adherence [9]. Since the patient receiving aggressive therapy may see results more quickly, this may further increase their trust in the medication and their adherence. Ultimately, route of medication administration, severity of disease, patient preference, and lifestyle should all be considered when

Table 4.2 Comparison of biologic medications used to treat psoriasis [30] [data derived from Treatment Comparison. In: treatments BtaTsato, editor. https://wwwpsoriasis.org/sites/default/files/treatment_comparison_chart_1pdf: National Psoriasis Foundation; 2016]

Treatment	Common side effects	Other risks	Monitoring
Certolizumab pegol (Cimzia)	Rash Upper respiratory infection Urinary tract infection	Hepatitis B reactivation Lupus-like syndrome Neurologic symptoms	Complete blood count Hepatic function Tuberculosis (TB) screening
Secukinumab (Cosentyx)	Upper respiratory infection Cold symptoms Diarrhea	Inflammatory bowel disease Reactivation of latent infections	Tuberculosis (TB) screening Hypersensitivity reactions
Etanercept (Enbrel)	Injection-site reaction Upper respiratory infection	Blood dyscrasias Hepatitis B reactivation Lupus-like syndrome Neurologic symptoms New or worsening heart failure	Complete blood count Hepatic function Tuberculosis (TB) screening
Adalimumab (Humira)	Headache Injection-site reaction Upper respiratory infection	Blood dyscrasias Hepatitis B reactivation Lupus-like syndrome Neurologic symptoms New or worsening heart failure	Complete blood count Hepatic function Tuberculosis (TB) screening
Infliximab (Remicade)	Abdominal pain Headache Upper respiratory infection	Blood dyscrasias Hepatitis B reactivation Lupus-like syndrome Neurologic symptoms New or worsening heart failure Lymphoma and other malignancies	Complete blood count Hepatic function Tuberculosis (TB) screening
Golimumab (Simponi)	Injection-site reaction Upper respiratory infection Cold symptoms	Blood dyscrasias Hepatitis B reactivation Lupus-like syndrome Neurologic symptoms New or worsening heart failure Lymphoma and other malignancies	Complete blood count Hepatic function Tuberculosis (TB) screening
Ustekinumab (Stelara)	Fatigue Headache Upper respiratory infection	Reversible posterior leukoencephalopathy syndrome Malignancies	Tuberculosis (TB) screening
Ixekizumab (Taltz)	Fungal infections Injection-site reaction Nausea	Hepatitis B reactivation	Hypersensitivity reactions

Table 4.3 Comparison of nonbiologic oral medications used to treat psoriasis [30] [data derived by Treatment Comparison. In: treatments BtaTsato, editor. https://wwwpsoriasis.org/sites/default/files/treatment_comparison_chart_1pdf: National Psoriasis Foundation; 2016]

Psoriasis systemic and targeted oral treatments [30]

Treatment	Common side effects	Other risks	Monitoring
Cyclosporine	Flu-like symptoms Headache High blood pressure High cholesterol Gastrointestinal upset Skin sensitivity	Birth defects Excess hair growth Gum hyperplasia (overgrowth) Kidney damage Liver damage Skin malignancies Tremor	Blood pressure Kidney function
H.P. Acthar Gel	Behavioral and mood changes Changes in glucose tolerance Fluid retention High blood pressure Increased appetite Weight gain	Birth defects Eye problems Hypersensitivity reactions Serious infection Unpredictable response to vaccines Worsening of other medical problems	Adrenal insufficiency Bone density Cushing's syndrome Physical development
Methotrexate	Difficulty sleeping Headache Light-headedness Mouth ulcers Nausea Tiredness Vomiting	Birth defects Fertility impairment Liver damage Lymphoma and other malignancies Blood dyscrasias Serious infection Serious toxicity	Hepatic function Kidney function Complete blood count Occasional liver biopsies
Apremilast (Otezla)	Diarrhea Headache Nausea	Depression Unexplained weight loss	None
Acitretin (Soriatane)	Chapped lips Depression Dry skin Alopecia Headache Joint pain	Birth defects Liver damage	Lipid panel Hepatic function

determining how to treat the patient most effectively while minimizing their fear of side effects. It is important to make sure that when getting informed consent from a patient the physician presents information in a way that the patient will understand it. A human characteristic that can affect patients' perception of side effects of treatment is the "Dumb and Dumber phenomenon," in which someone is told that there is a very small chance of something happening and they automatically think, "So you are saying there's a chance." For example, for rare but severe side effects, if you tell a patient that they have 1 out of 1000 chance of suffering side effects they will likely fear developing that issue. However, if a patient is told that there is 999 out of 1000 chance of not suffering a side effect, they will then feel more comfortable taking that medication because they will picture themselves as one of the people not getting the side effect. When these fears are minimized, increasing patient adherence and persistence to treatment are observed [3].

Route of Administration

Biologic and systemic medications can be administered via various routes, including intravenous infusion and intramuscular or subcutaneous injection. Each route carries with it different degrees of convenience, patient fear, and side effects that consequently affect patient adherence to treatment. Just as patients may prefer the most convenient topical treatments with the fewest tolerability issues, patients generally prefer biologic medications with the lowest frequency of administration and greatest ease and comfort of use [3].

Therefore, in addition to understanding which biologic would ideally treat the patient's disease, healthcare providers must consider what medication the patient would actually use. In international studies of psoriatic patients treated with biologic agents, patients had greater persistence to treatment with medications requiring in-office administration by a healthcare professional, versus self-administration at home. For example, ustekinumab (an injection administered by healthcare professional) has better persistence than etanercept (an injection that is self-administered at home) [19].

Medication Cost

Treating psoriasis can be expensive, and due to the cost of some therapies, some patients elect to live with their disease rather than paying copayments for their medications. Moderate-to-severe psoriasis is most inexpensively treated with methotrexate, the cost of which ranges from 1200 to 1700 dollars annually [17, 32]. Home phototherapy units are more cost effective in the long-term management of disease compared to the long-term costs of biologics.

The most expensive psoriasis medications are biologics, which can cost greater than $50,000 annually [17, 33]. Despite the higher cost of the medication, the total healthcare costs for moderate-to-severe psoriasis patients prior to and after starting biologics can be less overall when the lower need for hospitalization and ER visits for severe flares are considered [17]. Since these medications are highly effective, they may reduce the utilization of healthcare services overall, thus lowering rates of outpatient, inpatient, and emergency department visits [2, 17]. Increased efficacy of biologic therapy may lead to greater adherence due to fewer hospitalizations and ER visits. Increased efficacy rates, as indicated by a greater reduction in PASI scores, may lead to greater adherence to biologic therapy in the future. Patients taking biologic medication have fewer hospitalizations and ED visits than those taking nonbiologic medications [17].

Patient Demographics

While age is not a reason for nonadherence, it may be a helpful factor to consider when determining how to help a patient adhere to their medications. Poorer adherence is seen in those who are less than 30 years of age than those who are 41–50 [13, 17]. Older age generally corresponds with greater adherence, an effect that is observed until around the age of 70 [7]. This may be observed because older patients typically have more comorbidities and take more medications, and have thus developed a routine to assist them with taking their medications. Younger people who take fewer medications have not developed such a routine. However, both the very old (over 70) and the very young (less than 10) have poorer adherence because they typically require assistance with medication administration. Factors such as other caretaker responsibilities, discomfort with the task, and forgetfulness are out of these patients' control, and influence adherence and persistence [23].

Other demographic characteristics that impact adherence include gender, access to care, and employment. One study showed a 5% increase in adherence in females relative to their male counterparts [7]. However, more recent international data has shown that men with psoriasis taking TNF-alpha inhibitors or ustekinumab actually have a longer time to discontinuation of treatment than women [19]. These are not reasons for nonadherence; rather they are factors to consider in each individual patient and reemphasize the need for physicians to personalize their approach to increasing patient adherence.

Lifestyle Patterns

Weekends commonly provide a temporary deviation from the weekday routine, and predictably, patients miss more medication doses on the weekends than on weekdays [7]. Treatment gaps represent a behavioral pattern in drug usage. When medication is restarted after a full day or more of missed doses, baseline disease can reappear [7]. To help avoid this, doctors can advise patients on pitfalls that can occur with therapy (such as increased difficulty in continuation of therapy on weekends). This may help patients be more aware of possible difficulties and to be more adherent [7]. However, more studies need to be completed to test this hypothesis adequately.

Physicians value health more highly than does the general population [9, 34]. Patients, on the other hand, may follow the "live for today, save for tomorrow" mentality. Physicians must consider a patient's value system when developing a rational counseling strategy. Simply educating a patient on physician viewpoints is not likely to change patient behaviors [4]. This is why it is important to form a strong physician-patient relationship so that you can adequately understand your patient's lifestyle and what will motivate them the best to take their medications.

Poor Physician-Patient Relationship

When patients perceive their care to be high quality, their trust in their providers is maintained or even improved; the more a patient trusts his or her physician, the more likely he or she is to comply with the physician's instructions. Patient perception of the quality of their care is driven by the context of their visits [15]. A well-kept, efficient office with empathetic staff helps give patients the impression that they are receiving high-quality care. Despite busy office schedules, small, systematic gestures and patient education serve to express quality without backing up the day's schedule. Touch is well received by patients and takes little time. Encouraging patients with psoriasis to join the National Psoriasis Foundation can help address many of patients' psychosocial needs. Questions on these patient satisfaction surveys included "time physician spent with you," "physician's concern for your questions," "how well the physician kept you informed," and "friendliness/courtesy of physician." A well-kept office, empathetic staff, and encouraging involvement in support groups are simple techniques that will improve patient satisfaction and can make 5 min feel like 15 to a patient. It is the quality of the appointment that is more important to patients than the actual time spent with them.

Other Factors

Other factors that are related to persistence in biologic therapy regimens in psoriasis patients include body mass index, familial psoriasis history, smoking status, alcohol status, duration of psoriasis, age at psoriasis diagnosis, diagnosis of psoriatic arthritis, study site/geographic region, history of immunomodulator use, types of insurance, prior biologic therapies used, reasons for discontinuation of prior biologic therapies, and Physician's Global Assessment [19].

Methods of Combating Nonadherence

The goal of physicians is to improve the lives of our patients. Making the right diagnosis and prescribing the right medication may be necessary, but they aren't sufficient to affect patient outcomes. In addition to making the right diagnosis and prescribing the right therapy, physicians must get patients to take the medication. Getting patients to use the recommended treatment is one leg of a three-legged stool, and an essential component of successful treatment that physicians need to address. There are many approaches! The following strategies are discussed in this section: the timing of follow-up visits, motivational interviewing, cost reduction, simplifying therapeutic regimens, patient education, cues to action, patient accountability, incentivizing healthy lifestyle choices, avoidance of physician assumptions and biases, and building a trusting patient-physician relationship (Table 4.4).

The Timing of Follow-Up Visits

Complex and daunting treatment regimens for patients can adversely affect adherence; adherence is poor even to simple regimens. The common approach to prescribing treatment—giving patients a prescription to fill, expecting them to use the treatment regularly, and seeing them back for follow-up in 8–12 weeks—borders on ridiculous; if a piano teacher gave students sheet music (or worse, a prescription to fill at a music shop for sheet music) and said, "Practice every day, and I'll see you at the recital in 8–12 weeks," what kind of outcome would we expect? Visits drive behavior, for piano

Table 4.4 Health belief model as a structure for thinking about adherence interventions [permission acquired by Christine M. Zoro, Customer Account Specialist, Copyright Clearance Center in association with Wolters Kluwer Publishing]

Health belief model as a structure for thinking about adherence interventions [5]	
Concept 1: Perceived susceptibility/severity of disease	Educate patient on nature of disease
Concept 2: Perceived benefit	Educate patient about importance of treatment Confirm patient understanding of treatment Physician-patient relationship Written action plans
Concept 3: Self-efficacy	Timing of office visits Motivational interviewing
Concept 4: Perceived barriers to treatment (e.g., time, money)	Affordable treatment options, decreased copays Simplifying treatment regimens
Concept 5: Cues to action	Telephone call/text message reminders for office appointment Medication reminder software for smartphone Reminder packaging Memory strategies

lessons, for flossing teeth, and for getting patients to use medication. Scheduling a follow-up contact a few days after an initial visit (typically within 3–7) creates accountability to treatment. The request to assess patients' response shortly after initiating treatment drives home to the patient how much the doctor cares about the patient and is concerned about the patient's condition [17]. When patients are diligent about using their medications initially, good treatment results are observed, and when a patient finds a medication that works well for them, their need and motivation to continue treatment increase [12]. An early follow-up visit/contact may seem to mean more visits; however, by increasing adherence and improving treatment outcomes, that early contact may reduce the need for additional visits and medication changes, along with reducing patients' burden of disease [17].

When the first follow-up appointment occurs less than 2 weeks after the initial visit, greater adherence to therapy is observed [7]. Termed "white coat effect" or "white coat compliance," adherence tends to increase around physician visits; the visit is a powerful tool for influencing patients' adherence behavior [7, 35]. Patients taking ustekinumab and infliximab, treatments that can be administered by clinic staff, have longer persistence compared with patients treated with self-administered biologic therapies [19]. Psoriasis patients using topical salicylic acid and tacrolimus have increased adherence on the day of their clinic visit or within 3 days prior, as measured by weight-based evaluation of medication tubes, self-reporting data, and

MEMS caps [6, 7]. Patients ≤12 years of age treated with topical corticosteroids have the greatest adherence on the visit date, doubled adherence during an interval close to the visit, decreased adherence in the first few days after visit date, and a progressive decrease after [23, 36]. Moderate-to-severe atopic dermatitis patients <15 years of age treated with tacrolimus ointment and subsequent follow-up grouped into a control and extra-visit group had a considerable increase in absolute and relative adherence to therapy with an extra visit [35].

Intermediate treatment follow-up—at 1, 2, 4, 6, and 8 weeks— is a common design feature in clinical drug trials that doesn't happen in clinical practice. While patients may be seen every 2 weeks for a total of 8 weeks in a clinical trial, often patients are given a new medication in practice and not seen for 3–6 months. This may help explain why so many drugs are more effective in clinical trials than they are in clinical practice. As would be expected, patients with an early office visit have greater compliance and better treatment outcomes [12].

Motivational Interviewing

Motivational interviewing (MI) is a method of counseling that aims to produce behavioral change through the implementation of four key principles [17]. These principles are used in sequence during patient discussions to help patients accurately judge and report the barriers affecting their use of treatment. After recognition of these barriers, solutions and changes can be made to increase their persistency and adherence to physician instructions.

The four key principles of MI are as follows (Table 4.5). First, empathy or concern for the patient's struggles is expressed. The physician listens to the patient without interruption, and periodically responds with summary statements. Second, discrepancy is developed. This establishes that the patient's goal is to feel better and helps the patient realize

that nonadherence is detrimental to that goal. This principle is difficult to discuss with patients, and the physician must be ready for patient resistance to discrepancy acknowledgement [17]. Third, the physician must adjust their approach depending on their patient's resistance, reflect, rephrase patient arguments against change, and then redirect the conversation to generate solutions. By utilizing resistance, the physician draws upon solution-generating dialog, allowing patients to arrive at their own conclusions, in their own time. Lastly, the physician supports self-efficacy, reassuring patients of their abilities and praising their progress.

MI techniques can improve adherence to medications, as well as produce behavioral changes such as improved diet and exercise [5]. Motivational interviewing is a mechanism for achieving greater insight into one's disease, identifying barriers to treatment, and overcoming them [17].

Here's a concrete example of the use of motivational interviewing. You care about your patients, right? You want them to get well, don't you? Do you find it frustrating when they don't? Do you think that poor use of their medication may explain part of why they don't get better? Is it important to you to get them to use their medications well? What might you do to help them to be more adherent to treatment? Do you think any of the approaches suggested here would help? How might you incorporate them into your practice? Perhaps you could contact me next week to let me know what techniques you tried with them and how well they seem to be working for you.

Cost Reduction

The increasing cost of healthcare and the greater insurance copayments and deductibles can force patients with life-altering chronic disease to de-prioritize therapy in place of other more urgent costs [5]. Physicians and other healthcare professionals are working to address the financial burden that therapy exerts on their patients, and helping them obtain the treatment they need.

Healthcare professionals can act as financial advocates for their patients by identifying patients with financial constraints early on and providing resources for affordable drugs and coverage programs. Online resources (such as www.GoodRx.com) can increase price transparency and help patients find affordable treatment. When using electronic prescribing, a standardized message can be included with the prescription sent to the pharmacist permitting/encouraging substitution of comparable but more affordable treatments. Aside from finding less expensive drugs or better financial assistance programs, simplifying the complexity of treatment regimens may be the best method to decrease cost and increase adherence, persistency, and efficacy of treatment [10].

Table 4.5 Four principles of motivational interviewing [permission acquired by Christine M. Zoro, Customer Account Specialist, Copyright Clearance Center in association with Wolters Kluwer Publishing]

Four principles of motivational interviewing [5]	
Express empathy	Express concern regarding patient's struggles, listen without interrupting, and periodically respond with summary statements
Develop discrepancy	Establish that patient's goal is to feel better and guide patient to realization that nonadherence is counteracting that goal
Roll with the resistance	Reflect/rephrase patients' arguments against change; redirect conversation to generate solutions
Support self-efficacy	Reassure patients of their abilities and praise them on their progress

Simplifying Therapeutic Regimens

Treatments that are complex in terms of number of medications and frequency of dosing are difficult for patients to adhere to [5]. Drug failure commonly results from combining topical therapies with more expensive systemic agents, which in turn decreases therapeutic adherence and persistence. Drug regimens can be simplified by using combination medications [5], educating patients that multiple medications are a "single-treatment program" rather than individual treatments [37], and cautiously using shorter courses of higher potency topical and systemic medications rather than longer courses of lower potency medication [9].

Simplifying therapy is an effective way to increase therapeutic adherence and persistency. Psoriasis patients taking one to three medications versus those taking four or more medications have much better compliance [7]. Elderly patients taking multiple medications have poorer adherence and persistence to treatment with more medications [6]. The more doses that patients must take per day, the greater the likelihood they will make mistakes or forget to take their medications [5]. Combination medications and simplified treatment regimens reduce the risk of nonadherence in all realms of medicine [5].

Combination products may be costlier at times than the separate monotherapy components. Whether the potential for improving adherence justifies the cost can be determined on a patient-to-patient basis, incorporating patients' individual preferences in this regard.

Patient Education

Increased patient education improves patient understanding of disease and is generally associated with improved adherence (though the side effects described in commercial advertising may at times reduce patients' willingness to take medication) [5]. Medical education can be overwhelming for patients, especially those without a medical background or higher education. Information should be provided in a clear and concise manner, and in a format that reduces the burden of memorizing instructions and other information. Patient education should be focused on methods to guide treatment use, and sensitize patients to the benefits and risks of treatment as well as the risks of not treating their condition [5].

Resources for patient education that are both efficient for patients and providers include websites such as www.psoriasis.org, YouTube videos, informational community-based sessions, instructional CDs, and informational brochures. Another option for effective patient education is allowing patients access to their online electronic medical record (EMR). When allowed to view their EMR, patients gain access to a plethora of instructional and informational handouts, after-visit summaries, and a written "action plan." For patients with chronic diseases, local and national advocacy groups such as the National Psoriasis Foundation are also excellent resources [3].

Patient education materials such as informational workbooks and mnemonics increase compliance and understanding of treatment risks and benefits. These methods of patient education encourage patients to adhere to physician recommendations and be more self-aware of skin concerns. For example, reports show that education programs make patients more inclined to adhere to the recommendations for self-exam and to make an appointment with a dermatologist if they find a concerning lesion [5]. Action plans, single-sheet guides that clearly explain to patients how to treat a disease flare in a step-by-step fashion, increase adherence by decreasing the need to memorize instructions [3]. Patients who do not receive instruction regarding therapies are treated longer without remission than those who do [3]. With increased education, adherence and persistence to treatment, as well as patient satisfaction with treatment and provider, increase [3].

Cues to Action

Methods that remind patients to take their medications are called "cues to action" and effectively increase adherence and persistency to treatment [5]. Tying treatment to an activity that is already routine is a powerful way to help assure better adherence. Many of the "cues to action" discussed here are gathered from U.S. Department of Human Services Campaign *Script Your Future,* which asked patients to create videos to demonstrate helpful health information technology. These include patient reminder systems on cell phones in the form of cell phone alarms, calendars, and downloadable third-party applications designed by pharmacies [1].

Websites, like rememberitnow.com, allow patient reminders to be sent via phone or e-mail. Mymedschedule.com schedules refill dates and organizes drug history. Scriptyourfuture.org creates medication lists. Other helpful websites include pillbox.nlm.nih.gov/, dailymed.nlm.nih.gov/, and Healthit.gov. Electronic health information reminder tools include E-prescriptions and online pharmacies that ship directly to patients' homes.

Although modern technology is an excellent tool that can be used to improve adherence and persistency of medication use, there are many "cues to action" that are more simple and do not require access to a computer or smartphone (Table 4.6). Organizational cues include inexpensive weekly pillboxes and multidrug punch cards. Multidrug punch cards are plastic cards with 28 cavities, each filled with day's worth of prescribed patient medications. Memory-based techniques are simple habits that can be included in a patient's daily routine. For example, a consistent, visible location should be selected to store medications that are to be taken (e.g., a nightstand or bedside table). Medications can also be paired with specific items/activities (such as placing tubes of antifungal cream for tinea pedis in the sock drawer on top of the socks), and partners can be enlisted to give or apply the medication [17]. "Cues to action" and their roles in increasing

Table 4.6 Cues to action [permission acquired by Christine M. Zoro, Customer Account Specialist, Copyright Clearance Center in association with Wolters Kluwer Publishing]

Cues to action [5]	
Technological	Telephone call/text message reminder for office appointment Medication reminder application for smartphones
Organizational	Pill boxes Multidrug punch cards
Memory	Place medicine in visible location (bedside nightstand, dining table) Pair medicine with item (antifungal cream on top of socks)

adherence and persistence have been tested and proven [38]. SMS text message reminders as a "cue to action" increased doses taken (18%) within 1 and 4 h after receiving reminders [5, 20, 21, 39]. Employing these cues for a patient is a great way to aid patients who have trouble with medication adherence due to memory issues or busy schedules.

Incentivizing a Healthy Lifestyle

Many stakeholders have an interest in enhancing patients' adherence. Nurses, nutritionists, health insurance companies, employers, pharmaceutical companies, and pharmacists are all directly affected by patient adherence. Workplaces are now implementing workplace wellness programs designed to increase health awareness. These programs may involve personalized health coaching and incentives such as reduced insurance premiums if weight loss and blood pressure goals are achieved, as well as consequences for poor health behaviors, such as smoking and increased BMI [5]. An increasing culture of health awareness in all realms of society is incentivizing healthy living and well-being, and in turn has the potential to increase adherence. Ways that other "stakeholders" can improve adherence are numerous and varied depending upon one's area of expertise, and each professional's role is equally vital to improving adherence (Table 4.7) [5]. For example, information communicated to patients by pharmacists in copay assistance programs and synchronization of prescription refills increase adherence (if patients are on multiple chronic medications, having them refill the different medications at different times of the month is a truly needless barrier to treatment persistence) [5].

Trusting Patient-Physician Relationship

In order for physicians to help their patients take their medications, the importance of building a strong patient-physician relationship must not be ignored [5]. For a patient to take a

Table 4.7 Strategies for stakeholders to improve adherence [permission acquired by Christine M. Zoro, Customer Account Specialist, Copyright Clearance Center in association with Wolters Kluwer Publishing]

Strategies for stakeholders to improve adherence [5]	
Nurses and nutritionists	Patient education
Health insurance companies	Reduced copayments Reward adherence
Employers	Health coaching that emphasizes importance of adherence Incentives for improving blood pressure, cholesterol, and weight Incentives for regular physicians' visits
Pharmaceutical companies	Develop medications with fewer adverse effects Cost-effective treatments Combination therapies
Pharmacists	Simplify dosing regimens Recommend copayment assistance programs Patient education Synchronize prescription refills for same day

Table 4.8 Strategies for building a healthy, strong patient-physician relationship [data derived from Aslam I, Feldman SR. Practical Strategies to Improve Patient Adherence to Treatment Regimens. South Med J 2015 Jun;108(6):325–31]

Strategies for building a healthy, strong patient-physician relationship [5]	
1. Make a good first impression	All areas, from reception to exam room, are clean and comfortable. All personnel, including office staff, nurses, and physicians, are friendly and considerate
2. Do not interrupt	Patients are allowed to tell their stories
3. Ask questions	Patient understanding is affirmed
4. Explain	Diagnosis and treatment plan are explained in a manner that patient can't comprehend, without rushing
5. Encourage sharing information	Patient feelings and expectations are solicited regarding their condition, and patients are asked to evaluate physician performance, empowering them to participate in quality improvement

medication, they have to trust it—trust that it is safe to use, that any potential side effects will be monitored for and caught early, and that it is the best option for their disease state. A patient is not going to take a mediation because they trust the insurance company or the drug company. Their trust in their medication is almost wholly on their trust in their provider. This ties to accountability in that if a patient is being held accountable to someone that they believe cares about them, the patient will then have very strong motivation to adhere to their medications (Table 4.8).

Conclusion

Medication adherence and persistence are very important to patients and healthcare professionals alike. With the current emphasis on patient-centered care and measurement of health outcomes in light of a growing preference for the use of biologic and systemic medications in chronic, recalcitrant disease, a team approach to patient management is key. It may be helpful for physicians and healthcare professionals to focus on understanding barriers to adherence, methods of overcoming them, and practice of evidence-based medicine in order to achieve greater treatment efficacy, rather than simply adhering to commonly held assumptions. It is not necessarily a physician's role to devise a new treatment plan when receiving a new patient, but rather to first determine methods by which to help patients adhere to their previously prescribed medication regimens.

Conflicts of Interest *Disclosures*: The above authors have no conflicts of interest and/or financial disclosures to report.

References

1. Laffer MS, Feldman SR. Improving medication adherence through technology: analyzing the managing meds video challenge. Skin Res Technol. 2014;20(1):62–6.
2. Feldman SR. Improving adherence, improving outcomes: an expert interview with Steven R. Feldman, MD, PhD. Medscape. 2009.
3. Brown KK, Rehmus WE, Kimball AB. Determining the relative importance of patient motivations for nonadherence to topical corticosteroid therapy in psoriasis. J Am Acad Dermatol. 2006;55(4):607–13.
4. Dabade TS, Feldman SR. We must think outside the box to understand nonadherence. Pediatr Dermatol. 2011;28(3):353.
5. Aslam I, Feldman SR. Practical strategies to improve patient adherence to treatment regimens. South Med J. 2015;108(6):325–31.
6. Kim G, Barner JC, Rascati K, Richards K. Examining time to initiation of biologic disease-modifying antirheumatic drugs and medication adherence and persistence among Texas Medicaid recipients with rheumatoid arthritis. Clin Ther. 2016;38(3):646–54.
7. Carroll CL, Feldman SR, Camacho FT, Manuel JC, Balkrishnan R. Adherence to topical therapy decreases during the course of an 8-week psoriasis clinical trial: commonly used methods of measuring adherence to topical therapy overestimate actual use. J Am Acad Dermatol. 2004;51(2):212–6.
8. Feldman SR. What you should do when people don't get well. J Dermatolog Treat. 2007;18(4):196.
9. Hix E, Gustafson CJ, O'Neill JL, Huang K, Sandoval LF, Harrison J, et al. Adherence to a five day treatment course of topical fluocinonide 0.1% cream in atopic dermatitis. Dermatol Online J. 2013;19(10):20029.
10. Yentzer BA, Wood AA, Sagransky MJ, O'Neill JL, Clark AR, Williams LL, et al. An internet-based survey and improvement of acne treatment outcomes. Arch Dermatol. 2011;147(10):1223–4.
11. Nieuwlaat R, Wilczynski N, Navarro T, Hobson N, Jeffery R, Keepanasseril A, et al. Interventions for enhancing medication adherence (review). Cochrane Database Syst Rev. 2014;1:1–732.
12. Kim IH, Feldman SR. The compliance pyramid. J Dermatolog Treat. 2011;22(4):185–6.
13. Feldman SR. Tachyphylaxis to topical corticosteroids: the more you use them, the less they work? Clin Dermatol. 2006;24(3):229–30. discussion 30
14. West C, Narahari S, O'Neill J, Davis S, Huynh M, Clark A, et al. Adherence to adalimumab in patients with moderate to severe psoriasis. Dermatol Online J. 2013;19(5):18182.
15. Feldman SR. Looking beyond the borders of our specialty: the 2006 Clarence S. Livingood MD Lecture. Dermatol Online J. 2007;13(4):20.
16. Hilton L. Compliance is shockingly understudied. Dermatology Times. 2014.
17. Bhosle MJ, Feldman SR, Camacho FT, Timothy Whitmire J, Nahata MC, Balkrishnan R. Medication adherence and health care costs associated with biologics in Medicaid-enrolled patients with psoriasis. J Dermatolog Treat. 2006;17(5):294–301.
18. Pearce DJ, Higgins KB, Stealey KH, Balkrishnan R, Crane MM, Camacho F, et al. Adverse events from systemic therapies for psoriasis are common in clinical practice. J Dermatolog Treat. 2006;17(5):288–93.
19. Menter A, Papp KA, Gooderham M, Pariser DM, Augustin M, Kerdel FA, et al. Drug survival of biologic therapy in a large, disease-based registry of patients with psoriasis: results from the Psoriasis Longitudinal Assessment and Registry (PSOLAR). J Eur Acad Dermatol Venereol. 2016;30(7):1148–58.
20. Strowd LC, Yentzer BA, Fleischer AB, Feldman SR. Increasing use of more potent treatments for psoriasis. J Am Acad Dermatol. 2009;60(3):478–81.
21. Horn EJ, Fox KM, Patel V, Chiou CF, Dann F, Lebwohl M. Are patients with psoriasis undertreated? Results of National Psoriasis Foundation survey. J Am Acad Dermatol. 2007;57(6):957–62.
22. Rapp SR, Feldman SR. The promise and challenge of new biological treatments for psoriasis: how do they impact quality of life? Dermatol Ther. 2004;17(5):376–82.
23. Krejci-Manwaring J, Tusa MG, Carroll C, Camacho F, Kaur M, Carr D, et al. Stealth monitoring of adherence to topical medication: adherence is very poor in children with atopic dermatitis. J Am Acad Dermatol. 2007;56(2):211–6.
24. Feldman S. Modest innovations in psoriasis treatment? J Dermatolog Treat. 2003;14(4):198–9.
25. Nair RP, Duffin KC, Helms C, Ding J, Stuart PE, Goldgar D, et al. Genome-wide scan reveals association of psoriasis with IL-23 and NF-kappaB pathways. Nat Genet. 2009;41(2):199–204.
26. Sandoval LF, Pierce A, Feldman SR. Systemic therapies for psoriasis: an evidence-based update. Am J Clin Dermatol. 2014;15(3):165–80.
27. Gupta R, Levin E, JJ W, Koo J, Liao W. An update on drug-drug interactions with biologics for the treatment of moderate-to-severe psoriasis. J Dermatolog Treat. 2014;25(1):87–9.
28. Kalb RE, Fiorentino DF, Lebwohl MG, Toole J, Poulin Y, Cohen AD, et al. Risk of serious infection with biologic and systemic treatment of psoriasis: results from the Psoriasis Longitudinal Assessment and Registry (PSOLAR). JAMA Dermatol. 2015;151(9):961–9.
29. Becker I, Horneff G. Risk of serious infection in juvenile idiopathic arthritis patients associated with TNF-inhibitors and disease activity in the German BIKER registry. Arthritis Care Res (Hoboken). 2017;69(4):552–60.
30. National Psoriasis Foundation. Treatment comparison. In: Treatments BtaTsato. 2016. https://wwwpsoriasis.org/sites/default/files/treatment_comparison_chart_1pdf
31. Nielsen D, Ryg J, Nielsen W, Knold B, Nissen N, Brixen K. Patient education in groups increases knowledge of osteoporosis and adherence to treatment: a two-year randomized controlled trial. Patient Educ Couns. 2010;81(2):155–60.
32. D'Souza LS, Payette MJ. Estimated cost efficacy of systemic treatments that are approved by the US Food and Drug Administration for the treatment of moderate to severe psoriasis. J Am Acad Dermatol. 2015;72(4):589–98.

33. Chastek B, White J, van Voorhis D, Tang D, Stolshek BS. A retrospective cohort study comparing utilization and costs of biologic therapies and JAK inhibitor therapy across four common inflammatory indications in adult US managed care patients. Adv Ther. 2016;33(4):626–42.

34. Feldman SR, Chen GJ, JY H, Fleischer AB. Effects of systematic asymmetric discounting on physician-patient interactions: a theoretical framework to explain poor compliance with lifestyle counseling. BMC Med Inform Decis Mak. 2002;2:8.

35. Sagransky MJ, Yentzer BA, Williams LL, Clark AR, Taylor SL, Feldman SR. A randomized controlled pilot study of the effects of an extra office visit on adherence and outcomes in atopic dermatitis. Arch Dermatol. 2010;146(12):1428–30.

36. Feldman SR. Let's not presuppose that patients take their medications. J Dermatolog Treat. 2012;23(5):317.

37. Feldman SR. Perhaps programs are a better way to go. J Dermatolog Treat. 2010;21(6):325.

38. Strandbygaard U, Thomsen SF, Backer V. A daily SMS reminder increases adherence to asthma treatment: a three-month follow-up study. Respir Med. 2010;104(2):166–71.

39. Vervloet M, van Dijk L, Santen-Reestman J, van Vlijmen B, van Wingerden P, Bouvy ML, et al. SMS reminders improve adherence to oral medication in type 2 diabetes patients who are real time electronically monitored. Int J Med Inform. 2012;81(9):594–604.

Quality of Life in the Dermatology Practice

5

Jennifer Cather, J. Christian Cather, and Melodie Young

Introduction

Dermatologic disease can create significant burden, interfering with relationships, daily activities, work environments, personal well-being, and physical functioning. The impact of these diseases on quality of life (QOL) can be significant, and the psychosocial impact of many dermatologic diseases is often more impactful than the physical appearance or symptoms alone. We now know that many chronic dermatologic conditions are more than skin deep, and the impact once believed to be merely superficial is as complex physiologically as it is psychosocially. Any patients that have diseases with external features may have feelings of anxiety, depression, and social isolation. Fortunately, we are learning to evaluate and treat the whole person and not just a patient's skin. Expert dermatologic care is much more than assessing and treating the physical appearance or symptoms. Dermatologic conditions such as acne, alopecia, atopic dermatitis, psoriasis, and rosacea are unique, with differing presentations, symptoms, and psychosocial impacts. These conditions have a myriad of therapies available; however, selecting the most appropriate therapy for a given patient at a given time can be challenging, oftentimes more challenging than just establishing the correct diagnosis. In this chapter we explore how quality of life may impact dermatology patients, and how incorporating quality-of-life assessment can help providers select appropriate therapy, improving patient adherence and outcomes.

Measuring Quality of Life

Skin diseases can cause significant burden to patients and families affected by them. The 2013 Global Burden of Skin Disease Study measured the impact of skin diseases in 188 countries, and found that skin diseases were the fourth most common cause of disability worldwide [1]. In another large study across 13 European countries, patients with skin diseases, including hidradenitis suppurativa, blistering diseases, leg ulcers, infections, and most chronic skin diseases, had reduced health-related quality of life compared to patients with other serious medical conditions such as chronic obstructive lung disease, diabetes mellitus, cardiovascular disease, and cancers [2]. Adolescents and adults with acne, psoriasis, atopic dermatitis, and other visible dermatologic conditions have described impacts on appearance, self-consciousness, confidence, and social withdrawal. These conditions have also been linked to depression, ostracism, difficulty in finding and maintaining employment, as well as impacting intimate relationships. Historically, providers may have underestimated the psychosocial impact of these conditions in their patients.

Quality of life (QOL) is a broad, multidimensional concept that includes domains such as physical well-being, psychological well-being, functional status, social functioning, and health perceptions [3]. Health-related quality of life (HRQoL) is a complementary term that incorporates QOL from the perspective of health, disease, and its treatment. The Centers for Disease Control define Health Related Quality of Life (HRQoL) as "an individual's or group's perceived physical and mental health over time" [4]. However, HRQoL can mean different things to different people, which contributes to making it imprecise and difficult to define. Individual perceptions of the impact of a disease may differ due to each person's unique values, cultural influences, social situations, work experiences, religious beliefs, family and relationships, and other experiences and influences. Additionally, patients and their providers may have differing perceptions of HRQoL, particularly as it relates to treatment

J. Cather, MD (✉) • J.C. Cather, MD
M. Young, RN, ANP-C
Modern Research Associates, Dallas, TX, USA
e-mail: jennifercather@mac.com

© Springer International Publishing AG 2018
P.S. Yamauchi (ed.), *Biologic and Systemic Agents in Dermatology*, https://doi.org/10.1007/978-3-319-66884-0_5

and treatment success. Clinical success for treatment as defined by a provider may not equate to success as defined by their patient, and the burden of a disease and its impact on QOL can be a driver for this discrepancy. Assessing HRQoL at every visit can help close this gap and improve patient-provider communication.

HRQoL can be measured with generic, dermatology-specific, or disease-specific questionnaires. For example the Short Form 36 (SF-36) is a commonly used, validated, generic instrument used to measure quality of life that is easily administered [5]. The SF-36 has been used in many disease areas, and SF-36 scores have highlighted the impact of many dermatologic conditions compared to other well-known, chronic health conditions. In the field of dermatology, the Dermatology Life Quality Index (DLQI) is the most commonly used, validated instrument to measure HRQoL [6]. The DLQI was designed to be administered in a busy clinic setting, and DLQI scores of the common dermatologic disorders eczema and psoriasis are 4.2 and 4.5, respectively, compared to 0.3 of the normal population, indicating the impact of these diseases [7]. The DLQI has been used extensively in clinical trials, and has also been used to measure changes in HRQoL before and after treatment in a variety of dermatologic conditions, including acne, eczema, psoriasis, and others [7]. Disease-specific instruments have also been developed for a variety of dermatologic conditions and used in clinical trials, particularly in studies of psoriasis and eczema [8–10].

Treatment Selection and HRQoL

Significant therapeutic advances have occurred in dermatology in recent years, and this is probably most pronounced with advancements in the psoriasis treatment landscape. Here we use psoriasis as an example of how information about HRQoL can help improve treatment selection and shared decision making between providers and patients. In psoriasis, clinical trials have consistently shown improvements in both the Psoriasis Area Severity Index (PASI) and HRQoL in patients treated with biologics, with correlation between improvements of >75% in PASI scores and significant improvements in HRQoL [11]. Patients with clear skin are more likely to report no impact of psoriasis on their HRQoL compared to those with almost clear skin after treatment with biologics or systemics, suggesting that clear skin is an important outcome for patients, and limited disease can have significant impact [12]. It is worth noting that in patients with limited disease, objective disease severity measures like the PASI may not correlate well with HRQoL measures—especially when lesions are in high-impact areas such as the hands and feet, face, nails, scalp, and genitalia [13–15]. Additionally, itch, skin pain, joint pain, sleep disturbances,

and comorbidities all contribute to a reduction in HRQoL regardless of body surface area involvement. Despite advances in the treatment landscape, >80% of patients with moderate-to-severe psoriasis are receiving no therapy or topical therapy alone, suggesting that this population continues to be undertreated [16].

As dermatologists, we should ensure that our patients are receiving evidence-based treatments appropriate for their disease. There are often several appropriate therapies for a given disease, and selecting the best one should be a shared decision made with our patients. To improve patient-provider communication and foster shared decision making, it is helpful to ask patients about their goals for therapy and their expectations of therapy. Oftentimes, they have been misinformed about risks or toxicities of systemic therapies, and asking them about their biggest concerns for a specific therapy can be helpful. As dermatologists, it is not our job to talk our patients onto therapies, but rather we want to provide education and the opportunity to help our patients make informed decisions. When therapies do not work or do not meet the expectations of our patients, a solid foundation of communication and collaboration helps with the transition to other therapies. Shared treatment decision making may contribute to improved treatment satisfaction and adherence and thus improved clinical outcomes [17].

Treatment guidelines for dermatologic conditions have been revised in recent years; however evidence-based guidelines which define therapeutic success from both the clinical and HRQoL perspectives are not standardized and are inconsistent. It has been suggested that HRQoL can be used as a metric for success for treatment. Currently, many therapies may be tailored to individual patient's HRQoL demands; however, in the future, healthcare resources may be allocated based on how a particular disease impacts patients' HRQoL relative to other disease states. For example, in several European countries, national reimbursement for systemics for both psoriasis and atopic dermatitis has been based on disease severity and HRQoL measured by DLQI scores [18–20]. Maintenance of biologic therapy for psoriasis patients has also been tied to improvements in DLQI. However, recent research suggests that DLQI scores may differ with different therapies, and may or may not be generalizable across patient populations [21]. Further research is needed to understand the utility of using DLQI scores to guide coverage and reimbursement decisions.

Assessing HRQoL in the Dermatology Clinic

Many of our dermatologic diseases exhibit extraordinarily noticeable external manifestations and have complex and far-reaching impacts on HRQoL. Providers are oftentimes confronted with difficult diseases, but what is even more cumbersome are the difficult situations that result from the disease itself. Here we provide several examples to illustrate challenging situations. For example, young adults may still be on their parents' insurance, and a parent's opinion about treatment may not be in alignment with the young adult patient's opinion. By exploring the impact the disease has on the patient in front of the parent, it may be possible to start appropriate therapy, especially when parents are hesitant to start systemic or biologic therapy. Oftentimes the parent will look in disbelief and ask why their child never discussed the impact of the disease with them. Another scenario is the child with acne who will not go to the pool or take off their shirt due to their lesions, and having this discussion in front of a parent can help them understand the true impact of the disease. These childhood or adolescent traumatic experiences can have a lasting impact on self-esteem. We should also acknowledge that these challenges aren't limited to children and young adults. For example, men and women with hidradenitis suppurativa or severe psoriasis are often socially isolated and may have never engaged in age-appropriate interpersonal relationships.

It is difficult to measure the true impact of a disease in the clinic, as the impact of a disease can be influenced by multiple factors, including the impact on daily life, relationships, and financial costs. Costs include both direct costs such as medications, personal care supplies, and required doctor visits or procedures and indirect costs such as time missed from work. It has been suggested that measuring HRQoL in the clinic may be helpful in assessing the impact of disease, both on the patient and on society. Providers and patients acknowledge a disease's impact on HRQoL and the shared medical decision making that is needed to foster the desired improvement. However, instruments originally designed for clinical trials may not perform well in a clinical setting and are often too time consuming for the patient and the provider, and may not provide value to third-party payers. The question then becomes this: How can we quantify these impacts without using a variety of impersonal questionnaires, and match patient and provider goals to an appropriate therapy?

In an attempt to fully understand a disease's impact upon a patient, we have found it helpful to create a relationship between the patient and their family, the provider, and the full healthcare team. It is essential to start this relationship in a collaborative, positive fashion, with goal and agenda setting at the very first visit. At each subsequent visit, we revaluate the goals and our agenda, and how we are working together to meet these goals. We have found that this approach builds trust between patients and the extended healthcare team. This approach can be used for all dermatology patients—from the 10-year-old who has their whole life ahead of them to the patient who is terminally ill. Patients' agendas are personal and must be known to the healthcare team to improve care and outcomes. Without a collaborative relationship, patients may not reveal the full extent of their disease—physically or psychologically. This is illustrated with genital psoriasis. Approximately 30% of psoriasis patients have genital involvement, however, over 45% of the patients did not discuss genital involvement with their dermatologist and only 25% of patients thought that their dermatologist paid sufficient attention to their genital lesions [22, 23]. If challenging aspects of a disease are not discussed, it is impossible to create a plan to mitigate those challenges.

HrQOL should be assessed at each and every visit. During the initial visit, however, it may be challenging to accurately assess because many facets influencing HRQoL are personal. At every visit, we ask our patients "Is there anything your disease keeps you from doing?" This simple question helps us begin to understand the true impact of the disease on their daily lives. We can then ask a follow-up question "Is there anything your current treatment keeps you from doing?" This follow-up helps us understand how well they perceive that their disease is being controlled and helps guide treatment selection. Generally, symptoms that are not emotionally charged, such as itch or pain, are easier to elicit from patients compared to topics such as sexual dysfunction or social isolation. Trust can play an important role in eliciting these more private topics. Additionally, the landscape of a patient's life changes continually—psychosexual and social roles are ever changing and helping patients navigate thru these changes may be necessary. This may require refining our goals based on additional information and changing situations. Finally, asking patients what is the worse part of their disease at every visit helps with agenda setting—the answer may be related to the disease itself (e.g., symptoms of itch), the medication (e.g., cost or interval), or even the clinic office hours. The goal of this question is to understand if there are any barriers to continuing therapy. Even if the disease is under control, it is easy for minor things to disrupt continued dosing.

We should also acknowledge that many changes are beyond the control of the provider or even the patient. One role we have as medical providers is to help educate patients so they can make informed decisions and facilitate healthier lifestyles. Goal and agenda setting helps frame this conversation and is recommended at every visit. As providers, we share knowledge of their disease(s) and therapies, and our concern for their well-being, and we continually discuss their personal health goals as it pertains to the totality of their dermatologic disease. When possible, dermatology providers should encourage general wellness including smoking cessation, weight control, and exercise and activity, in addition to sun avoidance and appropriate skin care. Not all dermatology patients will have a primary care physician, and most of our patients would greatly benefit from discussions regarding health and wellness.

Conclusion

All future dermatologic therapies should be safe and effective, and show positive impacts on patients' social, emotional, and physical well-being. Providers must consider multiple aspects of a condition and its impact on a patient. Collaborative decision making is required to select the best therapy for any given patient. Whether or not the condition is stable or flaring, the age and life status of the patient, current symptoms, their support system, educational level, occupation, general health, and therapeutic success to this point are all factors in how an individual patient's HRQoL will be influenced. The impact a disease has on a patient's HRQoL is as important as is the effect a therapy has on the HRQoL. We must use our assessment skills and the bonds of the patient-provider relationship to help us evaluate how the disease is affecting our patients at that moment in time and what we can do to improve their overall life by alleviating as much of the disease as possible. When patients, families, providers, and the healthcare team collaborate through shared decision making to create an individualized treatment plan, clinical outcomes improve, and more importantly, hopefully, lives will change. Healthcare resources are not limitless, and therefore, it is important to consider allocating resources to dermatologic diseases based on their impact on our patients' lives, which can be significant.

References

1. Karimkhani C, Dellavalle RP, Coffeng LE, Flohr C, Hay RJ, Langan SM, et al. Global skin disease morbidity and mortality: an update from the global burden of disease study 2013. JAMA Dermatol. 2017;153(5):406–12. https://doi.org/10.1001/jamadermatol.2016.5538. [Epub ahead of print]
2. Balieva F, Kupfer J, Lien L, Gieler U, Finlay AY, Tomas-Aragones L, et al. The burden of common skin diseases assessed with the EQ 5D: a European multi-centre study in 13 countries. Br J Dermatol. 2017;176(5):1170–8. https://doi.org/10.1111/bjd.15280. [Epub ahead of print]
3. Basra MK, Shahrukh M. Burden of skin diseases. Expert Rev Pharmacoecon Outcomes Res. 2009;9:271–83. https://doi.org/10.1586/erp.09.23.
4. Centers for Disease Control. HRQOL Concepts. 2017. https://www.cdc.gov/hrqol/concept.htm. Accessed March 6, 2017.
5. RAND Corporation. 36-Item short form survey instrument (SF-36). 2017. http://www.rand.org/health/surveys_tools/mos/36-item-short-form/survey-instrument.html. Accessed March 6, 2017.
6. Basra MK, Fenech R, Gatt RM, Salek MS, Finlay AY. The dermatology life quality index 1994-2007: a comprehensive review of validation data and clinical results. Br J Dermatol. 2008;159:997–1035. https://doi.org/10.1111/j.1365-2133.2008.08832.x. Epub 2008 Sep 15
7. Lewis V, Finlay AY. 10 years experience of the dermatology life quality index (DLQI). J Investig Dermatol Symp Proc. 2004;9:169–80.
8. Ali FM, Cueva AC, Vyas J, Atwan AA, Salek MS, Finlay AY, et al. A systematic review of the use of quality-of-life instruments in randomized controlled trials for psoriasis. Br J Dermatol. 2017;176:577–93. https://doi.org/10.1111/bjd.14788. Epub 2016 Oct 12
9. Chalmers JR, Simpson E, Apfelbacher CJ, Thomas KS, von Kobyletzki L, Schmitt J, et al. Report from the fourth international consensus meeting to harmonize core outcome measures for atopic eczema/dermatitis clinical trials (HOME initiative). Br J Dermatol. 2016;175:69–79. https://doi.org/10.1111/bjd.14773. Epub 2016 Jul 19
10. Chernyshov PV, Tomas-Aragones L, Manolache L, Marron SE, Salek MS, Poot F, et al. Quality of life measurement in atopic dermatitis. Position paper of the European Academy of Dermatology and Venereology (EADV) task force on quality of life. J Eur Acad Dermatol Venereol. 2017;31(4):576–93. https://doi.org/10.1111/jdv.14058. [Epub ahead of print]
11. Mattie PL, Corey KC, Kimball AB. Psoriasis area severity index (PASI) and the dermatology life quality index (DLQI): the correlation between disease severity and psychological burden in patients treated with biological therapies. J Eur Acad Dermatol Venereol. 2014;28:333–7. https://doi.org/10.1111/jdv.12106. Epub 2013 Feb 21
12. Takeshita J, Callis Duffin K, Shin DB, Krueger GG, Robertson AD, Troxel AB, et al. Patient-reported outcomes for psoriasis patients with clear versus almost clear skin in the clinical setting. J Am Acad Dermatol. 2014;71:633–41. https://doi.org/10.1016/j.jaad.2014.05.001. Epub 2014 Jun 11
13. Chung J, Callis Duffin K, Takeshita J, Shin DB, Krueger GG, Robertson AD, et al. Palmoplantar psoriasis is associated with greater impairment of health-related quality of life compared with moderate to severe plaque psoriasis. J Am Acad Dermatol. 2014;71:623–32. https://doi.org/10.1016/j.jaad.2014.04.063. Epub 2014 Jun 2
14. Ryan C, Sadlier M, De Vol E, Patel M, Lloyd AA, Day A, et al. Genital psoriasis is associated with significant impairment in quality of life and sexual functioning. J Am Acad Dermatol. 2015;72:978–83. https://doi.org/10.1016/j.jaad.2015.02.1127. Epub 2015 Mar 29
15. Wade AG, Crawford GM, Young D, Leman J, Pumford N. Severity and management of psoriasis within primary care. BMC Fam Pract. 2016;17:145.
16. Lebwohl MG, Bachelez H, Barker J, Girolomoni G, Kavanaugh A, Langley RG, et al. Patient perspectives in the management of psoriasis: results from the population-based Multinational Assessment of Psoriasis and Psoriatic Arthritis Survey. J Am Acad Dermatol. 2014;70:871–81.e1-30. https://doi.org/10.1016/j.jaad.2013.12.018. Epub 2014 Feb 24
17. Belinchon I, Rivera R, Blanch C, Comellas M, Lizan L. Adherence, satisfaction and preferences for treatment in patients with psoriasis in the European Union: a systemic review of the literature. Patient Prefer Adherence. 2016;10:2357–67. eCollection 2016
18. Hagg D, Sundstrom A, Eriksson M, Schmitt-Egenolf M. Decision for biological treatment in real life is more strongly associated with the psoriasis area and severity index (PASI) than with the dermatology life quality index (DLQI). J Eur Acad Dermatol Venereol. 2015;29:452–6. https://doi.org/10.1111/jdv.12576. Epub 2014 Jun 9
19. Rencz F, Kemeny L, Gajdacsi JZ, Owczarek W, Arenberger P, Tiplica GS, et al. Use of biologics for psoriasis in Central and Eastern European countries. J Eur Acad Dermatol Venereol. 2015;29(11):2222–30. https://doi.org/10.1111/jdv.13222. Epub 2015 Sep 14
20. Basra MK, Chowdhury MM, Smith EV, Freemantle N, Piguet V. Quality of life in psoriasis and chronic hand eczema: the discrepancy in the definition of severity in NICE guidelines and its implications. Br J Dermatol. 2012;166:462–3. https://doi.org/10.1111/j.1365-2133.2011.10601.x. Epub 2011 Dec 5

21. Rencz F, Baji P, Gulacsi L, Karpati S, Pentek M, Poor AK, et al. Discrepancies between the dermatology life quality index and utility scores. Qual Life Res. 2016;25:1687–96. https://doi.org/10.1007/s11136-015-1208-z. Epub 2015 Dec 18

22. Meeuwis KA, de Hullu JA, van de Nieuwenhof HP, Evers AW, Massuger LF, van de Kerkhof PC, et al. Quality of life and sexual health in patients with genital psoriasis. Br J Dermatol. 2011;164:1247–55. https://doi.org/10.1111/j.1365-2133.2011.10249.x. Epub 2011 May 13

23. Meeuwis KA, van de Kerkhof PC, Massuger LF, Massuger LF, de Hullu JA, van Rossum MM. Patients experience of psoriasis in the genital area. Dermatology. 2012;224:271–6. https://doi.org/10.1159/000338858. Epub 2012 Jun 4

Medical Legal Issues with Biologic Agents in the Treatment of Psoriasis

David J. Goldberg and Allan Gibofsky

Introduction

There are several classes of biologics and systemic agents used in dermatology. The use of all of these may be associated with certain legal issues; however some of these may be unique to the use of biologic agents.

This chapter focuses on the use of biologic agents used in dermatologic diseases, in particular, psoriasis, as that is where they are most commonly used.

Although biologic drugs have changed the face of psoriasis treatment, affording greater efficacy and enhancing quality of life in most patients, with time safety issues have been reported and the warning labels have expanded. A variety of issues are now linked to biologic associated tumor necrosis factor-alpha (TNF-α) blocker use. Litigation has occurred with the use of a variety of biologics. These include adalimumab, etanercept, and infliximab, members of a category known as TNF-α inhibitors, because of their mechanism of inhibiting a specific cytokine, TNFa. The published risks of these agents include the development of lupus and autoimmune-like syndromes, squamous cell cancer (SCC), and opportunistic infections. While to our knowledge there are no reported litigation claims involving the biologic ustekinumab, an interleukin (IL) 12/IL23 inhibitor, current practice suggests that patients should be screened for infections before patients on this biologic.

This chapter focuses on litigation related to the use of biologics in dermatology, approaches to reducing physician liability, and hypothetical lawsuits against a dermatologist using biologics.

In general, biologic agents are safe and well-tolerated therapies. However, despite the fact that biologic drugs have changed the face of psoriasis treatment, with each passing year the updates in the package insert have expanded to such as additional infections and non-melanoma skin cancers.

Monitoring of psoriasis patients on biologics has been discussed comprehensively, and dermatologists should monitor patients carefully for adverse events that could be a potential source of litigation. Scheinfeld provided an extensive review of the litigation climate in regard to biologic use [1].

For the treatment of psoriasis, the package inserts indicate that the biologics are for patients who are candidates for other systemic agents (e.g., methotrexate) or phototherapy. Adalimumab is indicated for the treatment of adult patients with moderate-to-severe chronic plaque psoriasis who are candidates for systemic therapy or phototherapy, and when other systemic therapies are medically less appropriate. Adalimumab's package insert states that it should only be administered to patients who will be closely monitored and have regular follow-up visits with a physician. Etanercept is indicated for the treatment of adult and pediatric patients with chronic moderate-to-severe plaque psoriasis who are candidates for systemic therapy or phototherapy. Infliximab is indicated for the treatment of adult patients with chronic severe (i.e., extensive and/or disabling) plaque psoriasis who are candidates for systemic therapy and when other systemic therapies are medically less appropriate. Infliximab should be administered to patients who will be closely monitored and have regular follow-up visits with a physician. Ustekinumab is indicated for the treatment of adult patients (18 years or older) with moderate-to-severe plaque psoriasis who are candidates for phototherapy or systemic therapy.

Boxed warnings are included on the labeling for adalimumab, etanercept, and infliximab for tuberculosis. Ustekinumab, secukinumab, ixekizumab, and brodalumab do not have any

D.J. Goldberg, MD, JD (✉)
Icahn School of Medicine at Mt. Sinai,
New York, NY 10029, USA

Fordham Law School, New York, NY 10023, USA
e-mail: drdavidgoldberg@skinandlasers.com

A. Gibofsky, MD, JD
Fordham Law School, New York, NY 10023, USA

Weill Medical College of Cornell University,
New York, NY 10065, USA

Hospital for Special Surgery, New York, NY 10021, USA

© Springer International Publishing AG 2018
P.S. Yamauchi (ed.), *Biologic and Systemic Agents in Dermatology*, https://doi.org/10.1007/978-3-319-66884-0_6

boxed warning for tuberculosis; nevertheless, much like with the aforementioned biologic agents, it is necessary to check patients taking these other agents to screen for tuberculosis per the package insert. Periodic screening for tuberculosis after initiation of therapy is recommended. In addition, brodalumab has a boxed warning for depression and suicide. Patients on TNF-α inhibitors should also be screened for active hepatitis B before starting therapy, and periodically during the course of therapy. Some relative contraindications to TNF-α inhibitors are multiple sclerosis and moderate-to-severe congestive heart failure.

There is a warning about increased risk of SCC with TNF-α inhibitors and ustekinumab. However, many patients with psoriasis have undergone treatment with PUVA that puts them at higher risk of developing SCC. In addition, due to their immunosuppressive properties, the risk for lymphoma has been of potential concern, leading patients to believe that biologics cause cancer. The risk of some cancers, including some solid cancers, hematologic cancers, and skin cancers, appears to be increased in patients with psoriasis, possibly associated with chronic inflammation.

Despite the above, most studies have supported a favorable safety profile for biologics in terms of the risk for developing malignancy. In a 2015 analysis of 12,093 patients enrolled in PSOLAR (Psoriasis Longitudinal Assessment and Registry), none of the biologics were found to be associated with increased risk for malignancy [2].

In psoriasis patients with existing or prior malignancies, the benefits of biologic therapy to improve quality of life often outweigh the negligible risks for malignancy. However, coordinated care with oncology is recommended for psoriasis patients with a history of prior malignancies.

General recommendations from the American Academy of Dermatology indicate that one should carefully consider the decision to use a TNF-α inhibitor in patients with a history of malignancy, particularly lymphoma. Short-term treatment with biologics (up to 4 years) appears to be safe with respect to lymphoma risk, especially with TNF-α inhibitors. The potential risk for melanoma, cutaneous T-cell lymphoma, and non-melanoma skin cancer in patients treated with TNF inhibitors has also been raised. In reality, it is not clear that there is a direct association between biologics and other malignancies [3, 4].

Another study, the OBSERVE-5, was a 5-year phase 4, prospective, multicenter surveillance registry of 6059 psoriasis patients with at least a baseline dose of etanercept (Kimble et al., 2015). There was no increased risk for malignancy when compared to the Truven Health MarketScan database, which is a proxy for the general population [5].

ESPRIT is an ongoing, 10-year, international, prospective, observational registry of 6059 psoriasis patients with at least a baseline dosage of adalimumab. These patients also showed no increased risk of malignancies [6].

There are not enough numbers of psoriasis patients on secukinumab or ixekizumab yet, but their phase 3 trials also do not seem to indicate an increased risk for cancer or opportunistic infections [1].

In most biologic related lawsuits, the litigation is invariably brought against the drug maker. The dermatologist in the end may have some protection because [1] dermatologists generally obtained informed consent listing the risks of biologic agents and [2] the drug maker is a much deeper pocket than the dermatologist. Below is an example of a dermatologic biologic related case of litigation.

Plaintiff Cynthia DiBartolo ("DiBartolo" or "plaintiff") brought an action against defendant Abbott Laboratories ("Abbott" or "defendant"—now called "AbbVie") to recover from injuries she allegedly suffered as a result of her use of defendant's drug adalimumab to treat her psoriasis. After treatment with adalimumab for approximately 6 months, plaintiff was diagnosed with non-melanoma skin cancer, specifically SCC of the tongue, and underwent two surgeries that have allegedly left her with permanent disabilities.

In her First Amended Complaint (the "amended complaint"), filed against Abbott on May 8, 2012, DiBartolo asserted causes of action sounding in strict liability, negligence, and breach of warranty based on theories of design defect, failure to warn, and misrepresentation. This means that she claimed adalimumab as an inherently defective product. Such causes of action are common when a defendant sues regarding what they think is a defective product that has caused them harm.

Abbott filed a motion to dismiss plaintiff's amended complaint on May 25, 2012. DiBartolo filed her response to Abbot's motion to dismiss on June 15, 2012, and Abbott filed its reply in support of its motion to dismiss plaintiff's amended complaint on June 29, 2012. Abbott's motion was eventually granted to the extent that plaintiff alleged strict liability design defect, negligent design defect, strict liability misrepresentation, negligent misrepresentation, and breach of express warranty as the FDA had approved the product and it had been used in millions of people without incident.

Because DiBartolo has filed already one amended complaint and not demonstrated good cause why the Court should grant DiBartolo leave to file a second amended complaint, DiBartolo's claims were dismissed with prejudice to the extent stated above [7–9].

What becomes obvious is that although most lawsuits involving biologics are against the manufacturer of the drug, dermatologists can potentially be sued if their risk and benefit information does not provide patients with the relevant risks of drugs in general and biologics in particular (Tables 6.1, 6.2, and 6.3).

The basis of such a lawsuit will be one related to the tort of professional liability or, more specifically, medical malpractice. The tort of professional liability has for major elements: duty, breach, causation, and damages.

Table 6.1 Drug reactions: general

Predictable reactions	Unpredictable reactions
• Overdose	• Intolerance
• Side effects	• Idiosyncrasy
• Secondary effects	• Allergy or hypersensitivity
• Drug interactions	

Table 6.2 Risks to be documented

• Boxed warning
• Increased risk of fungal and other infections
• Potential increased risk of malignancies
• Potential increased risk of liver-related issues
• Potential risk of collagen vascular disease
• Potential risk of depression and suicide (unique to brodalumab)

Table 6.3 Informed consent: doctrine and elements

Doctrine:
• Most courts require that at a minimum, physicians disclose risks and benefits of a procedure or therapy as well as alternative procedures or therapies and their benefits and risks.

Duty

Duty is defined as the obligation to do or the obligation to refrain from doing. If a professional has no duty, there can be no liability for the outcome. A duty occurs when one contracts for a duty, assumes a duty, or is party in certain relationships with legally *recognized* inherent duty as in the physician-patient relationship.

Damages

The final element of the tort of professional liability is damages, which may be economic or noneconomic or both. Economic damages refer to pair of compensable monetary losses resulting from an injury or complaint, such as lost wages or medical costs. Setting limits on compensation for noneconomic damages (i.e., "pain and suffering") has been a major focus of efforts to reform the US legal system.

According to the doctrine of informed consent (Table 6.2), the clinician must disclose the risks and benefits of a procedure or therapy as well as alternative procedures or therapies and their benefits and risks. The information must be given to a competent patent who understands and voluntarily makes a decision.

The obligation to provide care and to provide information about alternatives is independent of whether payment will be provided. In the event of adverse drug reaction, a physician cannot avoid responsibility for care of the decision was based solely on cost considerations. In one important case, a court held: [T]he physician who complies without protest with the limitations imposed by a third-party payer, when his medical judgment dictates otherwise, cannot avoid his ultimate responsibility for his patient's care … "He cannot point to the healthcare payer as the liability scapegoat when the consequences of his own determinative medical decisions go sour."

Hypothetical Case #1

Dr. Plaque, although practicing in a small town, is a well-renowned expert in psoriasis. He has practiced for 20 years, has been involved in numerous FDA trials for biologic agents used to treat psoriasis, and offers every known treatment for psoriasis. His expertise is clearly in the use of biologics. Such patients are often difficult to treat; some have a variety of other medical issues. He often treats psoriatic patients who are eligible for phototherapy with biologics. Such patients are often difficult to treat; some have a variety of other medical issues. He often treats those psoriatic patients who are eligible for phototherapy with biologics. He routinely does a variety of blood tests and carefully follows his patients.

Dr. Plaque initiated therapy with a TNF-α inhibitor on a 54-year-old male with severe plaque psoriasis who had features of metabolic syndrome that included obesity, hypertension, type 2 diabetes, and hyperlipidemia. The patient had a good response to the biologic agent for 2 years and was monitored yearly by Dr. Plaque. Subsequently, the patient sustained a myocardial infarction and underwent emergent coronary artery bypass surgery. However, the patient became septic following the surgery and passed away.

The estate of this patient has now brought million dollar lawsuit against Dr. Plaque claiming that the TNF-α inhibitor caused the infection and that the patient should have never been put on the biologic agent because of his cardiovascular comorbidities. In addition, the plaintiff claimed that because the patient had a heart condition, congestive heart failure is a contraindication to the TNF-α inhibitor. Is there any basis for such a lawsuit?

Hypothetical Case #2

Dr. Psoriasis is an internationally respected expert in the treatment of psoriasis. He has published peer-reviewed manuscripts and books on the topic, and lectures both nationally and internationally on biologic therapy. In fact his dermatology practice in the southern portion of the United States is limited almost exclusively to patients with psoriasis. All his patients are warned about the risk of infections, potential increased risk of malignancies, and liver failure while on biologics. Five years ago, Dr. Psoriasis began to see a 52-year-old male, Fitzpatrick II skin phenotype with severe plaque psoriasis who had been unresponsive to all standard psoriasis treatments including years of both total body UVB PUVA treatments. Dr. Psoriasis discussed using biologics and provided his patient with his standard biologic consent form detailing the risks of infections, possible liver-related issues, and increased risk of malignancies.

One year after starting treatment, the patient developed numerous cutaneous basal and squamous cell carcinoma. Two years after starting treatment with biologics, the patient developed a rapidly enlarging poorly differentiated SCC on his scalp. The lesion was removed with Mohs micrographic surgery and adjuvant radiation therapy. Unfortunately, 6 months after treatment, the patient developed seizures and was found with numerous foci of metastatic SCC both in his brain and lungs. 9 months later the patient died.

Two years ago, Dr. Psoriasis was sued by the estate of the now-deceased patient. The gravamen of the lawsuit is that although the patient was warned about a potential increase in malignancies in patients on biologics, he also assured his patient that the scientific literature has not shown this risk to be real.

Dr. Psoriasis is certain that the SCC were related to his patient's lighter skin type and years of PUVA and UVB treatment as he prepares for his initial meeting with his insurance-company-assigned defense counsel. What will happen?

The package insert for biologics indicates that these drugs are for patients who are candidates for other systemic agents (e.g., methotrexate) or phototherapy. In general biologics, as described above, are indicated for the treatment of adult patients with moderate-to-severe chronic plaque psoriasis who are candidates for systemic therapy or phototherapy, and when other systemic therapies are medically less appropriate. Patients are to be closely monitored and have regular follow-up visits with their physician.

Dr. Psoriasis contends that his warnings and treatment protocol were consistent with the standard of care. He is certain that the skin cancers were related to his patient's years of sun exposure, PUVA, and UVB exposure and had nothing to do with the use of biologics. He will have his expert; the plaintiff's estate will have theirs. In the end, a jury will need to decide.

Conclusion

Biologic agents have resulted in enhanced efficacy and significantly improved the quality of life for patients who have psoriasis, psoriatic arthritis, rheumatoid arthritis, Crohn's disease, ulcerative colitis, ankylosing spondylitis, and juvenile rheumatoid arthritis, among other conditions. At the same time, however, all of these agents have risks as well as benefits. The dermatologist should provide a full explanation of the risks and benefits of these agents and then carefully document that this information was provided. This documentation could include at a minimum a standard chart entry or more appropriately the patient's signature on a form that outlines and specifies the risks and benefits of the selected therapy. Further, the dermatologist should perform appropriate pre-initiation laboratory studies and infection screening, and monitor the patient carefully for adverse events throughout the course of therapy. Understanding the risks associated with the use of biologics in dermatology and practicing according to the reasonable standard of care will markedly reduce the risk of litigation against dermatologists who choose to use biologic agents.

References

1. Scheinfeld N. Biologics and malpractice. Dermatologist. 2014;22:2.
2. Papp K, Gottlieb AB, Naldi L, et al. Safety surveillance for ustekinumamb and other psoriasis treatments from the Psoriasis Longitudinal Assessment and Registry (PSOLAR). J Drugs Dermatol. 2015;14:706–14.
3. American Academy of Dermatology. Psoriasis: TNF inhibitors general recommendations. 2016. https://www.aad.org/pratice-tools/quality-care/clinical-guidelines/psoriais/biologigs/tnf-inhibiyots-recommendations. Accessed June 14, 2016.
4. Dommasch E, Gelfand JM. Is there truly a risk of lymphoma from biologic therapies? Dermatol Ther. 2009;22:418–30.
5. Kimball AB, Rothman KJ, Kricorian G, et al. OBSERVE-5: observational postmarketing safety surveillance registry of etanercept for the treatment of psoriasis final 5-year results. J Am Acad Dermatol. 2015;72:115–22.
6. Menter A, Thaci D, Papp KA, et al. Five-year analysis from the ESPRIT 10-year postmarketing surveillance registry of adalimumab treatment for moderate to severe psoriasis. J Am Acad Dermatol. 2015;73:410–9. E6.
7. Larson v Abbott. Civil Action No. ELH-13-00554, United States District Court for the District of Maryland. 2016. http://www.mdd.uscourts.gov/Opinions/Opinions/Larson-AbbottMemo.pdf, Accessed November 17, 2016.
8. DiBartolo v Abbott Laboratories, 914 F. Supp. 2d 601 (Southern District NY). 2012.
9. Humira lawsuit filed by a man with fungal infection. AboutLawsuits.com website. 2014. http://www.aboutlawuits.com/humira-fungal-infection-law suit-18807/. Accessed January 28, 2014.

Patient and Physician Perspectives on Traditional Systemic and Biologic Therapies for Psoriasis

Margaretta Midura and Amit Garg

Introduction

Given the prevalence of psoriasis in the United States and its significant impact on the quality of life of those with the disease, appropriate treatment for psoriasis patients has been a long-standing topic for discussion in medical and public sectors. Over the past 15 years, the development of new systemic treatments, including targeted biologic therapies, has brought hope to patients and physicians alike of a more safe, effective, and convenient approach to managing psoriasis. Nonetheless there remain a number of therapeutic dilemmas and barriers for patients and their providers in addressing the burden of psoriatic disease. This chapter explores treatment trends with respect to systemic and biologic agents in the context of physician and patient perspectives related to these medications.

Assessing Disease Severity

Selection of appropriate treatment in psoriasis involves several considerations including at least disease severity, safety of the proposed medication in the context of patient comorbidities, long-term efficacy, likelihood of ongoing tolerability, patient preferences and conveniences, as well as payer-mandated restrictions. The decision on therapy is often a complex one that must be customized to the individual. Herein we provide a brief discussion on disease severity as the initial determinant of therapy.

M. Midura, BA
MSIII, Zucker School of Medicine at Hofstra/Northwell,
500 Hofstra Blvd, Hempstead, NY 11549, USA
e-mail: mmidura1@pride.hofstra.edu

A. Garg, MD (✉)
Department of Dermatology, Zucker School of Medicine at Hofstra/Northwell, SVP, Dermatology Service Line, Northwell Health, 1991 Marcus Avenue, Suite 300, Lake Success, NY 11042, USA
e-mail: amgarg@Northwell.edu

According to the National Psoriasis Foundation (NPF), mild disease is defined by involvement of less than 3% of a patient's body surface area (BSA), whereas moderate and severe psoriasis is defined by BSAs of 3–10% and >10%, respectively [1]. Indeed, the most preferred instrument by dermatologists to measure disease activity is body surface area [2]. However, dermatologists and patients have long since appreciated that severity of disease cannot be entirely captured by measurement of BSA alone, and that impact on quality of life in some instances may be an equally relevant determinant of disease severity. Psoriasis involving the scalp, genitals, palms, or soles of the feet, for example, may be particularly debilitating while only involving <3% of the BSA [3]. Nonetheless, discrepancies often exist between how patients and providers assess disease severity. In a multinational survey, dermatologists estimated the percentage of their patients having severe psoriasis to be 20%, while patients assessed their psoriasis to be severe in 27% of cases [4]. Differing quantitative and qualitative methods by which patients and physicians assess disease severity is a likely contributor to the discrepancy. For example, patients reported that itch and anatomic location, as opposed to surface area, of plaques were the most important contributors to severity of disease. Indeed, over a fifth of psoriasis patients with mild disease based on BSAs rated their disease as severe [5]. Dermatologists on the other hand most often prioritized size and anatomic location of plaques when determining disease severity [4]. It is our opinion that the most appropriate initial strategy in determining whether a patient is a candidate for systemic therapy should involve an objective assessment of severity coupled with a patient-centered discussion on the impact of the disease, regardless of BSA of involvement, and satisfaction with existing treatments.

Existing Treatment Trends

Experts from the medical board of the National Psoriasis Foundation agreed that the acceptable response to initiation of new therapy at 3 months was either a BSA of 3% or less or an improvement in BSA of 75% or more from baseline. The target response at 3 months post-initiation was a BSA of 1% or less. During the maintenance period, the target response evaluated at 6-month intervals was also a BSA 1% or less [2]. This construct, when applied to existing treatment trends, indicates that there are opportunities to reduce the burden of disease among patients living with psoriasis.

While it is understood that assessment of disease severity and determination of need to advance therapy may be complex, there remain a significant proportion of psoriasis patients who may be on no prescription treatments, even when their psoriasis is moderate to severe. These patients often self-treat with over-the-counter agents which have minimal comparative efficacy in psoriasis, and this may prolong suffering from the disease [6]. A large-scale national survey of 1657 patients conducted by the NPF in 2007 showed that 37 and 39% of respondents who had moderate and severe psoriasis, respectively, were not receiving any form of prescription treatment for their disease [7]. From 2003 through 2011, these percentages seemed to improve with 23.6–35.5% of patients with moderate psoriasis and only 9.4–29.7% of patients with severe psoriasis remaining untreated [8]. Based on data from a population-based survey of 3426 patients in both North America and Europe, patients with moderate psoriasis were on no treatment or on topical treatment alone in 32% and 55% of cases, respectively. Similar proportions of patients with severe psoriasis were on no treatment or on topical treatment alone [5]. Other studies have also described similar trends in under-treatment of psoriasis [9, 10].

There is also data to suggest that among patients that do receive treatment, management strategies are conservative, which carries risk of under-treating signs and symptoms of disease with a corresponding impact on quality of life and function. The 2007 survey report from the NPF indicated that 73% and 57% of patients with moderate and severe psoriasis, respectively, were receiving topical therapy alone [7]. In the follow-up NPF survey, under-treatment appeared to once again improve with 29.5% and 21.5% of patients with moderate and severe psoriasis, respectively, receiving topical agents alone [8].

Among patients that received conventional systemic treatments, methotrexate was used more frequently (10–15%) than either cyclosporine (0.5–2.3%) or acitretin [8]. The proportion of patients treated with phototherapy ranged from 8.5 to 33.2%, with ultraviolet-B therapy being utilized far more frequently than psoralen and ultraviolet-A treatments. The usage of phototherapy has dropped significantly since 2005, likely owing to treatment inconvenience and cost of care for patients, along with an increasing availability of highly effective biologic-based treatment options [11].

Coupled with widespread under-treatment of disease, over half (52.3%) of psoriasis patients are dissatisfied with their treatments [8]. Many patients do not comply with their treatment plans, likely at least in part due to low expectations they have for their existing therapies [12, 13]. Others do not see a healthcare professional as often as they should because they feel that the provider would not be of further assistance [5]. These sentiments of dissatisfaction with therapies are further reflected in the significant discontinuation rates of systemic therapies.

Thus, it appears on the surface that patients have highly conservative treatment strategies, including no treatment, across disease severities, and yet they are seemingly disappointed with their existing treatments. Several topics warrant further exploration in evaluating possible explanations for systemic and biologic agent underutilization, including patient-physician perspectives on these treatments that may account for conservative approaches, and therapeutic directions which will satisfy unmet needs to improve real-world outcomes for patients with psoriasis.

Patient Perspectives on Systemic and Biologic Agents

The importance of a patient-centered approach to management, inclusive of shared decision making and with specific considerations for safety, efficacy, convenience, and affordability, is increasingly recognized. An improved understanding of patients' complete perspective on systemic and biologic treatment initiation as well as maintenance is essential to achieving optimal long-term outcomes for patients with moderate-to-severe psoriasis.

When psoriasis patients using topical therapy were asked why they were not taking systemic or biologic agents as well, the top three reasons cited were that topical treatments had less adverse effects, their disease was not serious enough to warrant more advanced treatment, and their physicians would not prescribe any other treatments [8]. These findings suggest that patients are still weary of potential side effects related to biologic and systemic therapy. The data also reinforces the importance of the role of physicians in determining therapeutic strategies involving systemic medications. In a rather dynamic and rapidly evolving drug development environment for psoriasis, it is important for dermatologists to maintain a current and practical awareness of new systemic treatments, a critical evaluation of their safety and relative efficacy profiles, monitoring guidelines when they exist, and a willingness to appropriately prescribe or perhaps refer.

Approximately half of patients experience oral or biologic therapies to be burdensome because of adverse effects, inconvenience, or need for laboratory monitoring, and most feel that better treatment options are needed. Biologic agents were burdensome because of anxiety related to the injection, inconvenience, and their potential for adverse effects [5]. Half (50%) of those treated with oral systemic agents and

53% of those treated with biologics were concerned with the long-term health risks of their respective therapies [5]. Costs associated with treatment also appear to have an impact on patient use and adherence to medications [5].

Overall, less than half (45%) of patients who receive biologic therapy are very satisfied with the therapy, and only 29% are very satisfied with their long-term safety. Only 25% of patients who received oral therapies are very satisfied with treatment [5]. According to 2003–2011 NPF survey data, discontinuation of systemic and biologic agents was common among patients. Among those surveyed, 24% of patients had been on a systemic agent and 57% of these patients discontinued using it. Among patients on systemic agents, 11% had been on a biologic agent, and 45% of these patients discontinued using it [5]. Patients discontinue oral systemic treatments and phototherapy after medians of 6–12 months and biologic therapies after medians of 12–20.5 months [11]. The most common reasons patients discontinue biologic therapy included safety and tolerability issues (25%), a lack or loss of effectiveness (22%), anxiety or fear related to the injection, and difficulty with adequate insurance coverage [5, 11]. Over half (53%) of patients are concerned with the long-term health risks of biologic exposure. While discontinuation rates are higher for traditional oral therapies than for biologic therapies, the reasons for discontinuation are similar in both. Patients most often discontinue oral therapies for safety and tolerability issues (43%) and for a lack or loss of efficacy (30%). Half (50%) of patients express concern about the long-term health risks of oral systemic therapy.

Overall, NPF data suggests that 85% of patients feel that there is a need for improvement in therapies for psoriasis, and this sentiment likely translates into implications for use and adherence to these therapies [5]. No treatments are perfect for everyone, and the significant augmentation in efficacies of newer systemic treatments for psoriasis may balance some concerns such as the inconvenience of monitoring and perhaps even the anxiety, often initial, related to self-injections. Nonetheless, there should be continued focus on addressing patients' concerns related to near- and long-term safety, long-term efficacy, as well as access and overall costs.

Physician Perspectives on Systemic and Biologic Agents

As noted earlier, treatment strategies for the psoriasis patient can be complex, and partnered decision making between patients and physicians is essential to safe and effective long-term management. From the dermatologist's perspective, treatment goals most frequently include keeping signs and symptoms controlled, improving usual function and activities, and improving one's self-esteem [4].

In exploring physician perspectives on treatment strategies, over half (54%) of dermatologists surveyed stated they prescribe topical treatment as monotherapy for their patients with moderate-to-severe psoriasis [4]. Nonetheless, they also acknowledged the challenges related to topical monotherapy which include a lack of, a partial, or a waning response, poor compliance, patient inconvenience, and impracticality of application on larger surface areas [4]. Approximately half of dermatologists surveyed felt comfortable with prescription of conventional oral DMARD therapy, but about one-fifth reported prescribing them only sparingly. Most common limitations to initiating conventional oral therapy included physician concerns over long-term safety, tolerability, contraindications to therapy, and patient concerns related to the treatment option. The most commonly cited limitations to continuing oral systemic therapy included concerns over long-term safety, tolerability, and a lack or loss of response [4].

Citing concerns related to cost, long-term safety, and tolerability, only 65.5% of dermatologists surveyed said that they would initiate and manage psoriasis patients on biologic therapy. Most commonly cited limitations to initiating biologic therapy included concerns over cost, long-term safety, and contraindications. Limitations to continuing patients on biologic therapy also included physician concerns over a lack/loss of response [4]. In exploring additional challenges in management for psoriasis patients, approximately 60% of dermatologists surveyed feel that management with biologic therapy requires significant time in order to discuss risks and benefits associated with treatment, complete prior authorization paperwork, ensure patient compliance with monitoring results, respond to patient phone calls related to additional questions or concerns, and train patients on self-injections [4]. Nonetheless, despite limitation and barriers to management with systemic agents, over 80% of dermatologists are somewhat or very satisfied with these treatment options [4].

Reflections on Existing Trends in the Management of Psoriasis

Even with the multitude of systemic treatment options available for psoriasis, both patients and physicians believe that there is an unmet need for less burdensome, more safe, and more efficacious drugs. Perhaps the principal hurdles, albeit some based in perception only, to overcome appear to be related to efficacy and safety, as these were the top two characteristics physicians provided when asked what comprise an ideal therapy. Other frequently cited concerns included new mechanisms of action, options for oral administration, and improved access to therapy [4].

While working towards optimizing these goals, patient and physicians must maintain an open communication that will facilitate a customized strategy that for moderate-to-severe psoriasis patients should include an appropriate systemic or biologic agent. Choosing a systemic agent must be patient centered, having considered his/her goals as well as the apprehensions associated with treatment. When such trepidations may be overcome by explanation and discussion, which may require more time with patients, physicians can take the opportunity to elaborate on risk/benefit profiles of the now numerous available systemic options. Dermatologists less familiar with newer agents have numerous resources to further support their practices, and other colleagues with whom a collaboration in care may also further support their patients. At a grassroots level, patients and dermatologists may partner with other stakeholders, including advocacy organizations, regulatory agencies, payers, and policy makers, to advance access to the medications which have been shown to improve several disease-related outcomes for psoriasis.

References

1. "About Psoriasis." National Psoriasis Foundation, 1996–2016. 2017. www.psoriasis.org/about-psoriasis. Accessed 9 Mar 2017.
2. Armstrong AW, Siegel MP, Bagel J, Boh EE, Buell M, Cooper KD, Callis Duffin K, Eichenfield LF, Garg A, Gelfand JM, Gottlieb AB, Koo JYM, Korman NJ, Krueger GG, Lebwohl MG, Leonardi CL, Mandelin AM, Menter MA, Merola JF, Pariser DM, Prussick RB, Ryan C, Shah KN, Weinberg JM, Williams MJOU, JJ W, Yamauchi PS, Van Voorhees AS. From the Medical Board of the National Psoriasis Foundation: treatment targets for plaque psoriasis. J Am Acad Dermatol. 2017;76(2):290–8.
3. Menter A, Korman NJ, Elmets CA, Feldman SR, Gelfand JM, Gordon KB, et al. Guidelines of care for the management of psoriasis and psoriatic arthritis: section 4. Guidelines of care for the management and treatment of psoriasis with traditional systemic agents. J Am Acad Dermatol. 2009;61(3):451–85.
4. van de Kerkhof PCM, Reich K, Kavanaugh A, et al. Physician perspectives in the managment of psoriasis and psoriatic arthritis: results from the population-based multinational assessment of psoriasis and psoriatic arthritis survey. J Eur Acad Dermatol Venereol. 2015;29(10):2002.
5. Lebwohl MG, Bachelez H, Barker J, et al. Patient perspectives in the management of psoriasis: results from the population-based multinational assessment of psoriasis and psoriatic arthritis survey. J Am Acad Dermatol. 2014;70:871–81.
6. Kivelevitch DN, Tahhan PV, Bourren P, Kogan NN, Gusis SE, Rodríguez EA. Self-medication and adherence to treatment in psoriasis. Int J Dermatol. 2012;51(4):416–9.
7. Horn EJ, Fox KM, Patel V, et al. Are patients with psoriasis undertreated? Results of National Psoriasis Foundation survey. J Am Acad Dermatol. 2007;57:957–62.
8. Armstrong AW, Robertson AD, Wu J, Schupp C, Lebwohl MG. Undertreatment, treatment trends, and treatment dissatisfaction among patients with psoriasis and psoriatic arthritis in the United States: findings from the National Psoriasis Foundation surveys, 2003–2011. JAMA Dermatol. 2013;149(10):1180–5.
9. Nast A, Reytan N, Rosumeck S, Erdmann R, Rzany B. Low prescription rate for systemic treatments in the management of severe psoriasis vulgaris and psoriatic arthritis in dermatological practices in Berlin and Brandenburg, Germany: results from a patient registry. J Eur Acad Dermatol Venereol. 2008;22:1337–42.
10. Maza A, Richard MA, Aubin F, et al. Significant delay in the introduction of systemic treatment of moderate to severe psoriasis: a prospective multicentre observational study in outpatients from hospital dermatology Departments in France. Br J Dermatol. 2012;167:643–8.
11. Yeung H, Wan J, Van Voorhees AS, et al. Patient-reported reasons for the discontinuation of commonly used treatments for moderate to severe psoriasis. J Am Acad Dermatol. 2013;68:64–72.
12. Richards HL, Fortune DG, O'Sullivan TM, Main CJ, Griffiths CE. Patients with psoriasis and their compliance with medication. J Am Acad Dermatol. 1999;41(4):581–3.
13. Augustin M, Holland B, Dartsch D, Langenbruch A, Radtke MA. Adherence in the treatment of psoriasis: a systematic review. Dermatology. 2011;222(4):363–74.

Outcomes of Comorbidities with Biologic and Systemic Agents

Megan H. Noe and Joel M. Gelfand

Abbreviations

CHF   Congestive heart failure
CI   Confidence interval
CRP   C-reactive protein
HDL   High-density lipoprotein
IL   Interleukin
LDL   Low-density lipoprotein
MACE   Major adverse cardiovascular event
MI   Myocardial infarction
MTX   Methotrexate
NR   Not reported
RA   Rheumatoid arthritis
RCT   Randomized control trial
TCI   T-cell inhibitors (efalizumab, alefacept)
TNFi   Tumor necrosis factor alpha inhibitor

Introduction

Psoriasis is a chronic inflammatory disease that affects about 3% of the population [1]. In addition to inflammation in the skin, patients with psoriasis have been shown to have evidence of systemic inflammation [2] and increased rates of many other comorbidities including obesity [3], hypertension [4], diabetes [5], and major adverse cardiovascular events (MACE), including myocardial infarction and stroke [6–8]. The risk of MACE in patients with psoriasis treated

M.H. Noe, MD, MPH
Department of Dermatology, University of Pennsylvania,
3400 Civic Center Blvd, South Tower, Office 773, Philadelphia,
PA 19104, USA
e-mail: Megan.Noe@uphs.upenn.edu

J.M. Gelfand, MD, MSCE (✉)
Department of Dermatology, University of Pennsylvania,
3400 Civic Center Blvd, South Tower, Office 730, Philadelphia,
PA 19104, USA
e-mail: Joel.Gelfand@uphs.upenn.edu

with systemic agents and/or phototherapy is similar to the risk in those with rheumatoid arthritis, a systemic chronic inflammatory disorder [9]. Severe psoriasis confers an additional 6.2% absolute risk of a 10-year rate of cardiac events [10]. Most importantly, several large population-based studies have demonstrated an increased rate of cardiovascular mortality in people with severe psoriasis, even after controlling for traditional risk factors [6, 11–13].

Recent evidence in the cardiovascular literature has suggested that treating cardiovascular disease with anti-inflammatory drugs may improve outcomes [14]. Because of this it is important to understand how the treatment of psoriasis will affect its associated systemic comorbidities. We focus this review on the treatment outcomes of cardiometabolic comorbidities that have the best evidence of an effect on morbidity and mortality.

Methotrexate

Cardiovascular Events

Most of the information regarding methotrexate and cardiovascular outcomes comes from studies in patients with rheumatoid arthritis. A systematic literature review of 18 observational studies concluded that treatment with methotrexate can decrease cardiovascular events and cardiovascular mortality when used in patients with RA [15]. A meta-analysis of ten studies concluded that methotrexate use was associated with 21% lower risk of cardiovascular disease (95% CI 0.73–0.87) [16]. A subsequent meta-analysis published in 2015 confirmed these results, showing a decreased risk of cardiovascular events in adults with RA treated with methotrexate (RR: 0.72; 95% CI: 0.57–0.91) [17]. Few studies have specifically examined the risk of MACE in individuals with psoriasis (Table 8.1). Veterans with psoriasis and RA treated with methotrexate had significantly reduced risk of cardiovascular disease (RR = 0.73, 95% CI = 0.55–0.98) [18]. This risk was further reduced by the addition of folic acid [18]. In adults from a large

Table 8.1 Studies examining the risk of major cardiovascular events in psoriasis patients treated with methotrexate

Author	Year	Patients (patients and controls)	Average follow-up	Outcome	Comparison	Effect OR/RR/HR (95% CI)
Meta-analyses						
None						
Cohort studies						
Prodanovich [18]	2005	7615	NR	Any CVD	MTX vs. no MTX use	RR: 0.72 (0.55–0.98)
Wu [19]	2012	8445	4.3 years	MI only	MTX vs. topicals	HR: 0.52 (0.31–0.85)
Ahlehoff [20]	2013	2400	18 months	MACE	MTX vs. retinoids/cyclosporine/phototherapy	HR: 0.58 (0.29–1.15)
Ahlehoff [21]	2015	6902	2.3 years	MACE	MTX vs. topicals/phototherapy	HR: 0.53 (0.34–0.83)

healthcare system in the USA, methotrexate was associated with a decreased hazard of incident MI compared to topical therapy (HR: 0.52, 95% CI: 0.31–0.85) [19]. A population-based Danish cohort found that the risk of MACE decreased in those treated with methotrexate compared to other nonbiologic agents, including oral retinoids, cyclosporine, and phototherapy (HR: 0.41; 95% CI: 0.21–0.80) [20]. However, after adjusting for age, sex, baseline comorbidities, and socioeconomic status, the risk was no longer statistically significant (HR: 0.58: 0.29–1.15) [20]. In a 5-year follow-up on the Danish cohort, the decreased risk remained significant (compared to topicals and phototherapy) after controlling for age, sex baseline comorbidities, and year of inclusion (HR: 0.53, 95% CI: 0.34–0.83) [21].

A single, population-based study in Taiwan found a decreased hazard of cerebrovascular disease in psoriasis patients on methotrexate compared to those not on methotrexate (HR: 0.50, 95% CI: 0.27–0.92) [22].

Heart Failure

A single case-control study examined the impact of methotrexate on congestive heart failure (CHF) in adults with RA. Individuals on methotrexate monotherapy had a decreased risk of CHF (RR: 0.8, 95% CI: 0.6–1.0) compared to people not taking methotrexate [23]. The effects of methotrexate on CHF in adults with psoriasis have not been examined.

Metabolic Syndrome and Biomarkers

Metabolic syndrome is a cluster of classic cardiovascular risk factors including central obesity, dyslipidemia, glucose intolerance, and hypertension, and it is identified as a predictor of cardiovascular disease and MACEs. Methotrexate was found to be associated with a significant reduction in insulin resistance compared to treatment with topical coal-tar, after 12 weeks of therapy [24]. In a separate analysis, no effect was seen on the incidence of diabetes in patients on

methotrexate in adults with RA or psoriasis in a cohort study with a mean follow-up of 5.8 months [25]. Body weight is another important cardiometabolic risk factor. Several studies did not show significant changes in weight in patients treated with methotrexate [24, 26, 27].

There is limited evidence regarding the effect of methotrexate on lipid profile. In 495 patients recently diagnosed with RA, therapy with methotrexate or methotrexate combination therapy resulted in an increase in mean total cholesterol, low-density lipoprotein-C, and high-density lipoprotein cholesterol at 24 weeks compared to baseline ($p < 0.001$) [28]. Previous research suggests that systemic inflammation is associated with a reduction in serum lipids and treatment of this inflammation increases serum lipid levels and nonintuitively decreases the risk of cardiovascular disease [29].

C-reactive protein (CRP) is a biomarker of systemic inflammation and therefore has been used as a proxy endpoint for examining systemic inflammation. A decreased high-sensitivity-CRP (hs-CRP) was seen in psoriasis patients treated with methotrexate compared to those treated with topical coal tar, after 12 weeks of treatment [24, 30]. However, no change was seen in 32 patients from a single institution after 8–10 weeks of treatment with methotrexate [31].

TNF Inhibitors

Cardiovascular Events

In RA patients, a meta-analysis of six cohort studies found that treatment with a TNF inhibitor was associated with a reduced risk for all cardiovascular events (RR 0.46, 95% CI: 0.28–0.77), MI (RR 0.81, 95% CI: 0.68–0.96), and stroke (RR 0.69, 95% CI 0.53–0.89) [32]. Subsequently, a second meta-analysis of 16 observational studies or RCTs with more than 400 patients and at least 1 year of follow-up confirmed a decreased risk of any cardiovascular event (RR: 0.70, 95% CI: 0.57–0.91) in those treated with TNF inhibitors [17].

In psoriasis, a meta-analysis of five observational cohort studies published in 2016 found that compared to psoriasis patients treated with topicals and phototherapy, those treated with TNF inhibitors were at a significantly lower risk of cardiovascular events (RR: 0.58, 95% CI: 0.43–0.77) [33]. Treatment with TNF inhibitors was also associated with a decreased risk of cardiovascular events when compared to those treated with methotrexate (RR: 0.67, 95% CI: 0.52–0.88) [33]. Two meta-analyses including only RCTs, limited to an average of 12 weeks of follow-up, did not find a statistically significant difference in the rate of MACE. One analysis calculated a risk difference of −0.0005 events/person-year in patients receiving TNF inhibitors compared to those receiving placebo (95% CI: −0.10–0.009) [34]. The second analysis found a nonsignificant trend towards a decreased rate of MACE in those treated with TNF inhibitors (pooled OR: 0.67, 95% CI: 0.10–4.63) [35]. A subsequent cohort study of claims data concluded that after 12 months of treatment, individuals treated with TNF inhibitors had fewer cardiovascular events than those on methotrexate (HR: 0.55, 95% CI: 0.45–0.67) [36]. Also, total cumulative exposure to TNF inhibitors was associated with a reduced risk for MACE [36]. The details of all these studies can be found in Table 8.2.

When examining MI separately, the results are mixed. The meta-analysis of cohort studies previously discussed found a lower rate of MI in patients treated with TNF inhibitors compared to topicals/phototherapy (RR: 0.73, 95% CI: 0.59–0.90) and methotrexate (RR: 0.65, 95% CI: 0.48–0.89) [33]. A combined cohort of 3602 biologic-treated patients and 13,023 nonbiologic-treated patients from Danish [20], US [19], Canadian [37], and Kuwaiti cohorts (unpublished data) found a 44% decrease in the rate of MI in patients with psoriasis treated with biological therapy (OR: 0.56; 95% CI: 0.42–0.76) [38]. A cohort study of claims data from the United States found a trend towards an increased risk of MI in patients on any systemic treatment (methotrexate, cyclosporine, alefacept, efalizumab, adalimumab, etanercept, and infliximab) compared to those receiving phototherapy (HR: 1.33, 95% CI: 0.90–1.96) [39]. A retrospective cohort of patients on TNF inhibitors and IL-12/23 agents in Canada found a nonsignificant trend towards decreased MI risk (RR: 0.18, 95% CI: 0.24–1.34) [40]. Looking at the TNF inhibitors individually, etanercept, a soluble receptor, was associated

Table 8.2 Studies examining the risk of major cardiovascular events in psoriasis patients treated with TNF inhibitors

Author	Year	Patients (patients and controls)	Average follow-up	Outcome	Comparison(s)	Effect OR/RR/HR (95% CI)
Meta-analyses						
Ryan [34]	2011	1572 person-years (15 RCTs)	12 weeks	MACE	TNFi vs. placebo	RD[a]: −0.0005 events/person-year (−0.01–0.0009 events/person-yr)
Yang [33]	2016	49,795 (5 cohort studies)	38 months	MACE	TNFi vs. topicals/phototherapy TNFi vs. MTX	RR: 0.58 (0.43–0.77) RR: 0.67 (0.52–0.88)
Rungapiromnam [35]	2016	5,966 (23 RCTs)	12 weeks	MACE	TNFi vs. placebo/nonbiologic tx	OR: 0.67 (0.10–4.63)
Gulliver [38]	2016	16,085 (4 cohort studies)	NR	MI only	TNFi/IL 12/23 vs. nonbiologic tx	OR: 0.56 (0.42–0.76)
Cohort studies						
Ahlehoff[b,c] [20]	2013	2400	18 months	MACE	TNFi vs. retinoids, cyclosporine, phototherapy	HR: 0.48 (0.17–1.38)
Ahlehoff[b] [21]	2015	6902	2.3 years	MACE	TNFi vs. topicals and phototherapy	HR: 0.46 (0.22–0.98)
Abuabara[b] [39]	2011	24,314	3.6 years	MI only	Systemic tx[d] vs. phototherapy TNFi/TCI vs. MTX/cyclosporine	HR: 1.33 (0.90–1.96) HR: 1.03 (0.79–1.35)
Wu[b,c] [19]	2012	8445	4.3 years	MI only	TNFi vs. topicals TNFi vs. oral agents, phototherapy, and topicals	HR: 0.45 (0.30–0.68) HR: 0.79 (0.49–1.28)
Wu[b] [41]	2013	14,750	NR	MI only	Etanercept vs. topicals Infliximab/adalimumab vs. topicals	HR: 0.53 (0.31–0.92) HR: 0.25 (0.06–1.03)
Gulliver [40]	2016	739	49.0 months	MI only	TNFi/IL-12/23 vs. nonbiologic tx	HR: 0.18 (0.24–1.34)
Wu [36]	2017	9148	12 months	MACE MI	TNFi vs. MTX TNFi vs. MTX	HR: 0.55 (0.45–0.67) HR: 0.49 (0.34–0.71)

[a]Mantel-Haenszel risk difference
[b]Included in Yang (2016)
[c]Included in Gulliver (2016)
[d]TNFi, TCI, MTX, or cyclosporine

with a significant reduction in the risk of MI compared to topical therapy (HR: 0.53, 95% CI: 0.31–0.92), but that reduction was not seen with the monoclonal antibodies: adalimumab and infliximab (HR: 0.25, 95% 0.006–1.03) [41]. However, all TNF inhibitors were associated with a decreased risk of MI (HR: 0.49, 95% CI: 0.34–0.71) in a recently publish US cohort [36].

Most of the above studies included cerebrovascular disease as a component of MACE and did not examine the risk separately; however one separate cohort study from the United States found a decreased risk of stroke or transient ischemic attack in those treated with TNF inhibitors as compared to methotrexate (HR: 0.55, 95% CI: 0.42–0.71) [36].

Heart Failure

In a meta-analysis of seven studies performed in adults with RA, all with at least 1 year of follow-up, treatment with TNF inhibitors was not associated with a significant effect on heart failure (RR: 0.75, 95% CI: 0.49–1.15) [17]. In psoriasis, a Cochrane review of 24 studies (RCTs and associated open-label extension trials) concluded that there was no significant difference in the incidence of CHF between psoriasis patients treated with any biologic (abatacept, adalimumab anakinra, certolizumab, etanercept, golimumab, infliximab, rituximab, or tocilizumab) and controls (OR: 0.69, 0.18–2.69) [42]. A pooled analysis of data on etanercept only found no increased risk of CHF [43], but a single study showed increased hospitalization and mortality in patients with preexisting heart failure treated with infliximab [44].

Metabolic Syndrome and Biomarkers

Many studies have also investigated the effects of TNF inhibitors on cardiometabolic risk factors. A 2-year study in patients with psoriatic arthritis found a trend towards a reduction in the prevalence of metabolic syndrome in patients treated with adalimumab and etanercept, but no statistically significant reduction in prevalence was seen after treatment [45].

Looking at the components of metabolic syndrome individually, a multivariate analysis concluded that the use of a TNF inhibitor was associated with a reduced incidence of diabetes compared to other systemic therapies, among patients with both RA and psoriasis [25]. Several smaller studies have shown a reduction in fasting insulin after treatment with etanercept [46, 47].

A meta-analysis examined the effect of TNF inhibitors on lipid profile in patients with RA [48]. Combining data from six previously published studies, total cholesterol, HDL cholesterol, and triglycerides increased after 6–12 months of treatment with TNF inhibitors, but LDL cholesterol did not change significantly [48]. In 70 adults with psoriatic arthritis, a trend towards an increase in HDL cholesterol was seen after 24 months of treatment with etanercept and adalimumab compared to methotrexate [45]; however, a statistically significant difference was not seen in the lipid profile after 24 weeks of treatment in 45 patients with chronic plaque psoriasis that responded to etanercept [49]. Finally, TNF inhibitors have been shown to have small (1–3 kg) but statistically significant increases in weight gain after 24 weeks of treatment with a TNF inhibitor in several observational studies [26, 27, 50].

Many small, single-institution studies have shown statistically significant decreases in hs-CRP after 3–6 months of treatment with a TNF inhibitor [51–54]. Two additional case series failed to show a significant reduction in CRP after 3–6 months of treatment [46, 55]. Several larger studies examining the effect of treatment with a TNF inhibitor on CRP have also been published. A study of 134 Japanese patients, treated with infliximab and adalimumab and followed for 1 year, found a statistically significant decrease in CRP [56]. An analysis of 486 patients on etanercept and 166 controls receiving placebo from RCTs found a statistically significant decrease (1.0 mg/L) in CRP in those receiving etanercept that was not seen in control patients ($p < 0.001$) [57]. This larger analysis provides prospective evidence that etanercept is effective at decreasing systemic inflammation, as measured by serum CRP.

IL 12/23 Inhibitors

Cardiovascular Events

Three meta-analyses were conducted using the data from the Phase II/III clinical trials to examine the risk of MACE in patients treated with IL 12/23 inhibitors (Table 8.3). The first used a Mantel-Haenszel risk difference and found no significant increase or decrease in MACEs during the placebo-controlled portions of the trials (Mantel-Haenszel risk difference: 0.012 events/person-year, 95% CI: −0.001–0.026) [34]. The second used a Peto odds ratio and found an increased risk of MACEs in patients treated with IL 12/23 biologics compared to those receiving placebo (OR = 4.23, 95% CI: 1.07–16.75) [58]. The third used a Peto odds ratio again, but only used data on ustekinumab (not briakinumab), and found a nonsignificant trend towards an increased rate of MACE (OR: 4.48, 95% CI: 0.24–84.77) [35]. When examining these meta-analyses together, it is important to consider that the Peto OR method may lead to overestimation of the true relative risk because it effectively excludes trials with zero events from the analysis [59]. Moreover, there was substantially more dropout in the placebo group of these trials

Table 8.3 Studies examining the risk of major cardiovascular events in psoriasis patients treated with IL-12/23 inhibitors

Author	Year	Patients	Average follow-up time	Outcome	Comparison(s)	Effect OR/RR/HR (95% CI)
Meta-analyses						
Ryan[a] [34]	2011	1121 person-years (9 RCTs)	12 weeks	MACE	Ustekinumab/briakinumab vs. placebo	RD[b]: 0.0012 events/person-year (−0.001–0.026 events/person-year)
Tzellos[a] [58]	2013	4753 (9 RCTs)	12 weeks	MACE	Ustekinumab/briakinumab vs. placebo	OR: 4.23 (1.07–16.75)
Rungapiromnam[a] [35]	2016	3862 (8 RCTs)	12 weeks	MACE	Ustekinumab vs. placebo	OR: 4.48 (0.24–84.77)
Cohort studies						
Ahlehoff [21]	2015	178	2.3 years	MACE	TNFi vs. topicals/phototherapy	HR: 1.52 (0.47–4.94)

[a]Mantel-Haenszel risk difference
[b]Analysis of the same clinical trial data, using different meta-analysis techniques

and time-to-event analyses were not conducted which introduces additional bias in detecting an association when none truly exists.

A single population-based cohort study from Denmark found a nonsignificant trend towards an increased risk of cardiac events (HR: 1.52, 95% CI: 0.47–4.94) in people treated with ustekinumab compared to topicals and phototherapy [21]. Long-term pooled data from RCTs of over 3000 patients treated with ustekinumab, with up to 5 years of follow-up, found that the rate of MACE (0.44/100 person-years) was lower than historical data rates from psoriasis patients receiving nonbiologic, systemic treatments [10, 60].

Metabolic Syndrome and Biomarkers

There is no published data regarding the effect of ustekinumab on diabetes, insulin resistance, or serum lipids. A single study of 78 Japanese patients with psoriasis and psoriatic arthritis found no change in CRP after 1 year of treatment with ustekinumab [56].

IL-17 Inhibitors

Cardiovascular Events

A meta-analysis of three RCTs found no effect of treatment with IL-17 inhibitors on MACE (OR: 1.00, 95% CI: 0.09–11.09) [35]. A pooled analysis of ten Phase II/III RCTs of secukinumab with 52 weeks of follow-up, including 3993 individuals with 2725 person-years of exposure, found that the incidence of adjudicated MACEs in subjects receiving secukinumab 300 mg was 0.42 per 100 person-years [61], similar to what was reported for ustekinumab above.

Metabolic Syndrome and Biomarkers

There is no published data regarding the effect of IL-17 inhibitors on diabetes, insulin resistance, serum lipids, or CRP.

Conclusions

Psoriasis is a chronic inflammatory disease, and those with more severe disease have been shown to have higher rates of cardiometabolic comorbidities including myocardial infarction, stroke, and cardiovascular mortality. Current evidence from large observational studies suggests that treatment with both methotrexate and TNF inhibitors may reduce the risk of major cardiovascular events; however, prospective randomized control trials are necessary to better understand the full benefits of systemic therapy. Continued research is also needed to understand how newer biologics (IL-12/23 inhibitors, IL-17 inhibitors) alter cardiovascular disease and cardiometabolic risk factors.

References

1. Rachakonda TD, Schupp CW, Armstrong AW. Psoriasis prevalence among adults in the United States. J Am Acad Dermatol. 2014;70(3):512–6.
2. Mehta NN, Yu Y, Saboury B, Foroughi N, Krishnamoorthy P, Raper A, et al. Systemic and vascular inflammation in patients with moderate to severe psoriasis as measured by [18F]-fluorodeoxyglucose positron emission tomography-computed tomography (FDG-PET/CT): a pilot study. Arch Dermatol. 2011;147(9):1031–9.
3. Baeta IG, Bittencourt FV, Gontijo B, Goulart EM. Comorbidities and cardiovascular risk factors in patients with psoriasis. An Bras Dermatol. 2014;89(5):735–44.
4. Takeshita J, Wang S, Shin DB, Mehta NN, Kimmel SE, Margolis DJ, et al. Effect of psoriasis severity on hypertension control: a population-based study in the United Kingdom. JAMA Dermatol. 2015;151(2):161–9.

5. Azfar RS, Seminara NM, Shin DB, Troxel AB, Margolis DJ, Gelfand JM. Increased risk of diabetes mellitus and likelihood of receiving diabetes mellitus treatment in patients with psoriasis. Arch Dermatol. 2012;148(9):995–1000.

6. Gu WJ, Weng CL, Zhao YT, Liu QH, Yin RX. Psoriasis and risk of cardiovascular disease: a meta-analysis of cohort studies. Int J Cardiol. 2013;168(5):4992–6.

7. Gelfand JM, Neimann AL, Shin DB, Wang X, Margolis DJ, Troxel AB. Risk of myocardial infarction in patients with psoriasis. JAMA. 2006;296(14):1735–41.

8. Horreau C, Pouplard C, Brenaut E, Barnetche T, Misery L, Cribier B, et al. Cardiovascular morbidity and mortality in psoriasis and psoriatic arthritis: a systematic literature review. J Eur Acad Dermatol Venereol. 2013;27(Suppl 3):12–29.

9. Ogdie A, Yu Y, Haynes K, Love TJ, Maliha S, Jiang Y, et al. Risk of major cardiovascular events in patients with psoriatic arthritis, psoriasis and rheumatoid arthritis: a population-based cohort study. Ann Rheum Dis. 2015;74(2):326–32.

10. Mehta NN, Yu Y, Pinnelas R, Krishnamoorthy P, Shin DB, Troxel AB, et al. Attributable risk estimate of severe psoriasis on major cardiovascular events. Am J Med. 2011;124(8):775.e1–6.

11. Mehta NN, Azfar RS, Shin DB, Neimann AL, Troxel AB, Gelfand JM. Patients with severe psoriasis are at increased risk of cardiovascular mortality: cohort study using the general practice research database. Eur Heart J. 2010;31(8):1000–6.

12. Abuabara K, Azfar RS, Shin DB, Neimann AL, Troxel AB, Gelfand JM. Cause-specific mortality in patients with severe psoriasis: a population-based cohort study in the UK. Br J Dermatol. 2010;163(3):586–92.

13. Svedbom A, Dalen J, Mamolo C, Cappelleri JC, Mallbris L, Petersson IF, et al. Increased cause-specific mortality in patients with mild and severe psoriasis: a population-based Swedish register study. Acta Derm Venereol. 2015;95(7):809–15.

14. Taleb S. Inflammation in atherosclerosis. Arch Cardiovasc Dis. 2016;109(12):708–15.

15. Westlake SL, Colebatch AN, Baird J, Kiely P, Quinn M, Choy E, et al. The effect of methotrexate on cardiovascular disease in patients with rheumatoid arthritis: a systematic literature review. Rheumatology (Oxford). 2010;49(2):295–307.

16. Micha R, Imamura F, Wyler von Ballmoos M, Solomon DH, Hernan MA, Ridker PM, et al. Systematic review and meta-analysis of methotrexate use and risk of cardiovascular disease. Am J Cardiol. 2011;108(9):1362–70.

17. Roubille C, Richer V, Starnino T, McCourt C, McFarlane A, Fleming P, et al. The effects of tumour necrosis factor inhibitors, methotrexate, non-steroidal anti-inflammatory drugs and corticosteroids on cardiovascular events in rheumatoid arthritis, psoriasis and psoriatic arthritis: a systematic review and meta-analysis. Ann Rheum Dis. 2015;74(3):480–9.

18. Prodanovich S, Ma F, Taylor JR, Pezon C, Fasihi T, Kirsner RS. Methotrexate reduces incidence of vascular diseases in veterans with psoriasis or rheumatoid arthritis. J Am Acad Dermatol. 2005;52(2):262–7.

19. Wu JJ, Poon KY, Channual JC, Shen AY. Association between tumor necrosis factor inhibitor therapy and myocardial infarction risk in patients with psoriasis. Arch Dermatol. 2012;148(11):1244–50.

20. Ahlehoff O, Skov L, Gislason G, Lindhardsen J, Kristensen SL, Iversen L, et al. Cardiovascular disease event rates in patients with severe psoriasis treated with systemic anti-inflammatory drugs: a Danish real-world cohort study. J Intern Med. 2013;273(2):197–204.

21. Ahlehoff O, Skov L, Gislason G, Gniadecki R, Iversen L, Bryld LE, et al. Cardiovascular outcomes and systemic anti-inflammatory drugs in patients with severe psoriasis: 5-year follow-up of a Danish nationwide cohort. J Eur Acad Dermatol Venereol. 2015;29(6):1128–34.

22. Lan CC, Ko YC, Yu HS, Wu CS, Li WC, Lu YW, et al. Methotrexate reduces the occurrence of cerebrovascular events among Taiwanese psoriatic patients: a nationwide population-based study. Acta Derm Venereol. 2012;92(4):349–52.

23. Bernatsky S, Hudson M, Suissa S. Anti-rheumatic drug use and risk of hospitalization for congestive heart failure in rheumatoid arthritis. Rheumatology (Oxford). 2005;44(5):677–80.

24. Rajappa M, Rathika S, Munisamy M, Chandrashekar L, Thappa DM. Effect of treatment with methotrexate and coal tar on adipokine levels and indices of insulin resistance and sensitivity in patients with psoriasis vulgaris. J Eur Acad Dermatol Venereol. 2015;29(1):69–76.

25. Solomon DH, Massarotti E, Garg R, Liu J, Canning C, Schneeweiss S. Association between disease-modifying antirheumatic drugs and diabetes risk in patients with rheumatoid arthritis and psoriasis. JAMA. 2011;305(24):2525–31.

26. Gisondi P, Cotena C, Tessari G, Girolomoni G. Anti-tumour necrosis factor-alpha therapy increases body weight in patients with chronic plaque psoriasis: a retrospective cohort study. J Eur Acad Dermatol Venereol. 2008;22(3):341–4.

27. Saraceno R, Schipani C, Mazzotta A, Esposito M, Di Renzo L, De Lorenzo A, et al. Effect of anti-tumor necrosis factor-alpha therapies on body mass index in patients with psoriasis. Pharmacol Res. 2008;57(4):290–5.

28. Navarro-Millan I, Charles-Schoeman C, Yang S, Bathon JM, Bridges SL Jr, Chen L, et al. Changes in lipoproteins associated with methotrexate or combination therapy in early rheumatoid arthritis: results from the treatment of early rheumatoid arthritis trial. Arthritis Rheum. 2013;65(6):1430–8.

29. Robertson J, Peters MJ, McInnes IB, Sattar N. Changes in lipid levels with inflammation and therapy in RA: a maturing paradigm. Nat Rev Rheumatol. 2013;9(9):513–23.

30. Rajappa M, Shanmugam R, Munisamy M, Chandrashekar L, Rajendiran KS, Thappa DM. Effect of antipsoriatic therapy on oxidative stress index and sialic acid levels in patients with psoriasis. Int J Dermatol. 2016;55(8):e422–30.

31. Gyldenlove M, Jensen P, Lovendorf MB, Zachariae C, Hansen PR, Skov L. Short-term treatment with methotrexate does not affect microvascular endothelial function in patients with psoriasis. J Eur Acad Dermatol Venereol. 2015;29(3):591–4.

32. Barnabe C, Martin BJ, Ghali WA. Systematic review and meta-analysis: anti-tumor necrosis factor alpha therapy and cardiovascular events in rheumatoid arthritis. Arthritis Care Res (Hoboken). 2011;63(4):522–9.

33. Yang ZS, Lin NN, Li L, Li Y. The effect of TNF inhibitors on cardiovascular events in psoriasis and psoriatic arthritis: an updated meta-analysis. Clin Rev Allergy Immunol. 2016;51(2):240–7.

34. Ryan C, Leonardi CL, Krueger JG, Kimball AB, Strober BE, Gordon KB, et al. Association between biologic therapies for chronic plaque psoriasis and cardiovascular events: a meta-analysis of randomized controlled trials. JAMA. 2011;306(8):864–71.

35. Rungapiromnan W, Yiu ZZ, Warren RB, Griffiths CE, Ashcroft DM. Impact of biologic therapies on risk of major adverse cardiovascular events in patients with psoriasis: systematic review and meta-analysis of randomised controlled trials. Br J Dermatol. 2017;176(4):890–901.

36. Wu JJ, Guerin A, Sundaram M, Dea K, Cloutier M, Mulani P. Cardiovascular event risk assessment in psoriasis patients treated with tumor necrosis factor-alpha inhibitors versus methotrexate. J Am Acad Dermatol. 2017;76(1):81–90.

37. Gulliver W, Young H, Gulliver S, Randell S. HLA-Cw6 status predicts efficacy of biologic treatment in psoriais patients. Glob Dermatol. 2015;2(6):228–31.

38. Gulliver WP, Young HM, Bachelez H, Randell S, Gulliver S, Al-Mutairi N. Psoriasis patients treated with biologics and methotrexate have a reduced rate of myocardial infarction: a

collaborative analysis using international cohorts. J Cutan Med Surg. 2016;20(6):550–4.

39. Abuabara K, Lee H, Kimball AB. The effect of systemic psoriasis therapies on the incidence of myocardial infarction: a cohort study. Br J Dermatol. 2011;165(5):1066–73.

40. Gulliver WP, Randell S, Gulliver S, Connors S, Bachelez H, MacDonald D, et al. Do biologics protect patients with psoriasis from myocardial infarction? A retrospective cohort. J Cutan Med Surg. 2016;20(6):536–41.

41. Wu JJ, Poon KY, Bebchuk JD. Association between the type and length of tumor necrosis factor inhibitor therapy and myocardial infarction risk in patients with psoriasis. J Drugs Dermatol. 2013;12(8):899–903.

42. Singh JA, Wells GA, Christensen R, Tanjong Ghogomu E, Maxwell L, Macdonald JK, et al. Adverse effects of biologics: a network meta-analysis and Cochrane overview. Cochrane Database Syst Rev. 2011;(2):Cd008794.

43. Pariser DM, Leonardi CL, Gordon K, Gottlieb AB, Tyring S, Papp KA, et al. Integrated safety analysis: short- and long-term safety profiles of etanercept in patients with psoriasis. J Am Acad Dermatol. 2012;67(2):245–56.

44. Behnam SM, Behnam SE, Koo JY. TNF-alpha inhibitors and congestive heart failure. Skinmed. 2005;4(6):363–8.

45. Costa L, Caso F, Atteno M, Del Puente A, Darda MA, Caso P, et al. Impact of 24-month treatment with etanercept, adalimumab, or methotrexate on metabolic syndrome components in a cohort of 210 psoriatic arthritis patients. Clin Rheumatol. 2014;33(6):833–9.

46. Marra M, Campanati A, Testa R, Sirolla C, Bonfigli AR, Franceschi C, et al. Effect of etanercept on insulin sensitivity in nine patients with psoriasis. Int J Immunopathol Pharmacol. 2007;20(4):731–6.

47. Martinez-Abundis E, Reynoso-von Drateln C, Hernandez-Salazar E, Gonzalez-Ortiz M. Effect of etanercept on insulin secretion and insulin sensitivity in a randomized trial with psoriatic patients at risk for developing type 2 diabetes mellitus. Arch Dermatol Res. 2007;299(9):461–5.

48. Daien CI, Duny Y, Barnetche T, Daures JP, Combe B, Morel J. Effect of TNF inhibitors on lipid profile in rheumatoid arthritis: a systematic review with meta-analysis. Ann Rheum Dis. 2012;71(6):862–8.

49. Lestre S, Diamantino F, Veloso L, Fidalgo A, Ferreira A. Effects of etanercept treatment on lipid profile in patients with moderate-to-severe chronic plaque psoriasis: a retrospective cohort study. Eur J Dermatol. 2011;21(6):916–20.

50. Ehsani AH, Mortazavi H, Balighi K, Hosseini MS, Azizpour A, Hejazi SP, et al. Changes in body mass index and lipid profile in psoriatic patients after treatment with standard protocol of infliximab. Acta Med Iran. 2016;54(9):570–5.

51. Piaserico S, Osto E, Famoso G, Zanetti I, Gregori D, Poretto A, et al. Treatment with tumor necrosis factor inhibitors restores coronary microvascular function in young patients with severe psoriasis. Atherosclerosis. 2016;251:25–30.

52. Leonardi CL, Unnebrink K, Valdecantos WC. Reduction in C-reactive-protein levels with Adalimumab therapy in patients with moderate-to-severe hand and/or foot psoriasis. J Drugs Dermatol. 2016;15(5):562–6.

53. Kanelleas A, Liapi C, Katoulis A, Stavropoulos P, Avgerinou G, Georgala S, et al. The role of inflammatory markers in assessing disease severity and response to treatment in patients with psoriasis treated with etanercept. Clin Exp Dermatol. 2011;36(8):845–50.

54. Campanati A, Ganzetti G, Di Sario A, Damiani A, Sandroni L, Rosa L, et al. The effect of etanercept on hepatic fibrosis risk in patients with non-alcoholic fatty liver disease, metabolic syndrome, and psoriasis. J Gastroenterol. 2013;48(7):839–46.

55. Gkalpakiotis S, Arenbergerova M, Gkalpakioti P, Potockova J, Arenberger P, Kraml P. Impact of adalimumab treatment on cardiovascular risk biomarkers in psoriasis: results of a pilot study. J Dermatol. 2017;44(4):363–9.

56. Asahina A, Umezawa Y, Yanaba K, Nakagawa H. Serum C-reactive protein levels in Japanese patients with psoriasis and psoriatic arthritis: long-term differential effects of biologics. J Dermatol. 2016;43(7):779–84.

57. Strober B, Teller C, Yamauchi P, Miller JL, Hooper M, Yang YC, et al. Effects of etanercept on C-reactive protein levels in psoriasis and psoriatic arthritis. Br J Dermatol. 2008;159(2):322–30.

58. Tzellos T, Kyrgidis A, Zouboulis CC. Re-evaluation of the risk for major adverse cardiovascular events in patients treated with anti-IL-12/23 biological agents for chronic plaque psoriasis: a meta-analysis of randomized controlled trials. J Eur Acad Dermatol Venereol. 2013;27(5):622–7.

59. Dommasch ED, Troxel AB, Gelfand JM. Major cardiovascular events associated with anti-IL 12/23 agents: a tale of two meta-analyses. J Am Acad Dermatol. 2013;68(5):863–5.

60. Papp KA, Griffiths CE, Gordon K, Lebwohl M, Szapary PO, Wasfi Y, et al. Long-term safety of ustekinumab in patients with moderate-to-severe psoriasis: final results from 5 years of follow-up. Br J Dermatol. 2013;168(4):844–54.

61. van de Kerkhof PC, Griffiths CE, Reich K, Leonardi CL, Blauvelt A, Tsai TF, et al. Secukinumab long-term safety experience: a pooled analysis of 10 phase II and III clinical studies in patients with moderate to severe plaque psoriasis. J Am Acad Dermatol. 2016;75(1):83–98.e4.

Pharmacovigilance

Robert E. Kalb

Introduction

Pharmacovigilance refers to "the activities involved in the detection, assessment, understanding, and prevention of adverse effects or any other drug related problems [1]." All medications have the potential for adverse effects. As a product is under development, a rigorous and thorough analysis of possible risks is conducted; however, it is very difficult to identify all possible safety issues during clinical trials. This is especially true for rare adverse events particularly when there is a slightly higher risk of such adverse events in the treated population [2]. Once a product is approved, significantly more patients are exposed, including those with multiple comorbidities as well as those being treated with other medications or medical products that may have been exclusion criteria in the original studies. As a result, data collected from post-marketing safety studies can better aid in risk assessment and may better identify a medication's risk profile. Unfortunately post-marketing reporting is voluntary and may not be accurate. Therefore prospective long-term registries are better suited to obtain this information. These data will allow physicians and patients to make better informed decisions on risk minimization.

Pharmacovigilance principally involves the identification and evaluation of safety signals, concerning an increased risk of therapy-related adverse events compared to the incidence of the adverse event in the background population. These signals can arise from data obtained from post-marketing surveillance as well as other sources, such as preclinical data and events associated with other medications in the same pharmacologic class. A single well-documented case report can be viewed as a potential safety signal, especially if the report describes a positive event upon rechallenging or if the event is extremely rare when the drug is not used [3]. When these signals appear, further investigation is required, which may or may not lead to the conclusion that the medication caused the event. After a signal is identified, it should be further assessed to determine whether it represents a potential safety risk and whether other actions should be taken.

Psoriasis is a chronic disease, which usually requires long-term therapy. Often these medications are immunomodulatory in nature. It is increasingly vital that both patients and physicians are aware of the safety of these medications. Better long-term safety will allow physicians to select a therapy with a decreased likelihood of adverse events based on the patient's history and comorbid factors.

Adverse Events

Various studies have investigated post-marketing adverse effects throughout a variety of registries. These registries have collected information regarding potential medication-related side events including major cardiovascular adverse events (MACE), serious infections, and rates of malignancy. Initial registry publications have focused on these possible serious adverse events, as this data is vital for patients and physicians.

Biologics and Pharmacovigilance

There are many examples in medicine when drugs that were thought to be relatively safe were found to have unknown adverse events that become apparent after a drug has been on the market and used by a wider population for many years. One example in dermatology was efalizumab, which was FDA approved for treatment of moderate-to-severe plaque psoriasis based on studies in approximately 2700 patients

R.E. Kalb, MD
Suny At Buffalo School of Medicine, Buffalo, NY, USA
e-mail: kalb@buffalo.edu

© Springer International Publishing AG 2018
P.S. Yamauchi (ed.), *Biologic and Systemic Agents in Dermatology*, https://doi.org/10.1007/978-3-319-66884-0_9

[4]. Of note, approximately 200 were exposed to the drug for over 1 year. The drug had been in clinical trials for a few years and on the market for nearly 5 years, with more than 46,000 patients taking the medication. It was withdrawn in 2009 after one suspected and three confirmed cases of progressive multifocal leukoencephalopathy (PML) were reported [4, 5]. As PML is very rare, it was deemed that it was extremely unlikely that the four reported cases were due to chance alone. Additionally, as PML occurs primarily in immunosuppressed patients, the association was biologically plausible and likely causal. This situation raised questions on adverse event reporting and shed light on the importance of long-term safety monitoring particularly for rare events.

Multiple registries have been developed to track serious adverse events occurring in patients taking biologics. Many of these registries fulfill post-marketing commitments to the FDA for the individual approved agent. These include ESPRIT and OBSERVE-5, for monitoring adverse events in patients taking adalimumab and etanercept, respectively. These individual agent registries do not include a comparison group so it is difficult to compare rates of adverse events in similar psoriasis patients receiving other therapies. Other registries are country based and are disease specific including psoriasis patients on multiple therapies over time [6]. These registries include the Spanish Registry of Adverse Events Associated With Biologic Drugs in Dermatology also known as BIOBADADERM (Spain, 1956 patients, 5-year follow-up period), Bio-Capture (the Netherlands), PsoCare (Italy, 10,539 patients, 5-year follow-up period), DERMBIO (Denmark, 1277 patients, 10-year follow-up period), BADBIR (United Kingdom and Ireland, British Association of Dermatologists, 8399 patients) [7], and the German Psoriasis Registry PsoBest (Germany, 2556 patients, 5-year follow-up period).

The largest registry is the Psoriasis Longitudinal Assessment and Registry (PSOLAR), with over 12,000 patients at multiple clinical sites worldwide. This registry also fulfills post-marketing FDA commitment with respect to infliximab and ustekinumab. It is a unique post-marketing registry including psoriasis patients on multiple other therapies including other biologics, conventional systemic therapy, phototherapy, and topical therapy alone. The advantage is that patients on various treatments can be compared over time. Multiple studies have been reported analyzing post-marketing adverse events.

Infliximab

A 2014 study analyzing 1394 patients taking infliximab as the index agent enrolled in the PSOLAR registry from 2007 through 2013 revealed that the rate of major adverse cardiovascular events (MACE) was similar for infliximab

Table 9.1 Comparison of biologic agents with incidence and incidence rates of select serious adverse events from previously published PSOLAR studies [7, 8, 15]

	Infliximab	Adalimumab	Etanercept	Ustekinumab
MACE	0.38			0.32
Malignancy, excluding NMSC	0.58			0.48
Serious infection	2.73			0.93
	2.49[a]	1.97[a]	1.47[a]	0.83[a]
[a]Cellulitis	0.40[a]	0.19[a]	0.37[a]	0.19[a]
[a]Pneumonia	0.44[a]	0.39[a]	0.27[a]	0.19[a]

Notated in events/100 patient-years. Data from secukinumab and ixekizumab have not been published in PSOLAR studies
[a]Denotes data from PSOLAR study investigating the risk of serious infection [8]

Table 9.2 Overall rate of serious infections for biologics and nonbiologics according to PSOLAR registry [8]

Ustekinumab	Infliximab	Adalimumab	Etanercept	No Biologic	Combined
0.83	2.49	1.97	1.47	1.11	1.45

Expressed in events/100 PY

at 0.38 events per 100 patient-years (0.38/100 PY) (Tables 9.1 and 9.2) compared to other biologics (0.33/100 PY) [8]. Rates of malignancy (excluding nonmelanoma skin cancers) were 0.58/100 PY (Table 9.4), which was also similar to other biologics (0.74/100 PY). The rate of serious infections was 2.73/100 PY, suggestive of significant association between exposure to infliximab and development for serious infection. A recently published analysis for serious risk of infection of PSOLAR registrants showed an incidence rate of 2.49/100 PY (Table 9.5) in patients taking infliximab (1151 patients representing 2253 PY) [9]. The most common infections were pneumonia (0.44/100 PY) and cellulitis (0.40/100PY) (Table 9.1). Other reported infections in the PSOLAR registry included sepsis, diverticulitis, urinary tract infection, abscess, skin infection, bronchitis, pyelonephritis, gastroenteritis, colitis, osteomyelitis, meningitis, necrotizing fasciitis, viral infection, and herpes zoster. A recently reported analysis of the BIOBADADERM registry revealed that the rate of serious infections was 1.89/100 PY for patients taking infliximab [10]. The most commonly reported infections were upper respiratory tract infections, acute tonsillitis/pharyngotonsillitis, and urinary tract infection.

Additional safety data was published from the German Psoriasis Registry PsoBest [11]. The rate of MACE in patients taking infliximab was approximately 0.6/100 PY (Table 9.2). The rate of malignancy (excluding NMSC) was <0.1/100 PY (Table 9.3). The rate of serious infection was approximately 1.4/100 PY (Table 9.4). The study did not delineate which infections were most reported.

Table 9.3 Comparison of rates of MACE for biologics across registries

	Ustekinumab	Infliximab	Adalimumab	Etanercept
PSOLAR	0.32	0.38	–	–
BIOBADADERM	–	–	–	–
PsoBest	1.2	0.6	0.4	0.9

Expressed in events/100 PY

Table 9.4 Comparison of rates of malignancy (excluding NMSC) for biologics across registries

	Ustekinumab	Infliximab	Adalimumab	Etanercept
PSOLAR	0.48	0.58	–	–
BIOBADADERM	–	–	–	–
PsoBest	0.75	<0.1	0.5	0.2

Expressed in events/100 PY

Adalimumab

ESPRIT is an ongoing, multicenter, post-marketing, 10-year, international, observational registry with the objective of evaluating long-term safety and effectiveness of adalimumab in patients treated for chronic psoriasis in routine clinical practice. Data from the first 5 years were analyzed and reported recently [12]. The overall rate of serious treatment-emergent adverse events was 4.3/100 PY of total adalimumab exposure. The most common adverse event was infection (1.0/100 PY) (Table 9.1), and no patterns were identified across any exposure categories. The rates for adverse events leading to discontinuation from the registry or from adalimumab overall were 0.4/100 PY and 2.0/100 PY, respectively. The incidence of events leading to death regardless of etiology was 0.1/100PY. The most common event leading to death was MI (<0.1/100PY, four events). The rates of other cause of death were less than <0.1/100 PY (one event) for each of CHF, acute cardiac failure, cardiac arrest, arrhythmia, staphylococcal infection, staphylococcal sepsis, road traffic accident, metastatic breast cancer, metastatic gastric cancer, metastatic neoplasm, papillary thyroid cancer, sarcoma, small-cell lung cancer, squamous cell carcinoma of the lung, subarachnoid hemorrhage, COPD, and pneumonia aspiration. Cardiovascular-related adverse events of special interest included cerebrovascular accident (0.1/100PY), MI (0.1/100PY), and congestive heart failure (<0.1/100PY). The overall incidence rate for malignancy was 0.9/100PY (<0.1/100PY for melanoma, <0.1/100PY for lymphoma, and 0.6/100PY for nonmelanoma skin cancer) and 0.3/100PY for other malignancies, excluding NMSC (Table 9.4). The overall incidence rate of serious infections was 1.0/100PY. Cellulitis and pneumonia were the most common serious infections found in the ESPRIT study. The overall rate of cellulitis (including anorectal, staphylococcal, external-ear, infusion-site, and periorbital cellulitis) was 0.1/100 PY. The overall rate of pneumonia was 0.1/100 PY. Analysis of the PSOLAR registry revealed a rate for serious infections of 1.97/100 PY (Table 9.2) for patients taking adalimumab, suggesting that adalimumab exposure may be associated with an increased risk of developing serious infections [9]. The most common infections were pneumonia and cellulitis (rates of 0.39/100 PY and 0.19/100 PY, respectively). A recently published meta-analysis revealed that adalimumab was associated with a higher risk of serious infection compared to retinoid and/or phototherapy in adults (hazard ratio: 2.52, 95% confidence interval: 1.47–4.32) [13]. Analysis of the BIOBADADERM registry revealed a rate for serious infection of 0.98/100 PY (Table 9.5) [10]. The most commonly reported infections were upper respiratory tract infections (viral/adenoviral), urinary tract infections, and bronchitis. Analysis of the German Psoriasis Registry PsoBest reported the rates of serious adverse events [11]. The rate of serious infections was 0.5/100 PY (Table 9.5). The rate of MACE was approximately 0.4/100 PY (Table 9.3). The rate of malignancy (excluding NMSC) was approximately 0.5/100 PY (Table 9.4).

Observed adverse events in the first 5 years of ESPRIT registry were consistent with the adalimumab safety profile, with no new safety signals observed. Interestingly, rates of serious adverse events and serious infections decreased with increasing adalimumab exposure [12]. For patients exposed to adalimumab for less than 1 year, the rates for serious adverse events and serious infections were 23.5/100 PY and 6.1/100 PY, respectively. However, for patients exposed to adalimumab for greater than 5 years, the rates for serious adverse events and serious infections were 2.7/100 PY and 0.6/100 PY, respectively. This is supported by clinical experience in that patients remaining on long-term therapy are those who respond well and do not experience treatment-related side effects, which necessitate discontinuation of therapy.

Table 9.5 Comparison of rates of serious infections for biologics across select registries

	Ustekinumab	Infliximab	Adalimumab	Etanercept
PSOLAR	0.83	2.49	1.97	1.47
BIOBADADERM	0.59	1.89	0.98	0.16
PsoBest	0.5	1.47	0.5	1.0

Expressed in events/100 PY

Etanercept

The observational post-marketing safety surveillance registry of etanercept (OBSERVE-5) collected data regarding the incidence of adverse effects for patients taking etanercept over a 5-year period [14]. Approximately 2500 people were enrolled in the registry. It revealed a 5-year cumulative incidence of 22.2% for serious adverse effects (95% CI 20.3–24.2%). There was a 6.5% incidence for serious infections (95% CI 5.4–7.7%); the most common serious infections were pneumonia (incidence of 1.2%) and cellulitis (0.9%). The 5-year cumulative incidence for serious infectious events requiring hospitalization was 5.2% (95% CI 4.1–6.2%). An analysis of patients taking etanercept on the PSOLAR registry revealed a rate of 1.47/100 PY (Table 9.1). The most commonly reported infections were cellulitis (0.37/100PY) and pneumonia (0.27/100PY). An analysis of the BIOBADADERM registry revealed a rate for serious infection as 0.16/100 PY (Table 9.5) [10]. This rate was lower than that from the PSOLAR registry. The most commonly reported infections were upper respiratory tract infection, nasopharyngitis, and urinary tract infection.

The most commonly reported noninfectious serious adverse event in the OBSERVE-5 registry was MI with a reported incidence of 0.7%. A 3.2% incidence rate was reported for malignancies excluding nonmelanoma skin cancer (95% CI 2.3–4.1%); 3.6% incidence for nonmelanoma skin cancer (95% CI 2.7–4.5%); 2.8% incidence for coronary artery disease (95% CI 2.0–3.6%); 0.7% incidence for psoriasis worsening (95% CI 0.3–1.2%); 0.2% incidence for central nervous system demyelinating disorder (95% CI 0.0–0.4%); 0.1% incidence for lymphoma and for tuberculosis (95% CI 0.0–0.3%); and 0.1% incidence for opportunistic infection and for lupus (95% CI 0.0–0.2%); Of note, 55 fatal events were reported. Of these, 17 were of unknown cause. Four deaths were considered by the investigator to be related to etanercept: brain cancer and lung cancer, heart failure, osteomyelitis and sepsis, and idiopathic pulmonary fibrosis. Incidence rates for hospitalization-associated infections, malignancies (excluding NMSC), lymphoma, and NMSC were not higher than the rates of the psoriasis population using nonbiologic systemic therapies relative to administrative claims data. Also, the incidence of serious adverse events decreased with increased exposure. Analysis of the German Psoriasis Registry PsoBest reported the rates of serious adverse events [11]. The rate of serious

infections was approximately 1.0/100 PY. The rate of MACE was approximately 0.9/100 PY (Table 9.2). The rate of malignancy (excluding NMSC) was approximately 0.2/100 PY (Table 9.3).

Ustekinumab

A 5-year analysis of safety data pooled from prior studies reported the rates of serious adverse events in patients taking biologics [15]. The rate of serious adverse events was 7.0/100 PY and 7.2/100 PY in patients receiving ustekinumab 45 mg and 90 mg, respectively. The rates of serious adverse events were similar between dose groups. The rate of serious infections was 0.98/100 PY and 1.19/100 PY. The patient of other malignancies (excluding NSMC) was 0.59/100 PY and 0.61/100 PY). The rate of MACE was 0.56/100PY and 0.36/100 PY. The most common adverse events were nasopharyngitis, upper respiratory tract infection, headache, and arthralgia. The most frequently reported serious infections were diverticulitis, cellulitis, and pneumonia, which each occurred in <0.4% of patients receiving ustekinumab.

A recently published report analyzed the cumulative incidence rates of adverse events of special interests for patients taking ustekinumab as the index medication [16]. Multivariate analyses revealed that ustekinumab was not associated with an increased risk of malignancy, MACE, serious infections, or mortality. The rates of MACE and malignancy (excluding NMSC) for ustekinumab were 0.32/100 PY and 0.48/100 PY, respectively according to PSOLAR registry (Tables 9.3 and 9.4, respectively). Rates of serious infection for ustekinumab (0.93/100 PY) (Table 9.1) were lower compared to other biologics (1.91/100 PY), with exposures to other biologics associated with serious infections (HR = 1.96). A separate analysis of the PSOLAR registry investigating the risk of serious infections for patients taking ustekinumab revealed an incidence rate of serious infections of 0.83/100 PY (3474 patients representing 5923 PY) (Table 9.5). The most commonly reported serious infections were pneumonia and cellulitis (0.19/100 PY for both). There was no increased risk of serious infection compared to nonmethotrexate/nonbiologic or methotrexate/nonbiologic cohorts (incidence rates of 1.05/100 PY and 1.28/100 PY, respectively) [9]. The BIOBADADERM registry revealed that the rate of serious infections is 0.59/100 PY [10]. The most common reported infections were upper respiratory tract infection, urinary tract infection, and acute tonsillitis. Analysis of the German Psoriasis Registry PsoBest reported that the rate of serious infections was 0.5/100 PY [11]. The rate of MACE was approximately 1.2/100 PY. The rate of malignancy (excluding NMSC) was approximately 0.75/100 PY.

Patients who are genetically deficient in IL-1/23p40 and IL-12Rb have shown an increased susceptibility to infections of weakly virulent mycobacterial and salmonella [17–19]. No infections with salmonella or mycobacteria were reported in the studies.

Secukinumab

No registry data exists for secukinumab and long-term results have not been published. However safety data collected from ten phase II and III studies were recently reported [20]. Analysis of patients receiving secukinumab over 52 weeks included 3993 subjects; 3430 received secukinumab, representing 2725 patient-years of exposure. Over 52 weeks, for secukinumab 300 mg, 150 mg, and etanercept (comparator), respectively, exposure-adjusted incidence rates were comparable across treatments. The rates of total adverse events were 236.1/100 PY, 239.9/100 PY, and 243.4/100 PY, respectively; the rates of infections were 91.1/100 PY, 85.3/100 PY, and 93.7/100 PY, respectively; the most commonly reported adverse events reported were nasopharyngitis, headache, upper respiratory tract infections, arthralgias, hypertensions, diarrhea, back pain, pruritus, and cough.

The incidence rates of serious adverse events were 7.4/100 PY, 6.8/100 PY, and 7.0/100 PY for patients taking secukinumab 300 mg, 150 mg, and etanercept, respectively); the rates for serious infections were 1.4/100 PY, 1.1/100 PY, and 1.4/100 PY, respectively; the incidence rates of malignant or unspecified tumors were 0.77/100 PY, 0.97/100 PY, and 0.68/100 PY, respectively; and adjudicated major adverse cardiovascular events were 0.42/100 PY, 0.35/100 PY, and 0.34/100 PY, respectively. The aforementioned adverse events were not dose related. However, they were dose related for nonserious, mild/moderate, skin/mucosal candidiasis; the incidence rates were 3.55/100 PY for patients taking secukinumab 300 mg and 1.85/100 PY for patients taking secukinumab 150 mg. The rate of candidiasis for patients taking etanercept in the study was 1.37/100 PY. Candidal infections were mild and easily treated and did not lead to the discontinuation of therapy. There were no systemic candida infections. Once long-term safety data has been collected post-marketing, more information can be gleaned in identifying any new potential safety signals.

Ixekizumab

Similar to secukinumab, which was also recently approved, no long-term registry information has been reported. A recently published article reported integrated safety analysis from seven psoriasis clinical trials involving ixekizumab [21]. In total, 4209 patients received ixekizumab representing 6480 patient-years. In the combined ixekizumab data set the five most commonly reported treatment-emergent adverse events were nasopharyngitis, upper respiratory infection, injection-site reaction, headache, and arthralgia. The incidence rates were 14.1/100 PY, 7.9/100 PY, 6.8/100 PY, 4.8/100 PY, and 4.2/100 PY, respectively. There were no invasive fungal infections involving candidiasis or other deep organ infection reported. Of 165 (2.5/100 PY) reported Candida cases, 5 (0.1% of all patients) were found to be severe. It was not reported if it was vulvovaginal, oral, or other form of candidiasis. The most frequently occurring Candida infections included vulvovaginal candidiasis (2.4/100 PY) and oral candidiasis (1.2/100 PY). Ixekizumab was not associated with an increased risk of serious infection. The most common serious adverse event reported was cellulitis (0.3/100 PY). The rate of malignancies excluding NMSC among ixekizumab-treated patients was comparable with etanercept-treated patients during the induction period. The rates of malignancy and MACE were 0.3/100 PY and 0.4/100 PY; however the total duration of the trials was relatively low (60 weeks), limiting further conclusions.

Brodalumab

Brodalumab is currently undergoing clinical trials for safety and efficacy in the treatment of moderate-to-severe plaque psoriasis [22]. A recently published interim analysis at treatment week 120 of a 264-week open-label extension of the previously reported brodalumab study reported common adverse events [23, 24]. Approximately 180 patients were included in the analysis. The most commonly reported adverse events were nasopharyngitis (26.5%), upper respiratory tract infection (19.9%), arthralgia (16.0%), and back pain (11.0%). Serious adverse events were reported in 15 (8%) patients. The reported treatment-emergent serious adverse events, each with one event, were abscess, viral meningitis, streptococcal necrotizing fasciitis, pyelonephritis, septic shock, atrial fibrillation, congestive cardiac failure, supraventricular tachycardia, bile duct stone, cholecystitis, intervertebral disc protrusion, lumbar spinal stenosis, osteoarthritis, esophageal adenocarcinoma, benign parathyroid tumor, constipation, nephrolithiasis, toxic skin eruption, and aortic aneurysm rupture [24]. Four (2%) patients had grade 2 absolute neutrophil count (<1500 × 10 [9]/L) laboratory abnormalities; all were transient and resolved without changes to treatment. Five (3%) patients had low-grade (grade 2 or less) oral candidiasis. Five patients reported an AE of depression during the open-label extension. No reports of suicidal behavior were reported.

A paper investigating the long-term safety of brodalumab in the treatment of Japanese patients with moderate-to-severe psoriasis was recently reported [25]. Approximately 130 patients received brodalumab for 52 weeks and were monitored for serious adverse events. The most commonly reported adverse events were nasopharyngitis (35.2%), upper respiratory tract inflammation (10.3%), and contact dermatitis (9.7%). Serious adverse events were observed in eight patients; they included allergy to arthropod sting, cellulitis, osteoarthritis, varicose vein, myocardial ischemia, cellulitis, infection, and contact dermatitis in one patient each. One patient had grade 1 neutropenia (absolute neutrophil count 1482 × 10 [9]/L); seven patients had low-grade (grade 2 or less) oral candidiasis; and one had grade 2 skin candidiasis. Grade 3 infections occurred in three patients (two with cellulitis and one with a suspected severe infection [not a candidiasis]). Two patients reported injection-site reactions. There was no reported suicidal ideation and suicidal behavior.

During the AMAGINE-1 phase III trial, two cases of suicide were reported [26]. The exposure-adjusted event rate for depression was 1.2/100 PY. The aforementioned studies did not reveal an increased risk of suicidal behavior. Additionally, a recently published analysis revealed no association linking brodalumab treatment to the risk of suicidal behavior [27].

Cardiovascular Disease

Psoriasis is associated with significant comorbid conditions, such as diabetes, hyperlipidemia, obesity, and hypertension, all of which raise the risk of cardiovascular disease and lead to increased morbidity and mortality [28–30]. There were initial concerns that biologic therapy may increase the risk of cardiovascular events in psoriasis patients. As noted above the current data suggests that there is no increased risk. This again emphasizes the difficulty in identifying an increased risk of a rare event in a patient population with a slightly increased risk of that event.

More recent data have suggested that there may be a cardiovascular disease benefit in treating psoriasis patients with biologic therapy. Since coronary artery disease is felt to be primarily an inflammatory process it is possible that decreasing the significant degree of systemic inflammation in patients with severe psoriasis may be beneficial. One recently reported analysis [31] compiled patient data from previously published studies [32, 33] and found that the risk of MI in patients taking biologics compared to patients receiving

nonbiologic therapy (included methotrexate and topical therapies) was reduced by 44%. The rate of MI in patients taking biologics was 1.36/100 PY while the rate in those receiving nonbiologics was 2.39/100 PY. The study did not delineate among the biologics, precluding further analysis. Other studies have shown a decreased risk of cardiovascular events in patients receiving biologics/methotrexate compared to other systemic therapies [32–34].

A separate analysis of 9148 patients prescribed anti-TNF agents and 8813 patients on methotrexate was performed to measure the impact of major cardiovascular event risk [35]. It was found that those treated with anti-TNF agents had fewer cardiovascular events compared to patients receiving methotrexate (hazard ratio: 0.55). It was also reported that every 6 months of cumulative exposure to anti-TNF agents was associated with an 11% cardiovascular event risk reduction.

A recent analysis investigated the role of biologic agents affecting the progression of coronary artery disease in patients with severe psoriasis [36]. Fifty-six patients (28 biologic-treated patients and 28 controls) underwent noncontrast coronary artery calcium (CAC) CT and contrast-enhanced CT angiography. It was found that, in follow-up of 13 months, treatment with biologic agents was associated with reduced coronary artery disease progression; biologic-treated patients showed reduced progression of CAC scores and reduced progression of luminal abnormalities/narrowing as compared with controls. These findings may point to a role of biologic agents in preventing cardiovascular disease progression in patients with severe psoriasis.

A crucial issue in psoriasis is whether early intervention with effective therapy will decrease the risk of comorbid factors such as cardiovascular disease and joint destruction secondary to psoriatic arthritis. Hopefully these questions can be answered with further long-term follow-up.

Depression/Suicide

Another comorbidity that has been reported in psoriasis patients is the increased risk of suicide and depression [37]. Whether treatment will change this risk is unknown. No long-term registry follow-up has been published as of yet. There have not been significant signals identified based on the current published literature. A recent addition to the psoriasis armamentarium is the oral therapy apremilast. There is a package insert warning regarding a possible increased risk of depression. This potential issue has also been raised with brodalumab therapy and anti-IL-17 treatment as mentioned above. Whether this is a true association or simply the increased risk in the background psoriasis population is unknown [27].

Other Registry Data

Numerous publications from the BIOBADADERM registry have reported long-term safety data; however, these papers did not delineate the rates of serious adverse events among the different biologics [38–41]. One study revealed the rate of developing serious adverse events in patients taking biologics as 3.7/100 PY [40]. The comparator used in the study was the use of classic systemic drugs, which included methotrexate, acitretin, and cyclosporine. The rate of serious adverse events was 4.0/100 PY, indicating no difference in the rate of developing serious adverse events in patients receiving biologics and those treated with classic systemic therapies. A separate BIOBADADERM study revealed no difference in the risk of adverse events between young and elderly (age ≥65) patients receiving biologics [41].

The Psocare project was developed within the Italian National Health System as a nationwide outcome study of patients receiving a new systemic treatment for psoriasis for the first time. Numerous publications have investigated the use of biologics in this population [42–44]. It was noted that infliximab was associated with a risk of more than doubling the upper normal aspartate amino transferase (AST) and alanine amino transferase (ALT) [43]. It is unclear if this increase had a clinical impact on the patients. Adalimumab and etanercept were not associated with an increased risk of developing metabolic abnormalities. Ustekinumab was not included in the analysis.

The German Psoriasis Registry PsoBest records long-term safety as well as efficacy of psoriasis treatment regimens [45]. The overall rate of serious adverse events was 1.5/100 PY in patients treated with biologics compared to 1.3/100 PY in those treated with other systemic treatments [11]. The rate for serious infections was 0.65/100 PY in patients receiving biologics and 0.33/100 in patients receiving other systemic treatments. The rate of MACE was 0.77/100 PY for those receiving biologic treatments and 0.56/100 PY for patients receiving other systemic treatments. The rate of malignancy (excluding NMSC) was 0.49/100 PY in those on biologics and 0.46/100 PY in patients receiving other systemic therapies. Overall, no significant difference was noted between biologic and systemic treatments.

Registry data from the Netherlands reported 5-year safety data [46] with 173 patients enrolled in the registry. The rate of MACE was 1.95/100 PY for patients taking biologics. The rate of malignancy (excluding NMSC) was 0.73/100 PY in those receiving biologics. The rate of serious infection was 0.73/100 PY. It is difficult to draw conclusions based on the small cohort size. The Biologics Continuous Assessment of Psoriasis Treatment Use Registry (Bio-CAPTURE) database is a registry collecting information regarding patients on biologics in the Netherlands population [47, 48]. No rigorous investigation regarding the risk of serious adverse events has been reported.

The DERMBIO database is a Danish registry collecting information regarding safety and efficacy in patients receiving biologic therapy. A published report [49] revealed six serious adverse events: one case of ovarian cancer in a patient taking adalimumab and three cases of serious infection (pneumonia, abscess, urinary tract infection) in patients taking adalimumab. Two cases were reported in etanercept-treated patients: one case of vertigo and one case of sepsis. The cohort size may have been too small and the follow-up time (approximately 3 years) may have been too short to detect other serious adverse events. A larger analysis from the DERMBIO registry revealed 33 serious adverse events among the 1277 patients treated with biologics [50]. Nine events were related to infection, nine events related to cancer, and six events related to MACE.

Other registries include Child-CAPTURE, which contains information regarding 125 pediatric patients with psoriasis in the Netherlands [51, 52]. No long-term safety information regarding biologic use in this population has been published. The Malaysian Psoriasis Registry (MPR) has collected data from 2267 patients in a cross-sectional study spanning 2 years [53]; however, no long-term safety data has been published.

The Psonet initiative is a prospective observational cohort study that integrates data from independent psoriasis registries of nine European countries [54]. The registries include Psocare (Italy), PsoReg (Sweden), BIOBADADERM (Spain), BADBIR (United Kingdom/Ireland), Clalit Health Services (CHS, Israel), PsoBest (Germany), Bio-Capture (the Netherlands), as well as registries from France and Portugal. It includes 20,232 and will assess patients for 5 years. A recent Psonet prospective meta-analysis reported the risk of serious infections in patients taking anti-TNF therapy compared to nonbiologics (acitretin, methotrexate, cyclosporine) [55]. The adjusted hazard ratio of exposure to anti-TNF agents compared with nonbiologics was 0.98; for bacterial cutaneous infections, it was 1.00; for granulomatous infections it was 1.23. This suggests that treatment with anti-TNF medications was not associated with an increased risk of serious infections compared to nonbiologics. The study did not discriminate between different biologics.

Drug Persistence

Drug persistence rates have been measured to assess real-world utilization of biologics. A recent study revealed persistence rates of 19.0% for etanercept, 53.4% for adalimumab, and 70.8% for ustekinumab after a 12-month period [56]. The rates of discontinuation were 34.5, 27.2, and 15.9% for etanercept, adalimumab, and ustekinumab, respectively.

The most commonly reported reason for drug discontinuation was drug ineffectiveness. A separate report investigating drug utilization rates in patients taking ustekinumab revealed a persistence rate of 81.4% and a discontinuation (with/without a restart or switch to another biologic agent) rate of 11.9% [57]. A recently published retrospective analysis revealed a persistence rate of 53.2% from 13 months up to 6.8 years for patients taking adalimumab [58].

A recent PSOLAR analysis investigating drug survival revealed, for first-line use, discontinuation rates of 25.4% for patients taking infliximab, 37.6% for those taking adalimumab, 43.9% for those taking etanercept, and 8.6% for those taking ustekinumab [59]. A report analyzing drug survival for patients in the BADBIR registry revealed a 1-year survival rate of 65% for patients taking infliximab, 70% for those taking etanercept, 79% for those taking adalimumab, and 89% for those taking ustekinumab [60]. The most common reason for discontinuation among all biologics was drug ineffectiveness seen in 13%, followed by adverse events. The most common adverse event reported after 1 year of drug utilization was infections/infestations, which were seen in 0.9, 3/1, 1.3, and 1.3% in those patients taking etanercept, infliximab, adalimumab, and ustekinumab, respectively [60]. A report investigating drug discontinuation in the DERMBIO registry revealed discontinuation rates between approximately 40 and 55% in patients taking etanercept, adalimumab, or infliximab. The discontinuation of ustekinumab was approximately 20% [50]. A published analysis of the Bio-CAPTURE investigating drug survival in patients taking adalimumab revealed a rate of 76% after 1 year and 52% after 4.5 years [47].

Limitations

Observational data are subject to outcome reporting bias. For patients not enrolled in long-term registries, post-marketing reporting of adverse events via the FDA system is voluntary. Adverse events may be underreported during data collection. At entry into the registry, some patients were biologic naïve while others may have been on previous biologic therapy. For patients with long-term biologic treatment before registry enrollment, the total exposure-adjusted incidence rate of treatment-emergent adverse events may be underestimated.

Conclusions

Long-term safety data reported for biologic therapy is reassuring. There does not appear to be an increased risk of malignancy and MACE events over the risk in the background psoriasis population. For all biologics, no new safety signals were identified in reported registry studies. There may be a slightly higher risk for serious infections for patients receiving adalimumab and infliximab. No increased risk was reported for patients taking ustekinumab and etanercept. One meta-analysis revealed no increased risk of serious adverse events in patients taking adalimumab, etanercept, or infliximab compared to placebo [61]. Long-term data is limited but also reassuring for patients taking secukinumab and ixekizumab and real-world registry data is being collected. No psoriasis treatment was identified as a predictor of death. Further data collection is under way to identify long-term safety signals and better guide physicians in treating patients.

References

1. US Food and Drug Administration. Guidance for industry: good pharmacovigilance practices and pharmacoepidemiologic assessment. Rockville, MD: US Food and Drug Administration; 2005.
2. Ryan C, Kirby B. Psoriasis is a systemic disease with multiple cardiovascular and metabolic comorbidities. Dermatol Clin. 2015;33(1):41–55.
3. Arnaiz JA, Carne X, Riba N, Codina C, Ribas J, Trilla A. The use of evidence in pharmacovigilance. Case reports as the reference source for drug withdrawals. Eur J Clin Pharmacol. 2001;57(1):89–91.
4. Seminara NM, Gelfand JM. Assessing long-term drug safety: lessons (re) learned from raptiva. Semin Cutan Med Surg. 2010;29(1):16–9.
5. Nijsten T, Spuls PI, Naldi L, Stern RS. The misperception that clinical trial data reflect long-term drug safety: lessons learned from Efalizumab's withdrawal. Arch Dermatol. 2009;145(9):1037–9.
6. Eissing L, Rustenbach SJ, Krensel M, Zander N, Spehr C, Radtke MA, et al. Psoriasis registries worldwide: systematic overview on registry publications. J Eur Acad Dermatol Venereol. 2016;30(7):1100–6.
7. Iskandar IY, Ashcroft DM, Warren RB, Yiu ZZ, McElhone K, Lunt M, et al. Demographics and disease characteristics of patients with psoriasis enrolled in the British Association of Dermatologists Biologic Interventions Register. Br J Dermatol. 2015;173(2):510–8.
8. Gottlieb AB, Kalb RE, Langley RG, Krueger GG, de Jong EM, Guenther L, et al. Safety observations in 12095 patients with psoriasis enrolled in an international registry (PSOLAR): experience with infliximab and other systemic and biologic therapies. J Drugs Dermatol. 2014;13(12):1441–8.
9. Kalb RE, Fiorentino DF, Lebwohl MG, Toole J, Poulin Y, Cohen AD, et al. Risk of serious infection with biologic and systemic treatment of psoriasis: results from the Psoriasis Longitudinal Assessment and Registry (PSOLAR). JAMA Dermatol. 2015;151(9):961–9.
10. Davila-Seijo P, Dauden E, Descalzo MA, Carretero G, Carrascosa JM, Vanaclocha F, et al. Infections in moderate to severe psoriasis patients treated with biological drugs compared to classic systemic drugs: findings from the BIOBADADERM Registry. J Invest Dermatol. 2017;137(2):313–21.
11. Reich K, Mrowietz U, Radtke MA, Thaci D, Rustenbach SJ, Spehr C, et al. Drug safety of systemic treatments for psoriasis: results from the German Psoriasis Registry PsoBest. Arch Dermatol Res. 2015;307(10):875–83.
12. Menter A, Thaci D, Papp KA, Wu JJ, Bereswill M, Teixeira HD, et al. Five-year analysis from the ESPRIT 10-year postmarketing surveillance registry of adalimumab treatment for moderate to severe psoriasis. J Am Acad Dermatol. 2015;73(3):410–9. e6
13. Yiu ZZ, Exton LS, Jabbar-Lopez Z, Mohd Mustapa MF, Samarasekera EJ, Burden AD, et al. Risk of serious infections in

patients with psoriasis on biologic therapies: a systematic review and meta-analysis. J Invest Dermatol. 2016;136(8):1584–91.

14. Kimball AB, Rothman KJ, Kricorian G, Pariser D, Yamauchi PS, Menter A, et al. OBSERVE-5: observational postmarketing safety surveillance registry of etanercept for the treatment of psoriasis final 5-year results. J Am Acad Dermatol. 2015;72(1):115–22.

15. Papp KA, Griffiths CE, Gordon K, Lebwohl M, Szapary PO, Wasfi Y, et al. Long-term safety of ustekinumab in patients with moderate-to-severe psoriasis: final results from 5 years of follow-up. Br J Dermatol. 2013;168(4):844–54.

16. Papp K, Gottlieb AB, Naldi L, Pariser D, Ho V, Goyal K, et al. Safety surveillance for ustekinumab and other psoriasis treatments from the Psoriasis Longitudinal Assessment and Registry (PSOLAR). J Drugs Dermatol. 2015;14(7):706–14.

17. Fieschi C, Casanova JL. The role of interleukin-12 in human infectious diseases: only a faint signature. Eur J Immunol. 2003;33(6):1461–4.

18. van de Vosse E, Ottenhoff TH. Human host genetic factors in mycobacterial and salmonella infection: lessons from single gene disorders in IL-12/IL-23-dependent signaling that affect innate and adaptive immunity. Microbes Infect. 2006;8(4):1167–73.

19. Filipe-Santos O, Bustamante J, Chapgier A, Vogt G, de Beaucoudrey L, Feinberg J, et al. Inborn errors of IL-12/23- and IFN-gamma-mediated immunity: molecular, cellular, and clinical features. Semin Immunol. 2006;18(6):347–61.

20. van de Kerkhof PC, Griffiths CE, Reich K, Leonardi CL, Blauvelt A, Tsai TF, et al. Secukinumab long-term safety experience: a pooled analysis of 10 phase II and III clinical studies in patients with moderate to severe plaque psoriasis. J Am Acad Dermatol. 2016;75(1):83–98. e4

21. Strober B, Leonardi C, Papp KA, Mrowietz U, Ohtsuki M, Bissonnette R, et al. Short and long-term safety outcomes with ixekizumab from 7 clinical trials in psoriasis: etanercept comparisons and integrated data. J Am Acad Dermatol. 2017;76(3):432–440.e17.

22. Farahnik B, Beroukhim K, Abrouk M, Nakamura M, Zhu TH, Singh R, et al. Brodalumab for the treatment of psoriasis: a review of phase III trials. Dermatol Ther (Heidelb). 2016;6(2):111–24.

23. Papp KA, Leonardi C, Menter A, Ortonne JP, Krueger JG, Kricorian G, et al. Brodalumab, an anti-interleukin-17-receptor antibody for psoriasis. N Engl J Med. 2012;366(13):1181–9.

24. Papp K, Leonardi C, Menter A, Thompson EH, Milmont CE, Kricorian G, et al. Safety and efficacy of brodalumab for psoriasis after 120 weeks of treatment. J Am Acad Dermatol. 2014;71(6):1183–90. e3

25. Umezawa Y, Nakagawa H, Niiro H, Ootaki K. Long-term clinical safety and efficacy of brodalumab in the treatment of Japanese patients with moderate-to-severe plaque psoriasis. J Eur Acad Dermatol Venereol. 2016;30(11):1957–60.

26. Papp KA, Reich K, Paul C, Blauvelt A, Baran W, Bolduc C, et al. A prospective phase III, randomized, double-blind, placebo-controlled study of brodalumab in patients with moderate-to-severe plaque psoriasis. Br J Dermatol. 2016;175(2):273–86.

27. Chiricozzi A, Romanelli M, Saraceno R, Torres T. No meaningful association between suicidal behavior and the use of IL-17A-neutralizing or IL-17RA-blocking agents. Expert Opin Drug Saf. 2016;15(12):1653–9.

28. Gelfand JM, Troxel AB, Lewis JD, Kurd SK, Shin DB, Wang X, et al. The risk of mortality in patients with psoriasis: results from a population-based study. Arch Dermatol. 2007;143(12):1493–9.

29. Benson MM, Frishman WH. The heartbreak of psoriasis: a review of cardiovascular risk in patients with psoriasis. Cardiol Rev. 2015.

30. Gulliver WP, Macdonald D, Gladney N, Alaghehbandan R, Rahman P, Adam Baker K. Long-term prognosis and comorbidities associated with psoriasis in the Newfoundland and Labrador founder population. J Cutan Med Surg. 2011;15(1):37–47.

31. Gulliver WP, Young HM, Bachelez H, Randell S, Gulliver S, Al-Mutairi N. Psoriasis patients treated with biologics and methotrexate have a reduced rate of myocardial infarction: a collaborative analysis using international cohorts. J Cutan Med Surg. 2016;20(6):550–4.

32. Ahlehoff O, Skov L, Gislason G, Lindhardsen J, Kristensen SL, Iversen L, et al. Cardiovascular disease event rates in patients with severe psoriasis treated with systemic anti-inflammatory drugs: a Danish real-world cohort study. J Intern Med. 2013;273(2):197–204.

33. Wu JJ, Poon KY, Channual JC, Shen AY. Association between tumor necrosis factor inhibitor therapy and myocardial infarction risk in patients with psoriasis. Arch Dermatol. 2012;148(11):1244–50.

34. Ahlehoff O, Skov L, Gislason G, Gniadecki R, Iversen L, Bryld LE, et al. Cardiovascular outcomes and systemic anti-inflammatory drugs in patients with severe psoriasis: 5-year follow-up of a Danish nationwide cohort. J Eur Acad Dermatol Venereol. 2015;29(6):1128–34.

35. Wu JJ, Guerin A, Sundaram M, Dea K, Cloutier M, Mulani P. Cardiovascular event risk assessment in psoriasis patients treated with tumor necrosis factor-alpha inhibitors versus methotrexate. J Am Acad Dermatol. 2017;76(1):81–90.

36. Hjuler KF, Bottcher M, Vestergaard C, Botker HE, Iversen L, Kragballe K. Association between changes in coronary artery disease progression and treatment with biologic agents for severe psoriasis. JAMA Dermatol. 2016;152(10):1114–21.

37. Kurd SK, Troxel AB, Crits-Christoph P, Gelfand JM. The risk of depression, anxiety, and suicidality in patients with psoriasis: a population-based cohort study. Arch Dermatol. 2010;146(8):891–5.

38. Sanchez-Moya AI, Garcia-Doval I, Carretero G, Sanchez-Carazo J, Ferrandiz C, Herrera Ceballos E, et al. Latent tuberculosis infection and active tuberculosis in patients with psoriasis: a study on the incidence of tuberculosis and the prevalence of latent tuberculosis disease in patients with moderate-severe psoriasis in Spain. BIOBADADERM registry. J Eur Acad Dermatol Venereol. 2013;27(11):1366–74.

39. Garcia-Doval I, Carretero G, Vanaclocha F, Ferrandiz C, Dauden E, Sanchez-Carazo JL, et al. Risk of serious adverse events associated with biologic and nonbiologic psoriasis systemic therapy: patients ineligible vs eligible for randomized controlled trials. Arch Dermatol. 2012;148(4):463–70.

40. Carretero G, Ferrandiz C, Dauden E, Vanaclocha Sebastian F, Gomez-Garcia FJ, Herrera-Ceballos E, et al. Risk of adverse events in psoriasis patients receiving classic systemic drugs and biologics in a 5-year observational study of clinical practice: 2008-2013 results of the Biobadaderm registry. J Eur Acad Dermatol Venereol. 2015;29(1):156–63.

41. Medina C, Carretero G, Ferrandiz C, Dauden E, Vanaclocha F, Gomez-Garcia FJ, et al. Safety of classic and biologic systemic therapies for the treatment of psoriasis in elderly: an observational study from national BIOBADADERM registry. J Eur Acad Dermatol Venereol. 2015;29(5):858–64.

42. Piaserico S, Cazzaniga S, Chimenti S, Giannetti A, Maccarone M, Picardo M, et al. Efficacy of switching between tumor necrosis factor-alfa inhibitors in psoriasis: results from the Italian Psocare Registry. J Am Acad Dermatol. 2014;70(2):257–62. e3

43. Gisondi P, Cazzaniga S, Chimenti S, Giannetti A, Maccarone M, Picardo M, et al. Metabolic abnormalities associated with initiation of systemic treatment for psoriasis: evidence from the Italian Psocare Registry. J Eur Acad Dermatol Venereol. 2013;27(1):e30–41.

44. Gisondi P, Cazzaniga S, Chimenti S, Maccarone M, Picardo M, Girolomoni G, et al. Latent tuberculosis infection in patients with chronic plaque psoriasis: evidence from the Italian Psocare Registry. Br J Dermatol. 2015;172(6):1613–20.

45. Augustin M, Spehr C, Radtke MA, Boehncke WH, Luger T, Mrowietz U, et al. German psoriasis registry PsoBest: objectives,

methodology and baseline data. J Dtsch Dermatol Ges. 2014;12(1):48–57.

46. van Lumig PP, Driessen RJ, Berends MA, Boezeman JB, van de Kerkhof PC, de Jong EM. Safety of treatment with biologics for psoriasis in daily practice: 5-year data. J Eur Acad Dermatol Venereol. 2012;26(3):283–91.

47. van den Reek JM, Tummers M, Zweegers J, Seyger MM, van Lumig PP, Driessen RJ, et al. Predictors of adalimumab drug survival in psoriasis differ by reason for discontinuation: long-term results from the Bio-CAPTURE registry. J Eur Acad Dermatol Venereol. 2015;29(3):560–5.

48. van den Reek JM, Zweegers J, Kievit W, Otero ME, van Lumig PP, Driessen RJ, et al. 'Happy' drug survival of adalimumab, etanercept and ustekinumab in psoriasis in daily practice care: results from the BioCAPTURE network. Br J Dermatol. 2014;171(5):1189–96.

49. Gniadecki R, Kragballe K, Dam TN, Skov L. Comparison of drug survival rates for adalimumab, etanercept and infliximab in patients with psoriasis vulgaris. Br J Dermatol. 2011;164(5):1091–6.

50. Gniadecki R, Bang B, Bryld LE, Iversen L, Lasthein S, Skov L. Comparison of long-term drug survival and safety of biologic agents in patients with psoriasis vulgaris. Br J Dermatol. 2015;172(1):244–52.

51. van Geel MJ, Oostveen AM, Hoppenreijs EP, Hendriks JC, van de Kerkhof PC, de Jong EM, et al. Methotrexate in pediatric plaque-type psoriasis: long-term daily clinical practice results from the child-CAPTURE registry. J Dermatolog Treat. 2015;26(5):406–12.

52. van Geel MJ, Mul K, Oostveen AM, van de Kerkhof PC, de Jong EM, Seyger MM. Calcipotriol/betamethasone dipropionate ointment in mild-to-moderate paediatric psoriasis: long-term daily clinical practice data in a prospective cohort. Br J Dermatol. 2014;171(2):363–9.

53. Mazlin MB, Chang CC, Baba R. Comorbidities associated with psoriasis - data from the Malaysian Psoriasis Registry. Med J Malaysia. 2012;67(5):518–21.

54. Lecluse LL, Naldi L, Stern RS, Spuls PI. National registries of systemic treatment for psoriasis and the European 'Psonet' initiative. Dermatology. 2009;218(4):347–56.

55. Garcia-Doval I, Cohen AD, Cazzaniga S, Feldhamer I, Addis A, Carretero G, et al. Risk of serious infections, cutaneous bacterial infections, and granulomatous infections in patients with psoriasis treated with anti-tumor necrosis factor agents versus classic therapies: prospective meta-analysis of Psonet registries. J Am Acad Dermatol. 2017;76(2):299–308. e16

56. Feldman SR, Zhao Y, Navaratnam P, Friedman HS, Lu J, Tran MH. Patterns of medication utilization and costs associated with the use of etanercept, adalimumab, and ustekinumab in the management of moderate-to-severe psoriasis. J Manag Care Spec Pharm. 2015;21(3):201–9.

57. Cao Z, Carter C, Wilson KL, Schenkel B. Ustekinumab dosing, persistence, and discontinuation patterns in patients with moderate-to-severe psoriasis. J Dermatolog Treat. 2015;26(2):113–20.

58. Reddy SP, Lin EJ, Shah VV, Wu JJ. Persistence and failure rates of adalimumab monotherapy in biologic-naive patients with psoriasis: a retrospective study. J Am Acad Dermatol. 2016;74(3):575–7.

59. Menter A, Papp KA, Gooderham M, Pariser DM, Augustin M, Kerdel FA, et al. Drug survival of biologic therapy in a large, disease-based registry of patients with psoriasis: results from the Psoriasis Longitudinal Assessment and Registry (PSOLAR). J Eur Acad Dermatol Venereol. 2016;30(7):1148–58.

60. Warren RB, Smith CH, Yiu ZZ, Ashcroft DM, Barker JN, Burden AD, et al. Differential drug survival of biologic therapies for the treatment of psoriasis: a prospective observational cohort study from the British Association of Dermatologists Biologic Interventions Register (BADBIR). J Invest Dermatol. 2015;135(11):2632–40.

61. Nast A, Jacobs A, Rosumeck S, Werner RN. Efficacy and safety of systemic long-term treatments for moderate-to-severe psoriasis: a systematic review and meta-analysis. J Invest Dermatol. 2015;135(11):2641–8.

Pharmacoeconomics of Systemic and Biologic Therapy in Dermatology

Martina L. Porter and Alexa B. Kimball

Introduction

With continued rising costs of healthcare in the United States, the application of an economic framework to the health system is unavoidable. Data published on the CDC website estimates total national health expenditures to be $3.0 trillion, accounting for 17.5% of the United States' gross domestic product based on 2014 data [1]. These costs were further broken down into hospital care (32.1%), physician and clinical services (19.9%), and prescription drugs (9.8%) amongst others [1]. Given we have finite resources, we must choose how to best allocate these resources to gain the greatest health benefits overall. Pharmaceutical products, or medications, make up a significant portion of our national healthcare expenditures, and as such, they are becoming more heavily scrutinized for their safety and efficacy as well as their associated costs. With this focus on value-based health care, where value can be defined as patient health outcomes achieved per dollar spent [2], medications now need to prove that they are more than just an effective and tolerable treatment.

Pharmacoeconomics and pharmacoeconomic research first gained traction in the medical literature in the 1980s. Broadly, pharmacoeconomics can be defined as the cost of the pharmaceutical good to the healthcare system or society as a whole, and its goal is to identify the true value of a medication to justify its use in clinical practice [3]. Pharmacoeconomics is unique in that it seeks to quantify not only the economic but also the humanistic and clinical outcomes of pharmacotherapy. In doing so, perspectives of policy makers, payers, physicians, and, most importantly, patients must be considered.

In dermatology, we see the impact of these pharmacoeconomic decisions on a daily basis in our clinical practice. Attempts to curb medication costs, including the prior authorization process, medication tiering, step therapy, and narrowed insurance formularies, are numerous. These strategies are intended for cost containment, but many physicians and patients may view them as impediments to care. In addition to clinical practice, research is also impacted by economics. Clinical trials are often designed to evaluate not only the efficacy of a medication but also their impact directly on patients as reported through patient-reported outcomes (PROs). This additional step of collecting data on patients' experiences is necessary to help justify the true value of a medication beyond its safety, efficacy, or currency cost alone. Thus, understanding the methodology for determining this overall value of pharmaceutical medications may be helpful for dermatologists and may inform treatment decisions or allow dermatologists to better advocate for their patients' care.

From this chapter, we hope to impart a very basic understanding of pharmacoeconomics as it applies to dermatology and, we use systemic therapy with biologic agents for psoriasis as an example to illustrate these concepts.

Basic Principles of Pharmacoeconomics

In order to understand the framework for estimating value of a medication, familiarity with the variables that go into this determination is crucial. As discussed earlier, these variables can be divided into economic, such as costs, versus humanistic and clinical outcomes, including clinical effectiveness and personal effects on patients (Fig. 10.1). Each of these concepts is reviewed in the subsequent text. These three inputs, economic, humanistic, and clinical, are then applied to a cost analysis model to calculate a final output, or value.

M.L. Porter, MD
Department of Dermatology, Clinical Laboratory for Epidemiology and Applied Research in Skin (CLEARS), Beth Israel Deaconess Medical Center, 330 Brookline Avenue, Boston, MA 02215, USA

A.B. Kimball, MD, MPH (✉)
Department of Dermatology, Harvard Medical School, Beth Israel Deaconess Medical Center, 375 Longwood Ave, Boston, MA 02215, USA
e-mail: harvardskinstudies@gmail.com; kimballmdresearch@gmail.com

© Springer International Publishing AG 2018
P.S. Yamauchi (ed.), *Biologic and Systemic Agents in Dermatology*, https://doi.org/10.1007/978-3-319-66884-0_10

Fig. 10.1 Framework of pharmacoeconomics

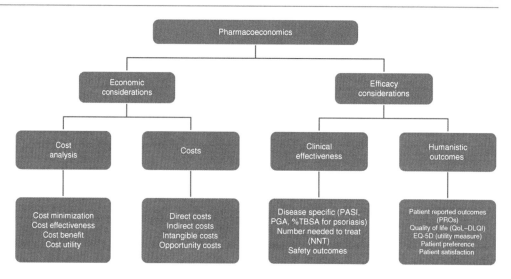

Depending on the perspective of the analysis or the desired final endpoint, some costs and/or outcomes may be prioritized over others, and different pharmacoeconomic cost analyses can be employed.

Costs

In order to compute the total costs, we must first know the costs for which we need to account. Definitions of these different costs are as follows and are also outlined in Fig. 10.2.

Direct costs are the costs incurred directly to the healthcare system for payment of medical products and services [4]. Examples include medications, laboratory and diagnostic testing, radiology services, medical supplies, durable medical equipment, physician fees, medical personnel fees, hospitalizations, rehabilitation, and long-term care. Theoretically, these transactional costs should be the easiest to measure, but pricing for many of these services and even pharmaceuticals is not always transparent as exemplified by drug pricing, which is detailed below.

Indirect costs are those that often result from morbidity or mortality, such as loss of productivity, loss of livelihood, or loss of life. These costs can result from premature death, disability, missed work, or decreased earning potential [4]. Also included in this is "presenteeism" where the patient may be present at work but still unable to perform his or her job functions, leading to lost productivity [5]. For a patient, presenteeism may allow the patient to avoid lost wages from being absent from work. However, in contrast, the estimated cost to society of presenteeism may be greater than absenteeism [6]. As an aside, this exemplifies the idea that costs can be different based on the perspective of those incurring the costs. Indirect costs, in general, are much more difficult to measure as they often require some conversion factor to quantify currency lost, but these may have a greater impact on patients and society as a whole.

In clinical trials, measurement of the indirect costs, such as absenteeism or presenteeism, can be estimated through patient-reported productivity scales, such as the Work Productivity and Activity Impairment (WPAI) Questionnaire, the Work Limitation Questionnaire (WLQ), the Sheehan Disability Scale (SDS), or the Health and Work Performance Questionnaire (HPQ). These are commonly employed in trials to better describe the impact of medications. For example, in the CLEAR trial, which compared secukinumab to ustekinumab, the WPAI was employed to estimate the indirect costs of psoriasis in Germany as correlated with Psoriasis Area Severity Index (PASI) scores. This study found that improvements in psoriasis of PASI ≥90 were associated with significantly decreased productivity loss (less than 2 h per week) compared to patients with poorly controlled moderate-to-severe psoriasis who lost >8 h of productivity per week due to psoriasis symptoms [7].

Intangible costs may be even more difficult to measure than indirect costs as they represent the costs of pain, suffering, grief, or other distresses that patients or their family members may suffer as a result of disease and medical care.

Opportunity cost is essentially a measure of the benefits lost when selecting one therapeutic option over another. For example, if one only had time to either go shopping or to the gym, then the opportunity cost of going shopping is any benefit that may have been derived from going to the gym for exercise. In our healthcare system, the opportunity cost of allocation of funds towards medications is the potential health gain that is foregone had those funds been applied elsewhere, such as towards social services or inpatient hospital care.

One of the difficulties with pharmacoeconomic analyses, specifically, is figuring out what a medication actually costs. The supply chain for pharmaceuticals grossly follows the order of pharmaceutical manufacturer to wholesaler or direct purchaser to pharmacy and then consumer or patient. With each step, price markups, rebates, or discounts may be applied, which can make pricing difficult to interpret. Wholesale

Fig. 10.2 Breakdown of costs associated with pharmacoeconomic modeling

Direct costs	Indirect costs	Intangible costs	Opportunity costs

• Medical
  • Medications
  • Lab tests
  • Radiology
  • Inpatient
   hospitalization
  • Durable
   medical
   equipment
  • Physician fees
  • Personnel fees
  • Medical
   supplies
• Nonmedical
  • Transportation
  • Food
  • Home help
	• Lost wages
	• Lost income due
	  to premature
	  death
	• Loss of
	  livelihood
	• Loss of life
	• Loss of
	  productivity
		• Pain
		• Suffering
		• Grief
		• Inconvenience
			• Lost opportunity
			• Revenue
			  forgone

acquisition costs (WAC) are often used in pharmacoeconomic modeling. The WAC is often published in price guides and is an estimate of the manufacturer's direct price without any rebates or discounts [8]. We will use this cost in our example of biologic therapy later in this chapter. Other costs that may be used in modeling are the average wholesale price (AWP), which is an estimate of the average price at which wholesalers sell drugs, often likened to the "list price" [8]. The average manufacturer price (AMP), which is defined by federal law and is the price charged by the manufacturer to wholesalers or pharmacies after discounts, is often not published [8].

Humanistic Outcomes

Humanistic outcomes often attempt to capture the emotional status of patients, and are sometimes considered to be under the umbrella of clinical effectiveness as well. Psychological stress and disability due to disease can have profound impact on patients' self-esteem, well-being, and health-related quality of life (HRQoL) and can be quantified. Other measures of humanistic outcomes include patient satisfaction and patient preference. In pharmaceutical clinical trials, patient-reported outcomes (PROs) are often used as endpoints in addition to physician-reported assessments of disease severity. The Food and Drug Administration (FDA) sets forth recommendations for the specific methodology of development of new PROs. These PROs measure patients' daily abilities and feelings in response to therapy as reported by patients, often in the form of questionnaires.

The Dermatology Life Quality Index (DLQI) is a routinely employed PRO in dermatology and is often used as a meaningful endpoint in clinical trials. The DLQI is a skin-specific HRQoL measure that was originally developed in 1994. Within 10 years of its initial publication, it was employed in over 85 peer-reviewed articles covering a wide range of skin diseases and dermatologic medications [9]. It consists of ten questions about daily activities, relationships, work, school, leisure, symptoms, and feelings. Responses are measured on a Likert scale and scored out of a total of 30, with higher scores suggesting greater levels of impairment. The DLQI is unique to dermatology in that it evaluates skin-related symptoms; however, this prevents these scores from being compared to QoL scores in other non-dermatologic diseases.

Utility scores in health economic analyses aim to measure the value of different health states based on patient preference [10]. As patients transition from one health state to another, often as a result of therapy, the utility score attempts to capture the patient satisfaction as patients go to a more or less desirable health state [11]. Scores range from zero to one where one side of the spectrum is as bad as death versus the other side being full health or no problems. In practice, these utility scores are often based on standardized instruments completed by patients that evaluate HRQoL. The EuroQol-5 Dimension (EQ-5D) is a generic QoL instrument that measures mobility, self-care, usual activities, pain, discomfort, anxiety, and depression across multiple diseases, and it is regularly used in cost analyses [10]. The EQ-5D is not commonly employed in dermatology though and may not be sensitive enough to show disease. Use of some components of the EQ-5D has been reported in psoriasis, hidradenitis suppurativa, chronic leg ulcers, and hand eczema [12]. Few studies though have evaluated the relationship between EQ-5D, PASI, and DLQI and found a moderate correlation amongst scores [10]. During the secukinumab randomized controlled trials, EQ-5D and PASI were measured simultaneously. The National Institute for Health and Care Excellence (NICE) publishes guidelines for medication use after evaluating clinical effectiveness and cost-effectiveness for new medications in the United Kingdom. The NICE technology assessment for secukinumab directly converted PASI scores into utility scores based on the EQ-5D and PASI data from the trial for evaluation in cost-effectiveness models. This conversion has been cited in other cost analyses for biologic medications in the United States as detailed in the example at the end of this chapter.

Measurements of Clinical Effectiveness

Clinical effectiveness aims to capture the safety and efficacy of pharmaceuticals in treating a medical condition. Safety data related to medications is described initially in clinical trials where adverse events are reported and evaluated. This data is relatively limited in nature by the small, selected sample size and short duration of the study as compared to widespread adoption of the medication following FDA approval. Therefore, post-marketing surveillance is also essential for determining the true safety outcomes of a medication.

Clinical effectiveness data is usually acquired from a physician evaluation of patient disease. One method for measuring clinical efficacy is through a disease-specific endpoint. For clinical trials, the FDA often requires a physician's global assessment, which is the investigator's overall assessment of extent of disease improvement or worsening compared to baseline. In psoriasis, affected total body surface area, PASI, and the Physicians Global Assessment (PGA) are the most commonly used disease-specific endpoint in clinical practice and clinical trials. Improvements in scores

for these validated measures are acceptable for quality reporting guidelines for reimbursement as well as FDA approval for new systemic psoriasis medications. Disease-specific endpoints though are not generalizable and do not allow for comparisons in clinical effectiveness amongst different diseases.

A second method of measuring clinical effectiveness is through a calculation of number needed to treat (NNT), which is relatively easy to calculate from dermatology clinical trial data, and the NNT can be compared across various diseases or treatments. NNT can be defined as the number of patients on average that need to be treated to achieve one additional gain as compared to standard therapy or placebo [13]. NNT is the inverse of the absolute risk reduction (Fig. 10.3). Assuming that the therapy is better than placebo, low NNTs are desirable with the ideal NNT equal to one. NNT can be used to compare efficacy across disease states and specialties.

The phase III clinical trials for the biologic agents used to treat psoriasis usually compared these agents to placebo with more recently approved agents compared to placebo, methotrexate, and/or etanercept. PASI 75 was generally employed as a clinically meaningful endpoint for these trials, and this endpoint was evaluated after the standard dosing for the first 10–16 weeks of treatment. The percentage of patients that achieved PASI 75 as compared to placebo can be used to calculate and compare the NNT for each individual agent against placebo (Table 10.1) [14–19]. As evidenced from these trials, biologic therapy

Calculation of NNT

$NNT = 1/ARR$

$ARR = Pt - Pc$

NNT: Number needed to treat, usually rounded to nearest whole number
ARR: Absolute Risk Reduction, Difference in events rate between control (Pc) and treatment (Pt) groups

Example

In a clinical trial of moderate to severe psoriasis, Systemic Drug X was compared to placebo for achievement of PASI 75 as the primary endpoint. A total of 103 patients received systemic drug X and 107 received placebo. Of those receiving Systemic Drug X, 45.6% (43/107) achieved PASI 75 compared to 12.1% (13/107) who received placebo. What is the NNT?

	Achieved PASI 75	Did not achieve PASI 75	Total patients	Event rate of those achieving PASI 75 (%)
Systemic drug X	47	56	103	45.6
Placebo	13	94	107	12.1

$NNT = 1/(0.456 - 0.121) = 2.99$

Thus, NNT is 3. This implies that 3 patients need to be treated with systemic drug X in order for 1 additional patient to achieve PASI 75.

Fig. 10.3 Calculation of number needed to treat (NNT) [13]

Table 10.1 Example of efficacy and number needed to treat of biologic agents

Biologic agent (dosing, clinical trial time endpoint)	PASI 75 of treated group (%)	PASI 75 of control group (%)	Number needed to treat (NNT)
Methotrexate (7.5 mg PO q week, increased as tolerated to 25 mg weekly, after 16 weeks) [16]	35.5	19	6.1
Etanercept (50 mg BIW, after 12 weeks) [14]	49	4	2.2
Infliximab (5 mg/kg, after 10 weeks) [15]	88	6	1.2
Adalimumab (40 mg q every other week) [16] (CHAMPION Trial)	80	19	1.6
Ustekinumab (90 mg q 3 months, after 12 weeks) [17]	67	3	1.6
Secukinumab (300 mg q 4 weeks, after 12 weeks) [19]	82	5	1.3
Ixekizumab (80 mg, after 12 weeks) [18]	90	2	1.1

is far more effective than methotrexate, and the newer agents were better able to achieve PASI 75 as evidenced by the lower NNT. The NNT for secukinumab is 1.1, meaning that we need to treat 11 patients in order for 10 to have a positive response, which was defined as PASI 75 in our scenario.

For clinicians, NNT is a relatively straightforward representation of the effect of treatment, but it still does not directly quantify costs.

Types of Cost Analyses

Once inputs (costs, humanistic outcomes, and clinical effectiveness) are defined for the cost analysis, the next step in conducting a cost analyses is choosing the specific model. The most common cost analyses are cost identification, cost-benefit, and cost-effectiveness analyses.

A *cost identification*, or cost minimization, analysis of drug therapy looks solely at the costs of a pharmaceutical agent or intervention without evaluating any benefits. The final output is in currency or dollars. Through a cost identification model, a price per service can be calculated. Since health outcomes are not factored into this equation, a cost identification analysis is best suited for the comparison of two therapies where the health outcomes, such as therapeutic efficacy and safety, are assumed to be equal or better for the drug that is of lower cost agent [4].

Cost-benefit analyses also use currency or dollars as its unit of measurement. The total cost of the treatment is compared to the total benefits (converted into dollar equivalents) and expressed as a ratio of benefits to costs. Because both units are in dollars, explicit net benefits or net costs can be calculated. The difficulty with this model may be quantifying the total benefits into a unit of currency.

Cost-effectiveness analyses compare costs to outcomes of the proposed pharmaceutical intervention. Because costs are measured in dollars, or other currency, and outcomes tend to be measured in or converted into non-currency units, such as utilities or years of life, the final output is a ratio of cost per unit outcome. The cost-effectiveness analysis allows for comparisons of treatments with different safety or efficacy outcomes, but it does not directly compare the costs of each treatment. It is best utilized to assess cost optimization or incremental improvements in clinical effectiveness for unit cost but does not determine the lowest cost treatment. When the outcomes are measured in utilities, the model is called a *cost utility* analysis.

The Markov model is a particular model used for cost-effectiveness analyses and is well suited for the modeling of chronic diseases over time. In this model, defined disease states are established within the greater context of the disease of interest, and the probability of transitioning between each disease state over a set time period is established. Healthcare costs and outcomes are attached to both the disease states and the transitions, which allows for estimation of cost-effectiveness [20].

Two cost-effectiveness ratios exist, the average cost-effectiveness ratio (ACER) and the incremental cost-effectiveness ratio (ICER). The ACER is calculated as healthcare cost per clinical outcome. The ICER is calculated as the difference between the costs in treatment over the difference in effect. Thus, ICER is used to answer the question of whether the increased benefit is worth the increased cost.

The quality-adjust life year (QALY) is a common unit of measurement of health improvement used in cost-effectiveness analyses. On the simplest level, the QALY assigns a weighted value to health benefits over a particular time period [21]. If utility scores are used as measure of the health state, then a psoriasis patient with a utility score of 0.7 would be expected to have 7 QALYs over a 10-year time horizon (0.7×10) [22].

In addition, a sensitivity analysis may be employed after results are obtained from a cost-effectiveness model. Because a certain amount of uncertainty is inherent in assumptions made in designing the model, the goal of a sensitivity analysis is to determine the significance of this uncertainty and the overall robustness of the final conclusion of the model [4]. Various types of sensitivity analyses, with increasing levels of sophistication, can be employed [23].

Psoriasis and Health Economic Analyses

Psoriasis is a chronic skin condition that causes significant morbidity but is generally not thought to cause mortality. As such, it requires lifelong therapy to control the symptoms or skin manifestations of the disease, but no cure currently exists for psoriasis. It is well known that psoriasis patients report significant impact of their disease on QoL and that improvement of disease through systemic treatment can improve QoL for these patients [24]. Over the last decade, targeted biologic therapies for psoriasis have been developed with ever-increasing efficacy, and many patients can now achieve and maintain clearance of their skin disease, which was unfathomable many years ago. These new treatments though come at considerably greater direct cost as compared to previous, non-targeted treatments for psoriasis. Because of this cost, many patients and providers experience difficulty obtaining these medications despite their great efficacy. This is a classic example of costs versus clinical effectiveness, making it well suited for demonstrating the role for pharmacoeconomic modeling.

In psoriasis clinical trials for systemic agents, we are fortunate that the design of the clinical trials for most agents is similar with employment of identical clinical assessment tools and patient-reported outcome measures. This allows for general comparability between psoriasis trials, and subsequent cost analyses are greatly enabled by this comparability.

A 2016 review of the literature for psoriasis and health economic analyses by Gutknecht et al. summarized the available published data [25]. They found a recent increase in studies focused on biologic agents. They also identified cost-effectiveness models as the most commonly employed, but these studies used varying methods and outcome measures, limiting the ability to compare results. Also, direct costs were generally included whereas indirect costs were neglected in the majority of the studies. Finally, a disproportionate number of studies came from the United Kingdom where NICE independently examines the cost-effectiveness of pharmaceuticals, suggesting that standardization of methods and outcome measures may lead to more interpretable and directly comparable results.

Pharmacoeconomics in Practice: Targeted Systemic Therapy for Psoriasis

As noted previously, the use of standardized measurements in psoriasis clinical trials, such as PASI, PGA, and DLQI scoring, allows for straightforward comparability, and as a result, cost-effectiveness is relatively easy to model. Around 2005, evaluations of cost-effectiveness of systemic therapy started to get published, likely due to the increased prevalence, uptake, and cost of biologic agents for systemic psoriasis

therapy. Since then, multiple studies looking at NNT and cost-effectiveness have been published for psoriasis. In 2008, Nelson et al. published a cost-effectiveness analysis for biologic agents (adalimumab, etanercept, and infliximab) over a 12-week period. The authors initially performed a literature review and meta-analysis and looked at the efficacy of the biologic agents at 12 weeks based on DLQI improvement and PASI 75 scores. Costs were estimated for the drugs, and an ICER was calculated with a sensitivity analysis to determine the most cost-effective biologic agents [26]. D'Souza and Payette performed a cost-effectiveness analysis for all systemic agents used in psoriasis in 2015. They also conducted a literature review to find the efficacy of medications achieving PASI 75. Using this data, NNT was calculated as were the direct costs associated with PASI 75 achievement for each therapy, and total costs for each systemic therapy were defined and compared [27]. Armstrong et al. also explored a cost analysis for methotrexate versus apremilast and used data from previous clinical trials for apremilast and adalimumab that compared these medications to methotrexate and/or placebo. Through their analysis, the incremental drug cost per responder and NNT were calculated using direct medication costs only, and the authors concluded that a significant cost was associated with apremilast without greater efficacy as compared to methotrexate [28].

With a basic understanding of pharmacoeconomics, we can now evaluate, or at least better understand, if these systemic biologic agents fill an important need or demonstrate a value relative to their cost that may better justify their use in treating moderate-to-severe plaque psoriasis. Unfortunately, no government-sponsored equivalent to NICE exists in the United States, but the Institute for Clinical and Economic Review (also ICER), an independent nonprofit organization that receives funding from various sources, including industry, published their health economic analysis focusing on effectiveness and value of targeted immunomodulators as compared to non-targeted therapy for the treatment of moderate-to-severe plaque psoriasis [29]. Independent of their findings, the cost-effectiveness model designed and employed to evaluate their endpoints will serve as a suitable example for demonstration of the role of these types of models in the valuation of pharmaceutical medications. The steps performed by ICER as part of the model are outlined in Fig. 10.4.

The ICER model examined each systemic agent as first-line therapy for efficacy [29]. Agents that were examined included adalimumab, etanercept, infliximab, ustekinumab, secukinumab, ixekizumab, brodalumab, and apremilast. Measurements of clinical effectiveness included PASI scores, the DLQI, and adverse events. All were found to be superior to placebo for achievement of PASI 75 with the newer agents, ixekizumab, secukinumab, and ustekinumab, also being superior to etanercept. Secukinumab, ixekizumab,

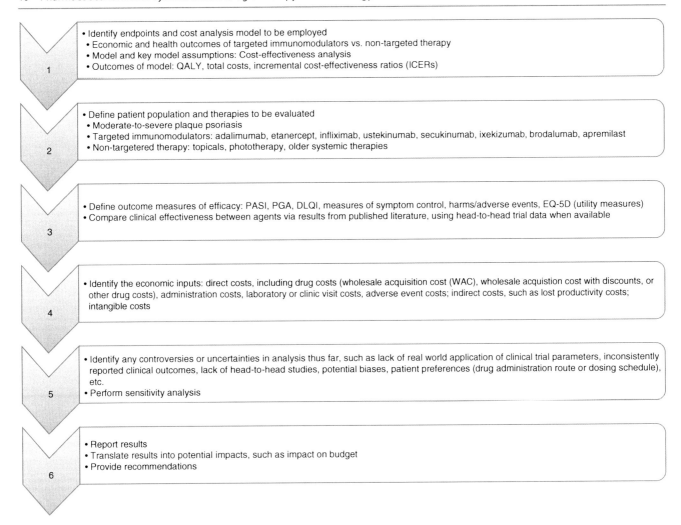

1
- Identify endpoints and cost analysis model to be employed
- Economic and health outcomes of targeted immunomodulators vs. non-targeted therapy
- Model and key model assumptions: Cost-effectiveness analysis
- Outcomes of model: QALY, total costs, incremental cost-effectiveness ratios (ICERs)

2
- Define patient population and therapies to be evaluated
- Moderate-to-severe plaque psoriasis
- Targeted immunomodulators: adalimumab, etanercept, infliximab, ustekinumab, secukinumab, ixekizumab, brodalumab, apremilast
- Non-targetered therapy: topicals, phototherapy, older systemic therapies

3
- Define outcome measures of efficacy: PASI, PGA, DLQI, measures of symptom control, harms/adverse events, EQ-5D (utility measures)
- Compare clinical effectiveness between agents via results from published literature, using head-to-head trial data when available

4
- Identify the economic inputs: direct costs, including drug costs (wholesale acquisition cost (WAC), wholesale acquistion cost with discounts, or other drug costs), administration costs, laboratory or clinic visit costs, adverse event costs; indirect costs, such as lost productivity costs; intangible costs

5
- Identify any controversies or uncertainties in analysis thus far, such as lack of real world application of clinical trial parameters, inconsistently reported clinical outcomes, lack of head-to-head studies, potential biases, patient preferences (drug administration route or dosing schedule), etc.
- Perform sensitivity analysis

6
- Report results
- Translate results into potential impacts, such as impact on budget
- Provide recommendations

Fig. 10.4 Detailed steps of a cost-effectiveness analysis

and brodalumab were also identified as superior to ustekinumab. Identified sources of uncertainty were application to real-world situations, specifically that trials limited concurrent use of topicals, dosing of medications in practice may not follow package inserts, and long-term efficacy and safety data may not be available.

Subsequently, a cost-effectiveness analysis was performed, and cost per QALY gained was determined through calculation of the incremental cost-effectiveness ratio of each therapy compared to non-targeted therapy. For QALY determination, PASI scores were converted to utility scores using the NICE data from the secukinumab trial. Costs were chosen based on the WAC with discounts factored in that were assumed to better reflect actual prices, and non-targeted therapy costs were estimated. All of systemic medications were found to be within or below the cited "reasonable" value in the US cost per QALY range of $100,000–$150,000. Of note though, only adalimumab, apremilast, and infliximab fell into this range without drug discounts applied. In conclusion, ICER stated that all targeted immunomodulators

demonstrated good value, and as such, they recommended abolishing step therapy or amending it to decrease higher out-of-pocket expenses for different targeted therapies [29].

A second article by Shahwan and Kimball presented a cost identification analysis that evaluated dose escalation of biologic agents for treatment of psoriasis [30]. They presented costs, based on WAC obtained from Redbook, and speculated that increased dosing of biologic therapy, often a doubling of dosage, essentially increases the WAC twofold. Thus, since the WAC of maintenance dosing of biologic agents is similar, it may be more cost effective to switch to a more efficacious agent rather than increasing the dosing of the current biologic medication. WAC costs of selected biologic agents are presented in Table 10.2.

One of the biggest limitations of both of these studies was the lack of transparency of drug pricing. Since neither study could ascertain the prices being paid by wholesalers or pharmacies, inherent inaccuracies will continue to exist for such pharmacoeconomic models.

Table 10.2 Costs of annual biologic therapy and clinical effectiveness

	Initial dosing	Maintenance dosing	Total cost for first year of therapy (initial dose + maintenance dosing)[a]	Annual cost after first year (maintenance dosing only)[a]	Clinical effectiveness
Etanercept	50 mg twice weekly × 3 months	50 mg weekly, starting at week 12	Initial (3 months) + maintenance: $67,386	$53,909	PASI 75: 34–49%
Adalimumab	80 mg once at week 0	40 mg every other week, starting at week 2	Initial (2 weeks) + maintenance: $58,045	$53,899	PASI 75: 68–80%
Ustekinumab	≤100 kg 45 mg at weeks 0 and 4	45 mg q12 weeks, starting at week 16	Initial (16 weeks) + maintenance: $58,966	$39,311	PASI 75: 66–76%
	> kg 90 mg at weeks 0 and 4	90 mg q12 weeks, starting at week 16	Initial (16 weeks) + maintenance: $117,933	$78,622	PASI 75: 66–76%
Secukinumab	300 mg weekly × 5 weeks	300 mg q4 weeks, starting at week 9 (option to decrease to 150 mg q4 weeks)	Initial (9 weeks) + maintenance: $70,195	$57,033 $28,517[b]	PASI 75: 67–82%
Ixekizumab	160 mg at week 0, then 80 mg q2 weeks for weeks 2–12	80 mg q4 weeks, starting at week 16	Initial (16 weeks) + maintenance: $83,714	$59,093	PASI 75: 81–89%

Adapted from "Managing the dose escalation of biologics in an era of cost containment: the need for a rational strategy," by K.T. Shahwan and A.B. Kimball, 2016, *International Journal of Women's Dermatology*, p. 151–153
[a]Prices are based on wholesale acquisition prices (WAC) and do not include any rebates or discounts
[b]Price based on the 300 mg package split into two 150 mg doses

Conclusion

We hope that a basic understanding of the principles underlying pharmacoeconomic evaluation of systemic therapy will allow dermatologists to better evaluate cost analysis studies and to make informed treatment decisions in regard to value of medications. Unfortunately, there is no absolute standard cutoff for medication pricing or value, and costs and benefits of medications are different from the perspective of society, payers, patients, and providers, which makes cost analyses more difficult to perform and interpret. As we continue to see healthcare costs rise, we will find that pharmaceutical decisions may be based upon the best overall value treatment regardless of total cost, or that these decisions may be based upon meeting cost containment benchmarks, leaving providers to find the best therapy within a price range. As a specialty, we should continue to provide updated treatment guidelines, such as for systemic therapy in psoriasis, that reflect both treatment efficacy and value.

References

1. Statistics CNCfH. Health expenditures CDC. 2016. https://www.cdc.gov/nchs/fastats/health-expenditures.htm.
2. Porter ME. What is value in health care? N Engl J Med. 2010;363(26):2477–81.
3. Trask LS. Chapter 1: Pharmacoeconomics: principles, methods, and applications. In: JT DP, Talbert RL, Yee GC, Matzke GR, Wells BG, Posey LM, editors. Pharmacotherapy: a pathophysiologic approach, 8e. New York, NY: McGraw-Hill; 2011.
4. Eisenberg JM. Clinical economics. A guide to the economic analysis of clinical practices. JAMA. 1989;262(20):2879–86.
5. Schmitt JM, Ford DE. Work limitations and productivity loss are associated with health-related quality of life but not with clinical severity in patients with psoriasis. Dermatology. 2006;213(2):102–10.
6. Hemp P. Presenteeism: at work—but out of it. Harv Bus Rev. 2004;82(10):49–58. 155
7. Graham CN, McBride D, Miles L, Kneidl J, Mollon P. Estimation of indirect (work-related productivity) costs associated with moderate-to-severe plaque psoriasis in Germany. Value Health. 2015;18(7):A419.
8. Gencarelli DM. One pill, many prices: variation in prescription drug prices in selected government programs. Issue Brief George Wash Univ Natl Health Policy Forum. 2005;807:1–20.
9. Lewis V, Finlay AY. 10 years experience of the dermatology life quality index (DLQI). J Investig Dermatol Symp Proc. 2004;9(2):169–80.
10. Herédi E, Rencz F, Balogh O, Gulácsi L, Herszényi K, Holló P, et al. Exploring the relationship between EQ-5D, DLQI and PASI, and mapping EQ-5D utilities: a cross-sectional study in psoriasis from Hungary. Eur J Health Econ. 2014;15(Suppl 1):S111–9.
11. Walley T, Haycox A. Pharmacoeconomics: basic concepts and terminology. Br J Clin Pharmacol. 1997;43(4):343–8.
12. Riis PT, Vinding GR, Ring HC, Jemec GB. Disutility in patients with hidradenitis suppurativa: a cross-sectional study using EuroQoL-5D. Acta Derm Venereol. 2016;96(2):222–6.
13. Manriquez JJ, Villouta MF, Williams HC. Evidence-based dermatology: number needed to treat and its relation to other risk measures. J Am Acad Dermatol. 2007;56(4):664–71.
14. Leonardi CL, Powers JL, Matheson RT, Goffe BS, Zitnik R, Wang A, et al. Etanercept as monotherapy in patients with psoriasis. N Engl J Med. 2003;349(21):2014–22.
15. Gottlieb AB, Evans R, Li S, Dooley LT, Guzzo CA, Baker D, et al. Infliximab induction therapy for patients with severe plaque-type

psoriasis: a randomized, double-blind, placebo-controlled trial. J Am Acad Dermatol. 2004;51(4):534–42.

16. Saurat JH, Stingl G, Dubertret L, Papp K, Langley RG, Ortonne JP, et al. Efficacy and safety results from the randomized controlled comparative study of adalimumab vs. methotrexate vs. placebo in patients with psoriasis (CHAMPION). Br J Dermatol. 2008;158(3):558–66.

17. Leonardi CL, Kimball AB, Papp KA, Yeilding N, Guzzo C, Wang Y, et al. Efficacy and safety of ustekinumab, a human interleukin-12/23 monoclonal antibody, in patients with psoriasis: 76-week results from a randomised, double-blind, placebo-controlled trial (PHOENIX 1). Lancet. 2008;371(9625):1665–74.

18. Griffiths CE, Reich K, Lebwohl M, van de Kerkhof P, Paul C, Menter A, et al. Comparison of ixekizumab with etanercept or placebo in moderate-to-severe psoriasis (UNCOVER-2 and UNCOVER-3): results from two phase 3 randomised trials. Lancet. 2015;386(9993):541–51.

19. Langley RG, Elewski BE, Lebwohl M, Reich K, Griffiths CE, Papp K, et al. Secukinumab in plaque psoriasis--results of two phase 3 trials. N Engl J Med. 2014;371(4):326–38.

20. Briggs A, Sculpher M. An introduction to Markov modelling for economic evaluation. Pharmacoeconomics. 1998;13(4):397–409.

21. Weinstein MC, Torrance G, McGuire A. QALYs: the basics. Value Health. 2009;12(Suppl 1):S5–9.

22. Whitehead SJ, Ali S. Health outcomes in economic evaluation: the QALY and utilities. Br Med Bull. 2010;96:5–21.

23. Jain R, Grabner M, Onukwugha E. Sensitivity analysis in cost-effectiveness studies: from guidelines to practice. Pharmacoeconomics. 2011;29(4):297–314.

24. Mease PJ, Menter MA. Quality-of-life issues in psoriasis and psoriatic arthritis: outcome measures and therapies from a dermatological perspective. J Am Acad Dermatol. 2006;54(4):685–704.

25. Gutknecht M, Krensel M, Augustin M. Health economic analyses of psoriasis management: a systematic literature search. Arch Dermatol Res. 2016;308(9):601–16.

26. Nelson AA, Pearce DJ, Fleischer AB, Balkrishnan R, Feldman SR. Cost-effectiveness of biologic treatments for psoriasis based on subjective and objective efficacy measures assessed over a 12-week treatment period. J Am Acad Dermatol. 2008;58(1):125–35.

27. D'Souza LS, Payette MJ. Estimated cost efficacy of systemic treatments that are approved by the US Food and Drug Administration for the treatment of moderate to severe psoriasis. J Am Acad Dermatol. 2015;72(4):589–98.

28. Armstrong AW, Betts KA, Sundaram M, Thomason D, Signorovitch JE. Comparative efficacy and incremental cost per responder of methotrexate versus apremilast for methotrexate-naïve patients with psoriasis. J Am Acad Dermatol. 2016;75(4):740–6.

29. (ICER) IfCaER. Targeted immunomodulators for the treatment of moderate-to-severe plaque psoriasis: effectiveness and value. 2016. https://icer-review.org/wp-content/uploads/2016/12/NE_CEPAC_Psoriasis_Evidence_Report_FINAL_120216.pdf.

30. Shahwan K, Kimball A. Managing the dose escalation of biologics in an era of cost containment: the need for a rational strategy. Int J Womens Dermatol. 2016;2(4):151–3.

Immunogenicity of Biologic Agents in Psoriasis

11

Alexandra G. Florek and Kennethk B. Gordon

Psoriasis is a common, chronic, immune-mediated disease that requires long-term treatment and has considerable impact on the quality of life of patients. Through the expanding knowledge of psoriasis pathogenesis, therapy has evolved from topical agents to phototherapy, to oral systemic therapies, and finally to biological therapies including fusion proteins and monoclonal antibodies.

Biological therapies have revolutionized the treatment of moderate-to-severe psoriasis. Over the last decade, a number of systemic biologic agents (including etanercept, infliximab, adalimumab, ustekinumab, secukinumab, ixekizumab) have been approved by the United States Food and Drug administration for the treatment of moderate-to-severe plaque psoriasis. They have become the gold standard for psoriasis in terms of efficacy, safety, and quality of life for the patients [1, 2]. Nevertheless, a significant number of patients fail to respond to these agents (primary nonresponse) or they experience a loss of efficacy over time following an initial response (secondary nonresponse or loss of response). In particular, while the reasons for the loss of response may be varied, one of the most often considered is the development of an immune reaction to the biologic medication itself. A review of the nature of these immune responses, referred to as immunogenicity and its potential effect on therapy, is the subject of this chapter.

Immunogenicity: An Introduction

In the recent years, immunogenicity has been implicated as one of the key mechanisms leading to reduced clinical efficacy and adverse events with biologic drugs [3–5].

A.G. Florek, MD
Department of Dermatology, Feinberg School of Medicine, Northwestern University, Chicago, IL, USA

K.B. Gordon, MD (✉)
Department of Dermatology, Medical College of Wisconsin, 9200 W. Wisconsin Ave., Milwaukee, WI 53226, USA
e-mail: kegordon@mcw.edu; gordon.kenneth@att.net

Immunogenicity is the development of antidrug antibodies (ADAs) against a specific antigen or epitope of the biologic protein. As a result, the biologic agent's full therapeutic effect may be blocked, potentially leading to reduced clinical efficacy and/or adverse events [3, 4, 6, 7]. Consequently, patients initially responding to a biologic agent may develop acquired drug resistance and gradual drug failure, and other patients may need to discontinue the biologic agent due to allergic reactions that at worst can result in infusion reactions or anaphylaxis [8].

The impact of immunogenicity on clinical outcomes remains to be fully elucidated, as only a fraction of the primary or secondary failures may be attributable to ADA development. A clinically significant reduction in therapeutic efficacy is observed in patients developing ADAs, but whether other mechanisms could be potentially responsible for the decline in the therapeutic response is not yet fully known. For instance, some patients who are not responders do not have any detectable levels of ADAs. In other words, these patients may be experiencing therapeutic failure due to a mechanism other than ADA development. Moreover, some patients show detectable levels of ADAs despite the fact that they have excellent clinical response.

Mechanisms of Immunogenicity of Biologics

ADAs targeted towards monoclonal antibodies may reduce their efficacy by one of the two mechanisms: by binding to the cytokine-binding site of the monoclonal antibody (neutralizing antibodies) or by promoting immune-complex clearance (neutralizing and non-neutralizing antibodies) [9]. Additionally, the presence of ADAs does not necessarily signal treatment failure, provided that the concentration of unbound active drug does not decrease below the therapeutic levels [10].

Biologic therapies are of two basic types. Receptor fusion proteins that bind to the target through the naturally occurring receptors and monoclonal antibodies that acquire their

© Springer International Publishing AG 2018
P.S. Yamauchi (ed.), *Biologic and Systemic Agents in Dermatology*, https://doi.org/10.1007/978-3-319-66884-0_11

93

specificity for the target based on an antibody-binding site. Monoclonal antibodies are categorized into four groups based on their molecular structure: murine, chimeric, humanized, or fully human. It is now known that all fusion proteins and monoclonal antibodies, including those that are fully human, are immunogenic, that is, they have the ability to induce an immune response in the treated patient [7, 11–13]. The first therapeutic antibodies were of mouse origin and were highly immunogenic as they represented xenogeneic proteins, or proteins that originated from other organisms. Murine biological drugs induced antidrug antibodies against the murine variable and constant domains, which consequently limited their therapeutic efficacy [14]. Chimeric antibodies, such as infliximab, in contrast, are composed of human constant domains and murine variable domains, making them less immunogenic than murine antibodies [15, 16]. Humanized antibodies contain murine components in the antigen-binding parts. Finally, fully human antibodies, such as adalimumab and ustekinumab, are synthesized with fully human sequences. The ADAs against fully human monoclonal antibodies usually bind to the idiotype, the part of the variable region of the antibody molecule that confers antigenic specificity. Unlike the monoclonal antibody-based agents, the biologic agent etanercept is a fusion protein made up of the extracellular domain of the p75 TNF receptor and the hinge and Fc domains of human IgG1 but still can induce low level of ADAs primarily at the hinge region of the molecule [17].

Testing for Immunogenicity and Biologic Drug Levels

One of the major obstacles in assessing the clinical relevance of immunogenicity is the complexity of measuring antibodies against biological therapies. A major disadvantage is the lack of standardization between various ADA assays which prohibits reliable data interpretation between various laboratories [9]. The ADAs are a heterogeneous population and they differ according to affinity, isotype, and neutralizing ability. No single assay is able to detect the different forms and isotypes of ADAs, and these assays differ in sensitivity and specificity. The majority of the ADA assays only detect ADAs if their production in serum exceeds the amount of drug that is present in the serum, and they ignore the ADAs that are bound to the drug [9]. Because of that, many studies may have actually underestimated the number of patients producing ADAs [9].

There are a number of different assays used to detect ADAs, including enzyme-linked immunosorbent assay (ELISA), radioimmunoassay antigen-binding test (RIA), reporter-gene assay, and pH-shift anti-idiotype antigen-binding tests. Table 11.1 illustrates the main assays for

Table 11.1 Methods used to detect ADAs and their potential advantages and disadvantages

Test used to detect presence of ADAs	Advantages	Disadvantages
Standard ELISA	Sensitive	Not very specific, and prone to false-positive results and nonspecific binding. Only detects free ADAs (not ADAs bound in immune complexes to the drug, thus resulting in false negatives) [18]
Two-site (bridging) ELISA	Both sensitive and specific	Highly susceptible to drug interference and does not detect IgG4 antibodies which comprise much of the immune response in RA with adalimumab [7, 20] Thus it can only detect ADAs in absence of detectable amounts of circulating drug
Solid-phase ELISA	Very sensitive	Not specific, thus resulting in false positives [19]
Radioimmunoassay antigen-binding test	Low background and can detect clinically relevant antibodies	Only detects free ADAs (not ADAs bound in immune complexes to the drug, thus resulting in false negatives) [18] Use of radioactivity is a disadvantage [7]
pH-shift anti-idiotype antigen-binding test	Overcomes drug interference to detect ADAs in complexes by using acid treatment to dissociate the complexes [21], and thus reveals "hidden immunogenicity" of bound and unbound ADAs	
Reporter gene essay		

detecting ADAs, and shows the advantages and disadvantages of each assay. ELISAs and radioimmunoassays detect mainly free ADAs but do not detect the ADAs that have formed immune complexes with the drug; thus they are limited by the presence of the drug in the serum samples [9, 18]. Solid-phase ELISAs are mainly used in the randomized clinical trials, and while being highly sensitive they are not as specific, and are prone to false-positive results [19]. A novel ELISA assay called two-site (bridging) ELISA has been designed, and while being both highly specific and sensitive, this test is very susceptible to interference by drugs present in the patient's serum, and it results in immune complex formation [7]. Furthermore, the two-site bridging assay does not detect IgG4 antibodies, which compose a major part of the immune response in adalimumab, and therefore is prone to false negatives [7, 20]. The radioimmunoassay antigen-binding test (RIA) has higher specificity than ELISAs and has less drug interference; however, its major disadvantage is the radioactivity which it contains. The pH-shift anti-idiotype antigen-binding test, although used in a limited number of studies, overcomes drug interference and detects ADAs which are found in drug complexes. Thus, this test has been able to detect the "hidden" or bound ADAs not detected with the prior tests in many of the RA patients treated with adalimumab [9, 21]. Finally, the timing of the sampling also needs to be standardized across the various assays [9].

Factors Which Affect Immunogenicity

Several factors influence development of ADAs, given that not all patients who lose therapeutic efficacy develop ADAs [22]. Moreover, the frequency of ADA development varies from one biologic to another [22]. Knowledge of factors affecting the immunogenicity of biologic agents could help in the development of treatment strategies to prevent loss of efficacy and to improve safety.

Both treatment and patient-related factors contribute to ADA formation. Some the various factors which influence immunogenicity include the molecular structure of the drug, treatment regimen including drug dosing intervals, route of administration, pharmacokinetics of the drug, concomitant medications, and lastly patient characteristics such as genetics of the patient and disease type [12].

Treatment-Related Factors Affecting Immunogenicity: Molecular Structure of the Drug

Primary molecular structure of the biologic and its posttranslational modifications are one of the key determinants of immunogenicity. The initial biologic agents were of mouse origin and were highly immunogenic. However, even the fully human antibodies including adalimumab and ustekinumab may also lead to production of ADAs [7, 9]. Etanercept, on the other hand, is a fusion protein, and antibodies against etanercept appear to be non-neutralizing as

they bind to epitopes outside of the drug-binding site and thus may have a lesser effect on clinical activity [7, 23, 24]. Non-neutralizing antibodies can also contribute to reduced efficacy of the drug, as they may form immune complexes with the drug and favor increased clearance [7]. Neutralizing antibodies, on the other hand, contribute to reduced therapeutic efficacy in one of the two ways: either by forming immune complexes with the biologic agent or by blocking the binding site of the biologic drug [7]. For example, anti-TNF antibodies including infliximab and adalimumab are neutralizing as they bock the binding of the therapeutic agents to its target, i.e., TNF-alpha [10]. Neutralizing antibodies have also been shown to develop in response to ustekinumab [25].

Treatment-Related Factors Affecting Immunogenicity: Treatment Regimen

Treatment regimen may also affect immunogenicity. Factors that may influence immunogenicity include the drug dose, serum concentration, administration route, frequency of administration, and duration of treatment. In the studies with infliximab in patients with plaque psoriasis, patients who were receiving the smaller dose of infliximab were more likely to develop ADAs compared to patients receiving the higher dose [26]. Similarly in the studies investigating ustekinumab, patients receiving the 45 mg dose were more likely to develop ADAs than the patients receiving the 90 mg dose. Low dose of drug administered intermittently is more likely to evoke an immunogenic response compared to a higher dose administered nonstop without taking drug breaks [9, 27]. For example, a study showed that the long-term continuous, uninterrupted therapy is less likely to cause ADA formation in patients receiving infliximab for psoriasis compared to intermittent treatment [28]. The administration route has also been shown to influence development of ADAs. Specifically, intramuscular and subcutaneous routes have been shown to be more immunogenic than intravenous administration [23].

Factors Affecting Immunogenicity: Concomitant Medications

Data, mostly from studies in rheumatoid arthritis and other chronic inflammatory diseases, suggests that the concomitant use of methotrexate may either prevent or diminish the rate of development of ADAs. A recent meta-analysis conducted in 936 patients with immune-mediated inflammatory diseases (rheumatoid arthritis, spondyloarthritis, psoriasis, and inflammatory bowel disease) treated with adalimumab or infliximab showed that concomitant methotrexate or azathioprine/mercaptopurine reduced detectable levels of ADA by about 47% [5]. However, due to its many undesirable side effects, methotrexate is infrequently co-administered with biological agents in psoriasis patients. The level of evidence whether to use concomitant immunosuppressive agents varies between the various inflammatory diseases, and current guidelines do not recommend preventative methotrexate in plaque psoriasis just to avoid immunogenicity. Nevertheless, the role of these agents in preventing or diminishing immunogenic response remains to be vital among these inflammatory diseases [22, 29, 30].

Factors Affecting Immunogenicity: Patient-Related Factors

Patient characteristics are also a key factor affecting immunogenicity. According to the currently used assays, not all patients receiving the same biologic under similar conditions will develop ADAs. Patients who have more severe disease at baseline, longer disease, or increased C-reactive protein have been shown to have higher immunogenicity [4]. Also, patients who have developed ADAs against a first TNF inhibitor are more likely to develop ADAs against a second TNF inhibitor [31, 32]. Importantly, there is no evidence that ADAs can cross-react between the various anti-TNF alpha agents. Therefore, the presence of an ADA does not contraindicate switching to another drug of the same class [33, 34]. Patients with infections that may trigger natural immunity and thus enhance immune response may also be prone to developing ADAs [9].

Immunogenicity Variability Among Various Biologic Agents

Infliximab

Immunogenicity against antitumor necrosis factor (TNF) monoclonal antibodies has been extensively studied. The reported extent of ADA development in psoriasis patients treated with infliximab ranges from 15 to 50% [26, 35]. Antibody-positive patients treated with infliximab were less likely to maintain response to treatment and had a greater risk of infusion reactions than the antibody-negative patients [35]. A recent systematic review and meta-analysis concluded that the presence of antibodies against antitumor necrosis factor monoclonal antibodies including adalimumab and infliximab confers a risk of discontinuation of treatment in rheumatoid arthritis patients only, and a risk of development of hypersensitivity reactions in all immune-mediated inflammatory diseases (rheumatoid arthritis, plaque psoriasis, juvenile idiopathic arthritis, inflammatory bowel disease, and spondyloarthritis)

[8]. For example, development of infusion reactions, serum sickness, and anaphylactic reactions may occur with infliximab [23]. Another recent systematic review found decreased treatment efficacy with infliximab and adalimumab, but not with etanercept [22].

Adalimumab

The extent of ADA development in psoriasis patients receiving adalimumab ranges from 6 to 45% [23, 36–39]. For example, Menter et al. found ADAs in 8.8% of patients [37], and Papp et al. found ADAs in 6% of patients [38]. ADAs were associated with an increased risk of failure to re-achieve efficacy following treatment discontinuation and relapse [38]. Lecluse et al. found ADAs among 45% of treated patients; however, their sample size consisted of only 29 patients [39]. ADAs to adalimumab were associated with lower serum drug concentration [22, 30, 40]. Takahashi et al. found that trough levels were positively associated with clinical response and were significantly lower in patients with ADAs [40].

Ustekinumab

The extent of ADA developing in psoriasis patients on ustekinumab is about 5% [23, 36]. Antibodies to ustekinumab have been shown to increase drug clearance by 35% [25].

A group by Zhu et al. showed that 76% of these antibodies were neutralizing, and patients with ADAs tended to have lower serum drug concentrations and lower therapeutic response to treatment [25].

Etanercept

Compared to antibodies against anti-TNF monoclonal antibodies, the incidence of antibodies against etanercept is low (1.1–1.6%) [41–44], and these ADAs are not neutralizing [22, 24, 45]. These ADAs are not associated with a decrease in therapeutic response [42–44]. Another study found 18.3% of patients developing ADAs; however, these were non-neutralizing and had no effect on efficacy or safety of the drug [46]. Majority of the data on immunogenicity comes from studies in rheumatoid arthritis and inflammatory bowel disease, and the existing data is incomplete [8].

Secukinumab

Several studies found minimal ADA development in patients treated with secukinumab. For instance, 0.4% of 980 patients treated with secukinumab developed ADAs [47]. In another study, 0.3% of 780 secukinumab-treated patients developed ADAs. No patient had neutralizing antibodies, and these were not associated with adverse events or loss of efficacy.

Ixekizumab

Antidrug antibodies against ixekizumab developed in 9.0% of 1150 patients treated with the biologic in the 2-week dosing group during the induction period [48]. 1.7% of these patients had high titers of the antidrug antibodies, and these were accompanied by a lower clinical response than the patients who had either no or low-to-moderate titers of antidrug antibodies [48]. The patients who initially responded to ixekizumab and continued in the long-term safety portion did not have high titers of ADAs and maintained a high-level clinical response, with no significant difference among patients with no, low, or moderate titers [48].

Immunogenicity Among Biosimilar Agents

Biosimilars are products that are similar in terms of quality, safety, and efficacy to an already licensed reference biotherapeutic product. The process for manufacturing the reference biologic is unique and proprietary. Thus, without access to the proprietary information, biosimilar manufacturers cannot duplicate the cell line or manufacturing process. Instead, they can only make a product that resembles the reference product. No two companies begin with the same master cell line or have the same manufacturing process. As a result, changes occur during manufacturing proteins, including glycosylation, which may have an impact on immunogenicity. Other chemical modifications include oxidation, deamidation, aldehyde modification, and deamination, and all of these may trigger an immune response [9]. All of these modifications create additional substrates for an immune response and thus pose a threat to increased ADA development and decreased therapeutic response. Moreover, due to the high level of similarities to the reference product, antibodies developed to either the parent compound or the biosimilar could reduce response to either agent. The magnitude of these theoretical effects will only be understood with widespread use of biosimilar agents.

Clinical Implications of Immunogenicity

Immunogenicity has critical clinical implications, including impact on efficacy, safety, and drug survival of biologic agents. Most of the data on clinical significance of antidrug antibodies comes from rheumatoid arthritis and spondyloarthritis. In these disease entities, development of ADAs in 19–26% of patients treated with infliximab has been shown to be associated with lower drug trough levels (the drug concentration measured just before the next dose), poor clinical response, infusion reactions, and greater likelihood of drug discontinuation [49, 50]. In RA, development of ADAs in 28% of patients has been associated with lower drug concentrations and lower clinical efficacy [4].

Impact on Efficacy

In plaque psoriasis, immunogenicity is vital in terms of loss response to biologic drugs. Clinical response has been shown to be reduced in psoriasis patients who developed ADAs to infliximab [28, 35], adalimumab [30, 37, 39], and in psoriasis patients using ustekinumab [25]. For example, in a recent systematic review and meta-analysis of patients with immune-mediated inflammatory diseases, ADAs against infliximab or adalimumab reduced drug response rate by 68% [5]. Anti-etanercept antibodies were not detected [5]. Several studies found a positive association between trough drug levels and clinical response, and trough drug levels were significantly lower in patients who developed ADAs [30, 40].

Interestingly, patients who discontinued adalimumab and who simultaneously developed ADAs to adalimumab were not able to regain a good clinical response [38]. Some patients, on the other hand, were able to regain the original clinical efficacy [38]. This conflicting data on the role of ADAs is also present in trials with etanercept with a low rate of ADA formation. In phase III studies, patients who were responders to etanercept for plaque psoriasis and then were retreated had less than 100% response rate upon retreatment with the drug [51].

Impact on Safety

The likely impact of immunogenicity on safety is quite limited though the development of ADAs has been associated with the development of infusion reactions, serum sickness, or anaphylactic reactions, along with other allergic type including headache, pruritus, hypotension, nausea, fever, skin rash, and arthralgias [27]. A causal effect of ADAs on these reactions has only been demonstrated with infliximab [26, 35]. Data from studies in patients with rheumatoid arthritis shows that rheumatoid arthritis patients with ADAs are more likely to develop arterial and venous thromboembolic events [52].

Impact on Drug Survival

In addition to efficacy and safety of therapies, immunogenicity also has an impact on drug survival. A study by Menter et al. has shown that psoriasis patients without ADAs treated with infliximab are more likely to sustain clinical efficacy compared to the patients with ADAs [35]. A recent review by Noiles et al. has found that etanercept has had the highest retention rates of treatment in psoriasis patients [53]. Similarly, Esposito et al. showed that psoriasis patients treated with etanercept experienced longer drug survival compared to those treated with infliximab and adalimumab [54].

Conclusions

Immunogenicity has been proven to play a significant role in the variability of clinical responses among patients with plaque psoriasis. ADAs may decrease the efficacy of drugs by either neutralizing them or modifying their clearance, and they may also account for adverse events including hypersensitivity reactions. While knowledge of immunogenicity of biologic agents is crucial for development of strategies for treatment of plaque psoriasis, it is imperative to remember that many of these responses will have no clinical impact. In fact, as has been suggested by the ixekizumab data, in very-high-performing biologic agents, the absolute impact of ADAs may be negligible when examining a large treatment population. Identification of key factors that influence the clinical impact of drug immunogenicity is useful for the optimization and personalization of biologic therapies. In patients who have a good clinical response, the issue of immunogenicity should also be taken into the account. Reducing drug dosage or frequency of infusions may appear to be economically rational; however, doing so may increase the risk of ADA development and secondary failure. Once an ideal clinical response is achieved, physicians should consider continued treatment with the biologic. To date, therapeutic drug monitoring remains to be the best predictor of clinical response, and has been successfully used in rheumatoid arthritis and Crohn's disease [55]. More studies are needed to evaluate the usefulness of such drug monitoring in plaque psoriasis. To date, an international consensus is needed to determine the therapeutic range of serum drug concentrations in plaque psoriasis. Further studies are needed to understand better the pathophysiology of ADA development along with improvement in methods for optimal ADA detection.

References

1. Gottlieb A, Korman NJ, Gordon KB, et al. Guidelines of care for the management of psoriasis and psoriatic arthritis: section 2. Psoriatic arthritis: overview and guidelines of care for treatment with an emphasis on the biologics. J Am Acad Dermatol. 2008;58(5):851–64.
2. Christophers E, Segaert S, Milligan G, Molta CT, Boggs R. Clinical improvement and satisfaction with biologic therapy in patients with severe plaque psoriasis: results of a European cross-sectional observational study. J Dermatolog Treat. 2013;24(3):193–8.
3. Baert F, Noman M, Vermeire S, et al. Influence of immunogenicity on the long-term efficacy of infliximab in Crohn's disease. N Engl J Med. 2003;348(7):601–8.
4. Bartelds GM, Krieckaert CL, Nurmohamed MT, et al. Development of antidrug antibodies against adalimumab and association with disease activity and treatment failure during long-term follow-up. JAMA. 2011;305(14):1460–8.
5. Garces S, Demengeot J, Benito-Garcia E. The immunogenicity of anti-TNF therapy in immune-mediated inflammatory diseases: a systematic review of the literature with a meta-analysis. Ann Rheum Dis. 2013;72(12):1947–55.
6. Bendtzen K, Geborek P, Svenson M, Larsson L, Kapetanovic MC, Saxne T. Individualized monitoring of drug bioavailability and immunogenicity in rheumatoid arthritis patients treated with the tumor necrosis factor alpha inhibitor infliximab. Arthritis Rheum. 2006;54(12):3782–9.
7. Wolbink GJ, Aarden LA, Dijkmans BA. Dealing with immunogenicity of biologicals: assessment and clinical relevance. Curr Opin Rheumatol. 2009;21(3):211–5.
8. Maneiro JR, Salgado E, Gomez-Reino JJ. Immunogenicity of monoclonal antibodies against tumor necrosis factor used in chronic immune-mediated inflammatory conditions: systematic review and meta-analysis. JAMA Intern Med. 2013;173(15):1416–28.
9. Jullien D, Prinz JC, Nestle FO. Immunogenicity of biotherapy used in psoriasis: the science behind the scenes. J Invest Dermatol. 2015;135(1):31–8.
10. van Schouwenburg PA, Rispens T, Wolbink GJ. Immunogenicity of anti-TNF biologic therapies for rheumatoid arthritis. Nat Rev Rheumatol. 2013;9(3):164–72.
11. Carrascosa JM. Immunogenicity in biologic therapy: implications for dermatology. Actas Dermosifiliogr. 2013;104(6):471–9.
12. Schellekens H. Immunogenicity of therapeutic proteins: clinical implications and future prospects. Clin Ther. 2002;24(11):1720–40. discussion 1719
13. Harding FA, Stickler MM, Razo J, DuBridge RB. The immunogenicity of humanized and fully human antibodies: residual immunogenicity resides in the CDR regions. MAbs. 2010;2(3):256–65.
14. Saravolatz LD, Wherry JC, Spooner C, et al. Clinical safety, tolerability, and pharmacokinetics of murine monoclonal antibody to human tumor necrosis factor-alpha. J Infect Dis. 1994;169(1):214–7.
15. Boulianne GL, Hozumi N, Shulman MJ. Production of functional chimaeric mouse/human antibody. Nature. 1984;312(5995):643–6.
16. LoBuglio AF, Wheeler RH, Trang J, et al. Mouse/human chimeric monoclonal antibody in man: kinetics and immune response. Proc Natl Acad Sci U S A. 1989;86(11):4220–4.
17. Scallon B, Cai A, Solowski N, et al. Binding and functional comparisons of two types of tumor necrosis factor antagonists. J Pharmacol Exp Ther. 2002;301(2):418–26.
18. Hart MH, de Vrieze H, Wouters D, et al. Differential effect of drug interference in immunogenicity assays. J Immunol Methods. 2011;372(1-2):196–203.
19. Radstake TR, Svenson M, Eijsbouts AM, et al. Formation of antibodies against infliximab and adalimumab strongly correlates with functional drug levels and clinical responses in rheumatoid arthritis. Ann Rheum Dis. 2009;68(11):1739–45.
20. van Schouwenburg PA, Krieckaert CL, Nurmohamed M, et al. IgG4 production against adalimumab during long term treatment of RA patients. J Clin Immunol. 2012;32(5):1000–6.
21. van Schouwenburg PA, Bartelds GM, Hart MH, Aarden L, Wolbink GJ, Wouters D. A novel method for the detection of antibodies to adalimumab in the presence of drug reveals "hidden" immunogenicity in rheumatoid arthritis patients. J Immunol Methods. 2010;362(1-2):82–8.

22. Hsu L, Snodgrass BT, Armstrong AW. Antidrug antibodies in psoriasis: a systematic review. Br J Dermatol. 2014;170(2):261–73.

23. Carrascosa JM, van Doorn MB, Lahfa M, Nestle FO, Jullien D, Prinz JC. Clinical relevance of immunogenicity of biologics in psoriasis: implications for treatment strategies. J Eur Acad Dermatol Venereol. 2014;28(11):1424–30.

24. Hsu L, Armstrong AW. Anti-drug antibodies in psoriasis: a critical evaluation of clinical significance and impact on treatment response. Expert Rev Clin Immunol. 2013;9(10):949–58.

25. Zhu Y SG, Yeilding N, et al. Immunogenicity assessment of ustekinumab in phase 3 studies in patients with moderate to severe plaque psoriasis. 19th annual congress of the European academy of dermatology and venereology; 6–10 Oct 2010; Gothenburg, Sweden.

26. Gottlieb AB, Evans R, Li S, et al. Infliximab induction therapy for patients with severe plaque-type psoriasis: a randomized, double-blind, placebo-controlled trial. J Am Acad Dermatol. 2004;51(4):534–42.

27. Parenky A, Myler H, Amaravadi L, et al. New FDA draft guidance on immunogenicity. AAPS J. 2014;16(3):499–503.

28. Reich K, Nestle FO, Papp K, et al. Infliximab induction and maintenance therapy for moderate-to-severe psoriasis: a phase III, multicentre, double-blind trial. Lancet. 2005;366(9494):1367–74.

29. Jani M, Barton A, Warren RB, Griffiths CE, Chinoy H. The role of DMARDs in reducing the immunogenicity of TNF inhibitors in chronic inflammatory diseases. Rheumatology (Oxford). 2014;53(2):213–22.

30. Menting SP, van Lumig PP, de Vries AC, et al. Extent and consequences of antibody formation against adalimumab in patients with psoriasis: one-year follow-up. JAMA Dermatol. 2014;150(2):130–6.

31. Bartelds GM, de Groot E, Nurmohamed MT, et al. Surprising negative association between IgG1 allotype disparity and anti-adalimumab formation: a cohort study. Arthritis Res Ther. 2010;12(6):R221.

32. Chirmule N, Jawa V, Meibohm B. Immunogenicity to therapeutic proteins: impact on PK/PD and efficacy. AAPS J. 2012;14(2):296–302.

33. van der Bijl AE, Breedveld FC, Antoni CE, et al. An open-label pilot study of the effectiveness of adalimumab in patients with rheumatoid arthritis and previous infliximab treatment: relationship to reasons for failure and anti-infliximab antibody status. Clin Rheumatol. 2008;27(8):1021–8.

34. Jamnitski A, Bartelds GM, Nurmohamed MT, et al. The presence or absence of antibodies to infliximab or adalimumab determines the outcome of switching to etanercept. Ann Rheum Dis. 2011;70(2):284–8.

35. Menter A, Feldman SR, Weinstein GD, et al. A randomized comparison of continuous vs. intermittent infliximab maintenance regimens over 1 year in the treatment of moderate-to-severe plaque psoriasis. J Am Acad Dermatol. 2007;56(1):31.e31–15.

36. De Simone C, Amerio P, Amoruso G, et al. Immunogenicity of anti-TNFalpha therapy in psoriasis: a clinical issue? Expert Opin Biol Ther. 2013;13(12):1673–82.

37. Menter A, Tyring SK, Gordon K, et al. Adalimumab therapy for moderate to severe psoriasis: a randomized, controlled phase III trial. J Am Acad Dermatol. 2008;58(1):106–15.

38. Papp K, Crowley J, Ortonne JP, et al. Adalimumab for moderate to severe chronic plaque psoriasis: efficacy and safety of retreatment and disease recurrence following withdrawal from therapy. Br J Dermatol. 2011;164(2):434–41.

39. Lecluse LL, Driessen RJ, Spuls PI, et al. Extent and clinical consequences of antibody formation against adalimumab in patients with plaque psoriasis. Arch Dermatol. 2010;146(2):127–32.

40. Takahashi H, Tsuji H, Ishida-Yamamoto A, Iizuka H. Plasma trough levels of adalimumab and infliximab in terms of clinical efficacy during the treatment of psoriasis. J Dermatol. 2013;40(1):39–42.

41. de Vries MK, van der Horst-Bruinsma IE, Nurmohamed MT, et al. Immunogenicity does not influence treatment with etanercept in patients with ankylosing spondylitis. Ann Rheum Dis. 2009;68(4):531–5.

42. Leonardi CL, Powers JL, Matheson RT, et al. Etanercept as monotherapy in patients with psoriasis. N Engl J Med. 2003;349(21):2014–22.

43. Papp KA, Tyring S, Lahfa M, et al. A global phase III randomized controlled trial of etanercept in psoriasis: safety, efficacy, and effect of dose reduction. Br J Dermatol. 2005;152(6):1304–12.

44. Tyring S, Gottlieb A, Papp K, et al. Etanercept and clinical outcomes, fatigue, and depression in psoriasis: double-blind placebo-controlled randomised phase III trial. Lancet. 2006;367(9504):29–35.

45. Dore RK, Mathews S, Schechtman J, et al. The immunogenicity, safety, and efficacy of etanercept liquid administered once weekly in patients with rheumatoid arthritis. Clin Exp Rheumatol. 2007;25(1):40–6.

46. Tyring S, Gordon KB, Poulin Y, et al. Long-term safety and efficacy of 50 mg of etanercept twice weekly in patients with psoriasis. Arch Dermatol. 2007;143(6):719–26.

47. Langley RG, Elewski BE, Lebwohl M, et al. Secukinumab in plaque psoriasis--results of two phase 3 trials. N Engl J Med. 2014;371(4):326–38.

48. Gordon KB, Blauvelt A, Papp KA, et al. Phase 3 trials of Ixekizumab in moderate-to-severe plaque psoriasis. N Engl J Med. 2016;375(4):345–56.

49. Ducourau E, Mulleman D, Paintaud G, et al. Antibodies toward infliximab are associated with low infliximab concentration at treatment initiation and poor infliximab maintenance in rheumatic diseases. Arthritis Res Ther. 2011;13(3):R105.

50. Plasencia C, Pascual-Salcedo D, Nuno L, et al. Influence of immunogenicity on the efficacy of longterm treatment of spondyloarthritis with infliximab. Ann Rheum Dis. 2012;71(12):1955–60.

51. Gordon KB, Gottlieb AB, Leonardi CL, et al. Clinical response in psoriasis patients discontinued from and then reinitiated on etanercept therapy. J Dermatolog Treat. 2006;17(1):9–17.

52. Korswagen LA, Bartelds GM, Krieckaert CL, et al. Venous and arterial thromboembolic events in adalimumab-treated patients with antiadalimumab antibodies: a case series and cohort study. Arthritis Rheum. 2011;63(4):877–83.

53. Noiles K, Vender R. Biologic survival. J Drugs Dermatol. 2009;8(4):329–33.

54. Esposito M, Gisondi P, Cassano N, et al. Survival rate of antitumour necrosis factor-alpha treatments for psoriasis in routine dermatological practice: a multicentre observational study. Br J Dermatol. 2013;169(3):666–72.

55. Chen DY, Chen YM, Tsai WC, et al. Significant associations of antidrug antibody levels with serum drug trough levels and therapeutic response of adalimumab and etanercept treatment in rheumatoid arthritis. Ann Rheum Dis. 2015;74(3):e16.

Manufacturing of Biologics

12

Jared J. Nathan, Monica Ramchandani, and Primal Kaur

Introduction

Since ancient times, humans have used cell biology to create products of interest, most notably the fermentation of yeast to efficiently make bread and alcohol. In 1919, agricultural engineer Karl Ereky envisioned a future time when more applications of biology could be utilized for making other useful products for human use [1]. He referred to this idea as "biotechnology," a portmanteau of biology and technology. Although there are many different subject areas that fall under the general term biotechnology, this chapter focuses on its application to the creation of human therapeutics from the fermentation of living cells—the manufacturing of biotechnology-derived biologics.

Through successive achievements in biology, such as microbiology, genetics, cell cloning, and recombinant DNA technology, Ereky's vision has come to fruition, and biotechnology is used every day by innumerable companies and research laboratories to make highly complex drugs known as biologics. Biologics are derived from genetically modified living organisms and have improved the treatment of many chronic diseases including diabetes, arthritic and dermatologic conditions, multiple sclerosis, and many cancers. For example, human insulin produced using biotechnology resulted in the first US Food and Drug Administration (FDA)-approved biologic in 1982 [2]. In 2003, alefacept (Amevive) was the first dermatologic biologic to receive FDA approval for the treatment of psoriasis, although the manufacturer, Astellas Pharma USA (Northbrook, IL) stopped sales in 2011 not because of supply or safety issues but due to business concerns [3]. Since then, many other biologics have been approved by the FDA either specifically for the treatment of psoriasis or as an additional indication to those originally approved (Table 12.1).

J.J. Nathan, BS chemistry
M. Ramchandani, BS, MS pharmacy, PhD pharmaceutical sciences
P. Kaur, MD, MBA (✉)
Biosimilars Development, Amgen Inc, Thousand Oaks, CA, USA
e-mail: pkaur@amgen.com

Perhaps the most familiar drugs are small-molecular-weight chemical compounds. Common examples include acetyl salicylic acid, nonsteroidal inflammatory drugs, antidepressants, antihypertensive drugs, and corticosteroids. Biologics, on the other hand, are larger and more structurally complex molecules with molecular weights that can be greater than 150,000 Da, such as monoclonal antibodies (Fig. 12.1) [4]. Small-molecule drugs are produced by chemical synthesis and are ultimately sold as homogenously pure substances. These substances are pure because the processes used to manufacture them involve thermodynamically predictable chemical reactions that can be optimized to produce high yields with minimal impurities. Furthermore, the purification steps (e.g., recrystallization) following such syntheses are relatively straightforward, with both the desired end product and any impurities easily separated and well characterized using established analytical techniques.

Biologics are sensitive to their environment in both solid form and when in solution [5]. The manufacturing process for biologics is therefore more complex than one used for small molecules. Since the desired product is made from individual living cells, and each can have a slight variation in synthesizing the complex protein, the final product is generally a mixture of structurally similar substances (this is known as microheterogeneity). This mixture of structurally related molecules makes biologics difficult to fully characterize using standard analytical techniques.

Development and Manufacturing of Biologics

The development and manufacturing of biologics entails a complex process. Since biologics are made using living cellular systems that are sensitive to their environmental conditions, the synthesis of biologics requires precise control and monitoring of many variables to ensure a consistent product from batch to batch. Manufacturing of biologics involves a

© Springer International Publishing AG 2018
P.S. Yamauchi (ed.), *Biologic and Systemic Agents in Dermatology*, https://doi.org/10.1007/978-3-319-66884-0_12

series of development, culturing, and purification steps that can be summarized in the following four stages:

1. *Cell Line Development*: Engineering a cell line that contains the gene that will transcribe for the desired biologic (i.e., the gene of interest)
2. *Expansion and Cell Culture*: Growing a large number of cells from the cell line to produce the biologic
3. *Recovery and Purification*: Separating the biologic from impurities
4. *Formulation*: Preparing the biologic for use by patients

Cell Line Development

The manufacturing of a biologic begins after a disease target has been identified and a protein (i.e., the biologic product) has been designed to interact with the target. During this first step, cells are transfected, screened, and cloned; a cell line that can produce the desired protein product with desired yields is then selected [6].

Transfection is a process used in recombinant DNA technology wherein the gene that encodes for synthesis of the protein product of interest is combined with an expression vector and is inserted into the cell (Fig. 12.2).

Table 12.1 Approved biologics for the treatment of psoriasis

Biologic	Class	Original approval date	Manufacturer
Adalimumab (Humira®)	TNFα inhibitors	12/31/2002	AbbVie
Adalimumab-atto (AMJEVITA™)[a]		9/23/2016	Amgen
Etanercept (Enbrel®)		11/2/1998	Amgen
Etanercept-szzs (Erelzi™)[a]		8/30/2016	Sandoz
Infliximab (Remicade®)		8/24/1998	Centocor
Infliximab-dyyb (INFLECTRA™)[a]		4/5/2016	Celltrion
Ixekizumab (Taltz®)	IL-17 inhibitors	3/22/2016	Eli Lilly
Secukinumab (COSENTYX®)		1/21/2015	Novartis
Usterkinumab (STELARA®)		9/25/2009	Centocor

TNFα = tumor necrosis factor alpha; IL-17 = Interleukin 17
[a]Biosimilar products

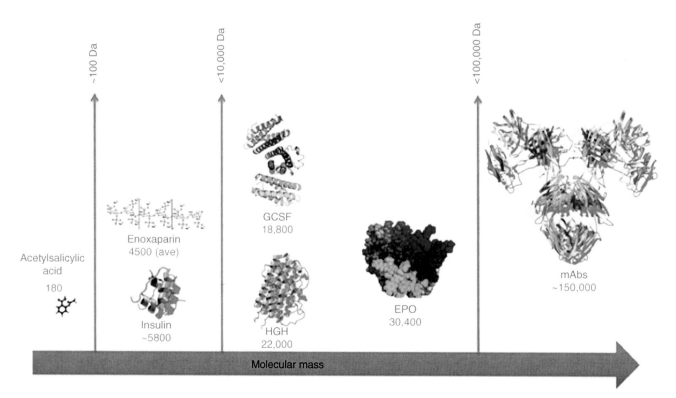

* Not drawn to scale.

Fig. 12.1 Biologics are larger and structurally more complex than chemically synthesized drugs. *Ave* average; *DA* Daltons; *EPO* erythropoeitin; *GCSF* granulocyte colony-stimulating factor; *HGH* human growth hormone; *mAbs* monoclonal antibodies

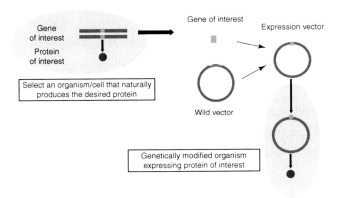

Fig. 12.2 Representation of the transfection process

The transfected cells are then grown, screened, and evaluated to identify those capable of producing the desired product, including the ability to grow in reproducible conditions. The detailed method is described in Fig. 12.3 [7]. Selected cells are then cloned, cultured, and evaluated to identify the clone that can produce the desired protein product with desired yields. After many iterations of the selection process, a final cell bank that consists of cells with a uniform genetic makeup (the clonal population) is established. Pools of the final clone are frozen, thereby creating cell banks (master and working cell banks) from which future batches of the biologic can be made. The cell line development process can take up to a few years to complete and is key to ensuring that a consistent product can be reliably made and supplied to consumers.

Many factors are considered when selecting the cell line. Some biologics can be made using common bacteria such as *E. coli*, yeast, or plant cells. However, many biologics have complex structural features that can be created only in mammalian cells. For example, certain biologics have saccharide units attached to them (i.e., glycosylation); and the biofunctional properties of the biologic are dependent on the glycosylation pattern [8]. Additionally, the potential for an immune response to the biologic could be increased when using non-mammalian derived cell lines [9].

Glycosylation is a posttranslational modification (PTM) that occurs in mammalian or mammalian derived cell lines and is paramount to yielding the correct structural and biofunctional characteristics of a particular biologic [10]. Most PTMs occur in the final stages of the cellular protein synthesis when the protein is secreted from the endoplasmic reticulum into the cytosol during the upstream process (Sect. "Expansion and Cell Culture"); some PTMs can occur in the downstream process, e.g., product recovery, purification, storage, and formulation (Sect. "Product Recovery and Purification"). Table 12.2 illustrates potential in vivo effects that different glycans attached to a monoclonal antibody can have [11]. The effector functions, such as antibody-dependent cell-mediated cytotoxicity (ADCC)

and complement-mediated cytotoxicity (CDC), may be part of the mechanism of action for biologics, and thus can be directly related to drug efficacy.

To add to the complexity of selecting a cell line, any given cell line type, such as Chinese hamster ovary (CHO), has innumerable variations. The most commonly used cells for a cell line are CHO cells, although some older biologics are manufactured using murine hybridoma (SP2) expression systems. Properties of CHO cells that make them versatile and more desired in biologic manufacturing include the following [7]:

- Growth in suspension culture which is ideal for large-scale manufacturing.
- Growth in serum-free and chemically defined media which ensures reproducibility between different batches of cell culture.

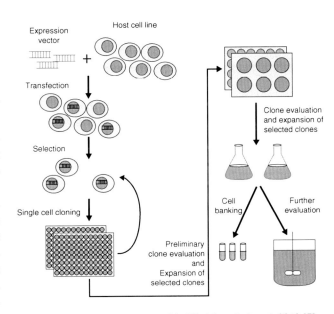

Fig. 12.3 Cell line development. Modified from Lai et al, 2013 [7]

Table 12.2 Potential impact of glycosylation on the pharmacokinetics and pharmacodynamics of monoclonal antibodies

Glycan species	Potential impact
None	No ADCC, no CDC
Mannose	Clearance, ADCC, FcγRIIIa, C1q, CDC
Fucose	ADCC. FcγRIIIa
Galactose	Clearance, CDC
GlcNAc	ADCC. FcγRIIIa
Sialic acid NANA	Anti-inflammatory activity
Sialic acid NGNA	ADCC. FcγRIIIa, immunogenicity

ADCC antibody-dependent cell-mediated cytotoxicity, *CDC* complement-dependent cytotoxicity, *C1q* a subcomponent (q) of complement C1, *FcγRIIIa* Fc gamma receptor, type IIIa (a receptor found on certain cell surfaces, having affinity for the Fc region of the antibody); *GlcNAc* N-Acetylglucosamine, *NANA* N-acetylneuraminic acid, *NGNA* N-glycolyneuraminic acid

- Allowance of PTMs, such as glycosylation, to recombinant proteins which are biologically active in humans. For example, SP2 cells tend to express specific glycoforms that are not present in humans and can therefore trigger immunogenicity. However, CHO cells do not express these glycoforms.
- Having a lower safety risk since few human viruses can propagate in them.
- Establishment of host cell lines for regulatory approval.

Cell banks of the selected cell line are necessary to guarantee that the biologic can be manufactured for years to come. Regulatory drug agencies require that cell banks be transferred to other geographic locations, as a precautionary step to protect against catastrophes so that the integrity of the unique cell line developed by the manufacturer can be maintained. The agencies require this because no two cells lines are alike, and cell lines can influence the quality, safety, and efficacy of the product. Therefore it is critical to protect them from loss for the life of the product as replacing them and achieving a similar biologic would be a profound undertaking. This further illustrates the complexity of the cell line development process. The cell banks are tested to ensure sterility (i.e., free of bacteria and fungi), absence of adventitious agents (i.e., viruses), and genetic stability. After the cell line has been chosen and banked, the cells can now be grown to manufacture large quantities of the biologic.

Expansion and Cell Culture

The next step in the biologics manufacturing process begins with cell culture (fermentation), or growing cells from the cell bank in the laboratory [12]. Cells are thawed from a storage tube and initially placed in Petri dishes or flasks containing a liquid medium that contains the nutrients required for the cell to grow. As more cells are obtained via mitosis (the expansion process), the cells are sequentially transferred to larger production-size vessels called bioreactors (Fig. 12.4)

[13]. The media and growth conditions used in biologic manufacturing are proprietary to the manufacturer of the biologic and may affect the growth of the cells and the structural and functional properties of the biologic they express.

At every step of this cell culture process, it is crucial to maintain the specific environment that the cells need to reproduce [14]. In the earlier stages of the expansion process, conditions are typically optimized to promote the cell growth. During later stages in bioreactors, the conditions are also optimized to promote the production of the desired protein. Even subtle environmental changes can affect the cells and alter the proteins they produce. For that reason, strict controls during the bioreactor stage are needed to ensure the quality, consistency, and safety of the final product. These controls include checks performed during production to monitor and, if appropriate, to specify corrective adjustments to certain process parameters. Scientists carefully monitor variables such as temperature, pH, nutrient concentration, cell density, and oxygen levels to achieve this required control. They also run frequent tests to safeguard against potential contamination from bacteria, yeast, and other microorganisms. The expansion and cell culture process can take from days to weeks, depending on the productivity of the cell line and other factors.

Product Recovery and Purification

When the growth process is complete, the desired biologic must be isolated from the cells and the growth media, also known as the downstream process. Various separation techniques (in multiple steps) are used to recover the biologic from cell debris based on the size, molecular weight, and/or electrical charge of the biologic molecule. Additionally, virus inactivation/removal steps are included to ensure that the final product is free of contaminants and safe for human use. Each of these steps also have strict in-process controls to ensure the delivery of a consistent, potent, and safe product.

The initial product obtained after the isolation and purification steps has a distribution of molecules with similar size,

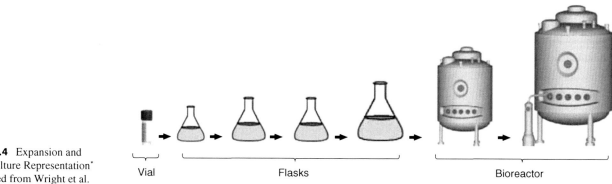

Fig. 12.4 Expansion and Cell Culture Representation* Modified from Wright et al. 2015 [13]

Vial   Flasks   Bioreactor

* Not drawn to scale.

molecular weight, and charge (i.e., the product contains microheterogeneity). This initial product is known as the drug substance or active pharmaceutical ingredient. Minor changes during isolation and purification can affect the structure and composition of the final product, and therefore the clinical outcomes [14]. Each of the steps leading to the drug substance are also proprietary to the manufacturer of the biologics. An example of the isolation and purification steps for a typical monoclonal antibody is shown in Fig. 12.5 [15].

Before moving on to the next stage in the manufacturing process, analytical testing is performed to ensure the drug substance identity, quality, purity, and potency. Guidances from regulatory authorities are available which specify the minimum requirements for tests that must be performed before moving to the next step in the manufacturing process. Additional tests specific to a biologic product may also be conducted if the attributes being measured are known to influence the consistency, safety, or efficacy of the final product [14]. The list of tests that are performed, and prespecified acceptance criteria of the product characteristics, is called the drug substance specification. Every batch of drug substance must conform to the specification if it is intended for human use. To ensure stability and shelf life, a drug substance lot is periodically tested after storage at different temperature conditions for prespecified time intervals, and is referred to as stability testing.

Each test has a predefined quality acceptance criterion to which the results are compared [14]. These predefined criteria can be based on results for the test on previously made biologic batches, generally accepted values for meeting quality and safety limits in the scientific literature, requirements provided by regulatory agencies, or direct

comparisons to a reference standard. The reference standard is a standardized substance which is used as a measurement base for future batches of product. The reference standard also provides a calibrated level of biological effects against which new sample preparations of the drug are compared. The standardization is a result of thorough characterization as well as knowledge gained during testing in the clinical setting. Of note, these characterization studies examine many more characteristics than are typically included in a product specification.

Formulation

The final step in the biologic manufacturing process, frequently referred to as fill/finish, involves the formulation of the drug substance into a suitable dosage form, most often an injectable since biologics cannot usually be administered orally [14]. Formulation of an injectable typically involves mixing the drug substance with a sterile solution with or without a buffer and other excipients that can enhance the drug delivery properties and the biologic's stability. The formulation excipients are also chosen to ensure their suitability with the desired route of administration (e.g., using excipients that do not cause local irritation at the injection site). The mixture is then transferred to vials or syringes.

Analytical testing is then performed to provide quality assurance of the drug product, in a manner similar to the drug substance testing, to ensure that the structure and function of the drug substance are not affected by the formulation. Additionally, package compatibility studies are also

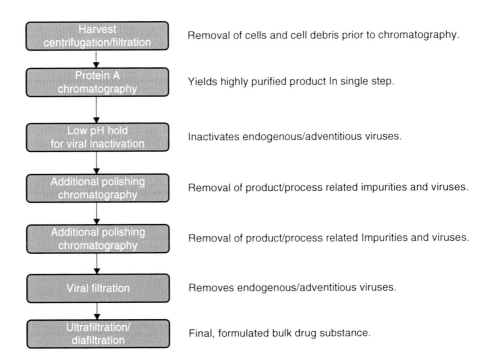

Fig. 12.5 Typical isolation and purification steps in the manufacturing of a monoclonal antibody. From Liu HF, Ma J, Winter C, et al. Recovery and purification process development for monoclonal antibody production. MAbs. 2010;2(5):480-499. Reprinted by permission of Taylor & Francis Ltd. http://www.tandfonline.com [15]

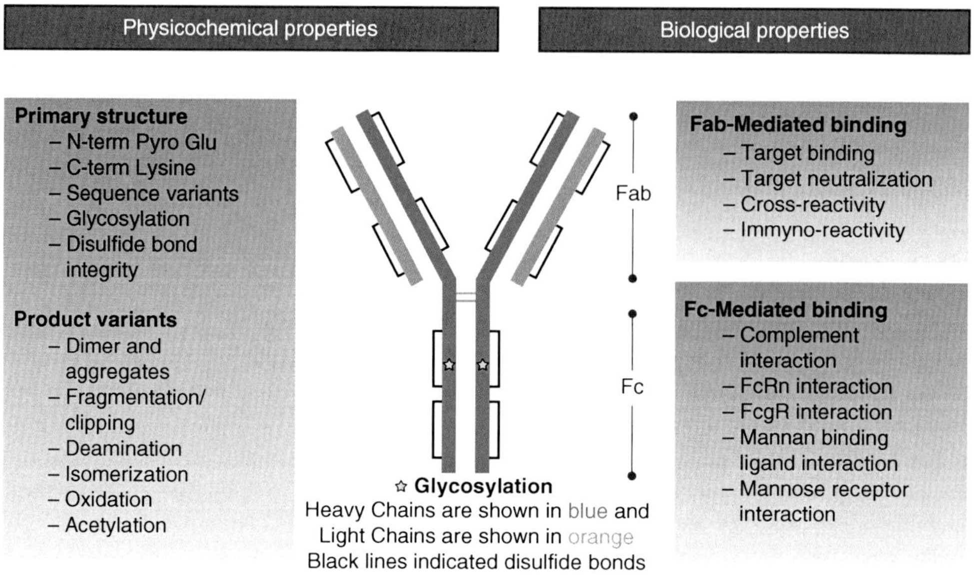

Fig. 12.6 Typical properties evaluated for a monoclonal antibody during the development of a manufacturing process. From Markus R, et al. BioDrugs. 2017;31:175-187

Physicochemical properties

Primary structure
 – N-term Pyro Glu
 – C-term Lysine
 – Sequence variants
 – Glycosylation
 – Disulfide bond
   integrity

Product variants
 – Dimer and
   aggregates
 – Fragmentation/
   clipping
 – Deamination
 – Isomerization
 – Oxidation
 – Acetylation

Fab

Fc

☆ **Glycosylation**
Heavy Chains are shown in blue and
Light Chains are shown in orange
Black lines indicated disulfide bonds

Biological properties

Fab-Mediated binding
 – Target binding
 – Target neutralization
 – Cross-reactivity
 – Immyno-reactivity

Fc-Mediated binding
 – Complement
   interaction
 – FcRn interaction
 – FcgR interaction
 – Mannan binding
   ligand interaction
 – Mannose receptor
   interaction

undertaken to ensure that no interactions exist between the active ingredient and the components of the delivery system (e.g., syringes or vials). After meeting the drug product specifications, the product is labeled, packaged, and released for distribution. Experience in all stages of the manufacturing process is critical to ensure that a manufacturer can deliver a reliable, high-quality supply of the biologic to the market place.

To illustrate the comprehensiveness of the analytical testing performed throughout the overall development of the manufacturing process (including characterization studies, in-process control testing, drug substance testing, and drug product testing), the structure of an IgG1 monoclonal antibody is shown in Fig. 12.6. The complex structure of this type of biologic gives rise to known physicochemical and biological properties that can affect the safety and efficacy of the product. Therefore, each of these properties are assessed using a variety of analytical and biological techniques that can measure and characterize these attributes. Frequently, different techniques measuring the same attribute from different scientific perspectives (i.e., orthogonal testing) are performed.

Biosimilars

While biosimilars are covered in detail in a separate chapter, this chapter would not be complete without discussing biosimilars at least briefly. A biosimilar is a biologic product that is highly similar to an already approved biologic product (originator/reference product) [16]. In the USA, the FDA defines a biosimilar as a product that is "highly similar" to the reference product, notwithstanding minor differences in clinically inactive components, and with no clinically meaningful differences between the proposed biosimilar and the reference product.

Today, biologics represent a large proportion of approved therapies for several conditions, including cancer and chronic inflammatory diseases. These products represent a significant growing portion of the healthcare expenditure. To improve access to biologics, the US Congress passed the Biologics Price Competition and Innovation Act (BPCIA) of 2009, which authorized the US FDA to oversee an abbreviated pathway for the approval of biosimilars [16]. Biosimilars of biologic products are intended to increase patient access by potentially lowering the cost of biologic treatments.

A major milestone since the enactment of BPCIA came with the US FDA's approval of its first biosimilar, Zarxio® (filgrastim-sndz), in March 2015 [17]. Since then, the US FDA has approved its first monoclonal antibody biosimilar, Inflectra® (infliximab-dyyb; April 2016) [18] followed by the first fusion protein, Erelzi™ (etanercept-szzs; August 2016) [19], and another monoclonal antibody, AMJEVITA™ (adalimumab-atto; September 2016) [20]. Additional approvals are expected in the near future. The European Union, through the European Medicines Agency (EMA), has also previously created guidelines for the development and approval of biosimilars, with their first biosimilar approval in 2006 for human growth hormone [21].

Understanding the differences between originator and biosimilars as well as between biosimilars and generics is essential. To that end, it is important to understand the science behind biosimilars. Biosimilars are not analogous to generics because, unlike generics, they are not "copies" of originator products [22]. As already discussed, the manufacturing of biologics is complex as these living systems are highly sensitive to manufacturing processes and therefore each biosimilar is expected to differ from the originator as well as from other biosimilars for the same reference product.

Manufacturing of Biosimilars

For a biosimilar, the structural and biofunctional property targets are already known based on the reference product. However, the cell line and manufacturing process development has to be created anew since the cell line and process of a reference product are proprietary to the originator of the drug. Therefore, a biosimilar manufacturer will have its own unique cell line and process; it is the uniqueness of the cell line that ultimately defines a biologic (reference product or biosimilar) and thus makes it difficult to replicate [16].

The complexities and steps of manufacturing biologics also apply to biosimilars, and each manufacturing step must be developed and performed to meet regulatory expectations for quality. In attempting to develop a product that is highly similar to an originator product, biosimilar manufacturers independently design their own cell line, expansion and cell culture steps, isolation and purification steps, and final formulations. A summary of all the steps in a biologic and biosimilar manufacturing process is shown in Fig. 12.7 [23]. The key differences between the reference product and biosimilar during each step are shown.

The biosimilar manufacturer begins with the final reference product and must develop its own manufacturing parameters to make a highly similar product. During this process, a concept often referred to as the knowledge gap becomes evident and further distinguishes biosimilars and their respective reference products (Fig. 12.8) [14]. This knowledge gap, which will be further explained later (Sect. "Comparability Versus Biosimilarity") [24], renders it impossible for biosimilar manufacturers to precisely replicate the manufacturing process of the original biologic. Therefore the biosimilar product eventually has to be tested in controlled clinical studies to verify that no clinically meaningful differences are observed with the biosimilar under the biosimilar regulatory approval pathway.

FDA Regulation of Biologics

Before a new drug/biologic can be sold for use in the treatment of patients, the manufacturer must receive approval from local regulatory authorities (e.g., FDA in the USA; EMA in the EU). In the USA, for new small molecules, the

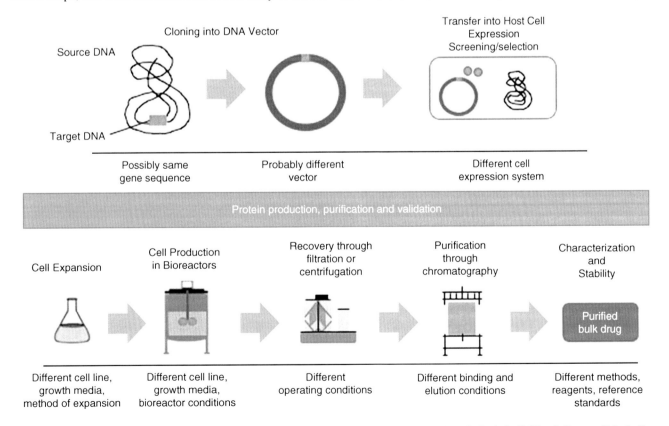

Fig. 12.7 Summary of a typical biological manufacturing process From Mellstedt H, Niederwieser D, Ludwig H. The challenge of biosimilars. Ann Oncol 2008;19:412-419, by permission of Oxford University Press [23]

Fig. 12.8 Representation of the biosimilars knowledge gap. From Lee JF, Litten JB, Grampp G. Comparability and biosimilarity: considerations for the healthcare provider. Curr Med Res Opin. 2012;28(6):1053-1058. Reprinted by permission of Taylor & Francis Ltd http://www.tandfonline.com [14]

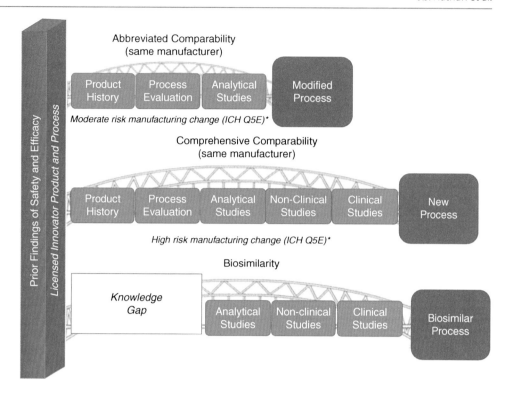

approval process involves submitting a New Drug Application (NDA) demonstrating that the drug is safe and effective based on a full complement of nonclinical data (animal studies), chemistry, manufacturing, and controls (CMC) data and information, and results from controlled clinical studies [25].

Generic versions of small-molecule drugs are also produced. As noted earlier, because of the relatively simple structure of small molecules, the ease of analytical characterization, and the predictability of its manufacturing process to produce a homogenous chemical substance, generic versions of reference small molecules are relatively easily manufactured by other companies. Furthermore, since these generic versions are exact replicas of the reference listed drug (RLD), it is not necessary to fully establish the safety and efficacy profile for the generic drug. Therefore, the sponsor submits an abbreviated NDA (ANDA), which relies on the FDA's finding that the RLD is safe and effective, if bioequivalence has been demonstrated. The ANDA application includes, among other things, CMC data and information that demonstrate that the manufacturing methods are adequate to ensure the identity, strength, quality, and purity of the drug. The result of this requirement is that the level of CMC detail that must be provided for approval of an NDA and an ANDA is to the same extent. The regulatory approval process is quite similar in the EU, Japan, and most of the world.

The regulatory approval process for a biologic is different from that of small-molecule drugs [16]. In the USA, biologics that are regulated under the Federal Food, Drug,

and Cosmetics Act are approved for use under Section 351(a) of the Public Health Service (PHS) Act; the application is termed a Biologics Licensing Application (BLA). Similar to an NDA, the BLA must contain information demonstrating that the drug is safe and effective based on a full complement of nonclinical data (animal studies), CMC data and information, and results from controlled clinical studies.

Guidances have been issued that allow for the development of biosimilars to originator biologics [16]. To expedite the approval process for biosimilars the US FDA has developed an abbreviated pathway under Section 351(k) of the PHS act. Section 351(k) allows a biosimilar sponsor to rely on existing scientific knowledge about the safety and efficacy of the reference product, and consequently enables a biosimilar biologic product to be licensed based on less than a full complement of product-specific nonclinical and clinical data typically required under the Section 351(a) regulatory pathway. Therefore, a biosimilar manufacturer typically focuses on (1) demonstrating the similarity of the proposed biosimilar to the reference product based on comprehensive analytical and functional assessments; (2) pharmacokinetic similarity in a phase 1 study; and (3) a confirmatory comparative clinical study in a representative indication to ensure that no clinically meaningful differences exist between the proposed biosimilar and the reference product. A key feature of the biosimilar approval process is that a product may be approved for use in indications that were not evaluated as part of its clinical development program; this is referred to as extrapolation. Extrapolation to additional indications that the reference product is approved for is based on scientific justification. Once again, the regulatory approval process for biosimilars is quite similar in the EU and Japan and most regions of the world.

Understand that once a new drug (or biologic) has been approved for use, all processes used in its manufacture and characterization are locked based on the procedures submitted in the regulatory application (NDA/ANDA/BLA, etc.). Any changes made to the process, major or minor, such as the manufacturing site, raw material supplier, and parts and equipment used, must be communicated to the authorities; the risk potential that the change may have on the final product and its performance identifies how the change must be communicated. In the USA, for small-molecule drugs and pharmaceuticals, the FDA has provided Scale-up and Post-approval Changes (SUPAC) guidance, to allow for the communication of such modifications [26]. For example, a minor change could allow the sponsor to make the change and continue production with only a notification to the FDA after the change is made effective. Changes considered to be major require FDA approval before the change can be implemented. Due to the complexity of biologics manufacturing, and their heterogeneous nature, more caution is required when making any manufacturing changes. Therefore, a change in the manufacturing process for a biologic is accompanied by a comparability study using analytical techniques that assess attributes known to have a potential to affect the safety and/or efficacy of the product. Of note, any changes affected during a comparability evaluation are backed by the extensive knowledge and understanding of the product manufacturing by the sponsor.

Comparability Versus Biosimilarity

An important discussion with respect to the manufacture of biologics and biosimilars is an understanding of comparability of a biologic product and how this differs from biosimilarity. Comparability refers to the comparative assessment of

characteristics of the biologic product after a specific change in the manufacturing process and is implemented by a manufacturer for their product. The implementation of such a change is supported by their comprehensive knowledge and history of the development of the product. The International Committee on Harmonization (ICH) guidance provides the degrees of risk associated with certain changes, and what types of testing should be performed to support these changes [27]. Note that this guidance does not apply to assessing biosimilarity. The reason regulatory authorities have distinguished the concepts of biosimilarity and comparability is because of the knowledge gap between the biosimilar manufacturer and the manufacturer of the originator product (Fig. 12.8) [14].

Some examples of comparability are shown in Fig. 12.9 [14]. Note that the high-risk changes, requiring more data to support the change, are the exact changes a biosimilar manufacturer must make. Also of note is that an originator manufacturer will rarely perform any other changes when implementing a major change, and will also limit the number of changes when even implementing changes with moderate risk. When a biosimilar manufacturer makes additional changes, no matter how minor, a clinical study may be simultaneously needed.

The comparability exercises conducted after completing process changes or manufacturing site changes to show that a comparable product is being produced pre- and post-change are different from a biosimilarity assessment that assesses the degree to which a biosimilar is similar to a reference product. A biosimilar product can be thought of as implementing every change in Fig. 12.9 at once. The analytical similarity assessment performed for biosimilarity typically involves the assessment of approximately 100 assay attribute combinations. In comparison, a post-approval change to an originator product may only need to evaluate ten assay attributes. Unlike comparability assessments, biosimilarity assessments require the manufacturer to demonstrate similar quality, safety, and efficacy without the reference product's history or knowledge of the manufacturing process.

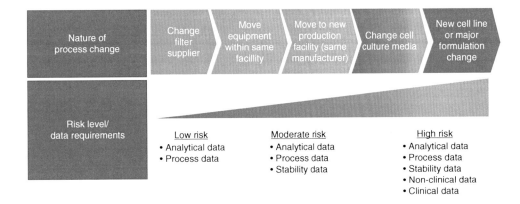

Fig. 12.9 Examples of post-approval manufacturing changes [14]

Conclusions

- Biologics have brought a new armamentarium for the treatment of several grievous diseases. However, the manufacturing of biologics is complex and follows a multistep approach.
- Biologics are large molecules that are difficult to fully characterize.
- Biologics are created in living cells that are sensitive to the manufacturing process.
- The approval pathway for biologics is different from that for small molecules. The regulatory agencies tightly control the manufacturing processes of biologics since small changes in the process may alter the structure or function of the final product.
- Biosimilars are not generics. However, recent regulations have allowed for the development of biosimilars.
- The manufacturing of a biosimilar is as complex as manufacturing an originator biologic.

References

1. Ereky K. Biotechnology of meat, fat and milk production in an agricultural large-scale farm. Berlin, Germany: P. Parey; 1919.
2. USFDA. Celebrating a milestone: FDA's approval of first genetically-engineered product. http://www.fda.gov/AboutFDA/WhatWeDo/History/ProductRegulation/SelectionsFromFDLIUpdateSeriesonFDAHistory/ucm081964.htm (2009). Accessed 9 Feb 2017.
3. Astellas Pharm US announces discontinuation of manufacturing for Amevive [press release]. Available at http://www.the-dermatologist.com/content/astellas-pharma-us-announces-discontinuation-manufacturing-amevive. Accessed 1 Feb 2017.
4. Amgen Inc. The power of biologics. Avaialble at http://www.amgenbiosimilars.com/the-basics/the-power-of-biologics/. Accessed 6 Feb 2017.
5. Rathore N, Rajan RS. Current perspectives on stability of protein drug products during formulation, fill and finish operations. Biotechnol Prog. 2008;24(3):504–14.
6. Ho K. Manufacturing process of biologics. International conference on harmonisation of technical requirements for registration of Pharmaceuticals for Human Use; May 30, 2011; Kuala Lumpur, Malaysia.
7. Lai T, Yang Y, Ng SK. Advances in mammalian cell line development technologies for recombinant protein production. Pharmaceuticals (Basel). 2013;6(5):579–603.
8. Arnold JN, Wormald MR, Sim RB, et al. The impact of glycosylation on the biological function and structure of human immunoglobulins. Annu Rev Immunol. 2007;25:21–50.
9. Dumont J, Euwart D, Mei B, et al. Human cell lines for biopharmaceutical manufacturing: history, status, and future perspectives. Crit Rev Biotechnol. 2016;36(6):1110–22.
10. Walsh G, Jefferis R. Post-translational modifications in the context of therapeutic proteins. Nat Biotechnol. 2006;24(10):1241–52.
11. Liu L. Antibody glycosylation and its impact on the pharmacokinetics and pharmacodynamics of monoclonal antibodies and fc-fusion proteins. J Pharm Sci. 2015;104(6):1866–84.
12. Lubiniecki A, Volkin DB, Federici M, et al. Comparability assessments of process and product changes made during development of two different monoclonal antibodies. Biologicals. 2011;39(1):9–22.
13. Wright B, Bruninghaus M, Vrabel N, et al. A novel seed-train process: using high-density cell banking, a disposable bioreactor, and perfusion technologies. Available at: http://www.bioprocessintl.com/upstream-processing/upstream-single-use-technologies/novel-seed-train-process-using-high-density-cell-banking-disposable-bioreactor-perfusion-technologies/ Accessed 4 Feb 2017: BioProcess International; 2015.
14. Lee JF, Litten JB, Grampp G. Comparability and biosimilarity: considerations for the healthcare provider. Curr Med Res Opin. 2012;28(6):1053–8.
15. Liu HF, Ma J, Winter C, et al. Recovery and purification process development for monoclonal antibody production. MAbs. 2010;2(5):480–99.
16. US Department of Health and Human Services Food and Drug Administration, Center for Drug Evaluation and Research (CDER), Center for Biologics Evaluation and Research (CBER). Scientific considerations in demonstrating biosimilarity to a reference product: guidance for industry. Available at http://www.fda.gov/downloads/DrugsGuidanceComplianceRegulatoryInformation/Guidances/UCM291128.pdf (2015). Accessed 4 Feb 2017.
17. FDA approves first biosimilar product Zarxio [press release]. Silver Spring, MD: Available at: http://www.fda.gov/NewsEvents/Newsroom/PressAnnouncements/ucm436648.htm. (2015). Accessed 4 Feb 2017.
18. FDA approves Inflectra, similar to Remicade [press release]. Silver Spring, MD: Available at: http://www.fda.gov/NewsEvents/Newsroom/PressAnnouncements/ucm494227.htm. (2016). Accessed 4 Feb 2017.
19. FDA approves Erelzi, a biosimilar to Enbrel [press release]. Silver Spring, MD: Available at: http://www.fda.gov/NewsEvents/Newsroom/PressAnnouncements/ucm518639.htm. (2016). Accessed 8 Feb 2017.
20. FDA approves amjevita, a biosimilar to Humira [press release]. Silver Spring, MD: Available at: http://www.fda.gov/NewsEvents/Newsroom/PressAnnouncements/ucm522243.htm. (2016). Accessed 4 Feb 2017.
21. Pro Pharma Communications International. GaBI online-generics and biosimilars initiative. Biosimilars use in Europe Mol, Belgium: Available at: http://www.gabionline.net/Reports/Biosimilars-use-in-Europe. (2011). Accessed 4 Feb 2017.
22. Zelenetz A, Ahmed I, Braud EL, et al. NCCN biosimilars white paper: regulatory, scientific, and patient safety perspectives. J Natl Compr Canc Netw. 2011;9(Suppl 4):S1–S22.
23. Mellstedt H, Niederwieser D, Ludwig H. The challenge of biosimilars. Ann Oncol. 2008;19:412–9.
24. Declerck P, Farouk-Rezk M, Rudd PM. Biosimilarity versus manufacturing change: two distinct concepts. Pharm Res. 2016;33(2):261–8.
25. US FDA. New Drug Application (NDA). Silver Spring, MD: Available at: http://www.fda.gov/Drugs/DevelopmentApprovalProcess/HowDrugsareDevelopedandApproved/ApprovalApplications/NewDrugApplicationNDA/default.htm. (2016). Accessed 4 Feb 2017.
26. Federal Register. Guidance for industry on scale-up post-approval changes: manufacturing equipment Addendum. Available at: https://www.gpo.gov/fdsys/pkg/FR-2014-12-02/pdf/2014-28256.pdf. (2014). Accessed 4 Feb 2017.
27. International Conference on Harmonisation. International conference on harmonisation of technical requirements for registration of pharmaceuticals for human use. ICH Harmonised Tripartite Guideline. Comparability of Biotechnological/Biological Products Subject to Changes in their Manufacturing Process. Avaialble at http://www.ich.org/fileadmin/Public_Web_Site/ICH_Products/Guidelines/Quality/Q5E/Step4/Q5E_Guideline.pdf. (2004). Accessed 8 Feb 2017.

K.A. Papp and Mathew N. Nicholas

Introduction

We now know tumor necrosis factor (TNF), formerly identified as TNF-alpha and cachexin, to be one member of the TNF superfamily of highly homologous proteins [1, 2]. Produced primarily by macrophages, less so by neutrophils, and still less by T-cells and other cell types [3], TNF presents at the cell surface where it undergoes enzymatic separation by a metalloprotease TACE (tumor necrosis factor-alpha-converting enzyme) [4, 5]. Once cleaved from the cell wall, TNF enters the extracellular milieu in predominantly dimerized or trimerized soluble TNF. Pervasive activity of TNF in inflammatory as well as metabolic and hematopoietic processes reflects the constitutive expression of TNF-R1 receptors by most tissues [3]. In its role as a pro-inflammatory cytokine, the activity of TNF is mediated by NF-kappa B [3].

Biologically and immunologically, TNF and its cousins are highly integrated into numerous physiologic functions as intercellular signals [6] and as drivers of inflammation [6, 7]. The TNF superfamily, with more than 20 members, has yet to be fully characterized [1, 8–11]. As a pivotal cytokine connecting the innate and adaptive immune systems, it is not surprising that TNF-alpha blockade is effective in treating a number of inflammatory conditions having disparate pathogenic pathways.

TNF was identified in 1975 [12] as a substance engaged in the necrosis of tumors. Not surprisingly, TNF was rapidly developed as a potential treatment for cancers [13–16]. However, patients treated with IV or IM TNF experienced significant dose-limiting effects: pyrexia; fatigue; headaches; granulocytopenia; thrombocytopenia; and elevated triglycerides without reduction in tumor burden. Parallel to testing TNF in cancer was exploration of its biological activity in septicemia. Profound production of TNF is a consequence of septicemia. Blockade of TNF reduced mortality in animal models [17]. In humans, clinical trials suggested marginal improvement in survival or decreased survival in patients with septic shock [18–21]. Multiple sclerosis, another condition with high unmet needs and mouse models suggesting a role for tumor necrosis factor therapy, saw progression of plaques when patients were treated with a lymphotoxin (TNF-beta) antagonist [22]. Another therapeutic opportunity where TNF levels were markedly elevated in humans and animal models was congestive heart failure. Three concurrent studies evaluating a TNF-fusion protein and an anti-TNF monoclonal antibody were terminated for futility (etanercept) or a trend to increased morbidity or mortality in patients treated at the highest dose of the monoclonal antibody (infliximab) [23–26]. Totally unanticipated was an observed increase in production of collagenase by synovial cells exposed to TNF [27, 28]. The successful treatment of rheumatoid arthritis with TNF blockade provided the first glimmer of hope for therapies targeting TNF [29].

TNF Inhibitors in Psoriasis

Psoriasis was an afterthought. Dermatology was certainly an afterthought largely because animal models at the time were not suggesting an important role for TNF in dermatologic conditions. Getting from rheumatoid arthritis [30, 31] to psoriasis required a creative clinical leap of faith. Philip Mease and Bob Goffe conducted a small study with etanercept in patients with psoriatic arthritis. Their results demonstrated the effectiveness of TNF blockade in the treatment of psoriatic arthritis with coincidental and clinically meaningful improvement in psoriasis [32]. Thus the adventure of exploring TNF in dermatologic conditions began.

Two pivotal studies of etanercept for the treatment of psoriasis showed consistent dose-related responses [33, 34]. PASI-75 response was achieved in 14%, 34%, and 49% of patients receiving weekly etanercept at doses of 25 mg,

K.A. Papp, MD, PhD (✉)
K Papp Clinical Research and Probity Medical Research,
135 Union Street East, Waterloo, ON, Canada, N2J 1C4
e-mail: kapapp@probitymedical.com

M.N. Nicholas, BMSc
Faculty of Medicine, University of Toronto, Toronto, ON, Canada

© Springer International Publishing AG 2018
P.S. Yamauchi (ed.), *Biologic and Systemic Agents in Dermatology*, https://doi.org/10.1007/978-3-319-66884-0_13

50 mg, and 100 mg, respectively [33]. Peak response did not occur until after week 16 with week 24 results of 25%, 44%, and 59%. A contemporaneous "global" study in 583 patients produced PASI-75 values of 34% and 49% in the respective 50 mg weekly and 100 mg weekly dosing arms [34]. Responses were so consistent that the medical monitor for both studies, Ralph Zitnik, thought that the statisticians had forwarded the wrong files when reviewing results from the global study (personal communication). Safety signals were comparable across all dose arms and remained similar to placebo in both studies.

Side bar: A novice investigator, CL was working closely with a still novice but more experienced investigator KAP during the US trial. The "global" study (042) was initiated several months following the USA-based phase III study (039). It was the shared experiences of CL and KAP that introduced routine clinical photography and long-term extensions into the clinical trial arena for psoriasis.

The etanercept psoriasis studies explored the lowest clinically relevant dose (25 mg weekly), continuous treatment for 24 weeks followed by randomized withdrawal [33], and ability to maintain or improve response when dosing was fixed at 50 mg weekly after week 12 [34]. With hindsight, the concept of "induction" followed by a lower maintenance dose is wrong minded. True, some patients maintained or even improved after switching from 100 mg weekly to 50 mg weekly but many lost response. Given the nature of population-based studies of clinical interventions, three lessons were learned from the pivotal etanercept-psoriasis studies. Higher exposure to TNF antagonism does not appear to result in appreciable changes in safety. Response to treatment correlates with drug exposure. Higher doses of drug result in greater therapeutic benefit.

An interesting incidental finding from the "global" study was rapid improvement in depression scores [35]. An observation made by KAP and other investigators is the abrupt improvement in mood experienced by patients receiving effective therapies. Patients often report feeling "better" soon after receiving therapy for their psoriasis. When asked what they mean by "feeling better," a significant proportion of patients state, "I don't hurt anymore." The latter is likely a manifestation of occult psoriatic arthropathy: these selfsame patients are not often those reporting joint symptoms prior to introduction of treatment. However, an increasing body of evidence, including in part results from the "global" etanercept study, supports a central role for TNF in the mediation of depression in patients experiencing chronic inflammatory conditions [36–38].

Underscoring TNF's central role in the inflammatory cascade is the fact that no other class of biologic agent has seen a larger number of related products: adalimumab, certolizumab pegol, etanercept, golimumab, and infliximab which are all commercially available; lenercept, onercept, and others which had their clinical development terminated [39, 40]

and dozens of additional compounds targeting the TNF superfamily [41]. At the same time, TNF antagonism demonstrates efficacy across as broad a range of therapeutic indications. Notably, adalimumab has availed therapeutic challenges most successfully having ten indications: rheumatoid arthritis, juvenile idiopathic arthritis, psoriatic arthritis, ankylosing spondylitis, adult Crohn's disease, pediatric Crohn's disease, ulcerative colitis, plaque psoriasis, hidradenitis suppurativa, and uveitis [42]. From a dermatologist's perspective, psoriasis and hidradenitis suppurativa are the most relevant of the foregoing list.

Listed in Table 13.1 are primary studies of TNF inhibitors for the treatment of plaque psoriasis. Historic values for PASI-75 results for etanercept are consistent with recent comparator studies against secukinumab [46] and ixekizumab [47]. One exception is a study comparing the response of patients with plaque psoriasis treated with ustekinumab or etanercept. PASI-75 response was higher at 65.8% of patients who received etanercept [58].

Problematic when discussing clinical trials results is the assumption that response will be maintained over time. A decrease in effectiveness is anticipated in long-term studies as a result of attrition but evidence of loss of efficacy between the fiducial date of the primary end point through week 48 is apparent for all TNF antagonists but possibly pronounced with infliximab (PASI-75 response decrease of 15–20%) [49] and adalimumab [59], both of which display a loss of PASI-75 response of 15–20% compared to a few percent for etanercept [60]. Consistent across all studies with biologics for the treatment of psoriasis, patients achieving high levels of response, between PASI-90 and PASI-100, tend to maintain this response throughout the first year of treatment [34, 49, 54, 60, 61].

TNF Inhibitors and Psoriatic Arthritis

Psoriasis as a disease effectively treated with TNF antagonists should not be considered as a disorder in isolation. Many of the indications listed above are comorbidities associated with psoriasis [62, 63], the most common of which is psoriatic arthritis. A study assessing the point prevalence of psoriatic arthritis in a population of patients with psoriasis seen by dermatologists confirmed that 30% had psoriatic arthritis [64]. Of the 30%, almost half, 41%, had not been diagnosed. The foregoing reiterates the importance and necessity for dermatologists to be aware of the presence of psoriatic arthritis in the psoriasis population, as the presence or absence of psoriatic arthritis is a significant point in the decision tree when selecting an appropriate therapy. Table 13.2 lists pivotal clinical trials evaluating TNF antagonists for the treatment of psoriatic arthritis. Relatively consistent across all the TNF antagonists is the rule of thumb for response 60, 40, and 20: 60% achieve an ACR-20, 40%

Table 13.1 TNF inhibitors and psoriasis

Trial (Author Journal Year)	Etanercept after 12 weeks										Infliximab after 10 weeks			Adalimumab after 16 weeks					Certolizumab after 12 weeks
	Leonardi NEJM 2003 [33]	Papp BJD 2005 [34]	Tyring Lancet 2006 [35]	Van de Kerkhof BJD 2008 [43]	Strober BJD 2011 [44]	Gottlieb BJD 2011 [45]	Langley NEJM 2014—fixture [46]	Griffiths Lancet 2015 UNCOVER-2 [47]	Griffiths Lancet 2015 UNCOVER-3 [47]	Bachelez Lancet 2015 [48]	Reich Lancet 2005 [49]	Menter JAAD 2007 [50]	Yang CMJ 2012 [51]	Gordon JAAD 2006 [52]	Saurat BJD 2008 [53]	Menter JAAD 2008 [54]	Asahina JD 2010 [55]	Gordon NEJM 2015 [56]	Reich Br J Dermatol 2C12 [57]
Dose	25 mg weekly; 25 mg twice/week; 50 mg twice/week	50 mg twice/week; 25 mg twice/week	50 mg twice/week	50 mg weekly	50 mg twice/week	50 mg twice/week	50 mg twice/week	50 mg twice/week	50 mg twice/week	50 mg twice/week	5 mg/kg infusion at week 0, 2, and 6	5 mg/kg infusion at week 0, 2, and 6; 3 mg/kg infusion at week 0, 2, and 6	5 mg/kg infusion at week 0, 2, and 6	80 mg on week 0 then 40 mg EOW; 80 mg on week 0 then 40 mg weekly	80 mg on week 0 then 40 mg EOW	80 mg on week 0 then 40 mg EOW	40 mg EOW; 80 mg on week 0 then 40 mg EOW; 80 mg EOW	80 mg on week 0 then 40 mg EOW	400 mg on week 0 then 200 mg EOW; 400 mg EOW
Study size (n)	160; 162; 164	194; 196	311	96	139	141	326	358	382	335	301	314; 313	84	46; 44	108	814	38; 43; 42	43	59 58
PASI 50 (%)	41; 58; 74	77; 64	74	68.8	NR	NR	NR	NR	NR	80.3	91.0	NR	94.0	76[b]; 80[b]	88.0	NR	73.7; 81.4; 90.5	NR	86 93
PASI 75 (%)	14; 34; 49	49; 34	47	37.5	39.6	56.0	44.0	41.6	53.4	58.8	80.4	70.3; 75.5	81.0	53[b]; 80[b]	79.6	71	57.9; 62.8; 81.0	69.8	74.6; 82.8
PASI 90 (%)	3; 12; 22	21; 11	21	13.5	13.7	22.7[a]	20.7	18.7	25.7	32.2	57.1	45.2; 37.1	57.1	24[b]; 48[b]	51.3	45	36.8; 39.5; 61.9	44.2	39.0; 46.6
PASI 100 (%)	NR	NR	NR	NR	5.8	7.1[a]	4.3	5.3	7.3	NR	NR	NR	NR	11[b]; 26[b]	16.7	20	NR	25.6	NR

NR not reported,
EOW every other week
[a]Approximated from graphs provided
[b]Primary end point at 12 weeks

achieve an ACR-50, and 20% achieve an ACR-70. KAP asserts that the consistency in response among anti-TNF agents with profoundly different avidities, affinities, and dosing regimens is a testament to the lack of realistic dynamic range of the outcome measure, ACR, rather than a fundamental result of TNF blockade.

TNF Inhibitors and Other Dermatological Conditions

Long after approvals for the treatment of psoriasis, anti-TNFs were explored for other dermatologic indications. Case reports hinted that TNF blockade was unlikely to be effective in the treatment of atopic dermatitis [77] while the results of a clinical study remain undisclosed. A small open-labell study yielded contrary yet mixed results treating atopic dermatitis patients with infliximab [78]. Significant improvement was observed but not sustained through 46 weeks of treatment with the exception of two of the nine patients.

A small open-label study in patients with chronic urticaria implied that treatment with etanercept or adalimumab could be effective in almost half of patients refractory to then current standard of care [79]. Lack of a control population and uncertain attribution of adverse events render the use of TNF antagonists for the treatment of urticaria more than suspect.

Case studies assessing a potpourri of inflammatory mucocutaneous disorders [80–82] running the gamut of neutrophilic dermatoses, bullous disorders, granulomatous diseases, autoimmune connective tissue diatheses, graft-versus-host disease, and pityriasis rubra pilaris have generated interesting but uncertain to more often negative results. Lack of proficient outcome measures may be to blame for some of the conflicting or negative results.

Another high-needs inflammatory condition, hidradenitis suppurativa (HS) was a therapeutic target for three of the anti-TNFs. Treatment with etanercept provided no clinical benefit in a small study of 20 patients [83]. Interestingly, infliximab used at the standard dermatologic dose of 5 mg/kg yielded amazing photographic evidence of effectiveness but failed to meet the primary endpoint [84]. Methodical and systemic development of a treatment regimen and clinically relevant outcome measures produced successful results for treating HS with adalimumab [85–87].

From the author's perspective (KAP), there are three lessons learned from the anti-TNF-HS story. Firstly, in diseases with high inflammatory burden such as HS [88] or Crohn's [89], high loading doses are necessary to quench inflammation. Secondly, in order to maintain response, high exposures must be maintained [90]. Finally, a clinically relevant measure of disease severity is essential for the assessment of disease activity.

In many ways that are reminiscent of the association of multiple comorbidities with psoriasis, we see a similar spectrum of comorbidities associated with HS [91]. Possibly the comorbidity of greatest concern is cardiovascular disease and the associated increased risk of major adverse cardiovascular events (MACE). It has been believed for some time that the severity of psoriasis is associated with MACE. More specifically, the risk of myocardial infarction is greatest in those with more severe disease [92, 93]. Suffice it to say that results are mixed regarding the attribution of cardiovascular risk to psoriasis. Using the same data as Gelfand [93], Brauchli was unable to find a convincing association between psoriasis or the severity of psoriasis and myocardial infarction risk [94].

Collateral Benefits

More contention should be applied to reports suggesting that TNF blockers decrease the risk of myocardial infarction (MI). Some studies fail to find a decreased risk of MI in patients treated with systemic therapies [95, 96] while others claim to identify significant benefit associated with TNF antagonists [97]. Other studies suggest that methotrexate alone decreases cardiovascular morbidity and mortality [98]. For all retrospective studies estimating cardiovascular risk reduction, the dominant driver of risk, age [99, 100], and modifiable risk factors [101–103] must be correctly accounted for. Smoking, obesity, and similar lifestyle-associated risk factors are frequently underdiagnosed or undertreated [104]. Thoughtful, careful, and critical deliberation is essential to every statistical analysis. For example, dichotomizing age [97] is not analytically sound [105]. Finally, the opportunity for bias to evade scrutiny is of more than a passing concern [106–108]. Well-designed, randomized, prospective studies in high-risk populations evaluating the effect of methotrexate (CIRT) [109] and canakinumab (CANTOS) [110] are under way. CIRT is following 7000 high-risk patients for 5 years in an effort to detect a 25% reduction in cardiovascular outcomes [109]. CANTOS will follow over 17,000 patients for up to 4 years in an attempt to identify a 20% hazard reduction for at least one of the three dosing regiments for canakinumab [110]. With the foregoing in mind, it is challenging to believe that short-term intervention (of months to a few years) will appreciably reduce underlying cardiovascular risk by more than a few percentage points in a low-to-moderate risk population such as that seen in patients with moderate-to-severe plaque psoriasis.

Safety of TNF Inhibition

Early safety concerns regarding TNF-alpha blockade with obvious exceptions have largely withered if not senesced [111–114]. Risk of lymphoma noted in the rheumatoid arthritis population appears to be associated with the severity of the underlying condition [115, 116]. Likewise, congestive heart failure was only deemed a concern because of a single

Table 13.2. TNF inhibitors and psoriatic arthritis (randomized clinical trials placebo controlled)

	Etanercept	Golimumab				Infliximab			Adalimumab				Certolizumab
Trial (Author Journal Year)	Mease 2000 Lancet [32]	Mease 2004 Arthritis Rheum [65]	Kavanaugh 2009 Arthritis Rheum [66]	Kavanaugh 2013 Ann Rheum Dis (GO-REVEAL) [67]	Kavanaugh 2014 Annals of Rheum (GO-REVEAL) [68]	Antoni 2005 Arthritis Rheum (IMPACT) [69, 70]	Antoni 2005 Ann Rheum Dis (IMPACT-2) [69, 70]	Baranauskaite 2012 Ann Rheum Dis (RESPOND) [71]	Mease 2005 Arthritis Rheum (ADEPT) [72]	Gladman 2007 Arthritis Rheum (ADEPT) [73]	Mease 2009 Ann Rheum Dis (ADEPT) [74]	Genovese 2007 J Rheumatol [75]	Mease 2014 Ann Rheum Dis (RAPID-PsA) [76]
Dose	25 mg BIW	25 mg BIW	50 mg every 4 weeks; 100 mg every 4 weeks	50 mg every 4 weeks; 100 mg every 4 weeks	50 mg every 4 weeks; 100 mg every 4 weeks	5 mg/kg infusion at week 0, 2, 6, and 14	5 mg/kg infusion at week 0, 2, 6, 14, and 22	5 mg/kg infusion at week 0, 2, 6, and 14 + 15 mg MTX/week	40 mg EOW	40 mg EOW	40 mg EOW	40 mg EOW	200 mg q2weeks; 400 mg q4weeks
Time points	12 weeks	12 weeks; 24 weeks	24 weeks	104 weeks	256 weeks	16 weeks	24 weeks	16 weeks	12 weeks; 24 weeks	48 weeks	104 weeks	12 weeks	12 weeks; 24 weeks
Study size (n)	30	101	146; 146	146; 146	146; 146	52	100	57	151	151	298	51	138; 135
ACR 20 (%)	73	12 weeks: 59 24 weeks: 55[a]	52; 61	67.1; 69.9	65.8; 69.9	65.4	54	86.3	12 weeks: 58 24 weeks: 57	56	57.3	39	12 weeks: 58.0; 51.9 24 weeks: 63.8; 56.3
ACR 50 (%)	50	12 weeks: 40[a] 24 weeks: 42[a]	36[a]; 35[a]	46.6; 51.4	47.9; 50.7	46.2	41	72.5	12 weeks: 36 24 weeks: 39	44	45.2	25	12 weeks: 36.2; 32.6 24 weeks: 44.2; 40.0
ACR 70 (%)	13	12 weeks: 15[a] 24 weeks: 13[a]	10[a]; 18[a]	28.8; 35.6	30.8; 35.6	28.8	27	49.0	12 weeks: 20 24 weeks: 23	30	29.9	14	12 weeks: 24.6; 12.6 24 weeks: 28.3; 23.7
PsARC (%)	87	12 weeks: 72 24 weeks: 70	73; 72	NR	NR	75	70	NR	12 weeks: 62 24 weeks: 60	NR	63.5	51	24 weeks: 78.3; 77.0
Enthesitis (scoring system)	NR	NR	Non-statistically significant improvement	Maastricht Ankylosing spondylitis Enthesitis score 2.4 ± 3.6; 2.6 ± 3.9 (NS) placebo: 2.9 ± 3.8	1.9 ± 3.3; 5.4 ± 6.7 Placebo	25.0 at baseline to 13.5 (%) (presence of enthesopathy in feet)	42% at baseline to 20% (presence of enthesopathy in feet)	(Maastricht ankylosing spondylitis enthesitis score) Median reduction of two sites	Non-statistically significant improvement	NR	−0.4 ± 3.4	Non-statistically significant improvement (present or absent of proximal insertion of Achilles tendon and plantar fascia, total score 0–4) (mean change −2.4)	Leeds Enthesitis index 24 weeks Mean change: −2.0; −1.8
Dactylitis (scoring system)	NR	NR	Non-statistically significant improvement	Graded 0–3 for each digit on hand and foot (/60) 1.3 ± 4.1; 0.8 ± 2.4	Graded 0–3 for each digit on hand and foot (/60) 1.3 ± 4.9; 0.8 ± 2.1	2.3 ± 3.5 at baseline to 84.5 ± 10.1 (0–60 scale) 51.9% at baseline with score of 0–72%	40% at baseline to 12% (patients with 1 or more dactylitis digits)	Number of digits with dactylitis Median reduction of two digits	Non-statistically significant improvement	NR	Graded 0–3 for each digit on hand and foot (/60) −1.3 ± 3.4	Non-statistically significant improvement Graded 0–3 for each digit on hand and foot (/60)	Leeds Dactylitis index 24 weeks Mean change: −40.7; −53.5

NR not reported

[a] Approximated from graphs provided

study in which there was an increased risk of worsening clinical status and death in congestive heart failure patients receiving 10 mg/kg of infliximab compared to placebo [23–26]. We do not see swaths of patients on TNF antagonists developing congestive heart failure. A multiple sclerosis study and numerous case reports have taught us that TNF-alpha blockade may exacerbate signs or symptoms of multiple sclerosis though the clinical reality is that TNF-induced onset of demyelinating disorders is very uncommon [117]. Notable is that patients receiving TNF antagonists who are exposed to tuberculosis appear to have a greater chance of developing active tuberculosis than those who are not [118]. And at least in the case of anti-TNFs that are monoclonal antibodies, the risk of activating latent tuberculosis is increased significantly compared to etanercept [118–125]. The best guess as to why is that etanercept does not engage membrane-bound TNF [119].

Registries in rheumatoid arthritis implicate TNF antagonists being responsible for a modest increased risk of zoster [126–128]. A much larger claim cohort evaluating the risk of zoster in psoriasis patients failed to find a strong association with TNF antagonists with the exception of patients receiving concomitant methotrexate [129, 130].

Rare lupus-like syndromes and vasculitis are associated with TNF antagonists [131]. Consistency of the foregoing presenting in patients with rheumatoid arthritis suggests that these two rare adverse events may be much less common in patients with psoriasis. Nonetheless, a certain degree of vigilance and clinical awareness should be maintained. Two patients in the infliximab phase III program developed profoundly elevated liver function tests yet remained clinically unaffected (KAP personal communication). One of the two patients underwent a liver biopsy which demonstrated liver toxicity consistent with drug-induced lupus [132].

Prudent episodic monitoring of patients receiving TNF antagonists is essential to maintain safe treatment.

Future Directions

Newer anti-TNF agents, ATROSAB, a TNFR antagonist [133–135]; MDS5541 a TNFR1 antagonist with one variable region specific to albumin [136, 137]; a trivalent nanobody TROS [138]; and TNF analogues (TNF muteins) [139, 140] such as R1antTNF [141, 142], XENP345 [143, 144], and XPro1595 [145], point to development of more selective and novel strategies to block TNF.

A complete story of TNF would require volumes—an annually increasing number of volumes. From intellectual property rights [146] to the challenges associated with drug development, TNF has played and will continue to play an important role in the treatment of inflammatory disorders.

Case Report

A 32-year-old white male developed psoriatic plaques on his elbows and knees 4 years ago which was managed with topical agents. His psoriasis worsened 6 months ago after his father passed away suddenly. The patient had undergone phototherapy for a few months but he had minimal response. He complains of severe itching and burning due to his psoriasis. There is no family history of psoriasis. He does not present with psoriatic arthritis symptoms.

Past Medical History:
- Hypertension
- Hyperlipidemia
- Obesity (BMI–31)

Social History:
- Drinks socially (a few glasses of wine per week)
- Smokes 1 ppd
- Married
- Manager of a restaurant

Previous Therapies:
- Topical steroids
- Narrowband UVB

Physical Exam:
- Psoriatic plaques on the scalp, trunk, upper, and lower extremities covering 18% of the body surface area
- No features of psoriatic arthritis (dactylitis, enthesitis, tender and swollen joints, etc.)

Management:
Because of the severity of his psoriasis, the biologic agent adalimumab was chosen. Methotrexate was not considered because he was a social drinker and he was obese which are risk factors for liver toxicity. The QuantiFERON gold assay test was negative and he had negative hepatitis B serologies. Other baseline laboratory monitoring was normal including compete blood count and liver function tests, and his HIV status was negative. The standard dose of adalimumab was used starting at 80 mg at day 0, 40 mg 1 week later, and then 40 mg every other week continuously. Within 3 months, his body surface area decreased to 1% and his itching and burning had disappeared. The patient has remained on adalimumab for 2 years and he is satisfied with the treatment.

References

1. Aggarwal BB. Signalling pathways of the TNF superfamily: a double-edged sword. Nat Rev Immunol. 2003;3:745–56.
2. Sun M, Fink PJ. A new class of reverse signaling costimulators belongs to the TNF family. J Immunol. 2007;179:4307–12.
3. Wajant H, Pfizenmaier K, Scheurich P. Tumor necrosis factor signaling. Cell Death Differ. 2003;10:45–65.
4. Black RA, Rauch CT, Kozlosky CJ, Peschon JJ, Slack JL, Wolfson MF, Castner BJ, Stocking KL, Reddy P, Srinivasan S, Nelson N, Boiani N, Schooley KA, Gerhart M, Davis R, Fitzner JN, Johnson RS, Paxton RJ, March CJ, Cerretti DP. A metalloproteinase disintegrin that releases tumour-necrosis factor-alpha from cells. Nature. 1997;385:729–33.
5. Mohan MJ, Seaton T, Mitchell J, Howe A, Blackburn K, Burkhart W, Moyer M, Patel I, Waitt GM, Becherer JD, Moss ML, Milla ME. The tumor necrosis factor-alpha converting enzyme (TACE): a unique metalloproteinase with highly defined substrate selectivity. Biochemistry. 2002;41:9462–9.
6. Ware CF. Network communications: lymphotoxins, LIGHT, and TNF. Annu Rev Immunol. 2005;23:787–819.
7. Locksley RM, Killeen N, Lenardo MJ. The TNF and TNF receptor superfamilies: integrating mammalian biology. Cell. 2001;104:487–501.
8. Aggarwal BB, Gupta SC, Kim JH. Historical perspectives on tumor necrosis factor and its superfamily: 25 years later, a golden journey. Blood. 2012;119:651–65.
9. Bodmer JL, Schneider P, Tschopp J. The molecular architecture of the TNF superfamily. Trends Biochem Sci. 2002;27:19–26.
10. Mikkola ML. TNF superfamily in skin appendage development. Cytokine Growth Factor Rev. 2008;19:219–30.
11. Sedy J, Bekiaris V, Ware CF. Tumor necrosis factor superfamily in innate immunity and inflammation. Cold Spring Harb Perspect Biol. 2015;7:a016279.
12. Carswell EA, Old LJ, Kassel RL, Green S, Fiore N, Williamson B. An endotoxin-induced serum factor that causes necrosis of tumors. Proc Natl Acad Sci U S A. 1975;72:3666–70.
13. Blick M, Sherwin SA, Rosenblum M, Gutterman J. Phase I study of recombinant tumor necrosis factor in cancer patients. Cancer Res. 1987;47:2986–9.
14. Feinberg B, Kurzrock R, Talpaz M, Blick M, Saks S, Gutterman JU. A phase I trial of intravenously-administered recombinant tumor necrosis factor-alpha in cancer patients. J Clin Oncol. 1988;6:1328–34.
15. Fukushima T, Yamamoto M, Ikeda K, Tsugu H, Kimura H, Soma G, Tomonaga M. Treatment of malignant astrocytomas with recombinant mutant human tumor necrosis factor-alpha (TNF-SAM2). Anticancer Res. 1998;18:3965–70.
16. Kimura K, Taguchi T, Urushizaki I, Ohno R, Abe O, Furue H, Hattori T, Ichihashi H, Inoguchi K, Majima H, Al ET. Phase I study of recombinant human tumor necrosis factor. Cancer Chemother Pharmacol. 1987;20:223–9.
17. Tracey KJ, Fong Y, Hesse DG, Manogue KR, Lee AT, Kuo GC, Lowry SF, Cerami A. Anti-cachectin/TNF monoclonal antibodies prevent septic shock during lethal bacteraemia. Nature. 1987;330:662–4.
18. Abraham E. Therapies for sepsis. Emerging therapies for sepsis and septic shock. West J Med. 1997;166:195–200.
19. Abraham E, Laterre PF, Garbino J, Pingleton S, Butler T, Dugernier T, Margolis B, Kudsk K, Zimmerli W, Anderson P, Reynaert M, Lew D, Lesslauer W, Passe S, Cooper P, Burdeska A, Modi M, Leighton A, Salgo M, van der Auwera P, Lenercept Study G. Lenercept (p55 tumor necrosis factor receptor fusion protein) in severe sepsis and early septic shock: a randomized, double-blind, placebo-controlled, multicenter phase III trial with 1,342 patients. Crit Care Med. 2001;29:503–10.
20. Abraham E, Wunderink R, Silverman H, Perl TM, Nasraway S, Levy H, Bone R, Wenzel RP, Balk R, Allred R, Al ET. Efficacy and safety of monoclonal antibody to human tumor necrosis factor alpha in patients with sepsis syndrome. A randomized, controlled, double-blind, multicenter clinical trial. TNF-alpha MAb sepsis study Group. JAMA. 1995;273:934–41.
21. Reinhart K, Karzai W. Anti-tumor necrosis factor therapy in sepsis: update on clinical trials and lessons learned. Crit Care Med. 2001;29:S121–5.
22. TNF neutralization in MS: results of a randomized, placebo-controlled multicenter study. The Lenercept Multiple Sclerosis Study Group and The University of British Columbia MS/MRI Analysis Group. Neurology. 1999: 53:457–65.
23. Chung ES, Packer M, Lo KH, Fasanmade AA, Willerson JT, Anti-TNF Therapy Against Congestive Heart Failure Investigators. Randomized, double-blind, placebo-controlled, pilot trial of infliximab, a chimeric monoclonal antibody to tumor necrosis factor-alpha, in patients with moderate-to-severe heart failure: results of the anti-TNF therapy against congestive heart failure (ATTACH) trial. Circulation. 2003;107:3133–40.
24. Coletta AP, Clark AL, Banarjee P, Cleland JG. Clinical trials update: Renewal (RENAISSANCE and RECOVER) and ATTACH. Eur J Heart Fail. 2002;4:559–61.
25. Deswal A, Bozkurt B, Seta Y, Parilti-Eiswirth S, Hayes FA, Blosch C, Mann DL. Safety and efficacy of a soluble P75 tumor necrosis factor receptor (Enbrel, etanercept) in patients with advanced heart failure. Circulation. 1999;99:3224–6.
26. Mann DL, Mcmurray JJ, Packer M, Swedberg K, Borer JS, Colucci WS, Djian J, Drexler H, Feldman A, Kober L, Krum H, Liu P, Nieminen M, Tavazzi L, Van Veldhuisen DJ, Waldenstrom A, Warren M, Westheim A, Zannad F, Fleming T. Targeted anti-cytokine therapy in patients with chronic heart failure: results of the randomized etanercept worldwide evaluation (RENEWAL). Circulation. 2004;109:1594–602.
27. Dayer JM, Beutler B, Cerami A. Cachectin/tumor necrosis factor stimulates collagenase and prostaglandin E2 production by human synovial cells and dermal fibroblasts. J Exp Med. 1985;162:2163–8.
28. Dayer JM, Breard J, Chess L, Krane SM. Participation of monocyte-macrophages and lymphocytes in the production of a factor that stimulates collagenase and prostaglandin release by rheumatoid synovial cells. J Clin Invest. 1979;64:1386–92.
29. Elliott MJ, Maini RN, Feldmann M, Long-Fox A, Charles P, Katsikis P, Brennan FM, Walker J, Bijl H, Ghrayeb J, Al ET. Treatment of rheumatoid arthritis with chimeric monoclonal antibodies to tumor necrosis factor alpha. Arthritis Rheum. 1993;36:1681–90.
30. Moreland LW, Baumgartner SW, Schiff MH, Tindall EA, Fleischmann RM, Weaver AL, Ettlinger RE, Cohen S, Koopman WJ, Mohler K, Widmer MB, Blosch CM. Treatment of rheumatoid arthritis with a recombinant human tumor necrosis factor receptor (p75)-Fc fusion protein. N Engl J Med. 1997;337:141–7.
31. Moreland LW, Schiff MH, Baumgartner SW, Tindall EA, Fleischmann RM, Bulpitt KJ, Weaver AL, Keystone EC, Furst DE, Mease PJ, Ruderman EM, Horwitz DA, Arkfeld DG, Garrison L, Burge DJ, Blosch CM, Lange ML, Mcdonnell ND, Weinblatt ME. Etanercept therapy in rheumatoid arthritis. A randomized, controlled trial. Ann Intern Med. 1999;130:478–86.

32. Mease PJ, Goffe BS, Metz J, Vanderstoep A, Finck B, Burge DJ. Etanercept in the treatment of psoriatic arthritis and psoriasis: a randomised trial. Lancet. 2000;356:385–90.

33. Leonardi CL, Powers JL, Matheson RT, Goffe BS, Zitnik R, Wang A, Gottlieb AB. Etanercept as Monotherapy in patients with psoriasis. N Engl J Med. 2003;349:2014–22.

34. Papp KA, Tyring S, Lahfa M, Prinz J, Griffiths CE, Nakanishi AM, Zitnik R, van de Kerkhof PC, Melvin L, Etanercept Psoriasis Study, G. A global phase III randomized controlled trial of etanercept in psoriasis: safety, efficacy, and effect of dose reduction. Br J Dermatol. 2005;152:1304–12.

35. Tyring S, Gottlieb A, Papp K, Gordon K, Leonardi C, Wang A, Lalla D, Woolley M, Jahreis A, Zitnik R, Cella D, Krishnan R. Etanercept and clinical outcomes, fatigue, and depression in psoriasis: double-blind placebo-controlled randomised phase III trial. Lancet. 2006;367:29–35.

36. Berthold-Losleben M, Himmerich H. The TNF-alpha system: functional aspects in depression, narcolepsy and psychopharmacology. Curr Neuropharmacol. 2008;6:193–202.

37. Miller AH, Raison CL. The role of inflammation in depression: from evolutionary imperative to modern treatment target. Nat Rev Immunol. 2016;16:22–34.

38. Schmidt FM, Kirkby KC, Himmerich H. The TNF-alpha inhibitor etanercept as monotherapy in treatment-resistant depression—report of two cases. Psychiatr Danub. 2014;26:288–90.

39. Papp K. Clinical development of onercept, a tumor necrosis factor binding protein, in psoriasis. Curr Med Res Opin. 2010;26:2287–300.

40. Stevens SR, Chang TH. History of development of TNF inhibitors. In: Weinberg JM, Buchholz R, editors. TNF-alpha inhibitors. Birkhäuser Basel: Basel; 2006.

41. Croft M, Benedict CA, Ware CF. Clinical targeting of the TNF and TNFR superfamilies. Nat Rev Drug Discov. 2013;12:147–68.

42. Highlights of prescribing information 125057s397lbl. In: ADMINISTRATION, F. A. D. (ed.). U.S Department of Health and Human Services. 2016.

43. van de Kerkhof PC, Segaert S, Lahfa M, Luger TA, Karolyi Z, Kaszuba A, Leigheb G, Camacho FM, Forsea D, Zang C, Boussuge MP, Paolozzi L, Wajdula J. Once weekly administration of etanercept 50 mg is efficacious and well tolerated in patients with moderate-to-severe plaque psoriasis: a randomized controlled trial with open-label extension. Br J Dermatol. 2008;159:1177–85.

44. Strober BE, Crowley JJ, Yamauchi PS, Olds M, Williams DA. Efficacy and safety results from a phase III, randomized controlled trial comparing the safety and efficacy of briakinumab with etanercept and placebo in patients with moderate to severe chronic plaque psoriasis. Br J Dermatol. 2011;165:661–8.

45. Gottlieb AB, Leonardi C, Kerdel F, Mehlis S, Olds M, Williams DA. Efficacy and safety of briakinumab vs. etanercept and placebo in patients with moderate to severe chronic plaque psoriasis. Br J Dermatol. 2011;165:652–60.

46. Langley RG, Elewski BE, Lebwohl M, Reich K, Griffiths CE, Papp K, Puig L, Nakagawa H, Spelman L, Sigurgeirsson B, Rivas E, Tsai TF, Wasel N, Tyring S, Salko T, Hampele I, Notter M, Karpov A, Helou S, Papavassilis C, ERASURE Study Group; FIXTURE Study Group. Secukinumab in plaque psoriasis—results of two phase 3 trials. N Engl J Med. 2014;371:326–38.

47. Griffiths CE, Reich K, Lebwohl M, van de Kerkhof P, Paul C, Menter A, Cameron GS, Erickson J, Zhang L, Secrest RJ, Ball S, Braun DK, Osuntokun OO, Heffernan MP, Nickoloff BJ, Papp K, UNCOVER-2 and UNCOVER-3 investigators. Comparison of ixekizumab with etanercept or placebo in moderate-to-severe psoriasis (UNCOVER-2 and UNCOVER-3): results from two phase 3 randomised trials. Lancet. 2015;386:541–51.

48. Bachelez H, van de Kerkhof PC, Strohal R, Kubanov A, Valenzuela F, Lee JH, Yakusevich V, Chimenti S, Papacharalambous J, Proulx J, Gupta P, Tan H, Tawadrous M, Valdez H, Wolk R, OPT Compare Investigators. Tofacitinib versus etanercept or placebo in moderate-to-severe chronic plaque psoriasis: a phase 3 randomised non-inferiority trial. Lancet. 2015;386:552–61.

49. Reich K, Nestle FO, Papp K, Ortonne JP, Evans R, Guzzo C, Li S, Dooley LT, Griffiths CE, EXPRESS study investigators. Infliximab induction and maintenance therapy for moderate-to-severe psoriasis: a phase III, multicentre, double-blind trial. Lancet. 2005;366:1367–74.

50. Menter A, Feldman SR, Weinstein GD, Papp K, Evans R, Guzzo C, Li S, Dooley LT, Arnold C, Gottlieb AB. A randomized comparison of continuous vs. intermittent infliximab maintenance regimens over 1 year in the treatment of moderate-to-severe plaque psoriasis. J Am Acad Dermatol. 2007;56(31):e1–15.

51. Yang HZ, Wang K, Jin HZ, Gao TW, Xiao SX, Xu JH, Wang BX, Zhang FR, Li CY, Liu XM, Tu CX, Ji SZ, Shen Y, Zhu XJ. Infliximab monotherapy for Chinese patients with moderate to severe plaque psoriasis: a randomized, double-blind, placebo-controlled multicenter trial. Chin Med J. 2012;125:1845–51.

52. Gordon KB, Langley RG, Leonardi C, Toth D, Menter MA, Kang S, Heffernan M, Miller B, Hamlin R, Lim L, Zhong J, Hoffman R, Okun MM. Clinical response to adalimumab treatment in patients with moderate to severe psoriasis: double-blind, randomized controlled trial and open-label extension study. J Am Acad Dermatol. 2006;55:598–606.

53. Saurat JH, Stingl G, Dubertret L, Papp K, Langley RG, Ortonne JP, Unnebrink K, Kaul M, Camez A. Efficacy and safety results from the randomized controlled comparative study of adalimumab vs. methotrexate vs. placebo in patients with psoriasis (CHAMPION). Br J Dermatol. 2008;158:558–66.

54. Menter A, Tyring SK, Gordon K, Kimball AB, Leonardi CL, Langley RG, Strober BE, Kaul M, Gu Y, Okun M, Papp K. Adalimumab therapy for moderate to severe psoriasis: a randomized, controlled phase III trial. J Am Acad Dermatol. 2008;58:106–15.

55. Asahina A, Nakagawa H, Etoh T, Ohtsuki M, Adalimumab MSG. Adalimumab in Japanese patients with moderate to severe chronic plaque psoriasis: efficacy and safety results from a phase II/III randomized controlled study. J Dermatol. 2010;37:299–310.

56. Gordon KB, Duffin KC, Bissonnette R, Prinz JC, Wasfi Y, Li S, Shen Y-K, Szapary P, Randazzo B, Reich K. A phase 2 trial of Guselkumab versus adalimumab for plaque psoriasis. N Engl J Med. 2015;373:136–44.

57. Reich K, Ortonne JP, Gottlieb AB, Terpstra IJ, Coteur G, Tasset C, Mease P. Successful treatment of moderate to severe plaque psoriasis with the PEGylated Fab' certolizumab pegol: results of a phase II randomized, placebo-controlled trial with a re-treatment extension. Br J Dermatol. 2012;167:180–90.

58. Griffiths CE, Strober BE, van de Kerkhof P, Ho V, Fidelus-Gort R, Yeilding N, Guzzo C, Xia Y, Zhou B, Li S, Dooley LT, Goldstein NH, Menter A, ACCEPT Study Group. Comparison of ustekinumab and etanercept for moderate-to-severe psoriasis. N Engl J Med. 2010;362:118–28.

59. 125057s110_MedR_P1: Medical Reviews sBLA125057/110: Humira—adalimumab for adults who are candidates for systemic therapy or phototherapy. In: RESEARCH, C. F. D. E. A. (ed.). U.S. Food and Drug Administration. 2008.

60. Papp KA. The long-term efficacy and safety of new biological therapies for psoriasis. Arch Dermatol Res. 2006;298:7–15.

61. Papp K, Menter A, Poulin Y, Gu Y, Sasso EH. Long-term outcomes of interruption and retreatment vs. continuous therapy with adalimumab for psoriasis: subanalysis of REVEAL and the open-label extension study. J Eur Acad Dermatol Venereol. 2013;27:634–42.

62. Ni C, Chiu MW. Psoriasis and comorbidities: links and risks. Clin Cosmet Investig Dermatol. 2014;7:119–32.

63. Reich K. The concept of psoriasis as a systemic inflammation: implications for disease management. J Eur Acad Dermatol Venereol. 2012;26(Suppl 2):3–11.

64. Mease PJ, Gladman DD, Papp KA, Khraishi MM, Thaci D, Behrens F, Northington R, Fuiman J, Bananis E, Boggs R, Alvarez D. Prevalence of rheumatologist-diagnosed psoriatic arthritis in patients with psoriasis in European/North American dermatology clinics. J Am Acad Dermatol. 2013;69:729–35.

65. Mease PJ, Kivitz AJ, Burch FX, Siegel EL, Cohen SB, Ory P, Salonen D, Rubenstein J, Sharp JT, Tsuji W. Etanercept treatment of psoriatic arthritis: safety, efficacy, and effect on disease progression. Arthritis Rheum. 2004;50:2264–72.

66. Kavanaugh A, Mcinnes I, Mease P, Krueger GG, Gladman D, Gomez-Reino J, Papp K, Zrubek J, Mudivarthy S, Mack M, Visvanathan S, Beutler A. Golimumab, a new human tumor necrosis factor alpha antibody, administered every four weeks as a subcutaneous injection in psoriatic arthritis: twenty-four-week efficacy and safety results of a randomized, placebo-controlled study. Arthritis Rheum. 2009;60:976–86.

67. Kavanaugh A, Mcinnes IB, Mease PJ, Krueger GG, Gladman DD, Van Der Heijde D, Xu W, Mack M, Xu Z, Beutler A. Clinical efficacy, radiographic and safety findings through 2 years of golimumab treatment in patients with active psoriatic arthritis: results from a long-term extension of the randomised, placebo-controlled GO-REVEAL study. Ann Rheum Dis. 2013;72:1777–85.

68. Kavanaugh A, Mcinnes IB, Mease P, Krueger GG, Gladman D, Van Der Heijde D, Zhou Y, Lu J, Leu JH, Goldstein N, Beutler A. Clinical efficacy, radiographic and safety findings through 5 years of subcutaneous golimumab treatment in patients with active psoriatic arthritis: results from a long-term extension of a randomised, placebo-controlled trial (the GO-REVEAL study). Ann Rheum Dis. 2014;73(9):1689–94.

69. Antoni C, Krueger G, De Vlam K, Birbara C, Beutler A, Guzzo C, Zhou B, Dooley L, Kavanaugh A, IMPACT 2 Trial Investigators. Infliximab improves signs and symptoms of psoriatic arthritis: results of the IMPACT 2 trial. Ann Rheum Dis. 2005b;64:1150–7.

70. Antoni CE, Kavanaugh A, Kirkham B, Tutuncu Z, Burmester GR, Schneider U, Furst DE, Molitor J, Keystone E, Gladman D, Manger B, Wassenberg S, Weier R, Wallace DJ, Weisman MH, Kalden JR, Smolen J. Sustained benefits of infliximab therapy for dermatologic and articular manifestations of psoriatic arthritis: results from the infliximab multinational psoriatic arthritis controlled trial (IMPACT). Arthritis Rheum. 2005a;52:1227–36.

71. Baranauskaite A, Raffayova H, Kungurov NV, Kubanova A, Venalis A, Helmle L, Srinivasan S, Nasonov E, Vastesaeger N, RESPOND investigators. Infliximab plus methotrexate is superior to methotrexate alone in the treatment of psoriatic arthritis in methotrexate-naive patients: the RESPOND study. Ann Rheum Dis. 2012;71:541–8.

72. Mease PJ, Gladman DD, Ritchlin CT, Ruderman EM, Steinfeld SD, Choy EH, Sharp JT, Ory PA, Perdok RJ, Weinberg MA, Adalimumab Effectiveness in Psoriatic Arthritis Trial Study, G. Adalimumab for the treatment of patients with moderately to severely active psoriatic arthritis: results of a double-blind, randomized, placebo-controlled trial. Arthritis Rheum. 2005;52:3279–89.

73. Gladman DD, Mease PJ, Ritchlin CT, Choy EH, Sharp JT, Ory PA, Perdok RJ, Sasso EH. Adalimumab for long-term treatment of psoriatic arthritis: forty-eight week data from the adalimumab effectiveness in psoriatic arthritis trial. Arthritis Rheum. 2007;56:476–88.

74. Mease PJ, Ory P, Sharp JT, Ritchlin CT, Van Den Bosch F, Wellborne F, Birbara C, Thomson GT, Perdok RJ, Medich J, Wong RL, Gladman DD. Adalimumab for long-term treatment of psoriatic arthritis: 2-year data from the adalimumab effectiveness in psoriatic arthritis trial (ADEPT). Ann Rheum Dis. 2009;68:702–9.

75. Genovese MC, Mease PJ, Thomson GT, Kivitz AJ, Perdok RJ, Weinberg MA, Medich J, Sasso EH, M02-570 Study Group. Safety and efficacy of adalimumab in treatment of patients with psoriatic arthritis who had failed disease modifying antirheumatic drug therapy. J Rheumatol. 2007;34:1040–50.

76. Mease PJ, Fleischmann R, Deodhar AA, Wollenhaupt J, Khraishi M, Kielar D, Woltering F, Stach C, Hoepken B, Arledge T, Van Der Heijde D. Effect of certolizumab pegol on signs and symptoms in patients with psoriatic arthritis: 24-week results of a phase 3 double-blind randomised placebo-controlled study (RAPID-PsA). Ann Rheum Dis. 2014;73:48–55.

77. Buka RL, Resh B, Roberts B, Cunningham BB, Friedlander S. Etanercept is minimally effective in 2 children with atopic dermatitis. J Am Acad Dermatol. 2005;53:358–9.

78. Jacobi A, Antoni C, Manger B, Schuler G, Hertl M. Infliximab in the treatment of moderate to severe atopic dermatitis. J Am Acad Dermatol. 2005;52:522–6.

79. Sand FL, Thomsen SF. TNF-alpha inhibitors for chronic Urticaria: experience in 20 patients. J Allergy (Cairo). 2013;2013:130905.

80. Graves JE, Nunley K, Heffernan MP. Off-label uses of biologics in dermatology: rituximab, omalizumab, infliximab, etanercept, adalimumab, efalizumab, and alefacept (part 2 of 2). J Am Acad Dermatol. 2007;56:e55–79.

81. Sanchez-Cano D, Callejas-Rubio JL, Ruiz-Villaverde R, Rios-Fernandez R, Ortego-Centeno N. Off-label uses of anti-TNF therapy in three frequent disorders: Behcet's disease, sarcoidosis, and noninfectious uveitis. Mediat Inflamm. 2013;2013:286857.

82. Wolverton SE. Comprehensive dermatologic drug therapy. Edinburgh: Saunders/Elsevier; 2013.

83. Adams DR, Yankura JA, Fogelberg AC, Anderson BE. Treatment of hidradenitis suppurativa with etanercept injection. Arch Dermatol. 2010;146:501–4.

84. Grant A, Gonzalez T, Montgomery MO, Cardenas V, Kerdel FA. Infliximab therapy for patients with moderate to severe hidradenitis suppurativa: a randomized, double-blind, placebo-controlled crossover trial. J Am Acad Dermatol. 2010;62:205–17.

85. Kimball AB, Jemec GB, Yang M, Kageleiry A, Signorovitch JE, Okun MM, Gu Y, Wang K, Mulani P, Sundaram M. Assessing the validity, responsiveness and meaningfulness of the Hidradenitis Suppurativa clinical response (HiSCR) as the clinical endpoint for hidradenitis suppurativa treatment. Br J Dermatol. 2014;171:1434–42.

86. Kimball AB, Kerdel F, Adams D, Mrowietz U, Gelfand JM, Gniadecki R, Prens EP, Schlessinger J, Zouboulis CC, Van Der Zee HH, Rosenfeld M, Mulani P, Gu Y, Paulson S, Okun M, Jemec GB. Adalimumab for the treatment of moderate to severe Hidradenitis suppurativa: a parallel randomized trial. Ann Intern Med. 2012a;157:846–55.

87. Kimball AB, Okun MM, Williams DA, Gottlieb AB, Papp KA, Zouboulis CC, Armstrong AW, Kerdel F, Gold MH, Forman SB, Korman NJ, Giamarellos-Bourboulis EJ, Crowley JJ, Lynde C, Reguiai Z, Prens EP, Alwawi E, Mostafa NM, Pinsky B, Sundaram M, Gu Y, Carlson DM, Jemec GB. Two phase 3 trials of adalimumab for Hidradenitis Suppurativa. N Engl J Med. 2016;375:422–34.

88. Hessam S, Sand M, Gambichler T, Bechara FG. Correlation of inflammatory serum markers with disease severity in patients with hidradenitis suppurativa (HS). J Am Acad Dermatol. 2015;73:998–1005.

89. Vermeire S, Van Assche G, Rutgeerts P. C-reactive protein as a marker for inflammatory bowel disease. Inflamm Bowel Dis. 2004;10:661–5.

90. Thomsen SF, Sand FL. Adherence to TNF-alpha inhibitors in patients with hidradenitis suppurativa. J Dermatolog Treat. 2015;26:97–8.

91. Crowley JJ, Mekkes JR, Zouboulis CC, Scheinfeld N, Kimball A, Sundaram M, Gu Y, Okun MM, Kerdel F. Association of hidradenitis suppurativa disease severity with increased risk for systemic comorbidities. Br J Dermatol. 2014;171:1561–5.

92. Ahlehoff O, Gislason GH, Charlot M, Jorgensen CH, Lindhardsen J, Olesen JB, Abildstrom SZ, Skov L, Torp-Pedersen C, Hansen PR. Psoriasis is associated with clinically significant cardiovascular risk: a Danish nationwide cohort study. J Intern Med. 2011;270:147–57.

93. Gelfand JM, Neimann AL, Shin DB, Wang X, Margolis DJ, Troxel AB. Risk of myocardial infarction in patients with psoriasis. JAMA. 2006;296:1735–41.

94. Brauchli YB, Jick SS, Miret M, Meier CR. Psoriasis and risk of incident myocardial infarction, stroke or transient ischaemic attack: an inception cohort study with a nested case-control analysis. Br J Dermatol. 2009;160:1048–56.

95. Abuabara K, Lee H, Kimball AB. The effect of systemic psoriasis therapies on the incidence of myocardial infarction: a cohort study. Br J Dermatol. 2011;165:1066–73.

96. Abuabara K, Lee H, Kimball AB. Association of systemic psoriasis therapies and incidence of myocardial infarction: reply from authors. Br J Dermatol. 2012;166:233.

97. Wu JJ, Poon KY, Channual JC, Shen AY. Association between tumor necrosis factor inhibitor therapy and myocardial infarction risk in patients with psoriasis. Arch Dermatol. 2012;148:1244–50.

98. Ahlehoff O, Skov L, Gislason G, Gniadecki R, Iversen L, Bryld LE, Lasthein S, Lindhardsen J, Kristensen SL, Torp-Pedersen C, Hansen PR. Cardiovascular outcomes and systemic anti-inflammatory drugs in patients with severe psoriasis: 5-year follow-up of a Danish nationwide cohort. J Eur Acad Dermatol Venereol. 2015;29:1128–34.

99. Bolland MJ, Avenell A, Baron JA, Grey A, Maclennan GS, Gamble GD, Reid IR. Effect of calcium supplements on risk of myocardial infarction and cardiovascular events: meta-analysis. BMJ. 2010;341:c3691.

100. Lind L, Vessby B, Sundstrom J. The apolipoprotein B/AI ratio and the metabolic syndrome independently predict risk for myocardial infarction in middle-aged men. Arterioscler Thromb Vasc Biol. 2006;26:406–10.

101. O'Donnell MJ, Chin SL, Rangarajan S, Xavier D, Liu L, Zhang H, Rao-Melacini P, Zhang X, Pais P, Agapay S, Lopez-Jaramillo P, Damasceno A, Langhorne P, Mcqueen MJ, Rosengren A, Dehghan M, Hankey GJ, Dans AL, Elsayed A, Avezum A, Mondo C, Diener HC, Ryglewicz D, Czlonkowska A, Pogosova N, Weimar C, Iqbal R, Diaz R, Yusoff K, Yusufali A, Oguz A, Wang X, Penaherrera E, Lanas F, Ogah OS, Ogunniyi A, Iversen HK, Malaga G, Rumboldt Z, Oveisgharan S, Al Hussain F, Magazi D, Nilanont Y, Ferguson J, Pare G, Yusuf S, INTERSTROKE investigators. Global and regional effects of potentially modifiable risk factors associated with acute stroke in 32 countries (INTERSTROKE): a case-control study. Lancet. 2016;388:761–75.

102. Yusuf S, Hawken S, Ounpuu S, Bautista L, Franzosi MG, Commerford P, Lang CC, Rumboldt Z, Onen CL, Lisheng L, Tanomsup S, Wangai PJR, Razak F, Sharma AM, Anand SS, INTERHEART Study Investigators. Obesity and the risk of myocardial infarction in 27,000 participants from 52 countries: a case-control study. Lancet. 2005;366:1640–9.

103. Yusuf S, Hawken S, Ounpuu S, Dans T, Avezum A, Lanas F, Mcqueen M, Budaj A, Pais P, Varigos J, Lisheng L, INTERHEART Study Investigators. Effect of potentially modifiable risk factors associated with myocardial infarction in 52 countries (the INTERHEART study): case-control study. Lancet. 2004;364:937–52.

104. Kimball AB, Szapary P, Mrowietz U, Reich K, Langley RG, You Y, Hsu MC, Yeilding N, Rader DJ, Mehta NN. Underdiagnosis and undertreatment of cardiovascular risk factors in patients with moderate to severe psoriasis. J Am Acad Dermatol. 2012b;67:76–85.

105. Kleinbaum DG, Kupper LL, Nizam A, Rosenberg ES. Applied regression analysis and other multivariable methods. Boston, MA: Cengage Learning; 2013.

106. Davies HT, Crombie IK. Bias in case-control studies. Hosp Med. 2000a;61:279–81.

107. Davies HT, Crombie IK. Bias in cohort studies. Hosp Med. 2000b;61:133–5.

108. Utley M, Gallivan S, Young A, Cox N, Davies P, Dixey J, Emery P, Gough A, James D, Prouse P, Williams P, Winfield J, Devlin JA. Potential bias in Kaplan-Meier survival analysis applied to rheumatology drug studies. Rheumatology (Oxford). 2000;39:1–2.

109. Everett BM, Pradhan AD, Solomon DH, Paynter N, Macfadyen J, Zaharris E, Gupta M, Clearfield M, Libby P, Hasan AA, Glynn RJ, Ridker PM. Rationale and design of the cardiovascular inflammation reduction trial: a test of the inflammatory hypothesis of atherothrombosis. Am Heart J. 2013;166(199–207):e15.

110. Ridker PM, Thuren T, Zalewski A, Libby P. Interleukin-1beta inhibition and the prevention of recurrent cardiovascular events: rationale and design of the Canakinumab anti-inflammatory thrombosis outcomes study (CANTOS). Am Heart J. 2011;162:597–605.

111. Burmester GR, Landewe R, Genovese MC, Friedman AW, Pfeifer ND, Varothai NA, Lacerda AP. Adalimumab long-term safety: infections, vaccination response and pregnancy outcomes in patients with rheumatoid arthritis. Ann Rheum Dis. 2017;76:414–7.

112. Burmester GR, Panaccione R, Gordon KB, Mcilraith MJ, Lacerda AP. Adalimumab: long-term safety in 23 458 patients from global clinical trials in rheumatoid arthritis, juvenile idiopathic arthritis, ankylosing spondylitis, psoriatic arthritis, psoriasis and Crohn's disease. Ann Rheum Dis. 2013;72:517–24.

113. Papp KA. The safety of etanercept for the treatment of plaque psoriasis. Ther Clin Risk Manag. 2007;3:245–58.

114. Scheinfeld N. A comprehensive review and evaluation of the side effects of the tumor necrosis factor alpha blockers etanercept, infliximab and adalimumab. J Dermatolog Treat. 2004;15:280–94.

115. Mercer LK, Galloway JB, Lunt M, Davies R, Low AA, Dixon WG, Watson KD, Symmons DP, Hyrich KL. Response to: 'Does the risk of lymphoma in patients with RA treated with TNF inhibitors differ according to the histological subtype and the type of TNF inhibitor?' by nocturne et al. Ann Rheum Dis. 2017;76:e4.

116. Mercer LK, Galloway JB, Lunt M, Davies R, Low AL, Dixon WG, Watson KD, Consortium BCC, Symmons DP, Hyrich KL. Risk of lymphoma in patients exposed to antitumour necrosis factor therapy: results from the British Society for Rheumatology biologics register for rheumatoid arthritis. Ann Rheum Dis. 2016;76(3):497–503.

117. Dreyer L, Magyari M, Laursen B, Cordtz R, Sellebjerg F, Locht H. Risk of multiple sclerosis during tumour necrosis factor inhibitor treatment for arthritis: a population-based study from DANBIO and the Danish multiple sclerosis registry. Ann Rheum Dis. 2016;75:785–6.

118. Solovic I, Sester M, Gomez-Reino JJ, Rieder HL, Ehlers S, Milburn HJ, Kampmann B, Hellmich B, Groves R, Schreiber S, Wallis RS, Sotgiu G, Scholvinck EH, Goletti D, Zellweger JP, Diel R, Carmona L, Bartalesi F, Ravn P, Bossink A, Duarte R, Erkens C, Clark J, Migliori GB, Lange C. The risk of tuberculosis related to tumour necrosis factor antagonist therapies: a TBNET consensus statement. Eur Respir J. 2010;36:1185–206.

119. Furst DE, Wallis R, Broder M, Beenhouwer DO. Tumor necrosis factor antagonists: different kinetics and/or mechanisms of action may explain differences in the risk for developing granulomatous infection. Semin Arthritis Rheum. 2006;36:159–67.

120. Tubach F, Salmon D, Ravaud P, Allanore Y, Goupille P, Breban M, Pallot-Prades B, Pouplin S, Sacchi A, Chichemanian RM, Bretagne S, Emilie D, Lemann M, Lortholary O, Mariette X, Research Axed on Tolerance of Biotherapies, G. Risk of tuberculosis is higher with anti-tumor necrosis factor monoclonal antibody therapy than with soluble tumor necrosis factor receptor therapy: The three-year prospective French Research Axed on Tolerance of Biotherapies registry. Arthritis Rheum. 2009;60:1884–94.

121. Wallis RS. Reactivation of latent tuberculosis by TNF blockade: the role of interferon gamma. J Investig Dermatol Symp Proc. 2007;12:16–21.

122. Wallis RS. Tumour necrosis factor antagonists: structure, function, and tuberculosis risks. Lancet Infect Dis. 2008;8:601–11.

123. Wallis RS. Mathematical models of tuberculosis reactivation and relapse. Front Microbiol. 2016;7:669.

124. Wallis RS, Broder M, Wong J, Lee A, Hoq L. Reactivation of latent granulomatous infections by infliximab. Clin Infect Dis. 2005;41(Suppl 3):S194–8.

125. Wallis RS, Broder MS, Wong JY, Hanson ME, Beenhouwer DO. Granulomatous infectious diseases associated with tumor necrosis factor antagonists. Clin Infect Dis. 2004;38:1261–5.

126. Winthrop KL, Baddley JW, Chen L, Liu L, Grijalva CG, Delzell E, Beukelman T, Patkar NM, Xie F, Saag KG, Herrinton LJ, Solomon DH, Lewis JD, Curtis JR. Association between the initiation of anti-tumor necrosis factor therapy and the risk of herpes zoster. JAMA. 2013;309:887–95.

127. Winthrop KL, Furst DE. Rheumatoid arthritis and herpes zoster: risk and prevention in those treated with anti-tumour necrosis factor therapy. Ann Rheum Dis. 2010;69:1735–7.

128. Yun H, Yang S, Chen L, Xie F, Winthrop K, Baddley JW, Saag KG, Singh J, Curtis JR. Risk of herpes zoster in autoimmune and inflammatory diseases: implications for vaccination. Arthritis Rheumatol. 2016;68:2328–37.

129. Dreiher J, Kresch FS, Comaneshter D, Cohen AD. Risk of herpes zoster in patients with psoriasis treated with biologic drugs. J Eur Acad Dermatol Venereol. 2012;26:1127–32.

130. Shalom G, Zisman D, Bitterman H, Harman-Boehm I, Greenberg-Dotan S, Dreiher J, Feldhamer I, Moser H, Hammerman A, Cohen Y, Cohen AD. Systemic therapy for psoriasis and the risk of herpes zoster: a 500,000 person-year study. JAMA Dermatol. 2015;151:533–8.

131. Brenner D, Blaser H, Mak TW. Regulation of tumour necrosis factor signalling: live or let die. Nat Rev Immunol. 2015;15:362–74.

132. Poulin Y, Therien G. Drug-induced hepatitis and lupus during infliximab treatment for psoriasis: case report and literature review. J Cutan Med Surg. 2010;14:100–4.

133. Landauer K, Unutmaz C, Egli S, Berger V, Lais S, Liebig T, Steiner D, Maier J, Rostalski I, Forcellino F, Herrmann A. Process development of ATROSAB, an anti TNFR1 monoclonal antibody: in three steps from research to GMP. BMC Proc. 2011;5(Suppl 8):P42.

134. Richter F, Liebig T, Guenzi E, Herrmann A, Scheurich P, Pfizenmaier K, Kontermann RE. Antagonistic TNF receptor one-specific antibody (ATROSAB): receptor binding and in vitro bioactivity. PLoS One. 2013;8:e72156.

135. Zettlitz KA, Lorenz V, Landauer K, Munkel S, Herrmann A, Scheurich P, Pfizenmaier K, Kontermann R. ATROSAB, a humanized antagonistic anti-tumor necrosis factor receptor one-specific antibody. MAbs. 2010;2:639–47.

136. Mccann FE, Perocheau DP, Ruspi G, Blazek K, Davies ML, Feldmann M, Dean JL, Stoop AA, Williams RO. Selective tumor necrosis factor receptor I blockade is antiinflammatory and reveals immunoregulatory role of tumor necrosis factor receptor II in collagen-induced arthritis. Arthritis Rheumatol. 2014;66:2728–38.

137. Schmidt EM, Davies M, Mistry P, Green P, Giddins G, Feldmann M, Stoop AA, Brennan FM. Selective blockade of tumor necrosis factor receptor 1 inhibits proinflammatory cytokine and chemokine production in human rheumatoid arthritis synovial membrane cell cultures. Arthritis Rheum. 2013;65:2262–73.

138. Steeland S, Puimege L, Vandenbroucke RE, Van Hauwermeiren F, Haustraete J, Devoogdt N, Hulpiau P, Leroux-Roels G, Laukens D, Meuleman P, De Vos M, Libert C. Generation and characterization of small single domain antibodies inhibiting human tumor necrosis factor receptor 1. J Biol Chem. 2015;290:4022–37.

139. Ameloot P, Brouckaert P. Production and characterization of receptor-specific TNF muteins. Methods Mol Med. 2004;98:33–46.

140. Steed PM, Tansey MG, Zalevsky J, Zhukovsky EA, Desjarlais JR, Szymkowski DE, Abbott C, Carmichael D, Chan C, Cherry L, Cheung P, Chirino AJ, Chung HH, Doberstein SK, Eivazi A, Filikov AV, Gao SX, Hubert RS, Hwang M, Hyun L, Kashi S, Kim A, Kim E, Kung J, Martinez SP, Muchhal US, Nguyen DH, O'brien C, O'keefe D, Singer K, Vafa O, Vielmetter J, Yoder SC, Dahiyat BI. Inactivation of TNF signaling by rationally designed dominant-negative TNF variants. Science. 2003;301:1895–8.

141. Kitagaki M, Isoda K, Kamada H, Kobayashi T, Tsunoda S, Tsutsumi Y, Niida T, Kujiraoka T, Ishigami N, Ishihara M, Matsubara O, Ohsuzu F, Kikuchi M. Novel TNF-alpha receptor 1 antagonist treatment attenuates arterial inflammation and intimal hyperplasia in mice. J Atheroscler Thromb. 2012;19:36–46.

142. Shibata H, Yoshioka Y, Ohkawa A, Minowa K, Mukai Y, Abe Y, Taniai M, Nomura T, Kayamuro H, Nabeshi H, Sugita T, Imai S, Nagano K, Yoshikawa T, Fujita T, Nakagawa S, Yamamoto A, Ohta T, Hayakawa T, Mayumi T, Vandenabeele P, Aggarwal BB, Nakamura T, Yamagata Y, Tsunoda S, Kamada H, Tsutsumi Y. Creation and X-ray structure analysis of the tumor necrosis factor receptor-1-selective mutant of a tumor necrosis factor-alpha antagonist. J Biol Chem. 2008;283:998–1007.

143. Mcalpine FE, Lee JK, Harms AS, Ruhn KA, Blurton-Jones M, Hong J, Das P, Golde TE, Laferla FM, Oddo S, Blesch A, Tansey MG. Inhibition of soluble TNF signaling in a mouse model of Alzheimer's disease prevents pre-plaque amyloid-associated neuropathology. Neurobiol Dis. 2009;34:163–77.

144. Mccoy MK, Martinez TN, Ruhn KA, Szymkowski DE, Smith CG, Botterman BR, Tansey KE, Tansey MG. Blocking soluble tumor necrosis factor signaling with dominant-negative tumor necrosis factor inhibitor attenuates loss of dopaminergic neurons in models of Parkinson's disease. J Neurosci. 2006;26:9365–75.

145. Sama DM, Mohmmad Abdul H, Furman JL, Artiushin IA, Szymkowski DE, Scheff SW, Norris CM. Inhibition of soluble tumor necrosis factor ameliorates synaptic alterations and Ca²⁺ dysregulation in aged rats. PLoS One. 2012;e38170:7.

146. Yung RL. Etanercept Immunex. Curr Opin Investig Drugs. 2001;2:216–21.

Dual Inhibition of IL-12/IL-23 and Selective Inhibition of IL-23 in Psoriasis

Andrew Blauvelt

Introduction

The etiology of psoriasis is unknown, although it is generally believed to be a complex T cell-mediated inflammatory disease with a genetic basis [1, 2]. CD4+ T helper cells, called T helper (Th) 17 cells, are important in the pathogenesis of psoriasis [2–5]. Interleukin (IL)-23 stimulates survival and proliferation of Th17 cells and thus serves as a key upstream cytokine regulator for this disease. Within psoriatic skin lesions, IL-23 is overproduced by activated dermal dendritic cells, and this in turn stimulates Th17 cells within the skin to survive and produce cytokines, including IL-17A. IL-17A and other pro-inflammatory cytokines drive keratinocyte activation and hyperproliferation in psoriasis. This review will focus on the role of IL-23 in psoriasis pathogenesis and the therapeutic targeting of IL-23 by monoclonal antibodies in patients with psoriasis.

Basic Biology of IL-23

IL-23 is the key cytokine involved in the survival and proliferation of Th17 cells (Fig. 14.1) [6, 7]. It is a heterodimeric protein that consists of a unique p19 subunit that is paired with a second subunit called p40 (Fig. 14.2). IL-12 is a related heterodimer consisting of p40 and a unique subunit

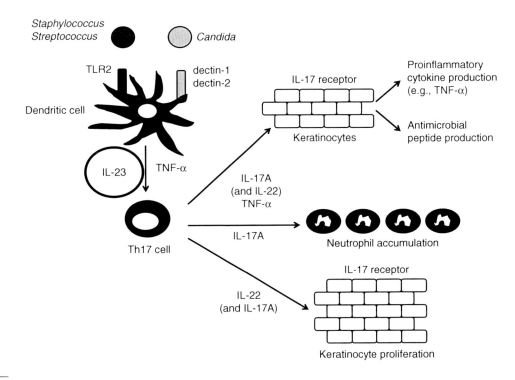

Fig. 14.1 Simplified schematic designed to emphasize the key cells and cytokines involved in the pathogenesis of psoriasis

A. Blauvelt, MD, MBA
Oregon Medical Research Center, 9495 SW Locust Street, Suite G, Portland, OR 97223, USA
e-mail: ablauvelt@oregonmedicalresearch.com

© Springer International Publishing AG 2018
P.S. Yamauchi (ed.), *Biologic and Systemic Agents in Dermatology*, https://doi.org/10.1007/978-3-319-66884-0_14

called p35 and promotes development of Th1 cells (Fig. 14.2) [8]. The IL-23 receptor is also a heterodimer consisting of IL-12Rβ1 and IL-23R subunits, whereas the IL-12 receptor is composed of IL-12Rβ1 and IL-12Rβ2 subunits (Fig. 14.2). IL-23 is produced by dendritic cells and other antigen-presenting cells [6, 9]. It also is produced, albeit at low levels, by keratinocytes [10].

Interestingly, dendritic cells produce IL-23 when stimulated by infection with *Candida albicans*, and this event is mediated by dectin-1, a C-type lectin receptor [11, 12]. IL-23-deficient mice are susceptible to chronic *Candida* infections [13]. In addition, activation through other innate receptors can trigger IL-23 production by dendritic cells, including toll-like receptor 4 signaling induced by lipopolysaccharide from *Bordetella pertussis* and other sources [14, 15]. It is unknown whether *C. albicans* and toll-like receptor ligands stimulate keratinocytes to make IL-23, although this is an intriguing possibility since microorganisms have long been postulated to be triggers for some types of psoriasis.

Role of IL-23 in Psoriasis Pathogenesis

In transgenic mice, overexpression of individual subunits of IL-23 leads to inflammation. Ubiquitous expression of p19 causes severe multi-organ inflammation, runting, infertility, high circulating levels of TNF-α and IL-1, and premature death [16]. Overexpression of p40 in basal keratinocytes induces psoriasis-like inflammatory skin disease [17]. These investigators suggested that transgenic p40 combined with endogenous p19 to form IL-23, which in turn caused cutaneous inflammation.

In other mouse studies, recombinant IL-23 injected into normal-appearing skin produced erythematous, thick, scaly skin, with histologic features reminiscent of psoriasis [18–20]. Recombinant IL-12 injected in a similar manner did not [18, 19]. Interestingly, acanthosis induced by injection of

IL-23 is dependent upon two key Th17 cytokines: IL-17A and IL-22 [20]. When IL-23 was injected into IL-17A knockout or IL-22 knockout mice, no keratinocyte hyperproliferation was observed [19, 20]. Thus, these studies directly demonstrated that both cytokines are critical downstream mediators of IL-23-induced psoriasis-like inflammation in the skin.

In humans, IL-23 is clearly elevated in psoriasis lesions as indicated by increased levels of both *p19* and *p40* mRNA in lesional skin as compared to non-lesional skin, whereas mRNA levels of *p35* are not elevated [18, 21–24]. This implies that IL-23, but not IL-12, is increased in the skin affected by psoriasis. Furthermore, immunohistochemical analyses have revealed p40 and p19 protein expression in dermal dendritic cells [23–25] and keratinocytes [26] in lesions of psoriasis. Importantly, IL-23 levels (assessed by either mRNA or protein) decrease with clinical improvement of psoriasis following effective treatment, providing a direct correlation between overproduction of IL-23 and active psoriasis [18, 21–23, 26–28].

The importance of IL-23 in psoriasis pathogenesis has also been strengthened by genetic studies. Tsunemi et al. found that a single nucleotide polymorphism in *p40* was associated with psoriasis [29]. This polymorphism was confirmed using genome-wide association studies and gene sequencing techniques in additional independent cohorts [30–32]. The association was independent of *HLA-Cw*0602*, another gene linked to psoriasis [33]. Polymorphisms in the gene encoding the IL-23-specific subunit, *p19*, are also associated with psoriasis development [30–32]. In addition, a common risk haplotype was identified for the gene encoding the receptor subunit that is specific for IL-23, *IL-23R*, with proline at amino acid 310 and arginine at amino acid 381 [30–32]. Conversely, a change in *IL-23R* at 381 from arginine to glutamine was found to be *protective* against psoriasis [30–32]. This amino acid is in the JAK2 kinase-binding domain of IL-23R, which transmits intracellular signals that are triggered following ligation of IL-23R. This change to glutamine inhibits the IL-23R signaling cascade and prevents inflammatory responses mediated by Th17 cells [34]. Of importance, no polymorphisms specific to IL-12, e.g., *p35* or *IL-12Rβ2*, are associated with psoriasis susceptibility.

Large numbers of recent reports suggest that IL-23 is critically involved in psoriasis pathogenesis (Table 14.1). Taken together, hypotheses can be generated as to how this cytokine could cause psoriasis. Perturbation of resident keratinocytes and dendritic cells by trauma and/or stimulation of pattern recognition receptors (e.g., dectin-1, TLR 2 and TLR 4) by microbes on the skin surface may trigger conditions that promote IL-23 production [11, 12] and thus lead to survival and proliferation of Th17 cells within the skin. Th17 cells may migrate into the skin via chemokine receptors [11, 35]. CCR6, whose chemokine ligand CCL20 is secreted by keratinocytes, is found in abundance on Th17 cells; CCR4 is

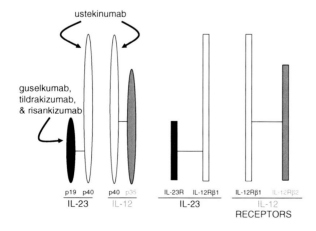

Fig. 14.2 Schematic showing the subunits of IL-23, IL-12, and their respective receptors, including p40 (the shared subunit targeted by ustekinumab) and p19 (the subunit targeted by guselkumab, tildrakizumab, and risankizumab)

Table 14.1 Summary of scientific evidence supporting a major role for Il-23 in psoriasis pathogenesis[a]

p19 (the IL-23-specific subunit) elevated in lesional psoriatic skin
p40 (the subunit shared by both IL-23 and IL-23) elevated in lesional psoriatic skin
Polymorphisms in *p19* associated with susceptibility to psoriasis
Polymorphisms in *p40* associated with susceptibility and protection from psoriasis, depending on the genetic change
Polymorphisms in *IL-23R* (IL-23 receptor-specific subunit) associated with susceptibility and protection from psoriasis, depending on the genetic change
Anti-p40 monoclonal antibodies markedly efficacious in psoriasis
Anti-p19 monoclonal antibodies efficacious in psoriasis
p19 transgenic mice develop a widespread inflammatory disease
p40 transgenic expression in the skin causes inflammatory skin disease
IL-23 injected into mouse skin causes psoriasis-like disease

[a]See text for specific references

also expressed on Th17 cell surfaces [11, 35]. Interestingly, these chemokine receptors are also characteristically found on resident skin T cells [36]. Thus, it is possible that skin preferentially recruits Th17 cells in resting or noninflammatory states and that perturbations that enhance local IL-23 production would allow for expansion of these cells and thus produce inflammation. CCL20 is overexpressed in psoriasis [37], and researchers have also demonstrated recently that IL-17A induces keratinocytes to produce CCL20 in vitro [38]. This may be important in maintenance of psoriasis lesions by stimulating ongoing chemotaxis of new CCR6+ Th17 cells and CCR6+ dendritic cells from blood. Genetic alterations that augment IL-23 signaling may increase the susceptibility to psoriasis [29–32]. By contrast, other mutations that result in decreased IL-23 production and receptor-mediated signaling [30, 31] confer protection from psoriasis [34]. Finally, since IL-23 is now believed to be a key "upstream" or effector cytokine in psoriasis pathogenesis (Table 14.1), it is also predicted that IL-23 inhibition would lead to death of Th17 cells and abrogation of psoriasis.

Dual Inhibition of IL-12 and IL-23 by Ustekinumab

Ustekinumab is a fully human IgG1κ monoclonal antibody directed against p40 and thus will inhibit functions of both IL-23 and IL-12 (Fig. 14.2). As discussed, inhibition of IL-23 is predicted to induce death of Th17 cells, since these cells are dependent upon IL-23 for survival and proliferation. Blocking IL-12 is predicted to cause loss of Th1 cells, since IL-12 stimulates function of these cells. Thus, although ustekinumab does not directly act upon T cells, the most likely result of its pharmacologic action is to cause T cell death by inhibition of two major T cell growth factors, IL-23 and IL-12.

Apoptosis of Th17 and Th1 cells has not been directly evaluated in patients receiving either ustekinumab. If this

mechanism of action is proven to be true, this would explain the prolonged clinical effects of this drug long after they have been cleared from serum, because a relatively lengthy series of immunologic events would be required to repopulate Th17 and Th1 cells into the skin.

Cooper and colleagues showed that ustekinumab therapy rapidly decreased expression of a variety of pro-inflammatory cytokine genes in lesional psoriatic skin, including *p19*, *p40*, and *IL-17A* [22]. TNF-α blocking agents do the same, and it appears that genes associated with the IL-23/Th17 inflammatory pathway are downregulated earlier than genes associated with the IL-12/Th1 inflammatory pathway [27, 39]. This finding suggests that IL-23 and Th17 cells are more primary, or earlier, targets for these biologic therapies when compared to IL-12 and Th1 cells. TNF-α is made by numerous cell types, including Th17 cells [40], and has pleiotropic inflammatory effects. Although TNF-α antagonists likely have anti-inflammatory effects on multiple cell types and tissues, recent data suggest that these agents also work, at least in part, by blocking the IL-23/Th17 inflammatory pathway.

Ustekinumab Efficacy

In early phase I clinical trials, ustekinumab use led to demonstrable clinical effects on psoriasis after intravenous and subcutaneous administration of single doses of the drug [41, 42]. These early trials led to a phase II study that produced promising clinical results [43]. In a classic dose-response manner, 52% of low-dose patients, 59% of low-medium-dose patients, 67% of medium-high-dose patients, and 81% of high-dose patients achieved PASI 75 at week 12, which means a reduction in the psoriasis area and severity index of at least 75%.

These early phase studies were confirmed by three major phase III studies, PHOENIX I and II, and one etanercept comparator trial, which in total had combined enrollment of over 3500 individuals from over 100 sites in the USA and Europe [44–46]. These three studies evaluated doses of 45 and 90 mg of ustekinumab given subcutaneously at weeks 0 and 4 (initiation therapy) and then dosing given every 8 or 12 weeks (maintenance therapy). Psoriasis responded well to ustekinumab; at week 12, PASI 75 ranged from 67% to 76% [44–46] (Table 14.2). By comparison, the etanercept response rate given at a dose of 50 mg twice weekly was 57% at week 12 [46]. Interestingly, the highest PASI 75 rates were recorded between weeks 20 and 24 and were approximately 75% with the 45-mg dose and 85% with the 90-mg dose [44, 45]. The majority of patients treated with either 45 or 90 mg every 12 weeks maintained clinical responses to ustekinumab for up to 76 weeks of therapy [44]. When a subset of patients were switched from ustekinumab to placebo at week 40, most individuals demonstrated long-lasting clinical effects on their psoriasis, with gradual, not abrupt, return of disease over the course of 24 weeks following discontinuation of the drug [44].

Table 14.2 Summary of PASI 75 phase III short-term and long-term efficacy results for ustekinumab

Conditions (mg)	PASI 75 (%)[a]	References
Week 12, 45	67	[44–46]
Week 12, 90	66–76	[44–46]
Weeks 20–24, 45	75–76	[44, 45]
Weeks 20–24, 90	84–85	[44, 45]
Maintenance among initial responders (>PASI 75), week 244, 45	79	[47]
Maintenance among initial responders (>PASI 75), week 244, 90	81	[47]
Maintenance among initial partial responders (PASI 50–PASI 75), week 244, 45	58	[47]
Maintenance among initial partial responders (PASI 50–PASI 75), week 244, 90	55	[47]

[a]PASI 75 = percentage of patients that improved their Psoriasis Area and Severity Index scores by at least 75% when compared to baseline index scores

Not all psoriasis patients responded well to ustekinumab in the phase III studies. Of note, partial responders at week 28 (PASI 50–PASI 75) were compared with responders (greater than PASI 75) in a variety of ways. Partial responders were more likely than responders to demonstrate the following historical, clinical, or immunologic features: (1) higher body weight, (2) inadequate response to at least one biologic agent in the past, (3) longer duration of psoriasis, (4) history of psoriatic arthritis, and (5) presence of neutralizing antibodies to ustekinumab [44, 45]. For the latter assay, antibodies to ustekinumab were detected in 12.7% of partial responders and in 2% of responders. Partial responders at week 28 tended to fare best when subsequently given doses of 90 mg every 8 weeks when compared to partial responders who received either 45 mg or dosing every 12 weeks [45]. Thus, the ability to give ustekinumab at higher doses (90 mg instead of 45 mg) and for shorter intervals (every 8 weeks instead of every 12 weeks) may prove clinically meaningful for certain patients that do not respond well at lower and/or less frequent doses. These trials proved that regular dosing of ustekinumab over the course of 1.5 years is a highly efficacious therapy for individuals with psoriasis. Based upon these phase III results, the US Food and Drug Administration (FDA) recommended approval of ustekinumab for moderate-to-severe plaque psoriasis in 2009.

Importantly, the PHOENIX I and II ustekinumab trials were continued for a 5-year period [47]. Sixty-nine percent of patients originally placed onto ustekinumab in these phase III studies completed the entire trial. Approximately 80% of initial responders maintained PASI 75 responses over the course of 5 years, and approximately 55% of initial partial responders (i.e., those who first reached PASI 50–PASI 75) achieved PASI 75 by week 244 (Table 14.2) [47]. These results demonstrate that clinical efficacy of ustekinumab is robust over an extended period.

Ustekinumab has also been shown to be effective in psoriatic arthritis, and has FDA approval for this indication, although efficacy is not as great as that observed with TNF blockers in this disease 48–51. In off-label usage, individuals with erythrodermic psoriasis [52–55], palmoplantar psoriasis [56–59], and TNF blocker-induced psoriasis/psoriasiform dermatitis [60, 61] have also been reported to respond well to ustekinumab. One common theme from these reports is that higher dosages of ustekinumab, i.e., 90 mg every 8 weeks, may be necessary to treat patients with more refractory or unusual forms of disease. While initial results are hopeful, further controlled studies are needed to assess the usefulness of ustekinumab in these conditions.

Ustekinumab Safety

Safety results from both short-term [44–46] and longer-term [62–65] clinical trials are highly encouraging. Rates of infection were not higher in ustekinumab-treated patients when compared to placebo-treated patients over a 12-week period [44, 45]. These rates remain very low with chronic use of ustekinumab (i.e., up to 5 years), and there does not appear to be any increase in infection rate with higher drug doses [44–46, 62–65].

Insight on infection risk can also be gleaned from other diseases. Humans that have genetic defects in p40 or in the IL-12 receptor subunit, IL-12Rβ1, and thus either cannot produce IL-12 or signal through the IL-12 receptor, are susceptible to intracellular bacterial infections like those caused by mycobacteria and *Salmonella enteritidis* [66–68]. However, there have not been cases of tuberculosis, atypical mycobacterial infection, or *Salmonella* infection reported with ustekinumab to date [44–46, 62–65]. In fact, patients diagnosed with latent tuberculosis upon screening were allowed into the phase III ustekinumab trials as long as they received appropriate antituberculous therapy; none of these individuals experienced worsening pulmonary disease [44, 45, 69]. Patients with a history of tuberculosis or those with potential to reactivate latent disease should either avoid treatment with ustekinumab or be treated with concomitant antituberculous medication [69].

Regarding the potential for ustekinumab-treated patients to develop malignancies, 5-year studies show no significant signals [63, 65]. In particular, the number of cases of lymphoma and squamous cell carcinomas, two cancers often associated with immunosuppression, is lower than what would be expected in the general population over a 5-year period [63, 65].

In early studies, five major adverse cardiovascular events (MACE) were reported in patients receiving ustekinumab within the first 12 weeks of therapy, whereas no cases in placebo-treated patients were noted during this time period

[44, 45]. These results were not statistically significant by standard methodology [70], but some have expressed concern with these numbers [71, 72]. Of major importance, this possible initial signal has not been borne out in follow-up studies to date [46, 64, 65, 72–74]. In fact, promising data emerging from long-term studies indicate that ustekinumab may actually *decrease* the likelihood of cardiovascular disease over time [65, 74].

Guselkumab, Tildrakizumab, and Risankizumab Efficacy

Guselkumab is a fully human IgG1κ monoclonal antibody directed against p19 and thus will inhibit functions of IL-23 alone. In early phase clinical trials, guselkumab use led to demonstrable clinical effects on psoriasis after subcutaneous administration of single ascending doses of the drug [75, 76]. This early trial led was further supported by results of a phase II study, which used adalimumab as a comparator [77]. In a classic dose-response manner, 44% of patients treated with 5 mg, 76% of patients treated with 15 mg, and 81% treated with higher doses of guselkumab (50–200 mg) achieved PASI 75 responses at week 16. By contrast, 70% of adalimumab-treated patients, used as active comparator in this study, achieved a PASI 75 at week 16.

Results from two major phase III guselkumab studies, VOYAGE 1 and 2, have recently been published [78, 79]. Over 2000 individuals from over 200 sites in the USA and Europe participated. These studies evaluated doses of 100 mg of guselkumab given subcutaneously at weeks 0 and 4 (initiation therapy) and then dosing given every 8 weeks thereafter (maintenance therapy). Psoriasis responded dramatically to guselkumab; at week 16, PASI 75 was 91% and 86% in VOYAGE 1 and 2, respectively [78, 79] (Table 14.3). By comparison, response rates for adalimumab, used as a comparator, were 73% and 69% at week 16. Interestingly, the highest PASI 90 rates were recorded at week 24 (80% and 75%), and the highest PASI 100 responses were recorded at week 48 (47%), indicating that guselkumab therapy tends to continually improve psoriasis over the course of the first year of treatment [78, 79]. Furthermore, difficult-to-treat regions of the body affected by psoriasis, including the scalp,

nails, and palms/soles, responded well to guselkumab, superior to response rates observed in adalimumab-treated patients [78]. When a subset of patients was switched from guselkumab to placebo at week 16, most individuals demonstrated long-lasting clinical effects on their psoriasis, with gradual, not abrupt, return of disease over the course of 24 weeks following discontinuation of the drug [79]. Long-term efficacy studies with guselkumab will be forthcoming, since the VOYAGE 1 and 2 trials will be extended for 3 years.

Tildrakizumab is a humanized IgG1κ monoclonal antibody directed against p19 and thus selectively targets IL-23. In an early phase I clinical trial, tildrakizumab use led to demonstrable clinical effects on psoriasis after three intravenous administrations of ascending doses of drug [80]. In a classic dose-response phase II study, 33% of patients treated with 5 mg, 64% of patients treated with 25 mg, 66% treated with 100 mg, and 74% treated with 200 mg achieved PASI 75 responses at week 16 [81].

Data from two major phase III studies, reSURFACE 1 and reSURFACE 2, have now been published [82]. Together, these studies included over 1800 individuals from 250 sites in the USA and Europe. These studies evaluated doses of 100 and 200 mg of tildrakizumab given subcutaneously at weeks 0 and 4 (initiation therapy) and then dosing given every 12 weeks thereafter (maintenance therapy). Etanercept was used as a comparator. At week 12, PASI 75 ranged 61–66%, with no clear differences observed between the 100 and 200-mg doses at this early timepoint [82] (Table 14.4). By comparison, the etanercept response rate was 48% at week 12. Interestingly, the highest PASI 75 rates were recorded at week 28 (73–79%) [82], indicating that tildrakizumab, like other IL-23 blockers, tends to improve psoriasis over time. Also, at week 28, the 200-mg group seemed to fare better than the 100-mg group, i.e., PASI 90 and PASI 100 response rates were highest in the 200-mg group (57% and 26–31%, respectively) [82]. reSURFACE 1 and reSURFACE 2 are ongoing and are planned to continue for 5 years.

Risankizumab is a fully human IgG1 anti-p19 antibody, which selectively blocks IL-23. In a phase I trial, psoriasis patients received single ascending intravenous or subcutaneous doses of the drug. Patients receiving higher doses

Table 14.3 Summary of phase III PASI 75, PASI 90, and PASI 100 efficacy results for guselkumab

Time	PASI 75 (%)[a]	PASI 90 (%)[a]	PASI 100 (%)[a]	References
Week 16	86–91	70–73	34–37	[78, 79]
Week 24	89–91	75–80	44	[78, 79]
Week 48	88	76	47	[78]

[a]PASI 75/90/100 = percentage of patients that improved their Psoriasis Area and Severity Index by at least 75%, 90%, or 100% when compared to baseline score

Table 14.4 Summary of phase III PASI 75, PASI 90, and PASI 100 efficacy results for tildrakizumab

Conditions (mg)	PASI 75 (%)[a]	PASI 90 (%)[a]	PASI 100 (%)[a]	References
Week 12, 100	61–64	35–39	12–14	[82]
Week 12, 200	62–66	35–37	12–14	[82]
Week 28, 100	74–77	49–55	22	[82]
Week 28, 200	73–79	57	26–31	[82]

[a]PASI 75/90/100 = percentage of patients that improved their Psoriasis Area and Severity Index by at least 75%, 90%, or 100% when compared to baseline score

experienced rapid, substantial, and durable improvements in psoriasis, with several patients who received higher doses achieving and maintaining PASI for up to 24 weeks [83]. In a phase II study, patients received subcutaneous risankizumab at doses of 18, 90, and 180 mg at weeks 0, 4, and 16. At week 12, PASI 75/PASI 90/PASI 100 was 98%/73%/41% for the 90-mg dose group and 88%/79%/48% for the 180-mg group [84]. At week 24, PASI 75/PASI 90 was 90%/63% for the 90-mg dose group and 88%/81% for the 180-mg group [84]. Phase III studies for risankizumab are ongoing, and results have not yet been revealed at the time of publication of this chapter.

Guselkumab, Tildrakizumab, and Risankizumab Safety

Thus far, no safety signals have emerged with selective IL-23 blockers with up to 48 weeks of use [75–84]. Specifically, higher rates of serious infections, tuberculosis, reactivation, hepatitis B reactivation, cancer, congestive heart failure, multiple sclerosis, major adverse cardiovascular events, candidiasis, inflammatory bowel disease, suicide, and laboratory/EKG abnormalities have not been observed. Long-term safety studies are needed to better assess the safety of these agents. Of note, long-term safety of ustekinumab, a less specific blocker, likely means that IL-23 inhibitors will also be safe with prolonged use.

Summary

Numerous recent studies demonstrate that psoriasis is a Th17 cell-mediated disease driven by IL-23 (Table 14.1). Indeed, most scientists involved in studying psoriasis pathogenesis now believe that ustekinumab principally acts through IL-23 inhibition, whereas the specific role that IL-12 plays in psoriasis pathogenesis is now unclear. Thus, it is not surprising that therapeutic targeting of IL-23 by ustekinumab and other more selective drugs (e.g., guselkumab, tildrakizumab, risankizumab) demonstrates considerable efficacy in psoriatics (Tables 14.2, 14.3, and 14.4). In most cases, the newer more selective IL-23 blockers are more efficacious than ustekinumab, while demonstrating no worrisome safety signals to date. These drugs are now several years into phase III clinical trial programs and may be on the market for general use as early as the third quarter of 2017. In summary, identification of IL-23 as a key "upstream" mediator of psoriatic inflammation and the blocking of IL-23 by ustekinumab and newer more selective drugs have represented major advances in the understanding of psoriasis and in the development of highly safe and effective targeted therapies.

Case

A 42-year-old female professional presents with a 5-year history of moderate psoriasis, with no history of psoriatic arthritis. She is otherwise healthy. The patient is anxious about safety of systemic medications, so she was initially given topical corticosteroids and was recommended for phototherapy by another dermatologist. Biologics were not initially discussed. Disease control was inadequate and phototherapy proved to be too time-consuming for her busy schedule.

Past Medical History
- None

Social History
- Drinks socially (a few glasses of wine per week)
- Married
- Busy professional

Previous Therapies
- Topical corticosteroids

Physical Exam
- Psoriatic plaques on the scalp, trunk, upper, and lower extremities covering 11% of the body surface area
- No features of psoriatic arthritis (dactylitis, enthesitis, tender and swollen joints, etc.)
- 150 pounds

Management

The patient is a candidate for systemic therapy because of the extent of her psoriasis and because she has failed topical corticosteroids. She is not a candidate for phototherapy given her busy schedule. She is anxious about safety of systemic therapy. Thus, methotrexate would not be a good choice for this patient given its poor efficacy and its possible liver toxicity. Similarly, apremilast would not be a good choice for this patient given its poor efficacy and poor short-term tolerability. Ustekinumab was chosen for several reasons. First, it has high efficacy when compared to older systemic therapies. Second, it has the best long-term safety record of any biologic, which would be important for this patient. Third, it is the most convenient systemic therapy for psoriasis, which would make it fit well into her busy schedule.

Baseline PPD was performed and was negative. No other baseline routine labs were checked, as these are not required nor necessary with ustekinumab therapy. The standard dose of ustekinumab was used starting at 45 mg SC at weeks 0, 4, and 16. At her week 28 visit, her skin was clear and she was having no side effects. Her quality of life had improved dramatically, and she stated that she was not aware that obtaining clear skin so easily was even a possibility until she had presented 7 months earlier.

References

1. Nestle FO, Kaplan DH, Barker J. Psoriasis. N Engl J Med. 2009;361(5):496–509.
2. Di Cesare A, Di Meglio P, Nestle FO. The IL-23/Th17 axis in the immunopathogenesis of psoriasis. J Invest Dermatol. 2009;129:1339–50.
3. Blauvelt A. New concepts in the pathogenesis and treatment of psoriasis: key roles for IL-23, IL-17A and TGF-b1. Expert Rev Dermatol. 2007;2(1):1–10.
4. Fitch E, Harper E, Skorcheva I, Kurtz SE, Blauvelt A. Pathophysiology of psoriasis: recent advances on IL-23 and Th17 cytokines. Curr Rheumatol Rep. 2007;9(6):461–7.
5. Blauvelt A. T-helper 17 cells in psoriatic plaques and additional genetic links between IL-23 and psoriasis. J Invest Dermatol. 2008;128(5):1064–7.
6. Oppmann B, Lesley R, Blom B, Timans JC, Xu Y, Hunte B, et al. Novel p19 protein engages IL-12p40 to form a cytokine, IL-23, with biological activities similar as well as distinct from IL-12. Immunity. 2000;13(5):715–25.
7. Stockinger B, Veldhoen M. Differentiation and function of Th17 T cells. Curr Opin Immunol. 2007;19(3):281–6.
8. Tesmer LA, Lundy SK, Sarkar S, Fox DA. Th17 cells in human disease. Immunol Rev. 2008;223:87–113.
9. Gerosa F, Baldani-Guerra B, Lyakh LA, Batoni G, Esin S, Winkler-Pickett RT, et al. Differential regulation of interleukin 12 and interleukin 23 production in human dendritic cells. J Exp Med. 2008;205(6):1447–61.
10. Piskin G, Sylva-Steenland RM, Bos JD, Teunissen MB. In vitro and in situ expression of IL-23 by keratinocytes in healthy skin and psoriasis lesions: enhanced expression in psoriatic skin. J Immunol. 2006;176(3):1908–15.
11. Acosta-Rodriguez EV, Rivino L, Geginat J, Jarrossay D, Gattorno M, Lanzavecchia A, et al. Surface phenotype and antigenic specificity of human interleukin 17-producing T helper memory cells. Nat Immunol. 2007;8(6):639–46.
12. LeibundGut-Landmann S, Gross O, Robinson MJ, Osorio F, Slack EC, Tsoni SV, et al. Syk- and CARD9-dependent coupling of innate immunity to the induction of T helper cells that produce interleukin 17. Nat Immunol. 2007;8(6):630–8.
13. Kagami S, Rizzo HL, Kurtz SE, Miller LS, Blauvelt A. IL-23 and IL-17A, but not IL-12 and IL-22, are required for optimal skin host defense against Candida albicans. J Immunol. 2010;185(9):5453–62.
14. Re F, Strominger JL. Toll-like receptor 2 (TLR2) and TLR4 differentially activate human dendritic cells. J Biol Chem. 2001;276(40):37692–9.
15. Higgins SC, Jarnicki AG, Lavelle EC, Mills KH. TLR4 mediates vaccine-induced protective cellular immunity to Bordetella pertussis: role of IL-17-producing T cells. J Immunol. 2006;177(11):7980–9.
16. Wiekowski MT, Leach MW, Evans EW, Sullivan L, Chen SC, Vassileva G, et al. Ubiquitous transgenic expression of the IL-23 subunit p19 induces multiorgan inflammation, runting, infertility, and premature death. J Immunol. 2001;166(12):7563–70.
17. Kopp T, Lenz P, Bello-Fernandez C, Kastelein RA, Kupper TS, Stingl G. IL-23 production by cosecretion of endogenous p19 and transgenic p40 in keratin 14/p40 transgenic mice: evidence for enhanced cutaneous immunity. J Immunol. 2003;170(11):5438–44.
18. Chan JR, Blumenschein W, Murphy E, Diveu C, Wiekowski M, Abbondanzo S, et al. IL-23 stimulates epidermal hyperplasia via TNF and IL-20R2-dependent mechanisms with implications for psoriasis pathogenesis. J Exp Med. 2006;203(12):2577–87.
19. Zheng Y, Danilenko DM, Valdez P, Kasman I, Eastham-Anderson J, Wu J, et al. Interleukin-22, a T(H)17 cytokine, mediates IL-23-induced dermal inflammation and acanthosis. Nature. 2007;445(7128):648–51.
20. Rizzo HL, Kagami S, Phillips KG, Kurtz SE, Jacques SL, Blauvelt A. IL-23-mediated psoriasis-like epidermal hyperplasia is dependent on IL-17A. J Immunol. 2011;186(3):1495–502.
21. Chamian F, Lowes MA, Lin SL, Lee E, Kikuchi T, Gilleaudeau P, et al. Alefacept reduces infiltrating T cells, activated dendritic cells, and inflammatory genes in psoriasis vulgaris. Proc Natl Acad Sci U S A. 2005;102(6):2075–80.
22. Toichi E, Torres G, McCormick TS, Chang T, Mascelli MA, Kauffman CL, et al. An anti-IL-12p40 antibody down-regulates type 1 cytokines, chemokines, and IL-12/IL-23 in psoriasis. J Immunol. 2006;177(7):4917–26.
23. Lee E, Trepicchio WL, Oestreicher JL, Pittman D, Wang F, Chamian F, et al. Increased expression of interleukin 23 p19 and p40 in lesional skin of patients with psoriasis vulgaris. J Exp Med. 2004;199(1):125–30.
24. Wilson NJ, Boniface K, Chan JR, McKenzie BS, Blumenschein WM, Mattson JD, et al. Development, cytokine profile and function of human interleukin 17-producing helper T cells. Nat Immunol. 2007;8(9):950–7.
25. Lillis JV, Guo CS, Lee JJ, Blauvelt A. Increased IL-23 expression in palmoplantar psoriasis and hyperkeratotic hand dermatitis. Arch Dermatol. 2010;146(8):918–9.
26. Piskin G, Tursen U, Sylva-Steenland RM, Bos JD, Teunissen MB. Clinical improvement in chronic plaque-type psoriasis lesions after narrow-band UVB therapy is accompanied by a decrease in the expression of IFN-gamma inducers—IL-12, IL-18 and IL-23. Exp Dermatol. 2004;13(12):764–72.
27. Gottlieb AB, Chamian F, Masud S, Cardinale I, Abello MV, Lowes MA, et al. TNF inhibition rapidly down-regulates multiple proinflammatory pathways in psoriasis plaques. J Immunol. 2005;175(4):2721–9.
28. Lowes MA, Chamian F, Abello MV, Fuentes-Duculan J, Lin SL, Nussbaum R, et al. Increase in TNF-alpha and inducible nitric oxide synthase-expressing dendritic cells in psoriasis and reduction with efalizumab (anti-CD11a). Proc Natl Acad Sci U S A. 2005;102(52):19057–62.
29. Tsunemi Y, Saeki H, Nakamura K, Sekiya T, Hirai K, Fujita H, et al. Interleukin-12 p40 gene (IL12B) 3'-untranslated region polymorphism is associated with susceptibility to atopic dermatitis and psoriasis vulgaris. J Dermatol Sci. 2002;30(2):161–6.
30. Cargill M, Schrodi SJ, Chang M, Garcia VE, Brandon R, Callis KP, et al. A large-scale genetic association study confirms IL12B and leads to the identification of IL23R as psoriasis-risk genes. Am J Hum Genet. 2007;80(2):273–90.
31. Capon F, Di Meglio P, Szaub J, Prescott NJ, Dunster C, Baumber L, et al. Sequence variants in the genes for the interleukin-23 receptor (IL23R) and its ligand (IL12B) confer protection against psoriasis. Hum Genet. 2007;122:201–6.
32. Nair RP, Ruether A, Stuart PE, Jenisch S, Tejasvi T, Hiremagalore R, et al. Polymorphisms of the IL12B and IL23R genes are associated with psoriasis. J Invest Dermatol. 2008;128(7):1653–61.
33. Nair RP, Stuart PE, Nistor I, Hiremagalore R, Chia NV, Jenisch S, et al. Sequence and haplotype analysis supports HLA-C as the psoriasis susceptibility 1 gene. Am J Hum Genet. 2006;78(5):827–51.
34. Di Meglio P, Di Cesare A, Laggner U, Chu CC, Napolitano L, Villanova F, et al. The IL23R R381Q gene variant protects against immune-mediated diseases by impairing IL-23-induced Th17 effector response in humans. PLoS One. 2011;6(2):e17160.
35. Annunziato F, Cosmi L, Santarlasci V, Maggi L, Liotta F, Mazzinghi B, et al. Phenotypic and functional features of human Th17 cells. J Exp Med. 2007;204(8):1849–61.

36. Clark RA, Chong B, Mirchandani N, Brinster NK, Yamanaka K, Dowgiert RK, et al. The vast majority of CLA+ T cells are resident in normal skin. J Immunol. 2006;176(7):4431–9.

37. Homey B, Dieu-Nosjean MC, Wiesenborn A, Massacrier C, Pin JJ, Oldham E, et al. Up-regulation of macrophage inflammatory protein-3 alpha/CCL20 and CC chemokine receptor 6 in psoriasis. J Immunol. 2000;164(12):6621–32.

38. Harper EG, Guo C, Rizzo H, Lillis JV, Kurtz SE, Skorcheva I, et al. Th17 cytokines stimulate CCL20 expression in keratinocytes in vitro and in vivo: implications for psoriasis pathogenesis. J Invest Dermatol. 2009;129(9):2175–83.

39. Zaba LC, Cardinale I, Gilleaudeau P, Sullivan-Whalen M, Suarez Farinas M, Fuentes-Duculan J, et al. Amelioration of epidermal hyperplasia by TNF inhibition is associated with reduced Th17 responses. J Exp Med. 2007;204(13):3183–94.

40. Kagami S, Rizzo HL, Lee JJ, Koguchi Y, Blauvelt A. Circulating Th17, Th22, and Th1 cells are increased in psoriasis. J Invest Dermatol. 2010;130(5):1373–83.

41. Kauffman CL, Aria N, Toichi E, McCormick TS, Cooper KD, Gottlieb AB, et al. A phase I study evaluating the safety, pharmacokinetics, and clinical response of a human IL-12 p40 antibody in subjects with plaque psoriasis. J Invest Dermatol. 2004;123(6):1037–44.

42. Gottlieb AB, Cooper KD, McCormick TS, Toichi E, Everitt DE, Frederick B, et al. A phase 1, double-blind, placebo-controlled study evaluating single subcutaneous administrations of a human interleukin-12/23 monoclonal antibody in subjects with plaque psoriasis. Curr Med Res Opin. 2007;23(5):1081–92.

43. Krueger GG, Langley RG, Leonardi C, Yeilding N, Guzzo C, Wang Y, et al. A human interleukin-12/23 monoclonal antibody for the treatment of psoriasis. N Engl J Med. 2007;356(6):580–92.

44. Leonardi CL, Kimball AB, Papp KA, Yeilding N, Guzzo C, Wang Y, et al. Efficacy and safety of ustekinumab, a human interleukin-12/23 monoclonal antibody, in patients with psoriasis: 76-week results from a randomised, double-blind, placebo-controlled trial (PHOENIX 1). Lancet. 2008;371(9625):1665–74.

45. Papp KA, Langley RG, Lebwohl M, Krueger GG, Szapary P, Yeilding N, et al. Efficacy and safety of ustekinumab, a human interleukin-12/23 monoclonal antibody, in patients with psoriasis: 52-week results from a randomised, double-blind, placebo-controlled trial (PHOENIX 2). Lancet. 2008;371(9625):1675–84.

46. Griffiths CE, Strober BE, van de Kerkhof P, Ho V, Fidelus-Gort R, Yeilding N, et al. Comparison of ustekinumab and etanercept for moderate-to-severe psoriasis. N Engl J Med. 2010;362(2):118–28.

47. Kimball AB, Papp KA, Wasfi Y, Chan D, Bissonnette R, Sofen H, et al. Long-term efficacy of ustekinumab in patients with moderate-to-severe psoriasis treated for up to 5 years in the PHOENIX 1 study. J Eur Acad Dermatol Venereol. 2013;27(12):1535–45.

48. McInnes IB, Kavanaugh A, Gottlieb AB, Puig L, Rahman P, Ritchlin C, et al. Efficacy and safety of ustekinumab in patients with active psoriatic arthritis: 1 year results of the phase 3, multicentre, double-blind, placebo-controlled PSUMMIT 1 trial. Lancet. 2013;382(9894):780–9.

49. Kavanaugh A, Ritchlin C, Rahman P, Puig L, Gottlieb AB, Li S, et al. Ustekinumab, an anti-IL-12/23 p40 monoclonal antibody, inhibits radiographic progression in patients with active psoriatic arthritis: results of an integrated analysis of radiographic data from the phase 3, multicentre, randomised, double-blind, placebo-controlled PSUMMIT-1 and PSUMMIT-2 trials. Ann Rheum Dis. 2014;73(6):1000–6.

50. Ritchlin C, Rahman P, Kavanaugh A, McInnes IB, Puig L, Li S, et al. Efficacy and safety of the anti-IL-12/23 p40 monoclonal antibody, ustekinumab, in patients with active psoriatic arthritis despite conventional non-biological and biological anti-tumour necrosis factor therapy: 6-month and 1-year results of the phase 3, multicentre, double-blind, placebo-controlled, randomised PSUMMIT 2 trial. Ann Rheum Dis. 2014;73(6):990–9.

51. de Souza A, Ali-Shaw T, Reddy SM, Fiorentino D, Strober BE. Inflammatory arthritis following ustekinumab treatment for psoriasis: a report of two cases. Br J Dermatol. 2013;168(1):210–2.

52. Santos-Juanes J, Coto-Segura P, Mas-Vidal A, Galache OC. Ustekinumab induces rapid clearing of erythrodermic psoriasis after failure of antitumour necrosis factor therapies. Br J Dermatol. 2010;162(5):1144–6.

53. Wang TS, Tsai TF. Clinical experience of ustekinumab in the treatment of erythrodermic psoriasis: a case series. J Dermatol. 2011;38(11):1096–9.

54. Castineiras I, Fernandez-Diaz L, Juarez Y, Lueiro M. Sustained efficacy of ustekinumab in refractory erythrodermic psoriasis after failure of antitumor necrosis factor therapies. J Dermatol. 2012;39(8):730–1.

55. Buggiani G, D'Erme AM, Krysenka A, Pescitelli L, Lotti T, Prignano F. Efficacy of ustekinumab in sub-erythrodermic psoriasis: when TNF-blockers fail. Dermatol Ther. 2012;25(3):283–5.

56. Gerdes S, Franke J, Domm S, Mrowietz U. Ustekinumab in the treatment of palmoplantar pustulosis. Br J Dermatol. 2010;163(5):1116–8.

57. Bulai Livideanu C, Lahfa M, Mazereeuw-Hautier J, Paul C. Efficacy of ustekinumab in palmoplantar psoriasis. Dermatology. 2010;221(4):321–3.

58. Au SC, Goldminz AM, Kim N, Dumont N, Michelon M, Volf E, et al. Investigator-initiated, open-label trial of ustekinumab for the treatment of moderate-to-severe palmoplantar psoriasis. J Dermatol Treatment. 2013;24(3):179–87.

59. Morales-Munera C, Vilarrasa E, Puig L. Efficacy of ustekinumab in refractory palmoplantar pustular psoriasis. Br J Dermatol. 2013;168(4):820–4.

60. Chu DH, Van Voorhees AS, Rosenbach M. Treatment of refractory tumor necrosis factor inhibitor-induced palmoplantar pustulosis: a report of 2 cases. Arch Dermatol. 2011;147(10):1228–30.

61. Puig L, Morales-Munera CE, Lopez-Ferrer A, Geli C. Ustekinumab treatment of TNF antagonist-induced paradoxical psoriasis flare in a patient with psoriatic arthritis: case report and review. Dermatology. 2012;225(1):14–7.

62. Lebwohl M, Leonardi C, Griffiths CE, Prinz JC, Szapary PO, Yeilding N, et al. Long-term safety experience of ustekinumab in patients with moderate-to-severe psoriasis (part I of II): results from analyses of general safety parameters from pooled phase 2 and 3 clinical trials. J Am Acad Dermatol. 2012;66(5):731–41.

63. Gordon KB, Papp KA, Langley RG, Ho V, Kimball AB, Guzzo C, et al. Long-term safety experience of ustekinumab in patients with moderate to severe psoriasis (part II of II): results from analyses of infections and malignancy from pooled phase II and III clinical trials. J Am Acad Dermatol. 2012;66(5):742–51.

64. Papp KA, Griffiths CE, Gordon K, Lebwohl M, Szapary PO, Wasfi Y, et al. Long-term safety of ustekinumab in patients with moderate-to-severe psoriasis: final results from 5 years of follow-up. Br J Dermatol. 2013;168(4):844–54.

65. Papp KA, Strober B, Augustin M, Calabro S, Londhe A, Chevrier M, et al. PSOLAR: design, utility, and preliminary results of a prospective, international, disease-based registry of patients with psoriasis who are receiving, or are candidates for, conventional systemic treatments or biologic agents. J Drugs Dermatol. 2012;11(10):1210–7.

66. de Jong R, Altare F, Haagen IA, Elferink DG, Boer T, van Breda Vriesman PJ, et al. Severe mycobacterial and salmonella infections in interleukin-12 receptor-deficient patients. Science. 1998;280 (5368):1435–8.

67. Altare F, Lammas D, Revy P, Jouanguy E, Doffinger R, Lamhamedi S, et al. Inherited interleukin 12 deficiency in a child with bacille Calmette-Guerin and salmonella enteritidis disseminated infection. J Clin Invest. 1998;102(12):2035–40.

68. Altare F, Jouanguy E, Lamhamedi S, Doffinger R, Fischer A, Casanova JL. Mendelian susceptibility to mycobacterial infection in man. Curr Opin Immunol. 1998;10(4):413–7.

69. Tsai TF, Ho V, Song M, Szapary P, Kato T, Wasfi Y, et al. The safety of ustekinumab treatment in patients with moderate-to-severe psoriasis and latent tuberculosis infection. Br J Dermatol. 2012;167(5):1145–52.

70. Ryan C, Leonardi CL, Krueger JG, Kimball AB, Strober BE, Gordon KB, et al. Association between biologic therapies for chronic plaque psoriasis and cardiovascular events: a meta-analysis of randomized controlled trials. JAMA. 2011;306(8):864–71.

71. Tzellos T, Kyrgidis A, Trigoni A, Zouboulis CC. Association of ustekinumab and briakinumab with major adverse cardiovascular events: an appraisal of meta-analyses and industry sponsored pooled analyses to date. Dermato-Endocrinology. 2012;4(3):320–3.

72. Dommasch ED, Troxel AB, Gelfand JM. Major cardiovascular events associated with anti-IL 12/23 agents: a tale of two meta-analyses. J Am Acad Dermatol. 2013;68(5):863–5.

73. Reich K, Langley RG, Lebwohl M, Szapary P, Guzzo C, Yeilding N, et al. Cardiovascular safety of ustekinumab in patients with moderate to severe psoriasis: results of integrated analyses of data from phase II and III clinical studies. Br J Dermatol. 2011;164(4):862–72.

74. Reich K, Papp KA, Griffiths CE, Szapary PO, Yeilding N, Wasfi Y, et al. An update on the long-term safety experience of ustekinumab: results from the psoriasis clinical development program with up to four years of follow-up. J Drugs Dermatol. 2012;11(3):300–12.

75. Zuang Y, Calderon C, Marciniak SJ, Bouman-Thio E, Szapary P, Yang TW, et al. First-in-human study to assess guselkumab (anti-IL-23 mAb) pharmacokinetics/safety in healthy subjects and patients with moderate-to-severe psoriasis. Eur J Clin Pharmacol. 2016;72:1303–10.

76. Sofen H, Smith S, Matheson RT, Leonardi CL, Calderon C, Brodmerkel C, et al. Guselkumab (an IL-23-specific mAb) demonstrates clinical and molecular response in patients with moderate-to-severe psoriasis. J Allergy Clin Immunol. 2014;133:1032–40.

77. Gordon KB, Callis Duffin K, Bissonnette R, Prinz JC, Wasfi Y, Li S, et al. A phase 2 trial of guselkumab versus adalimumab for plaque psoriasis. N Engl J Med. 2015;373:136–44.

78. Blauvelt A, Papp KA, Griffiths CE, Randazzo B, Wasfi Y, Shen YK, et al. Efficacy and safety of guselkumab, an anti-interleukin-23 monoclonal antibody, compared with adalimumab for the continuous treatment of patients with moderate to severe psoriasis: results from the phase III, double-blinded, placebo- and active comparator-controlled VOYAGE 1 trial. J Am Acad Dermatol. 2017;76(3):405–17.

79. Reich K, Armstrong AW, Foley P, Song M, Wasfi Y, Randazzo B, et al. Efficacy and safety of guselkumab, an anti-interleukin-23 monoclonal antibody, compared with adalimumab for the treatment of patients with moderate to severe psoriasis with randomized withdrawal and retreatment: results from the phase III, double-blind, placebo- and active comparator-controlled VOYAGE 2 trial. J Am Acad Dermatol. 2017;76(3):418–31.

80. Kopp T, Riedl E, Bangert C, Bowman EP, Greisenegger E, Horowitz A, et al. Clinical improvement in psoriasis with specific targeting of interleukin-23. Nature. 2015;521:222–6.

81. Papp K, Thaci D, Reich K, Riedl E, Langley RG, Krueger JG, et al. Tildrakizumab (MK-3222), an anti-interleukin-23 monoclonal antibody, improves psoriasis in a phase IIb randomized placebo-controlled trial. Br J Dermatol. 2015;173:930–9.

82. Reich K, Papp KA, Blauvelt A, Tyring SK, Sinclair R, Thaçi D, et al. Tildrakizumab, a selective IL-23p19 antibody, in the treatment of chronic plaque psoriasis: results from two randomised, controlled, phase 3 trials (reSURFACE 1 and reSURFACE 2). Lancet. 2017;390:276–8.

83. Krueger JG, Ferris LK, Menter A, Wagner F, White A, Visvanathan S, et al. Anti–IL-23A mAb BI 655066 for treatment of moderate-to-severe psoriasis: safety, efficacy, pharmacokinetics, and biomarker results of a single-rising-dose, randomized, double-blind, placebo-controlled trial. J Allergy Clin Immunol. 2015;136:116–24.

84. Papp KA, Blauvelt A, Bukhalo M, Gooderham M, Krueger J, Lacour JP, et al. Risankizumab versus ustekinumab for moderate-to-severe plaque psoriasis. N Engl J Med. 2017;376:1551–60.

Interleukin-17 Inhibition for the Treatment of Inflammatory Skin Disease

15

Jason E. Hawkes, Jose A. Gonzalez, and James G. Krueger

Abbreviations

ACR	American College of Rheumatology
AD	Atopic dermatitis
ADAMTSL5	A disintegrin-like and metalloprotease domain containing thrombospondin type 1 motif-like 5
AMPs	Antimicrobial peptides
C/EBP	CCAAT-enhancer-binding protein
DLE	Discoid lupus erythematosus
EAE	Experimental autoimmune encephalomyelitis
IBD	Inflammatory bowel disease
IL	Interleukin
ILC	Innate lymphoid cells
PASI	Psoriasis Area and Severity Index
SCLE	Subacute cutaneous lupus erythematosus
SLE	Systemic lupus erythematosus
STAT1	Signal transducer and activator of transcription 1
T17	Interleukin-17-producing T cells
Tc17	Interleukin-17-producing CD8+ T cells
Th	T helper

Introduction

Psoriasis is a chronic, T cell-mediated inflammatory skin disease that affects approximately 2–3% of the Caucasian population [1]. It is commonly characterized by inflamed, thickened, scaly plaques on the scalp and extensor surfaces of the extremities. Less common disease variants include erythrodermic, pustular, palmoplantar, guttate, inverse, and

Jason E. Hawkes and Jose A. Gonzalez contributed equally to this work.

J.E. Hawkes, MD • J.A. Gonzalez, BS
J.G. Krueger, MD, PhD (✉)
The Laboratory for Investigative Dermatology, The Rockefeller University, New York, NY 10065, USA
e-mail: kruegej@rockefeller.edu

psoriatic arthritis. The etiology of psoriasis is highly complex and involves an interplay between psoriasis-associated genes, the environment, and several distinct immune cell populations and their secreted pro-inflammatory signals [2].

Our understanding of the immune mechanisms contributing to the pathophysiology of psoriasis has been considerably expanded due to the recent discovery of pathogenic T cells that produce large amounts of interleukin (IL)-17 (also known as T17 cells) in response to IL-23 [3, 4]. Evidence for the central role of the IL-23/T17 axis in psoriatic disease has since become more evident with the recent development of highly efficacious treatments that selectively target IL-17 or disrupt the IL-23/T17 signaling pathway. In this review, we will outline the research that led to the discovery of the IL-23/T17 pathway in psoriasis, as well as provide an overview of the ongoing development and testing of novel IL-17 inhibitors for the treatment of psoriasis and other chronic inflammatory skin conditions.

History of the Dissection of Psoriasis Immune Pathways

Through the use of broad T cell targeting drugs in psoriasis clinical trials (e.g., cyclosporine [5, 6], DAB$_{389}$ IL-2 (denileukin diftitox) [7], CTLA4-Ig (abatacept) [8], anti-CD11a (efalizumab) [9], and LFA3-Ig (alefacept) [10]), psoriasis emerged as a T cell-mediated inflammatory or autoimmune disease. This represented an important advance over earlier pathogenic concepts that proposed primary dysregulation of epidermal growth and differentiation driven by excess production of growth factors, such as transforming growth factor alpha and keratinocyte growth factor which regulate keratinocyte hyperplasia. However, when alefacept and efalizumab were approved as new biologic drugs to treat psoriasis, little was known about the specific T cell subsets mediating psoriasis. How specific immune-derived cytokines and other inflammatory factors altered the biology of resident skin cells to create cellular and molecular disease features was also poorly understood.

Work over the next decade focused on phenotyping the specific subsets of T cells, dendritic (antigen-presenting) cells, and associated cytokines in psoriasis, along with demonstrations of how these cells and inflammatory molecules altered the biology of skin cells and associated psoriasis molecular phenotypes. Initially, T cells were primarily categorized by class-defining cytokines. CD4+ T cells that made interferon-γ (IFN-γ) were classified as type 1 T helper (Th1) cells, whereas CD4+ T cells that made IL-4, IL-5, or IL-13 ("allergic" cytokines) were classified as Th2. These two T cell subsets were considered "polar" phenotypes, as common skin diseases had differential expression of Th1 vs. Th2 cells (e.g., psoriasis was defined as a Th1-related disease, whereas atopic dermatitis (AD) was mainly associated with activated Th2 cells). Thus, concepts of disease associations with "polar" T cell subsets were established. IFN-γ, the defining cytokine of Th1 cells, binds to surface receptors on target cells and then activates the transcription factor signal transducer and activator of transcription 1 (STAT1). Activation of STAT1 in turn increases synthesis of hundreds of genes that control cell growth, differentiation, production of antiviral proteins, and other inflammatory molecules that regulate ongoing interactions between antigen-presenting cells, T cells, leukocytes, and other somatic cells. Indeed, tissue profiling studies in psoriasis showed increased production of IFN-γ, activation of STAT1, and increased production of hundreds of IFN-induced genes. Plausible arguments were made that psoriasis could be driven by Th1 cells through activating effects of IFN-γ with upstream regulation of T cells by the "master" cytokine, IL-12, which controls activation and differentiation of the Th1 subset [11, 12].

In the earlier part of this decade, IL-23 was discovered by "gene-hunting" technologies. This discovery was highly intriguing since it is a dimeric (two subunit) cytokine that contains a shared p40 subunit with IL-12, as well as a unique p19 subunit [13]. Having the association with IL-12 gave it the potential to also be a "master" regulatory cytokine for T cells. The murine model commonly used to study multiple sclerosis, experimental autoimmune encephalomyelitis (EAE), was shown to be critically dependent on IL-23 [14]; subsequent work showed that this cytokine regulated a new T cell subset termed Th17, which was defined by coproduction of IL-17 and IL-22 cytokines by CD4+ cells in mice [15]. This finding was ground-breaking, as EAE had been assumed to be a Th1-mediated disease, much like psoriasis. However, with gene knockouts in mice, IL-23 was identified as a "driver" cytokine of EAE, whereas the IL-12/Th1 axis was actually shown to be relatively protective [15]. The question then arose whether any T cell-associated human diseases might be associated with this new Th17 subset. For the following work, it is important to note that the Th17 cell subset as defined by IL-17 and IL-22 production in mice has diverged in humans to different cells producing IL-17 vs. IL-22. CD4+ T cells producing IL-17, which has IL-17A and

IL-17F isomers, are classified as Th17, whereas those producing IL-22 are classified as Th22. IL-23 is a master regulator of human Th17 cells, and it likely regulates Th22 T cells to a significant extent [16].

While psoriasis had been identified as a disease with strong upregulation of the IL-12 p40 subunit and thus presumed IL-12 overproduction, the other IL-12 subunit (p35) did not show increased production in psoriasis lesions. With the recognition that IL-12 p40 could be associated with the p19 chain of IL-23 to make functional IL-23, a series of publications starting in 2004 found that psoriasis lesions had consistent upregulation of both p40 and p19 IL-23 subunits [17] and increased Th17 cells [3], which were highly activated based on mRNA profiling [18]. Th22 cells were also identified as a component of the T cell infiltrate, along with increased production of IL-22 mRNA. IL-22 was found to induce key psoriasis-related molecules in keratinocytes, including S100A7 (psoriasin), S100A8, and S100A9, while IFN-γ had no effect on these molecules [19]. IL-22, found to activate STAT3 in keratinocytes, also served as an inducer of epidermal hyperplasia in transgenic mouse models and in reconstructed human skin models in vitro [20]. IL-17 was also shown to serve as a transcriptional inducer of specific S100 genes, leukocyte chemokines, and a set of antimicrobial peptides (AMPs) that were previously associated with psoriasis. Thus, immune models for psoriasis began to consider that multiple subtypes of T cells (i.e., Th1, Th17, and Th22) were increased and activated in psoriasis lesions with a hypothesis that the sum of genes activated in psoriasis might be produced by distinct actions of "polar" T cell cytokines on keratinocytes and other tissue-resident cells [21].

Pathogenic concepts and models in psoriasis began to be tested by both broad and "narrow" immune antagonists. An early study with cyclosporine showed disease improvement paralleling reductions in Th1, Th17, and Th22 T cell cytokines, which was consistent with the "multiple pathogenic T cell subset" model [18]. Ustekinumab, a selective antagonist of the p40 subunit shared by IL-12 and IL-23, was shown to have high activity in suppressing psoriasis, typically inducing a 75% reduction in the Psoriasis Area and Severity Index (PASI75) score in ~70% of patients after 12 weeks of treatment compared to only 3–4% of patients in the placebo group [22]. As expected from blockade of both IL-12 and IL-23, its effects in psoriasis lesions included parallel reductions in the activity of Th1, Th17, and Th22 T cell subsets, data that is highly consistent with the existing pathogenic model. However, the testing of other more "narrow" or selective cytokine antagonists began to challenge the "multiple pathogenic subset" model, which required co-activation of Th1, Th17, and Th22 T cell subsets to produce a tissue, cellular, and molecular disease phenotype. Another cytokine antagonist that emerged as an effective treatment for psoriasis was etanercept, a fusion protein that binds tumor necrosis factor alpha (TNF-α) and thus restricts it from activating cells with cognate receptors. In performing studies with etanercept in psoriasis, it was found that etanercept was a strong modulator of both IL-23 and IL-17 production in psoriasis skin lesions and that patients who responded to this agent were only those that had suppressed production of IL-23 and IL-17. These data thus suggested that the IL-23/Th17 axis might be selectively important for disease pathogenesis [23]. Conversely, selective targeting of IFN-γ [24] or IL-22 with monoclonal antibodies in psoriasis patients produced little benefit, consistent with the lack of cytokine inhibition seen in study tissues. Hence, by the process of elimination, IL-17 remained untested as the cytokine which might be most critical for induction of psoriasis.

By 2010, three selective IL-17 antagonists became available for clinical studies in psoriasis patients. These agents targeted either IL-17 or its receptor. IL-17 is a dimeric cytokine which consists of IL-17A or IL-17F subunits, organized as homodimers or an A/F heterodimer [25]. IL-17 dimers bind to a receptor composed of IL-17RA and IL-17RC subunits. Two monoclonal antibodies (secukinumab, ixekizumab) were developed to IL-17A, and one antibody (brodalumab) was developed to the receptor subunit IL-17RA. The first report of IL-17 antagonism in psoriasis was in early 2010 at a presentation during the Society for Investigative Dermatology using brodalumab [26]. This presentation described a proof of concept study in which 8 patients were treated with 700 mg of intravenous drug 7/8 patients in this study had a PASI75 response and 8/8 had PGA scores of 0 or 1 after 6 weeks of initial treatment. The study also obtained skin biopsies from all patients, and this showed histologic disease reversal over 6 weeks. More importantly, normalization of 95% of disease-associated mRNA transcripts was observed within only 2 weeks of treatment [27]. Thus, while the study was small, it strongly implicated IL-17 as the key pathogenic T cell-associated cytokine in psoriasis. Later in 2010, a study published with secukinumab showed a major change in disease activity by selective antagonism of IL-17A, confirming the concept that IL-17 was a likely driver cytokine in psoriasis pathogenesis [28]. At the same time, an early proof of concept study was conducted with ixekizumab where 8/8 patients treated with a 150 mg dose of the antibody had PASI75 responses within 6 weeks and corresponding reductions in histologic and molecular markers of psoriasis [29]. Larger phase II studies with brodalumab and ixekizumab showing rapid and high-level disease improvements in psoriasis were published as back-to-back reports in the *New England Journal of Medicine* in 2012 [30, 31]. Consistent disease improvements with secukinumab were also shown in phase III studies [32] after different dose and administration schedules were explored in phase II studies. Subsequent FDA approval of each of these IL-17 antagonists was based on demonstrated efficacy and safety in phase III trials discussed in more detail below.

Updating IL-17 Biology in Psoriasis and the Pathogenic Disease Model

There is now a much better mechanistic understanding of how IL-17 can function to activate the many cellular and molecular changes in the skin that collectively produce psoriasis. With the recent demonstration of new autoantigens that activate Th17 cells in psoriasis, we now face a need to update the psoriasis pathogenic model to one that is centered on psoriasis as a T17 cell disease, which includes the possibility that cells other than CD4+ "helper" T cells make IL-17 after activation. Other cell types that can make IL-17 and are potentially implicated in psoriasis include CD8+ T cells (Tc17), innate lymphoid cells (ILC3 subset), and γδ T cells. Each of these IL-17-producing cells has upstream regulation by IL-23, so our new pathogenic model focuses on the IL-23/T17 axis as the main pathogenic driver of psoriasis [33]. Many different cell types, including leukocytes, have IL-17 receptors and functional responses to IL-17, but the keratinocyte response is really key for induction of psoriasis. A point of early confusion about the role of IL-17 in psoriasis is that exposure of cultured keratinocytes to IL-17 induced a limited response in which ~40 genes were induced, whereas similar exposure to TNF-α or IFN-γ induced hundreds of genes, many of which are found to be upregulated in psoriasis lesions. Thus, an IL-17 signature in the overall psoriasis transcriptome (defined as mRNAs differentially expressed in psoriasis plaques vs. background skin) was very small in comparison to TNF-α or IFN-γ [34]. However, treatment with two IL-17 inhibitors—ixekizumab and brodalumab—produced early changes in hundreds of genes in the psoriasis transcriptome, suggesting IL-17 had much broader effects on keratinocytes (as well as other cell types) than identified through *in vitro* models. In fact, *in vivo*, ixekizumab was shown to have faster and broader suppression of psoriasis-related gene products than the TNF-α antagonist etanercept [29]. We now know that the initial *in vitro* models for exposure of keratinocytes to IL-17 were too simple, since keratinocytes undergo a complex differentiation program *in vivo* that divides the epidermis into basal, spinous, granular, and cornified layers. While all of the viable cell layers of the epidermis have IL-17 receptors, transcriptional activation of target genes by IL-17 requires activation of the transcription factors CCAAT-enhancer-binding protein beta (C/EBPβ) or CCAAT-enhancer-binding protein delta (C/EBPδ). Keratinocytes synthesize C/EBPβ and δ in a differentiation-dependent fashion, such that granular layer keratinocytes have the highest expression of this factor. In turn, the highest expression of many IL-17-regulated products is in the upper and granular layers of the epidermis (Fig. 15.1). When IL-17 is added to keratinocyte cultures that form all differentiated epidermal layers, there is a robust response of keratinocytes such that several hundred mRNAs are induced or repressed [35]. The IL-17-regulated gene products are highly represented in the psoriasis transcriptome, and they also correspond

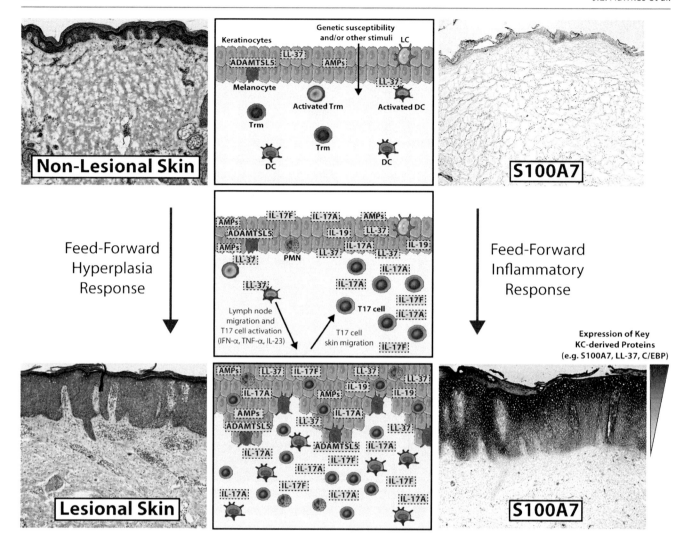

Fig. 15.1 IL-17 induces key proteins (e.g., S100A7, LL-37, IL-19) in keratinocytes that drive the psoriatic tissue response. Continuous IL-17 production is required to sustain psoriasis plaques, as therapeutic inhibition of IL-17 reverses the epidermal response to the non-lesional skin phenotype (Abbreviations: *ADAMTSL5* a disintegrin-like and metalloprotease domain containing thrombospondin type 1 motif-like 5, *AMPs* antimicrobial peptides, *C/EBP* CCAAT-enhancer-binding protein beta, *DC* mature dendritic cell, *IFN* interferon, *IL* interleukin, *KC* keratinocyte, *LC* Langerhans cell, *LL-37* cathelicidin, *PMNs* polymorphonuclear leukocytes or neutrophils, *T17* interleukin-17-producing T cells, *TNF* tumor necrosis factor, *Trm* tissue-resident memory cell)

to genes that are rapidly modulated by IL-17 antagonism with *in vivo* treatment of psoriasis. Hence, with this new "gene map" for IL-17 effects, one can appreciate a high IL-17 signature within the overall psoriasis transcriptome. Another biological pathway that increases the effect of IL-17 on epidermal keratinocytes is that IL-17 synergizes with TNF-α for regulation of many inflammation-related genes [36], a finding that is likely explained by co-utilization of the transcription factor nuclear factor kappa beta (NFκB) with C/EBPβ or δ in promoters of IL-17-responsive genes.

If psoriasis is an autoimmune disease driven by activation of T17 cells to autoantigens, then one must be able to explain how this response can create overall disease features of psoriasis that includes skin infiltration by Th1, Th17, and Th22 T cell subsets, myeloid dendritic cells, and neutrophils, as well as epidermal hyperplasia and other alterations in skin architecture.

A new disease model recently put forward explains how many of these features can be explained by cellular responses to cytokines of T17 cells, which include IL-17A, IL-17F, IL-26, and IL-29 [33]. Thus, these cytokines on epidermal keratinocytes create a "feed-forward" molecular inflammatory response (i.e., recruitment of leukocyte subsets associated with psoriasis, amplification of keratinocyte-produced proteins, and regulation of epidermal cell proliferation), can amplify expression of many specific molecules associated with psoriasis, and can regulate keratinocyte proliferation and differentiation (Fig. 15.1). IL-17 also directly or indirectly increases expression of the psoriasis autoantigens, such as disintegrin-like and metalloprotease domain containing thrombospondin type 1 motif-like 5 (ADAMTSL5) and cathelicidin (LL-37), thus setting the stage for chronic T cell activation by cutaneous dendritic cells. Emerging work indicates that these newly identified autoantigens are upregulated in psoriasis lesions in a pattern that generally matches the pattern of T cell and dendritic cell infiltrates [37–40] and that dendritic antigen-presenting cells contain the relevant antigens for stimulating a T17 cell response. For the future, studies will be needed to determine how tolerance is "broken" to these antigens to trigger initiation of psoriasis and whether tolerance can be restored to control psoriasis by approaches not requiring long-term treatment with immune-modulating drugs.

A Key Role for IL-23 in Psoriasis

Given the role of IL-23 as a master regulator of T17 cells, the role of this cytokine in psoriasis has also been tested by the use of antibodies against the p19 subunit that uniquely defines IL-23. Clinical studies coupled with skin biopsies and blood measures in psoriasis have shown that IL-23 is a key regulator of IL-17 production in psoriasis lesions. When sufficient anti-p19 antibody is given to affect IL-17 production, there is histological and molecular resolution of psoriasis that is overall very similar to disease improvements attainted with IL-12/23 or IL-17 antagonists [41]. Interestingly, the clinical effects of IL-23 inhibition appear to be superior to effects attained with IL-12/23p40 or TNF-α inhibition in terms of the frequency of patients that attain PASI90 and PASI100 responses. Since the IL-12/IFN-γ pathway is not suppressed by blocking IL-23 with these p19 selective antibodies, one can question whether IL-12/IFN-γ might actually serve as a negative regulator of the IL-23/T17 response pathway, as suggested by gene knockouts in the EAE model described earlier [14]. Another feature of T17 cell biology that could be impacted by IL-23 treatments is that this cell differentiation pathway is not completely fixed and irreversible. In model systems where T17 cell fate can be tracked by genetic modification of these cells, T17 cells have transdifferentiated into regulatory T(Treg) and Th1 cell lineages [42, 43]. By blocking IL-23 signals to T17 cells, transdifferentiation might also be possible in humans, and this could be another reason why relatively long-term treatment responses have been observed with single

doses of IL-23 inhibitors in two early studies in psoriasis [41, 44]. The significance of IL-23 signaling and blockade for the treatment of psoriasis is discussed in greater detail in another chapter of this publication.

A Review of Phase III Clinical Trials

Several phase III clinical trials have demonstrated a high efficacy and good safety profile for secukinumab, ixekizumab, and brodalumab in the treatment of moderate-to-severe psoriasis (Table 15.1). Here, we will provide a brief summary of the efficacy and safety information for these novel agents.

Secukinumab

Secukinumab is a fully human monoclonal antibody against IL-17A approved for the treatment of moderate-to-severe plaque psoriasis, psoriatic arthritis, and ankylosing spondylitis. For plaque psoriasis, it is administered subcutaneously with a loading dose of 300 mg at weeks 0, 1, 2, 3, and 4, followed by monthly injections of 300 mg. The treatment dose for psoriatic arthritis is 150 mg at weeks 0, 1, 2, 3, and 4, followed by monthly injections of 150 mg. However, the treatment dose may be increased to 300 mg every 4 weeks for patients with persistent arthritis symptoms.

Three, 52-week, double-blind, phase III placebo-controlled clinical trials provided pivotal evidence supporting the use of secukinumab for the treatment of moderate-to-severe plaque psoriasis [32]. The ERASURE trial ($n = 738$) compared secukinumab to placebo, whereas the FIXTURE trial ($n = 1306$) compared secukinumab to etanercept and placebo. In the ERASURE trial, 82% (300 mg every 4 weeks) and 72% (150 mg every 4 weeks) of patients treated with secukinumab achieved a PASI75 at week 12 compared to only 4.5% of patients in the placebo arm. In the FIXTURE trial, 77% (300 mg every 4 weeks) and 67% (150 mg every 4 weeks) of patients treated with secukinumab achieved a PASI75 response at week 12 compared to 44% in

Table 15.1 Approved IL-17 inhibitors or investigational products in early development

Medication	Target	Manufacturer	Approved clinical indication
Secukinumab	IL-17A	Novartis	Plaque psoriasis, psoriatic arthritis, and ankylosing spondylitis
Ixekizumab		Eli Lilly	Plaque psoriasis
Brodalumab	IL-17RA	Valeant/AstraZeneca	Plaque psoriasis
ALX-0761/M1095	IL-17A	Ablynx/Merck Serono	None
Bimekizumab	IL-17F	UCB	None
NI-1401		Novimmune/Genentech	None
ABT-122	IL-17A	AbbVie	None
COVA322	TNF-A	Janssen/Covagen	None

the etanercept (50 mg twice weekly) and 5% placebo groups. In a subsequent 52-week, double-blind, randomized controlled, prospective trial of 676 patients with moderate-to-severe plaque psoriasis (CLEAR trial), secukinumab (300 mg every 4 weeks) was shown to be superior to ustekinumab [45]. At week 16, 79% of patients in the secukinumab group achieved a PASI90 response compared to 58% from the ustekinumab (45 mg or 90 mg dosing based on body weight) group; similar results were observed at 1 year [46]. The Dermatology Life Quality Index was also significantly higher for secukinumab (72%) compared to ustekinumab (57%). Additional support for the efficacy and safety of secukinumab administered by auto-injector/pen and prefilled syringes was also provided by the JUNCTURE [47] and FEATURE [48] clinical trials, respectively.

Two phase III clinical trials have evaluated the efficacy of secukinumab for the treatment of psoriatic arthritis. In the first double-blind, placebo-controlled trial (FUTURE-1), 606 patients with psoriatic arthritis were randomized to treatment with secukinumab (150 or 75 mg every 4 weeks) or placebo [49]. At week 24, 50% (150 mg every 4 weeks) and 51% (75 mg every 4 weeks) of patients treated with secukinumab achieved an ACR20 response compared to 17% in the placebo group. A significant decrease in joint symptoms was sustained through 52 weeks of treatment. In the FUTURE-2 trial, 397 psoriatic arthritis patients were randomized to receive secukinumab (300, 150, or 75 mg every 4 weeks) or placebo [50]. After 24 weeks of treatment, 54% (300 mg every 4 weeks), 51% (150 mg every 4 weeks), and 29% (75 mg every 4 weeks) of patients treated with secukinumab achieved an ACR20 compared to 15% of patients treated with placebo.

Ixekizumab

Ixekizumab is a humanized IgG4 monoclonal antibody that binds the IL-17A cytokine and is approved for the treatment of moderate-to-severe plaque psoriasis. For plaque psoriasis, ixekizumab is administered subcutaneously with a loading dose of 160 mg at week 0, followed by 80 mg at weeks 2, 4, 6, 8, 10, and 12. Subsequently 80 mg injections are given every 4 weeks thereafter. Ixekizumab is not currently approved for the treatment of psoriatic arthritis.

In three double-blind, placebo-controlled, randomized phase III studies, ixekizumab for the treatment of moderate-to-severe plaque psoriasis was compared to placebo alone (UNCOVER-1) [51] or etanercept (50 mg twice weekly) and placebo (UNCOVER-2 and UNCOVER-3) [52]. In the UNCOVER-1 trial (n = 1296), 89% (80 mg every 2 weeks) and 83% (80 mg every 4 weeks) of patients treated with ixekizumab achieved a PASI75 response at week 12 compared to 4% in the placebo group. In the UNCOVER-2 and UNCOVER-3 trials, patients were randomized to receive placebo, etanercept, or a subcutaneous injection of 80 mg

ixekizumab every 2 weeks or every 4 weeks. In the UNCOVER-2 trial (n = 1224), 90% (80 mg every 2 weeks) and 78% (80 mg every 4 weeks) of patients treated with ixekizumab achieved a PASI75 response at week 12 compared to 42% and 2% in the etanercept and placebo groups, respectively. In the UNCOVER-3 trial (n = 1346), 87% (80 mg every 2 weeks) and 84% (80 mg every 4 weeks) of patients treated with ixekizumab achieved a PASI75 response at week 12 compared to 53% and 7% in the etanercept and placebo groups, respectively. 75% and 73% of patients treated with ixekizumab every 2 weeks and every 4 weeks, respectively, remained clear or had minimal psoriasis after 60 weeks of treatment [51]. To date, one double-blind, placebo-controlled, randomized trial (SPIRIT-P1) evaluating the use of ixekizumab for the treatment of psoriatic arthritis has been completed [53]. In this trial, biologic-naïve patients were randomized to subcutaneous injection of ixekizumab (80 mg every 2 or 4 weeks), adalimumab (40 mg every 2 weeks), and placebo. After 24 weeks of treatment with ixekizumab, 62% (80 mg every 2 weeks) and 58% (80 mg every 4 weeks) of patients achieved an ACR20 compared to 30% in the placebo arm. However, a statistically significant improvement in joint disease activity was demonstrated as early as week 12. Additional studies evaluating the efficacy of ixekizumab for the treatment of psoriatic arthritis are ongoing, including the SPIRIT-P2 trial (ClinicalTrials.gov Registration Number: NCT02349295).

Brodalumab

Brodalumab is a human IgG2 monoclonal antibody that inhibits IL-17RA. It is approved for the treatment of moderate-to-severe plaque psoriasis. For plaque psoriasis, brodalumab is administered subcutaneously with a loading dose of 210 mg at weeks 0, 1, and 2 followed by 210 mg every 2 weeks.

In three prospective, phase III, randomized, double-blind, placebo-controlled studies, brodalumab for the treatment of moderate-to-severe plaque psoriasis was compared to placebo alone (AMAGINE-1) [54] or ustekinumab (45 or 90 mg dosing based on body weight) and placebo (AMAGINE-2 and AMAGINE-3) [55]. In the AMAGINE-1 trial (n = 661), 83% (210 mg every 2 weeks) and 60% (140 mg every 2 weeks) of patients achieved a PASI75 response at week 12 compared to 3% in the placebo group. Very similar PASI75 responses at week 12 were observed in the subsequent AMAGINE-2 (n = 1831) and AMAGINE-3 (n = 1881) trials, and the 140 and 210 mg doses of brodalumab were shown to be superior to placebo (P-value < 0.001 for both groups) [55]. Of note, 44% (210 mg every 2 weeks) and 37% (140 mg every 2 weeks) of patients in the AMAGINE-2 and AMAGINE-3 trials, respectively, experienced complete clearance (PASI100) of their psoriasis at week 12 [55].

Brodalumab is not currently approved for the treatment of psoriatic arthritis. Following promising phase II clinical trial results for this indication, two phase III clinical trials were initiated (AMVISION-1 and AMVISION-2). However, results from these studies are not publicly available at this time.

Adverse Events of Secukinumab, Ixekizumab, and Brodalumab

Good safety has been demonstrated for secukinumab, ixekizumab, and brodalumab, and their side effect profiles are largely overlapping. The most common reported adverse events include nasopharyngitis, headache, upper respiratory infection, mucocutaneous candidiasis, and mild, transient neutropenia without associated infections. Interestingly, humans with inborn errors of IL-17RA or IL-17F are also associated with recurrent candida infections, upper respiratory infections, and mild skin infections [56]. Less common adverse events of IL-17 inhibition included diarrhea, inflammatory bowel disease (IBD), arthralgias, and injection site reactions. Brodalumab and secukinumab were tested for clinical efficacy in patients with IBD and no comorbid inflammatory skin disease, and these trials reported some worsening of gastrointestinal symptoms with IL-17 blockade [57, 58]. These agents should, therefore, be used cautiously in psoriasis patients that may have early, comorbid gastrointestinal disease. Lastly, four suicides out of ~4000 psoriasis patients were reported in the AMAGINE trials, though a causal relationship with brodalumab was not demonstrated. However, this concern has led to the additional requirement that brodalumab only be prescribed in conjunction with a Risk Evaluation and Mitigation Strategy (REMS).

Newer IL-17 Target Drugs in the Pipeline

The approval and commercialization of IL-17 inhibitors have transformed the way psoriasis is treated. However, nonresponders to IL-17 blockade continue to highlight the complexity of disease. Basic and translational research has shown insights into why this may be, including the role of IL-17F and the integrated TNF-α pathway [36, 59, 60]. New advances in antibody engineering may overcome these complexities through the development of bispecific antibodies allowing simultaneous targeting of two molecules with a single antibody [61].

A closer look at the mechanisms of currently approved IL-17 inhibitors shows possible limitations in this treatment modality. Ixekizumab and secukinumab only target the IL-17A homodimer without impacting IL-17F dimers. Brodalumab blocks IL-17RA and subsequent downstream activity of all IL-17 isoforms, including IL-17E (IL-25)

which inhibits IL-17-mediated inflammation. Novel bispecific antibodies, which are currently being developed, permit dual targeting of IL-17A and IL-17F without suppressing the beneficial effects of IL-17E. Doing so should theoretically result in an improved treatment response over current IL-17 therapies. However, it remains to be seen if there is a more severe risk of infection and other side effects in these dual inhibitors.

A common method of developing bispecific antibodies has been to design antibodies to have dual variable domains such that each antibody arm has a distinct epitope. This can be used for a wide variety of molecules and is best exemplified in developing bispecific antibodies for dual inhibition of IL-17A/IL-17F, or IL-17A/TNF-α [61]. An iteration of this includes the Ablynx Nanobody® technology in which trivalent antibodies only contain truncated heavy chain components allowing for better targeting and improved pharmacokinetics. Alternatively, Covagen FynomAb® technology designs fynomer proteins capable of binding a specific molecule and attaches it to the amino or carboxyl-terminal end of the antibody heavy or light chains [62]. These technologies have led to the development of dual IL-17A/IL-17F inhibitors including ALX-0761/M1095, bimekizumab, and NI-1401. Additionally, IL-17A/TNF-α dual inhibitors including ABT-122 and COVA322 are also in development.

Several of these next-generation IL-17 inhibitors have already entered and completed early phase clinical trials; however, results of these studies are limited and not yet published. Most notably, a small phase Ib trial of ALX-0761/M1095 in psoriasis has shown PASI90 in 100% of patients, with PASI100 being reached in 56% of patients (unpublished data presented at the 2017 American Academy of Dermatology Annual Meeting in Orlando, FL). A small phase Ib trial of bimekizumab in psoriatic arthritis showed that 80% of patients achieved an ACR20 at week 8 compared to 17% in the placebo group, whereas 40% of patients achieved an ACR50 compared to 8% in the placebo group [63, 64]. The remaining aforementioned bispecific antibodies have completed preclinical and early phase I trials but have yet to report results of PASI or ACR treatment response [61, 62, 65, 66].

While these IL-17 dual inhibitors are still early in development, early phase clinical trial data is encouraging. The technology to design antibodies that simultaneously target two or even three distinct molecules holds much promise but has yet to be mastered, particularly in the context of treating psoriasis and psoriatic arthritis. Further basic and translational research could identify currently unknown molecules important to the development of psoriatic disease, which could be co-targeted using these antibodies. Doing so could lead to improved therapies in which not only PASI75 is achieved, but in which it becomes the standard to achieve responses of PASI90 and PASI100.

Future Directions: IL-17 Targeting for Other Skin Conditions

While psoriasis may be the most well-known of the IL-17-mediated skin diseases, there are several others which might benefit from anti-IL-17 therapy [67]. These diseases can be broadly classified into the noninfectious neutrophilic dermatoses and the lymphocyte-mediated dermatoses. The potential association of neutrophilic dermatoses with IL-17 is driven by the concept that IL-17 induces multiple chemokines (e.g., CXCL1, CXCL2, CXCL3, and CXCL8) that attract neutrophils to sites of inflammation.

Some notable noninfectious neutrophilic dermatoses include Sweet syndrome, pyoderma gangrenosum, and Behçet disease [68–70]. These diseases can be characterized as having recurrent inflammation with a cutaneous neutrophilic infiltrate. Recent studies have found increased levels of IL-17A and IL-17R in the skin of both Sweet syndrome and pyoderma gangrenosum [71]. Likewise, Behçet disease has been found to have increased levels of IL-17A in the skin and plasma during acute flares of mucocutaneous and ocular disease [72]. Although not classified as a neutrophilic dermatosis, hidradenitis suppurativa has been found to display many of the same disease characteristics including increased levels of IL-17 in lesional and uninvolved skin with an accompanying neutrophilic infiltrate [73].

Neutrophils are an additional cellular source for IL-17A and are capable of recruiting additional neutrophils to sites of inflammation through the production of IL-17 in a paracrine fashion [74]. Thus, it has been postulated that improvement in neutrophilic dermatoses can be accomplished by interrupting this self-propagating cycle. There is currently limited data regarding these diseases and IL-17 inhibition in both humans and *in vitro* models. Results from a clinical trial evaluating secukinumab for the treatment of uveitis in Behçet disease were disappointing, failing to reach its primary endpoints [75]. However, the effect of IL-17 inhibition on mucocutaneous lesions of Behçet disease remains unknown.

The lymphocyte-mediated dermatoses in which IL-17 is implicated encompass a wide array of diseases, including AD and lupus. In AD, subsets of patients (e.g., pediatric, intrinsic disease in adults, and adult Asian populations) [76–78] have prominent IL-17 expression. Similarly, studies have found increased staining of IL-17A in lesional skin of subacute cutaneous lupus erythematosus (SCLE), discoid lupus erythematosus (DLE), and non-lesional skin of systemic lupus erythematosus (SLE). When looking at plasma, only SLE and DLE had increased levels of IL-17A relative to healthy controls. In contrast, plasma IL-17F was found to be increased in SCLE, DLE, and SLE [79], and serum IL-17 correlates poorly with disease activity [80]. Though IL-17 expression is increased in AD and lupus, it is unclear if this cytokine drives disease pathogenesis or is simply the by-product of the primary immune response. The role of IL-17 in these complex diseases remains unclear and must be further elucidated through selective inhibition of inflammatory cytokines.

Conclusion

The identification of the central role for the IL-23/T17 axis in psoriatic disease broadened our understanding of the pathogenic immune events driving this chronic inflammatory condition. Further evidence that this signaling pathway is the predominant immune axis in psoriasis is supported by the substantial proportion of patients achieving a PASI90 or PASI100 following IL-17 inhibition compared to other systemic biologic medications. It will be interesting to explore the clinical efficacy of IL-17 antagonists in combination with other biologic therapies, such as TNF-α or IL-22 antagonists. Further, the role of IL-17 inhibition for the treatment of other inflammatory or autoimmune conditions is not entirely clear. However, preclinical and translational research studies suggest that IL-17 blockade may represent a promising treatment modality for noninfectious conditions with a prominent neutrophilic infiltrate or high levels of S100A7 expression in the skin. Additional studies are needed to fully understand the molecular mechanisms of IL-17 signaling in the skin and the implications of IL-17 blockade in patients with chronic inflammatory conditions.

Case Presentation

A 65-year-old Caucasian female presents to the dermatology clinic with a more than 10-year history of recalcitrant plaque psoriasis with prominent joint involvement. Her psoriatic arthritis was confirmed by her rheumatologist. She rates the severity of her skin disease as 5 out of 10, which has been unsuccessfully treated with high-potency topical steroids and multiple systemic agents. She endorses severe joint pain and swelling in her hands, along with morning stiffness in the large joints that lasts longer than 30 min. She reports mild improvement in her skin lesions following treatment with multiple systemic therapies, but has had persistent worsening of her joint symptoms.

Past Medical History
- Hypertension
- Hyperlipidemia
- Obesity
- Mild renal insufficiency

Social and Family History
- Single
- Denies a history of alcohol or tobacco use
- No family history of psoriasis

Previous Therapies

- High-potency topical steroids and NBUVB
- Cyclosporine and methotrexate
- Etanercept, infliximab, ustekinumab, and apremilast

Physical Examination

- Well-demarcated, erythematous, scaly plaques with thin scale on the scalp, trunk, and bilateral extremities
- Body surface area involvement of approximately 7%
- Joint swelling and tenderness noted on the second and third metacarpal joints, as well as pain with palpation of the sacroiliac joint and Achilles tendon

Management

Given the patient's failure to respond to multiple biologic therapies and progressive joint disease, the patient was started on secukinumab. Secukinumab was administered subcutaneously with a loading dose of 300 mg at weeks 0, 1, 2, 3, and 4, followed by monthly injections of 300 mg. Within 3 weeks, the patient experienced a dramatic improvement in her skin lesions and rated her skin disease severity as 2. After 6 weeks of treatment, the patient reported significant improvement in her joint swelling and pain, as well as complete resolution of her morning stiffness. Her body surface area involvement at 2 months was less than 1%, and the patient endorsed only mild joint tenderness in her sacroiliac joint. She denied any adverse events other than mild irritation of the skin following each injection. This particular case highlights the utility of secukinumab for the simultaneous treatment of plaque psoriasis and psoriatic arthritis that is resistant to two TNF-α inhibitors.

Acknowledgments JEH, JAG, and JGK are supported in part by grant # UL1TR001866 and # KL2TR001865 from the National Center for Advancing Translational Sciences (NCATS), National Institutes of Health (NIH) Clinical and Translational Science Award (CTSA) program.

Conflict of Interest JEH and JAG declare that they have no conflict of interest. JGK has been a consultant to and has received research support from companies that have developed or are developing therapeutics for psoriasis: AbbVie, Amgen, Boehringer, Bristol-Myers Squibb, Celgene, Dermira, Idera, Janssen, Leo, Lilly, Merck, Novartis, Pfizer, Regeneron, Sanofi, Serono, Sun, Valeant, and Vitae.

References

1. Rachakonda TD, Schupp CW, Armstrong AW. Psoriasis prevalence among adults in the United States. J Am Acad Dermatol. 2014;70(3):512–6. https://doi.org/10.1016/j.jaad.2013.11.013.
2. Martin DA, Towne JE, Kricorian G, Klekotka P, Gudjonsson JE, Krueger JG, et al. The emerging role of IL-17 in the pathogenesis of psoriasis: preclinical and clinical findings. J Invest Dermatol. 2013;133(1):17–26. https://doi.org/10.1038/jid.2012.194.
3. Lowes MA, Kikuchi T, Fuentes-Duculan J, Cardinale I, Zaba LC, Haider AS, et al. Psoriasis vulgaris lesions contain discrete populations of Th1 and Th17 T cells. J Invest Dermatol. 2008;128(5):1207–11. https://doi.org/10.1038/sj.jid.5701213.
4. Res PC, Piskin G, de Boer OJ, van der Loos CM, Teeling P, Bos JD, et al. Overrepresentation of IL-17A and IL-22 producing CD8 T cells in lesional skin suggests their involvement in the pathogenesis of psoriasis. PLoS One. 2010;5(11):e14108. https://doi.org/10.1371/journal.pone.0014108.
5. Ellis CN, Gorsulowsky DC, Hamilton TA, Billings JK, Brown MD, Headington JT, et al. Cyclosporine improves psoriasis in a double-blind study. JAMA. 1986;256(22):3110–6.
6. Mozzanica N, Cattaneo A, Pigatto PD, Finzi AF. Cyclosporine a in psoriasis: an immunohistological study. Transplant Proc. 1988;20(3 Suppl 4):78–84.
7. Gottlieb SL, Gilleaudeau P, Johnson R, Estes L, Woodworth TG, Gottlieb AB, et al. Response of psoriasis to a lymphocyte-selective toxin (DAB389IL-2) suggests a primary immune, but not keratinocyte, pathogenic basis. Nat Med. 1995;1(5):442–7.
8. Abrams JR, Lebwohl MG, Guzzo CA, Jegasothy BV, Goldfarb MT, Goffe BS, et al. CTLA4Ig-mediated blockade of T-cell costimulation in patients with psoriasis vulgaris. J Clin Invest. 1999;103(9):1243–52. https://doi.org/10.1172/JCI5857.
9. Lebwohl M, Tyring SK, Hamilton TK, Toth D, Glazer S, Tawfik NH, et al. A novel targeted T-cell modulator, efalizumab, for plaque psoriasis. N Engl J Med. 2003;349(21):2004–13. https://doi.org/10.1056/NEJMoa030002.
10. Krueger GG, Callis KP. Development and use of alefacept to treat psoriasis. J Am Acad Dermatol. 2003;49(2 Suppl):S87–97. https://doi.org/10.1016/mjd.2003.552.
11. Austin LM, Ozawa M, Kikuchi T, Walters IB, Krueger JG. The majority of epidermal T cells in psoriasis vulgaris lesions can produce type 1 cytokines, interferon-gamma, interleukin-2, and tumor necrosis factor-alpha, defining TC1 (cytotoxic T lymphocyte) and TH1 effector populations: a type 1 differentiation bias is also measured in circulating blood T cells in psoriatic patients. J Invest Dermatol. 1999;113(5):752–9. https://doi.org/10.1046/j.1523-1747.1999.00749.x.
12. Yawalkar N, Karlen S, Hunger R, Brand CU, Braathen LR. Expression of interleukin-12 is increased in psoriatic skin. J Invest Dermatol. 1998;111(6):1053–7. https://doi.org/10.1046/j.1523-1747.1998.00446.x.
13. Oppmann B, Lesley R, Blom B, Timans JC, Xu Y, Hunte B, et al. Novel p19 protein engages IL-12p40 to form a cytokine, IL-23, with biological activities similar as well as distinct from IL-12. Immunity. 2000;13(5):715–25.
14. Li J, Gran B, Zhang GX, Ventura ES, Siglienti I, Rostami A, et al. Differential expression and regulation of IL-23 and IL-12 subunits and receptors in adult mouse microglia. J Neurol Sci. 2003;215(1-2):95–103.
15. Cua DJ, Sherlock J, Chen Y, Murphy CA, Joyce B, Seymour B, et al. Interleukin-23 rather than interleukin-12 is the critical cytokine for autoimmune inflammation of the brain. Nature. 2003;421(6924):744–8. https://doi.org/10.1038/nature01355.
16. Lowes MA, Suarez-Farinas M, Krueger JG. Immunology of psoriasis. Annu Rev Immunol. 2014;32:227–55. https://doi.org/10.1146/annurev-immunol-032713-120225.
17. Lee E, Trepicchio WL, Oestreicher JL, Pittman D, Wang F, Chamian F, et al. Increased expression of interleukin 23 p19 and p40 in lesional skin of patients with psoriasis vulgaris. J Exp Med. 2004;199(1):125–30. https://doi.org/10.1084/jem.20030451.
18. Haider AS, Lowes MA, Suarez-Farinas M, Zaba LC, Cardinale I, Khatcherian A, et al. Identification of cellular pathways of "type 1," Th17 T cells, and TNF- and inducible nitric oxide synthase-producing dendritic cells in autoimmune inflammation through pharmacogenomic study of cyclosporine a in psoriasis. J Immunol. 2008;180(3):1913–20.
19. Wolk K, Witte E, Wallace E, Docke WD, Kunz S, Asadullah K, et al. IL-22 regulates the expression of genes responsible for

antimicrobial defense, cellular differentiation, and mobility in keratinocytes: a potential role in psoriasis. Eur J Immunol. 2006;36(5):1309–23. https://doi.org/10.1002/eji.200535503.

20. Ma HL, Liang S, Li J, Napierata L, Brown T, Benoit S, et al. IL-22 is required for Th17 cell-mediated pathology in a mouse model of psoriasis-like skin inflammation. J Clin Invest. 2008;118(2):597–607. https://doi.org/10.1172/JCI33263.

21. Lowes MA, Bowcock AM, Krueger JG. Pathogenesis and therapy of psoriasis. Nature. 2007;445(7130):866–73. https://doi.org/10.1038/nature05663.

22. Leonardi CL, Kimball AB, Papp KA, Yeilding N, Guzzo C, Wang Y, et al. Efficacy and safety of ustekinumab, a human interleukin-12/23 monoclonal antibody, in patients with psoriasis: 76-week results from a randomised, double-blind, placebo-controlled trial (PHOENIX 1). Lancet. 2008;371(9625):1665–74. https://doi.org/10.1016/S0140-6736(08)60725-4.

23. Zaba LC, Cardinale I, Gilleaudeau P, Sullivan-Whalen M, Suarez-Farinas M, Fuentes-Duculan J, et al. Amelioration of epidermal hyperplasia by TNF inhibition is associated with reduced Th17 responses. J Exp Med. 2007;204(13):3183–94. https://doi.org/10.1084/jem.20071094.

24. Harden JL, Johnson-Huang LM, Chamian MF, Lee E, Pearce T, Leonardi CL, et al. Humanized anti-IFN-gamma (HuZAF) in the treatment of psoriasis. J Allergy Clin Immunol. 2015;135(2):553–6. https://doi.org/10.1016/j.jaci.2014.05.046.

25. Gaffen SL. Structure and signalling in the IL-17 receptor family. Nat Rev Immunol. 2009;9(8):556–67. https://doi.org/10.1038/nri2586.

26. Russell C, Kerkof K, Bigler J, Timour M, Welcher A, Novitskaya I, et al. Blockade of the IL-17R with AMG 827 leads to rapid reversal of gene expression and histopathologic abnormalities in human psoriatic skin (abstract 273). J Invest Dermatol. 2010;130(Suppl 1):S46. https://doi.org/10.1038/jid.2010.71.

27. Russell CB, Rand H, Bigler J, Kerkof K, Timour M, Bautista E, et al. Gene expression profiles normalized in psoriatic skin by treatment with brodalumab, a human anti-IL-17 receptor monoclonal antibody. J Immunol. 2014;192(8):3828–36. https://doi.org/10.4049/jimmunol.1301737.

28. Hueber W, Patel DD, Dryja T, Wright AM, Koroleva I, Bruin G, et al. Effects of AIN457, a fully human antibody to interleukin-17A, on psoriasis, rheumatoid arthritis, and uveitis. Sci Transl Med. 2010;2(52):52ra72. https://doi.org/10.1126/scitranslmed.3001107.

29. Krueger JG, Fretzin S, Suarez-Farinas M, Haslett PA, Phipps KM, Cameron GS, et al. IL-17A is essential for cell activation and inflammatory gene circuits in subjects with psoriasis. J Allergy Clin Immunol. 2012;130(1):145–54.e9. https://doi.org/10.1016/j.jaci.2012.04.024.

30. Leonardi C, Matheson R, Zachariae C, Cameron G, Li L, Edson-Heredia E, et al. Anti-interleukin-17 monoclonal antibody ixekizumab in chronic plaque psoriasis. N Engl J Med. 2012;366(13):1190–9. https://doi.org/10.1056/NEJMoa1109997.

31. Papp KA, Leonardi C, Menter A, Ortonne JP, Krueger JG, Kricorian G, et al. Brodalumab, an anti-interleukin-17-receptor antibody for psoriasis. N Engl J Med. 2012;366(13):1181–9. https://doi.org/10.1056/NEJMoa1109017.

32. Langley RG, Elewski BE, Lebwohl M, Reich K, Griffiths CE, Papp K, et al. Secukinumab in plaque psoriasis—results of two phase 3 trials. N Engl J Med. 2014;371(4):326–38. https://doi.org/10.1056/NEJMoa1314258.

33. Kim J, Krueger JG. Highly effective new treatments for psoriasis target the IL-23/type 17 T cell autoimmune axis. Annu Rev Med. 2017;68:255–69. https://doi.org/10.1146/annurev-med-042915-103905.

34. Suarez-Farinas M, Li K, Fuentes-Duculan J, Hayden K, Brodmerkel C, Krueger JG. Expanding the psoriasis disease profile: interrogation of the skin and serum of patients with moderate-to-severe psoriasis. J Invest Dermatol. 2012;132(11):2552–64. https://doi.org/10.1038/jid.2012.184.

35. Chiricozzi A, Nograles KE, Johnson-Huang LM, Fuentes-Duculan J, Cardinale I, Bonifacio KM, et al. IL-17 induces an expanded range of downstream genes in reconstituted human epidermis model. PLoS One. 2014;9(2):e90284. https://doi.org/10.1371/journal.pone.0090284.

36. Chiricozzi A, Guttman-Yassky E, Suarez-Farinas M, Nograles KE, Tian S, Cardinale I, et al. Integrative responses to IL-17 and TNF-alpha in human keratinocytes account for key inflammatory pathogenic circuits in psoriasis. J Invest Dermatol. 2011;131(3):677–87. https://doi.org/10.1038/jid.2010.340.

37. Arakawa A, Siewert K, Stohr J, Besgen P, Kim SM, Ruhl G, et al. Melanocyte antigen triggers autoimmunity in human psoriasis. J Exp Med. 2015;212(13):2203–12. https://doi.org/10.1084/jem.20151093.

38. Bonifacio KM, Kunjravia N, Krueger JG, Fuentes-Duculan J. Cutaneous expression of a disintegrin-like and metalloprotease domain containing thrombospondin type 1 motif-like 5 (ADAMTSL5) in psoriasis goes beyond melanocytes. J Pigment Disord. 2016;3(3):244. https://doi.org/10.4172/2376-0427.1000244.

39. Cheung KL, Jarrett R, Subramaniam S, Salimi M, Gutowska-Owsiak D, Chen YL, et al. Psoriatic T cells recognize neolipid antigens generated by mast cell phospholipase delivered by exosomes and presented by CD1a. J Exp Med. 2016;213(11):2399–412. https://doi.org/10.1084/jem.20160258.

40. Lande R, Botti E, Jandus C, Dojcinovic D, Fanelli G, Conrad C, et al. The antimicrobial peptide LL37 is a T-cell autoantigen in psoriasis. Nat Commun. 2014;5:5621. https://doi.org/10.1038/ncomms6621.

41. Sofen H, Smith S, Matheson RT, Leonardi CL, Calderon C, Brodmerkel C, et al. Guselkumab (an IL-23-specific mAb) demonstrates clinical and molecular response in patients with moderate-to-severe psoriasis. J Allergy Clin Immunol. 2014;133(4):1032–40. https://doi.org/10.1016/j.jaci.2014.01.025.

42. Gagliani N, Amezcua Vesely MC, Iseppon A, Brockmann L, Xu H, Palm NW, et al. Th17 cells transdifferentiate into regulatory T cells during resolution of inflammation. Nature. 2015;523(7559):221–5. https://doi.org/10.1038/nature14452.

43. Jager A, Kuchroo VK. Effector and regulatory T-cell subsets in autoimmunity and tissue inflammation. Scand J Immunol. 2010;72(3):173–84. https://doi.org/10.1111/j.1365-3083.2010.02432.x.

44. Krueger JG, Ferris LK, Menter A, Wagner F, White A, Visvanathan S, et al. Anti-IL-23A mAb BI 655066 for treatment of moderate-to-severe psoriasis: safety, efficacy, pharmacokinetics, and biomarker results of a single-rising-dose, randomized, double-blind, placebo-controlled trial. J Allergy Clin Immunol. 2015;136(1):116–24.e7. https://doi.org/10.1016/j.jaci.2015.01.018.

45. Thaci D, Blauvelt A, Reich K, Tsai TF, Vanaclocha F, Kingo K, et al. Secukinumab is superior to ustekinumab in clearing skin of subjects with moderate to severe plaque psoriasis: CLEAR, a randomized controlled trial. J Am Acad Dermatol. 2015;73(3):400–9. https://doi.org/10.1016/j.jaad.2015.05.013.

46. Blauvelt A, Reich K, Tsai TF, Tyring S, Vanaclocha F, Kingo K, et al. Secukinumab is superior to ustekinumab in clearing skin of subjects with moderate-to-severe plaque psoriasis up to 1 year: results from the CLEAR study. J Am Acad Dermatol. 2017;76(1):60–9.e9. https://doi.org/10.1016/j.jaad.2016.08.008.

47. Paul C, Lacour JP, Tedremets L, Kreutzer K, Jazayeri S, Adams S, et al. Efficacy, safety and usability of secukinumab administration by autoinjector/pen in psoriasis: a randomized, controlled trial (JUNCTURE). J Eur Acad Dermatol Venereol. 2015;29(6):1082–90. https://doi.org/10.1111/jdv.12751.

48. Blauvelt A, Prinz JC, Gottlieb AB, Kingo K, Sofen H, Ruer-Mulard M, et al. Secukinumab administration by pre-filled syringe: efficacy, safety and usability results from a randomized controlled

trial in psoriasis (FEATURE). Br J Dermatol. 2015;172(2):484–93. https://doi.org/10.1111/bjd.13348.

49. Mease PJ, McInnes IB, Kirkham B, Kavanaugh A, Rahman P, van der Heijde D, et al. Secukinumab inhibition of interleukin-17A in patients with psoriatic arthritis. N Engl J Med. 2015;373(14):1329–39. https://doi.org/10.1056/NEJMoa1412679.

50. McInnes IB, Mease PJ, Kirkham B, Kavanaugh A, Ritchlin CT, Rahman P, et al. Secukinumab, a human anti-interleukin-17A monoclonal antibody, in patients with psoriatic arthritis (FUTURE 2): a randomised, double-blind, placebo-controlled, phase 3 trial. Lancet. 2015;386(9999):1137–46. https://doi.org/10.1016/S0140-6736(15)61134-5.

51. Gordon KB, Blauvelt A, Papp KA, Langley RG, Luger T, Ohtsuki M, et al. Phase 3 trials of ixekizumab in moderate-to-severe plaque psoriasis. N Engl J Med. 2016;375(4):345–56. https://doi.org/10.1056/NEJMoa1512711.

52. Griffiths CE, Reich K, Lebwohl M, van de Kerkhof P, Paul C, Menter A, et al. Comparison of ixekizumab with etanercept or placebo in moderate-to-severe psoriasis (UNCOVER-2 and UNCOVER-3): results from two phase 3 randomised trials. Lancet. 2015;386(9993):541–51. https://doi.org/10.1016/S0140-6736(15)60125-8.

53. Mease PJ, van der Heijde D, Ritchlin CT, Okada M, Cuchacovich RS, Shuler CL, et al. Ixekizumab, an interleukin-17A specific monoclonal antibody, for the treatment of biologic-naive patients with active psoriatic arthritis: results from the 24-week randomised, double-blind, placebo-controlled and active (adalimumab)-controlled period of the phase III trial SPIRIT-P1. Ann Rheum Dis. 2017;76(1):79–87. https://doi.org/10.1136/annrheumdis-2016-209709.

54. Papp KA, Reich K, Paul C, Blauvelt A, Baran W, Bolduc C, et al. A prospective phase III, randomized, double-blind, placebo-controlled study of brodalumab in patients with moderate-to-severe plaque psoriasis. Br J Dermatol. 2016;175(2):273–86. https://doi.org/10.1111/bjd.14493.

55. Lebwohl M, Strober B, Menter A, Gordon K, Weglowska J, Puig L, et al. Phase 3 studies comparing brodalumab with ustekinumab in psoriasis. N Engl J Med. 2015;373(14):1318–28. https://doi.org/10.1056/NEJMoa1503824.

56. Puel A, Cypowyj S, Bustamante J, Wright JF, Liu L, Lim HK, et al. Chronic mucocutaneous candidiasis in humans with inborn errors of interleukin-17 immunity. Science. 2011;332(6025):65–8. https://doi.org/10.1126/science.1200439.

57. Hueber W, Sands BE, Lewitzky S, Vandemeulebroecke M, Reinisch W, Higgins PD, et al. Secukinumab, a human anti-IL-17A monoclonal antibody, for moderate to severe Crohn's disease: unexpected results of a randomised, double-blind placebo-controlled trial. Gut. 2012;61(12):1693–700. https://doi.org/10.1136/gutjnl-2011-301668.

58. Targan SR, Feagan B, Vermeire S, Panaccione R, Melmed GY, Landers C, et al. A randomized, double-blind, placebo-controlled phase 2 study of brodalumab in patients with moderate-to-severe Crohn's disease. Am J Gastroenterol. 2016;111(11):1599–607. https://doi.org/10.1038/ajg.2016.298.

59. Johansen C, Usher PA, Kjellerup RB, Lundsgaard D, Iversen L, Kragballe K. Characterization of the interleukin-17 isoforms and receptors in lesional psoriatic skin. Br J Dermatol. 2009;160(2):319–24. https://doi.org/10.1111/j.1365-2133.2008.08902.x.

60. van Baarsen LG, Lebre MC, van der Coelen D, Aarrass S, Tang MW, Ramwadhdoebe TH, et al. Heterogeneous expression pattern of interleukin 17A (IL-17A), IL-17F and their receptors in synovium of rheumatoid arthritis, psoriatic arthritis and osteoarthritis: possible explanation for nonresponse to anti-IL-17 therapy? Arthritis Res Ther. 2014;16(4):426. https://doi.org/10.1186/s13075-014-0426-z.

61. Torres T, Romanelli M, Chiricozzi A. A revolutionary therapeutic approach for psoriasis: bispecific biological agents. Expert Opin

Investig Drugs. 2016;25(7):751–4. https://doi.org/10.1080/13543784.2016.1187130.

62. Silacci M, Lembke W, Woods R, Attinger-Toller I, Baenziger-Tobler N, Batey S, et al. Discovery and characterization of COVA322, a clinical-stage bispecific TNF/IL-17A inhibitor for the treatment of inflammatory diseases. MAbs. 2016;8(1):141–9. https://doi.org/10.1080/19420862.2015.1093266.

63. Walker G, Croasdell G. The European league against rheumatism (EULAR)—17th annual European congress of rheumatology (June 8-11, 2016 - London, UK). Drugs Today (Barc). 2016;52(6):355–60. https://doi.org/10.1358/dot.2016.52.6.2516435.

64. Alexander W. European league against rheumatism and american diabetes association. P T. 2016;41(8):517–22.

65. 2016 ACR/ARHP. Annual meeting abstract supplement. Arthritis Rheum. 2016;68(Suppl 10):1–4550. https://doi.org/10.1002/art.39977.

66. Glatt S, Helmer E, Haier B, Strimenopoulou F, Price G, Vajjah P, et al. First-in-human randomized study of bimekizumab, a humanized monoclonal antibody and selective dual inhibitor of IL-17A and IL-17F, in mild psoriasis. Br J Clin Pharmacol. 2016. https://doi.org/10.1111/bcp.13185.

67. Speeckaert R, Lambert J, Grine L, Van Gele M, De Schepper S, van Geel N. The many faces of interleukin-17 in inflammatory skin diseases. Br J Dermatol. 2016;175(5):892–901. https://doi.org/10.1111/bjd.14703.

68. Sakane T, Takeno M, Suzuki N, Inaba G. Behcet's disease. N Engl J Med. 1999;341(17):1284–91. https://doi.org/10.1056/NEJM199910213411707.

69. Su WP, Davis MD, Weenig RH, Powell FC, Perry HO. Pyoderma gangrenosum: clinicopathologic correlation and proposed diagnostic criteria. Int J Dermatol. 2004;43(11):790–800. https://doi.org/10.1111/j.1365-4632.2004.02128.x.

70. Sweet RD. An acute febrile neutrophilic dermatosis. Br J Dermatol. 1964;76:349–56.

71. Marzano AV, Fanoni D, Antiga E, Quaglino P, Caproni M, Crosti C, et al. Expression of cytokines, chemokines and other effector molecules in two prototypic autoinflammatory skin diseases, pyoderma gangrenosum and Sweet's syndrome. Clin Exp Immunol. 2014;178(1):48–56. https://doi.org/10.1111/cei.12394.

72. Ekinci NS, Alpsoy E, Karakas AA, Yilmaz SB, Yegin O. IL-17A has an important role in the acute attacks of Behcet's disease. J Invest Dermatol. 2010;130(8):2136–8. https://doi.org/10.1038/jid.2010.114.

73. Lima AL, Karl I, Giner T, Poppe H, Schmidt M, Presser D, et al. Keratinocytes and neutrophils are important sources of proinflammatory molecules in hidradenitis suppurativa. Br J Dermatol. 2016;174(3):514–21. https://doi.org/10.1111/bjd.14214.

74. Cai S, Batra S, Langohr I, Iwakura Y, Jeyaseelan S. IFN-gamma induction by neutrophil-derived IL-17A homodimer augments pulmonary antibacterial defense. Mucosal Immunol. 2016;9(3):718–29. https://doi.org/10.1038/mi.2015.95.

75. Dick AD, Tugal-Tutkun I, Foster S, Zierhut M, Melissa Liew SH, Bezlyak V, et al. Secukinumab in the treatment of noninfectious uveitis: results of three randomized, controlled clinical trials. Ophthalmology. 2013;120(4):777–87. https://doi.org/10.1016/j.ophtha.2012.09.040.

76. Esaki H, Brunner PM, Renert-Yuval Y, Czarnowicki T, Huynh T, Tran G, et al. Early-onset pediatric atopic dermatitis is TH2 but also TH17 polarized in skin. J Allergy Clin Immunol. 2016;138(6):1639–51. https://doi.org/10.1016/j.jaci.2016.07.013.

77. Noda S, Suarez-Farinas M, Ungar B, Kim SJ, de Guzman SC, Xu H, et al. The Asian atopic dermatitis phenotype combines features of atopic dermatitis and psoriasis with increased TH17 polarization. J Allergy Clin Immunol. 2015;136(5):1254–64. https://doi.org/10.1016/j.jaci.2015.08.015.

78. Suarez-Farinas M, Dhingra N, Gittler J, Shemer A, Cardinale I, de Guzman SC, et al. Intrinsic atopic dermatitis shows similar TH2 and higher TH17 immune activation compared with extrinsic atopic dermatitis. J Allergy Clin Immunol. 2013;132(2):361–70. https://doi.org/10.1016/j.jaci.2013.04.046.

79. Tanasescu C, Balanescu E, Balanescu P, Olteanu R, Badea C, Grancea C, et al. IL-17 in cutaneous lupus erythematosus.
Eur J Intern Med. 2010;21(3):202–7. https://doi.org/10.1016/j.ejim.2010.03.004.

80. Vincent FB, Northcott M, Hoi A, Mackay F, Morand EF. Clinical associations of serum interleukin-17 in systemic lupus erythematosus. Arthritis Res Ther. 2013;15(4):R97. https://doi.org/10.1186/ar4277.

Systemic Therapies in Psoriasis

Gregory Peterson, Annika Silfast-Kaiser, and Alan Menter

Psoriasis is a chronic inflammatory skin disease with a significant negative impact on a patient's self-esteem, work productivity, quality of life, and indeed pocketbook [1–4]. Moderate-to-severe psoriasis has also been associated with multiple comorbidities including the metabolic syndrome, cardiovascular disease, depression, and psoriatic arthritis [5–9] (Fig. 16.1). For patients with moderate-to-severe psoriasis (>10% body surface area involvement), conventional systemic therapies can offer an effective, cost-effective, well-tolerated alternative treatment to topical treatments, light therapy, as well as the full spectrum of biologic agents [10].

Introduction

Although the pathogenesis of psoriasis is not yet fully understood, there is a great deal of evidence that points to psoriasis being an immune-mediated disease with T-cells playing a central role. Environmental factors, dendritic cells, cytokines, numerous gene loci, and T-cells all interact to induce the systemic inflammation essential for the creation of psoriatic plaques as well as psoriatic arthritis. Initially, dendritic cells are activated by affected keratinocytes. Dendritic cells then travel to local lymph nodes to release cytokines including IL-12 that activate type 1 helper T-cells, IL-23, and type 17 helper T-cells. These T-cells trigger the release of multiple cytokines including TNF-α, IL-22, and IL-17, producing a vicious cycle of inflammation of the skin and/or joints. For this reason, systemic agents play an important role in the treatment of moderate-to-severe psoriasis and psoriatic arthritis by specifically impacting T-cells or their products directly. Biologic agents

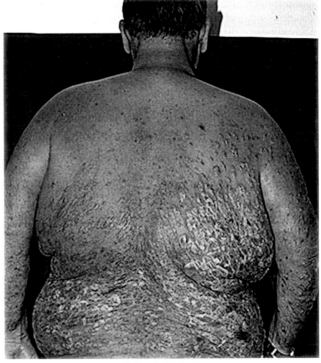

Patient's BMI- 41

Fig. 16.1 Psoriasis association with the metabolic syndrome. Patient's BMI-41

work by more specifically inhibiting the action of individual cytokines that mediate the production, maintenance, and development of T-cells within the immune system [7].

Treatment Eligibility

Systemic therapies are typically considered when a patient's psoriasis is defined as moderate to severe, i.e., greater than 10% body surface area involvement. Involvement of the face, palms, soles, or genitalia, i.e., disabling psoriasis, while frequently less than 5% involvement, has a major impact on

G. Peterson, MD • A. Menter, MD (✉)
Baylor University Medical Center, Dallas, TX, USA
e-mail: amderm@gmail.com; caitrionaryan80@gmail.com; chernandez@texasderm.com; Fortega@texasderm.com

A. Silfast-Kaiser, BS
Texas A&M Health Science Center College of Medicine, Temple, TX, USA

© Springer International Publishing AG 2018
P.S. Yamauchi (ed.), *Biologic and Systemic Agents in Dermatology*, https://doi.org/10.1007/978-3-319-66884-0_16

patients' quality of life (QOL) and thus frequently requires systemic therapies. In order to assess disease severity, the Psoriasis Area and Severity Index (PASI) is a common measure used to evaluate the extent of disease. It is traditionally used in clinical trials involving systemic agents, with a PASI score of greater than or equal to ten being required for patient inclusion in these trials. In forms of psoriasis where PASI is not applicable, both affected body surface area (BSA) and a DLQI (Dermatology Life Quality Index) greater than ten can be utilized.

When designing a treatment plan for a psoriatic patient it is important that clinicians take into account multiple variables other than simply severity of the disease. Treatment plans must be made while keeping quality-of-life issues, relevant comorbidities, safety, cost, efficacy of treatment, patient preference and accessibility, as well as patient's prior clinical responses in mind.

Traditional Systemic Agents in Psoriasis

Systemic treatment options prior to the revolution of biologics have focused on producing clinical improvement in psoriasis patients without necessarily targeting the specific causative factors. Although biologic therapy is now a clinician's more specific targeted treatment option, with less potential for organ toxicity and zero potential for teratogenicity, traditional systemic agents continue to play a major role in psoriasis therapies worldwide. Traditional systemic agents are significantly less expensive in comparison to biologics, and, for many patients, provide a more preferable route of administration by oral administration, rather than by injection.

Methotrexate

Methotrexate is the most common systemic therapy prescribed by dermatologists worldwide. Methotrexate is an antimetabolite that competitively inhibits dihydrofolate reductase and thymidylate reductase. In psoriasis, it is used for its anti-inflammatory properties—it increases the level of adenosine, an anti-inflammatory compound, released by fibroblasts and endothelial cells at sites of inflammation in the body. Neutrophil and monocyte chemotaxis is markedly inhibited in psoriasis with methotrexate therapy [32–34]. Methotrexate was approved in 1972 by the FDA for severe psoriasis before randomized clinical trials were the standard of determining drug efficacy. As a result, clinical experience rather than documentation of its efficacy is much greater. The usual starting dose for methotrexate is between 7.5 and 25 mg/week [35]. Patients are traditionally given an initial test dose of 5 mg with a blood count 5 days thereafter before

moving forward with the intended treatment dose which can thereafter be increased until an optimal response is achieved, not to exceed 30 mg/week. An excellent recent 1-year study of Methotrexate by subcutaneous injection, published in The Lancet, shows a 40% PASI-75 score. For the approximately 40% of patients who achieve PASI 75 about 75% of these patients will do so after 12 weeks of a 15 mg/week methotrexate dose. The only placebo-controlled trial of methotrexate treatment for psoriasis showed that 36% of patients on 7.5 mg/week, with gradual increases up to 25 mg/week, were able to achieve PASI 75 after 16 weeks of ongoing treatment [11]. The American Academy of Dermatology Guidelines on Psoriasis recommends a complete blood count and platelet counts every 2 weeks for the first month thereafter every 3–4 months in addition to renal and liver function tests at the same intervals [99].

For long-term methotrexate users, hepatotoxicity is the most important adverse effect, with myelosuppression and pulmonary fibrosis also of concern [36]. Mild elevations of transaminases to less than twice the upper limit of normal are not uncommon and do not correlate well with hepatic fibrosis. A systematic review of methotrexate trials assessing liver toxicity has shown extreme variability of the incidence of hepatic fibrosis, making the risk of fibrosis unquantifiable. Liver fibrosis is associated with type II diabetes, obesity, hepatitis, and alcohol use [37]. The fact that patients with psoriasis tend to have an increase in cardiovascular risk factors including the metabolic syndrome (obesity and type II diabetes) may serve, at least in part, as a confounding variable when it comes to the association of hepatic fibrosis and methotrexate use [37–39]. This hypothesis has been supported by the fact that the pathologic features of methotrexate-induced liver toxicity resemble nonalcoholic steatohepatitis, suggesting that methotrexate possibly aggravates preexisting nonalcoholic steatohepatitis [11]. When methotrexate-induced hepatic fibrosis does occur, and is identified in a timely manner, it is frequently reversible with discontinuation of the drug. The association between concomitant alcohol and methotrexate use with hepatotoxicity is well known and therefore physicians frequently instruct their patients to limit alcohol while on the medication. Prior American Academy of Dermatology guidelines do allow moderate alcohol consumption defined as 1–2 glasses of alcohol a day [100].

Prior to initiation of methotrexate treatment, patients need to be screened for risk factors including alcohol intake, obesity, diabetes, hyperlipidemia, and hepatitis B and C. The development of pulmonary symptoms such as a non-productive cough must also be carefully evaluated. Folic acid or folinic acid supplementation is essential in methotrexate patients both to reduce gastrointestinal side effects (nausea, vomiting, and diarrhea) and to reduce the risk of hepatotoxicity [40]. In addition to side effects and the potential for significant drug-drug interactions (eg. Sulfonamides), the physician must also be familiar with folinic acid rescue in case of methotrexate overdose. The total cumulative methotrexate dosage should always be calculated for patients on methotrexate therapy. It is recommended that physicians consider referral for hepatic evaluation in their patients (with no prior history of liver disease) after 3.5–4 g total cumulative methotrexate dosage [41]. Liver biopsies were the standard of care in the past, but data has shown the value of the serum amino-terminal propeptide type III collagen (PIIINP) test to detect early fibrosis without an invasive procedure [90] in addition to fibroelastography and other noninvasive imaging. PIIINP testing has led to a 75% decrease in liver biopsies and will be used in conjunction with other serum tests such as the elevated liver function test (ELF) to ensure a reduction in liver biopsies in the near future [107].

Although biologics including adalimumab and infliximab have shown significantly higher efficacy in head-to-head trials with methotrexate, methotrexate is still a largely affordable and effective option for many patients and is the most commonly used systemic agent for psoriasis worldwide [42, 43]. Based on published data, methotrexate treatment achieves PASI 75 in approximately 40% of cases and can be used even in cases of erythrodermic psoriasis (Fig. 16.2). Methotrexate is also used frequently in combination with biologic agents for psoriasis and psoriatic arthritis, especially as a tool to suppress acquired antibodies against TNF-alpha inhibitors including adalimumab and infliximab [44].

Recently, a new MTX molecule based on the initial pre-methotrexate compound, called aminopterin has been evaluated with phase I testing showing decreased side effects and comparable efficacy [106]. Phase II studies are imminent.

Acitretin

Acitretin is an oral retinoid and is the only synthetic form of vitamin A approved for the treatment of psoriasis in the USA. It is used for severe psoriasis, including pustular and erythrodermic forms (Figs. 16.3 and 16.4), as well as for psoriasis in HIV patients due to its lack of immunosuppressive effects [45]. The exact mechanism of action of acitretin in the treatment of psoriasis is not fully understood. However, as a retinoid, acitretin is known to modulate epidermal proliferation and differentiation while also having immunomodulatory and anti-inflammatory effects. Thus, hyperproliferation of keratinocytes is reduced along with the inhibition of inflammatory molecules that induce premature maturation of keratinocytes and neutrophil chemotaxis in psoriasis occurs [101].

Acitretin plays a role in long-term maintenance therapy for plaque psoriasis. In a long-term clinical trial, 89% of plaque psoriasis patients achieved a PASI 50 and 78.4% of these patients attained PASI 75 after 12 months of treatment [91]. Acitretin is frequently considered as a first-line treatment in pustular psoriasis, both generalized and in the localized palmoplantar variety [92] (Fig. 16.5).

Acitretin provides a rapid response in these patients with initial clearance of lesions seen in as little as 10 days in some patients. It is only moderately effective in the treatment of psoriatic nail disease. Acitretin is the least most effective systemic drug for plaque psoriasis when used as monotherapy. It is frequently used in smaller doses in combination with UVB or PUVA therapy as more effective higher doses of the drug as monotherapy are frequently not well tolerated by patients [93]. The combination of acitretin and UVB or PUVA has also been shown to be more effective than using either UVB, PUVA, or acitretin as monotherapy [102] (Fig. 16.6).

Combination therapy additionally reduces the number of necessary phototherapy sessions as well as the required dosage of acitretin, thus diminishing the amount of UV

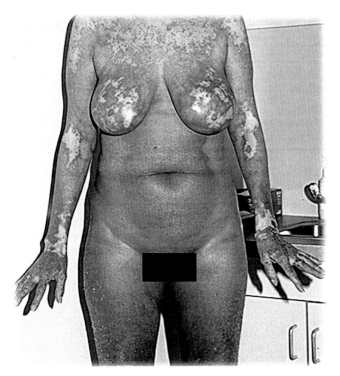

Fig. 16.2 Erythrodermic psoriasis

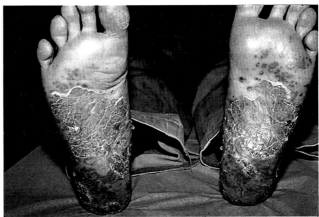

Fig. 16.3 Severe plantar psoriasis

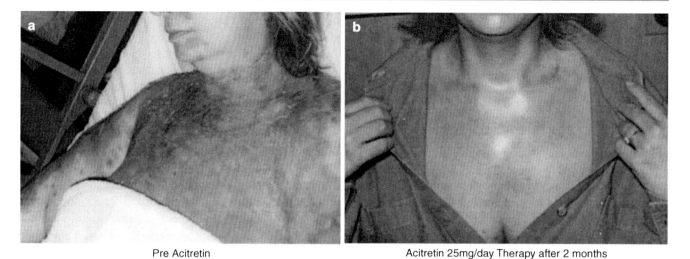

Pre Acitretin   Acitretin 25mg/day Therapy after 2 months

Fig. 16.4 (**a**) Erythrodermic: psoriasis with pustules; pre-acitretin. (**b**) Erythrodermic: psoriasis with pustules; acitretin 25 mg/day therapy after 2 months

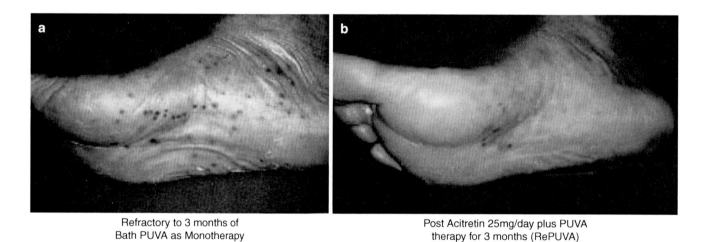

Refractory to 3 months of   Post Acitretin 25mg/day plus PUVA
Bath PUVA as Monotherapy   therapy for 3 months (RePUVA)

Fig. 16.5 (**a**) Pustular plantar psoriasis; refractory to 3 months of bath PUVA as monotherapy. (**b**) Pustular plantar psoriasis; post-acitretin 25 mg/day plus PUVA therapy for 3 months (RePUVA)

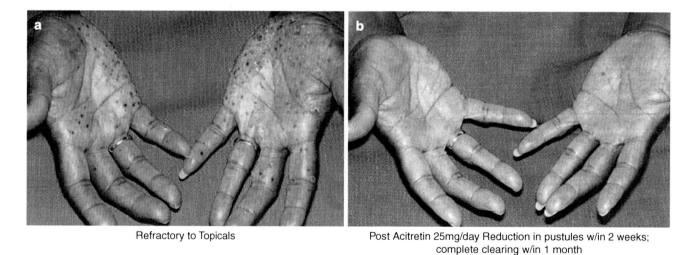

Refractory to Topicals   Post Acitretin 25mg/day Reduction in pustules w/in 2 weeks;
                                                                complete clearing w/in 1 month

Fig. 16.6 (**a**) Palmar pustular psoriasis; refractory to topicals. (**b**) Palmar pustular psoriasis; post-acitretin 25 mg/day reduction in pustules w/in 2 weeks; complete clearing w/in 1 month

exposure and intolerable side effects [94]. Acitretin monotherapy response is slow—with maximal response occurring at 3–6 months [11]. The usual dose for acitretin ranges from 10 to 50 mg daily, and can also be dosed by weight, i.e., 0.25–0.5 mg/kg daily. As with all oral retinoid therapies, monitoring for hypertriglyceridemia and hepatotoxicity is essential. Twenty five to fifty percentage of patients experience increases in triglycerides, while 13–16% of patients experience elevation of transaminases [103]. The majority of patients on acitretin will experience mucocutaneous side effects in the form of cheilitis, dry eyes or dry mouth, epistaxis, xerosis, and/or alopecia. Acitretin, as is the case for all retinoids, is a potent teratogen, leading to strict requirements for pregnancy prevention during and subsequent to their use, being only indicated in men and in females of nonreproductive potential [46]. Acitretin, in the presence of alcohol, converts to etretinate which can increase hepatotoxicity potential.

Acitretin is the active metabolite of etretinate, a second-generation retinoid approved for use in psoriasis in 1986. Etretinate has a long half-life of 120 days and was replaced in 1996 by the less lipophilic acitretin, which has a half-life of 50 h [103]. While still available in Japan, etretinate was removed from the European and American markets in 1996 and 1998, respectively.

Cyclosporine

Cyclosporine is an immunosuppressive drug originally used in transplantation to reduce graft rejection relating to interference of the growth and activity of T-cells. Published originally as a case reporting efficacy for psoriasis in a transplant patient, cyclosporine shifted the entire focus of psoriasis from an epidermal hyperproliferative disease to a T-cell-mediated disease [109]. By reducing lymphocytes and macrophages in the epidermis, cyclosporine inhibits not only the activation of T-cells, but also natural killer cells and antigen-presenting cells [12]. Cyclosporine has a rapid mode of action and is effective in the majority of psoriasis patients. Cyclosporine binds to a family of cytoplasmic proteins called cyclophilins, forming a drug-receptor complex that competitively inhibits calcineurin, which normally activates transcription of IL-2 and related cytokines [13, 14]. Ultimately, the drug leads to decreased transcriptional activation of cytokine genes for IL-2, IL-3, IL-4, TNF-alpha, CD40L, GM-CSF, IFN-gamma, and reduction in lymphocyte proliferation. Cyclosporine is frequently used in patients with severe psoriasis who are in need of a rapid response with quick symptomatic relief or as interventional therapy when other systemic medications have failed.

Cyclosporine is best used as an intermittent therapy in short courses of 3–4 months due to adverse effects with long-term treatment including renal toxicity, hypertension,

lymphoma, and an increase in cutaneous malignancies, especially in prior PUVA-treated patients. Renal impairment and hypertension occur due to cyclosporine's vasoconstrictive effects on afferent renal arterioles, whereas its immunosuppressive effects lead to concerns regarding malignancy [15]. A significant portion of patients on cyclosporine for up to 2–5 years will develop glomerulosclerosis, with subsequent loss of renal function. Loss of renal function also occurs when a patient is on greater than 5 mg/kg/day [16–19]. In one study, interstitial fibrosis and tubular atrophy were present in all biopsies after 1 year and continued to progress with further treatment. Additionally, these changes were not strongly correlated to renal function [20]. In another study, renal biopsies from patients on cyclosporine for 4 years all showed pronounced glomerular sclerosis [21]. Past studies have shown little to no correlation, however, with dose or treatment duration [19–22]. The best predictor in some studies has been a persistent increase in serum creatinine level 1 month after treatment has been discontinued [22].

Acute loss of renal function is usually reversible after discontinuation of cyclosporine. It has been suggested that if the serum creatinine increases 30% over the baseline creatinine level, after two consecutive blood draws, the dose of cyclosporine should be decreased by 1 m/kg/day or by 25–50% for a duration of at least 4 weeks. If, after 4 weeks, a patient's creatinine does not improve at the reduced dose, the cyclosporine dose should again be decreased by 25–50%. If the creatinine continues to remain elevated, the drug should be discontinued (Fig. 16.7). Because secretion of creatinine in the renal tubules can increase due to cyclosporine-induced nephropathy, serum creatinine levels as a sole determinant of kidney function is considered less reliable [22]. Annual measurement of GFR, in addition to the trending creatinine, is recommended for patients on long-term treatment [19]. A minimum of twice-weekly measurement of early morning blood pressure by the patient is essential and a reliable marker for early reported toxicity. If the patient begins to experience hypertension, the recommendation is to reduce

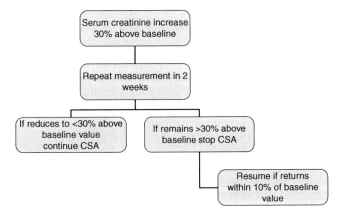

Fig. 16.7 Management of cyclosporine-induced renal dysfunction

the cyclosporine dose by 25–50% or introduce antihypertensive therapy either through initiation of a calcium channel blocker or of the dihydropyridine class. As a subset of patients are especially sensitive to cyclosporine's hypertensive effects, it has been proposed that rather than discontinuing therapy, adding an antihypertensive to a patient's regimen should be the initial step in management [19, 23] (Fig. 16.8).

The most common cutaneous side effect of cyclosporine is hypertrichosis which occurs in approximately 6% of patients [24].

Cyclosporine has limited oral bioavailability due to inadequate absorption and minimal metabolism of the drug by intestinal enzymes. The drug is extensively metabolized by CYP450 in the liver and is excreted in bile. Because bile salts are necessary for its absorption, cyclosporine microemulsion formulations have been created to increase its bioavailability without the need for bile salts or simultaneous intake of a fatty meal. Initial dosing of cyclosporine for the treatment of psoriasis ranges from 2.5 to 5 mg/kg/day with improvement frequently seen as early as 2 weeks and subsequent doses thereafter maintained at 2.5–3.5 mg/kg/day [11]. Numerous potential drug interactions exist with cyclosporine therapy and thus a detailed review of the patient's current medications must occur before initiating cyclosporine treatment. Patients should also be educated regarding the introduction of new drugs while taking cyclosporine.

There have been multiple studies showing cyclosporine to be a highly effective, rapid treatment option for psoriatic patients. In 12–16-week time periods it has been shown to dramatically improve up to 80–90% of patients [25–30]. In 1991, Ellis and colleagues concluded that the efficacy of cyclosporine is dose dependent [26]. This double-blind, placebo-controlled trial included doses of 3, 5, and 7.5 mg/kg of cyclosporine per day, and showed that after 8 weeks of treatment, 36%, 65%, and 85% of the respective patients were rated as clear or almost clear (PASI 75 to PASI 85). All three dosages were shown to be superior to placebo (Fig. 16.9). Fifty to seventy percentage of patients show a

PASI 75 response when cyclosporine is dosed at 3 mg/kg/day. When dosed at the same 3 mg/kg/day, a PASI 90 response in 30–50% of patients has been seen [30]. A study comparing MTX v CYA showed no statistically significant difference in reduction of PASI over 16 weeks of treatment between the two medications with perhaps most importantly no difference in duration of remission [96].

Due to its immunosuppressive effects, the physician must inquire about the presence of contraindications including malignancy, uncontrolled hypertension, renal insufficiency, uncontrolled infection, immune deficiency, high cumulative dose of previous phototherapy, especially PUVA, and lymphoma in a patient being considered for cyclosporine treatment. Because of the risk for gingival hyperplasia, patients should also be instructed to see a dentist every 6 months [19].

Fumaric Acid Esters

Fumaric acid esters (also known as fumarates) inhibit the pro-inflammatory cytokine production of molecules including TNF-alpha, IL-12, and IL-23 while also inducing T-cell apoptosis and T-helper type 2 cell differentiation, thus correcting the imbalance of cytokines produced by T-cells in psoriasis [56, 57]. Fumarate treatment has been shown to achieve PASI 75 in 50–70% of treated patients within 4 months [58]. In a year-long open clinical trial of 83 patients, a mean reduction of 76% of PASI occurred [59]. Fumarates are commonly used in Germany where they have been approved since 1994, as well as in other European countries, for the treatment of moderate-to-severe psoriasis. Fumarates are not currently approved for use in the USA.

In a systematic review of 19 articles on management of psoriasis with fumarates it was shown to be an effective and safe treatment option with few significant side effects [60]. The largest randomized controlled trial occurred in Germany in 1994 and involved 100 patients assigned to either fumarate treatment or placebo over 16 weeks. The patients exhibited a mean decrease in PASI score of 50% after 16 weeks of fumarate treatment [61]. In other randomized controlled trials, mean improvement of 42–76% in psoriasis severity after fumarate treatment has been shown [62–65]. A randomized control trial revealed that fumarates were equally as effective as methotrexate in the treatment of moderate-to-severe psoriasis [95]. A recent meta-analysis showed a 64% increase in PASI 50 response with fumaric esters compared to 14% with placebo [108]. Limiting side effects include gastrointestinal symptoms such as nausea, stomach cramps, and diarrhea, headaches, and skin flushing in 76% of patients receiving therapy [56, 108]. Up to 40% of patients discontinue fumarate treatment due to these intolerable side effects [66, 67]. Gastrointestinal side effects upon initiation of the drug can be minimized by slow titration of the drug. Lymphocytopenia,

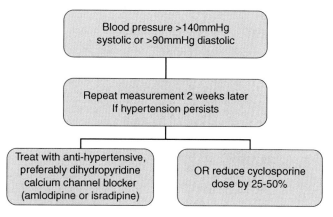

Fig. 16.8 Management of cyclosporine-induced hypertension

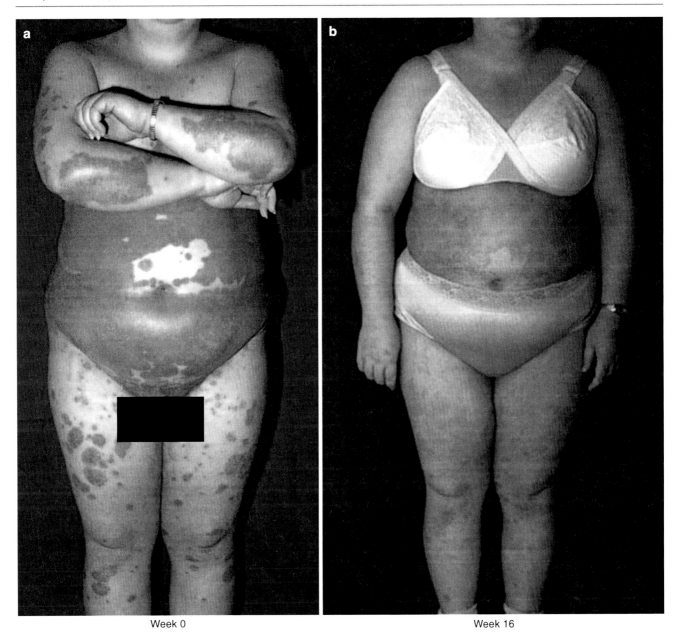

Week 0

Week 16

Fig. 16.9 (**a**) Erythrodermic psoriasis pretreatment with cyclosporine; week 0. (**b**) Erythrodermic psoriasis posttreatment with cyclosporine; week 16

eosinophilia, and proteinuria can also be seen during treatment, but these are usually not significant enough for discontinuation of treatment and can simply be observed [67, 68]. Despite no significant data showing an increased risk of infection or malignancy with fumarate therapy, long-term follow-up is still needed to confirm these observations.

Fumarate treatment is initially commenced with one tablet of Fumaderm® (made up of 120 mg dimethylfumarate, 87 mg calcium monoethylfumarate, 5 mg magnesium monoethylfumarate, and 3 mg zinc monoethylfumarate), with subsequent titrations over the ensuing 8 weeks. The maximum dose of Fumaderm® is six tablets daily [56].

Less Commonly Used Systemic Therapies in Psoriasis

Mycophenolate Mofetil

Mycophenolate Mofetil (MMF) is currently approved for the prevention of organ rejection, but is frequently used off-label in dermatology for the treatment of a variety of autoimmune diseases including psoriasis. MMF is a noncompetitive inhibitor of inosine monophosphate dehydrogenase (IMPDH) which inhibits de novo purine synthesis, inhibiting lymphocyte proliferation and antibody production [47]. By reversibly inhibiting guanine nucleotide synthesis, MMF specifically affects B and T lymphocytes. MMF also inhibits the glycosylation of lymphocyte and monocyte glycoproteins that serve endothelial cell adhesion [48].

MMF has been shown to be only moderately effective in the treatment of psoriasis. In 11 patients who received 1 g MMF twice daily for 3 weeks, and then 0.5 g twice daily, 7 patients showed a 40–70% reduction in their PASI score within 3 weeks. After 6 more weeks on the lower dose, six of these patients showed further improvement with four patients worsening after the decrease in dosage [49]. In another clinical trial, with doses of MMF ranging from 2 to 3 g daily, PASI reduction was observed to be 24% at 6 weeks and 47% at 12 weeks [50].

MMF is well tolerated compared to other psoriatic regimens including methotrexate and cyclosporine as it does not have the potential to cause kidney or liver toxicity [97]. The most common side effects experienced with MMF are gastrointestinal—nausea, vomiting, abdominal pain, diarrhea, constipation, and anorexia. Genitourinary side effects can also be experienced including urgency, frequency, dysuria, hematuria, and sterile pyuria [11]. While on MMF treatment, patients are at a greater risk for acquiring viral and bacterial infections, specifically herpes zoster, and cytomegalovirus [51]. Because this risk seems to be more common in transplant patients who receive MMF within a combination immunosuppressive regimen, it has been postulated that it is this treatment combination which increases the risk, and not treatment with MMF as monotherapy.

The long-term risk of carcinogenicity with MMF remains a controversial topic. In the field of dermatology, few malignancies have been reported in patients on MMF monotherapy [51]. There were no changes in the incidence of malignancy in renal and cardiac transplant patients over an observed 3-year period.

The initial daily dose of MMF is between 1 and 1.5 g orally, with an increase up to 3 g/day as needed [52].

Azathioprine

Azathioprine is a purine analog that blocks purine synthesis, i.e., a disease-modifying antirheumatic drug (DMARDs). It is an immunosuppressant that is approved for use in renal transplant patients and rheumatoid arthritis, but it is commonly used off-label for the treatment of autoimmune skin disease including psoriasis and atopic dermatitis. There are no randomized clinical trials for azathioprine use in psoriasis, with individual studies suggesting it to be beneficial. One open-label study showed that of 29 patients on 100–300 mg azathioprine daily, 19 patients showed improvement ranging from 50% to greater than 75% improvement [53]. In

another study of ten patients, five of these patients showed at least 25% improvement of their psoriasis [54].

Gastrointestinal side effects of azathioprine include nausea, vomiting and diarrhea, as well as elevations in serum transaminases and alkaline phosphatase. Anemia, leukopenia, thrombocytopenia, and pancytopenia can also occur [11]. An increased risk of myelotoxicity also exists in patients who have an inherited deficiency of thiopurine methyltransferase (TPMT). Thus, testing for TPMT is essential in patients prior to initiating azathioprine therapy.

The usual dose of azathioprine in the treatment of psoriasis ranges from 0.5 to 3 mg/kg. TPMT levels are typically used to guide dosing, with one schedule suggesting that at TPMT levels below five, one should not initiate azathioprine treatment [55]. Some physicians do initiate dosing at 0.5 mg/kg and monitor for cytopenia while then increasing dosing as necessary. Azathioprine has a slow onset of action, usually requiring 6–8 weeks of treatment before improvement is noticed.

Hydroxyurea

Hydroxyurea has been used as an off-label psoriatic treatment for many decades. It is an antimetabolite and cytotoxic agent that is approved for use in the treatment of hematologic diseases and various cancers. In psoriasis, it is hypothesized to work by inhibiting DNA replication within the basal cells of the epidermis. There are no randomized, controlled trials for psoriasis treatment with hydroxyurea but there have been studies showing it to be beneficial in psoriatic patients. In a retrospective study, using dosages of 0.5–1.5 g/day, 60% of patients achieved near-complete or complete clearance of their disease after an average of 16 months of treatment [69]. In a comparative study with methotrexate and hydroxyurea, a 48% reduction in mean PASI score was seen after 12 weeks of treatment with hydroxyurea. In comparison, methotrexate achieved 77% decrease in the mean PASI score [70]. A separate study showed a greater than 70% reduction in PASI score for 55% of 31 patients treated with 1–1.5 g/day of hydroxyurea [71].

Bone marrow toxicity is the most concerning side effect of hydroxyurea treatment. Leukopenia, anemia, thrombocytopenia, or pancytopenia can all occur but are reversible [72]. Most patients on hydroxyurea develop mild hematologic abnormalities and as many as 1/3 of these patients require dose adjustments [70]. Other significant side effects include lower leg ulcers, skin pigmentation, and diffuse alopecia, which are usually reversible with dose adjustment or discontinuation of the drug [71, 73].

Hydroxyurea is usually initiated at 500 mg orally twice daily, with subsequent increases as tolerated, to a maximum dose of 2 g/day [11].

Leflunomide

Leflunomide is another DMARD that works by inhibiting de novo pyrimidine synthesis, preventing lymphocyte proliferation, especially in regard to T-cells [74, 75]. It is thought to have both antiproliferative and anti-inflammatory activity. There is only one large randomized controlled trial of 190 patients using leflunomide for the treatment of psoriasis and psoriatic arthritis. In this trial, PASI 75 achievement was seen in 17% of leflunomide-treated patients vs. 8% of placebo-treated patients after 24 weeks of usual dosing. Of note, 15% of the leflunomide-treated group were concurrently allowed to use low-dose systemic corticosteroids for the treatment of their psoriatic arthritis [76].

Typical side effects of leflunomide include gastrointestinal symptoms such as diarrhea, nausea, and dyspepsia. Elevated liver enzymes and leukopenia have also been reported in higher frequency with leflunomide use than with placebo [76–78].

Leflunomide treatment is initiated with a loading dose of 100 mg/day for 3 days, and then decreased to a dose of 20 mg daily [11]. As treatment is more expensive than other DMARD treatments, leflunomide is typically reserved for patients who have tried and failed other therapies first. Rarely used in the field of dermatology as monotherapy, it is more commonly used by rheumatologists as combination therapy for severe joint disease.

Sulfasalazine

Although the exact mechanism of sulfasalazine is not known, it is thought to act as an anti-inflammatory agent. Sulfasalazine is used to treat inflammatory bowel disease and has also been used in the treatment of rheumatoid arthritis. There is only one double-blind, randomized controlled clinical trial of sulfasalazine in psoriasis where 50 patients with moderate-to-severe psoriasis were treated either with sulfasalazine for 8 weeks or with placebo [79]. The sulfasalazine-treated patients were dosed in escalation over time as tolerated, ranging from 1.5 to 4 g daily. Psoriasis severity was assessed at the end of 8 weeks and the patients were required to have tolerated sulfasalazine at least 2 g daily for 6 weeks. 26% of the sulfasalazine-treated group discontinued therapy due to side effects of rash or nausea with seven patients showing a 60–89% improvement and seven others showing 30–59% improvement in their psoriasis. Psoriasis treated with placebo was shown to worsen in all but one patient, who showed moderate improvement of their psoriasis. Sulfasalazine has been shown to be effective in the treatment of psoriatic arthritis in isolated studies but does not have the ability to prevent further joint damage [98].

Side effects of sulfasalazine include gastrointestinal intolerance such as nausea, vomiting, heartburn, and diarrhea. Although adverse effects with sulfasalazine are not generally serious, these adverse effects may be a limiting factor in treatment as they occur in up to 60% of patients treated with the drug [80].

Tacrolimus

Tacrolimus is a macrolide antibiotic that acts by inhibiting calcineurin which inhibits T-lymphocyte activation. It is approved for use in organ-transplant recipients to prevent organ rejection and is also commonly used in a topical formulation for atopic dermatitis and infrequently orally and off-label for psoriasis. The discovery of tacrolimus as an effective therapeutic option for psoriasis occurred fortuitously when four organ-transplant recipients were treated with the drug to prevent transplant rejection and showed significant improvement of their psoriasis as well. To date, the efficacy of oral tacrolimus for psoriasis is not well established.

In a randomized, placebo-controlled trial with 50 moderate-to-severe psoriasis patients, orally dosed tacrolimus reduced PASI scores by 83% compared with 47% reduction with placebo at the end of 9 weeks [81]. Tacrolimus was dosed at 0.05–0.15 mg/kg/day. It is important to note that after 3 weeks on 0.05 mg/kg/day there was no difference in improvement between tacrolimus and placebo. By 9 weeks, when dosed at 0.10–0.15 mg/kg/day, PASI improvement was significant in tacrolimus-treated patients when compared to placebo.

Side effects of tacrolimus in transplant patients have included hypertension, nephrotoxicity, diabetes mellitus, tremors, paresthesias, and gastrointestinal issues including diarrhea, nausea, vomiting, constipation, and abdominal pain.

6-Thioguanine

6-Thioguanine is a purine analog of guanine that functions by disrupting DNA and RNA. It is indicated for the treatment of acute myelogenous leukemia. It is the natural metabolite of azathioprine and is thought to induce apoptotic death in proliferating T lymphocytes. 6-Thioguanine has been used as an off-label treatment option for psoriasis since the 1950s and has shown effectiveness in both treating psoriasis and maintaining psoriatic improvement.

There are no randomized trials for the treatment of psoriasis with 6-thioguanine. However, many other studies and case reports advocate its use in psoriatic disease. In a retrospective, open-label study of 6-thioguanine in 40 patients, 78% of patients achieved complete or almost complete clearing of their disease. Eleven percentage of these patients showed moderate improvement and another 11% showed little to no improvement of their disease. The treatment course and dosage varied in this study [82]. Another study with a variable duration of therapy (maximum of 220 months) reported 49% of patients controlled on 6-thioguanine, with 51% of patients discontinuing therapy due to initial failure, side effects, or relapse of their disease [83]. In both studies, reversible myelosuppression was the most frequently observed side effect. One study proposed prescribing 6-thioguanine in a pulse dosing regimen. When given between 120 and 160 mg, 2–3 times/week, 10 out of 14 patients showed significant improvement in their recalcitrant psoriasis. This group also showed a clear decrease in bone marrow toxicity when compared to daily dosing [84].

Long-term use of 6-thioguanine is dose limited by the induction of myelosuppression, especially thrombocytopenia. However, it does not have significant hepatotoxic or renal effects as compared to methotrexate and cyclosporine, which makes it a useful addition to rotational therapy with these drugs.

Initial dosing with 6-thioguanine is 80 mg twice weekly with subsequent increases in 20 mg increments every 2–4 weeks. The maximum recommended dose is 160 mg given three times/week.

Novel Treatments in Psoriasis

New Oral Treatments

Apremilast

Apremilast (Otezla®) is the newest oral treatment indicated for psoriasis and psoriatic arthritis and the first oral agent approved for psoriatic arthritis. Apremilast exerts its effect intracellularly, regulating inflammation by specifically inhibiting phosphodiesterase 4 (PDE4), an enzyme that regulates inflammatory action intracellularly [85].

Unlike biologic agents that set their sights on targeting a specific pro-inflammatory cytokine like TNF-α, apremilast works early on the inflammatory cascade, affecting more than just one inflammatory mediator. By inhibiting the action of PDE4, the degradation of cAMP is prevented. Increased cAMP then downregulates production of pro-inflammatory cytokines like TNF-α, IL-17, IL-23, and interferon γ. cAMP also upregulates the anti-inflammatory mediator IL-10 [86] (Fig. 16.10).

Apremilast is dosed as a 30 mg tablet twice a day, with an initial 5-day period of gradually increasing dosage to eventually reach the recommended dose of 30 mg twice daily. In two phase III clinical trials, ESTEEM and PALACE, apremilast reduced the extent and severity of moderate-to-severe plaque psoriasis and psoriatic arthritis, respectively, when compared to placebo. In the ESTEEM trials, with a primary endpoint of PASI 75, 29–33% of patients on apremilast showed clinically and statistically significant improvement in their plaque psoriasis at 16 weeks when compared to 5–6% of placebo patients [86, 87]. There was significant improvement in nail psoriasis severity index (NPSI) with apremilast compared to placebo as well as significantly more patients achieving clear/almost clear scalp activity compared with placebo. These studies also showed significant improvement in the palmoplantar variant of psoriasis.

Common side effects noted in up to 17% of patients include diarrhea, nausea, headache, upper respiratory tract infections, and nasopharyngitis. The gastrointestinal side effects usually spontaneously remit after the initial 4–6 weeks of therapy. Apremilast has also been associated with rare instances of depression and mild degrees of weight loss in 10–12% of patients [88].

Tofacitinib

Tofacitinib (Xeljanz) is an inhibitor of the Janus kinase 1 and 3 enzymes (JAK1, 3), thereby influencing gene transcription in the nucleus. This family of tyrosine kinases are integral to the growth and differentiation of cells as well as the cytokine cascades. It is currently only FDA approved for the treatment of rheumatoid arthritis. Tofacitinib has been used off-label for treatment of alopecia areata, vitiligo, ulcerative colitis,

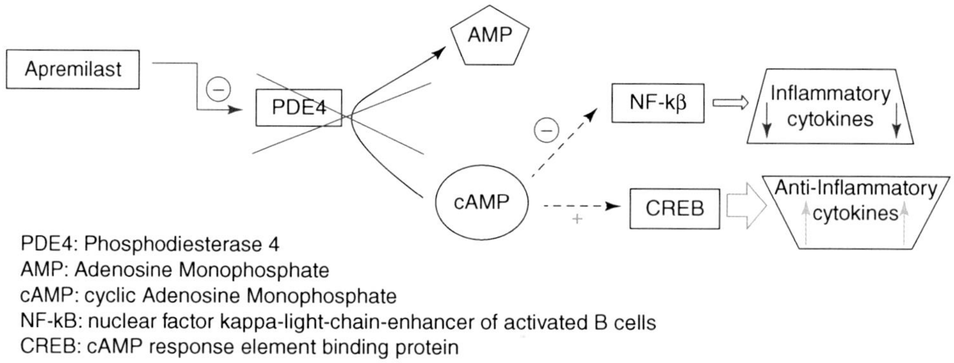

Fig. 16.10 Mechanism of action of apremilast

PDE4: Phosphodiesterase 4
AMP: Adenosine Monophosphate
cAMP: cyclic Adenosine Monophosphate
NF-kB: nuclear factor kappa-light-chain-enhancer of activated B cells
CREB: cAMP response element binding protein

and atopic dermatitis. Phase III trials have shown oral tofacitinib dosed at 10 mg twice daily to be noninferior to etanercept [104]. Increased rates of clearance were found in the 10 mg twice-daily groups compared to the 5 mg twice daily and placebo [105].

Side effects of tofacitinib include an increased risk of lymphoma, opportunistic infections, as well as URIs, headache, and diarrhea with one study showing 80% of patients having adverse effects [105]. Further investigation is required relating to its safety and efficacy data in the treatment of psoriasis.

Summary

Despite the major impact over the last decade with the introduction of injectable biologic agents for moderate-severe psoriasis, oral agents still remain an essential category of treatment for psoriasis patients. Methotrexate, with its 44-year history of use in psoriasis, and despite its side effect profile and only moderate efficacy compared to biologic agents, is likely to remain an important drug, either as monotherapy or in combination, in the treatment of all forms of psoriasis in the future.

Case Report

A 26-year-old female presented with a 14-year history of psoriatic plaques which started on her calves. She had no history of psoriatic arthritis symptoms and had no family history of psoriasis. Her medical history was otherwise noncontributory. She complained of significant itching as well as persistent scaling from her plaques. The patient's disease was refractory to many past treatments and she presented for a second opinion.

Past Medical History
- None

Social History
- Drinks socially (a few glasses of wine per week)
- Married

Previous Therapies
- Topical steroids
- Narrowband UVB
- Cyclosporine
- Methotrexate
- Bexarotene
- Infliximab

- Adalimumab
- Etanercept

Physical Exam
- Generalized small psoriatic plaques on the scalp, trunk, upper, and lower extremities covering over 50% of the body surface area
- No features of psoriatic arthritis (dactylitis, enthesitis, tender and swollen joints, etc.)

Management
As she had failed many prior therapies (see above) she was restarted on a combination of methotrexate and infliximab. However, the patient had to stop all systemic medications as she became pregnant a few months after resuming treatment. She was restarted on cyclosporine when she was 3 months pregnant due to significant flare. At week 24 of her pregnancy, the patient presented with marked improvement. Her upper extremities showed a few active areas and she was approximately 80% clear. There was some activity in her breast folds and on her rib margins. Her cyclosporine was tapered and discontinued during her eighth month of pregnancy. Despite her use of Methotrexate in the first 3 months of her pregnancy, she delivered a healthy baby boy and remains 90% clear to date after restarting adalimumab and home UVB treatments.

References

1. Rachakonda TD, Schupp CW, Armstrong AW. Psoriasis prevalence among adults in the United States. J Am Acad Dermatol. 2014;70(3):512–6.
2. Feldman SR, Malakouti M, Koo JY. Social impact of the burden of psoriasis: effects on patients and practice. Dermatol Online J. 2014;20(8.) pii: 13030/qt48r4w8h2
3. Fowler JF, Duh MS, Rovba L, et al. The impact of psoriasis on health care costs and patient work loss. J Am Acad Dermatol. 2008;59(5):772–80.
4. Edson-Heredia E, Zhu B, Guo J, Maeda-Chubachi T, Lebwohl M. Disease burden and quality of life in psoriasis patients with and without comorbid psoriatic arthritis: results from National Psoriasis Foundation panel surveys. Cutis. 2015;95(3):173–8.
5. Gisondi P, Galvan A, Idolazzi L, Girolomoni G. Management of moderate to severe psoriasis in patients with metabolic comorbidities. Front Med (Lausanne). 2015;2:1.
6. Armstrong AW, Harskamp CT, Armstrong EJ. The association between psoriasis and obesity: a systematic review and meta-analysis of observational studies. Nutr Diabetes. 2012;2:e54.
7. Menter A, Gottlieb G, Steven R, Van Voorhees AS, Leonardi CL, Gordon KB, et al. Guidelines of care for the management of psoriasis and psoriatic arthritis. Section 1. Overview of psoriasis and

guidelines of care for the treatment of psoriasis with biologics. J Am Acad Dermatol. 2008;58:826–50.

8. Armstrong EJ, Harskamp CT, Armstrong AW. Psoriasis and major adverse cardiovascular events: a systematic review and meta-analysis of observational studies. J Am Heart Assoc. 2013;2(2):e000062. https://doi.org/10.1161/JAHA.113.000062.

9. Ogdie A, Yu YD, Haynes K, Love TJ, Maliha S, Jiang Y, Troxel AB, Hennessy S, Kimmel SE, Margolis DJ, Choi H, Mehta NN, Gelfand JM. Risk of major cardiovascular events in patients with psoriatic arthritis, psoriasis and rheumatoid arthritis: a population-based cohort study. Ann Rheum Dis. 2015;74(2):326–32.

10. Rustin MHA. Long-term safety of biologics in the treatment of moderate-to-severe plaque psoriasis: review of current data. Br J Dermatol. 2012;167(Suppl 3):3–11.

11. Menter A, Korman NJ, Elmets CA, et al. Guidelines of care for the management of psoriasis and psoriatic arthritis: section 4. Guidelines of care for the management and treatment of psoriasis with traditional systemic agents. J Am Acad Dermatol. 2009;61(3):451–85.

12. Gupta AK, Baadsgaard O, Ellis CN, Voorhees JJ, Cooper KD. Lymphocytes and macrophages of the epidermis and dermis in lesional psoriatic skin, but no epidermal Langerhans cells, are depleted by treatment with cyclosporine A. Arch Dermatol Res. 1989;281:219–26.

13. Gottlieb AB, Grossman RM, Khandke L, Carter DM, Sehgal PB, Fu SM, et al. Studies of the effect of cyclosporine in psoriasis in vivo: combined effects on activated T lymphocytes and epidermal regenerative maturation. J Invest Dermatol. 1992;98:302–9.

14. Prens EP, van Joost T, Hegmans JP, t Hooft-Benne K, Ysselmuiden OE, Benner R. Effects of cyclosporine on cytokines and cytokine receptors in psoriasis. J Am Acad Dermatol. 1995;33:947–53.

15. Taler SJ, Textor SC, Canzanello VJ, Schwartz L. Cyclosporin induced hypertension: incidence, pathogenesis and management. Drug Saf. 1999;20:437–49.

16. Lowe NJ, Wieder JM, Rosenbach A, Johnson K, Kunkel R, Bainbridge C, et al. Long-term low-dose cyclosporine therapy for severe psoriasis: effects on renal function and structure. J Am Acad Dermatol. 1996;35:710–9.

17. Markham T, Watson A, Rogers S. Adverse effects with long term cyclosporin for severe psoriasis. Clin Exp Dermatol. 2002;27:111–4.

18. Powles AV, Hardman CM, Porter WM, Cook T, Hulme B, Fry L. Renal function after 10 years' treatment with cyclosporin for psoriasis. Br J Dermatol. 1998;138:443–9.

19. Ryan C, Amor KT, Menter A. The use of cyclosporine in dermatology: Part II. J Am Acad Dermatol. 2010;63(6):949–72.

20. Young EW, Ellis CN, Messana JM, Johnson KH, Leichtman AB, Mihatsch MJ, et al. A prospective study of renal structure and function in psoriasis patients treated with cyclosporin. Kidney Int. 1994;46:1216–22.

21. Zachariae H, Kragballe K, Hansen HE, Marcussen N, Olsen S. Renal biopsy findings in long-term cyclosporin treatment of psoriasis. Br J Dermatol. 1997;136:531–5.

22. Tomlanovich S, Gobletz H, Periroth M, Stinson E, Myers BD. Limitations of creatinine in quantifying the severity of cyclosporine-induced nephropathy. Am J Kidney Dis. 1986;8:332–3.

23. Feutren G, Abeywickrama K, Friend D, Von Graffenried B. Renal function and blood pressure in psoriatic patients treated with cyclosporin A. Br J Dermatol. 1990;122(Suppl 36):57–69.

24. Lebwohl M, Ellis C, Gottlieb A, Koo J, Krueger G, Linden K, et al. Cyclosporine consensus conference: with emphasis on the treatment of psoriasis. J Am Acad Dermatol. 1998;39:464–75.

25. Berth-Jones J, Henderson CA, Munro CS, Rogers S, Chalmers RJ, Boffa MJ, et al. Treatment ofpsoriasis with intermittent short course cyclosporin (Neoral): a multicenter study. Br J Dermatol. 1997;136:527–30.

26. Ellis CN, Fradin MS, Messana JM, Brown MD, Siegel MT, Hartley AH, et al. Cyclosporine for plaque-type psoriasis: results of a multidose, double-blind trial. N Engl J Med. 1991;324:277–84.

27. Faerber L, Braeutigam M, Weidinger G, Mrowietz U, Christophers E, Schulze HJ, et al. Cyclosporine in severe psoriasis: results of a meta-analysis in 579 patients. Am J Clin Dermatol. 2001;2:41–7.

28. Ho VC, Griffiths CE, Albrecht G, Vanaclocha F, Leon-Dorantes G, Atakan N, et al. Intermittent short courses of cyclosporin (Neoral(R)) for psoriasis unresponsive to topical therapy: a 1-year multicenter, randomized study. The PISCES Study Group. Br J Dermatol. 1999;141:283–91.

29. Ho VC, Griffiths CE, Berth-Jones J, Papp KA, Vanaclocha F, Dauden E, et al. Intermittent short courses of cyclosporine microemulsion for the long-term management of psoriasis: a 2-year cohort study. J Am Acad Dermatol. 2001;44:643–51.

30. Nast A, Kopp I, Augustin M, Banditt KB, Boehncke WH, Follmann M, et al. German evidence-based guidelines for the treatment of psoriasis vulgaris (short version). Arch Dermatol Res. 2007;299:111–38.

31. Gilbert SC, Emmett M, Menter A, Silverman A, Klintmalm G. Cyclosporine therapy for psoriasis: serum creatinine measurements are an unreliable predictor of decreased renal function. J Am Acad Dermatol. 1989;21:470–4.

32. Ternowitz T, Herlin T. Neutrophil and monocyte chemotaxis in methotrexate-treated psoriasis patients. Acta Derm Venereol Suppl (Stockh). 1985;120:23–6.

33. Jeffes EW III, McCullough JL, Pittelkow MR, McCormick A, Almanzor J, Liu G, et al. Methotrexate therapy of psoriasis: differential sensitivity of proliferating lymphoid and epithelial cells to the cytotoxic and growth-inhibitory effects of methotrexate. J Invest Dermatol. 1995;104:183–8.

34. Saporito FC, Menter MA. Methotrexate and psoriasis in the era of new biologic agents. J Am Acad Dermatol. 2004;50:301–9.

35. Dogra S, Mahajan R. Systemic methotrexate therapy for psoriasis: past, present and future. Clin Exp Dermatol. 2013;38:573–88.

36. MacDonald A, Burden AD. Noninvasive monitoring for methotrexate hepatotoxicity. Br J Dermatol. 2005;152:405–8.

37. Montaudié H, Sbidian E, Paul C, Maza A, Gallini A, Aractingi S, Aubin F, Bachelez H, Cribier B, Joly P, Jullien D, Le Maître M, Misery L, Richard MA, Ortonne J-P. Methotrexate in psoriasis: a systematic review of treatment modalities, incidence, risk factors and monitoring of liver toxicity. J Eur Acad Dermatol Venereol. 2011;25:12–8.

38. Langman G, Hall PM, Todd G. Role of non-alcoholic steatohepatitis in methotrexate-induced liver injury. J Gastroenterol Hepatol. 2001;16:1395–401.

39. Rosenberg P, Urwitz H, Johannesson A, Ros AM, Lindholm J, Kinnman N, et al. Psoriasis patients with diabetes type 2 are at high risk of developing liver fibrosis during methotrexate treatment. J Hepatol. 2007;46:1111–8.

40. Strober BE, Menon K. Folate supplementation during methotrexate therapy for patients with psoriasis. J Am Acad Dermatol. 2005;53:652–9.

41. Kalb RE, Strober B, Weinstein G, Lebwohl M. Methotrexate and psoriasis: 2009 National Psoriasis Foundation consensus conference. J Am Acad Dermatol. 2009;60:824–37.

42. Saurat JH, Stingl G, Dubertret L, Papp K, Langley RG, Ortonne JP, et al. Efficacy and safety results from the randomized controlled comparative study of adalimumab vs methotrexate vs placebo in patients with psoriasis (CHAMPION). Br J Dermatol. 2008;158:558–66.

43. Barker J, Hoffmann M, Wozel G, et al. Efficacy and safety of infliximab vs. methotrexate in patients with moderate-to-severe plaque psoriasis: results of an open-label, active-controlled, randomized trial (RESTORE1). Br J Dermatol. 2011;165:1109–17.

44. Atzeni F, Sarzi-Puttini P. Autoantibody production in patients treated with anti-TNF. Expert Rev Clin Immunol. 2008;4:275–80.

45. Buccheri L, Katchen BR, Kart AJ, Her J, Cohen SR. Acitretin therapy is effective for psoriasis associated with human immunodeficiency virus infection. Arch Dermatol. 1997;133:711–5.

46. Katz HI, Waalen J, Leach EE. Acitretin in psoriasis: an overview of adverse effects. J Am Acad Dermatol. 1999;41:S7–S12.

47. Yamauchi PS, Rizk D, Kormeili T, et al. Current systemic therapies for psoriasis: where are we now? J Am Acad Dermatol. 2003;49:S66–77.

48. Allison AC, Eugui EM. Purine metabolism and immunosuppressive effects of mycophenolate mofetil (MMF). Clin Transplant. 1996;10(1 Pt 2):77–84.

49. Geilen CC, Arnold M, Orfanos CE. Mycophenolate mofetil as a systemic antipsoriatic agent: positive experience in 11 patients. Br J Dermatol. 2001;144(3):583–6.

50. Zhou Y, Rosenthal D, Dutz J, Ho V. Mycophenolate mofetil (CellCept(R)) for psoriasis: a two-center, prospective, open-label clinical trial. J Cutan Med Surg. 2003;7:193–7.

51. Orvis AK, Wesson SK, Breza TS, Church AA, Mitchell CL, Watkins SW. Mycophenolate mofetil in dermatology. J Am Acad Dermatol. 2009;60:183–99.

52. Assmann T, Ruzicka T. New immunosuppressive drugs in dermatology (mycophenolate mofetil, tacrolimus): unapproved uses, dosages, or indications. Clin Dermatol. 2002;20(5):505–14.

53. Du Vivier A, Munro DD, Verbov J. Treatment of psoriasis with azathioprine. Br Med J. 1974;1:49–51.

54. Greaves MW, Dawber R. Azathioprine in psoriasis. Br Med J. 1970;2:237–8.

55. Snow JL, Gibson LE. The role of genetic variation in thiopurine methyltransferase activity and the efficacy and/or side effects of azathioprine therapy in dermatologic patients. Arch Dermatol. 1995;131:193–7.

56. Roll A, Reich K, Boer A. Use of fumaric acid esters in psoriasis. Indian J Dermatol Venereol Leprol. 2007;73:133–7.

57. Mrowietz U, Christophers E, Altmeyer F. Treatment of severe psoriasis with fumaric acid esters: scientific background and guidelines for therapeutic use. The German Fumaric Acid Ester Consensus Conference. Br J Dermatol. 1999;141:424–9.

58. Mrowietz U, Christophers E, Altmeyer P. Treatment of psoriasis with fumaric acid esters: results of a prospective multicenter study; German multicenter study. Br J Dermatol. 1998;138:456–60.

59. Altmeyer P, Hartwig R, Matthes U. Efficacy and safety profile of fumaric acid esters in oral long-term therapy with severe treatment refractory psoriasis vulgaris. A study of 83 patients. Hautarzt. 1996;47(3):190–6.

60. Smith D. Fumaric acid esters for psoriasis: a systematic review. Ir J Med Sci. 2017;186(1):161–77.

61. Altmeyer PJ, Matthes U, Pawlak F, et al. Antipsoriatic effect of fumaric acid derivatives. Results of a multicenter double-blind study in 100 patients. J Am Acad Dermatol. 1994;30(6):977–81.

62. Nieboer C, de Hoop D, Langendijk PN, van Loenen AC, Gubbels J. Fumaric acid therapy in psoriasis: a double-blind comparison between fumaric acid compound therapy and monotherapy with dimethylfumaric acid ester. Dermatologica. 1990;181(1):33–7.

63. Fallah Arani S, Neumann H, Hop WC, Thio HB. Fumarates vs methotrexate in moderate to severe chronic plaque psoriasis: a multicentre prospective randomized controlled clinical trial. Br J Dermatol. 2011;164(4):855–61.

64. Gollnick H, Altmeyer P, Kaufmann R, et al. Topical calcipotriol plus oral fumaric acid is more effective and faster acting than oral fumaric acid monotherapy in the treatment of severe chronic plaque psoriasis vulgaris. Dermatology. 2002;205(1):46–53.

65. Balak DM, Fallah-Arani S, Venema CM, Neumann HA, Thio HB. Addition of an oral histamine antagonist to reduce adverse events associated with fumaric acid esters in the treatment of psoriasis: a randomized double-blind placebo-controlled trial. Br J Dermatol. 2015;172(3):754–9. https://doi.org/10.1111/bjd.13277. Epub 2016 Jan 18

66. Mrowietz U, Asadullah K. Dimethylfumarate for psoriasis: more than a dietary curiosity. Trends Mol Med. 2005;11:43–8.

67. Harries MJ, Chalmers RJ, Griffiths CE. Fumaric acid esters for severe psoriasis: a retrospective review of 58 cases. Br J Dermatol. 2005;153(3):549–51.

68. Kolbach DN, Nieboer C. Fumaric acid therapy in psoriasis: results and side effects of 2 years of treatment. J Am Acad Dermatol. 1992;27:769–71.

69. Layton AM, Sheehan-Dare RA, Goodfield MJ, Cotterill JA. Hydroxyurea in the management of therapy resistant psoriasis. Br J Dermatol. 1989;121:647–53.

70. Ranjan N, Sharma NL, Shanker V, Mahajan VK, Tegta GR. Methotrexate versus hydroxycarbamide (hydroxyurea) as a weekly dose to treat moderate-to-severe chronic plaque psoriasis: a comparative study. J Dermatolog Treat. 2007;18:295–300.

71. Kumar B, Saraswat A, Kaur I. Rediscovering hydroxyurea: its role in recalcitrant psoriasis. Int J Dermatol. 2001;40:530–4.

72. Sharma VK, Dutta B, Ramam M. Hydroxyurea as an alternative therapy for psoriasis. Indian J Dermatol Venereol Leprol. 2004;70:13–7.

73. Smith CH. Use of hydroxyurea in psoriasis. Clin Exp Dermatol. 1999;24:2–6.

74. Frieling U, Luger TA. Mycophenolate mofetil and leflunomide: promising compounds for the treatment of skin diseases. Clin Exp Dermatol. 2002;27(7):562–70.

75. Wozel G, Pfeiffer C. Leflunomide: a novel drug for pharmacological immunomodulation. Hautarzt. 2002;53(5):309–15.

76. Kaltwasser JP, Nash P, Gladman D, Rosen CF, Behrens F, Jones P, et al. Efficacy and safety of leflunomide in the treatment of psoriatic arthritis and psoriasis: a multinational, double-blind, randomized, placebo-controlled clinical trial. Arthritis Rheum. 2004;50:1939–50.

77. Prakash A, Jarvis B. Leflunomide: a review of its use in active rheumatoid arthritis. Drugs. 1999;58:1137–64.

78. Nguyen M, Kabir M, Ravaud P. Short-term efficacy and safety of leflunomide in the treatment of active rheumatoid arthritis in everyday clinical use: open-label, prospective study. Clin Drug Investig. 2004;24(2):103–12.

79. Gupta AK, Ellis CN, Siegel MT, Duell EA, Griffiths CE, Hamilton TA, et al. Sulfasalazine improves psoriasis: a double-blind analysis. Arch Dermatol. 1990;126:487–93.

80. Watkinson G. Sulphasalazine: a review of 40 years' experience. Drugs. 1986;32(Suppl 1):1–11.

81. Bos JD, Witkamp L, Zonneveld IM, Ruzicka T, Szarmach H, Szczerkowska-Dobosz A. Systemic tacrolimus (FK 506) is effective for the treatment of psoriasis in a double-blind, placebo-controlled study: the European FK 506 multicenter psoriasis study group. Arch Dermatol. 1996;132:419–23.

82. Zackheim HS, Maibach HI. Treatment of psoriasis with 6-thioguanine. Australas J Dermatol. 1988;29:163–7.

83. Zackheim HS, Glogau RG, Fisher DA, Maibach HI. 6-Thioguanine treatment of psoriasis: experience in 81 patients. J Am Acad Dermatol. 1994;30:452–8.

84. Silvis NG, Levine N. Pulse dosing of thioguanine in recalcitrant psoriasis. Arch Dermatol. 1999;135:433–7.

85. Duong R, Gilbert M. Psoriasis: overview, recent approvals, therapies on the horizon. Pharmacy Today. 2016;22(1):44–5.

86. Schafer P. Apremilast mechanism of action and application to psoriasis and psoriatic arthritis. Biochem Pharmacol. 2012;83:1583–90.

87. Papp K, Reich K, Leonardi CL, et al. Apremilast, an oral phosphodiesterase 4 (PDE4) inhibitor, in patients with moderate to severe plaque psoriasis: results of a phase III, randomized, controlled trial (Efficacy and Safety Trial Evaluating the Effects of Apremilast in Psoriasis [ESTEEM]1). J Am Acad Dermatol. 2015;73(1):37–49.

88. Paul C, et al. Efficacy and safety of apremilast, an oral phosphodiesterase 4 inhibitor, in patients with moderate-to-severe plaque psoriasis over 52 weeks: a phase III, randomized, controlled trial (ESTEEM 2). Br J Dermatol. 2015;173(6):1387–99.

89. Cauli A, Porru G, Piga M, Vacca A, Dessole G, Mathieu A. Clinical potential of apremilast in the treatment of psoriatic arthritis. Immunotargets Ther. 2014;3:91–6.

90. Barker J, Horn EJ, Lebwohl M, et al. Assessment and management of methotrexate hepatotoxicity in psoriasis patients: report from a consensus conference to evaluate current practice and identify key questions toward optimizing methotrexate use in the clinic. J Eur Acad Dermatol Venereol. 2011;25(7):758–64.

91. Murray HE, Anhalt AW, Lessard R, Schacter RK, Ross JB, Stewart WD. A 12-month treatment of severe psoriasis with acitretin: Results of a Canadian open multicentre trial. J Am Acad Dermatol. 1991;24:598–602.

92. Lassus A, Geiger JM. Acitretin and etretinate in the treatment of palmoplantar pustulosis. A double-blind comparative trial. Br J Dermatol. 1988;119:755–9.

93. Katugampola RP, Finlay AY. Oral retinoids therapy for disorders of keratinization: A single-centre retrospective 25 years' experience on 23 patients. Br J Dermatol. 2006;154:267–76.

94. Spuls PI, et al. J Dermatolog Treat. 2003;14(Suppl 2):17–20.

95. Barker JN. Methotrexate or fumarates: which is the best oral treatment for psoriasis? Br J Dermatol. 2011;164(4):695.

96. Heydendael VM, Spuls PI, Opmeer BC, et al. Methotrexate versus cyclosporine in moderate-to-severe chronic plaque psoriasis. N Engl J Med. 2003;349(7):658–65.

97. Pedraz J, Daudén E, Delgado-jiménez Y, et al. Sequential study on the treatment of moderate-to-severe chronic plaque psoriasis with mycophenolate mofetil and cyclosporin. J Eur Acad Dermatol Venereol. 2006;20(6):702–6.

98. Rahman P, Gladman DD, Cook RJ, Zhou Y, Young G. The use of sulfasalazine in psoriatic arthritis: a clinic experience. J Rheumatol. 1998;25(10):1957–61.

99. https://www.aad.org/practice-tools/quality-care/clinical-guidelines/psoriasis/systemic-agents/recommendations-for-methotrexate.

100. Menter A, Korman NJ, Elmets CA, et al. Guidelines of care for the management of psoriasis and psoriatic arthritis: section 4. Guidelines of care for the management and treatment of psoriasis with traditional systemic agents. J Am Acad Dermatol. 2009;61(3):451–85.

101. Raposo I, Torres T. Palmoplantar psoriasis and palmoplantar pustulosis: current treatment and future prospects. Am J Clin Dermatol. 2016;17(4):349–58.

102. Spuls PI, et al. J Dermatolog Treat. 2003;14(Suppl 2):17–20.

103. Chiricozzi A, Panduri S, Dini V, Tonini A, Gualtieri B, Romanelli M. Optimizing acitretin use in patients with plaque psoriasis. Dermatol Ther. 2017;30(2). https://doi.org/10.1111/dth.12453. Epub 2016 Dec 20

104. Valenzuela F, Paul C, Mallbris L, et al. Tofacitinib versus etanercept or placebo in patients with moderate to severe chronic plaque psoriasis: patient-reported outcomes from a Phase 3 study. J Eur Acad Dermatol Venereol. 2016;30(10):1753–9.

105. Papp KA, Menter MA, Abe M, et al. Tofacitinib, an oral Janus kinase inhibitor, for the treatment of chronic plaque psoriasis: results from two randomized, placebo-controlled, phase III trials. Br J Dermatol. 2015;173(4):949–61.

106. Menter A, Thrash B, Cherian C, et al. Intestinal transport of aminopterin enantiomers in dogs and humans with psoriasis is stereoselective: evidence for a mechanism involving the proton-coupled folate transporter. J Pharmacol Exp Ther. 2012;342(3):696–708.

107. Van der voort EA, Wakkee M, Veldt-kok P, Darwish murad S, Nijsten T. Enhanced liver fibrosis test (ELF) in psoriasis, psoriatic arthritis and rheumatoid arthritis patients: a cross-sectional comparison with procollagen-3 N-terminal peptide (P3NP). Br J Dermatol. 2017;176(6):1599–606. https://doi.org/10.1111/bjd.15220. Epub 2017 Apr 24

108. Atwan A, Ingram JR, Abbott R, et al. Oral fumaric acid esters for psoriasis: abridged Cochrane systematic review including GRADE assessments. Br J Dermatol. 2016;175(5):873–81.

109. Mueller W, Herrmann B. Cyclosporin A for psoriasis. N Engl J Med. 1979;301(10):555.

Nail, Scalp, and Palmoplantar Psoriasis

Jeffrey J. Crowley

Psoriasis can affect many areas of the body and treatments should target the areas of involvement. Nail disease is difficult to treat with topical therapy as the vehicle must be optimized to penetrate the nail and surrounding tissues. Some of the inflammation in nail disease is deep in the nail matrix and thus difficult for topical therapies to access. Scalp disease is difficult to treat with topical and phototherapy due to the presence of hair, bathing habits, and convenience issues. The palms and soles often have particularly thick plaques of psoriasis which may prevent absorption of topical therapy and resist phototherapy. Patients with primarily palmoplantar disease often do not respond to multiple therapies, and many require combination therapy for disease control. Collectively, nail, scalp, and palmoplantar psoriasis are considered "tough to treat" and often do not respond as well as plaque psoriasis elsewhere on the body. This chapter critically addresses the challenges posed by each condition and evaluates available treatment options.

Nail Psoriasis

Psoriasis is a chronic systemic inflammatory disease involving the skin, nails, and joints. Approximately 50% of psoriasis patients have some nail involvement and the lifetime incidence of nail disease is estimated at 80–90%. Nail disease may rarely be the only manifestation of psoriasis [1]. Nail psoriasis is associated with higher overall disease severity and male gender. Importantly, nail psoriasis can cause significant pain, discomfort, and embarrassment, leading to impairment in quality of life (QoL) and work function [2, 3].

There is a strong correlation of nail psoriasis and psoriatic arthritis [4]. Psoriatic arthritis patients have rates of nail disease as high as 70% and there is evidence that nail psoriasis may be a predictor of joint disease developing later in life [5].

Psoriatic arthritis may involve the distal interphalangeal joints and the anatomic link between these joints and the nail unit may result in nail changes. In fact, nail disease is one of the components of the CASPAR criteria, which is used to aid in the diagnosis of psoriatic arthritis [6]. Fingernail psoriasis, due to its visibility and impacts on function, is more problematic for many patients compared with toenail disease. Additionally, psoriatic toenails are often secondarily infected with dermatophytes which may complicate treatment assessment [7]. Treatment with immunosuppressive medications may even contribute to the development of onychomycosis in patients with toenail psoriasis. For these reasons, most studies evaluate fingernail psoriasis alone [8].

Clinically, nail disease has many different presentations which depend on the location of the inflammatory process. Nail pitting, the most common finding in nail psoriasis, nail dystrophy, and leukonychia (white discoloration of nails) are due to nail matrix involvement [9] (Fig. 17.1). Nail bed psoriasis is characterized by onycholysis (lifting of the distal nail from the nail bed), oil drop patches (yellow discolorations below the nail), subungual hyperkeratosis (thickening

J.J. Crowley, MS, MD, FAAD
Bakersfield Dermatology and Skin Cancer Medical Group, Bakersfield, CA, USA
e-mail: crowley415@aol.com

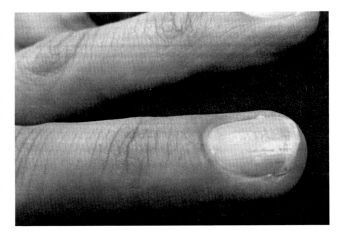

Fig. 17.1 Nail matrix psoriasis: note the extensive pitting in this nail. Some of the pits are linear and a splinter hemorrhage is also present. This patient has concomitant psoriatic arthritis and inflammatory bowel disease

© Springer International Publishing AG 2018
P.S. Yamauchi (ed.), *Biologic and Systemic Agents in Dermatology*, https://doi.org/10.1007/978-3-319-66884-0_17

of the nail), and splinter hemorrhages (linear streaks of dried blood in the nail) [1] (Fig. 17.2a, b). One recent study demonstrated that nail clippings of clinically uninvolved nails from patients with psoriasis may show abnormalities, and thus subclinical nail disease exists [10].

The methods of reporting changes in nail disease within clinical trials have not been standardized. The nail psoriasis and severity index (NAPSI) was developed to measure changes in nail disease over time [11]. When utilizing this measure each nail is divided into four quadrants and then assessed for the presence or absence of signs of both nail matrix and nail bed disease. Each quadrant of nail with disease present is given a score of "1" for signs of matrix disease and "1" for signs of nail bed disease. A normal nail is scored "0" and the maximum value for each nail is 8, 4 for matrix involvement and 4 for nail bed disease. Thus, the maximum NAPSI value for a study measuring fingernail disease is 80 and the maximum for a target nail is 8. NAPSI measures the extent of nail disease but not the severity of nail involvement, so a modified NAPSI (mNAPSI) has also been used as a clinical endpoint in some studies [12]. The mNAPSI has a maximum score of 13 for each nail. Some studies utilize a single-target nail or an overall nail severity score.

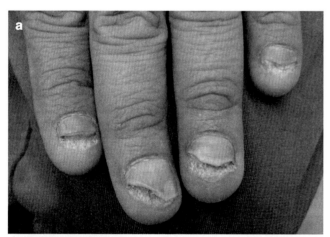

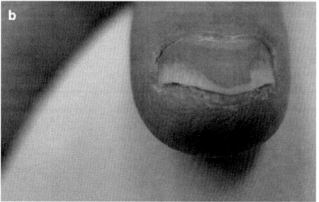

Fig. 17.2 (a) Nail bed psoriasis. Note the hyperkeratosis, onycholysis, oil droplet formation in the nail bed, and destruction of the distal nail. (b) Nail bed psoriasis. Note the onycholysis, oil droplet formation, and distal hyperkeratosis

Other scales have been used to measure nail involvement but most of the studies reviewed herein utilize some form of the NAPSI. The wide variety of objective measures used in psoriasis studies to measure nail disease and the variety of time points when the measurements are made make comparison of treatment outcomes for various interventions difficult.

Treatment of Nail Psoriasis

An array of treatment options are available for nail psoriasis including topical products, procedural interventions, and oral systemic and biologic agents. The challenges to treating nail disease are many: poor penetration of topical therapy into the nail and surrounding tissue, pain associated with intralesional injections, side effects and monitoring of systemic therapies, and patient adherence to therapy [13]. A Cochrane review has recently been published which reviewed the published literature on randomized double-blind placebo-controlled trials (RDBPCT) of nail psoriasis [14]. Unfortunately, many of the treatments most commonly used to treat psoriasis do not have published RDBPCT specifically addressing nail disease. Others have reviewed nail psoriasis treatments and the results of a Delphi consensus conference have also been published [15–17].

Topical agents are often the first-line option for treating patients with nail disease. These products are readily available, may have cost advantages, and rarely require laboratory monitoring. Although data are limited and placebo-controlled trials rare, there are data to support the efficacy of topical cyclosporine, topical tacrolimus, clobetasol nail lacquer, calcipotriol, calcipotriol plus betamethasone, tazarotene, and indigo naturalis extract [18–25]. Keratolytics such as urea and salicylic acid are also used in patients with nail psoriasis and, in particular, for nail debridement [26]. Topical preparations, in particular, take several months to show efficacy and adherence to therapy over months is challenging. In a study comparing calcipotriol twice daily with calcipotriol/betamethasone once daily, adherence to the twice-daily regimen was only 26% [21]. Therefore, topical therapy may not only be limited by penetration into the nail unit but also by adherence to lengthy treatment regimens lasting weeks or months.

Procedures have also been studied in the treatment of nail psoriasis. Phototherapy, a common treatment for skin disease, in the absence of psoralen or a retinoid, is not likely to improve nail disease and is therefore not a viable option for nail psoriasis. There is limited efficacy data showing improvement of NAPSI scores with psoralen plus UVA (PUVA), acitretin plus UVA (Re-PUVA), and acitretin plus UVB (Re-UVB) [27]. In a 1999 study of Grenz ray therapy (superficial X-ray therapy), 22 patients with nail psoriasis had one hand treated with weekly radiation and the other hand serve as an internal control. The treated hand showed significant but moderate improvement but the effect proved more limited with hyperkeratotic nails [28]. Limited access to Grenz ray therapy, a mostly historical therapy in the United States, may further inhibit the use of this modality. Several studies evaluated pulsed dye laser (PDL) in nail psoriasis. The studies noted that therapy is limited by pain, experienced by all patients, and an incidence of both petechiae and hyperpigmentation in one-third of patients [29, 30]. A combination of PDL and tazarotene cream was studied in two groups of nail psoriasis patients: those on stable doses of systemic medication and those on no systemic medication. The study showed efficacy in both groups but did not show any difference between the groups [30]. Another study evaluated PDL both with and without the addition of methylaminoleuvulinic acid (photodynamic therapy, PDT) and found no additional benefit of PDT over PDL [31]. Intralesional injection of corticosteroid is an accepted clinical treatment for localized nail psoriasis. Even though this technique has been used for many decades, published data to support the safety or efficacy of intralesional injections is extremely limited. Injection techniques vary but generally involve injection of 0.1–0.2 mL of 5–10 mg/mL triamcinolone acetonide suspension into the lateral nail folds [32]. Nerve blocks and/or topical anesthetics, to ease the pain associated with injection, may be performed prior to steroid injection [33]. Injections are repeated at various intervals. Side effects from intralesional steroids include pain on injection, skin atrophy, depigmentation, secondary infection, cyst formation, subungual hemorrhage, and tendon rupture [33]. Nonetheless, for a patient with one or two isolated psoriatic nails, intralesional injection after ring block anesthesia has been a useful method in the author's practice.

The systemic agents acitretin, methotrexate, and cyclosporine, which are effective in plaque psoriasis, are also effective in nail disease. Apremilast, a newer oral agent for psoriasis which targets phosphodiesterase 4, also has data showing efficacy in nail disease. Appropriate monitoring of both the patient and the laboratory values pertinent to the systemic therapy should be performed.

Supporting evidence for the efficacy of oral systemic therapies is detailed in Table 17.1. Cyclosporine and methotrexate, in a comparator trial, showed a 43.3% and 37.2% mean reduction in NAPSI, respectively, over a 24-week period [34]. The most robust efficacy data with methotrexate is from a randomized double-blind trial of methotrexate and the experimental anti-interleukin-12/23 antibody briakinumab (a drug no longer being studied). Methotrexate showed a 48% improvement in target nail NAPSI at 1 year [35]. In a 6-month open-label trial of acitretin for nail psoriasis there was a 41% mean reduction in NAPSI [36]. Apremilast, FDA approved for psoriasis and psoriatic arthritis, has been studied in nail disease. In the phase III ESTEEM 1 and 2 studies, 66.1 and 64.7% of patients had nail psoriasis (NAPSI ≥ 1). Mean percent change in target NAPSI score from baseline was −22.5% and −29% at week 16 and −43.6% and −60% at week 32 for ESTEEM 1 and 2, respectively [37]. These agents may be an excellent option for a patient who is otherwise a candidate for systemic therapy for psoriatic disease. Combination treatment for nail psoriasis, though widely used, is little studied. A 2004 study of oral cyclosporine and topical calcipotriol showed that at 12 weeks the combination group showed 79% of patients with improvement compared with 47% of patients on cyclosporine alone [38]. Combination therapy with topical agents and systemic therapy is frequently employed in clinical practice and is likely safe and may be more effective than systemic therapy alone.

Table 17.2 reviews the data on biologics in nail psoriasis. In a rare trial of a biologic, designed specifically to target only patients with nail psoriasis, adalimumab showed a modified NAPSI 75 response at 26 weeks in patients with and without psoriatic arthritis of 61.5% and 40.9%, respectively (placebo 0.5% and 4.6%) [39]. Adalimumab, in a RPCDBT

Table 17.1 Efficacy of systemic therapies in nail psoriasis

Agent	Dose	Length	Patients (n)	Trial type	NAPSI improvement	References
Methotrexate	15–20 mg/week	52 weeks	317	Randomized, double-blind, controlled trial (active comparator)	48%	[35]
Acitretin	0.2–0.3 mg/kg/day	24 weeks	36	Open label	41%	[36]
Cyclosporine	5.0 mg/kg/day	24 weeks	37	Comparator (vs. methotrexate)	43.3%	[34]
Apremilast	30 mg bid	52 weeks	558	Randomized, double-blind, placebo-controlled phase III trials, subanalysis of patients with baseline nail disease	60.2% (ESTEEM 1) 59.7% (ESTEEM 2)	[96]

Table 17.2 Efficacy of biologic therapies in nail psoriasis

Agent	Dosing	Patients (n)	Trial type	Weeks	Outcomes (note different primary outcome measures)	References
Adalimumab	80 mg/40 mg eow	72	RPCDBT in hand/foot psoriasis	16	50% reduction in NAPSI (8% for placebo)	[40]
Etanercept	50 mg biw/50 mg qw	711	Randomized dose comparison	24	82.3% NAPSI 50 response	[42]
Golimumab	100 mg q4 weeks	405	RPCDBT in psoriatic arthritis	24	54% reduction in NAPSI (0% for placebo)	[43]
Infliximab	5 mg/kg weeks 0,2, and 6 then q8 weeks	378	RPCDBT, data from the open-label extension	50	67.8% reduction in NAPSI (49.2% with complete nail clearance)	[45]
Ustekinumab	45 or 90 mg at weeks 0, 4, 16	545	RDBPCT	24	46.5%(45 mg), 48.7%(90 mg) reduction in NAPSI	[48]
Secukinumab	150 or 300 mg at weeks 1–5 then q4 weeks	198	RDBPCT of patients with nail disease, data from the open-label extension	32	52.6% (150 mg) and 63.2% (300 mg) reduction in NAPSI	[52]
Ixekizumab	80 mg q2 or q4 weeks for 12 weeks then 80 mg q4 weeks	1346	RDBPCT, retrospective analysis of open-label period	24	34% and 30% with no nail involvement (NAPSI = 0) on q2 and q4 doses, respectively	[51]

Legend: *eow* every other week, *NAPSI* nail area psoriasis severity index, *RDBPCT* randomized double-blind placebo-controlled trial

of patients with psoriasis involving the hands and/or feet, demonstrated 50% improvement in NAPSI at 16 weeks compared with 8% for placebo [40]. In a study evaluating both fingernails and toenails, open-label adalimumab showed improvements at 6 months in NAPSI of 85% and 72% in fingernails and toenails, respectively [41]. An open-label study of etanercept in nail psoriasis compared patients randomized to two dosing regimens: 50 mg twice weekly for 12 weeks followed by 50 mg weekly for 12 weeks, or 50 mg weekly for 24 weeks. A 50% improvement in NAPSI was demonstrated in 58.1% and 82.3% of patients in the twice-weekly/weekly group and 50.5% and 80.7% in the weekly group at 12 and 24 weeks, respectively [42]. In a RDBPCT patients with psoriatic arthritis were treated with placebo, golimumab 50 mg every 4 weeks, or golimumab 100 mg every 4 weeks for 24 weeks. Median percent change in NAPSI at weeks 14 and 24 was 0%, 25%, and 43% and 0%, 33%, and 54% for the placebo, golimumab 50 mg, and golimumab 100 mg groups, respectively. Patients in this trial for psoriatic arthritis were allowed to use stable doses of methotrexate and prednisone during the study [43]. Currently golimumab is FDA approved for psoriatic arthritis but not for psoriasis. In a RDBPCT of infliximab, patients were randomized to either placebo or infliximab 5 mg/kg at weeks 0, 2, 6, and every 8 weeks through week 46, with placebo crossover at week 24. Mean percentage improvement in target nail

NAPSI at weeks 10 and 24 was 26.8% and 57.2%, compared with −7.7% and −4.1% for infliximab and placebo, respectively [44]. In a retrospective analysis of patients from this same infliximab study, mean NAPSI improvement was 28.3%, 61.4%, and 67.8%, at weeks 10, 24, and 50, respectively [45].

No controlled comparisons of anti-TNF agents in nail psoriasis have been performed. However, an open-label prospective study showed that infliximab was superior to adalimumab and etanercept at 14 weeks [46]. A retrospective comparison of these agents also showed high efficacy of all the TNF-blocking agents in nail psoriasis with some greater improvement with infliximab [47]. The differences in efficacy of these agents in nail psoriasis may parallel the differences seen in skin response. Infliximab may also have an advantage in the speed to which clearance is achieved. However, after 4 months or more, all anti-TNF therapies are successful in improving nail disease by at least 50%, as measured by NAPSI.

Robust data is also available for IL-12/23 blockade in nail psoriasis. Data from a large phase III trial of ustekinumab showed significant improvement in NAPSI compared with placebo at 12 weeks. Additionally, the ustekinumab 45 mg and 90 mg groups showed 46.5% and 48.7% NAPSI improvement, respectively, at 24 weeks [48]. Long-term data with 68 weeks of ustekinumab in a Japanese study showed a

56.6% and 67.8% improvement from baseline NAPSI in patients treated with 45 mg or 90 mg of ustekinumab, respectively [49].

Antibodies to interleukin 17 and an interleukin 17 receptor antagonist are currently approved, or in late-stage development, for psoriasis. Data from a phase II dose finding trial of the anti-interleukin 17 antibody ixekizumab showed improvement of 57.1% and 49.3% in NAPSI scores at the 75 mg and 150 mg doses, respectively, at 16 weeks [50]. Further data with ixekizumab from the UNCOVER 3 phase III clinical trial has also been published [51]. At week 12, patients with baseline nail involvement showed reduction in NAPSI of 39%, 40%, 28%, and −4.7% in the ixekizumab every 2 weeks; ixekizumab every 4 weeks; etanercept 50 mg twice weekly; and placebo groups, respectively. Additionally, at 24 weeks, 34% and 30% of patients had no nail involvement on ixekizumab q2weeks/q4 weeks and ixekizumab q4 weeks/q4 weeks, respectively. At 60 weeks, half of the patients with initial nail disease had a NAPSI = 0 while on continuous ixekizumab. Secukinumab, another antibody to IL-17A, was studied in a clinical trial specifically designed to study patients with nail psoriasis. In the TRANSFIGURE study, mean improvement of NAPSI from baseline was 10.8, 37.9, and 45.3 at week 16 for placebo, secukinumab 150 mg, and secukinumab 300 mg, respectively. At week 32, in the open-label period, a 52.6% and 63.2% improvement in mean NAPSI was seen for secukinumab 150 mg and 300 mg, respectively [52]. The rapid onset of action and high levels of efficacy make these anti-IL-17 agents particularly attractive for patients with extensive nail disease.

Treatment Approach to Nail Disease

A treatment algorithm for nail psoriasis, based on published data for treatment of nail psoriasis and expert opinion where data is lacking, has been previously published by the Medical Board of the National Psoriasis Foundation [53] and is summarized here. All psoriasis patients should be evaluated for nail disease and the extent to which their nail disease contributes to overall disease burden. Nail disease should be classified as mild if it has minimal impact on QoL and poses no functional impact for the patient. Significant or extensive nail disease has real impact on daily activities, may be disfiguring, and may be associated with significant pain. Patients with significant nail disease need therapies to address their nail psoriasis. Patients with moderate-to-severe psoriasis and significant nail disease should be treated with appropriate therapy which addresses skin and nail disease. Previous consensus guidelines for the treatment of moderate-to-severe psoriasis also apply to the patient with nail disease [54]. Options include cyclosporine, methotrexate, acitretin, apremilast, and biologics. Patients with significant nail disease

and psoriatic arthritis (PsA) should be treated with an appropriate systemic treatment for PsA that has efficacy in nails. Data support the following options in this patient group: methotrexate, apremilast, the TNF inhibitors, IL-17 inhibitors, and IL-12/23 inhibitor. For the rare patient with nail disease as the primary manifestation of their psoriatic disease, a 3–6-month trial of topical therapy and/or intralesional injections may be appropriate. For patients with severe nail disease affecting QoL, systemic and biologic therapies may be needed. Patients who have their skin and/or joint disease well controlled but still have significant nail involvement may need combination topical therapy or intralesional injections. If this fails, a change in the systemic or biologic therapy may be warranted.

Improvements in nail psoriasis often trail the improvements in skin and joint disease. Fingernails grow at a rate of 3–4 mm/month; thus it takes 5–7 months for a nail to grow from matrix to distal fingertip [55]. Therefore, the length of a clinical trial must reflect this delay. Few studies, with the exception of the anti-IL 17 inhibitors and infliximab, demonstrate any significant improvement before 12 weeks and several studies with adalimumab, etanercept, infliximab, ustekinumab, ixekizumab, and secukinumab demonstrate continued improvement up to and even beyond 6 months [42, 45, 46, 56].

One of the problems in reviewing data on nail psoriasis is the lack of consistent outcome reporting among the studies. Even when NAPSI data is presented, it may be presented in different ways. Target nail NAPSI, mean improvement in NAPSI, percent of patients with no nail disease (NAPSI = 0), and modified NAPSI are some of the many outcomes reported. The dermatology life quality index (DLQI) contains some questions pertinent to nail signs and symptoms but does not specifically account for the influence of nail disease on QoL. Some researchers have used QoL measures validated in onychomycosis and applied these to psoriasis [57]. A validated measure specific to nail psoriasis, the NPQ10, has been published but not extensively utilized [58]. Additionally, the Nail Assessment in Psoriasis and Psoriatic Arthritis (NAPPA) may prove useful in evaluating response to therapy in nail disease [59]. Clearly there is a need for more uniform reporting of nail outcomes and adoption of a valid and easily performed QoL metric that is specific to nail disease.

Scalp Psoriasis

Is scalp psoriasis difficult to treat? Indeed, it may respond faster than other body regions to some biologic therapies but it remains a challenge to obtain good results with both topical and phototherapy. While the head and neck represent about 10% of the body surface area, the impact of psoriasis in this region may be disproportionate to the area, and may have social and emotional impacts on affected individuals. Most scalp psoriasis is treated with topical therapies including shampoos, oils, foams, liquids, and gels. Over-the-counter remedies, containing tar, salicylic acid, zinc, and others, are relatively inexpensive and widely available. One of the reasons that scalp psoriasis has been labeled "tough to treat" is the difficulty with using and complying with topical medications. Prescription topical therapy mainly involves the use of mid- to high-potency topical steroids and topical vitamin D analogues. Many larger trials for the biologics have had measures of scalp psoriasis as secondary endpoints. A few trials have been designed specifically to assess scalp disease and these will be highlighted in this chapter. Indeed, scalp psoriasis provides challenges to both practitioner and patient.

The incidence of scalp psoriasis in patients with psoriasis is estimated between 40% and 90%. In up to half of patients, psoriasis may initially present on the scalp [60, 61]. Some patients only have psoriasis on the scalp. The scalp is characterized by the presence of the prominent pilosebaceous unit and has a microbiome that differs from other skin sites. Both yeast and bacteria colonize the scalp [62]. Indeed *Malassezia furfur, M. globosa*, candida, and other commensal organisms are found on the scalp in significant numbers and may influence scalp diseases such as seborrheic dermatitis and psoriasis [63, 64]. The role of these organisms in psoriasis is not well established but they likely play a role. Treatments targeting these organisms have shown some efficacy in seborrheic dermatitis [65, 66]. Friction and trauma to the scalp from scratching and hair grooming my also contribute to scalp disease severity [67, 68].

Recent studies have shown that the hair in patients with scalp psoriasis may also be modified by the presence of psoriatic inflammation. Indeed, hair shafts evaluated in patients with psoriasis reveal pits, thought to be analogous to the pitting seen in nails [69]. Additionally, recent studies evaluating the transcriptome of both scalp and body psoriasis suggest that there may be differences in gene activation between the scalp and body [70].

Clinical Presentation of Scalp Psoriasis

Scalp lesions may vary from mild, with minimal erythema and scaling, to severe with thick well-defined plaques with silvery scale and an erythematous border (Fig. 17.3). Classic scalp lesions are asymmetric, sharply demarcated, covered with silvery-white or gray scale, and may extend beyond scalp margins to affect the forehead, ear, and neck [71]. Most patients with psoriasis of the face also have scalp disease [72]. Multiple surveys have cited itching and scaling as the most disturbing aspects of scalp psoriasis [73, 74]. This itch

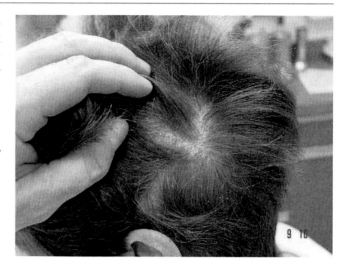

Fig. 17.3 Scalp psoriasis

may be so severe that it can interfere with sleep and lead to actual hair loss due to hair breakage and trauma.

Scalp psoriasis is usually not associated with significant hair loss; however, some patients may have alopecia due to the trauma of chronic itching leading to hair breakage. In an analysis of 47 patients with psoriatic alopecia followed for several years, many patients only had alopecia in some of the scalp plaques and indeed, as the psoriasis cleared, the hair regrew [75]. In some cases the differentiation of scalp psoriasis and seborrheic dermatitis can be difficult. Seborrheic dermatitis is characterized by diffuse thin scale that is localized to the hair-bearing scalp and may involve the central face and chest. Psoriasis, on the other hand, may extend beyond the scalp, is sharply marginated, and may occur elsewhere on the body [76].

Measuring Scalp Disease

A variety of measures have been developed to assess the extent and burden of scalp psoriasis (Table 17.3). The Psoriasis Scalp Severity Index (PSSI) and the Scalp-modified PASI (S-mPASI) are modifications of the standard PASI measurement of psoriasis [77, 78]. Both the PSSI and the S-mPASI measure erythema, induration, and desquamation of the plaques of psoriasis on the scalp only in contrast to PASI where the entire body is evaluated. Some studies, including one on the IL-17 inhibitor secukinumab, have utilized the head and neck portion of the PASI score (HN-PASI) as a proxy for scalp involvement [79]. Other measures have also been used for evaluation of scalp psoriasis including the Total Severity Scale (TSS), the Scalp-specific Physicians Global Assessment (S-PGA), and the Global Severity Scale (GSS) [80]. A recent study of 102 patients with predominately

Table 17.3 Measures of scalp psoriasis

Measure	Parameters measured	Max. score	Description	Reference
Psoriasis scalp severity index (PSSI)	Extent of involvement, erythema, induration, and desquamation of scalp	72	Sum of 3 parameter scores (0–4) multiplied by a score for the area of involvement (1–6)	[77]
Scalp-modified PASI (S-mPASI)	Extent of involvement, erythema, induration, desquamation of scalp	7.2	Sum of 3 parameter scores (0–4) multiplied by a score for the area of involvement (1–6) times a constant (0.1)	[78]
Head and neck PASI (HN-PASI)	Extent of involvement, erythema, induration, desquamation of head and neck	7.2	Sum of 3 parameter scores (0–4) multiplied by a score for the area of involvement (1–6) times a constant (0.1)	[79]
Total severity score (TSS)	Erythema, induration, desquamation of scalp	9	Sum of scores (0–3) for erythema, induration, and desquamation	[80]
Scalp-specific Patient's Global Assessment (SPaGA)	Overall scalp disease, as judged by the patient, as compared to baseline involvement	−2 to +2	Current scalp disease severity compared with baseline visit on a 5-point scale; "much worse" (−2) through "much improved" (+2)	[78]
Global Severity Score (GSS)	Overall scalp disease measured by investigator	5	Assessment of scalp disease from "none" (0) to "very severe" (5)	[80]
Scalpdex	Measure of symptoms, functioning, and emotions on scalp disease (23 items)	0 to 100	Measures may be combined to form subscores for symptoms, functioning, and emotions	[73]

scalp psoriasis treated with secukinumab or placebo utilized a 90% improvement of PSSI and a two-point improvement in Investigators Global Assessment as the two primary endpoints to the study [81].

Patient assessment tools have also been developed to evaluate scalp psoriasis. The Scalp-specific Patient's Global Assessment (S-PaGA) has been utilized to gauge patient assessment of disease change from baseline. Pruritus, a major issue for many scalp psoriasis patients, may be measured by a visual analogue scale (VAS) of itch. Scalpdex is a validated measure of quality of life for scalp conditions (not specific to psoriasis) that utilizes 23 questions that address symptoms, emotions, and functions surrounding the scalp condition [73].

Management of Scalp Psoriasis: Topical Therapies

Topical therapies are the foundation in the management of scalp psoriasis and utilized by approximately 60% of patients [61]. These therapies have been formulated into shampoos, gels, foams, oils, and solutions. Some of these products have been evaluated in large clinical trials. High costs limit the use of many of these proprietary products. Calcipotriol is a synthetic derivative of calcitriol (vitamin D3); calcipotriol binds to the vitamin D3 receptor, but, unlike calcitriol, is a poor regulator of calcium metabolism. The efficacy and safety of calcipotriol solution support its use as a first-line therapy as well as its use as maintenance therapy [82, 83]. This treatment, however, can be associated with some burning, redness, dryness, and itching in some patients. The combination of calcipotriol and topical steroids decreases some of the irritation of calcipotriol and is certainly more efficacious than calcipotriol monotherapy. There may also be an advantage to this combination due to the potential protective effect of calcipotriol on corticosteroid-induced skin atrophy.

Shampoos and foams containing high-potency topical steroids such as clobetasol propionate 0.05% have demonstrated improvement in scalp psoriasis in as little as 2 weeks. In these short, 2–4-week studies, skin atrophy, folliculitis, and telangiectasia were not observed [84, 85]. Clobetasol propionate 0.05% shampoo was superior in efficacy and tolerability compared with calcipotriol 0.005% solution [80]. In a study comparing 1% tar blend shampoo with clobetasol shampoo, the clobetasol product was cosmetically more acceptable to patients [85]. Betamethasone valerate 0.12% in a mousse (foam) vehicle was compared to topical corticosteroid solution and calcipotriol lotion and showed superior efficacy over 4 weeks. Most of these patients preferred the foam formulation [82]. An open-label study of the combination product (betamethasone/calcipotriene) in patients 12–17 years of age showed efficacy over 8 weeks with one patient demonstrating mild adrenal suppression and no patients demonstrating hypercalcemia [86]. The authors concluded that this treatment was safe and efficacious in adolescents with scalp psoriasis.

A 2016 Cochrane review of topical therapies reviewed 59 randomized controlled clinical trials in scalp psoriasis [87]. They concluded that a corticosteroid of high or very high potency or a combination of a corticosteroid and vitamin D (calcipotriol) was superior to vitamin D alone. The two-compound combination also led to fewer withdrawals from treatment compared to the other treatments. Further the authors concluded "Given the comparable safety profile and only slim benefit of the two-compound combination over the corticosteroid alone, monotherapy with generic topical steroids of high and very high potency may be fully acceptable for short term therapy."

However, do patients adhere to treatment with topical therapy? There is some evidence that optimizing the vehicle may improve adherence to scalp psoriasis treatments; however adherence to topical therapy for psoriasis is low [88]. Even with interventions to assist and remind patients to apply topical therapies, adherence is less than 50% after several weeks [89]. In clinical practice, the use of anti-dandruff shampoos is generally encouraged by dermatologists to help remove the scale from the plaques of psoriasis. The use of high-potency topical steroids is usually limited to a few weeks but patients may continue to use these products intermittently for months and even years. The use of topical vitamin D products, when available and when well tolerated, is also a reasonable approach to maintenance therapy. Many practitioners will utilize a high-potency topical steroid 1 or 2 days per week and a topical vitamin D analogue on the other days in an effort to minimize potential side effects of long-term topical steroid use [90].

Procedural Therapies for Scalp Psoriasis

Intralesional injection of corticosteroids has also been used by dermatologists to address localized treatment-resistant plaques of psoriasis with some success. Triamcinolone acetonide (5–10 mg/mL) is injected directly into the psoriatic plaques in small (0.1–0.2 mL) aliquots. The aim is to deliver the steroid directly into the area of inflammation in the dermis. This technique, however, has not been studied in a rigorous fashion [33].

Phototherapy for scalp psoriasis is limited due to hair blocking the penetration of the light. Devices have been designed and are available to help deliver phototherapy to the scalp. These devices use fiber optics that penetrate through the hair and deliver the phototherapy, broadband or narrowband UVB, directly to the scalp [91]. Additionally, the 308 nM laser can be used to treat scalp psoriasis. In one study, 17 of 35 patients had >95% clearance after a mean of 21 treatments [92]. In this study the hair was manually parted to gain access to the psoriatic plaques.

Notably, all patients demonstrated erythema and some blistering to treated sites. In another study, patients treated with the laser administered with a blow dryer to part the hair had significant improvement after twice-weekly treatments for up to 15 weeks [93]. Grenz ray therapy has also been efficacious in scalp psoriasis. The lack of availability of Grenz ray therapy units and the potential for skin cancer formation in the treated area significantly limit this modality [94, 95].

Systemic Therapy for Scalp Psoriasis

There are few studies that specifically address the efficacy of methotrexate, cyclosporine, and acitretin in scalp psoriasis. Nonetheless, these therapies may be effective in treating scalp disease. Appropriate monitoring of liver function (methotrexate, acitretin), creatinine (cyclosporine, methotrexate), complete blood counts (methotrexate), triglycerides (acitretin), and blood pressure (cyclosporine) should be maintained during treatment with these agents.

Apremilast, an oral phosphodiesterase 4 inhibitor, is approved for psoriasis and psoriatic arthritis. Scalp disease was evaluated as a secondary endpoint in the two phase III psoriasis programs for apremilast. Scalp disease was moderate or greater in about two-thirds of patients in these trials. Approximately half of those with baseline moderate scalp involvement achieved a clear or almost clear PGA at 16 weeks. Most patients who continued in trial maintained this response out to 1 year [37, 96]. Apremilast may be a reasonable option for patients with significant scalp disease.

Biologic Therapy for Scalp Psoriasis

The treatment of scalp psoriasis with biologics is summarized in Table 17.4. There have been some studies specifically designed to evaluate scalp psoriasis. Etanercept, a TNF-fusion protein that binds TNF-alpha, was used in a study specifically addressing patients with scalp disease [97]. In this placebo-controlled trial, PSSI at week 12 was improved by 86.8% and 20.4% in the etanercept 50 mg biw group and placebo group, respectively. Improvement continued in the open-label period to week 24. In a sub-analysis of a larger trial of adalimumab in psoriasis, PSSI was improved by a median of 100% (mean 77.2%) at 16 weeks [98].

Blockade of interleukin-17 has also been studied in scalp psoriasis. In a placebo-controlled study designed specifically for scalp disease patients, secukinumab 300 mg achieved 90% improvement in PSSI in 52.9% of patients compared with 2% on placebo at 12 weeks. Investigators Global

Table 17.4 Efficacy of systemic therapies in scalp psoriasis

Agent	Dosing	Patients (n)	Trial type	Weeks	Outcomes (note different primary outcome measures)	References
Apremilast	30 mg biw	558	RPCDBT, subanalysis of patients with moderate scalp involvement	16	Scalp PGA of clear or almost clear (0 or 1) of 46.5% (ESTEEM 1) and 40.9% (ESTEEM 2)	[37]
Etanercept	50 mg biw or placebo	124	Placebo-controlled study in moderate scalp disease	12	Improvement in PSSI from baseline 86.8% (vs. 20.4% for placebo)	[97]
Adalimumab	80 mg week 0, then 40 mg eow	730	RPCDBT, subanalysis of patients with baseline scalp disease	16	77.2% improvement in PSSI	[98]
Secukinumab	300 mg weeks 0–4, then 300 mg q4 weeks		RPCDBT in patients with scalp psoriasis	12	52.9% PSSI improvement (2% for placebo)	[81]
Ixekizumab	80 mg week 0, then 80 mg q2 or q4 weeks, also comparator arm with etanercept biw	3866	RDBPCT with etanercept comparator arm	12	PSSI 100 response of 74.6, 68.8, 48.1, and 6.7% in Ixe q2 week, Ixe q4 week, etanercept, and placebo, respectively	[99]

Legend: *biw* twice weekly, *eow* every other week, *RPCDBT* randomized placebo-controlled double-blind clinical trial, *PGA* physician's global assessment, *PSSI* psoriasis scalp severity index

Assessment of clear or almost clear was achieved by 56.9% on secukinumab and 5.9% on placebo at 12 weeks [81]. In a subanalysis of larger phase III trials for ixekizumab, scalp psoriasis was evaluated [99]. Of patients with baseline scalp psoriasis, PSSI 90 and PSSI 100 at 12 weeks were obtained by 81.7 and 74.6, 75.6 and 68.8, 55.5 and 48.1, and 7.6 and 6.7, in the ixekizumab q2 weeks, ixekizumab q4 weeks, etanercept 50 mg biw, and placebo groups, respectively. Thus, more than half of patients on etanercept and over three-quarters of patients on ixekizumab had complete clearance of scalp psoriasis at 12 weeks.

Treatment Algorithm for Scalp Psoriasis

For limited scalp disease, treatment with potent topical steroids with or without vitamin D derivatives is a reasonable initial treatment. This may be augmented by OTC shampoos to remove scale. For patients who fail to respond to a trial of topical therapy, phototherapy (if available) and oral treatment with methotrexate or apremilast may be appropriate. For patients who prove recalcitrant to these therapies or for patients with significant psoriasis elsewhere, biologic therapies that target TNF or interleukin-17 are recommended.

TNF-Induced Psoriasis

Paradoxically, treatment with anti-TNF agents may induce scalp psoriasis in patients who have not had a previous history of psoriasis [100, 101]. These cases have been reported with all the anti-TNF agents and the patients are often being treated for rheumatoid arthritis and inflammatory bowel disease. The scalp, palms, soles, and other body areas may be involved. Occasionally, these patients may have lesions consistent with pustular psoriasis [101]. Some patients can be treated with topical or phototherapy and remain on the TNF agent while others may require discontinuation of the TNF inhibitor to control the eruption. The incidence of this eruption is between 1 and 2% of patients treated with anti-TNF agents [102]. The cause of this phenomenon is not well elucidated but may involve compensatory increases in interferon in patients treated with anti-TNFs [103].

Palmoplantar Psoriasis

Psoriasis of the hands and feet may be one of the most difficult therapeutic dilemmas for the dermatologist. Palmoplantar psoriasis affects up to 5% of patients with psoriasis [104]. First, however, we need to define the spectrum of psoriatic disease that can affect the palms and soles. There are several distinct presentations of psoriasis on the palms and soles:

- Plaque psoriasis of the hands and feet with significant psoriasis elsewhere (Fig. 17.4).
- Plaque psoriasis of the hands and feet with little psoriasis elsewhere (palmoplantar psoriasis, PPP, Fig. 17.5).
- Pustular psoriasis of the hands and feet (palmoplantar pustulosis, PPPP, Fig. 17.6): This may also be called Acrodermatitis Continua of Hallopeau, particularly when it involves bony resorption of the distal phalanx [105].
- Psoriasiform dermatitis of the hands and feet—with features of hand dermatitis and psoriasis.

These presentations represent distinct patient populations that may respond differently to various therapies and may have differing genetic and environmental factors involved in their disease development. This review focuses on plaque psoriasis of the hands and feet (PPP) and pustular psoriasis of the hands and feet (PPPP).

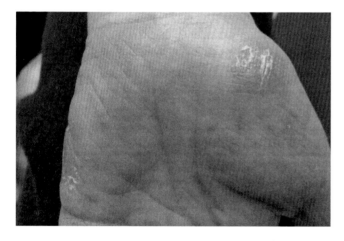

Fig. 17.4 Palm psoriasis in a patient with chronic plaque psoriasis

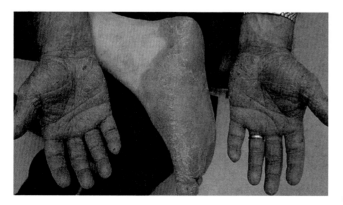

Fig. 17.5 Severe palmoplantar plaque psoriasis in a patient with minimal psoriasis on body

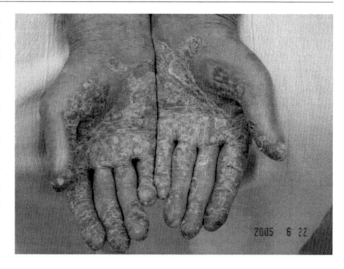

Fig. 17.6 Palmar pustular psoriasis. Note resorption of distal digits and extensive pustules. These are features of a variant of pustular psoriasis termed acrodermatitis continua of Hallopeau

A key factor in palmoplantar disease is disability. The use of the hands and feet may be significantly compromised by disease. The scale, fissures, cracking, and hyperkeratosis can lead to pain with movement. Chung et al. evaluated the quality of life (QoL) of patients with PPP and compared them with plaque psoriasis [106]. These patients were receiving treatment with systemic or phototherapy. The palmoplantar psoriasis patients had significantly more impairment in QoL characterized by limitations of mobility, self-care, and pursuing usual activities. Additionally, palmoplantar patients were more likely to be taking multiple topical and oral therapies for their disease. Others have reported on physical disability and discomfort associated with PPP [107]. Smoking appears to play a role in palmoplantar disease and there is some data suggesting that pustular disease severity may improve with smoking cessation [108].

There are few controlled clinical trials addressing treatments for palmoplantar disease. Most treatment has been based on case series, small clinical trials, and anecdotal clinical evidence. If you were to ask ten dermatologists for their top five treatments for hand and foot psoriatic disease, you would get dramatically different answers. Reviews of the literature have also yielded differing recommendations for treatment of palmoplantar psoriasis. Seravin et al. concluded in 2013 "Phototherapy, cyclosporine and topical corticosteroids seem to be able to control PPPP. However, the standard of care for PPPP remains an issue and there is a strong need for reliable RCTs to better define treatment strategies for PPPP" [109]. The National Psoriasis Foundation concluded in a 2012 review of treatments for pustular psoriasis that "acitretin, cyclosporine, methotrexate, and infliximab are considered to be first line therapies in generalized pustular disease" [110]. All sources conclude that better data is needed to guide clinical decisions regarding treatment.

Topical steroids, vitamin D analogues, tar and anthralin preparations, either by themselves or in combination, and under occlusion have all been reported to improve psoriasis and are regularly used in palmoplantar disease. In a comparative trial, in PPP, of clobetasol plus tar compared with topical psoralen plus UVA, both treatments were effective [111]. Phototherapy with psoralen plus UVA (PUVA), and narrowband UVB, has shown some efficacy in hand and foot disease [112]. Multiple small studies and case series have demonstrated the efficacy of the 308 nM laser in the treatment of palmoplantar disease [113–115]. A recent comparison of paint PUVA (psoralen not ingested but instead painted on the skin) and broadband UVB showed improvement with both treatments but more complete and longer remissions with paint PUVA [116]. Another study used a split-hand design to treat one side with narrowband UVB and the other with topical PUVA. The PUVA side fared better than the hand treated with narrowband UVB [117]. Thus, topical therapies and phototherapy may be beneficial in treating palmoplantar psoriasis.

Systemic treatments for palmoplantar disease have also been studied. Methotrexate (0.4 mg/kg weekly) and acitretin (0.5 mg/kg daily) were studied in an active comparator trial of 111 PPP patients [118]. Both treatments showed improvement but methotrexate significantly improved more patients. Wald et al. published a series of 48 hand/foot psoriasis patients treated with methotrexate, most in combination with other therapies, and concluded that methotrexate was effective in PPP [119]. In a study of cyclosporine in PPPP, most patients improved on relatively low doses (1–2 mg/kg/day) of cyclosporine [120]. In a pooled analysis of phase II and two phase III trials of apremilast, a phosphodiesterase 4 inhibitor, in psoriasis, patients with baseline palmoplantar physicians global assessment (PP-PGA) of moderate or greater were evaluated during the 16-week placebo-controlled period. At week 16, 46% and 25% of patients showed a PP-PGA of clear or almost clear for the apremilast and placebo groups, respectively [121]. Thus, acitretin, cyclosporine, and apremilast all demonstrate some efficacy in PPP and/or PPPP. However, there are no randomized placebo-controlled studies specifically addressing these systemic agents in PPP or PPPP.

The biologics have also been studied in PPP and PPPP. Adalimumab was studied in patients with at least moderate plaque psoriasis of the hands and feet and moderate-to-severe plaque psoriasis elsewhere [40]. In this placebo-controlled trial, 31% of patients in the adalimumab group were able to achieve a hand/foot PGA of clear or almost clear at week 16, compared to only 4% in the placebo group. In a study of 24 palmoplantar psoriasis patients randomized to placebo or infliximab infusions, more patients reached 75% improvement in palmoplantar PASI in the infliximab group (33.3% vs. 8.3%), but this did not reach statistical significance [122]. Success with treating PPP and PPPP has also been demonstrated in case reports with etanercept [123, 124]. The TNF inhibitors do appear to show some efficacy in treating PPP, but this efficacy is significantly attenuated compared with overall plaque psoriasis results.

Ustekinumab, in an open-label study of patients with PPP and PPPP, cleared 35% (7/20); however the 90 mg dose was superior to 45 mg [125]. The interleukin-17 inhibitors have been studied in both PPP and PPPP. In a subanalysis of the large phase III trials of ixekizumab in psoriasis, patients with significant palmoplantar disease (PP-PASI of ≥8) at baseline were evaluated [126]. This analysis involved 105 patients (total study $n = 1224$) and revealed PP-PASI 75 and PP-PASI-100 results of 16.7, 44.1, 81.8, and 74.2 and 5.6, 29.4, 45.5, and 51.6 in the placebo, etanercept 50 mg biw, ixekizumab q2 weeks, and ixekizumab q4 weeks, respectively. Thus, roughly half of the ixekizumab-treated patients achieved total clearance of their plaque psoriasis of the hands and feet. Secukinumab was studied in a placebo-controlled trial of patients with moderate-to-severe palmoplantar psoriasis [127]. Many of these patients would not have had enough psoriasis to meet enrollment criteria for typical phase III psoriasis trials and thus may better represent the vexing patients with primarily palmoplantar disease. Two hundred and five patients were randomized 1:1:1 to secukinumab 300 mg, secukinumab 150 mg, and placebo. In this study, palmoplantar IGA of clear or almost clear at week 16 was achieved by 33.3%, 22.1%, and 1.5% of patients treated with secukinumab 300 mg, secukinumab 150 mg, and placebo, respectively. These results are impressive but are not as robust as seen in the larger phase III trials of plaque psoriasis. An additional study of secukinumab in PPPP was also performed [128]. In this study 237 patients with palmoplantar pustulosis (PPPP) were randomized to placebo, secukinumab 150 mg, or secukinumab 300 mg. Forty percent of these patients did not have plaque psoriasis elsewhere. Change in PP-PASI was measured at week 16 and 29.7%, 30.2%, and 42.3% improvement was noted in the placebo, secukinumab 150 mg, and secukinumab 300 mg, respectively. Thus, there was minimal response of PPPP to IL-17 inhibition. More studies are needed to confirm this finding but it does appear that IL-17 is not a key target for PPPP.

PPP remains a difficult disease to treat. Multiple therapies are often necessary, and a trial of many treatments is often needed in order to achieve adequate control. There are some data to support topical therapy, phototherapy (especially PUVA), cyclosporine, methotrexate, acitretin, and apremilast. The anti-TNF antibodies may also improve some patients. The anti-IL-17 antibodies may offer some additional efficacy with PPP. Treatment options for PPPP are even more dismal, with few studies to guide treatment. Cyclosporine is likely the best oral option for pustular disease.

Case Study: Nail Psoriasis

A 31-year-old Indian-American man presented to clinic with nail changes for several years. He was treated previously for onychomycosis for 1 year with oral terbinafine and itraconazole. There was no improvement with this treatment.

Past Medical History
Unremarkable

Social History
No alcohol or tobacco use
Works in an office

Previous Therapies and Workup
Terbinafine, itraconazole
Negative exams for KOH of fingernail, fungal culture, nail clipping for histology
Negative PPD, liver function within normal limits

Physical Exam
8/10 fingernails with severe onychodystrophy: hyperkeratosis, distal nail loss, and oil droplet sign
No psoriasis on body (complete skin exam)
There is some pain in his distal fingers but no evidence of arthritis

Diagnosis and Management
He was initially treated with apremilast for 4 months along with topical clobetasol 0.05% solution. A trial of intralesional kenalog (10 mg/mL) into the lateral and distal aspects of several involved fingers was also performed. After 4-month apremilast/clobetasol therapy, there was minimal improvement in the nails. Additionally, very little improvement was seen with intralesional injections. In fact, the disease appeared to be progressing, with more nail destruction. Adalimumab was then initiated along with a topical two-compound product (betamethasone/calcipotriol). A 6-month trial of adalimumab revealed minimal improvement. In March of 2016, the patient began secukinumab 300 mg at the standard psoriasis dosing. After 6 months on secukinumab, he is significantly improved (Figs. 17.7 and 17.8).

Case Study: Palmoplantar Psoriasis

A 54-year-old man presented to clinic with severe palmoplantar psoriasis. He is a mechanic and his condition impairs his ability to perform his duties. He has tried numerous topical therapies including topical steroids, vitamin D analogues, crude coal tar, and anthralin. He was initially managed with acitretin 50 mg daily for 6 months with minimal improvement. Efalizumab therapy was effective and he remained on efalizumab until it was discontinued from the US market secondary to rare side effects. After discontinuation of efalizumab, he experienced a flare of his disease (Fig. 17.9).

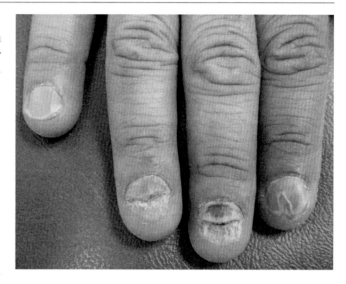

Fig. 17.7 Nail psoriasis on apremilast and topical therapy for 4 months

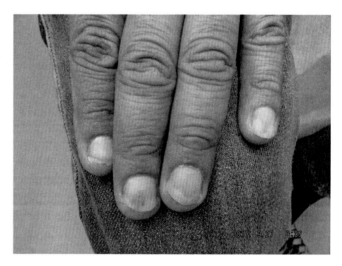

Fig. 17.8 Nails after 6 months of secukinumab

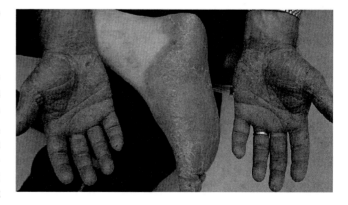

Fig. 17.9 Hands and foot of patient on acitretin 50 mg daily and topical therapy. Note deep red plaques with deep fissures.

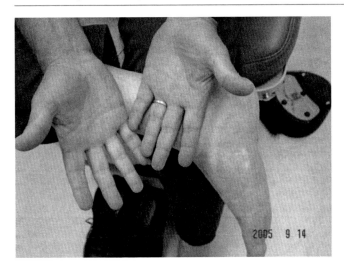

Fig. 17.10 Near complete resolution of hand and foot psoriasis with adalimumab and 50 mg acitretin daily.

Past Medical History

Hypertension

Hyperlipidemia

Social History

Thirty pack-year smoker, currently smoking, has tried numerous cessation treatments

Married

Employed as a high-end race car mechanic

Previous Therapies

Topicals

Acitretin 50 mg daily for 6 months

Efalizumab for 2 years with success

Cyclosporine was used to control the post-efalizumab flare. He had significant issues with cyclosporine including elevations in serum creatinine and severe headaches. Adalimumab and acitretin were started simultaneously and complete clearance was achieved over 3–4 months. Figure 17.10 shows the patient on adalimumab and acitretin 25 mg daily.

References

1. Jiaravuthisan MM, Sasseville D, Vender RB, Murphy F, Muhn CY. Psoriasis of the nail: anatomy, pathology, clinical presentation, and a review of the literature on therapy. J Am Acad Dermatol. 2007;57(1):1–27.
2. de Jong EM, Seegers BA, Gulinck MK, Boezeman JB, van de Kerkhof PC. Psoriasis of the nails associated with disability in a large number of patients: results of a recent interview with 1,728 patients. Dermatology. 1996;193(4):300–3.
3. van der Velden HM, Klaassen KM, van de Kerkhof PC, Pasch MC. The impact of fingernail psoriasis on patients' health-related and disease-specific quality of life. Dermatology. 2014;229(2):76–82.
4. Langenbruch A, Radtke MA, Krensel M, Jacobi A, Reich K, Augustin M. Nail involvement as a predictor of concomitant psoriatic arthritis in patients with psoriasis. Br J Dermatol. 2014;171(5):1123–8.
5. Armesto S, Esteve A, Coto-Segura P, Drake M, Galache C, Martinez-Borra J, et al. Nail psoriasis in individuals with psoriasis vulgaris: a study of 661 patients. Actas Dermosifiliogr. 2011;102(5):365–72.
6. Chandran V, Schentag CT, Gladman DD. Sensitivity and specificity of the CASPAR criteria for psoriatic arthritis in a family medicine clinic setting. J Rheumatol. 2008;35(10):2069–70; author reply 70.
7. Gupta AK, Lynde CW, Jain HC, Sibbald RG, Elewski BE, Daniel CR 3rd, et al. A higher prevalence of onychomycosis in psoriatics compared with non-psoriatics: a multicentre study. Br J Dermatol. 1997;136(5):786–9.
8. Al-Mutairi N, Nour T, Al-Rqobah D. Onychomycosis in patients of nail psoriasis on biologic therapy: a randomized, prospective open label study comparing Etanercept, infliximab and Adalimumab. Expert Opin Biol Ther. 2013;13(5):625–9.
9. Halprin KM. Afflictions of a vestigial appendage. II. Inflammatory processes affecting the nail matrix. (trauma, eczema, psoriasis, lichen planus, alopecia areata). JAMA. 1967;202(11):1045.
10. Werner B, Fonseca GP, Seidel G. Microscopic nail clipping findings in patients with psoriasis. Am J Dermatopathol. 2015;37(6):429–39.
11. Rich P, Scher RK. Nail psoriasis severity index: a useful tool for evaluation of nail psoriasis. J Am Acad Dermatol. 2003;49(2):206–12.
12. Cassell SE, Bieber JD, Rich P, Tutuncu ZN, Lee SJ, Kalunian KC, et al. The modified nail psoriasis severity index: validation of an instrument to assess psoriatic nail involvement in patients with psoriatic arthritis. J Rheumatol. 2007;34(1):123–9.
13. Radtke MA, Beikert FC, Augustin M. Nail psoriasis—a treatment challenge. J Dtsch Dermatol Ges. 2013;11(3):203–19; quiz 20.
14. de Vries AC, Bogaards NA, Hooft L, Velema M, Pasch M, Lebwohl M, et al. Interventions for nail psoriasis. Cochrane Database Syst Rev. 2013;31(1):CD007633.
15. Oram Y, Akkaya AD. Treatment of nail psoriasis: common concepts and new trends. Dermatol Res Pract. 2013;2013:180496.
16. Langley RG, Saurat JH, Reich K. Nail psoriasis Delphi expert P. Recommendations for the treatment of nail psoriasis in patients with moderate to severe psoriasis: a dermatology expert group consensus. J Eur Acad Dermatol Venereol. 2012;26(3):373–81.
17. Armstrong AW, Tuong W, Love TJ, Carneiro S, Grynszpan R, Lee SS, et al. Treatments for nail psoriasis: a systematic review by the GRAPPA nail psoriasis work group. J Rheumatol. 2014;41(11):2306–14.
18. Cannavo SP, Guarneri F, Vaccaro M, Borgia F, Guarneri B. Treatment of psoriatic nails with topical cyclosporin: a prospective, randomized placebo-controlled study. Dermatology. 2003;206(2):153–6.
19. De Simone C, Maiorino A, Tassone F, D'Agostino M, Caldarola G. Tacrolimus 0.1% ointment in nail psoriasis: a randomized controlled open-label study. J Eur Acad Dermatol Venereol. 2013;27(8):1003–6.
20. Nakamura RC, Abreu L, Duque-Estrada B, Tamler C, Leverone AP. Comparison of nail lacquer clobetasol efficacy at 0.05%, 1% and 8% in nail psoriasis treatment: prospective, controlled and randomized pilot study. An Bras Dermatol. 2012;87(2):203–11.
21. Tzung TY, Chen CY, Yang CY, Lo PY, Chen YH. Calcipotriol used as monotherapy or combination therapy with betamethasone dipropionate in the treatment of nail psoriasis. Acta Derm Venereol. 2008;88(3):279–80.
22. Rigopoulos D, Gregoriou S, Daniel Iii CR, Belyayeva H, Larios G, Verra P, et al. Treatment of nail psoriasis with a two-compound formulation of calcipotriol plus betamethasone dipropionate ointment. Dermatology. 2009;218(4):338–41.

23. Tosti A, Piraccini BM, Cameli N, Kokely F, Plozzer C, Cannata GE, et al. Calcipotriol ointment in nail psoriasis: a controlled double-blind comparison with betamethasone dipropionate and salicylic acid. Br J Dermatol. 1998;139(4):655–9.

24. Scher RK, Stiller M, Zhu YI. Tazarotene 0.1% gel in the treatment of fingernail psoriasis: a double-blind, randomized, vehicle-controlled study. Cutis. 2001;68(5):355–8.

25. Lin YK, See LC, Chang YC, Huang YH, Chen JL, Tsou TC, et al. Treatment of psoriatic nails with indigo naturalis oil extract: a non-controlled pilot study. Dermatology. 2011;223(3):239–43.

26. Farber EM, South DA. Urea ointment in the nonsurgical avulsion of nail dystrophies. Cutis. 1978;22(6):689–92.

27. Sanchez-Regana M, Sola-Ortigosa J, Alsina-Gibert M, Vidal-Fernandez M, Umbert-Millet P. Nail psoriasis: a retrospective study on the effectiveness of systemic treatments (classical and biological therapy). J Eur Acad Dermatol Venereol. 2011;25(5):579–86.

28. Lindelof B. Psoriasis of the nails treated with grenz rays: a double-blind bilateral trial. Acta Derm Venereol. 1989;69(1):80–2.

29. Treewittayapoom C, Singvahanont P, Chanprapaph K, Haneke E. The effect of different pulse durations in the treatment of nail psoriasis with 595-nm pulsed dye laser: a randomized, double-blind, intrapatient left-to-right study. J Am Acad Dermatol. 2012;66(5):807–12.

30. Huang YC, Chou CL, Chiang YY. Efficacy of pulsed dye laser plus topical tazarotene versus topical tazarotene alone in psoriatic nail disease: a single-blind, intrapatient left-to-right controlled study. Lasers Surg Med. 2013;45(2):102–7.

31. Fernandez-Guarino M, Harto A, Sanchez-Ronco M, Garcia-Morales I, Jaen P. Pulsed dye laser vs. photodynamic therapy in the treatment of refractory nail psoriasis: a comparative pilot study. J Eur Acad Dermatol Venereol. 2009;23(8):891–5.

32. Nantel-Battista M, Richer V, Marcil I, Benohanian A. Treatment of nail psoriasis with intralesional triamcinolone acetonide using a needle-free jet injector: a prospective trial. J Cutan Med Surg. 2014;18(1):38–42.

33. Bleeker JJ. Intralesional triamcinolone acetonide using the port-O-jet and needle injections in localized dermatoses. Br J Dermatol. 1974;91(1):97–101.

34. Gumusel M, Ozdemir M, Mevlitoglu I, Bodur S. Evaluation of the efficacy of methotrexate and cyclosporine therapies on psoriatic nails: a one-blind, randomized study. J Eur Acad Dermatol Venereol. 2011;25(9):1080–4.

35. Reich K, Langley RG, Papp KA, Ortonne JP, Unnebrink K, Kaul M, et al. A 52-week trial comparing briakinumab with methotrexate in patients with psoriasis. N Engl J Med. 2011;365(17):1586–96.

36. Tosti A, Ricotti C, Romanelli P, Cameli N, Piraccini BM. Evaluation of the efficacy of acitretin therapy for nail psoriasis. Arch Dermatol. 2009;145(3):269–71.

37. Rich P, Gooderham M, Bachelez H, Goncalves J, Day RM, Chen R, et al. Apremilast, an oral phosphodiesterase 4 inhibitor, in patients with difficult-to-treat nail and scalp psoriasis: results of 2 phase III randomized, controlled trials (ESTEEM 1 and ESTEEM 2). J Am Acad Dermatol. 2016;74(1):134–42.

38. Feliciani C, Zampetti A, Forleo P, Cerritelli L, Amerio P, Proietto G, et al. Nail psoriasis: combined therapy with systemic cyclosporin and topical calcipotriol. J Cutan Med Surg. 2004;8(2):122–5.

39. Elewski B. Phase 3 study: 26-week efficacy and safety of adalimumab in patients with nail psoriasis, with and without psoriatic arthritis. Journal of the European Academy of Dermatology and Venereology. 2016;EADV, Vienna, Austria, Poster 2061.

40. Leonardi C, Langley RG, Papp K, Tyring SK, Wasel N, Vender R, et al. Adalimumab for treatment of moderate to severe chronic plaque psoriasis of the hands and feet: efficacy and safety results from REACH, a randomized, placebo-controlled, double-blind trial. Arch Dermatol. 2011;147(4):429–36.

41. Rigopoulos D, Gregoriou S, Lazaridou E, Belyayeva E, Apalla Z, Makris M, et al. Treatment of nail psoriasis with adalimumab: an open label unblinded study. J Eur Acad Dermatol Venereol. 2010;24(5):530–4.

42. Ortonne JP, Paul C, Berardesca E, Marino V, Gallo G, Brault Y, et al. A 24-week randomized clinical trial investigating the efficacy and safety of two doses of etanercept in nail psoriasis. Br J Dermatol. 2013;168(5):1080–7.

43. Kavanaugh A, McInnes I, Mease P, Krueger GG, Gladman D, Gomez-Reino J, et al. Golimumab, a new human tumor necrosis factor alpha antibody, administered every four weeks as a subcutaneous injection in psoriatic arthritis: twenty-four-week efficacy and safety results of a randomized, placebo-controlled study. Arthritis Rheum. 2009;60(4):976–86.

44. Rich P, Griffiths CE, Reich K, Nestle FO, Scher RK, Li S, et al. Baseline nail disease in patients with moderate to severe psoriasis and response to treatment with infliximab during 1 year. J Am Acad Dermatol. 2008;58(2):224–31.

45. Reich K, Ortonne JP, Kerkmann U, Wang Y, Saurat JH, Papp K, et al. Skin and nail responses after 1 year of infliximab therapy in patients with moderate-to-severe psoriasis: a retrospective analysis of the EXPRESS trial. Dermatology. 2010;221(2):172–8.

46. Saraceno R, Pietroleonardo L, Mazzotta A, Zangrilli A, Bianchi L, Chimenti S. TNF-alpha antagonists and nail psoriasis: an open, 24-week, prospective cohort study in adult patients with psoriasis. Expert Opin Biol Ther. 2013;13(4):469–73.

47. Kyriakou A, Patsatsi A, Sotiriadis D. Anti-TNF agents and nail psoriasis: a single-center, retrospective, comparative study. J Dermatolog Treat. 2013;24(3):162–8.

48. Rich P, Bourcier M, Sofen H, Fakharzadeh S, Wasfi Y, Wang Y, et al. Ustekinumab improves nail disease in patients with moderate-to-severe psoriasis: results from PHOENIX 1. Br J Dermatol. 2014;170(2):398–407.

49. Igarashi A, Kato T, Kato M, Song M, Nakagawa H. Japanese Ustekinumab study G. Efficacy and safety of ustekinumab in Japanese patients with moderate-to-severe plaque-type psoriasis: long-term results from a phase 2/3 clinical trial. J Dermatol. 2012;39(3):242–52.

50. Leonardi C, Matheson R, Zachariae C, Cameron G, Li L, Edson-Heredia E, et al. Anti-interleukin-17 monoclonal antibody ixekizumab in chronic plaque psoriasis. N Engl J Med. 2012;366(13):1190–9.

51. Dennehy EB, Zhang L, Amato D, Goldblum O, Rich P. Ixekizumab is effective in subjects with moderate to severe plaque psoriasis with significant nail involvement: results from UNCOVER 3. J Drug Dermatol. 2016;15(8):958–61.

52. Reich K. TRANSFIGURE: secukinumab efficacy in nail psoriasis: NAPSI % change over 32 weeks. J Eur Acad Dermatol Venereol. 2016;EADV, Vienna, Austria, October, 2016.

53. Crowley JJ, Weinberg JM, Wu JJ, Robertson AD, Van Voorhees AS, National PF. Treatment of nail psoriasis: best practice recommendations from the medical Board of the National Psoriasis Foundation. JAMA Dermatol. 2015;151(1):87–94.

54. Hsu S, Papp KA, Lebwohl MG, Bagel J, Blauvelt A, Duffin KC, et al. Consensus guidelines for the management of plaque psoriasis. Arch Dermatol. 2012;148(1):95–102.

55. Yaemsiri S, Hou N, Slining MM, He K. Growth rate of human fingernails and toenails in healthy American young adults. J Eur Acad Dermatol Venereol. 2010;24(4):420–3.

56. Paul C, Reich K, Gottlieb AB, Mrowietz U, Philipp S, Nakayama J, et al. Secukinumab improves hand, foot and nail lesions in moderate-to-severe plaque psoriasis: subanalysis of a randomized, double-blind, placebo-controlled, regimen-finding phase 2 trial. J Eur Acad Dermatol Venereol. 2014;28(12):1670–5.

57. Rigopoulos D, Gregoriou S, Makris M, Ioannides D. Efficacy of ustekinumab in nail psoriasis and improvement in nail-associated

quality of life in a population treated with ustekinumab for cutaneous psoriasis: an open prospective unblinded study. Dermatology. 2011;223(4):325–9.

58. Ortonne JP, Baran R, Corvest M, Schmitt C, Voisard JJ, Taieb C. Development and validation of nail psoriasis quality of life scale (NPQ10). J Eur Acad Dermatol Venereol. 2010;24(1):22–7.

59. Augustin M, Blome C, Costanzo A, Dauden E, Ferrandiz C, Girolomoni G, et al. Nail assessment in psoriasis and psoriatic arthritis (NAPPA): development and validation of a tool for assessment of nail psoriasis outcomes. Br J Dermatol. 2014;170(3):591–8.

60. van de Kerkhof PC, de Hoop D, de Korte J, Kuipers MV. Scalp psoriasis, clinical presentations and therapeutic management. Dermatology. 1998;197(4):326–34.

61. van de Kerkhof PC, Franssen ME. Psoriasis of the scalp. Diagnosis and management. Am J Clin Dermatol. 2001;2(3):159–65.

62. Sommer B, Overy DP, Kerr RG. Identification and characterization of lipases from Malassezia restricta, a causative agent of dandruff. FEMS Yeast Res. 2015;15(7). https://doi.org/10.1093/femsyr/fov078.

63. Gomez-Moyano E, Crespo-Erchiga V, Martinez-Pilar L, Godoy Diaz D, Martinez-Garcia S, Lova Navarro M, et al. Do Malassezia species play a role in exacerbation of scalp psoriasis? J Mycol Med. 2014;24(2):87–92.

64. Gupta AK, Batra R, Bluhm R, Boekhout T, Dawson TL Jr. Skin diseases associated with Malassezia species. J Am Acad Dermatol. 2004;51(5):785–98.

65. Dobrev H, Zissova L. Effect of ketoconazole 2% shampoo on scalp sebum level in patients with seborrhoeic dermatitis. Acta Derm Venereol. 1997;77(2):132–4.

66. Faergemann J. Treatment of seborrhoeic dermatitis of the scalp with ketoconazole shampoo. A double-blind study. Acta Derm Venereol. 1990;70(2):171–2.

67. Gupta S. Many faces of Koebner phenomenon in psoriasis. Indian J Dermatol Venereol Leprol. 2002;68(4):222–4.

68. Kim KS, Shin MK, Ahn JJ, Haw CR, Park HK. A comparative study of hair shafts in scalp psoriasis and seborrheic dermatitis using atomic force microscopy. Skin Res Technol. 2013;19(1):e60–4.

69. Shin MK, Kim KS, Ahn JJ, Kim NI, Park HK, Haw CR. Investigation of the hair of patients with scalp psoriasis using atomic force microscopy. Clin Exp Dermatol. 2012;37(2):156–63.

70. Ruano J, Suarez-Farinas M, Shemer A, Oliva M, Guttman-Yassky E, Krueger JG. Molecular and cellular profiling of scalp psoriasis reveals differences and similarities compared to skin psoriasis. PLoS One. 2016;11(2):e0148450.

71. Elewski BE. Clinical diagnosis of common scalp disorders. J Investig Dermatol Symp Proc. 2005;10(3):190–3.

72. Woo SM, Choi JW, Yoon HS, Jo SJ, Youn JI. Classification of facial psoriasis based on the distributions of facial lesions. J Am Acad Dermatol. 2008;58(6):959–63.

73. Chen SC, Yeung J, Chren MM. Scalpdex: a quality-of-life instrument for scalp dermatitis. Arch Dermatol. 2002;138(6):803–7.

74. Amatya B, Wennersten G, Nordlind K. Patients' perspective of pruritus in chronic plaque psoriasis: a questionnaire-based study. J Eur Acad Dermatol Venereol. 2008;22(7):822–6.

75. Runne U, Kroneisen-Wiersma P. Psoriatic alopecia: acute and chronic hair loss in 47 patients with scalp psoriasis. Dermatology. 1992;185(2):82–7.

76. Schwartz RA, Janusz CA, Janniger CK. Seborrheic dermatitis: an overview. Am Fam Physician. 2006;74(1):125–30.

77. Thaci D, Daiber W, Boehncke WH, Kaufmann R. Calcipotriol solution for the treatment of scalp psoriasis: evaluation of efficacy, safety and acceptance in 3,396 patients. Dermatology. 2001;203(2):153–6.

78. Krell J, Nelson C, Spencer L, Miller S. An open-label study evaluating the efficacy and tolerability of alefacept for the treatment of scalp psoriasis. J Am Acad Dermatol. 2008;58(4):609–16.

79. Kircik L, Fowler J, Weiss J, Meng X, Guana A, Nyirady J. Efficacy of secukinumab for moderate-to-severe head and neck psoriasis over 52 weeks: pooled analysis of four phase 3 studies. Dermatol Ther (Heidelb). 2016;6(4):627–38.

80. Reygagne P, Mrowietz U, Decroix J, de Waard-van der Spek FB, Acebes LO, Figueiredo A, et al. Clobetasol propionate shampoo 0.05% and calcipotriol solution 0.005%: a randomized comparison of efficacy and safety in subjects with scalp psoriasis. J Dermatolog Treat. 2005;16(1):31–6.

81. Bagel J. Phase 3b study of secukinumab in moderate to severe scalp psoriasis: 12 week results. 2016; Contract No.: EADV, Vienna, 2016 FC04.09.

82. Andreassi L, Giannetti A, Milani M, Scale IG. Efficacy of betamethasone valerate mousse in comparison with standard therapies on scalp psoriasis: an open, multicentre, randomized, controlled, cross-over study on 241 patients. Br J Dermatol. 2003;148(1):134–8.

83. Green C, Ganpule M, Harris D, Kavanagh G, Kennedy C, Mallett R, et al. Comparative effects of calcipotriol (MC903) solution and placebo (vehicle of MC903) in the treatment of psoriasis of the scalp. Br J Dermatol. 1994;130(4):483–7.

84. Mazzotta A, Esposito M, Carboni I, Schipani C, Chimenti S. Clobetasol propionate foam 0.05% as a novel topical formulation for plaque-type and scalp psoriasis. J Dermatolog Treat. 2007;18(2):84–7.

85. Griffiths CE, Finlay AY, Fleming CJ, Barker JN, Mizzi F, Arsonnaud S. A randomized, investigator-masked clinical evaluation of the efficacy and safety of clobetasol propionate 0.05% shampoo and tar blend 1% shampoo in the treatment of moderate to severe scalp psoriasis. J Dermatolog Treat. 2006;17(2):90–5.

86. Eichenfield LF, Ganslandt C, Kurvits M, Schlessinger J. Safety and efficacy of calcipotriene plus betamethasone dipropionate topical suspension in the treatment of extensive scalp psoriasis in adolescents ages 12 to 17 years. Pediatr Dermatol. 2015;32(1):28–35.

87. Schlager JG, Rosumeck S, Werner RN, Jacobs A, Schmitt J, Schlager C, et al. Topical treatments for scalp psoriasis: summary of a cochrane systematic review. Br J Dermatol. 2017;176(3):604–14.

88. Feldman SR, Housman TS. Patients' vehicle preference for corticosteroid treatments of scalp psoriasis. Am J Clin Dermatol. 2003;4(4):221–4.

89. Alinia H, Moradi Tuchayi S, Smith JA, Richardson IM, Bahrami N, Jaros SC, et al. Long-term adherence to topical psoriasis treatment can be abysmal: a 1-year randomized intervention study using objective electronic adherence monitoring. Br J Dermatol. 2017;176(3):759–64.

90. White S, Vender R, Thaci D, Haverkamp C, Naeyaert JM, Foster R, et al. Use of calcipotriene cream (Dovonex cream) following acute treatment of psoriasis vulgaris with the calcipotriene/betamethasone dipropionate two-compound product (Taclonex): a randomized, parallel-group clinical trial. Am J Clin Dermatol. 2006;7(3):177–84.

91. Taneja A, Racette A, Gourgouliatos Z, Taylor CR. Broad-band UVB fiber-optic comb for the treatment of scalp psoriasis: a pilot study. Int J Dermatol. 2004;43(6):462–7.

92. Morison WL, Atkinson DF, Werthman L. Effective treatment of scalp psoriasis using the excimer (308 nm) laser. Photodermatol Photoimmunol Photomed. 2006;22(4):181–3.

93. Taylor CR, Racette AL. A 308-nm excimer laser for the treatment of scalp psoriasis. Lasers Surg Med. 2004;34(2):136–40.

94. Johannesson A, Lindelof B. Additional effect of grenz rays on psoriasis lesions of the scalp treated with topical corticosteroids. Dermatologica. 1987;175(6):290–2.

95. Lindelof B, Johannesson A. Psoriasis of the scalp treated with Grenz rays or topical corticosteroid combined with Grenz rays. A comparative randomized trial. Br J Dermatol. 1988;119(2):241–4.

96. Nguyen CM, Leon A, Danesh M, Beroukhim K, Wu JJ, Koo J. Improvement of nail and scalp psoriasis using apremilast in patients with chronic psoriasis: phase 2b and 3, 52-week randomized, placebo-controlled trial results. J Drugs Dermatol. 2016;15(3):272–6.

97. Bagel J, Lynde C, Tyring S, Kricorian G, Shi Y, Klekotka P. Moderate to severe plaque psoriasis with scalp involvement: a randomized, double-blind, placebo-controlled study of etanercept. J Am Acad Dermatol. 2012;67(1):86–92.

98. Thaci D, Unnebrink K, Sundaram M, Sood S, Yamaguchi Y. Adalimumab for the treatment of moderate to severe psoriasis: subanalysis of effects on scalp and nails in the BELIEVE study. J Eur Acad Dermatol Venereol. 2015;29(2):353–60.

99. Reich K, Leonardi C, Lebwohl M, Kerdel F, Okubo Y, Romiti R, et al. Sustained response with ixekizumab treatment of moderate-to-severe psoriasis with scalp involvement: results from three phase 3 trials (UNCOVER-1, UNCOVER-2, UNCOVER-3). J Dermatolog Treat. 2016;13:1–6.

100. Sfikakis PP, Iliopoulos A, Elezoglou A, Kittas C, Stratigos A. Psoriasis induced by anti-tumor necrosis factor therapy: a paradoxical adverse reaction. Arthritis Rheum. 2005;52(8):2513–8.

101. de Gannes GC, Ghoreishi M, Pope J, Russell A, Bell D, Adams S, et al. Psoriasis and pustular dermatitis triggered by TNF-{alpha} inhibitors in patients with rheumatologic conditions. Arch Dermatol. 2007;143(2):223–31.

102. Guerra I, Perez-Jeldres T, Iborra M, Algaba A, Monfort D, Calvet X, et al. Incidence, clinical characteristics, and management of psoriasis induced by anti-TNF therapy in patients with inflammatory bowel disease: a nationwide cohort study. Inflamm Bowel Dis. 2016;22(4):894–901.

103. Cuchacovich R, Espinoza CG, Virk Z, Espinoza LR. Biologic therapy (TNF-alpha antagonists)-induced psoriasis: a cytokine imbalance between TNF-alpha and IFN-alpha? J Clin Rheumatol. 2008;14(6):353–6.

104. Kurd SK, Gelfand JM. The prevalence of previously diagnosed and undiagnosed psoriasis in US adults: results from NHANES 2003–2004. J Am Acad Dermatol. 2009;60(2):218–24.

105. Puig L, Barco D, Vilarrasa E, Alomar A. Treatment of acrodermatitis continua of Hallopeau with TNF-blocking agents: case report and review. Dermatology. 2010;220(2):154–8.

106. Chung J, Callis Duffin K, Takeshita J, Shin DB, Krueger GG, Robertson AD, et al. Palmoplantar psoriasis is associated with greater impairment of health-related quality of life compared with moderate to severe plaque psoriasis. J Am Acad Dermatol. 2014;71(4):623–32.

107. Pettey AA, Balkrishnan R, Rapp SR, Fleischer AB, Feldman SR. Patients with palmoplantar psoriasis have more physical disability and discomfort than patients with other forms of psoriasis: implications for clinical practice. J Am Acad Dermatol. 2003;49(2):271–5.

108. Michaelsson G, Gustafsson K, Hagforsen E. The psoriasis variant palmoplantar pustulosis can be improved after cessation of smoking. J Am Acad Dermatol. 2006;54(4):737–8.

109. Sevrain M, Richard MA, Barnetche T, Rouzaud M, Villani AP, Paul C, et al. Treatment for palmoplantar pustular psoriasis: systematic literature review, evidence-based recommendations and expert opinion. J Eur Acad Dermatol Venereol. 2014;28(Suppl 5):13–6.

110. Robinson A, Van Voorhees AS, Hsu S, Korman NJ, Lebwohl MG, Bebo BF Jr, et al. Treatment of pustular psoriasis: from the medical Board of the National Psoriasis Foundation. J Am Acad Dermatol. 2012;67(2):279–88.

111. Khandpur S, Sharma VK. Comparison of clobetasol propionate cream plus coal tar vs. topical psoralen and solar ultraviolet a therapy in palmoplantar psoriasis. Clin Exp Dermatol. 2011;36(6):613–6.

112. Nistico SP, Saraceno R, Chiricozzi A, Giunta A, Di Stefani A, Zerbinati N. UVA-1 laser in the treatment of palmoplantar pustular psoriasis. Photomed Laser Surg. 2013;31(9):434–8.

113. Goldberg DJ, Chwalek J, Hussain M. 308-nm Excimer laser treatment of palmoplantar psoriasis. J Cosmet Laser Ther. 2011;13(2):47–9.

114. Gattu S, Rashid RM, Wu JJ. 308-nm excimer laser in psoriasis vulgaris, scalp psoriasis, and palmoplantar psoriasis. J Eur Acad Dermatol Venereol. 2009;23(1):36–41.

115. Nistico SP, Saraceno R, Stefanescu S, Chimenti S. A 308-nm monochromatic excimer light in the treatment of palmoplantar psoriasis. J Eur Acad Dermatol Venereol. 2006;20(5):523–6.

116. Lozinski A, Barzilai A, Pavlotsky F. Broad-band UVB versus paint PUVA for palmoplantar psoriasis treatment. J Dermatolog Treat. 2016;27(3):221–3.

117. Sezer E, Erbil AH, Kurumlu Z, Tastan HB, Etikan I. Comparison of the efficacy of local narrowband ultraviolet B (NB-UVB) phototherapy versus psoralen plus ultraviolet a (PUVA) paint for palmoplantar psoriasis. J Dermatol. 2007;34(7):435–40.

118. Janagond AB, Kanwar AJ, Handa S. Efficacy and safety of systemic methotrexate vs. acitretin in psoriasis patients with significant palmoplantar involvement: a prospective, randomized study. J Eur Acad Dermatol Venereol. 2013;27(3):e384–9.

119. Wald JM, Klufas DM, Strober BE. The use of methotrexate, alone or in combination with other therapies, for the treatment of palmoplantar psoriasis. J Drug Dermatol. 2015;14(8):888–92.

120. Erkko P, Granlund H, Remitz A, Rosen K, Mobacken H, Lindelof B, et al. Double-blind placebo-controlled study of long-term low-dose cyclosporin in the treatment of palmoplantar pustulosis. Br J Dermatol. 1998;139(6):997–1004.

121. Bissonnette R, Pariser DM, Wasel NR, Goncalves J, Day RM, Chen R, et al. Apremilast, an oral phosphodiesterase-4 inhibitor, in the treatment of palmoplantar psoriasis: results of a pooled analysis from phase II PSOR-005 and phase III efficacy and safety trial evaluating the effects of Apremilast in psoriasis (ESTEEM) clinical trials in patients with moderate to severe psoriasis. J Am Acad Dermatol. 2016;75(1):99–105.

122. Bissonnette R, Poulin Y, Guenther L, Lynde CW, Bolduc C, Nigen S. Treatment of palmoplantar psoriasis with infliximab: a randomized, double-blind placebo-controlled study. J Eur Acad Dermatol Venereol. 2011;25(12):1402–8.

123. Weinberg JM. Successful treatment of recalcitrant palmoplantar psoriasis with etanercept. Cutis. 2003;72(5):396–8.

124. Floristan U, Feltes R, Ramirez P, Alonso ML, De Lucas R. Recalcitrant palmoplantar pustular psoriasis treated with etanercept. Pediatr Dermatol. 2011;28(3):349–50.

125. Au SC, Goldminz AM, Kim N, Dumont N, Michelon M, Volf E, et al. Investigator-initiated, open-label trial of ustekinumab for the treatment of moderate-to-severe palmoplantar psoriasis. J Dermatolog Treat. 2013;24(3):179–87.

126. Menter A. UNCOVER-2: impact of ixekizumab on palmoplantar plaque psoriasis. J Am Acad Dermatol. 2016; Poster 3271, Presented at the American Academy of Dermaology, Wahsington DC.

127. Gottlieb A, Sullivan J, van Doorn M, Kubanov A, You R, Parneix A, et al. Secukinumab shows significant efficacy in palmoplantar psoriasis: results from GESTURE, a randomized controlled trial. J Am Acad Dermatol. 2017;76(1):70–80.

128. Mrowietz U. 2PRECISE: randomized, double-blind, placebo-controlled trial of secukinumab in moderate to severe pustular palmoplantar psoriasis. J Eur Acad Dermatol Venereol. 2016;Poster 2121, European Academy of Dermatology and Venereology, VIenna Austria, October, 2016.

Current and Emerging Treatments for Psoriatic Arthritis

Philip J. Mease

Introduction and Background

The introduction of the TNF inhibitors (TNFi), the first biologics used in the treatment of rheumatologic disease, in the late 1990s greatly strengthened the ability to achieve states of low disease activity or remission for conditions such as rheumatoid arthritis and the spondyloarthritides, including psoriatic arthritis (PsA) [1]. These agents have established a gold standard for management of these diseases and represent a significant advance over the modest effectiveness of Conventional oral disease-modifying drugs (DMARDs) such as methotrexate, sulfasalazine, and leflunomide. However, not all patients are able to achieve or maintain low disease activity or remission states due to lack or loss of effect or tolerability issues. Fortunately, as our understanding of disease pathogenesis deepens, there are appearing a number of different medicines with mechanisms of action which address core pathogenic pathways. These include medicines which inhibit the TH17 cell pathway, including inhibitors of IL17 and IL23 [2], intracellular signaling modulators that downregulate activation of immune cells such as phosphodiesterase 4 (PDE4) and janus kinase (JAK) inhibitors, and co-stimulatory blockade agents which modulate T cell function [1]. Reasons for loss of effect of the TNFi, as well as subsequently introduced biologics and targeted synthetic disease-modifying drugs (DMARDs), appear to be multifactorial. In some patients, intolerability or serious adverse effects may occur with time; in others, disease activity may change and increase despite the use of the TNFi; and in others, gradual loss of effect may occur. Loss of effect may be partly due to development of immunogenicity to the therapeutic protein, i.e., development of an antibody response which may wholly or partly neutralize treatment effect. This has most clearly been documented with chimeric antibody constructs such as infliximab, in which the antibody response may be directed against the murine portion of the molecule [3, 4]. Neutralizing antibodies appear to be more likely to occur in monoclonal antibody constructs compared to the soluble receptor construct exemplified by etanercept [3, 4]. It is known that concomitant use of methotrexate can inhibit antibody formation against biologics [3, 4]. There is an ongoing need for therapies with different mechanisms of action and demonstrated ability to modify disease activity. Furthermore, the development of therapies with different administration frequency and improved safety profile will appeal to patient and physician preference.

Conventional Oral DMARDS

Methotrexate: Methotrexate (MTX) is one of the most widely used oral immunomodulatory drugs for PsA, yet the evidence for its efficacy is scant. Kingsley et al. conducted the Methotrexate in Psoriatic Arthritis (MIPA) trial [5]. Over the course of 5 years, 221 subjects were enrolled. At 6 months, statistically significant improvement was observed in patient and physician global assessment and mean PASI score, but only a trend was seen (not statistically significant) in improvement of tender and swollen joint count, measures of pain or function, PASI75, or composite measures such as ACR20, DAS28, or Psoriatic Arthritis Response Criteria (PsARC). The authors concluded that MTX is not disease modifying in PsA and had "borderline" symptom-modifying properties. However, there were many problems with the study, including dropout of a third of patients in each arm, the possibility that investigators channeled less severely diseased patients to the study, and insufficient aggressiveness of dose increase. In contrast, an open-label study comparing MTX with MTX plus infliximab in a relatively early patient cohort [6], showed high joint and skin responses in the combination arm, but also substantial improvements in both

P.J. Mease, MD
Swedish Medical Center, Seattle, WA 98122, USA

University of Washington School of Medicine, Seattle, WA 98122, USA
e-mail: pmease@philipmease.com

© Springer International Publishing AG 2018
P.S. Yamauchi (ed.), *Biologic and Systemic Agents in Dermatology*, https://doi.org/10.1007/978-3-319-66884-0_18

joints and skin in the MTX monotherapy arm. Although it has been difficult to conduct a proper controlled trial to demonstrate its efficacy, MTX remains the most widely used systemic drug PsA in both monotherapy format and in combination with biologic therapy, the latter partly for inhibition of immunogenicity potential.

Although the largest number of controlled trials of conventional oral DMARD therapy in PsA has been conducted with sulfasalazine [1, 7], its utility remains limited because of lack of effect in the skin, and occasional gastrointestinal intolerability.

Leflunomide, a pyrimidine antagonist, has demonstrated effectiveness in PsA and is formally approved for PsA treatment in Europe at a dose of 20 mg per day [7, 8].

Although cyclosporine can achieve rapid improvement of the skin lesions of psoriasis, evidence for its effectiveness in musculoskeletal disease is scant, and its utility is limited by concerns regarding the adverse effects of hypertension and renal insufficiency [7, 8]. It has been used in combination with adalimumab [9].

TNF Inhibition

TNFα was one of the first pro-inflammatory cytokines to be implicated in the pathogenesis of numerous inflammatory/autoimmune diseases. It is produced by several types of immune cells and activates a number of key effector cells involved in tissue inflammation and destruction in psoriasis and PsA including lymphocytes, macrophages, chondroctyes, osteoclasts, and keratinoctyes. There are five approved agents for PsA which inhibit TNFα: etanercept, infliximab, adalimumab, golimumab, and certolizumab (Table 18.1) [10–14]. All are also approved for ankylosing spondylitis, an important consideration for PsA patients with spondylitis. Etanercept, infliximab, and adalimumab are approved for the treatment of psoriasis and all five have demonstrated effectiveness in psoriasis. All except for etanercept are classified as monoclonal antibodies and have demonstrated effectiveness in inflammatory bowel disease, whereas etanercept has not. It also appears that these agents are effective in treating an associated condition, uveitis, especially the monoclonal antibody constructs [1, 15, 16].

Table 18.1 Anti-TNF therapies in PsA: ACR responses

Trial	n	ACR20%		ACR50%		ACR70%	
		Rx	P	Rx	P	Rx	P
Adalimumab[a] [10]	315	58	14	36	4	20	1
Certolizumab[a] [11]	409	58	24	36	11	25	3
Etanercept[a] [12]	205	59	15	38	4	11	0
Golimumab[b] [13]	405	52	8	32	3.5	18	0.9
Infliximab[b] [14]	200	58	11	36	3	15	1

[a]12 weeks
[b]14 weeks

Etanercept

Etanercept is a soluble receptor antibody administered subcutaneously 50 mg per week. Its efficacy in PsA was first demonstrated in an investigator-initiated trial of 60 patients [17], later confirmed in a phase 3 trial in 205 patients (Table 18.1) [12]. Dosing in PsA is 50 mg subcutaneously weekly. This was the first TNFi to be approved for PsA and was the first of this class to demonstrate ability to inhibit progressive joint damage as measured by serial radiographs of hands and feet [12]. Ability to improve enthesitis and dactylitis with this agent was demonstrated in the PRESTA study [18], in which the 50 mg weekly regimen was compared to 50 mg twice weekly for 12 weeks followed by 50 mg weekly (dosage regimen approved for psoriasis) in patients with moderate-to-severe arthritis and severe skin disease. Etanercept can be administered with or without background methotrexate and durability of effectiveness does not appear to be affected by background methotrexate use, implying lesser tendency to immunogenicity [19].

Infliximab

Infliximab demonstrated effectiveness in a 200-patient study using 5 mg/kg intravenously every 2 months after a loading dose regimen [14]. All PsA clinical domains improved significantly (Table 18.1), including inhibition of structural damage. This agent has a murine component, and thus may generate more immunogenicity with subsequent neutralization of effect over time. Although it can be administered without background methotrexate, its efficacy may be more sustained with concomitant methotrexate [19].

Adalimumab

Adalimumab is a fully human subcutaneously administered TNFi given at a dose of 40 mg every other week. Its efficacy in PsA was established in the ADEPT trial of 313 patients (Table 18.1) [10]. Sustained effectiveness has been demonstrated in PsA clinical domains, including inhibition of structural damage and patient-reported outcomes of function, quality of life, and fatigue, as have other TNFis [20]. Durability of effectiveness has been demonstrated with or without background methotrexate [19].

Golimumab

Golimumab is a TNFi with a prolonged half-life, allowing for monthly subcutaneous administration, approved for PsA, in 50 mg dose based on a 405-patient study (Table 18.1) [13]. It is also available in intravenous formulation, although this formulation only approved for RA at the current time. Golimumab is effective in all clinical domains of PsA and demonstrates long-term efficacy through 5 years [13, 21].

Certolizumab

Certolizumab is a unique antibody composed of the Fab portion of an immunoglobulin molecule attached to two polyethylene glycol moieties to prolong half-life. It is administered subcutaneously at a dose of 200 mg every 2 weeks or 400 mg every 4 weeks. At 12 and 24 weeks In the RAPID-PsA trial, 405 patients were evaluated with both doses and placebo, showing statistically significant benefit in ACR responses (Table 18.1), as well as significant improvement in DAS28, HAQ-DI, enthesitis, dactylitis, skin and nail measures, inhibition of radiologic damage progression, as well as improvement in SF-36 and work productivity measures [11]. In this study, 20% of patients had been previously exposed to TNFi therapy and similar degrees of response were seen in this group compared to TNFi-naïve patients, suggesting that it can effectively be used after another TNFi. Safety results were similar to other agents of this class.

Safety of TNFi

Detailed safety review of the TNFi class of medications is beyond the scope of this chapter, but a few key points can be reinforced. As immunomodulatory medications, an increased risk for infection, including serious infections, can be observed. In addition to bacterial infections, this can include opportunistic infections such as tuberculosis, invasive fungal infections such as histoplasmosis and coccidioidomycosis, and listeria and legionella. Other more rare potential side effects include risk for lymphoma and non-melanoma skin cancer; autoimmune reactions such as drug-induced lupus, psoriasis, or multiple sclerosis; hypersensitivity reactions; skin reactions; congestive heart failure; and hematologic aplasias.

Targeting the Th17 Cell Axis in PsA

Studies conducted in the last few years have shown that IL-23, IL-17, and IL-22, key cytokines involved in the pathway of Th17 lymphocyte activation and effector activities (Fig. 18.1) [22], are upregulated in psoriatic skin lesions and the blood and synovium of PsA patients. Their roles in pathophysiology include hyperproliferation of keratinocytes, promotion of synovitis, and activation of a variety of effector cells involved in cartilage and bone destruction [23–27]. Trials of therapeutic agents which inhibit IL23 and IL17 demonstrate significant benefit in various clinical domains of psoriasis and PsA [2, 28, 29]. These agents have demonstrated effectiveness in patients naïve to TNFi therapy as well as patients who have experienced TNFis previously, with somewhat lesser efficacy in the latter group.

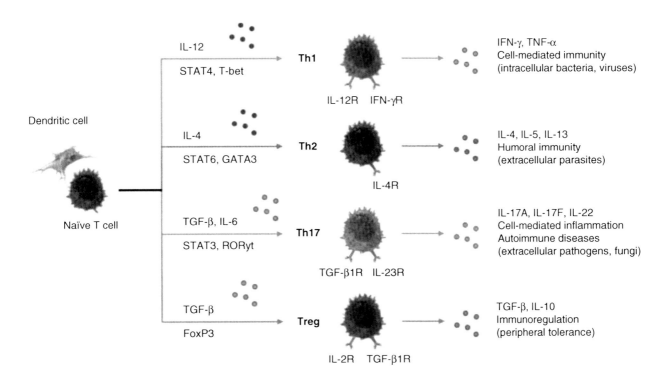

Fig. 18.1 T-cell differentiation pathways [22]

IL-12/23 Inhibition

Ustekinumab

Ustekinumab is a fully human monoclonal IgG1 antibody which binds to the common p40 subunit of IL-12 and IL-23, thus inhibiting the activity of those two cytokines and theoretically both Th1 and Th17 cell pathways. Ustekinumab is approved by the FDA for the treatment of psoriasis and PsA in a weight-based regimen: 45 mg for patients less than 100 kg and 90 mg for those greater than 100 kg. The drug is given subcutaneously at baseline, 4 weeks, and every 12 weeks thereafter. Efficacy in psoriasis is described elsewhere in this textbook.

Ustekinumab was studied in two phase 3 trials in PsA. In PSUMMIT 1, 615 patients who had inadequate response to methotrexate were randomized to receive 45 or 90 mg of ustekinumab vs. placebo [30]. At the primary endpoint, week 24, 42.4% and 49.5% of the 45 and 90 mg treated patients achieved ACR 20 response compared to 22.8% of placebo-treated patients, which was statistically significant. Other key measures of enthesitis, dactylitis, skin and nail disease, function, and quality of life also improved. Similar rates of adverse events were noted between treated and placebo groups and there were no opportunistic infections or major cardiovascular events. PSUMMIT 2 was similar in design but allowed two-thirds of its subject population to have previously been treated with TNFis [31]. ACR20 response was observed in 43.7%, 43.8%, and 20.2% of the 45, 90 mg, and placebo-treated patients in the overall population, and 36.7%, 34.5%, and 14.5% of the TNFi-experienced population. In a separate report in which radiographic data from the two trials was pooled, inhibition of structural damage was observed, primarily in the subjects in PSUMMIT 1 rather than subjects from PSUMMIT 2 who had been previously exposed to TNFi therapy [32].

IL-17 Inhibition

Three IL-17 inhibitors, secukinumab, ixekizumab, and brodalumab, have been studied for the treatment of psoriasis, psoriatic arthritis, and/or ankylosing spondylitis. Secukinumab and ixekizumab are now approved for psoriasis and secukinumab for PsA and AS.

Secukinumab

Secukinumab is a human monoclonal IgG1k antibody that targets IL-17A, which has recently gained FDA approval for psoriasis, PsA, and AS. Results of psoriasis trials are reported elsewhere in this textbook.

Two phase 3 trials in PsA have been conducted [33, 34]. FUTURE 1 enrolled 606 patients who were randomized to an IV loading dose of secukinumab, 10 mg/kg at baseline, weeks 2 and 4, and then either 150 or 75 mg every 4 weeks from week 8 vs. placebo. Thirty percent had received prior TNFi therapy and 60% were on concomitant MTX, randomized equally. At 24 weeks, the 150 mg dose arm demonstrated 50.0%, 34.7%, and 18.8% ACR 20/50/70 responses while the 75 mg arm demonstrated 50.5%, 30.7%, and 16.8% responses and placebo arm 17.3%, 7.4%, and 2.0% responses, respectively. Key secondary measures of enthesitis, dactylitis, skin disease, radiographic evidence of inhibition of X-ray progression, function, and quality of life all separated statistically from placebo in the treatment arms compared to placebo. FUTURE 2 [34] enrolled 397 patients to receive subcutaneous secukinumab 300, 150, and 75 mg and placebo at weeks 1, 2, 3, 4, and every 4 weeks thereafter. Thirty-five percent had received previous TNFi therapy. ACR, enthesitis, dactylitis, skin, function, and quality of life responses were similar to those seen in FUTURE 1. In both studies, the two-thirds of patients who had not had previous TNFi exposure demonstrated higher response rates than those who had previously been exposed to TNFi therapy. Overall serious adverse events were few and similar in frequency between the treatment and placebo arms through week 16 in both studies. In FUTURE 1, overall infection rate was slightly greater in the secukinumab arm than placebo; there were no opportunistic infections, including TB. Mild-to-moderate cases of cutaneous or oral candidiasis and infrequent episodes of neutropenia were noted. Both of these side effects are felt to be related mechanistically to the inhibition of IL-17. Infrequent events of flare of preexisting Crohn's disease or ulcerative colitis and more infrequent new-onset cases of inflammatory bowel disease (IBD) have been reported with secukinumab. It is not clear whether this is causally related to IL17 inhibition or due to IL17 inhibition not treating IBD, which is known to be associated with psoriasis, PsA, and AS. Patients should be queried about a history of IBD and this should be taken into account.

If a PsA patient has moderate-to-severe psoriasis, then the usual dose is 300 mg in a loading dose of 5 weekly injections followed by monthly administration. If the PsA patient has minimal or no psoriasis, the recommended dose is 150 mg. At the time of writing of this chapter, 3-year results of the FUTURE 1 trial and 2-year results of FUTURE 2 have been recently reported and showed sustained efficacy and no increase of adverse effects [33, 34].

Secukinumab has also demonstrated significant efficacy in the treatment of ankylosing spondylitis, using a 150 mg subcutaneous dose [35]. (It is appropriate to extrapolate the data for secukinumab in AS to the component of PsA.)

Results with secukinumab in RA have not been as robust; thus no further development of secukinumab for RA is anticipated.

Ixekizumab

Ixekizumab is an IL-17A inhibitor that has been approved for psoriasis and is in development for PsA and AS. As with secukinumab, this agent has shown a high degree of efficacy and similar safety profile in the treatment of psoriasis [36].

Phase 3 results through 1 year in PsA have recently been reported in 417 patients treated with ixekizumab 80 mg every 2 weeks or 4 weeks vs. an active control arm of adalimumab every 2 weeks vs. placebo [37]. At 24 weeks, ACR 20 responses were 62/58/57/30% for ixekizumab q 2 weeks/4 weeks/adalimumab/placebo; ACR 50 responses were 47/40/39/15% and ACR 70 responses were 34/23/26/6%, respectively. PASI 75 responses were 80/71/54/10%, respectively. Enthesitis, dactylitis, and function statistically improved with ixekizumab treatment and radiographic progression was inhibited. These results were maintained through week 52 [38]. A phase 3 trial in PsA patients previously treated with TNFi has not yet been reported at the time of writing of this chapter.

Brodalumab

Brodalumab is a human monoclonal antibody which blocks the IL17A receptor. As in the trials of the direct IL17A inhibitors, brodalumab has demonstrated significant efficacy in psoriasis [39].

Brodalumab was studied in a phase 2 study in 168 PsA patients [40]. At the 12-week primary endpoint, ACR20 response was experienced by 37 and 39% of 140 and 280 mg treated subjects vs. 18% in the placebo group, statistically superior for both treatment arms. As these same patients continued into open-label use of brodalumab on these same doses, ACR20 responses were observed in 51% and 64%, respectively, of the 140 and 280 mg treated patients. During the open-label extension, two events of Grade 2 neutropenia occurred.

Brodalumab was not effective in RA [41, 42].

At the time of writing of this chapter, clinical trial work with brodalumab has been put on hold as a result of infrequent events of suicidal ideation and suicide noted in psoriasis clinical trials, of uncertain causal relationship.

Bimekizumab

Bimekizumab is a humanized IgG1 monoclonal antibody that binds to IL-17A and IL-17F, instead of only IL-17A. The rationale is that inhibition of both of these forms of IL-17 may result in greater efficacy. Early data in psoriasis demonstrates excellent results (see elsewhere in this textbook). In a proof-of-concept trial in 42 PsA patients, the ACR 20

response in the aggregated top three doses (80, 160, 320 mg IV dosed once) at 8 weeks was 80% vs. 17% in placebo and the ACR 50 response was 40% vs. 8%, respectively, while PASI 75 was 100% [43]. Further development of this agent in psoriasis, PsA, and AS is anticipated.

Dual-TNF and -IL-17 Inhibitor

A novel approach to cytokine blockade is therapeutic antibodies which inhibit more than one cytokine. The idea is that such an antibody can be a "two for one," demonstrating additive or synergistic effect, and be less costly than administering two different cytokine blockers simultaneously. A key issue is determining whether there is also additive safety concern. Several dual-cytokine blockers are in development and data was recently presented in PsA and RA on one which blocks both TNF and IL-17, known as ABT-122. In a phase 2 trial in 240 PsA patients, ACR 20 results at 12 weeks showed ABT-122240 mg weekly/120 mg weekly/adalimumab 40 mg every other week/placebo results of 75/65/68/25% [44]. ACR 50 results were 53/37/38/13% and ACR 70 was demonstrated in 32/23/15/4%, respectively. PASI 75 was demonstrated in 78/74/58/27% of ABT-122240 mg/120 mg/adalimumab 40 mg/placebo, respectively. Importantly, there were no serious infections in any of the treatment arms. One case of Candida infection occurred in each of the ABT-122 arms, consistent with IL-17 inhibition effect. Unlike prior trials in RA in which two different cytokine blockers were employed and serious infection rate was increased, this was not observed, although the duration of observation was just 12 weeks. The high-dose ABT-122 achieved better ACR and psoriasis responses. In a parallel study in RA, the drug was similarly safe but there was less differentiation between the effect of ABT-122 and adalimumab [45]. At the time of writing, further development of this molecule is not progressing because it was considered not to be differentiated enough from adalimumab alone to warrant the expense and effort of a full development program. Despite this, the trial demonstrated that this novel approach to molecular development can work and be reasonably safe, thus paving the way for potential further development of dual inhibitors.

IL-23 Inhibitors

IL-23 is a key cytokine involved in the differentiation and proliferation of Th17 cells, thus acting upstream from IL-17 expression and potentially capable of inhibiting the production of several different types of cytokines, including both IL-17 and IL-22 [28, 29]. Data from psoriasis trials of three different IL-23i, guselkumab, tildrakizumab, and risankizumab, has been reported elsewhere in this text. Data from one trial in PsA with guselkumab has recently been reported [2] and trials with tildrakizumab and risankizumab are under way.

Guselkumab

Guselkumab is a human monoclonal antibody directed against the p19 subunit of IL-23. In a phase 2 study of 149 patients with PsA, 9% of whom had previously received TNFi, ACR 20/50/70 responses were seen in 58/34/14% vs. 18/10/2% in the placebo group. PASI 75 responses were 79% vs. 13% in guselkumab vs. placebo-treated patients. Resolution of enthesitis and dactylitis were 57% and 55% in guselkumab-treated vs. 29% and 17% in placebo-treated patients [46]. Further study of this agent is anticipated.

Co-stimulatory Blockade Modulating T-Lymphocyte Function

Abatacept

Abatacept is a co-stimulatory blockade agent which inhibits T-cell activation through second signal inhibition. The "first" signal of T-cell activation is the interaction between the major histocompatibility complex (MHC) and the T-cell receptor (TCR). A "second" signal is needed for full T-cell activation. A number of receptor-ligand pairs act as second signals, including CD80/86 on an antigen-presenting cell and CD28 on the T-cell surface. The natural inhibitor of this second signal interaction is CTLA4Ig. This molecule is mimicked by abatacept, which by binding to CD80/86 inhibits CD28 binding, thus inhibiting the second signal and reducing T-cell activation. Abatacept is approved for the treatment of rheumatoid arthritis. A phase 2 study of 170 PsA patients, using various doses of the intravenous formulation of abatacept, demonstrated significant improvement of ACR20 response [47]. Magnetic resonance imaging (MRI) study of hands or feet at 24 weeks demonstrated improved synovitis, erosion, and osteitis scores. Skin psoriasis responses were modest. A phase 3 study of subcutaneous abatacept in 424 PsA patients, 60% of whom had been treated with previous TNFi therapy, has been recently presented in abstract form [48]. At 24 weeks, statistically more abatacept-treated than placebo-treated patients (39% vs. 22%) achieved ACR 20 response. Greater responses were also seen in other musculoskeletal domains with abatacept treatment; however, only modest change in psoriasis was noted.

Alefacept

Alefacept, which blocks LFA3-CD2 signaling, was the first biologic developed and approved for treatment of psoriasis. Although efficacious, the modesty of skin response and need for laboratory monitoring of CD4 lymphocyte levels were among several factors which led to its voluntary withdrawal. A phase 2 trial showed modest efficacy in musculoskeletal aspects of PsA [49].

Efalizumab

Efalizumab, which blocks LFA1 second signaling, was transiently approved for the treatment of psoriasis, but withdrawn due to adverse effects of sepsis and progressive multifocal leukoencephalopathy which appeared post-approval. A phase 2 trial in PsA showed modest efficacy [50].

IL-6 Inhibition

Interleukin 6 (IL-6) is a pleiotropic pro-inflammatory cytokine which has a significant role in RA pathogenesis and has been demonstrated to be elevated in PsA synovitis and psoriasis skin lesions [51]. Tocilizumab, an IL-6 receptor blocker, is approved for RA. Case reports of its use in PsA have shown both positive and negative results [52].

Clazakizumab

Clazakizumab is a direct IL-6 inhibitor that has demonstrated efficacy in RA [53]. This agent was studied in a phase 2 trial with 165 PsA patients, 70% of whom were on background MTX [54]. ACR20 response was observed in 29/46/52/39% of patients in the placebo/25/100/200 mg monthly groups at the week 16 primary endpoint, which was statistically significant in the 100 mg group. PASI 75 responses were observed in 12/15/17/5% of placebo/25/100/200 mg groups. Improvements in enthesitis and dactylitis were most noted in the 100 mg group. The safety profile included issues expected for an IL-6-inhibiting agent, including increased risk for infection and elevation of hepatic transaminases and lipids. The demonstration of apparently greater effect in joints than skin suggests a differential role for IL-6 in the pathogenesis of synovitis as compared to psoriasis.

B-Lymphocyte Inhibition

Rituximab, which works by ablating B lymphocytes, is approved for the treatment of RA and vasculitis. Although some B-cell aggregation has been noted in PsA synovium [55], B lymphocytes are not considered to be as prominent a part of the pathophysiology of PsA as RA. Small cohorts of PsA patients have been treated with rituximab [56, 57] and modest effect on arthritis but virtually no effect on skin psoriasis has been noted [58].

Emerging Oral Therapies

Oral therapies which inhibit intracellular signaling pathways and decrease activation of pro-inflammatory immune cells and production of pro-inflammatory cytokines have been developed or are being developed.

Phosphodiesterase4 (PDE4) Inhibitor

Apremilast is an oral PDE4 inhibitor which appears to work in inflammatory conditions by decreasing the conversion of cyclic adenosine monophosphate (cAMP) to AMP by inhibiting the enzyme responsible for this conversion, PDE4. Increase of cAMP results in downregulation of expression of pro-inflammatory cytokines and upregulation of the expression of anti-inflammatory cytokines [59]. Apremilast was approved for treatment of PsA based on the results of three pivotal phase 3 studies, PALACE 1–3. In these trials, approximately 1500 patients with PsA were studied, randomized to apremilast 30 mg bid, 20 mg bid, or placebo, with primary endpoint of ACR20 response at 16 weeks [60, 61]. In PALACE 1, 38% of 30 mg bid-treated patients and 30% of 20 mg bid-treated patients achieved ACR20 response compared to 19% of placebo-treated patients, both statistically significant results. Statistical improvement was also seen in function and quality-of-life measures. Similar results were seen in the other trials. The prespecified analysis of enthesitis and dactylitis pooled data from all three trials also showed improvement. Other than tolerability issues, the overall safety profile of apremilast demonstrates essentially no issue of serious infection, malignancy, cardiovascular events, or laboratory abnormalities. Tolerability problems include nausea, diarrhea, and headache, which typically are mild to moderate, and, in the majority of patients, diminish and resolve even with continued use of the medicine. Patients should be advised that side effects of depressed mood and weight loss were noted more frequently in the apremilast than placebo-treated patients. Long-term observation of patients in the phase 3 clinical development program shows persistent efficacy in all clinical domains as well as very good safety and tolerability [61, 62].

Subsequent to the PsA approval, apremilast has also been approved for the treatment of psoriasis [63]. It appears that an optimal position for use of this agent would be early in the course of PsA, particularly for patients who prefer an oral therapy.

Janus Kinase (JAK) Inhibitors

An emerging class of compounds, the janus kinase (JAK) inhibitors, inhibit a number of different pro-inflammatory cytokines, including IL-6, -7, -10, -12, -15, -21, and -23 and IFNα and -β which utilize the JAK intracellular signaling pathway to activate immune cells to regulate inflammatory and immune responses [64]. JAK 1, 2, and 3 and TYK 2 form intracytoplasmic heterodimers in the receptor complex, which when phosphorylated activate STAT signaling to the cell nucleus. One JAK inhibitor, tofacitinib, is now approved for the treatment of rheumatoid arthritis, in a dose of 5 mg bid or 11 mg SR qd, and several others are in development.

Tofacitinib

Phase 3 studies of tofacitinib have been conducted in psoriasis which demonstrate its efficacy in that disease [65, 66]. However, as of this writing, tofacitinib has not been approved for the treatment of psoriasis. A phase 3 trial in PsA has been recently reported and showed significant efficacy in all clinical domains of PsA [67]. The ACR 20 responses at 12 weeks in the tofacitinib 5 mg bid, 10 mg bid, adalimumab, and placebo arms were 50%, 61%, 52%, and 33%, respectively. By a nonresponder imputation analysis, at 52 weeks the ACR 20 responses in the tofacitinib 5 mg bid, 10 mg bid, and adalimumab arms were 68%, 70%, and 58%, respectively. A similar profile of early-onset efficacy, maintained or increased at 12 months, was demonstrated for measures of enthesitis, dactylitis, psoriasis, function, and quality of life. The side effect potential of tofacitinib includes serious infection, herpes zoster, rare potential for malignancy, and need for laboratory monitoring for anemia, neutropenia, lymphopenia, thrombocytopenia, hyperlipidemia, and elevated hepatic transaminases.

Treating-to-Target and Treatment Algorithms

As in diseases such as diabetes and cancer, in rheumatology a treat-to-target approach has been advocated [68]. The key principle is that unrestrained disease activity yields current disabling symptomatology and long-term disability, joint damage, reduced quality of life, and potentially early mortality due to disease effects and comorbidities such as premature cardiovascular disease. Thus, clinicians are exhorted to assess disease activity quantitatively via history, physical exam (e.g., joint counts), laboratory (e.g., acute-phase reactants), and imaging (X-ray, ultrasound, or MRI) to determine disease activity. The aim is to treat active disease sufficiently to achieve a state of remission or low disease activity, as long as the patient can tolerate treatment. It is expected that through sensitive patient interaction and education the goals of treatment will be mutually shared by the patient and clinician. The TICOPA trial was the first treat-to-target trial in PsA [69]. This trial compared patients seen every 3 months, with no specific mandate to achieve a certain threshold of

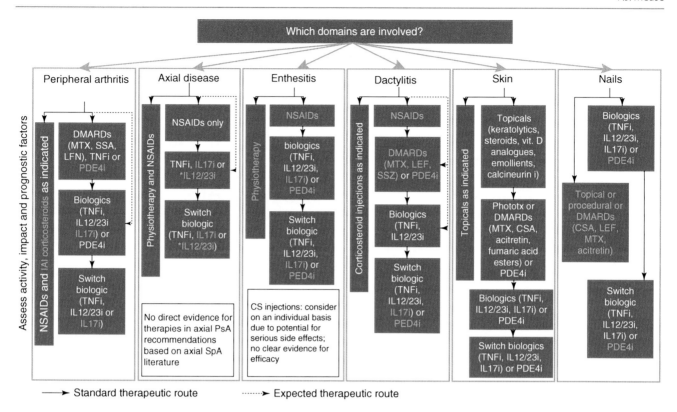

Fig. 18.2 Group for Research and Assessment of Psoriasis and Psoriatic Arthritis (GRAPPA) 2015 Treatment Recommendations for Psoriatic Arthritis [72]

minimal disease activity (MDA) with patients seen monthly, for whom lack of achievement of MDA led to mandated intensification of treatment—either addition of oral DMARDs or biologic therapy. After a year, there was a significantly different improvement in outcome for those treated in the more "tight control" fashion, albeit with slightly more side effects. These results support the importance of regularly assessing disease activity with the aim of achieving minimal disease activity.

Two different groups, the Group for Research and Assessment of Psoriasis and Psoriatic Arthritis (GRAPPA) and a task force of the European League Against Rheumatism (EULAR), have produced evidence-based treatment recommendations for PsA, most recently updated in 2016 [70, 71]. A third set of recommendations is in process by a working group of the American College of Rheumatology (ACR) in collaboration with the National Psoriasis Foundation (NPF) in the United States. The GRAPPA group has published a group of ten overarching principles of treatment, including treating to target, mutuality of patient and clinician decision making, comprehensive treatment of all involved clinical domains, and so forth. Separate task forces then evaluated the evidence for therapies within each of the key clinical domains of PsA: arthritis, enthesitis, dactylitis, spondylitis, psoriasis, and nail disease and, using standard methods for rigorous treatment recommendations, came up with

algorithms of treatment, establishing treatment "ladders" that make sense for clinicians and are tailored to the individual patient's clinical domain activities [72] (Fig. 18.2). In certain clinical domains, where there is little or no evidence for effectiveness of conventional oral DMARDS, such as for enthesitis, dactylitis, spondylitis, and nail disease, it is acceptable to move more quickly to biologic or targeted synthetic DMARD therapy in order to sooner achieve control of disease activity in that domain. Also, the GRAPPA group recognized that the coexistence of a variety of comorbid factors or associated conditions, e.g., the presence of cardiovascular disease, obesity, diabetes, liver disease, uveitis, inflammatory bowel disease, etc. could influence the choice of therapy [70, 71].

The EULAR recommendations are overall very similar to the GRAPPA recommendations, with some minor variations [71].

Conclusion

Our ability to achieve therapeutic benefit for the heterogeneous clinical aspects of PsA, including arthritis, enthesitis, dactylitis, spondylitis, and psoriasis, has been significantly improved by the introduction of parenteral biologic therapies. The first introduced biologic therapies which inhibit

TNFα have been able to achieve enduring states of low disease activity or remission in many, but not all, patients. Further, efficacy may be lost over time due to a number of factors including issues of tolerability and safety or development of immunogenicity. Thus, it has been important to develop and test biologic agents with a different mechanism of action than TNF inhibition. Agents which have shown effectiveness in psoriasis, as well as PsA thus far tested, and have been approved for use or are in development include those which inhibit IL-12/23 (ustekinumab), IL-17 (secukinumab, ixekizumab), IL-23 (guselkumab, tildraki-zumab, risankizumab), abatacept, apremilast, and tofacitinib, as well as more agents with novel mechanisms of action in the therapeutic pipeline.

Case Report

A 38-year-old white male developed psoriatic plaques on his scalp and elbows 10 years ago which was managed with topical agents. He also had psoriatic patches in the interglu-teal cleft and minor pitting of the fingernails. Recently, he noted one of his fingers becoming swollen even though there was no history of trauma. He also complained of low back and hip pain. There is no family history of psoriasis.

Past Medical History

- Recent diagnosis of multiple sclerosis

Social History

- Drinks socially (a few glasses of wine per week)
- Nonsmoker
- Married
- Sales representative

Previous Therapies

- Topical steroids
- Over-the-counter nonsteroidal anti-inflammatory agents

Physical Exam

- Psoriatic plaques on the scalp and elbows; pitting of the nails; erythema in the intergluteal cleft (5% BSA)
- Swelling of the entire left middle finger
- Tenderness to palpation at the left sacroiliac joint

Management

The patient was diagnosed with psoriatic arthritis based on the presence of dactylitis, pitting of the nails, tenderness at the sac-roiliac joint, and presence of psoriasis. The QuantiFERON gold assay test was negative and he had negative hepatitis B and C serologies. Other baseline laboratory monitoring was normal including compete blood count and liver function tests. Because of his history of multiple sclerosis, antitumor necrosis factor agents were not considered. The patient was initiated on secukinumab at 300 mg weekly for 5 weeks and then every

4 weeks afterwards. Within 3 months, the swelling of his left middle finger due to dactylitis improved by 80% and there was disappearance of the pits of his nails. His psoriasis had attained 90% clearance. The patient continues to remain on secukinumab to control his psoriasis and psoriatic arthritis.

Acknowledgments Catherine Loeffler, manuscript preparation assistance.

Disclosures Research grant, consultant, and/or speaker: AbbVie, Amgen, Bristol Myers Squibb, Celgene, Crescendo, Corrona, Demira, Genentech, Janssen, Lilly, Merck, Novartis, Pfizer, Sun, UCB, and Zynerba.

References

1. Mease PJ, Armstrong AW. Managing patients with psoriatic disease: the diagnosis and pharmacologic treatment of psoriatic arthritis in patients with psoriasis. Drugs. 2014;74(4):423–41.
2. Mease PJ. Inhibition of interleukin-17, interleukin-23 and the TH17 cell pathway in the treatment of psoriatic arthritis and psoriasis. Curr Opin Rheumatol. 2015;27(2):127–33.
3. Thomas SS, Borazan N, Barroso N, et al. Comparative immunogenicity of TNF inhibitors: impact on clinical efficacy and tolerability in the management of autoimmune diseases. A systematic review and meta-analysis. BioDrugs. 2015;29(4):241–58.
4. Zisapel M, Zisman D, Madar-Balakirski N, et al. Prevalence of TNF-alpha blocker immunogenicity in psoriatic arthritis. J Rheumatol. 2015;42(1):73–8.
5. Kingsley GH, Kowalczyk A, Taylor H, et al. A randomized placebo-controlled trial of methotrexate in psoriatic arthritis. Rheumatology (Oxford). 2012;51(8):1368–77.
6. Baranauskaite A, Raffayova H, Kungurov NV, et al. Infliximab plus methotrexate is superior to methotrexate alone in the treatment of psoriatic arthritis in methotrexate-naive patients: the RESPOND study. Ann Rheum Dis. 2012;71(4):541–8.
7. Nash P, Clegg DO. Psoriatic arthritis therapy: NSAIDs and traditional DMARDs. Ann Rheum Dis. 2005;64(Suppl 2):ii74–i7.
8. Mease PJ. Psoriatic arthritis assessment and treatment update. Curr Opin Rheumatol. 2009;21(4):348–55.
9. Karanikolas GN, Koukli EM, Katsalira A, et al. Adalimumab or cyclosporine as monotherapy and in combination in severe psoriatic arthritis: results from a prospective 12-month nonrandomized unblinded clinical trial. J Rheumatol. 2011;38(11):2466–74.
10. Mease PJ, Gladman DD, Ritchlin CT, et al. Adalimumab for the treatment of patients with moderately to severely active psoriatic arthritis: results of a double-blind, randomized, placebo-controlled trial. Arthritis Rheum. 2005;52(10):3279–89.
11. Mease PJ, Fleischmann R, Deodhar AA, et al. Effect of certoli-zumab pegol on signs and symptoms in patients with psoriatic arthritis: 24-week results of a phase 3 double-blind randomised placebo-controlled study (RAPID-PsA). Ann Rheum Dis. 2014;73(1):48–55.
12. Mease PJ, Kivitz AJ, Burch FX, et al. Etanercept treatment of psoriatic arthritis: safety, efficacy, and effect on disease progression. Arthritis Rheum. 2004;50(7):2264–72.
13. Kavanaugh A, McInnes I, Mease P, et al. Golimumab, a new human tumor necrosis factor alpha antibody, administered every four weeks as a subcutaneous injection in psoriatic arthritis: twenty-four-week efficacy and safety results of a randomized, placebo-controlled study. Arthritis Rheum. 2009;60(4):976–86.

14. Antoni C, Krueger GG, de Vlam K, et al. Infliximab improves signs and symptoms of psoriatic arthritis: results of the IMPACT 2 trial. Ann Rheum Dis. 2005;64(8):1150–7.

15. Acosta Felquer ML, Coates LC, Soriano ER, et al. Drug therapies for peripheral joint disease in psoriatic arthritis: a systematic review. J Rheumatol. 2014;41(11):2277–85.

16. Mease P. Psoriatic arthritis and spondyloarthritis assessment and management update. Curr Opin Rheumatol. 2013;25(3):287–96.

17. Mease PJ, Goffe BS, Metz J, et al. Etanercept in the treatment of psoriatic arthritis and psoriasis: a randomised trial. Lancet. 2000;356:385–90.

18. Sterry W, Ortonne JP, Kirkham B, et al. Comparison of two etanercept regimens for treatment of psoriasis and psoriatic arthritis: PRESTA randomised double blind multicentre trial. BMJ. 2010;340:c147.

19. Fagerli KM, Lie E, van der Heijde D, et al. The role of methotrexate co-medication in TNF-inhibitor treatment in patients with psoriatic arthritis: results from 440 patients included in the NOR-DMARD study. Ann Rheum Dis. 2014;73(1):132–7.

20. Mease PJ, Ory P, Sharp JT, et al. Adalimumab for long-term treatment of psoriatic arthritis: 2-year data from the Adalimumab effectiveness in psoriatic arthritis trial (ADEPT). Ann Rheum Dis. 2009;68(5):702–9.

21. Kavanaugh A, van der Heijde D, Beutler A, et al. Patients with psoriatic arthritis who achieve minimal disease activity in response to golimumab therapy demonstrate less radiographic progression: results through 5 years of the randomized, placebo-controlled, GO-REVEAL study. Arthritis Care Res. 2016;68(2):267–74.

22. Patel DD, Lee DM, Kolbinger F, et al. Effect of IL-17A blockade with secukinumab in autoimmune diseases. Ann Rheum Dis. 2013;72(Suppl 2):ii116–23.

23. Frleta M, Siebert S, McInnes IB. The interleukin-17 pathway in psoriasis and psoriatic arthritis: disease pathogenesis and possibilities of treatment. Curr Rheumatol Rep. 2014;16(4):414.

24. Nestle FO, Kaplan DH, Barker J. Psoriasis. N Engl J Med. 2009;361(5):496–509.

25. Raychaudhuri SP. Role of IL-17 in psoriasis and psoriatic arthritis. Clin Rev Allergy Immunol. 2013;44(2):183–93.

26. Jandus C, Bioley G, Rivals JP, et al. Increased numbers of circulating polyfunctional Th17 memory cells in patients with seronegative spondylarthritides. Arthritis Rheum. 2008;58(8):2307–17.

27. Suzuki E, Mellins ED, Gershwin ME, et al. The IL-23/IL-17 axis in psoriatic arthritis. Autoimmun Rev. 2014;13(4–5):496–502.

28. Tausend W, Downing C, Tyring S. Systematic review of interleukin-12, interleukin-17, and interleukin-23 pathway inhibitors for the treatment of moderate-to-severe chronic plaque psoriasis: ustekinumab, briakinumab, tildrakizumab, guselkumab, secukinumab, ixekizumab, and brodalumab. J Cutan Med Surg. 2014;18(3):156–69.

29. Leonardi CL, Gordon KB. New and emerging therapies in psoriasis. Semin Cutan Med Surg. 2014;33(2 Suppl 2):S37–41.

30. McInnes IB, Kavanaugh A, Gottlieb AB, et al. Efficacy and safety of ustekinumab in patients with active psoriatic arthritis: 1 year results of the phase 3, multicentre, double-blind, placebo-controlled PSUMMIT 1 trial. Lancet. 2013;382(9894):780–9.

31. Ritchlin C, Rahman P, Kavanaugh A, et al. Efficacy and safety of the anti-IL-12/23 p40 monoclonal antibody, ustekinumab, in patients with active psoriatic arthritis despite conventional non-biological and biological anti-tumour necrosis factor therapy: 6-month and 1-year results of the phase 3, multicentre, double-blind, placebo-controlled, randomised PSUMMIT 2 trial. Ann Rheum Dis. 2014;73(6):990–9.

32. Kavanaugh A, Ritchlin C, Rahman P, et al. Ustekinumab, an anti-IL-12/23 p40 monoclonal antibody, inhibits radiographic progression in patients with active psoriatic arthritis: results of an integrated analysis of radiographic data from the phase 3, multicentre, randomised, double-blind, placebo-controlled PSUMMIT-1 and PSUMMIT-2 trials. Ann Rheum Dis. 2014;73(6):1000–6.

33. Mease PJ, McInnes IB, Kirkham B, et al. Secukinumab inhibition of interleukin-17A in patients with psoriatic arthritis. N Engl J Med. 2015;373(14):1329–39.

34. McInnes IB, Mease PJ, Kirkham B, et al. Secukinumab, a human anti-interleukin-17A monoclonal antibody, in patients with psoriatic arthritis (FUTURE 2): a randomised, double-blind, placebo-controlled, phase 3 trial. Lancet. 2015;386(9999):1137–46.

35. Baeten D, Sieper J, Braun J, et al. Secukinumab, an interleukin-17A inhibitor, in Ankylosing spondylitis. N Engl J Med. 2015;373(26):2534–48.

36. Leonardi C, Matheson R, Zachariae C, et al. Anti-interleukin-17 monoclonal antibody ixekizumab in chronic plaque psoriasis. N Engl J Med. 2012;366(13):1190–9.

37. Mease PJ, van der Heijde D, Ritchlin CT, et al. Ixekizumab, an interleukin-17A specific monoclonal antibody, for the treatment of biologic-naive patients with active psoriatic arthritis: results from the 24-week randomised, double-blind, placebo-controlled and active (adalimumab)-controlled period of the phase III trial SPIRIT-P1. Ann Rheum Dis. 2017;76(1):79–87.

38. Mease P, Okada M, Kishimoto M, et al. Efficacy and safety of ixekizumab in patients with active psoriatic arthritis: 52 week results from a phase 3 study. Arthritis Rheum. 2016;68(Supplement S10)

39. Papp KA, Leonardi C, Menter A, et al. Brodalumab, an anti-interleukin-17-receptor antibody for psoriasis. N Engl J Med. 2012;366(13):1181–9.

40. Mease PJ, Genovese MC, Greenwald MW, et al. Brodalumab, an anti-IL17RA monoclonal antibody, in psoriatic arthritis. N Engl J Med. 2014;370(24):2295–306.

41. Martin DA, Churchill M, Flores-Suarez L, et al. A phase Ib multiple ascending dose study evaluating safety, pharmacokinetics, and early clinical response of brodalumab, a human anti-IL-17R antibody, in methotrexate-resistant rheumatoid arthritis. Arthritis Res Ther. 2013;15(5):R164.

42. Pavelka K, Chon Y, Newmark R, et al. A randomized, double-blind, placebo-controlled, multiple-dose study to evaluate the safety, tolerability, and efficacy of brodalumab (AMG 827) in subjects with rheumatoid arthritis and an inadequate response to methotrexate (abstract 831). Arthritis Rheum. 2012;64(S362)

43. Glatt S, Strimenopoulou F, Baeten D, et al. Bimekizumab, a monoclonal antibody that inhibits both IL-17A and IL-17F, produces a profound response in both skin and joints: results of an early-phase, proof-of-concept study in psoriatic arthritis. Ann Rheum Dis. 2016;75(Suppl 2, EULAR 2016)

44. Mease P, Genovese M, Weinblatt M, et al. Safety and efficacy of ABT-122, a TNF and IL-17–targeted dual variable domain (DVD)–Ig™, in psoriatic arthritis patients with inadequate response to methotrexate: results from a phase 2 trial. Arthritis Rheum. 2016;68(Supplement S10)

45. Genovese M, Weinblatt M, Aelion JA, et al. ABT-122, a TNF– and IL-17–targeted dual variable domain (DVD)–Ig™ in rheumatoid arthritis patients with inadequate response to methotrexate: results from a phase 2 trial. Arthritis Rheum. 2016;68(Supplement S10)

46. Deodhar A, Gottlieb A, Boehncke WH, et al. Efficacy and safety results of guselkumab, an anti-IL23 monoclonal antibody, in patients with active psoriatic arthritis over 24 weeks: a phase 2a, randomized, double-blind, placebo-controlled study. Arthritis Rheum. 2016;68(Supplement S10)

47. Mease P, Genovese MC, Gladstein G, et al. Abatacept in the treatment of patients with psoriatic arthritis: results of a six-month, multicenter, randomized, double-blind, placebo-controlled, phase II trial. Arthritis Rheum. 2011;63(4):939–48.

48. Mease P, Gottlieb A, Van der Heidje D, et al. Abatacept in the treatment of active psoriatic arthritis: 24-week results from a phase III study. Arthritis Rheum. 2016;68(Supplement S10)

49. Mease PJ, Gladman DD, Keystone EC. Alefacept in combination with methotrexate for the treatment of psoriatic arthritis: results of a randomized, double-blind, placebo-controlled study. Arthritis Rheum. 2006;54(5):1638–45.

50. Papp KA, Caro I, Leung HM, et al. Efalizumab for the treatment of psoriatic arthritis. J Cutan Med Surg. 2007;11(2):57–66.

51. Fonseca JE, Santos MJ, Canhao H, et al. Interleukin-6 as a key player in systemic inflammation and joint destruction. Autoimmun Rev. 2009;8(7):538–42.

52. Costa L, Caso F, Cantarini L, et al. Efficacy of tocilizumab in a patient with refractory psoriatic arthritis. Clin Rheumatol. 2014;33(9):1355–7.

53. Mease P, Strand V, Shalamberidze L, et al. A phase II, double-blind, randomised, placebo-controlled study of BMS945429 (ALD518) in patients with rheumatoid arthritis with an inadequate response to methotrexate. Ann Rheum Dis. 2012;71(7):1183–9.

54. Mease PJ, Gottlieb A, Berman A, et al. A phase IIb, randomized, double-blind, placebo-controlled, dose-ranging, multicenter study to evaluate the efficacy and safety of clazakizumab, an anti-IL-6 monoclonal antibody, in adults with active psoriatic arthritis. Arthritis Rheum. 2014;66(S10)

55. Veale D, Yanni G, Rogers S, et al. Reduced synovial membrane macrophage numbers, ELAM-1 expression, and lining layer hyperplasia in psoriatic arthritis as compared with rheumatoid arthritis. Arthritis Rheum. 1993;36(7):893–900.

56. Mease PJ. Is there a role for rituximab in the treatment of spondyloarthritis and psoriatic arthritis? J Rheumatol. 2012;39(12):2235–7.

57. Mease P, Kavanaugh A, Genovese M, et al. Rituximab in psoriatic arthritis provides modest clinical improvement and reduces expression of inflammatory biomarkers in skin lesions. Arthritis Rheum. 2010;62(10 (Supplement S818))

58. Wendling D, Dougados M, Berenbaum F, et al. Rituximab treatment for spondyloarthritis. A nationwide series: data from the AIR registry of the French Society of Rheumatology. J Rheumatol. 2012;39(12):2327–31.

59. Schafer P. Apremilast mechanism of action and application to psoriasis and psoriatic arthritis. Biochem Pharmacol. 2012;83(12):1583–90.

60. Kavanaugh A, Mease PJ, Gomez-Reino JJ, et al. Treatment of psoriatic arthritis in a phase 3 randomised, placebo-controlled trial with apremilast, an oral phosphodiesterase 4 inhibitor. Ann Rheum Dis. 2014;73(6):1020–6.

61. Mease P. Apremilast: a phosphodiesterase 4 inhibitor approved for treatment of psoriatic arthritis. Rheumatol Ther. 2014;1:1–20.

62. Raychaudhuri SP, Wilken R, Sukhov AC, et al. Management of psoriatic arthritis: early diagnosis, monitoring of disease severity and cutting edge therapies. J Autoimmun. 2017;76:21–37.

63. Papp K, Reich K, Leonardi CL, et al. Apremilast, an oral phosphodiesterase 4 (PDE4) inhibitor, in patients with moderate to severe plaque psoriasis: results of a phase III, randomized, controlled trial (efficacy and safety trial evaluating the effects of Apremilast in psoriasis [ESTEEM] 1). J Am Acad Dermatol. 2015;73(1):37–49.

64. O'Shea JJ. Targeting the Jak/STAT pathway for immunosuppression. Ann Rheum Dis. 2004;63(Suppl 2):ii67–71.

65. Papp KA, Menter MA, Abe M, et al. Tofacitinib, an oral Janus kinase inhibitor, for the treatment of chronic plaque psoriasis: results from two randomized, placebo-controlled, phase III trials. Br J Dermatol. 2015;173(4):949–61.

66. Bachelez H, van de Kerkhof PC, Strohal R, et al. Tofacitinib versus etanercept or placebo in moderate-to-severe chronic plaque psoriasis: a phase 3 randomised non-inferiority trial. Lancet. 2015;386(9993):552–61.

67. Mease P, Hall S, FitzGerald O, et al. Efficacy and safety of tofacitinib, an oral janus kinase inhibitor, or adalimumab in patients with active psoriatic arthritis and an inadequate response to conventional synthetic DMARDs: a randomized, placebo-controlled, phase 3 trial. Arthritis Rheum. 2016;68(Supple S10)

68. Smolen JS, Braun J, Dougados M, et al. Treating spondyloarthritis, including ankylosing spondylitis and psoriatic arthritis, to target: recommendations of an international task force. Ann Rheum Dis. 2014;73(1):6–16.

69. Coates LC, Moverley AR, McParland L, et al. Effect of tight control of inflammation in early psoriatic arthritis (TICOPA): a UK multicentre, open-label, randomised controlled trial. Lancet. 2015;386(10012):2489–98.

70. Coates LC, Kavanaugh A, Mease PJ, et al. Group for research and assessment of psoriasis and psoriatic arthritis: treatment recommendations for psoriatic arthritis. Arthritis Rheum. 2015:2016.

71. Gossec L, Smolen JS, Gaujoux-Viala C, et al. European league against rheumatism recommendations for the management of psoriatic arthritis with pharmacological therapies. Ann Rheum Dis. 2012;71(1):4–12.

72. Coates LC, Kavanaugh A, Mease PJ, et al. Group for research and assessment of psoriasis and psoriatic arthritis 2015 treatment recommendations for psoriatic arthritis. Arthritis Rheumatol. 2016;68(5):1060–71.

Janus Kinase Inhibitors

19

Andrew Kim and Bruce Strober

Introduction

Janus kinases (JAKs) were first discovered in a 1989 screen among a panel of other protein kinases [1]. Before their importance was readily known, some individuals lightheartedly referred to them as "just another kinase" given the abundance of other known protein kinases at the time. Subsequently, four distinct members of the JAK family were identified.

The Janus kinase-signal transducer and activation of transcription (JAK-STAT) signaling pathway has since been implicated in a myriad of inflammatory and hematologic conditions, with increased focus on its role in cutaneous disorders. Targeted cytokine inhibition (e.g., TNF inhibition) was a pivotal moment in the treatment of autoinflammatory disorders such as rheumatoid arthritis (RA), psoriasis, psoriatic arthritis (PsA), and inflammatory bowel disease (IBD). A natural evolution of this targeted therapy has been to look at the downstream signaling pathways of these cytokines, which presented new opportunities for targeted treatment within the JAK-STAT pathway. Two Jakinibs (short for JAK inhibitors) have already been approved for human use in the USA—tofacitinib for the treatment of RA in 2012 and ruxolitinib for myelofibrosis and polycythemia vera (PV) in 2011 and 2014, respectively [2–4]. Similarly, oclacitinib was approved for treating allergic dermatitis in canines in 2012 [5]. Further research continues to be done on other Jakinibs with no less than 20 other agents in the developmental pipeline [6].

The JAK-STAT pathway is believed to play a significant role in the pathogenesis of several dermatologic conditions, with current research efforts mainly being focused on psoriasis and alopecia areata. Early success in these arenas have led to additional investigative studies into using Jakinibs for atopic dermatitis, vitiligo, and dermatomyositis.

JAK-STAT Signaling Pathway

A broad range of cytokines and other extracellular messengers such as erythropoietin (EPO), thrombopoietin (TPO), colony stimulating factors (CSF), and growth hormone (GH) bind to transmembrane receptors associated with the JAK-STAT signaling pathway [6]. As the transmembrane receptors themselves lack any intrinsic ability for signal transduction, they depend on the cytosolic-bound JAK family of protein-tyrosine kinases to activate downstream STAT molecules for signal transduction.

A generalized overview of the JAK-STAT signaling pathway converting extracellular signals into a transcriptional response is illustrated in Fig. 19.1. Binding of an extracellular ligand engages its specific transmembrane receptor which subsequently undergoes a conformational change. Cytosolic-bound JAKs are brought together to catalyze an autophosphorylation reaction between one another. Next, the activated JAKs phosphorylate tyrosine residues of the transmembrane receptors which attract the STATs. Subsequent direct phosphorylation of the bound STATs by the JAKs allows the phosphorylated STATs to dimerize with one another. These dimers translocate to the nucleus and bind to promotor regions of DNA to ultimately modulate relevant gene transcription [7].

The JAK family of protein-tyrosine kinases are composed of the four structurally distinct members—JAK1, JAK2, JAK3, and TYK2—which selectively bind to the cytosolic portion of specific transmembrane receptors [8]. JAK1, JAK2, and TYK2 are expressed throughout the body, whereas JAK3 is predominantly found only in

A. Kim, MD
Department of Surgery, Division of Dermatology, Dartmouth-Hitchcock, Concord, NH 03301, USA
e-mail: andrew.kim@hitchcock.org

B. Strober, MD, PhD (✉)
Department of Dermatology, University of Connecticut Health Center, 21 South Road, 2nd Floor, Farmington, CT 06032, USA

Probity Medical Research, Waterloo, Ontario, Canada
e-mail: strober@uchc.edu

© Springer International Publishing AG 2018
P.S. Yamauchi (ed.), *Biologic and Systemic Agents in Dermatology*, https://doi.org/10.1007/978-3-319-66884-0_19

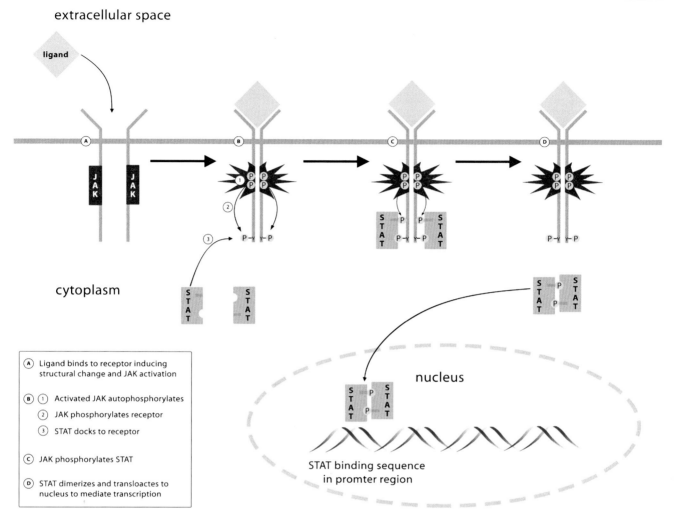

Fig. 19.1 JAK-STAT signaling pathway

hematopoietic cells [9]. The JAKs have seven distinct domains with sequence homology among the members, termed Janus homology domains (JH1 to JH7). The JH1 domain represents the active kinase domain with the adjacent JH2 being an inactive "pseudokinase" region possessing critical regulatory functions over JH1 [10, 11]. This unique dual kinase domain configuration differentiates JAKs from other protein kinases, and this is how they came to be named after the two-faced Roman goddess Janus [12]. Discovery of the seven downstream STAT family transcription factors—STATs 1, 2, 3, 4, 5a, 5b, and 6— occurred concurrently with JAKs, unveiling the direct pathway of extracellular signaling via transmembrane receptors to gene transcription in the nucleus. STAT transcription factors have six conserved domains including a transcriptional activation domain (TAD), an SH2 domain, and a DNA-binding domain [13]. The SH2 domain facilitates STAT docking to the phosphorylated tyrosine residues on the transmembrane receptor, while the TAD region serves as the site of direct phosphorylation by the JAK.

Among the cytokine receptor superfamilies, JAKs are essential to the type I and II cytokine family of transmembrane receptors. These receptors which employ the JAK-STAT pathway engage a wide range of extracellular messengers that have broad effects on immunity and inflammation. Different receptors of type I and II cytokines pair with different JAKs, giving rise to distinct effects when certain JAKs are preferentially targeted.

Type I cytokines are broadly broken down by the receptor types with the major constituents belonging to the common γ-chain (γc) cytokines (IL-2, IL-4, IL-7, IL-9, IL-15, and IL-21), common β-chain cytokines (IL-3, IL-5, and GM-CSF), gp130 receptor subunit cytokines (IL-6, IL-11, IL-27), and dimeric cytokines (IL-12, IL-23, IL-27, and IL-35) [7, 14]. Additionally, hormone-like cytokines—EPO, TPO, G-CSF, GF, and leptin—also are classified under this category as well. Type II cytokines fall under the INF family of cytokines (INF-α, INF-β, INF-γ, IL-28, IL-29) and the IL-10 family of cytokines (IL-10, IL-19, IL-20, IL-22) (Table 19.1) [7, 14, 15].

Table 19.1 Upstream and downstream JAK signaling

Cytokine/hormone	Downstream JAKs	Downstream STATs	Immune function, potential disease role
Type I cytokines			
Common γ-chain cytokines			
IL-2	JAK1, JAK3	3, 5	Enhances effector and regulatory responses
IL-4	JAK1, JAK3	6	T_H2-mediated diseases—allergies and asthma
IL-7	JAK1, JAK3	3, 5	T-cell development and homeostasis
IL-9	JAK1, JAK3	1, 3, 5	Atopic disease, IBD
IL-15	JAK1, JAK3	3, 5	Memory T cells, NK cells, induction of cell proliferation
IL-21	JAK1, JAK3	1, 3, 5	T_{FH} cells
Common β-chain cytokines			
GM-CSF	JAK2	3, 5	Macrophages, T cells, mast cells, NK cells, endothelial cells and fibroblasts, stem cell stimulation, and differentiation
IL-3	JAK2	3, 5, 6	Differentiation of multipotent hematopoietic stem cells, proliferation of all cells in the myeloid lineage
IL-5	JAK2	3, 5, 6	Allergies, asthma, eosinophilic disease
gp130 cytokines			
IL-6	JAK1, JAK2, TYK2	1, 3	Prototypic pro-inflammatory cytokine, broadly relevant for many autoimmune disease
IL-11	JAK1, JAK2, TYK2	3	Hematopoiesis, bone remodeling
IL-27	JAK1, JAK2, TYK2	1, 2, 3, 4, 5	Regulation of B and T lymphocytes
Heterodimeric cytokines			
IL-12	JAK2, TYK2	4	T_H1-associated disease
IL-23	JAK2, TYK2	3, 4	T_H17-mediated disease
IL-27	JAK1, TYK2	1, 3	Enhance T_H1 and inhibit T_H17 responses
IL-35	JAK1, TYK2	1, 4	Anti-inflammatory responses
Hormonelike cytokines			
EPO	JAK2	5	Control of erythropoiesis
TPO	JAK2	1, 3, 5	Regulation of the differentiation of megakaryocytes and platelets
G-CSF	JAK2	5	Bone marrow stimulation to produce stem cells and granulocytes
GH	JAK2	3, 5a	Stimulation of cell division of chondrocytes and IGF-1
Leptin	JAK2	3, 5a	Coordination of energy homeostasis, increases satiety
Type II cytokines			
IFN family cytokines			
INF-α/β	JAK1, TYK2	1, 2, 3, 4, 5	Enhance immunity against infections and drive autoimmunity
INF-γ	JAK1, TYK2	1	Enhance immunity against infections and drive autoimmunity
IL-28	JAK1, TYK2	1, 2, 3, 4, 5	Enhance immunity against infections
IL-29	JAK1, TYK2	1, 2, 3, 4, 5	Enhance immunity against infections
IL-10 family cytokines			
IL-10	JAK1, JAK2, TYK2	1, 3, 5	Anti-inflammatory actions
IL-19	JAK1, JAK2, TYK2	3	B-cell activation, antibody production
IL-20	JAK1, JAK2, TYK2	3	Synoviocyte migration, osteoclast formation
IL-22	JAK1, JAK2, TYK2	1, 3, 5	Promote barrier immunity, anti-inflammatory responses, augment IL-17 function
Growth factors [7]			
EGF	JAK1	1, 3, 5a	Stimulates cell growth, proliferation, and differentiation
PDGF	JAK1, JAK2	1, 2, 3, 5, 6	Angiogenesis, stem cell growth

Reproduced with permission and minor adaptations from: Schwartz DM, Bonelli M, Gadina M, O'Shea JJ. Type I/II cytokines, JAKs, and new strategies for treating autoimmune diseases. Nat Rev Rheumatol. 2016;12(1):25–36

Among the JAK family, JAK3 exclusively associates with the common γ-chain (γc) receptor and pairs with JAK1, whereas other JAKs do not exhibit the same degree of specificity to just a single receptor class [16]. However, JAK2 is solely responsible for signal transduction via common β-chain cytokines/receptors and signal transduction for hematopoietic cell-development hormones such as EPO, TPO, and G-CSF. These cytokines all flow exclusively through JAK2, thus making it an integral component of signal transduction for these molecules [17]. TYK2 is most often seen in concert with JAK1 and JAK2. Downstream STATs exhibit greater cross-reactivity to upstream JAKs since they do not demonstrate as much fidelity in the signaling pathways compared to JAK and their associated receptors. Some minor variance can be observed in the preferential JAK-STAT signaling depending on the specific cytokines and cell type being described (e.g., CD4 cells vs. monocytes vs. mast cells).

JAK-STAT Signaling in Disease

Over- or under-activation of the JAK-STAT pathway—from either somatic mutation in these components or abnormal receptor activation—has been demonstrated in a number of inflammatory disorders, primary immunodeficiency diseases, and malignancies (Table 19.2).

Table 19.2 Select diseases associated with JAK-STAT

JAK/STAT	Select associated diseases
JAK1	Somatic mutations in ALL, AML, ductal breast carcinoma, NSCLC (gain of function mutations) [7]
JAK2	Myeloproliferative disorders—PV, ET, myelofibrosis (gain of function mutation) [19]
JAK3	AR- and X-linked SCID variants (loss of function mutation) [20]
TYK2	AR-HIES (loss of function mutation) [92]
STAT1	Susceptibility to mycobacterial +/− viral infections (loss of function mutation) [93, 94] Chronic mucocutaneous candidiasis (gain of function mutation) [95]
STAT2	Increased susceptibility to viral illnesses (loss of function mutation) [96]
STAT3	AD-HIES (loss of function mutation) [97] Polymorphisms seen in UC and psoriasis [98]
STAT4	Polymorphisms associated with RA, SLE [99]
STAT5a/b	AR syndrome of dwarfism, autoimmunity, and immunodeficiency (loss of function mutation) [6]
STAT6	Polymorphisms associated with asthma, atopy, increased levels of IgE [100]

ALL acute lymphocytic leukemia, *AML* acute myeloid leukemia, *NSCLC* non-small cell lung cancer, *PV* polycythemia vera, *ET* essential thrombocytosis, *AR* autosomal recessive, *SCID* severe combined immunodeficiency, *HIES* hyper-immunoglobulin E syndrome, *AD* autosomal dominant, *UC* ulcerative colitis, *RA* rheumatoid arthritis, *SLE* systemic lupus erythematosus

Diseases with Direct JAK-STAT Pathway Mutations

Knockout murine models for individual components of JAK-STAT signaling as well as from our understanding of cytokine signaling in human diseases helps illustrate the critical role the JAK-STAT pathway serves in immune cell development and function. Specific diseases where the distinct functions of the JAK-STAT signaling have become relevant can be seen in cases such as with myeloproliferative disorders and severe combined immunodeficiency (SCID).

PV and essential thrombocytosis (ET) are characterized by clonal proliferation of red blood cells and platelets, respectively, whereas primary myelofibrosis results from the replacement of bone marrow by fibrotic scar tissue following the abnormal proliferation of hematopoietic stem cells. PV, ET, and primary myelofibrosis have all been linked to activating JAK2 V617F mutations in the regulatory JH2 pseudokinase domain resulting in a gain of function mutation [18]. This JAK2 mutation is seen in over 95% of PV patients and about half of all ET and myelofibrosis patients [19]. These three myeloproliferative diseases collectively share a common sensitivity of hematopoietic cells to growth factors given the integral role JAK2 plays in signal transduction for hematopoietic hormones like EPO, TPO, and G-CSF among others [17].

The immunologic function of JAK3 can be highlighted by many of the autosomal recessive variants of SCID. Mutations along the common γc JAK-STAT pathway include loss of function mutation in the γc receptor, JAK3 deficiency, or isolated IL-7 receptor deficiency. These three deficits all results in variants of SCID subtypes—the former two clinically manifest with absent T and natural killer (NK) cells along with impaired B-cell function, while the latter form manifests in a similar way except they have intact NK cells [20]. Correction of these cellular deficiencies and defective immune responses following hematopoietic stem cell transplant further highlights the limited role and functional distribution of JAK3.

Activating mutations in JAK1, JAK2, and JAK3 are seen in various malignancies, but it is most commonly reported in various lymphoma and leukemia subtypes [21].

Type I and II Cytokines and Dysregulation of JAK-STAT in Cutaneous Disease

Our understanding of the pathogenesis of various autoinflammatory diseases continue to evolve as additional targets are identified and selectively modulated.

Psoriasis

Psoriasis is a chronic, immune-mediated disease characterized by red scaly cutaneous plaques as well as, in some patients, a destructive psoriatic arthritis (PsA). While the pathogenesis of psoriasis involves interactions between genetics and the environment, an abnormal T-lymphocyte-mediated response causing release of pro-inflammatory cytokines is central to the disorder [22]. Elevated levels of numerous pro-inflammatory and proliferative cytokines are involved with psoriasis including the type I/II cytokines IL-2, IL-6, IL-12, IL-15, IL-19, IL-20, IL-22, IL-23, IL-24, IFN-α, and IFN-γ which signal through JAK-STAT [23]. In vitro studies of psoriatic skin have demonstrated upregulation of JAK3 in the epidermis, as well as JAK1 and JAK3 in the dermal infiltrates [24]. Likewise, upregulation of STAT1 and STAT3 signals are seen as well [25, 26]. Selective inhibition of JAK1/JAK3 signaling in murine models of psoriasis result in significant clinical and histologic improvement along with reductions in plasma levels of IL-17, IL-22, IL-23, and TNF-α [27]. Signal transduction of these cytokines through JAK-STAT is responsible for the production of other cytokines central to psoriasis pathogenesis such as with IL-17. While the IL-12 and IFN-γ signals driving a T_H1 response are elevated, the relevance of IL-23- and T_H17-mediated responses are currently the defining paradigm for the condition [28]. The IL-17 signature of psoriasis is not part of the group of type I or II cytokines signaling through JAK-STAT, but IL-17 production by T cells is dependent on IL-23 (which signals though STAT3), and thus, JAK-STAT signaling can be considered an upstream regulator for this pathway [29].

Alopecia Areata

Alopecia areata (AA) is a common autoimmune disease notable for causing a non-cicatricial alopecia that can vary from small discrete patches to total body hair loss (alopecia universalis). Like psoriasis, the etiology of AA appears to be multifactorial, but the condition is characterized by a cytotoxic T-cell-mediated inflammatory response along with upregulation of INF-γ and select γc cytokines (particularly IL-15 and IL-2) promoting the activation and survival of these INF-γ-producing CD8$^+$ T cells [30, 31]. INF-γ signaling though JAK1/2 and STAT1 mediates IL-15 expression, which in turn signals through the JAK1/3 pathway to upregulate IL-2 via STAT3 (and to a lesser extent STAT5) [31]. Analysis of AA skin in vitro shows strong expression of JAK3; however, JAK1 and JAK2 expression is also elevated to a lesser extent [24, 31]. Interestingly, a strong STAT2 signal was noted in one study involving seven AA skin biopsies bringing into question whether another signaling mechanism other than the INF-γ pathway may be implicated in the pathogenesis of the condition [24].

Atopic Dermatitis

Atopic dermatitis (AD), which may be more common than psoriasis, is considered the prototypical T_H2-mediated disease [32]. Like AA and psoriasis, AD is also a multifactorial condition stemming from complex interactions between environmental, genetic, and immunologic factors [33]. The immunologic profile for AD is characterized by a T_H2 predominant response with upregulation of IL-4, IL-5, IL-13, and IL-31, among others. IL-4 signals through JAK1/3 and STAT6 to propagate a T_H2 response by inducing further production of IL-4 as well as IL-5, IL-10, and IL-13 and other pro-inflammatory cytokines [34]. Recent developments with targeted therapies such as dupilumab, a monoclonal antibody against the IL-4 receptor alpha (IL-4Rα) subunit needed for IL-4 and IL-13 signaling, have shown effective modulation of the disease, pointing to the key roles these cytokines serve in AD [35]. JAK-STAT plays a critical role with these cytokines in AD development given its essential role in T_H2 cell differentiation [36].

Other Autoimmune Cutaneous Disorder

Jakinib use has been reported in smaller studies and case reports for vitiligo, dermatomyositis (DM), and cutaneous lupus erythematosus (CLE), but detailed information on the mechanism and affected signaling pathways have not yet been fully elucidated and are pending further study [37–39].

Janus Kinase Inhibitors in Cutaneous Disease

Discovery of the JAK-STAT pathway opened the doors for targeted treatment of a new class of mediators involved in inflammatory conditions. Currently, there are three FDA-approved Jakinibs for clinical use—tofacitinib for the treatment of RA [2], ruxolitinib for the treatment myelofibrosis [3] and polycythemia vera [4], and oclacitinib for the treatment of allergic dermatitis in canines [5]. The success of these agents has drawn interest in their use as immunomodulatory drugs to treat inflammatory disease, and in particular, cutaneous autoimmune disease. While currently there are no FDA-approved indications for Jakinibs in cutaneous disorders, several Jakinibs are in early and late stage testing in clinical trials (Table 19.3). Unlike targeted therapy with biologic medications such as those that block TNF-α, Jakinibs are small molecules that can be made into topical formulations given their ability to penetrate the epidermal barrier, opening up additional therapeutic delivery options [40].

Development of target specific Jakinibs is a significant challenge due to the degree of homology shared between the JAK family of protein-tyrosine kinases [14]. Target selectivity

Table 19.3 Jakinibs approved for clinical use and those under investigation for skin disease

Drug	Manufacturer	Target	Status and use
First-generation Jakinibs			
Tofacitinib (CP690550)	Pfizer	JAK3>JAK1>>(JAK2)	FDA approved—RA
			Phase III—psoriasis, PsA, UC
			Phase II—AS, JIA, CD
Ruxolitinib (INC424)	Incyte/Novartis	JAK1, JAK2	FDA approved—PV, myelofibrosis
			Phase II—psoriasis, AD, AA, vitiligo, various malignancies
Baricitinib (LY3009104)	Incyte/Eli Lilly	JAK1, JAK2	Under FDA review—RA
			Phase II—psoriasis, AD, SLE
Oclacitinib (PF03394197)	Zoetis	JAK1	FDA approved—canine allergic dermatitis
Second-generation Jakinibs			
Lestaurtinib (CEP-701)	TEVA	JAK2, FLT3	Phase III—AML (FDA approved under orphan drug status)
			Phase II—myelofibrosis, PV, ET, psoriasis
Peficitinib (ASP015K)	Astellas/Maruho	JAK1>JAK3>>JAK2	Phase III—RA
			Phase II—psoriasis
Solcitinib (GSK2586184)	Galapagos/GlaxoSmithKline	JAK1	Phase II—psoriasis, SLE
Upadacitinib (ABT-494)	Abbvie	JAK1	Phase III—RA, UC
			Phase II—CD, AD
Itacitinib (INCB039110)	Incyte	JAK1>JAK2	Phase II—RA, psoriasis, chronic pruritus, various malignancies
			Phase I—GVHD
PF-04965842	Pfizer	JAK1	Phase II—psoriasis, AD

Abbreviations: *RA* rheumatoid arthritis, *PsA* psoriatic arthritis, *UC* ulcerative colitis, *AS* ankylosing spondylitis, *JIA* juvenile idiopathic arthritis, *CD* Crohn's disease, *PV* polycythemia vera, *ET* essential thrombocytosis, *GVHD* graft versus host disease, *AA* alopecia areata, *AD* atopic dermatitis, *SLE* systemic lupus erythematosus, *FLT3* Fms-like tyrosine kinase 3, *AML* acute myeloid leukemia, *MDS* myelodysplastic syndrome, *NSCLC* non-small cell lung cancer

is a concern with systemic Jakinibs given the wide-reaching effects of potent signal modulation of multiple type I and II cytokines. Minor variations in the kinase domain of JAKs allow for more directed targeting, but often there is considerable cross-reactivity between Jakinibs and their intended JAK target. The first-generation Jakinibs (tofacitinib, ruxolitinib, baricitinib, and oclacitinib) demonstrate more broadly targeting effects, whereas second-generation Jakinibs are somewhat more specific (Table 19.4).

Tofacitinib

Tofacitinib is among the first of the Jakinibs put into clinical use. Initially designated for RA, it is now in trials for numerous other autoinflammatory conditions such as inflammatory bowel disease (IBD), psoriatic arthritis (PsA), juvenile idiopathic arthritis (JIA), ankylosing spondylitis (AS), and psoriasis.

Tofacitinib blocks JAK-STAT signaling by functioning as a reversible, competitive inhibitor at the ATP binding site on JAK, effectively inhibiting autophosphorylation and autoactivation [41]. JAK3 is preferentially targeted, but inhibitory effects are also seen with JAK1 and to a lesser extent with JAK2 while TYK2 is minimally affected [42]. IL-6 signaling through STAT1/3/5 is also attenuated [42, 43]. Broad downstream effects are seen in muted T_H1 and T_H17

Table 19.4 Jakinib selectivity indexed to their most selective receptor (IC_{50} values [nM])[a]

Drug	JAK1	JAK2	JAK3	TYK2
First-generation Jakinibs				
Tofacitinib [101] (CP690550)	6 (3)	2 (1)	1 (0.5)	22 (11)
Ruxolitinib [102] (INCB018424)	1 (3.3)	1 (2.8)	153 (428)	7 (19)
Baricitinib [103] (LY3009104)	1 (6)	1 (6)	67 (>400)	9 (53)
Oclacitinib [104] (PF03394197)	1 (10)	2 (18)	10 (99)	8 (84)
Second-generation Jakinibs				
Lestaurtinib [7] (CEP-701)	4 (8.8)	2 (3.7)	1 (2.3)	7 (15)
Peficitinib [74] (ASP015K)	5 (3.9)	7 (5)	1 (0.71)	7 (4.8)
Solcitinib [82] (GSK2586184)	1 (9.8)	11 (107.8)	55 (539)	23 (225.4)
Upadacitinib [78] ABT-494	1 (8, 40[b])	75 (600)	58 (2300[b])	–
Itacitinib (INCB039110)	–	–	–	–
PF-04965842	–	–	–	–

[a]Most IC_{50} data taken from in vitro cellular assay testing which may not accurately reflect in vivo receptor interactions and selectivity
[b]Extrapolated data based on ~58-fold higher IC_{50} in JAK1 versus JAK3 using a biochemical assay (40 nM and 2300 nM, respectively) compared to ~75-fold higher IC_{50} in JAK1 versus JAK2 from a cellular assay (8 nM versus 600 nM) [78]

CD4+ T-cell responses, the inhibition of antigen presentation in dendritic cells, and inhibition of B-cell differentiation and antibody production [44].

FDA-approved formulations of tofacitinib come as either 5 mg tablets taken twice daily or a single 11 mg extended release tablet taken once daily. Once orally ingested, peak plasma concentrations are reached around 1.1 h after administration. Clearance is predominantly via hepatic metabolism through CYP3A4 and CYP2C19 with the remaining 30% shuttling through renal clearance mechanisms. Mean half-life has been measured around 3.2 h. Recommendations for dose adjustments in moderate-to-severe renal impairment or moderate hepatic impairment is to reduce daily dosing to one 5 mg tablet. Tofacitinib is not recommended for use in severe hepatic impairment [41, 45]. Tofacitinib is considered a pregnancy category C medication due to the lack of sufficient data in pregnant women with caution being advised in breastfeeding women given findings from murine models where the drug was excreted into lactating milk [46].

Multiple phase 2 and 3 clinical trials of tofacitinib for RA established the drug as viable as monotherapy, combination treatment with standard DMARDs, or even as an alternative treatment for patients who have failed traditional biologics [47–51]. Treatment efficacy in trials with tofacitinib was demonstrated to have non-inferiority to the typical first-line biologic adalimumab and superiority to methotrexate in treatment naïve patients [49]. Radiologic monitoring also showed stabilization of destructive joint disease while on the drug as well [50, 52, 53].

Similar success has been seen in phase 2 and 3 psoriasis trials, though higher 10 mg twice daily dosing was required to match efficacy the efficacy of etanercept at its standard psoriasis dose [54, 55]. Lower dosing at 5 mg twice daily resulted in PASI 75 rates of only 39.5–46%, whereas the 10 mg twice daily dose achieved rates between 59.2 and 63.6% [54, 55]. Given the loss of response phenomenon often seen with biologic therapy, another study attempted to assess the durable response to tofacitinib following a withdrawal period. Data indicates that upward of 61% of patients resuming tofacitinib are able to recapture their initial PASI 75 response, but only 36.8% of patients at the lower RA dosing of 5 mg twice daily are able to achieve PASI 75 again [56]. Despite success in clinical trials, the FDA denied tofacitinib approval for psoriasis pending additional safety data given the higher 10 mg twice daily dose required to achieve acceptable clinical response.

A growing number of studies treating AA, alopecia totalis (AT), and alopecia universalis (AU) with tofacitinib have shown promising results in response to twice daily 5 mg tofacitinib treatment. After 3–4 months of treatment, as many as 77% of patients exhibit a relative improvement of at least >5% in hair growth with a slightly smaller subset of patients (ranging between 33 and 58%) having at least a 50% improvement [30, 57].

Topical formulations are also being actively assessed with promising results following therapeutic trials in many conditions. Results from a phase 2a study in psoriasis demonstrated efficacy at week 4 for a 2% topical formulation over plain vehicle [58]. Another phase 2a study in AD showed a significant change from the baseline eczema severity score compared to placebo after 4 weeks of treatment [59]. Meanwhile, murine studies of topical tofacitinib for AA have been highly effective in restoring hair growth [31]. While the FDA approval of topical tofacitinib is likely not forthcoming, the proof of concept opens the door for other similar topical medications to be tested.

Ruxolitinib

Ruxolitinib is a potent JAK1 and JAK2 inhibitor initially developed for the treatment of myeloproliferative disease. It has the distinction for being the first ever FDA-approved Jakinib for clinical use [6]. Dramatic results are observed in the treatment of polycythemia vera and myelofibrosis as ruxolitinib directly targets the aberrant signaling mechanism induced by the activating JAK2 V617F mutation [60].

Ruxolitinib has also found secondary usage in the treatment of cutaneous diseases for psoriasis, vitiligo, and alopecia areata. Topical treatment in a small phase 2 study of psoriasis patients demonstrated greater efficacy at the end of 4 weeks with ruxolitinib 1.5% cream applied twice daily compared to topical calcipotriene and betamethasone dipropionate cream [61]. In a larger phase 2 study of 200 participants, ruxolitinib 1% cream induced an average 40% PASI improvement compared to 1% PASI improvement in the placebo group [62]. Orally administered ruxolitinib in AA showed similar positive improvement with 75% of patients (9 of 12) experiencing significant scalp hair regrowth and improvement of average hair regrowth exceeding 90% at the end of 3–6 months of treatment [63]. Further topical studies in AA, AD, and vitiligo are currently ongoing [64–66].

Baricitinib

Baricitinib is another JAK1 and JAK2 selective inhibitor currently under FDA review for the treatment of RA. Data from several phase 3 studies reflect a strong positive response to baricitinib treatment. It is capable of halting joint disease and has also been used effectively to treat patients who are refractory to traditional DMARD or biologic treatment [67–70]. Comparisons in dosing regiments suggest a greater efficacy at the higher 4 mg daily dose over the 2 mg daily dose with only negligible effects on medication-related adverse events [71]. Similar to the case in tofacitinib, treatment in psoriatic patients requires higher doses to achieve comparable results. 8 and 10 mg daily dosing in the psoriasis trials were associated with PASI 75 rates of 43% and 54% at the 12-week endpoint [72]. Testing in AD is currently ongoing with a randomized, double-blind, placebo-controlled, phase 2 trial [73].

Select Second-Generation Jakinibs in Current Testing for Dermatologic Conditions

At the present time, six additional second-generation Jakinibs—lestaurtinib, ABT-494, peficitinib, itacitinib, PF-04965842, and solcitinib—are involved in clinical testing for dermatologic disorders, four of which have preliminary data available. Though still in early testing, the hope with some of the selective second-generation Jakinibs is that preferential targeting away from JAK2 will result in a milder adverse effect profile, particularly as it relates to hematologic abnormalities that are seen with pan-inhibiting Jakinibs.

Peficitinib, a novel oral JAK inhibitor with mild selectivity for JAK3, is in development for the treatment of RA and psoriasis [74]. Clinical testing at once daily dosing in a randomized, double-blind, placebo-controlled study is correlated with a dose-dependent improvement response for psoriasis [75]. Positive findings are also seen in RA testing where once daily dosing up to 150 mg of peficitinib showed effectiveness as monotherapy for RA [74].

Itacitinib is currently under investigation as a therapeutic agent for psoriasis as well as for chronic pruritus. Cell-assay testing demonstrates highly selective JAK1 inhibition with at least 420-fold selectivity over other JAKs [76]. Early clinical testing thus far is promising for psoriasis given notable efficacy during a dose-escalation study over 4 weeks during which the drug was well tolerated. A phase 2 study is currently pending to assess the effect of oral itacitinib administration for symptoms of chronic pruritus [77].

Like itacitinib, ABT-494 is a highly selective JAK1 inhibitor in testing against RA and AD, as well as other diseases [78]. ABT-494 is effective in controlling active RA patients with inadequate responses to MTX, and as such, further phase 3 studies are planned to better characterize the clinical and pharmacological profile of the drug [78]. In addition, a phase 2b randomized, placebo-controlled, dose-ranging study is currently planned for atopic dermatitis [79].

PF-04965842 is a novel JAK1 specific inhibitor currently in phase 2 testing for psoriasis and atopic dermatitis. Preliminary data from the psoriasis trial with 59 participants is notable for a dose-escalation response. PASI reduction of 33%, 58%, 68%, and 76% across the placebo, 200 mg daily, 400 mg daily, and 200 mg twice daily groups were seen with treatment [80]. Enrollment for a phase 2b study in severe atopic dermatitis is currently underway [81].

Early solcitinib data shows a JAK1 selective inhibition with minimal effect on JAK2. Recent phase 2 results for the drug in psoriasis realized a 57% PASI 75 and 36% PASI 90 at week 12 of treatment using the highest 400 mg twice daily dose in the study [82].

Minimal data relating to studies on cutaneous disorders is available for lestaurtinib. Phase 2 dose escalation trials for psoriasis were completed, but results of the trial have not yet been made available [83].

Adverse Effects of Jakinibs

Many adverse effects in the Jakinibs class can be linked to their ability to block cytokine signaling. The interest in cleaner JAK inhibition with newer second-generation Jakinibs stems from desire to avoid overly broad inhibition of cytokine signaling. Current safety data comes from both tofacitinib and baricitinib use, though tofacitinib is more heavily weighted in a review of adverse effects due to the more frequent use of this medication in clinical studies and post-marketing surveillance. Studies to date seem to indicate similar safety profiles for both of these medications [69, 70].

Laboratory Abnormalities

All first-generation Jakinibs signaling though JAK2 can cause cytopenias—most commonly anemia with neutropenia, though lymphopenias are not uncommon as well [6]. When it occurs, lymphocytosis typically starts around 1 month following exposure, before a slower gradual decline of another 10% over the following calendar year. In pooled data from long-term extension studies with tofacitinib, neutropenia was reported in 0.7% of cases (30/4095), anemia in 2.7% (109/4095), but lymphopenia in 53.7% (2197/4095) [84]. Recommended parameters from the tofacitinib product insert indicate that therapy should be held for hemoglobin less than 8 g/dL, ANC less than 1000 cells/mm^3, or lymphocyte counts less than 500 cells/mm^3 [45]. Increasing tofacitinib dosing to 15 mg twice daily did result in significantly more severe and frequent cytopenias demonstrating a dose-dependent response not seen at lower dosage levels [85].

Minor transaminitis was seen in over 30% of patients, but AST $\geq$ 2 times the upper limit of normal (ULN) was only noted in 3.8% (152/4102) and ALT $\geq$ 2 × ULN in 6% (244/4102) [84]. Increased levels of cholesterol, LDL, and HDL have also been noted among treated patients, suggesting a possible intertwining of immune and metabolic signaling, especially given that treatment of RA patients with tocilizumab, an IL-6R blocker, results in similar phenotypic hypercholesterolemia [86]. Pooled analysis from long-term extension data did not show any clinically relevant increase in incidence of major adverse cardiovascular events (MACE) [87]. Lipid levels typically peaked within 6 weeks of starting therapy.

Immunosuppression

Serious or opportunistic infections are a significant source of worry for both patients and physicians alike. The most common adverse effects reported were nasopharyngitis and upper respiratory infections at 12.7% and 10.5%, respectively [84]. Severe infection events from a meta-analysis of tofacitinib collectively estimated 3.19 events per 100 person-years across all long-term studies at the 10 mg twice daily dose [88]. Opportunistic infections (including tuberculosis) come out to 0.4 events per 100 person-years in a different combined long-term extension safety review [84]. Neutropenia with ANC <500 cells/mm^3 has been associated with an increased incidence of treated and serious infections; therefore, these individuals should not be treated with tofacitinib [45]. Of note, herpes zoster infection/reactivation occurs at 4.3 events per 100 person-years in Jakinib users compared to 2.4 events per 100 person-years in a similar comparator group not on Jakinibs [84, 89]. The effect of pretreatment varicella zoster vaccination is unclear.

A secondary concern of immunosuppression is the potential for malignancy development, due to JAK1 and JAK2 signal blockade, especially with regards to interferon signaling. However, short- and long-term study data do not show increased rates of malignancy [84, 90, 91]. Given the relative short term of available clinical data compared to some of the older biologics or DMARDs, caution should be exercised when considering treatment of individuals with a history of malignancy.

Future Considerations

The advent of targeted inhibition of the JAK-STAT pathway opens up new possibilities in treating and managing chronic inflammatory skin disease. Early efforts on selectively attenuating the cytokine signal transduction involved in autoinflammatory responses are already resulting in tangible clinical benefits. As newer Jakinibs continue to be developed based on JAK subgroup fidelity, additional benefits involving higher response rates, fewer adverse events and a broader choice of responsive disease states may be realized.

Case Scenario

A 52-year-old man is referred to the psoriasis clinic for severe widespread plaque psoriasis involving 60% of his body surface area (BSA). This follows the failure of numerous other medications. Methotrexate therapy was initially attempted with mild efficacy. However, the patient suffered from debilitating fatigue and marked transaminitis which limited ongoing use. Short courses of cyclosporine were very effective, but therapy was discontinued due to signs of medication induced renal toxicity. Adequate trials of both etanercept and adalimumab were ineffective. The patient had most recently been well controlled on ustekinumab and then subsequently ixekizumab over the past 18 months until clinical response was lost to both biologics. The patient was subsequently started on off-label therapy with tofacitinib 5 mg taken orally twice daily before escalation to 10 mg twice daily after 3 months to manage his severe psoriasis.

References

1. Wilks AF. Two putative protein-tyrosine kinases identified by application of the polymerase chain reaction. Proc Natl Acad Sci U S A. 1989;86(5):1603–7.
2. FDA. FDA approves Xeljanz for rheumatoid arthritis 2012 [updated Nov. 6, 2012]. http://www.fda.gov/NewsEvents/Newsroom/PressAnnouncements/ucm327152.htm.
3. FDA. FDA approves first drug to treat a rare bone marrow disease 2011 [updated Nov. 16, 2011]. http://www.fda.gov/NewsEvents/Newsroom/PressAnnouncements/ucm280102.htm.
4. FDA. FDA approves Jakafi to treat patients with a chronic type of bone marrow disease 2014 [updated December 4, 2014]. Available from: http://www.fda.gov/NewsEvents/Newsroom/PressAnnouncements/ucm425677.htm.
5. FDA. NADA 141–345 APOQUEL Oclacitinib Tablet Dogs 2013 [updated May 14, 2013]. http://www.fda.gov/downloads/AnimalV.../UCM363901.pdf.
6. O'Shea JJ, Schwartz DM, Villarino AV, Gadina M, McInnes IB, Laurence A. The JAK-STAT pathway: impact on human disease and therapeutic intervention. Annu Rev Med. 2015;66:311–28.
7. Roskoski R Jr. Janus kinase (JAK) inhibitors in the treatment of inflammatory and neoplastic diseases. Pharmacol Res. 2016;111:784–803.
8. Williams NK, Bamert RS, Patel O, Wang C, Walden PM, Wilks AF, et al. Dissecting specificity in the Janus kinases: the structures of JAK-specific inhibitors complexed to the JAK1 and JAK2 protein tyrosine kinase domains. J Mol Biol. 2009;387(1):219–32.
9. Kawamura M, McVicar DW, Johnston JA, Blake TB, Chen YQ, Lal BK, et al. Molecular cloning of L-JAK, a Janus family protein-tyrosine kinase expressed in natural killer cells and activated leukocytes. Proc Natl Acad Sci U S A. 1994;91(14):6374–8.
10. Candotti F, Oakes SA, Johnston JA, Giliani S, Schumacher RF, Mella P, et al. Structural and functional basis for JAK3-deficient severe combined immunodeficiency. Blood. 1997;90(10):3996–4003.
11. Chen M, Cheng A, Candotti F, Zhou YJ, Hymel A, Fasth A, et al. Complex effects of naturally occurring mutations in the JAK3 pseudokinase domain: evidence for interactions between the kinase and pseudokinase domains. Mol Cell Biol. 2000;20(3):947–56.
12. Stark GR, Darnell JE Jr. The JAK-STAT pathway at twenty. Immunity. 2012;36(4):503–14.
13. Chen X, Vinkemeier U, Zhao Y, Jeruzalmi D, Darnell JE Jr, Kuriyan J. Crystal structure of a tyrosine phosphorylated STAT-1 dimer bound to DNA. Cell. 1998;93(5):827–39.
14. Schwartz DM, Bonelli M, Gadina M, O'Shea JJ. Type I/II cytokines, JAKs, and new strategies for treating autoimmune diseases. Nat Rev Rheumatol. 2016;12(1):25–36.
15. Samadi A, Ahmad Nasrollahi S, Hashemi A, Nassiri Kashani M, Firooz A. Janus kinase (JAK) inhibitors for the treatment of skin and hair disorders: a review of literature. J Dermatolog Treat 2017:1–11.
16. Laurence A, Pesu M, Silvennoinen O, O'Shea J. JAK kinases in health and disease: an update. Open Rheumatol J. 2012;6:232–44.
17. Kisseleva T, Bhattacharya S, Braunstein J, Schindler CW. Signaling through the JAK/STAT pathway, recent advances and future challenges. Gene. 2002;285(1–2):1–24.

18. Bandaranayake RM, Ungureanu D, Shan Y, Shaw DE, Silvennoinen O, Hubbard SR. Crystal structures of the JAK2 pseudokinase domain and the pathogenic mutant V617F. Nat Struct Mol Biol. 2012;19(8):754–9.

19. Baxter EJ, Scott LM, Campbell PJ, East C, Fourouclas N, Swanton S, et al. Acquired mutation of the tyrosine kinase JAK2 in human myeloproliferative disorders. Lancet. 2005;365(9464):1054–61.

20. Buckley RH. Molecular defects in human severe combined immunodeficiency and approaches to immune reconstitution. Annu Rev Immunol. 2004;22:625–55.

21. O'Shea JJ, Holland SM, Staudt LM. JAKs and STATs in immunity, immunodeficiency, and cancer. N Engl J Med. 2013;368(2):161–70.

22. Chiricozzi A, Faleri S, Saraceno R, Bianchi L, Buonomo O, Chimenti S, et al. Tofacitinib for the treatment of moderate-to-severe psoriasis. Expert Rev Clin Immunol. 2015;11(4):443–55.

23. Lowes MA, Suarez-Farinas M, Krueger JG. Immunology of psoriasis. Annu Rev Immunol. 2014;32:227–55.

24. Alves de Medeiros AK, Speeckaert R, Desmet E, Van Gele M, De Schepper S, Lambert J. JAK3 as an emerging target for topical treatment of inflammatory skin diseases. PLoS One. 2016;11(10):e0164080.

25. Andres RM, Hald A, Johansen C, Kragballe K, Iversen L. Studies of Jak/STAT3 expression and signalling in psoriasis identifies STAT3-Ser727 phosphorylation as a modulator of transcriptional activity. Exp Dermatol. 2013;22(5):323–8.

26. Hald A, Andres RM, Salskov-Iversen ML, Kjellerup RB, Iversen L, Johansen C. STAT1 expression and activation is increased in lesional psoriatic skin. Br J Dermatol. 2013;168(2):302–10.

27. Chang BY, Zhao F, He X, Ren H, Braselmann S, Taylor V, et al. JAK3 inhibition significantly attenuates psoriasiform skin inflammation in CD18 mutant PL/J mice. J Immunol. 2009;183(3):2183–92.

28. Nakajima K. Critical role of the interleukin-23/T-helper 17 cell axis in the pathogenesis of psoriasis. J Dermatol. 2012;39(3):219–24.

29. Cho ML, Kang JW, Moon YM, Nam HJ, Jhun JY, Heo SB, et al. STAT3 and NF-kappaB signal pathway is required for IL-23-mediated IL-17 production in spontaneous arthritis animal model IL-1 receptor antagonist-deficient mice. J Immunol. 2006;176(9):5652–61.

30. Liu LY, Craiglow BG, Dai F, King BA. Tofacitinib for the treatment of severe alopecia areata and variants: a study of 90 patients. J Am Acad Dermatol. 2017;76(1):22–8.

31. Xing L, Dai Z, Jabbari A, Cerise JE, Higgins CA, Gong W, et al. Alopecia areata is driven by cytotoxic T lymphocytes and is reversed by JAK inhibition. Nat Med. 2014;20(9):1043–9.

32. DaVeiga SP. Epidemiology of atopic dermatitis: a review. Allergy Asthma Proc. 2012;33(3):227–34.

33. Leung DY, Bieber T. Atopic dermatitis. Lancet. 2003;361(9352):151–60.

34. O'Shea JJ, Plenge R. JAK and STAT signaling molecules in immunoregulation and immune-mediated disease. Immunity. 2012;36(4):542–50.

35. Beck LA, Thaci D, Hamilton JD, Graham NM, Bieber T, Rocklin R, et al. Dupilumab treatment in adults with moderate-to-severe atopic dermatitis. N Engl J Med. 2014;371(2):130–9.

36. Bao L, Zhang H, Chan LS. The involvement of the JAK-STAT signaling pathway in chronic inflammatory skin disease atopic dermatitis. JAKSTAT. 2013;2(3):e24137.

37. Craiglow BG, King BA. Tofacitinib citrate for the treatment of vitiligo: a pathogenesis-directed therapy. JAMA Dermatol. 2015;151(10):1110–2.

38. Klaeschen AS, Wenzel J. Upcoming therapeutic targets in cutaneous lupus erythematous. Expert Rev Clin Pharmacol. 2016:1–12.

39. Kurtzman DJ, Wright NA, Lin J, Femia AN, Merola JF, Patel M, et al. Tofacitinib citrate for refractory cutaneous dermatomyositis: an alternative treatment. JAMA Dermatol. 2016;152(8):944–5.

40. van de Kerkhof PC. An update on topical therapies for mild-moderate psoriasis. Dermatol Clin. 2015;33(1):73–7.

41. Dowty ME, Lin J, Ryder TF, Wang W, Walker GS, Vaz A, et al. The pharmacokinetics, metabolism, and clearance mechanisms of tofacitinib, a janus kinase inhibitor, in humans. Drug Metab Dispos. 2014;42(4):759–73.

42. Ghoreschi K, Jesson MI, Li X, Lee JL, Ghosh S, Alsup JW, et al. Modulation of innate and adaptive immune responses by tofacitinib (CP-690,550). J Immunol. 2011;186(7):4234–43.

43. Lindstrom TM, Robinson WH. A multitude of kinases—which are the best targets in treating rheumatoid arthritis? Rheum Dis Clin N Am. 2010;36(2):367–83.

44. Kubo S, Yamaoka K, Kondo M, Yamagata K, Zhao J, Iwata S, et al. The JAK inhibitor, tofacitinib, reduces the T cell stimulatory capacity of human monocyte-derived dendritic cells. Ann Rheum Dis 2014;73(12):2192–2198.

45. Xeljanz. package insert. New York, NY: Pfizer Laboratories; 2016.

46. Clowse ME, Feldman SR, Isaacs JD, Kimball AB, Strand V, Warren RB, et al. Pregnancy outcomes in the tofacitinib safety databases for rheumatoid arthritis and psoriasis. Drug Saf. 2016;39(8):755–62.

47. Fleischmann R, Kremer J, Cush J, Schulze-Koops H, Connell CA, Bradley JD, et al. Placebo-controlled trial of tofacitinib monotherapy in rheumatoid arthritis. N Engl J Med. 2012;367(6):495–507.

48. Burmester GR, Blanco R, Charles-Schoeman C, Wollenhaupt J, Zerbini C, Benda B, et al. Tofacitinib (CP-690,550) in combination with methotrexate in patients with active rheumatoid arthritis with an inadequate response to tumour necrosis factor inhibitors: a randomised phase 3 trial. Lancet. 2013;381(9865):451–60.

49. van Vollenhoven RF, Fleischmann R, Cohen S, Lee EB, Garcia Meijide JA, Wagner S, et al. Tofacitinib or adalimumab versus placebo in rheumatoid arthritis. N Engl J Med. 2012;367(6):508–19.

50. van der Heijde D, Tanaka Y, Fleischmann R, Keystone E, Kremer J, Zerbini C, et al. Tofacitinib (CP-690,550) in patients with rheumatoid arthritis receiving methotrexate: twelve-month data from a twenty-four-month phase III randomized radiographic study. Arthritis Rheum. 2013;65(3):559–70.

51. Lee EB, Fleischmann RM, Hall S, van Vollenhoven RF, Bradley J, et al. Radiographic, clinical and functional comparison of tofacitinib monotherapy versus methotrexate in methotrexate-nave patients with rheumatoid arthritis. Arthritis Rheum. 2012;(S):64, 1049.

52. Lee EB, Fleischmann R, Hall S, Wilkinson B, Bradley JD, Gruben D, et al. Tofacitinib versus methotrexate in rheumatoid arthritis. N Engl J Med. 2014;370(25):2377–86.

53. Conaghan PG, Ostergaard M, Bowes MA, Wu C, Fuerst T, van der Heijde D, et al. Effects of tofacitinib on MRI enpoints in methotrexate-naive early rheumatoid arthritis: a phase 2 MRI study with semi-quantitative and quantitative endpoints. Ann Rheum Dis. 2015;74(Suppl 2):738.

54. Papp KA, Menter MA, Abe M, Elewski B, Feldman SR, Gottlieb AB, et al. Tofacitinib, an oral Janus kinase inhibitor, for the treatment of chronic plaque psoriasis: results from two randomized, placebo-controlled, phase III trials. Br J Dermatol. 2015;173(4):949–61.

55. Bachelez H, van de Kerkhof PCM, Strohal R, Kubanov A, Valenzuela F, Lee J-H, et al. Tofacitinib versus etanercept or placebo in moderate-to-severe chronic plaque psoriasis: a phase 3 randomised non-inferiority trial. Lancet. 2015;386(9993):552–61.

56. Bissonnette R, Iversen L, Sofen H, Griffiths CE, Foley P, Romiti R, et al. Tofacitinib withdrawal and retreatment in moderate-to-severe chronic plaque psoriasis: a randomized controlled trial. Br J Dermatol. 2015;172(5):1395–406.

57. Kennedy Crispin M, Ko JM, Craiglow BG, Li S, Shankar G, Urban JR, et al. Safety and efficacy of the JAK inhibitor tofacitinib citrate in patients with alopecia areata. JCI Insight. 2016;1(15):e89776.

58. Ports WC, Khan S, Lan S, Lamba M, Bolduc C, Bissonnette R, et al. A randomized phase 2a efficacy and safety trial of the topical Janus kinase inhibitor tofacitinib in the treatment of chronic plaque psoriasis. Br J Dermatol. 2013;169(1):137–45.

59. Bissonnette R, Papp KA, Poulin Y, Gooderham M, Raman M, Mallbris L, et al. Topical tofacitinib for atopic dermatitis: a phase IIa randomized trial. Br J Dermatol. 2016;175(5):902–11.

60. Cervantes F, Vannucchi AM, Kiladjian JJ, Al-Ali HK, Sirulnik A, Stalbovskaya V, et al. Three-year efficacy, safety, and survival findings from COMFORT-II, a phase 3 study comparing ruxolitinib with best available therapy for myelofibrosis. Blood. 2013;122(25):4047–53.

61. Punwani N, Scherle P, Flores R, Shi J, Liang J, Yeleswaram S, et al. Preliminary clinical activity of a topical JAK1/2 inhibitor in the treatment of psoriasis. J Am Acad Dermatol. 2012;67(4):658–64.

62. Ortiz-Ibanez K, Alsina MM, Munoz-Santos C. Tofacitinib and other kinase inhibitors in the treatment of psoriasis. Actas Dermosifiliogr. 2013;104(4):304–10.

63. Mackay-Wiggan J, Jabbari A, Nguyen N, Cerise JE, Clark C, Ulerio G, et al. Oral ruxolitinib induces hair regrowth in patients with moderate-to-severe alopecia areata. JCI Insight. 2016;1(15):e89790.

64. Identifier NCT02809976. Topical Ruxolitinib for the Treatment of Vitiligo [Internet]. https://clinicaltrials.gov/ct2/show/NCT028099 76?term=Ruxolitinib&rank=11.

65. Identifier NCT03011892. A study to evaluate the safety and efficacy of INCB018424 phosphate cream applied topically to adults with atopic dermatitis [Internet]. https://clinicaltrials.gov/ct2/show/NCT03011892?term=Ruxolitinib&rank=87.

66. Identifier NCT02553330. A study with INCB018424 phosphate cream applied topically to subjects with alopecia areata (AA) [Internet]. https://clinicaltrials.gov/ct2/show/NCT02553330?term=Ruxolitinib&rank=92.

67. Keystone EC, Taylor PC, Drescher E, Schlichting DE, Beattie SD, Berclaz PY, et al. Safety and efficacy of baricitinib at 24 weeks in patients with rheumatoid arthritis who have had an inadequate response to methotrexate. Ann Rheum Dis. 2015;74(2):333–40.

68. Smolen JS, Kremer JM, Gaich CL, DeLozier AM, Schlichting DE, Xie L, et al. Patient-reported outcomes from a randomised phase III study of baricitinib in patients with rheumatoid arthritis and an inadequate response to biological agents (RA-BEACON). Ann Rheum Dis. 2017;76(4):694–700.

69. Genovese MC, Kremer J, Zamani O, Ludivico C, Krogulec M, Xie L, et al. OP0029-Baricitinib, an oral Janus Kinase (JAK)1/JAK2 inhibitor, in patients with active rheumatoid arthritis (RA) and an inadequate response to TNF inhibitors: results of the phase 3 RA-beacon study. Ann Rheum Dis. 2015;74(S2):75–6.

70. Dougados M, van der Heijde D, Chen YC, Greenwald M, Drescher E, Liu J, et al. Baricitinib, an oral Janus Kinase (JAK)1/JAK2 inhibitor, in patients with active rheumatoid arthritis (RA) and an inadequate response to cDMARD therapy: results of the phase 3 RA-BUILD Study. Ann Rheum Dis. 2015;74(S2)

71. Genovese MC, Kremer J, Zamani O, Ludivico C, Krogulec M, Xie L, et al. Baricitinib in Patients with Refractory Rheumatoid Arthritis. N Engl J Med. 2016;374(13):1243–52.

72. Papp KA, Menter MA, Raman M, Disch D, Schlichting DE, Gaich C, et al. A randomized phase 2b trial of baricitinib, an oral Janus kinase (JAK) 1/JAK2 inhibitor, in patients with moderate-to-severe psoriasis. Br J Dermatol. 2016;174(6):1266–76.

73. Identifier NCT02576938. A study of baricitinib (LY3009104) in participants with moderate-to-severe atopic dermatitis [Internet]. https://clinicaltrials.gov/ct2/show/NCT02576938?term=baricitinib+atopic+dermatitis&rank=1.

74. Takeuchi T, Tanaka Y, Iwasaki M, Ishikura H, Saeki S, Kaneko Y. Efficacy and safety of the oral Janus kinase inhibitor peficitinib (ASP015K) monotherapy in patients with moderate to severe rheumatoid arthritis in Japan: a 12-week, randomised, double-blind, placebo-controlled phase IIb study. Ann Rheum Dis. 2016;75(6):1057–64.

75. Papp K, Pariser D, Catlin M, Wierz G, Ball G, Akinlade B, et al. A phase 2a randomized, double-blind, placebo-controlled, sequential dose-escalation study to evaluate the efficacy and safety of ASP015K, a novel Janus kinase inhibitor, in patients with moderate-to-severe psoriasis. Br J Dermatol. 2015;173(3):767–76.

76. Bissonnette R, Luchi M, Fidelus-Gort R, Jackson S, Zhang H, Flores R, et al. A randomized, double-blind, placebo-controlled, dose-escalation study of the safety and efficacy of INCB039110, an oral janus kinase 1 inhibitor, in patients with stable, chronic plaque psoriasis. J Dermatolog Treat. 2016;27(4):332–8.

77. Identifier NCT02909569. Relieving chronic itch: oral medication (CIPS) [Internet]. https://clinicaltrials.gov/ct2/show/NCT029095 69?term=INCB039110&rank=15.

78. Genovese MC, Smolen JS, Weinblatt ME, Burmester GR, Meerwein S, Camp HS, et al. Efficacy and safety of ABT-494, a selective JAK-1 inhibitor, in a phase IIb study in patients with rheumatoid arthritis and an inadequate response to methotrexate. Arthritis Rheum. 2016;68(12):2857–66.

79. Identifier NCT02925117. A study to evaluate ABT-494 in adult subjects with moderate to severe atopic dermatitis [Internet]. https://clinicaltrials.gov/ct2/show/NCT02925117?term=ABt-494&rank=6.

80. Identifier NCT02201524. Study to evaluate PF-04965842 in patients with moderate to severe psoriasis [Internet]. https://clinicaltrials.gov/ct2/show/results/NCT02201524?sect=X70156&term=PF-04965842&rank=1 - outcome1.

81. Identifier NCT02780167. Study to evaluate Pf-04965842 in subjects with moderate to severe atopic dermatitis [Internet]. https://clinicaltrials.gov/ct2/show/NCT02780167.

82. Ludbrook VJ, Hicks KJ, Hanrott KE, Patel JS, Binks MH, Wyres MR, et al. Investigation of selective JAK1 inhibitor GSK2586184 for the treatment of psoriasis in a randomized placebo-controlled phase IIa study. Br J Dermatol. 2016;174(5):985–95.

83. Identifier NCT00236119. Study of the efficacy, safety and tolerability of oral CEP-701 in patients with severe psoriasis [Internet]. https://clinicaltrials.gov/ct2/show/NCT00236119?term=lestaurtinib&rank=8.

84. Wollenhaupt J, Silverfield J, Lee EB, Curtis JR, Wood SP, Soma K, et al. Safety and efficacy of tofacitinib, an oral janus kinase inhibitor, for the treatment of rheumatoid arthritis in open-label, longterm extension studies. J Rheumatol. 2014;41(5):837–52.

85. Strober B, Buonanno M, Clark JD, Kawabata T, Tan H, Wolk R, et al. Effect of tofacitinib, a Janus kinase inhibitor, on haematological parameters during 12 weeks of psoriasis treatment. Br J Dermatol. 2013;169(5):992–9.

86. Rao VU, Pavlov A, Klearman M, Musselman D, Giles JT, Bathon JM, et al. An evaluation of risk factors for major adverse cardiovascular events during tocilizumab therapy. Arthritis Rheum. 2015;67(2):372–80.

87. Wu JJ, Strober BE, Hansen PR, Ahlehoff O, Egeberg A, Qureshi AA, et al. Effects of tofacitinib on cardiovascular risk factors and cardiovascular outcomes based on phase III and long-term extension data in patients with plaque psoriasis. J Am Acad Dermatol. 2016;75(5):897–905.

88. Strand V, Ahadieh S, French J, Geier J, Krishnaswami S, Menon S, et al. Systematic review and meta-analysis of serious infections with tofacitinib and biologic disease-modifying antirheumatic drug treatment in rheumatoid arthritis clinical trials. Arthritis Res Ther. 2015;17:362.

89. Winthrop KL, Yamanaka H, Valdez H, Mortensen E, Chew R, Krishnaswami S, et al. Herpes zoster and tofacitinib therapy in patients with rheumatoid arthritis. Arthritis Rheum. 2014;66(10):2675–84.

90. Sivaraman P, Cohen SB. Malignancy and Janus Kinase inhibition. Rheum Dis Clin N Am. 2017;43(1):79–93.

91. Curtis JR, Lee EB, Kaplan IV, Kwok K, Geier J, Benda B, et al. Tofacitinib, an oral Janus kinase inhibitor: analysis of malignancies across the rheumatoid arthritis clinical development programme. Ann Rheum Dis. 2016;75(5):831–41.

92. Woellner C, Schaffer AA, Puck JM, Renner ED, Knebel C, Holland SM, et al. The hyper IgE syndrome and mutations in TYK2. Immunity. 2007;26(5):535; author reply 6.

93. Dupuis S, Dargemont C, Fieschi C, Thomassin N, Rosenzweig S, Harris J, et al. Impairment of mycobacterial but not viral immunity by a germline human STAT1 mutation. Science. 2001;293(5528):300–3.

94. Kong XF, Ciancanelli M, Al-Hajjar S, Alsina L, Zumwalt T, Bustamante J, et al. A novel form of human STAT1 deficiency impairing early but not late responses to interferons. Blood. 2010;116(26):5895–906.

95. O'Shea JJ, Kontzias A, Yamaoka K, Tanaka Y, Laurence A. Janus kinase inhibitors in autoimmune diseases. Ann Rheum Dis. 2013;72(Suppl 2):ii111–5.

96. Hambleton S, Goodbourn S, Young DF, Dickinson P, Mohamad SM, Valappil M, et al. STAT2 deficiency and susceptibility to viral illness in humans. Proc Natl Acad Sci U S A. 2013;110(8):3053–8.

97. Minegishi Y, Saito M, Tsuchiya S, Tsuge I, Takada H, Hara T, et al. Dominant-negative mutations in the DNA-binding domain of STAT3 cause hyper-IgE syndrome. Nature. 2007;448(7157):1058–62.

98. Ellinghaus D, Ellinghaus E, Nair RP, Stuart PE, Esko T, Metspalu A, et al. Combined analysis of genome-wide association studies for Crohn disease and psoriasis identifies seven shared susceptibility loci. Am J Hum Genet. 2012;90(4):636–47.

99. Remmers EF, Plenge RM, Lee AT, Graham RR, Hom G, Behrens TW, et al. STAT4 and the risk of rheumatoid arthritis and systemic lupus erythematosus. N Engl J Med. 2007;357(10):977–86.

100. Duetsch G, Illig T, Loesgen S, Rohde K, Klopp N, Herbon N, et al. STAT6 as an asthma candidate gene: polymorphism-screening, association and haplotype analysis in a Caucasian sib-pair study. Hum Mol Genet. 2002;11(6):613–21.

101. Farmer LJ, Ledeboer MW, Hoock T, Arnost MJ, Bethiel RS, Bennani YL, et al. Discovery of VX-509 (Decernotinib): a potent and selective Janus Kinase 3 inhibitor for the treatment of autoimmune diseases. J Med Chem. 2015;58(18):7195–216.

102. Quintas-Cardama A, Vaddi K, Liu P, Manshouri T, Li J, Scherle PA, et al. Preclinical characterization of the selective JAK1/2 inhibitor INCB018424: therapeutic implications for the treatment of myeloproliferative neoplasms. Blood. 2010;115(15): 3109–17.

103. Kim MK, Shin H, Park KS, Kim H, Park J, Kim K, et al. Benzimidazole derivatives as potent JAK1-selective inhibitors. J Med Chem. 2015;58(18):7596–602.

104. Gonzales AJ, Bowman JW, Fici GJ, Zhang M, Mann DW, Mitton-Fry M. Oclacitinib (APOQUEL((R))) is a novel Janus kinase inhibitor with activity against cytokines involved in allergy. J Vet Pharmacol Ther. 2014;37(4):317–24.

Katrina Lee, Amber Alcaraz, and Jennifer Soung

Abbreviations

Bath PUVA	Bath photochemotherapy
BSA	Body surface area
CLE	Cutaneous lupus erythematosus
DLE	Discoid lupus erythematosus
DMF	Dimethyl fumarate
DTIC	Dacarbazine; anticancer chemotherapy drug
FAE(s)	Fumaric acid ester(s)
GSH	Glutathione; antioxidant
MEF	Monoethylfumarate
MMF	Monomethylfumarate
NFkB	Nuclear factor-kappa B
NL	Necrobiosis lipoidica
PASI	Psoriasis Area and Severity Index
PGA	Physician's Global Assessment
PPP	Psoriasis pustulosa palmoplantaris
PPPASI	Palmo-plantar Pustular Psoriasis Area Severity Index
RCLASI	Revised Cutaneous Lupus Erythematosus Disease Area and Severity Index
SCID	Severe combined immunodeficiency
SCLE	Subacute cutaneous lupus erythematosus
VEGFR2	Vascular endothelial growth factor receptor 2

K. Lee, BS
School of Medicine, UC Irvine Medical Center,
University of California, Irvine, CA 92617, USA
e-mail: katrihl1@uci.edu

A. Alcaraz, BA • J. Soung, MD (✉)
Clinical Research, Southern California Dermatology, Inc,
Santa Ana, CA 92701, USA
e-mail: aalcaraz092@gmail.com; doctorsoung@gmail.com

Introduction and Pharmacology

History

Oral fumaric acid esters (FAEs) are simple dicarbonic acid molecules that demonstrate immune-modulating effects on the T-cell system [1]. Schweckendiek, a German chemist, first proposed FAEs as an oral treatment for psoriasis vulgaris in 1959 after a number of self-experiments reported positive improvement of his own psoriatic lesions. After developing several formulations of fumarates, a composed mixture of different FAEs with dimethyl fumarate (DMF) and monoethylfumarate (MEF) salts showed higher efficacy and bioavailability when compared against fumaric acid itself [2, 3].

After a renewed interest in FAEs during the 1980s by both patients and dermatologists, preliminary observational studies were conducted in Switzerland and the Netherlands. The results of these studies helped demonstrate the efficacy and safety profile of fumarates. This ultimately paved the way for the approval of a mixture of DMF with Ca, Mg, and Zn monoethyl ester salts in the treatment of psoriasis [4]. FAEs were approved in Germany in 1994 under the brand name Fumaderm® for use in cases of severe psoriasis vulgaris. Since its official approval, Fumaderm® has become the drug of choice for the systemic treatment of psoriasis in Germany, accounting for approximately 66% of the treatments prescribed for systemic psoriasis management [5].

In 2008, the formulation was approved to include treatment of both moderate and severe psoriasis. FAE/fumarate mixtures are currently prepared as Fumaderm® Initial and Fumaderm®, weaker and stronger strength formulas, respectively. These standardized drugs are now commonly used in Germany and the Netherlands for the management of moderate to severe psoriasis [6]. Despite their approval in Germany and the Netherlands, they lack approval and availability in most other countries, including the United States, due to a shortage of randomized controlled clinical trials and sound evidence regarding their use for psoriasis.

P.S. Yamauchi (ed.), *Biologic and Systemic Agents in Dermatology*, https://doi.org/10.1007/978-3-319-66884-0_20

Pharmacological Properties

FAEs are chemical compounds derived from fumaric acid, an intermediate in the citric acid cycle, also commonly found as a food additive that regulates acidity. Ester forms of fumaric acid, such as dimethyl fumarate (DMF), monomethylfumarate (MMF), and monoethylfumarate (MEF), were developed due to the poor oral bioavailability and absorption of fumaric acid. An experiment conducted in 1989 demonstrated that MEF monotherapy had no superior effect to placebo when compared to DMF monotherapy, making MEF less likely to be important in the therapeutic effects of FAEs [3]. The major active ingredient of Fumaderm®, DMF, was seemingly thought to act as a prodrug for its main metabolite MMF.

Following complete absorption in the small intestine, enteric-coated tablets containing DMF are rapidly metabolized to MEF by esterases and partial saponification in the alkaline intestines. After the metabolism of DMF in the intestine, MMF is absorbed, distributed throughout the body, and readily detectable in the plasma [7]. The plasma levels of DMF and fumaric acid are not as readily detectable [8]. Although DMF is not detected in vivo and was previously believed to be entirely metabolized in the intestine [9], results of a urine sample analysis study conducted by Rostami-Yazdi et al. suggest that a considerable portion of DMF escapes hydrolysis in the lumen and instead enters the circulation where it depletes intracellular glutathione (GSH) in immune cells. This may be associated with the release of anti-inflammatory cytokines and the induction of apoptosis [10]. Further recent studies contradict the idea of complete metabolism of DMF in the intestine and point more toward the notion that DMF may enter the pre-systemic circulation before it is broken down into MMF. The lack of DMF in the plasma may be due to its short half-life [8] and its delivery by the portal vein to the liver where it undergoes substantial first-pass metabolism by the liver. These findings better correlate with the increased effectiveness of DMF in a number of vitro assays than its suggested metabolite MMF.

Contrary to prior belief, DMF has been proposed as the primary active component of Fumaderm® that exerts its therapeutic effects on psoriasis patients [11]. Although there has been an increase in the amount of knowledge gained regarding the pharmacokinetic properties of FAEs, more studies must be conducted in order to work toward gaining a full understanding of the metabolism, absorption, and longevity of FAEs.

Mechanism of Action

Psoriasis is a chronic hyperplastic skin condition characterized by overabundant proliferation of keratinocytes resulting in raised, erythematous, pruritic, and scaly plaques through-out the body. It is known to be a complex condition resulting from an elaborate combination of genetic, epigenetic, and environmental triggers. Although the definitive pathogenesis of this clinical diagnosis remains largely elusive, it has been postulated that the condition is a result of immunological dysfunction [12]. FAEs have been theorized to improve psoriasis through a number of various mechanisms.

The Th1 subset of CD4+ T helper cells were originally considered the primary players in the pathogenesis of psoriasis; however, over the past two decades, many advances have been made regarding the understanding of the disease etiology. This has led to the identification of various subsets of CD4+ T helper immune cells that contribute to the manifestation of psoriasis. At present, it is generally accepted that Th17 cells and other T helper cell subsets play a pivotal role in propagating the inflammatory response of the disease [13]. The transmigration of Th17 and Th1 cells into the skin results in keratinocyte proliferation, recruitment of neutrophils, and increased generation of small vessels [14]. Despite recent progress in understanding the causes of the disease, there is currently no cure. Conventional treatments are administered with the goal of controlling symptoms and improving quality of life. In addition to methotrexate, cyclosporine, and acitretin, some countries outside of the United States have started to utilize FAEs as a systemic treatment for psoriasis [15].

The mechanism of action of FAEs and their specific effects on intracellular signaling pathways are not completely understood. FAEs contain a mixture of DMF and MMF. DMF, the most active component of FAEs, is a prodrug that is further metabolized into MMF, its in vivo bioactive metabolite, and S-(1,2-dimethoxycarbonylethyl) glutathione [7]. DMF has been demonstrated to be effective in the management of patients with psoriasis via its potential influence on pro-inflammatory signal transduction pathways and reduction in lesional T-cell subsets that normalize the epidermal hyperproliferation of keratinocytes [16].

As the understanding of the pathogenesis of psoriasis has molded over the past decades, a number of various postulations regarding the mechanism of action of FAEs have been proposed. Previous theories suggest that FAEs may act by directly inhibiting keratinocyte proliferation [17], reducing the production of chemokines involved in neutrophil recruiting and T-lymphocyte activation [18], and modulating the immune system by affecting adhesion molecule expression and leukocyte rolling [19]. Additionally, DMF may play a role in reducing endothelial expression of vascular endothelial growth factor receptor 2 (VEGFR2) and subsequent inhibition of endothelial cell proliferation and survival [20].

More recent studies have shifted toward the idea that DMF may exert its effects by increasing intracellular GSH levels that further inhibits nuclear factor-kappa B (NFkB) entry into the nucleus, where it normally acts in the production of pro- and anti-inflammatory cytokines, cell proliferation, and apoptosis; this is believed to effectively result in a reduction of pro-inflammatory signal transduction pathways [21, 22].

Additionally, FAEs have been noted to exert cytoprotective effects on the nervous system [23] and inhibit the production of interleukin-12 and interleukin-23 by dendritic cells during episodes of inflammation [24]. Accumulating evidence has demonstrated DMF's ability to promote lymphocyte count reduction, a Th$_2$ cell shift, and anti-inflammatory type II dendritic cell differentiation with relatively low toxicities. Although FAEs are not approved in the United States for the treatment of psoriasis, they have been permitted as first-line treatment of multiple sclerosis under the brand name Tecfidera® since February of 2014 [25].

Treatment Candidates

Patients being considered for treatment with FAEs should be formally diagnosed with moderate to severe psoriasis that is refractory to other forms of conventional treatment. FAEs are recommended for those over the age of 18. Although, FAEs have been effective in the treatment of a small set of pediatric cases, they should be used with caution in patients under the age of 18 due to the limitation of data and the lack of randomized controlled trials regarding this age group [26]. FAEs should not be used in patients with significant gastrointestinal diseases such as chronic gastritis or active or recent gastric or duodenal ulcers or severe liver or kidney diseases. Other contraindications include malignancy or history of malignancy, and leukopenia or other hematologic irregularities. Although there has been no evidence that FAEs are teratogenic, they should be avoided in pregnant or breast-feeding women due to limited data [27].

Clinical Uses

FAEs for Psoriasis

Plaque Psoriasis

Although there is limited data from controlled clinical trials regarding the efficacy of FAEs in treating psoriasis, available studies suggest that after 12–16 weeks of treatment 50% of patients achieve a reduction of at least 75% in their baseline "Psoriasis Area and Severity Index" (PASI) score [28, 29]. The first randomized, double-blind, placebo-controlled trial was conducted in which a total of 39 patients living with psoriasis between the ages of 20 and 73 were randomly assigned to 1 of 3 treatment groups. After 16 weeks of treatment, the group administered a combination of MEF and DMF showed an average 14% (21% at baseline to 6.7%) reduction of body surface area (BSA). Additionally, six of the subjects showed complete clearance. The improvement was statistically significant when compared to the groups

who were given octylhydrogen fumarate or placebo tablets. No complete clearance was observed in these groups. Of the 39 patients initially enrolled, 5 subjects withdrew from the trial due to undesired side effects or worsening of symptoms. The results of the study demonstrated the benefit of combination treatment with DMF and MEF in patients with psoriasis and provided preliminary support for the use of FAEs as a potential alternative treatment option [30].

A larger-scaled multicenter study consisting of 101 patients with severe psoriasis was conducted, in which an emphasis was placed on individual dose adjustment of fumarates. Of the initial 101 participants, 70 patients completed the study. The group showed a mean reduction in the PASI score of 80% after 16 weeks of monitored treatment with Fumaderm® Initial and Fumaderm®. The study revealed that systemic FAE treatment could be used as effective psoriasis treatment in a large group of people. Adverse symptoms were experienced by 69% of the cohort, including gastrointestinal complaints, flushing, and increased pruritus. A maximal dose of six tablets of Fumaderm® was required by 46% of patients of which 17% were able to reduce their dosing while maintaining therapeutic effects. Contrarily, 6% of patients were able to achieve satisfactory clinical response with only one high-strength tablet daily. Despite recommended guidelines regarding treatment with FAEs, this study indicates the importance of individual-based dosing. Each patient's response should be carefully monitored and his treatment appropriately adjusted in order to optimize response to FAE therapy [31].

A similar longer-term study was conducted in Italy where 40 patients received oral FAEs for a minimum of 6 months and were subsequently assessed for improvement in PASI scores. A majority of the patients achieved complete remission with the oral treatment as early as 3 months after the initiation of treatment. Many of the patients showed noticeable response to treatment after only the first month of treatment. The adverse side effects of diarrhea, itching, and abdominal cramping occurred mainly at the beginning of therapy and were reversible upon stopping the treatment. Twenty patients continued minimal maintenance therapy for 24 months with no recurrence of disease or serious adverse effects. In addition to confirming the efficacy of FAEs observed in previous studies, the results of this investigation suggest that DMF may be a well-tolerated and safe long-term option to consider when treating patients with moderate to severe psoriasis [32].

In 2009, Reich et al. conducted a retrospective study in which data was collected on the long-term (>2 years) safety and efficacy of FAEs. A total of 984 patients with Physician's Global Assessment (PGA) baseline scores ranging from mild to very severe from 163 dermatology offices were included in the study. The following data was collected: therapy duration, dosing, demographics, concurrent medications, comorbidities, subtype of psoriasis, PASI and PGA scores, noted serious adverse events, and any monitored laboratory parameters. The average duration of continuous treatment with FAEs was approximately 44 months. Patients with the following psoriasis classifications were included in the study: chronic stable type (plaque type) (87.3%), scalp psoriasis (38.3%), nail psoriasis (22.6%), exanthematous (guttate) psoriasis (15.6%), psoriatic arthritis (8.3%), inverse (intertriginous) psoriasis (7.4%), psoriasis pustulosa palmoplantaris (3.5%), psoriatic erythroderma (1.6%), and generalized pustular psoriasis (0.8%). After 6 months of treatment, 67% of patients experienced notable improvement or clearance of their psoriatic lesions. A larger proportion of patients experienced improvement as the treatment duration increased; 78% of patients experienced marked improvement after 24 months of therapy, and 82% after 36 months. Patients who experienced significant improvement or full clearance had a mean maintenance dose of 3 and 2.8 tablets per day, respectively; higher maintenance doses were seemingly required in patients with poorer responses to treatment. The most noted laboratory abnormalities after 24 months were leukopenia, lymphopenia, and increased serum creatinine. Elevated liver enzymes were recorded most frequently after 3 months and eosinophilia between the first and third months of treatment. Deviation in normal values was negligible in most cases allowing approximately 95% of patients to continue treatment without any alterations [33].

A prospective single-blind follow-up study conducted by Lijnen et al. revealed a 1.7 out of 5-point decrease in PGA score indicating significantly lower psoriasis activity in a total of 176 patients. The mean maintenance dose was 480 mg daily. On average, patients received DMF monotherapy for a duration of 28 months. It has been suggested that approximately half of all patients on high-dose monotherapy may benefit clinically. One hundred and fifty-two patients reported at least one adverse event due to the systemic treatment causing 24% of the patients to discontinue treatment. Despite the high rate of experiencing adverse effects, the authors concluded DMF monotherapy to be a safe and effective long-term psoriasis treatment alternative [34].

Psoriatic Arthritis

A study of 27 patients diagnosed with psoriatic arthritis split into two randomly assigned groups was conducted over the course of 16 weeks in order to assess efficacy of FAE treatment. The group of 13 patients treated with fumarates showed a moderate decrease in joint pain at the end of 16 weeks, quantified by the patient's global assessment and Ritchie articular index. One patient discontinued participation in the study due to diarrhea resistant to tapering doses and another due to proteinuria with elevated serum creatinine, which were both later reversed and normalized after discontinuation of the drug. These findings demonstrated the

potential benefit of fumarates in the management of psoriatic arthritis in addition to their previously studied effects on psoriasis with short-term treatment and strict monitoring of side effects [35]. However, FAEs are no longer recommended for the treatment of psoriatic arthritis because of a shortage in additional convincing studies regarding its effect on arthritis, dactylitis, and enthesitis [36].

Psoriasis Pustulosa Palmoplantaris

An open prospective clinical study of 13 patients ranging from the ages of 25 to 78 was conducted in order to assess the efficacy of FAEs in the management of psoriasis pustulosa palmoplantaris (PPP). Patients were placed on FAEs and closely monitored monthly for clinical examination and laboratory investigation. FAEs were an effective monotherapy treatment for PPP in eight of the patients with an average reduction in Palmo-plantar Pustular Psoriasis Area Severity Index (PPPASI) scores of 49% and 44% for palmar and plantar lesions, respectively. High doses of FAE, an average of 584.4 mg daily, were necessary to maintain positive therapeutic results. With additional studies and data, FAE may be considered as a possible treatment option for patients diagnosed with PPP [37].

Nail Psoriasis

There has been one documented case of nail psoriasis successfully treated with FAEs. Nail psoriasis is traditionally treated with topical and systemic compounds with little efficacious effect. Great improvement in nail onycholysis was noticed within 10 months of treatment in a patient on a gradually dose-increasing regimen of Fumaderm® [38].

FAE in the Treatment of Other Dermatological Diseases

Granuloma Annulare

FAEs may be considered for patients with various noninfectious uncontrolled granulomatous skin diseases. Fumarates have demonstrated effectiveness in the clearing of noninfectious granulomatous lesions in two small-scaled retrospective studies. FAEs faded, flattened, and/or improved the appearance of granulomatous skin lesions. A majority of the patients with granulomatous disease have shown therapeutic improvement with FAE monotherapy [39, 40]. FAEs may be considered as a possible treatment option for most noninfectious granulomatous skin conditions without severe and nonreversible side effects in most patients.

Granuloma annulare is a skin condition of unknown etiology that usually shows little improvement with topical treatments. A middle-aged female patient with erythematous annular plaques on her legs and abdomen achieved complete clearance after 3 months of treatment with FAE tablets [41].

A partial rapid response was also seen in an otherwise healthy patient with typical granuloma annulare who failed to show response with bath-photochemotherapy (bath PUVA) and topical corticosteroids. The drug was well tolerated and resulted in an initial resolution at just 3 weeks, followed by significant clearance at 12 weeks with only slightly hyperpigmented non-palpable lesion remnants [42].

Udaya et al. treated two granuloma annulare patients with standard dosing who failed to resolve with other treatments. One patient saw significant improvement after just 2 months of starting therapy. The patient's treatment was discontinued after 12 months due to satisfactory results. The other patient observed abdominal and upper extremity clearance within 3 months, followed by complete clearance of the legs within 6 months. After 2 months of discontinuing the medication, the lesions reappeared and the patient was restarted on the regimen. Continuous low-dose fumarates have been administered in order to keep her condition under control [43].

Sarcoidosis

Sarcoidosis is a condition characterized by noncaseating granulomas that may manifest in the lungs, lymph nodes, eyes, or skin. Some conventional therapies include corticosteroids and chloroquine. FAEs have been reported as an effective treatment option in cases that were refractory to a number of more traditional treatments. In a published case study, three patients diagnosed with conventional treatment resistant recalcitrant cutaneous sarcoidosis were placed on an increasing dose of fumarates. FAEs were administered in accordance with standard dosing and scheduling in the patients. All three patients achieved complete remission after 4–12 months of treatment and continued on an adjusted maintenance dose to prevent relapse [44].

Gutzmer et al. reported a 61-year-old female treated with FAEs for her cutaneous sarcoidosis. Improvements were seen after 12 months of treatment. Upon discontinuing treatment, her cutaneous and pulmonary lesions relapsed 18 months later. Fumarates successfully cleared her reoccurrence within 2 months of restarting the drug [45]. An additional retrospective study conducted by Breuer et al. analyzed various patients with granulomatous disease, including 11 patients with sarcoidosis (either systemic or cutaneous). Marked improvement or complete clearance was noticed in three patients, and moderate improvement observed in three patients. Five patients did not respond to the treatment [39]. A recent report of a 47-year-old woman with systemic sarcoidosis showed complete clinical recovery along with reduction in lung opacities and improved overall pulmonary function after 6 months of treatment with FAEs [46]. These preliminary results regarding the effectiveness of FAEs in sarcoidosis should be further confirmed in larger-scaled controlled studies.

Necrobiosis Lipoidica

Necrobiosis lipoidica (NL) is a rare disease often associated with diabetes mellitus. There has been no proven effective treatment for the management of this medical condition. Typically, symptoms are alleviated with topical corticosteroids and a number of different drugs with varying success. The efficacy of FAEs has been evaluated in a noncontrolled study of a small group of patients with NL. FAEs precipitated statistically significant positive clinical improvement in a majority of the treated patients with no documentation of unexpected adverse effects. This preliminary study indicates that FAEs may be safe and favorable in patients suffering with NL [47].

Cutaneous Lupus Erythematosus

Results from a prospective, open-label, phase II pilot study demonstrated FAEs as an effective treatment option for cutaneous lupus erythematosus (CLE). This study follows only three previously published case studies highlighting the treatment of CLE with FAEs [40, 48, 49]. Ten patients diagnosed with discoid lupus erythematosus (DLE) and one patient diagnosed with subacute cutaneous lupus erythematosus (SCLE) with a single DLE lesion were included in the study. Response to treatment was measured using the Revised Cutaneous Lupus Erythematosus Disease Area and Severity Index (RCLASI), which was measured at baseline, 12 weeks, 24 weeks, and 28 weeks after the follow-up period. Total activity RCLASI score, RCLASI activity score for skin lesions, and total RCLASI damage score were evaluated. A significant decrease in the mean total RCLASI activity score and mean RCLASI activity score for skin lesions was observed between baseline and at both 12 and 24 months of treatment. Total RCLASI activity scores decreased from a mean of 15.5 to 9.9 at 12 weeks and remained relatively decreased with a score of 10.1 at 24 weeks. The activity score for skin lesions decreased from 14.8 to 9.4 at 12 weeks and remained lowered at 9.5 at 24 weeks. Both scores remained lowered in comparison to the baseline values at 28 weeks after the follow-up period. Overall, off-label use of FAEs resulted in reduced activity of skin lesions in 7 patients (1 SCLE patient and 6 patients with chronic therapy resistance DLE) of 11. Reported adverse effects included abdominal cramps, headaches, diarrhea, tachycardia, and flushing. Lumbar discus prolapse and reimplantation of urinary bladder pacemaker were two reported serious adverse events reported during the study. However, these events were determined as unlikely secondary to the treatment. With further confirmation through randomized controlled trials, FAEs may be a safe and effective treatment in those with refractory CLE [50].

Alopecia Areata

Six out of ten patients with alopecia areata resistant to conventional treatment for at least 6 months showed positive results with FAE therapy in a small non-placebo-controlled pilot study. Three patients experienced nearly complete remission, one patient showed focal remission, while two patients displayed moderate improvement with diffuse regrowth of thin hair. Four of the patients within the cohort received no therapeutic benefit. FAEs may act by modulating pro-inflammatory processes in patients whose alopecia areata is due to an etiology where this process can be regulated. Future multicentered, placebo-controlled randomized trial may provide further convincing evidence regarding the efficacy and safety of FAE use in conventional treatment of refractory alopecia areata [51].

Melanoma

Preclinical testing studies on animal models have indicated DMF's antiproliferative and antiapoptotic effects and ability to reduce melanoma proliferation at primary sites and metastasis to lymph nodes. These effects were seen in severe combined immunodeficiency (SCID) mouse xenotransplantation models [52]. DMF's potential as an antimetastatic agent in the treatment of malignant melanoma was further validated in a study conducted by Yamazoe et al. The study deduced that DMF worked by inhibiting the nuclear entry of NFkB and subsequent invasion and metastasis of melanoma cells [53]. In a following study, intradermally injected melanoma cells showed delayed metastasis to sentinel nodes when treated with dacarbazine (DTIC) and DMF. This co-therapy also reduced the density of lymph vessels in the primary tumors when evaluated by real-time PCR and immunohistochemistry. In vitro, DTIC and DMF were able to impair migration of melanoma cells. Reduction of the mRNA expression and protein concentration of CXCL2 and CXCL1, pro-migratory chemokines, was observed in vivo [54].

Although there are currently no known human in vivo studies regarding the effect of FAEs on the progression of melanoma, DMF has become a compound of interest regarding malignant melanoma due to its previously mentioned effects on cell culture lines and animal models.

Contraindicative to FAEs possible antitumor effects, two cases of melanoma were diagnosed after initiation of therapy. No consensus has been made whether FAEs were the causative agent of the malignancy. Further reports and additional research may help to clarify this discrepancy [55].

Other Conditions

There is limited data indicating the possible usefulness of FAEs in treating the following conditions: lichen planus, pityriasis rubra pilaris [40], and collagenous colitis [56].

Dosing

Fumaderm® Initial and Fumaderm® are standardized enteric-coated tablets that have been used in Germany since 1994 as systemic therapies to treat "moderate to severe" forms of psoriasis. The current formulations consist of four active ingredients: 30 or 120 mg of DMF, respectively, along with a mixture of three MEF salts (MEF Ca-salt, MEF Mg-salt, and MEF Zn-salt). More specifically, Fumaderm® contains 120 mg of DMF, 87 mg of Ca-MEF, 5 mg of Mg-MEF, and 3 mg of zinc MEF. In accordance with the S-3 guideline for psoriasis therapy, FAEs are administered in gradually increasing doses, starting at lower doses in order to minimize possible side effects. Patients are commonly started on one tablet of Fumaderm® Initial daily for the first week. Doses are incrementally increased to Fumaderm® Initial twice a day the second week and three times daily the third. If the initial dosing is well tolerated, the patient is switched to the higher-dosed Fumaderm®. Thereafter, dose-escalation occurs every week to a maximum of six tablets daily (1.2 g/day). On average, most patients experience clinical benefit with three to four tablets daily and therefore do not reach the maximal dose during the course of their treatment. Clinically, the dose of Fumaderm is increased until the desired clinical effects are observed and is adjusted according to the individual after the desired treatment response has been achieved [29].

FAEs should be administered until a satisfactory improvement in psoriasis is seen. In patients suffering from severe disease, FAE therapy may be prolonged up to 2 years in order to prevent relapse of the disease. The treatment may also be used as a short-course therapeutic option and withdrawn once major improvement has been achieved. If a relapse of psoriasis is experienced, FAEs may be reintroduced. If a patient remains without disease while on treatment, the FAEs should be gradually decreased to the minimal dose that prevents the reoccurrence of lesions [57].

Side Effects/Toxicities

Side effects experienced due to treatment with FAEs are relatively common but mild. Adverse effects have been noted since the first randomized, double-blind, placebo-controlled study conducted in 1990 [30]. The most commonly observed side effects have included gastrointestinal issues (including gastric and esophageal pain), diarrhea, flushing, nausea, and stomach cramps [30, 32, 34, 35, 37]. These adverse events, mainly gastrointestinal effects, were frequently reported at the beginning of treatment between weeks 4 and 12 [31]. Flushing tended to be experienced 1/2 to 2 h after taking the tablet and would persist for up to ½ an hour [58]. In a systematic review conducted by Balak et al., 69–92% of patients enrolled in previous studies reported adverse events, with up to 100% percent reporting GI complaints and 92% experiencing flushing within individual studies. Overall, approximately between 8 and 39% of patients discontinued FAE therapy due to undesirable adverse events [59]. In most patients experiencing adverse responses, the side effects disappeared or lessened after decreasing or discontinuing FAE treatment [35].

Additionally, some patients have experienced hematological changes with FAEs including: transient leukopenia, lymphopenia, and eosinophilia [30, 60]. A subset of patients also experienced increases in liver enzymes, triglycerides, cholesterol, proteinuria, and serum potassium and creatinine [31, 34]. Organ function was normalized within 3 months of terminating treatment in patients that experienced renal insufficiency and abnormal liver function tests. Lymphopenia and leukopenia reversed within 6 months [3]. There have been reports of a small number of patients who experienced reversible acute renal failure during the use of fumarates; however, FAEs are not believed to be directly related to this abnormality; this has not been observed in any documented controlled trials [61].

Recently, a small number of cases have been reported regarding possible fumarate treatment-related progressive multifocal leukoencephalopathy (PML). PML is a rare viral condition characterized by progressive inflammation and degradation of the white matter in the brain often associated with severe lymphocytopenia. Nieuwkamp et al. reported a case of a 64-year-old woman being treated for psoriasis with glucocorticoids and delayed-release DMF who had presented with progressive apraxia. The patient was not known to be on any other immunosuppressive medications. Subsequent magnetic resonance imaging (MRI) of the patient's brain revealed multiple subcortical white matter lesions. The patient's leukocyte and lymphocyte counts dropped from normal to a level of 4000 leukocytes and 792 lymphocytes per cubic millimeter. The patient further deteriorated and died due to complications from PML. Later histological analysis of the brain and positive detection of JC virus DNA via PCR assay confirmed the diagnosis [62]. Rosenkranz et al. reported a similar case of a 54-year-old woman who was being treated with delayed-release DMF for multiple sclerosis. She had received DMF over the course of 4.5 years as a patient in an open-label extension study. She experienced severe lymphocytopenia 12 months after the initiation of her treatment. MRI imaging and positive detection of JC virus led to the diagnosis of PML [63]. Although rare, PML should be considered in patients who present with worsening neurological symptoms. Patients should receive careful monitoring of lymphocyte counts

and preventative measures to decrease the risk of developing immunosuppression while receiving FAE therapy. Regulatory authorities in the United Kingdom revised their recommendations to healthcare professionals in April 2016 to consider a baseline cranial MRI and MRI imaging for any patient with severe prolonged lymphopenia as part of increased vigilance for PML.

In total, there has been only one known report of a severe adverse event with FAE treatment. Adnexitis was observed in one patient who was receiving fumarate therapy in conjunction with calcipotriol. However, it was determined that the study medication was highly unlikely to be a contributing factor to this adverse inflammatory response [64]. Therefore, it is generally believed that the use of FAEs is not associated with the risk of experiencing serious toxicities.

To date, there has been no data published on the safety of FAEs during pregnancy and the possibility for teratogenicity in humans. Therefore, it is contraindicated in those who are pregnant or planning on conceiving. No data has been found regarding the transfer of FAE metabolites to breast milk; therefore, breastfeeding mothers should not be prescribed FAEs for their psoriasis. Although there has been no published data on the effect FAEs may have on male fertility or possible paternal teratogenicity, no known negative reports have been documented. Nonetheless, due to a lack of knowledge regarding this subject, FAEs are not recommended in males who are planning to conceive [65].

Monitoring

Patients under FAE therapy should be closely monitored for fluctuations in normal laboratory values. The following parameters should be followed: serum creatinine, blood urea nitrogen, alanine aminotransferases, aspartate aminotransferases, and gammaglutamyl transferase along with routine urine dip test and blood counts including white blood cells. These values should be taken before the initiation of therapy in order to establish a baseline profile of the patient. After the start of therapy with FAEs, laboratory values should be reevaluated monthly for the first 6 months. If laboratory parameters remain stable over the first 6 months, reassessment can be extended to every 8 weeks [31].

According to the most recently updated European S3-Guidelines on systemic treatment of psoriasis vulgaris, FAE treatment should be terminated if leukocytes are below 3000/μL or if lymphocytes are less than 500/μL. If lymphocytes fall below 700/μL, the patient's most recent dosage should be decreased by half for the following 2–4 weeks followed up by laboratory evaluation. If the patient's lymphocytes fail to normalize to above 700/mL over the adjusted period, the fumarates should be terminated. Alongside monitoring of laboratory values, the patients taking FAEs should be followed up with routine clinical examination, objective assessment of disease (such as PASI/BSA/PGA), and evaluation of health-related quality of life (DLQI/Skindex-29 or −17) [66].

Co-therapy and Drug Interactions

A study conducted by Gollnick et al. in 2002 aimed to determine the additive effect of topical calcipotriol with FAEs in patients with chronic plaque psoriasis found that combination treatment seemed to be significantly faster acting and efficacious. The data from the study demonstrated a noteworthy superior benefit/risk ratio because calcipotriol evoked a moderate dose-sparing effect of FAE. No statistically significant differences regarding the proportion of patients reporting adverse events were observed between the combination and monotherapy treatment groups. Benefits may be seen when using FAEs in conjunction with calcipotriol [64].

One report has been made regarding a possible drug interaction between DMF and acenocoumarol, a vitamin K agonist. The female patient required substantially higher doses of acenocoumarol after initiating treatment with DMF monotherapy. This dosing increase was reversible upon discontinuation of fumarate therapy. No other known similar reports have been found [34]. According to the European S3 Psoriasis Guidelines, FAEs should not be used in conjunction with infliximab or methotrexate. Expert opinion suggests that co-therapy with infliximab may cause increased risk of immunosuppression and a more exacerbated lymphocytopenia. Methotrexate may cause similar effects [66]. Co-administration of FAEs with other fumaric acid derivatives, cyclosporine, cytostatic drugs, or drugs that can cause renal insufficiency may potentiate toxicity.

Conclusion

Although FAEs are not currently approved in the United States for the treatment of psoriasis, further studies and investigation may allow them to be used as a treatment option. Since their discovery approximately 50 years ago, FAE derivatives have successfully treated a number of autoimmune-mediated dermatological diseases such as psoriasis, necrobiosis lipoidica, granulomatous disease, sarcoidosis, lupus erythematosus, and alopecia areata. Although side effects may be experienced quite often, proper dosing can improve tolerability. Common side effects include gastrointestinal discomfort, flushing, nausea, vomiting, and diarrhea. Minor hematological changes such as lymphopenia, leukopenia, and eosinophilia are also not commonly experienced. Some patients can experience an increase in liver enzymes, triglycerides, cholesterol, pro-

teinuria, and serum potassium and creatinine. With proper management and monitoring, most patients are able to continue therapy with minor fluctuations in these values. Some studies have provided insight on the safety and efficacy of fumarates in both the short and long-term treatment of a number of dermatological conditions. The results of ongoing and future clinical trials will provide more insight on this alternative treatment option.

Fictional Case Report

A 38-year-old female presents with a painful rash on the hands and feet. The patient also has plaques with micaceous scale on trunk and elbows and complains of severe itching and discomfort. She was diagnosed with psoriasis over 10 years ago and failed on apremilast and cyclosporine in the past. The patient does not have arthritis. The patient is negative for any liver, kidney, GI, or hematological abnormalities. The patient is not currently pregnant, is not breastfeeding, and is not actively planning conception.

Physical Exam

Psoriatic plaques on the left posterior upper arm, right pretibial region, posterior scalp, and anterior trunk as well as palms and soles.

Total BSA (%) = 30

Social History

- Social drinker (2–3 drinks per week)
- Nonsmoker

Past Medical History

- High cholesterol
- Family history of diabetes mellitus (mothers side)

Previous Therapies

- Clobetasol 0.05% Foam BID
- NBUVB three times weekly
- Otezla 30 mg BID
- Cyclosporine 100 mg BID

Management

Due to uncontrolled symptoms of psoriasis and previous failure of traditional oral systemic options, the patient was counseled on the use of fumaric acid esters, Fumaderm® for the treatment of moderate to severe or severe psoriasis. In this patient, it is necessary to consider treatment with alternative agents because of treatment-resistant disease and multiple intolerable adverse events. Acitretin is contraindicated in women of child-bearing age. The patient will start taking one tablet QD for the first week followed by weekly dose increases until a treatment response is seen. The maximum recommended dose of Fumaderm® is six tablets daily. Routine lab tests will be performed before administering first dose and at regularly scheduled periods of time. Once the psoriasis has cleared, the dose will be gradually reduced to the lowest possible dose to maintain clearance.

References

1. Roll A, Reich K, Boer A. Use of fumaric acid esters in psoriasis. Indian J Dermatol Venereol Leprol. 2007;73:133–7.
2. Schweckendiek W. Treatment of psoriasis vulgaris. Med Monatsschr. 1959;13:103–4. German.
3. Nieboer C, Hoop DD, Loenen AV, Langendijk P, Dijk EV. Systemic therapy with fumaric acid derivates: new possibilities in the treatment of psoriasis. J Am Acad Dermatol. 1989;20:601–8.
4. Gibson TS, Lambert C, Dinges J. Fumaric acid esters. In: Bioactive carboxylic compound classes: pharmaceuticals and agrochemicals, first edition. KGaA: Wiley-VCH Verlag GmbH & Co; 2016. p. 209–19.
5. Mrowietz U, Asadullah K. Dimethylfumarate for psoriasis: more than a dietary curiosity. Trends Mol Med. 2005;11:43–8.
6. Pathirana D, Ormerod AD, Saiag P, Smith C, Pl S, Nast A, et al. European S3-guidelines on the systemic treatment of psoriasis vulgaris. J Eur Acad Dermatol Venereol. 2009;23(Suppl 2):1–70.
7. Litjens NH, van Strijen E, van Gulpen C, Mattie H, van Dissel JT, Thio HB, et al. In vitro pharmacokinetics of anti-psoriatic fumaric acid esters. BMC Pharmacol. 2004;4:22.
8. Emre S. Review of the use of fumaric acid esters in dermatology. J Turk Acad Dermatol. 2016;10(4):16104r1.
9. Werdenberg D, Joshi R, Wolffram S, Merkle HP, Langguth P. Presystemic metabolism and intestinal absorption of antipsoriatic fumaric acid esters. Biopharm Drug Dispos. 2003;24(6):259–73.
10. Rostami-Yazdi M, Clement B, Schmidt TJ, Schinor D, Mrowietz U. Detection of metabolites of fumaric acid esters in human urine: implications for their mode of action. J Investig Dermatol. 2009;129:231–4.
11. Rostami-Yazdi M, Clement B, Mrowietz U. Pharmacokinetics of anti-psoriatic fumaric acid esters in psoriasis patients. Arch Dermatol Res. 2010;302:531–8.
12. Deng Y, Chang C, Lu Q. The inflammatory response in psoriasis: a comprehensive review. Clin Rev Allergy Immunol. 2016;50:377–89.
13. Diani M, Altomare G, Reali ET. Helper cell subsets in clinical manifestations of psoriasis. J Immunol Res. 2016:1–7.
14. Ghoreschi K, Weigert C, Röcken M. Immunopathogenesis and role of T cells in psoriasis. Clin Dermatol. 2007;25:574–80.
15. Boehncke W-H, Schön MP. Psoriasis. Lancet. 2015;386:983–94.
16. Bovenschen HJ, Langewouters AM, Kerkhof PCVD. Dimethylfumarate for psoriasis. Am J Clin Dermatol. 2010;11:343–50.
17. Sebök B, Bonnekoh B, Mahrle G. Il-1 alpha-induced expression of icam-1 on cultured hyperproliferative keratinocytes: suppression by antipsoriatic dimethyl-fumarate. Int J Dermatol. 1994;33:367–70.
18. Stoof T, Flier J, Sampat S, Nieboer C, Tensen C, Boorsma D. The antipsoriatic drug dimethylfumarate strongly suppresses chemokine production in human keratinocytes and peripheral blood mononuclear cells. Br J Dermatol. 2001;144:1114–20.
19. Rubant SA, Ludwig RJ, Diehl S, Hardt K, Kaufmann R, Pfeilschifter JM, et al. Dimethylfumarate reduces leukocyte rolling in vivo through modulation of adhesion molecule expression. J Investig Dermatol. 2008;128:326–31.
20. Meissner M, Doll M, Hrgovic I, Reichenbach G, König V, Hailemariam-Jahn T, et al. Suppression of VEGFR2 expression in human endothelial cells by dimethylfumarate treatment: evidence for anti-angiogenic action. J Investig Dermatol. 2011;131:1356–64.
21. Gold R, Linker RA, Stangel M. Fumaric acid and its esters: an emerging treatment for multiple sclerosis with antioxidative mechanism of action. Clin Immunol. 2012 Jan;142(1):44–8.
22. Loewe R, Holnthoner W, Groger M, et al. Dimethylfumarate inhibits TNF-induced nuclear entry of NF-kappa B/p65 in human endothelial cells. J Immunol. 2002;168:4781–7.
23. Linker RA, Lee DH, Ryan S, et al. Fumaric acid esters exert neuroprotective effects in neuroinflammation via activation of the Nrf2 antioxidant pathway. Brain. 2011;134:678–92.
24. Geisel J, Bruck J, Glocova I, et al. Sulforaphane protects from T cell-mediated autoimmune disease by inhibition of IL-23 and IL-12 in dendritic cells. J Immunol. 2014;192:3530–9.
25. Kretzschmar B, Pellkofer H, Weber MS. The use of oral disease-modifying therapies in multiple sclerosis. Curr Neurol Neurosci Rep. 2016. https://doi.org/10.1007/s11910-016-0639-4.
26. Steinz K, Gerdes S, Domm S, Mrowietz U. Systemic treatment with fumaric acid esters in six paediatric patients with psoriasis in a psoriasis centre. Dermatol. 2014;229:199–204.
27. Boer A, Roll A, Reich K. Use of fumaric acid esters in psoriasis. Indian J Dermatol Venereol Leprol. 2007;73:133.
28. Ormerod AD, Mrowietz U. Fumaric acid esters, their place in the treatment of psoriasis. Br J Dermatol. 2004;150:630–2.
29. Nast A, Kopp IB, Augustin M, Banditt KB, Boehncke WH, Follmann M, et al. S3-Leitlinie zur Therapie der Psoriasis vulgaris. J German Soc Dermatol. 2006;4:51–5.
30. Nugteren-Huying WM, Schroeff JGVD, Hermans J, Suurmond D. Fumaric acid therapy for psoriasis: a randomized, double-blind, placebo-controlled study. J Am Acad Dermatol. 1990;22:311–2.
31. Mrowietz U, Christophers E, Altmeyer P. Treatment of psoriasis with fumaric acid esters. Results of a prospective multicenter study. Br J Dermatol. 1999;138:456–60.
32. Carboni I, De Felice C, De Simoni I, Soda R, Chimenti S. Fumaric acid esters in the treatment of psoriasis: an Italian experience. J Dermatol Treatment. 2004;15(1):23–6.
33. Reich K, Thaci D, Mrowietz U, Kamps A, Neureither M, Luger T. Efficacy and safety of fumaric acid esters in the long-term treatment of psoriasis a retrospective study (FUTURE). J Dtsch Dermatol Ges. 2009;7:603–10.
34. Lijnen RCAB, Otters E, Balak D, Thio B. Long-term safety and effectiveness of high-dose dimethylfumarate in the treatment of moderate to severe psoriasis: a prospective single-blinded follow-up study. J Dermatol Treat. 2015;27:31–6.
35. Peeters AJ, Dukmans BAC, Schroeff JGVD. Fumaric acid therapy for psoriatic arthritis. A randomized, double-blind, placebo-controlled study. Rheumatology. 1992;31:502–4.
36. Wollina U, Unger L, Heinig B, Kittner T. Psoriatic arthritis. Dermatol Therap. 2010;23:123–36.
37. Stander H, Stadelmann A, Luger T, Traupe H. Efficacy of fumaric acid ester monotherapy in psoriasis pustulosa palmoplantaris. Br J Dermatol. 2003;149:220–2.
38. Vlachou C, Berth-Jones J. Nail psoriasis improvement in a patient treated with fumaric acid esters. J Dermatol Treatment. 2007;18:175–7.
39. Breuer K, Gutzmer R, Volker B, Kapp A, Werfel T. Therapy of non-infectious granulomatous skin diseases with fumaric acid esters. Br J Dermatol. 2005;152:1290–5.
40. Klein A, Coras B, Landthaler M, Babilas P. Off-label use of fumarate therapy for granulomatous and inflammatory skin diseases other than psoriasis vulgaris: a retrospective study. J Eur Acad Dermatol Venereol. 2011;26:1400–6.
41. Kreuter A, Gambichler T, Altmeyer P, Brockmeyer NH. Treatment of disseminated granuloma annulare with fumaric acid esters. BMC Dermatol. 2002. https://doi.org/10.1186/1471-5945-2-5.
42. Wollina U. Granuloma annulare disseminatum responding to fumaric acid esters. Dermatol Online J. 2008;14(12):12.
43. Acharya U. Successful treatment of disseminated granuloma annulare with oral fumaric acid esters. Int J Dermatol. 2013;52: 633–4.

44. Nowack U, Gambichler T, Hanefeld C, Kastner U, Altmeyer P. Successful treatment of recalcitrant cutaneous sarcoidosis with fumaric acid esters. BMC Dermatol. 2002. https://doi.org/10.1186/1471-5945-2-15.

45. Gutzmer R, Kapp A, Werfel T. Successful treatment of sarcoidosis with cutaneous and pulmonary involvement with fumaric acid ester. Hautarzt. 2004;55:553–7.

46. Zouboulis CC, Lippert U, Karagiannidis I. Multi-organ sarcoidosis treatment with fumaric acid esters: a case report and review of the literature. Dermatol. 2014;228:202–6.

47. Kreuter A, Knierim C, Stucker M, Pawlak F, Rotterdam S, Altmeyer P, Gambichler T. Fumaric acid esters in necrobiosis lipoidica: results of a prospective noncontrolled study. Br J Dermatol. 2005;153:802–7.

48. Balak D, Thio HB. Treatment of lupus erythematosus with fumaric acid esters: two case-reports. J Transl Med. 2011;9(Suppl 2):15.

49. Tsianakas A, Herzog S, Landmann A, et al. Successful treatment of discoid lupus erythematosus with fumaric acid esters. J Am Acad Dermatol. 2014;71:e15–7.

50. Kuhn A, Landmann A, Patsinakidis N, Ruland V, Nozinic S, Ortiz AMP, Sauerland C, Luger T, Tsianakas A, Bonsmann G. Fumaric acid ester treatment in cutaneous lupus erythematosus (CLE): a prospective, open-label, phase II pilot study. Lupus. 2016;25:1357–64.

51. Venten I, Hess N, Hirschmüller A, Altmeyer P, Brockmeyer N. Treatment of therapy-resistant alopecia areata with fumaric acid esters. Eur J Med Res. 2006;11:300–5.

52. Loewe R, Valero T, Kremling S, Pratscher B, Kunstfeld R, Pehamberger H, Petzelbauer P. Dimethylfumarate impairs melanoma growth and metastasis. Cancer Res. 2006;66:11888–96.

53. Yamazoe Y, Tsubaki M, Matsuoka H, Satou T, Itoh T, Kusunoki T, Kidera Y, Tanimori Y, Shoji K, Nakamura H. Dimethylfumarate inhibits tumor cell invasion and metastasis by suppressing the expression and activities of matrix metalloproteinases in melanoma cells. Cell Biol Int. 2009;33:1087–94.

54. Valero T, Steele S, Neumüller K, Bracher A, Niederleithner H, Pehamberger H, et al. Combination of dacarbazine and dimethylfumarate efficiently reduces melanoma lymph node metastasis. J Invest Dermatol. 2010;130:1087–94.

55. Barth D, Simon JC, Wetzig T. Malignant melanoma during treatment with fumaric acid esters—coincidence or treatment-related? J Dtsch Dermatol Ges. 2011;9:223–5.

56. Hoffmann K, Casetti F, Venzke T, Löckermann S, Schempp CM. Collagenous colitis during treatment with fumaric acid esters. J Dtsch Dermatol Ges. 2014;12:1138–40.

57. Mrowietz U, Cristophers E, Altmeyer P. Treatment of severe psoriasis with fumaric acid esters: scientific background and guidelines for therapeutic use. The German Fumaric acid Ester consensus conference. Br J Dermatol. 1999;141:424–9.

58. Altmeyer PJ, Mattlies U, Pawlak F, Hoffmann K, Frosch PJ, Ruppert P, et al. Antipsoriatic effect of fumaric acid derivatives. J Am Acad Dermatol. 1994;30:977–81.

59. Balak D, Arani SF, Hajdarbegovic E, Hagemans C, Bramer W, Thio H, Neumann H. Efficacy, effectiveness and safety of fumaric acid esters in the treatment of psoriasis: a systematic review of randomized and observational studies. Br J Dermatol. 2016;175:250–62.

60. Kolbach DN, Nieboer C. Fumaric acid therapy in psoriasis: results and side effects of 2 years of treatment. J Am Acad Dermatol. 1992;27:769–71.

61. Raschka C, Koch HJ. Longterm treatment of psoriasis using fumaric acid preparations can be associated with severe proximal tubular damage. Hum Exp Toxicol. 1999;18:738–9.

62. Nieuwkamp DJ, Murk J-L, Cremers CH, Killestein J, Viveen MC, Hecke WV, et al. PML in a patient without severe lymphocytopenia receiving dimethyl fumarate. New Engl J Med. 2015;372(15):1474–6.

63. Rosenkranz T, Novas M, Terborg C. PML in a patient with lymphocytopenia treated with dimethyl fumarate. N Engl J Med. 2015;372(15):1476–8.

64. Gollnick H, Altmeyer P, Kaufmann R, Ring J, Christophers E, Pavel S, Ziegler J. Topical calcipotriol plus oral fumaric acid is more effective and faster acting than oral fumaric acid monotherapy in the treatment of severe chronic plaque psoriasis vulgaris. Dermatology. 2002;205:46–53.

65. Yiu ZZN, Warren RB, Mrowietz U, Griffiths CEM. Safety of conventional systemic therapies for psoriasis on reproductive potential and outcomes. J Dermatol Treatment. 2015;26:329–34.

66. Nast A, Gisondi P, Ormerod A, et al. European S3-guidelines on the systemic treatment of psoriasis vulgaris—update 2015—short version—EDF in cooperation with EADV and IPC. J Eur Acad Dermatol Venereol. 2015;29:2277–94.

Phosphodiesterase (PDE) Inhibitors for the Treatment of Inflammatory Skin Conditions

Jordan Huber, Gerald G. Krueger, and Jason E. Hawkes

Abbreviations

cAMP   Cyclic adenosine monophosphate
cGMP   Cyclic guanosine monophosphate
CREB   Camp responsive element binding protein
ESTEEM   Efficacy and safety trials evaluating the effects of apremilast in psoriasis
IFN-γ   Interferon-gamma
IL   Interleukin
NF-κB   Nuclear factor kappa beta
PASI   Psoriasis Area and Severity Index
PDE   Phosphodiesterase
PDE4   Phosphodiesterase-4
PKA   Protein kinase A
Th   T helper
TNF-α   Tumor necrosis factor-alpha
PASI-75   75% Improvement in PASI scores
DLQI   Dermatology Life Quality Index
NB-UVB   Narrowband-ultraviolet B
PALACE   Psoriatic arthritis long-term assessment of clinical efficacy
DMARD   Disease-modifying antirheumatic drugs
ACR20   American College of Rheumatology criteria for 20% improvement
PPPGA   Palmoplantar Psoriasis Physician Global Assessment
NAPSI-50   50% Reduction in baseline Nail Psoriasis Severity Index
EASI   Eczema area and severity index

PRP   Pityriasis rubra pilaris
DLE   Discoid lupus erythematosus
CLASI   CLE Disease area and severity
SASI   Sarcoidosis Activity and Severity Index
ISGA   Investigator Static Global Assessment

J. Huber, MD • G.G. Krueger, MD (✉)
Department of Dermatology, University of Utah School of Medicine, Salt Lake City, UT, USA
e-mail: gerald.krueger@hsc.utah.edu

J.E. Hawkes, MD
Department of Dermatology, University of Utah School of Medicine, Salt Lake City, UT, USA

The Laboratory for Investigative Dermatology, The Rockefeller University, New York, NY, USA

Introduction

Phosphodiesterases (PDEs) are a family of enzymes that hydrolyze cyclic nucleotides and contribute to the intracellular regulation of cyclic adenosine monophosphate (cAMP) and cyclic guanosine monophosphate (cGMP) [1]. cAMP and cGMP are key secondary messengers central to numerous signaling pathways and normal cellular functions, including the neurotransmitter signaling and the intracellular effects of hormones [1]. The regulation of cAMP is also essential for immune cell homeostasis [2]. Therefore, PDE inhibitors represent a novel class of medications with broad therapeutic application [3].

In 2014, apremilast became the first FDA-approved PDE inhibitor for the treatment of moderate to severe plaque psoriasis and psoriatic arthritis. The anti-inflammatory properties of apremilast also have efficacy in the treatment of other chronic inflammatory skin diseases, such as atopic dermatitis, alopecia areata, and lupus erythematosus [4–6]. In this chapter, we provide a brief overview of the PDE family and their role in the regulation of the immune response. We will also discuss the use of oral and topical PDE inhibitors in the treatment of these conditions.

The PDE Family and Their Mechanism of Action

There are 11 PDE families, each family having a different tissue-expression pattern [7]. Eight of the eleven PDE families have the capacity to degrade intracellular cAMP [8].

© Springer International Publishing AG 2018
P.S. Yamauchi (ed.), *Biologic and Systemic Agents in Dermatology*, https://doi.org/10.1007/978-3-319-66884-0_21

The phosphodiesterase-4 (PDE4) family consists of 4 genes (*PDE4A-D*) that generate >20 different variants [9] and account for much of the cAMP-hydrolyzing activity of epithelial cells, chondrocytes, keratinocytes, dendritic cells, and inflammatory cells [10–15].

Inhibition of PDE leads to decreased degradation of cAMP, resulting in elevated cAMP levels. Subsequently, cAMP activates protein kinase A (PKA) [16], which phosphorylates a nuclear transcription factor named the cAMP responsive element binding protein (CREB) [17]. This sequence of events results in the inhibition of nuclear factor kappa beta (NF-κB) signaling and the transcription of pro-inflammatory cytokines, such as tumor necrosis factor-alpha (TNF-α) [18]. The mechanism by which activated CREB does this is by competing with the NF-κB p65 subunit for binding of the coactivator CREB-binding protein [19]. In other studies, inhibition of PDE has resulted in decreased levels of other pro-inflammatory cytokines such as interleukin (IL)-2 and interferon-γ (IFN-γ) [13]. Elevation of anti-inflammatory cytokines (e.g., IL-10) with inhibition of PDE has also been shown [20]. Therefore, regulation of cAMP signaling is essential for maintaining appropriate levels of inflammation.

Apremilast: General Information

Before the anti-inflammatory effects of PDE4 inhibitors were discovered, PDE4 inhibitors were being studied for the treatment of depression [21] and chronic obstructive pulmonary disease [22]. In 2014, the FDA approved apremilast for the treatment of moderate to severe plaque psoriasis and psoriatic arthritis. Apremilast is an oral, small molecule inhibitor that is highly selective for PDE4 with no appreciable effect on other cell enzymes or cell surface receptors [23]. Apremilast's specificity for PDE4 is attributed to its dialkoxyphenyl pharmacophore chemical group [24].

Schafer et al. showed that apremilast increases intracellular cAMP levels in peripheral blood monocytes and T cells [23] and inhibits the production of pro-inflammatory cytokines and chemokines, such as IL-2, IL-12, IL-17, IL-23, TNF-α, granulocyte-macrophage colony-stimulating factor (GMCSF), and IFN-γ [23, 25]. It has similar anti-inflammatory effects in dendritic cells, polymorphonuclear cells, natural killer cells, and keratinocytes [23, 25]. Apremilast also results in upregulation of IL-10, which has important anti-inflammatory properties [25]. The foregoing observations support the broad anti-inflammatory effects seen with apremilast [26].

Apremilast is absorbed rapidly and reaches its maximum concentration in the serum in less than 2 h [27]. The major route of elimination is hepatic metabolism with a lesser extent of excretion due to nonenzymatic hydrolysis and elimination of unchanged drug [27]. Its pharmacokinetic properties are affected by severe renal impairment, whereas moderate to severe hepatic impairment does not require dose adjustment. Apremilast is in pregnancy category C and has a similar efficacy in adult and elderly populations. The use of apremilast with strong CYP3A4 inducers (e.g., St. John's wort, phenytoin, rifampin, and carbamazepine) is not recommended as this combination may result in decreased serum levels of apremilast.

Common adverse events include diarrhea, nausea, and weight loss [28, 29]. While these adverse events affect approximately 20% of patients and often resolve within 1 month of starting apremilast [29], they may negatively affect patient compliance and/or the long-term treatment of chronic inflammatory conditions. In the authors' experience, antidiarrheal agents (e.g., loperamide or psyllium) seem to mitigate diarrhea symptoms and may improve compliance in patients affected by these symptoms. Less common side effects include upper respiratory infections, headaches, depression, suicidal ideation, and fatigue. The average wholesale acquisition cost for sixty 30 mg tablets is currently estimated to be $2221 [30]. Unfortunately, the high cost of apremilast may limit its use where cheaper medications with comparable efficacy are available, such as methotrexate [30–32].

Apremilast for the Treatment of Inflammatory Skin Disease

Apremilast is currently available in the USA, Canada, and Europe for the treatment of psoriasis and psoriatic arthritis. Strong evidence supports the use of apremilast for the treatment of psoriasis, and its potential benefits for the treatment of other chronic inflammatory conditions of the skin are rapidly increasing. Here, we provide a summary of the evidence supporting the use of this medication in the treatment of various inflammatory skin diseases.

Plaque Psoriasis

Psoriasis is a chronic, T-cell-mediated, inflammatory skin condition with several distinct clinical subtypes. The pathogenesis of this inflammatory skin disease is the result of a complex interplay between the skin, immune system, genetics, and environmental triggers. T helper (Th) cell populations (e.g., Th-1 and Th-17) and their respective cytokines (e.g., TNF-α, IFN-γ, IL-17, IL-12/23) are the primary effector cells in psoriasis [33–37].

Early phase clinical trials demonstrated a clear treatment response in psoriatic patients treated with apremilast (20–30 mg twice daily) [38–41]. In two of these early studies,

46.7–57% of patients experienced a >50% improvement in their Psoriasis Area and Severity Index (PASI) scores after 12 weeks of treatment [38, 41]. In two studies by Gottlieb et al., one demonstrated a 34% median reduction in epidermal thickness of psoriatic lesions at 12 weeks, and both had significant reductions of infiltrating inflammatory cells of psoriatic lesions [40, 41]. Two phase 3, randomized, controlled trials entitled the "Efficacy and Safety Trials Evaluating the Effects of Apremilast in Psoriasis" (e.g., ESTEEM 1 and 2) have evaluated the benefit of apremilast for moderate to severe plaque psoriasis [28, 42]. After 16 weeks, 28.8–33.1% of the 836 patients treated with apremilast 30 mg twice daily versus 5.3–5.8% of 419 patients on placebo achieved a PASI-75. Additionally, ~20% of patients achieved a Static Physician's Global Assessment (PGA) score of 0 or 1 (clear or almost clear) at week 16, and pruritus and skin discomfort were decreased by ~50% in the apremilast group by week 16. A decrease of ≥ 5 points in the Dermatology Life Quality Index (DLQI) was also seen in ~70% of patients with a baseline of DLQI >5 in the apremilast group [28, 42]. A phase 4 trial looking at apremilast for the treatment of moderate plaque psoriasis reported the mean percentage change in the product of sPGA and BSA scores (PGAxBSA) was -48.1% for apremilast versus only -10.2% for placebo Efficacy and Safety of Apremilast in Patients With Moderate Plaque Psoriasis With Lower BSA: Week 16 Results from the UNVEIL Study. J Drugs Dermatol. 2017 Aug 1;16(8):801-808. PMID 28809995].

Several studies have assessed the efficacy of apremilast in combination with other psoriatic therapies. In patients with chronic plaque psoriasis on narrowband ultraviolet B (NB-UVB), systemic medications (i.e., methotrexate, cyclosporine), and/or biologics for at least 16 weeks (i.e., etanercept, adalimumab, infliximab, ustekinumab), the addition of apremilast 30 mg twice daily resulted in 51 of 63 patients (81%) achieving PASI-75 after 12 weeks [43]. Additionally, two recent case reports describe recalcitrant psoriatic patients who failed treatment with secukinumab and adalimumab but experienced dramatic clinical improvement following the addition of apremilast [44, 45].

A recent meta-analysis of 13 studies comparing the effectiveness of apremilast with other systemic anti-psoriatic medications found apremilast to have the lowest response rates (18.7%) and maintenance of response in initial responders (61%) at 1 year [46]. A different meta-analysis compared methotrexate (7.5 mg weekly increased to 25 mg as tolerated or needed) and apremilast 30 mg twice daily. In this study, there was no statistically significant difference in PASI-75 between apremilast (36.6%) and methotrexate (36.4%) at week 16 [30]. Another study compared the efficacy and safety of apremilast 30 mg twice daily ($n = 83$) to etanercept 50 mg once a week ($n = 83$) or placebo ($n = 84$). Although the study was not designed to com-

pare apremilast with etanercept, 39.8% of patients taking apremilast achieved PASI-75 in comparison to 48.2% of patients taking etanercept at week 16 [47]. Both groups showed significant efficacy when compared to placebo. At week 16, the patients originally started on etanercept were switched to apremilast and had no significant adverse events [47].

Importantly, one case report demonstrated that apremilast 30 mg twice daily was effective in a 14-year-old patient. The patient achieved a meaningful improvement in his psoriasis at 6 months of treatment and experienced decreased plaque thickness and reductions in pruritus and scale as early as 1 month after treatment [48]. No significant adverse events were noted. This case report suggests that apremilast may be a safe systemic treatment for pediatric psoriasis. There is currently a phase 2 trial looking at apremilast in the treatment of moderate to severe plaque psoriasis in ages 6–17 years (ClinicalTrials.gov Identifier: NCT02576678).

Psoriatic Arthritis

The pathophysiological mechanisms leading to plaque psoriasis and psoriatic arthritis are largely shared, making apremilast a potential therapeutic option for both disease variants. The psoriatic arthritis long-term assessment of clinical efficacy (PALACE) clinical trial program was designed to further evaluate the safety and effectiveness of apremilast in psoriatic arthritis and consists of four phase 3 randomized, placebo-controlled clinical trials [49]. The PALACE 1–3 trials included psoriatic arthritis patients previously treated with disease-modifying antirheumatic drugs (DMARD) as well as those taking concomitant therapies like methotrexate [29, 50, 51]. In contrast, the PALACE 4 was designed to evaluate the efficacy of apremilast in DMARD-naïve patients [52].

In the PALACE 1–3 trials, the proportion of patients that achieved the American College of Rheumatology criteria for 20% improvement (ACR20) at week 16 ranged from 28– -37.4% for those taking apremilast 20 mg twice daily, 32.1–41% for apremilast 30 mg twice daily, and 18–19% for placebo [29, 50, 51]. For PALACE 4, ACR20 at week 16 was 29.2% for apremilast 20 mg twice daily, 32.3% for apremilast 30 mg twice daily, and 16.9% for placebo [52]. In all of the PALACE trials, ACR20 was achieved in a statistically significant number of psoriatic arthritis patients compared to placebo at week 16. At week 52, the PALACE 1–3 trials demonstrated that 52.6–63% of patients taking apremilast 30 mg twice daily met ACR20 [29, 50, 51]. Improvement was also seen with the number of swollen and tender joints at both 16 and 52 weeks with apremilast 30 mg twice daily. The mean percent change for the number of swollen joints ranged from -24.5– -42.2 at 16 weeks and -66.8– -73.6 at 52 weeks, and the number of tender joints ranged from -18.6– -32.1 at 16 weeks and -51.8– -53.5 at 52 weeks [29, 51]. Lastly, the proportion of patients in the PALACE 3 trial that reached the minimal clinically important difference in quality of life as measured by the Health Assessment Questionnaire Disability Index was 32% at week 16 and 52% at week 52 [29].

Long-term data for the PALACE 1 revealed that 65.3% of patients taking apremilast 30 mg twice daily and 60.9% of patients taking apremilast 20 mg twice daily achieved ACR20 at week 104 [53]. For the PALACE 4 trial at 104 weeks, 64.8% taking apremilast 20 mg twice daily and 57.3% taking apremilast 30 mg twice daily achieved ACR20 [54]. Interestingly, diarrhea and nausea occurred at lower rates after week 52 compared to week 52, and there were no significant differences in the type or severity of adverse events with apremilast exposure beyond 52 weeks [54].

Palmoplantar Psoriasis

Palmoplantar psoriasis has a spectrum of clinical phenotypes that can include pustular lesions and/or thick, hyperkeratotic plaques. This disease variant is often severe and difficult to manage. In a retrospective review of 150 patients with palmoplantar psoriasis, 48% of patients were categorized as having moderate psoriatic disease, whereas 34% had severe disease [55]. Another retrospective analysis of 114 patients with palmoplantar psoriasis demonstrated that less than one-third of patients had marked clinical improvement with topical therapies and the remaining patients required systemic therapy [56]. In the authors' experience, the quality of life for patients with palmoplantar disease is often equal to or lower than other disease variants. These observations underscore challenges associated with the management of this psoriasis and the need for better treatments.

Bissonnette et al. [57] performed a *post hoc* analysis of patients enrolled in the phase 2 and ESTEEM trials for chronic plaque psoriasis. A total of 427 patients were found to have palmoplantar psoriasis with a total of 274 patients in the apremilast 30 mg twice daily group and 153 patients in the placebo group. A significant number of the patients in the apremilast group with moderate to severe palmoplantar psoriasis, defined by a baseline Palmoplantar Psoriasis Physician Global Assessment (PPPGA) score ≥3, experienced significant improvement in the PPPGA score with 48% of these patients achieving a clear or almost clear score at 16 weeks compared to 27% of patients taking placebo ($P = 0.021$) [28, 39, 42, 57]. Apremilast was generally well tolerated, and most adverse events were mild in severity [28, 39, 42, 57]. There is currently a phase 4 trial looking at apremilast in the treatment of palmoplantar psoriasis (ClinicalTrials.gov Identifier: NCT02400749).

Nail and Scalp Psoriasis

Approximately two-thirds of patients in the ESTEEM 1 and 2 trials had moderate to severe scalp psoriasis and nail disease. In these patients, a significant proportion of patients taking apremilast 30 mg twice daily achieved a ≥50% reduction in their baseline Nail Psoriasis Severity Index (NAPSI-50) score at week 16 compared to baseline (33.3–44.6% vs. 14.9–18.7%, respectively). They also achieved a score of 0 (clear) or 1 (minimal) in the Scalp Physician Global Assessment compared to baseline (40.9–46.5% vs. 17.2–17.5%, respectively). Additionally, the apremilast group demonstrated a mean decrease of 0.7–1.3 nails involved at week 16. At week 32, those achieving NAPSI-50 in the apremilast group was as high as 55.4%, and the number of nails and nail bed/matrix scores continued to decrease. The improvements seen in nail and scalp psoriasis were maintained through 52 weeks [28, 42, 58]. Taken together, this clinical trial data suggests that apremilast has the ability to reverse the systemic effects of psoriasis including the inflammation at distant skin sites.

Atopic Dermatitis

Like psoriasis, atopic dermatitis (or eczema) is a common, chronic, inflammatory skin disease. Atopic dermatitis is mediated by pathogenic T-cell populations and the increased expression of Th-2, Th-17, and Th-22 cytokines [59, 60]. Two small studies have been performed to look at the efficacy of apremilast in adults with atopic dermatitis, and the results are conflicting [4, 61]. In one study, ten patients with atopic dermatitis received apremilast 30 mg twice daily. At 3 months, these patients experienced a 39% reduction in their Eczema Area and Severity Index (EASI) scores, a 25% reduction in itch as measured by a Visual Analog Scale, and a 58% improvement in quality of life scores as measured by the DLQI. Statistically significant clinical improvement in atopic dermatitis was seen within the first 2 weeks of the study, and improvements in quality of life, itch, and EASI scores remained statistically significant at 6 months [4]. In a separate study, ten adult patients with atopic dermatitis or allergic contact dermatitis received apremilast 20 mg twice daily. At 12 weeks, one patient achieved a 75% reduction in EASI, and two achieved a 50% reduction in EASI. The mean EASI score only decreased by 5% at 12 weeks. There was no statistically significant reduction in itch or improvement in quality of life in this specific study [61]. The majority of adverse events in these two studies were mild and were generally well tolerated [4, 61].

With regard to the treatment of atopic dermatitis in children, one case report describes an 8-year-old male with a history of severe and recalcitrant atopic dermatitis that was treated with apremilast 30 mg daily. The patient saw a drastic improvement in symptoms such as pruritus in as little as 2 weeks [62]. Given the limited number of atopic dermatitis patients treated with apremilast and the lack of randomized clinical trials, it is difficult to assess the efficacy of apremilast for this condition. Nevertheless, additional systematic studies are warranted and needed as PDE inhibitors may represent a safe alternative for atopic dermatitis patients who fail to respond to topical therapies and/or traditional immunosuppressant medications. A phase 2 trial is underway and is further investigating apremilast in the treatment of moderate to severe atopic dermatitis (ClinicalTrials.gov Identifier: NCT02087943).

Alopecia Areata

Alopecia areata is an autoimmune disorder characterized by the immune destruction of hair follicles and non-scarring alopecia. Lesional skin biopsies from the scalp of alopecia areata patients reveal robust activation of Th-1, Th-2, and IL-23 cytokine pathways as well as increased PDE4 levels [63]. Interestingly, atopic dermatitis is two to three times more likely to be found in patients with alopecia areata [64]. The overlapping cytokine profile of alopecia areata with other inflammatory skin disorders, its co-occurrence with atopic dermatitis, and the increased PDE levels in areas of hair loss support the notion that apremilast may represent an effective treatment modality for alopecia areata.

This hypothesis has been studied in a preclinical mouse model of alopecia areata. Using a humanized alopecia areata model where normal human scalp skin is transplanted onto mice with severe combined immunodeficiency, hair loss is induced in mice by injecting IL-2-stimulated peripheral blood mononuclear cells [65]. Oral apremilast abrogates this hair loss phenotype and is associated with reduced IFN-α, TNF-γ, and perifollicular inflammatory cells [5]. There is currently a randomized controlled trial looking at the treatment of apremilast in moderate to severe alopecia areata (ClinicalTrials.gov Identifier: NCT02684123).

Rosacea

Rosacea is a pleomorphic, inflammatory skin disease affecting the face. Common clinical manifestations include flushing, erythema, telangiectasia, and papules/pustules. The etiology of this condition is poorly understood and involves a complex interaction between the innate immune response, cutaneous microbiota, environmental factors, and adnexal structures of the skin. Traditional treatments are aimed at the prevention of symptoms or clinical manifestations (e.g., erythema or telangiectasia) by targeting the pilosebaceous units

and blood vessels [66]. However, the clinical symptoms of rosacea are bothersome to patients, and management of this condition can be challenging.

In a recent phase 2 study for moderate to severe erythematotelangiectatic and papulopustular rosacea, ten adult patients were treated with apremilast 20 mg twice daily for 12 weeks. While the primary endpoint of papule and pustule count did not reach statistical significance during the study, statistically significant improvements were seen in the following outcomes at the end of 12 weeks: the Physician Global 7-Point Assessment, Physician Overall Erythema Severity, the erythematotelangiectatic rating, and nontransient erythema. Affirmation of these findings in a larger controlled study is needed to determine the efficacy of apremilast for rosacea [67].

Pityriasis Rubra Pilaris

Pityriasis rubra pilaris (PRP) is a papulosquamous skin disease that is commonly mistaken for psoriasis. Clinical features of this disease may include follicular hyperkeratosis, palmoplantar keratoderma, and/or reddish-orange-colored scaling patches. The etiology of this disease is not clear; however, studies have shown increased neutrophils and lymphocytes [68] as well as increased TNF-α and CXCL-10 in the lesional skin of individuals with PRP [69].

A potential role for apremilast in the treatment of PRP is supported by one case report involving an elderly male with leukemia and refractory PRP [70]. This patient's disease was not responsive to acitretin, methotrexate, cyclosporine, or infliximab. His PRP worsened following chemotherapy, and apremilast 30 mg twice daily was started. Within 4 weeks, improvement was observed, and a near complete resolution was noted within 6–8 months of treatment; he remained disease-free at 12 months. The only adverse event reported by the patient was mild gastrointestinal upset [70].

Discoid Lupus Erythematosus

Discoid lupus erythematosus (DLE) is a chronic autoimmune condition characterized by scaly, disklike plaques commonly on the head and neck. Lesional biopsies have demonstrated increased levels of Th-1 cytokines (IFN-γ and IL-2) [71]. The presence of these cytokines and an associated inflammatory infiltrate in the biopsies of lesional skin make DLE a good target for apremilast. In a study of eight patients with active DLE, apremilast 20 mg twice daily was taken for 85 days [6]. The CLE Disease Area and Severity Index (CLASI) was used to evaluate treatment response and incorporates assessments of erythema, scale/hypertrophy, dyspigmentation, scarring/atrophy/panniculitis, location, mucous membrane involvement, and alopecia [72]. There was a statistically significant decrease in their CLASI scores after 85 days of treatment [6]. Two patients had complete regression of their scalp lesions following treatment. The most common side effects experienced were nausea, diarrhea, and headache.

Bechet's Disease

Similar to psoriasis, Bechet's disease has an immunologic and genetic basis, and response to apremilast has been assessed [73]. The disease is a systemic vasculitis with an unknown etiology and is characterized by mouth and genital ulcers [74]. TNF-α, IL-6, IL-1, and IL-8 have been shown to be increased in Bechet's disease [75]. A phase 2 study was conducted to assess the use of apremilast for the treatment of Bechet's syndrome. In this study, 111 patients were enrolled and randomized to apremilast 30 mg twice a day or placebo for 12 weeks. At week 12 (the primary endpoint), the mean number of ulcers for each patient was significantly lower in the apremilast group versus placebo (0.5 ulcers vs. 2.1). Clinical responses to apremilast were reported as early as 2 weeks. The mean change in pain from oral ulcers from baseline to week 12, measured by a 100 mm Visual Analog Scale, was −44.7 mm for the apremilast cohort versus -16.0 mm for placebo. All ten patients in the apremilast group that had genital ulcers at baseline were free of genital ulcers by week 12. Improvements in quality of life, as measured by the Bechet's Disease Quality of Life at week 12, were also statistically significant for the treatment group. There were no unique adverse events different from those commonly found with apremilast [76]. There is currently a phase 3 trial looking at apremilast in the treatment of Bechet's disease (ClinicalTrials.gov Identifier: NCT02307513).

Lichen Planus

Lichen planus is a T-cell-mediated process that results in painful, pruritic lesions of the skin or mucosal surfaces. The etiology of this condition is not entirely clear [77], though elevated levels of CD8$^+$ cells, TNF-α, and IFN-γ are present in lesional tissues [78]. In one study, ten patients that either had moderate to severe cutaneous lichen planus, lichen planus with severe itching and/or pain that significantly interfered with activities of daily living, or lichen planus that was refractory to topical corticosteroids were treated with apremilast 20 mg twice daily for 12 weeks [79]. At 12 weeks, 30% of patients had a $\geq$2 grade improvement and a significant decrease in lesion count from 35 at baseline to 20.5. A decrease in pruritus score from 67 to

18.5 at the end of 12 weeks was also noted, and two patients had complete clearance of their lesions at 12 weeks. Additionally, one patient with 40% involvement of her bilateral buccal mucosa at baseline improved to 12% involvement at the end of the study. No significant adverse effects were noted. This study demonstrates a potential role for apremilast in the treatment of lichen planus and might be considered for other related disease variants such as oral lichen planus or lichen planopilaris.

Sarcoidosis

Sarcoidosis, a systemic inflammatory disease characterized by noncaseating granulomas can be associated with a pleomorphic number of skin lesions [80]. Cutaneous sarcoidosis was found to have increased levels of IL-12 and upregulation of the IFN pathway [81]. The efficacy of apremilast 20 mg twice daily for 12 weeks was evaluated in a study of 15 patients with persistent, chronic cutaneous sarcoidosis [82]. For each patient, an index lesion was determined at baseline. Lesion induration was measured by the Sarcoidosis Activity and Severity Index (SASI) induration score. At weeks 4 and 12 of treatment, there were statistically significant decreases in index lesion induration compared to baseline with a median decrease of 1 point in the SASI score for both time points. Paired pre- and post-treatment photographs also supported a beneficial role for apremilast in this patient cohort. Interestingly, one patient required apremilast dosage reduction of 20 mg once daily due to "jitteriness." No mechanism for this adverse effect has been suggested, and additional studies are necessary to determine its validity.

Other PDE Inhibitors

Introduction

There are other formulations of PDE4 inhibitors aside from oral medications like apremilast that have been developed and studied. For example, inhaled PDE4 inhibitors have been studied in asthma [83], one of the components of the atopic triad. It is not known how the inhaled PDE4 inhibitors affect skin disease. However, topical PDE4 inhibitors have been developed and studied in skin disease.

Topical PDE Inhibitors

The development and study of topical PDE inhibitors are currently under way. In cell culture, benzoxaborole PDE4 inhibitors have been shown to inhibit the release of cytokines like TNF-α, IFN-g, IL-12, IL-23, and Th2 cytokines (e.g., IL-4, IL-5, IL-13) in human peripheral blood mononuclear cells and human monocytes [84]. This is similar to systemic PDE4 inhibitors such as apremilast; however, crisaborole is more active in inhibiting IL-4 release, while apremilast has better inhibition of TNF-α, IL-23, and IL-17 secretion. Apremilast and benzoxaborole PDE4 inhibitors have high infinity for the PDE4 isoforms and are not selective among PDE4 isozymes. However, unlike apremilast, the benzoxaborole PDE4 inhibitors showed moderate inhibitory activity on PDE enzymes outside the PDE4 family and were less selective for PDE4. It is thought that the inhibition of other PDE families in addition to PDE4 may lead to an enhanced anti-inflammatory effect [84].

Using a mouse model of atopic dermatitis, one study demonstrated that a single application of a topical PDE4 inhibitor (E6005) relieved dermatitis-associated pruritus. Hind-paw scratching of the rostral back was used as an index of itching, and the firing activity of the cutaneous nerves was electrophysiologically recorded to assess pruritus/itching. Additionally, cAMP concentration in the involved skin of these mice was markedly decreased and reversed by application of the topical PDE4 inhibitor [85]. Further, a study of Japanese children with atopic dermatitis reported decreased pruritus, erythema, immune cell infiltration, excoriation, and lichenification following topical application of E6005 for 2 weeks compared to vehicle alone [86].

Crisaborole 2% ointment is another topical benzoxaborole PDE4 inhibitor that has been studied in the treatment of atopic dermatitis and psoriasis. In December 2016, Crisaborole was approved by the FDA to be used in the treatment of mild to moderate atopic dermatitis. Phase 1b and 2a trials showed promising results for crisaborole 2% ointment applied twice daily to affected areas for 28 days in adolescents with atopic dermatitis [87, 88]. 35–47.1% of these patients achieved a clear or almost clear Investigator Static Global Assessment (ISGA) score with a ≥2 grade improvement in the score compared to baseline [87, 88].

Two phase 3 trials enrolled patients 2 years and older and assigned patients to crisaborole 2% ointment twice daily versus placebo vehicle twice daily for 28 days with a 2:1 randomization [89]. A combined total of 1522 patients were analyzed in these studies. The proportion of individuals that achieved an ISGA score of 1 or less (clear or almost clear) with ≥ 2 grade improvement versus baseline was 32.8% (vs. 25.4% for placebo) for the first trial and 31.4% (vs. 18.0% for placebo) for the second, demonstrating a significant improvement when compared to the vehicle group at day 29. Statistically significant reductions in mean severity at day 29 when compared to baseline were seen in erythema (-41%), exudation (-65%), excoriation (-52%), induration/papulation (-37%), and lichenification (-42%)

in a pooled analysis of the two trials. Disease severity improvement was seen as early as 8 days after the start of treatment. Additionally, the early and sustained improvement in pruritus was also noted with no significant adverse effects. Pain or burning/stinging at the site of application were the most common reported adverse effects.

The use of topical PDE inhibitors for the treatment of chronic inflammatory skin diseases shows tremendous promise. According to information obtained from clinicaltrials.org, the efficacy of crisaborole is currently being investigated in other inflammatory conditions, such as psoriasis. The results of these studies have not yet been published.

Conclusion and Future Directions

PDE4 inhibitors have been shown to be efficacious in a number of inflammatory skin diseases. It is interesting to note the mechanism by which these inhibitors work (i.e., inhibition of inflammatory pathways further upstream and within target cells). This is quite different than traditional immunosuppressants and biological agents (e.g., TNF-α inhibitors act primarily within the extracellular compartment). Additionally, the most common reasons for the discontinuation of conventional systemic and biological therapies include the safety concerns/contraindications, fear of injections, cost, loss of effectiveness, and need for routine lab monitoring [90–92]. It will be interesting to see whether the availability of oral and/or topical PDE inhibitors, which have fewer contraindications and require less monitoring, will displace the use of traditional systemic and biologic agents in specific subsets of patients and/or diseases.

Long-term safety data for PDE inhibitors, such as apremilast, is not yet available and will require the treatment of thousands of patients over the next 10–15 years. A 5-year extension study of the ESTEEM trial is currently ongoing and offers insight into the long-term safety of apremilast. However, the safety data that we do have indicates that this class of medication is safe and well tolerated, other than those affected by mild gastrointestinal complaints. Unfortunately, the high cost and low efficacy rates of apremilast compared to standard traditional systemic therapies and biologics will likely limit its use in psoriasis and possibly other inflammatory diseases. Randomized controlled trials in diseases other than psoriasis and psoriatic arthritis represent an unmet need, and the safety and efficacy of apremilast in the pediatric population are desperately needed. One clear use for apremilast in dermatology is in the treatment of palmoplantar psoriasis. For many clinicians, apremilast offers the potential of becoming the first-line therapy in this specific patient population. A careful evaluation of apremilast in specific subtypes of diseases is also needed and will offer additional insights into the role of PDE inhibitors in inflammatory skin disease [57].

Case Presentation

A 75-year-old Caucasian male presents to the dermatology clinic with a more than 10-year history of recalcitrant plaque and pustular palmoplantar psoriasis. He notes that he has been treated with multiple topical and systemic agents but with little success. He endorses intermittent joint pains, morning stiffness, and swelling/redness of his fingers or toes. Associated symptoms included decreased sleep, itch, pain, skin tightness, fissures, and bleeding.

Past Medical History

- Hypertension
- Hyperlipidemia
- Obesity

Social and Family History

- Married
- 35-pack-year history of tobacco use, quit smoking 18 years ago
- Mother, father, and other first-degree relatives with a history of psoriasis

Previous Therapies

- High-potency topical steroids, PUVA, NBUVB, and excimer laser
- Acitretin, cyclosporine, and methotrexate
- Infliximab, etanercept, ustekinumab, and efalizumab

Physical Examination

- Thick, well-demarcated, erythematous, scaly plaques with prominent scale on the bilateral palms, soles, scalp, elbows, trunk, lower extremities, and gluteal cleft
- Thick, scaly, plaques with pustules and fissures on the palms and soles
- Pitting of the nail plate noted on multiple nails of the bilateral hands
- No recent dactylitis, tender or swollen joints, or enthesitis
- Body surface area involvement of approximately 13%

Management

Given the patient's failure to respond to multiple biologic therapies and the prominent involvement of the palms and soles, apremilast 30 mg twice daily in combination with acitretin 25 mg once daily was started. Within several weeks, the patient experienced a dramatic improvement in his skin lesions and rated his disease severity as a 3. His body surface area involvement at 4 months was less than 1%, and the patient denied any joint symptoms. Adverse events included diarrhea that was problematic for the first 3 weeks of treatment but improved gradually thereafter. He denied any other significant adverse effects other than skin dryness. This particular case highlights the utility of apremilast for the treatment of palmoplantar psoriasis. It also demonstrates its usefulness when combined with other treatment modalities, such as acitretin or phototherapy.

Conflicts of Interest JH and JEH have no conflicts of interest to declare. JEH is supported in part by The Rockefeller University CTSA award grant # UL1TR001866 and # KL2TR001865 from the National Center for Advancing Translational Sciences (NCATS), National Institutes of Health (NIH) Clinical and Translational Science Award (CTSA) program. GGK has received honoraria and has served as a consultant for Celgene.

References

1. Boswell-Smith V, Spina D, Page CP. Phosphodiesterase inhibitors. Br J Pharmacol. 2006;147(Suppl 1):S252–7. https://doi.org/10.1038/sj.bjp.0706495.
2. Mosenden R, Tasken K. Cyclic AMP-mediated immune regulation—overview of mechanisms of action in T cells. Cell Signal. 2011;23(6):1009–16. https://doi.org/10.1016/j.cellsig.2010.11.018.
3. Maurice DH, Ke H, Ahmad F, Wang Y, Chung J, Manganiello VC. Advances in targeting cyclic nucleotide phosphodiesterases. Nat Rev Drug Discov. 2014;13(4):290–314. https://doi.org/10.1038/nrd4228.
4. Samrao A, Berry TM, Goreshi R, Simpson EL. A pilot study of an oral phosphodiesterase inhibitor (apremilast) for atopic dermatitis in adults. Arch Dermatol. 2012;148(8):890–7. https://doi.org/10.1001/archdermatol.2012.812.
5. Keren A, Shemer A, Ullmann Y, Paus R, Gilhar A. The PDE4 inhibitor, apremilast, suppresses experimentally induced alopecia areata in human skin in vivo. J Dermatol Sci. 2015;77(1):74–6. https://doi.org/10.1016/j.jdermsci.2014.11.009.
6. De Souza A, Strober BE, Merola JF, Oliver S, Franks AG Jr. Apremilast for discoid lupus erythematosus: results of a phase 2, open-label, single-arm, pilot study. J Drugs Dermatol. 2012;11(10):1224–6.
7. Omori K, Kotera J. Overview of PDEs and their regulation. Circ Res. 2007;100(3):309–27. https://doi.org/10.1161/01.RES.0000256354.95791.f1.
8. Houslay MD, Schafer P, Zhang KY. Keynote review: phosphodiesterase-4 as a therapeutic target. Drug Discov Today. 2005;10(22):1503–19. https://doi.org/10.1016/S1359-6446(05)03622-6.
9. Halpin DMABCD. Of the phosphodiesterase family: interaction and differential activity in COPD. Int J Chron Obstruct Pulmon Dis. 2008;3(4):543–61.
10. Wright LC, Seybold J, Robichaud A, Adcock IM, Barnes PJ. Phosphodiesterase expression in human epithelial cells. Am J Phys. 1998;275(4 Pt 1):L694–700.
11. Shepherd MC, Baillie GS, Stirling DI, Houslay MD. Remodelling of the PDE4 cAMP phosphodiesterase isoform profile upon monocyte-macrophage differentiation of human U937 cells. Br J Pharmacol. 2004;142(2):339–51. https://doi.org/10.1038/sj.bjp.0705770.
12. Heystek HC, Thierry AC, Soulard P, Moulon C. Phosphodiesterase 4 inhibitors reduce human dendritic cell inflammatory cytokine production and Th1-polarizing capacity. Int Immunol. 2003;15(7):827–35.

13. Claveau D, Chen SL, O'Keefe S, Zaller DM, Styhler A, Liu S, et al. Preferential inhibition of T helper 1, but not T helper 2, cytokines in vitro by L-826,141 [4-[2-(3,4-Bisdifluromethoxyphenyl)-2-[4-(1,1,1,3,3,3-hexafluoro-2-hydroxypropan- 2-yl)-phenyl]-ethyl]3-methylpyridine-1-oxide], a potent and selective phosphodiesterase 4 inhibitor. J Pharmacol Exp Ther. 2004;310(2):752–60. https://doi.org/10.1124/jpet.103.064691.

14. Tenor H, Hedbom E, Hauselmann HJ, Schudt C, Hatzelmann A. Phosphodiesterase isoenzyme families in human osteoarthritis chondrocytes—functional importance of phosphodiesterase 4. Br J Pharmacol. 2002;135(3):609–18. https://doi.org/10.1038/sj.bjp.0704480.

15. Tenor H, Hatzelmann A, Wendel A, Schudt C. Identification of phosphodiesterase IV activity and its cyclic adenosine monophosphate-dependent up-regulation in a human keratinocyte cell line (HaCaT). J Invest Dermatol. 1995;105(1):70–4.

16. Gill GN, Garren LD. A cyclic-3′,5′-adenosine monophosphate dependent protein kinase from the adrenal cortex: comparison with a cyclic AMP binding protein. Biochem Biophys Res Commun. 1970;39(3):335–43.

17. Montminy MR, Bilezikjian LM. Binding of a nuclear protein to the cyclic-AMP response element of the somatostatin gene. Nature. 1987;328(6126):175–8. https://doi.org/10.1038/328175a0.

18. Ollivier V, Parry GC, Cobb RR, de Prost D, Mackman N. Elevated cyclic AMP inhibits NF-kappaB-mediated transcription in human monocytic cells and endothelial cells. J Biol Chem. 1996;271(34):20828–35.

19. Parry GC, Mackman N. Role of cyclic AMP response element-binding protein in cyclic AMP inhibition of NF-kappa B-mediated transcription. J Immunol. 1997;159(11):5450–6.

20. Eigler A, Siegmund B, Emmerich U, Baumann KH, Hartmann G, Endres S. Anti-inflammatory activities of cAMP-elevating agents: enhancement of IL-10 synthesis and concurrent suppression of TNF production. J Leukoc Biol. 1998;63(1):101–7.

21. Wachtel H. Potential antidepressant activity of rolipram and other selective cyclic adenosine 3′,5′-monophosphate phosphodiesterase inhibitors. Neuropharmacology. 1983;22(3):267–72.

22. Fabbri LM, Calverley PM, Izquierdo-Alonso JL, Bundschuh DS, Brose M, Martinez FJ, et al. Roflumilast in moderate-to-severe chronic obstructive pulmonary disease treated with longacting bronchodilators: two randomised clinical trials. Lancet. 2009;374(9691):695–703. https://doi.org/10.1016/S0140-6736(09)61252-6.

23. Schafer PH, Parton A, Capone L, Cedzik D, Brady H, Evans JF, et al. Apremilast is a selective PDE4 inhibitor with regulatory effects on innate immunity. Cell Signal. 2014;26(9):2016–29. https://doi.org/10.1016/j.cellsig.2014.05.014.

24. Man HW, Schafer P, Wong LM, Patterson RT, Corral LG, Raymon H, et al. Discovery of (S)-N-[2-[1-(3-ethoxy-4-methoxyphenyl)-2-methanesulfonylethyl]-1,3-dioxo-2,3-dihy dro-1H-isoindol-4-yl] acetamide (apremilast), a potent and orally active phosphodiesterase 4 and tumor necrosis factor-alpha inhibitor. J Med Chem. 2009;52(6):1522–4. https://doi.org/10.1021/jm900210d.

25. Schafer PH, Parton A, Gandhi AK, Capone L, Adams M, Wu L, et al. Apremilast, a cAMP phosphodiesterase-4 inhibitor, demonstrates anti-inflammatory activity in vitro and in a model of psoriasis. Br J Pharmacol. 2010;159(4):842–55. https://doi.org/10.1111/j.1476-5381.2009.00559.x.

26. Schett G, Sloan VS, Stevens RM, Schafer P. Apremilast: a novel PDE4 inhibitor in the treatment of autoimmune and inflammatory diseases. Ther Adv Musculoskelet Dis. 2010;2(5):271–8. https://doi.org/10.1177/1759720X10381432.

27. Hoffmann M, Kumar G, Schafer P, Cedzik D, Capone L, Fong KL, et al. Disposition, metabolism and mass balance of [(14)C]apremilast following oral administration. Xenobiotica. 2011;41(12):1063–75. https://doi.org/10.3109/00498254.2011.604745.

28. Papp K, Reich K, Leonardi CL, Kircik L, Chimenti S, Langley RG, et al. Apremilast, an oral phosphodiesterase 4 (PDE4) inhibitor, in patients with moderate to severe plaque psoriasis: results of a phase III, randomized, controlled trial (efficacy and safety trial evaluating the effects of Apremilast in psoriasis [ESTEEM] 1). J Am Acad Dermatol. 2015;73(1):37–49. https://doi.org/10.1016/j.jaad.2015.03.049.

29. Edwards CJ, Blanco FJ, Crowley J, Birbara CA, Jaworski J, Aelion J, et al. Apremilast, an oral phosphodiesterase 4 inhibitor, in patients with psoriatic arthritis and current skin involvement: a phase III, randomised, controlled trial (PALACE 3). Ann Rheum Dis. 2016;75(6):1065–73. https://doi.org/10.1136/annrheumdis-2015-207963.

30. Armstrong AW, Betts KA, Sundaram M, Thomason D, Signorovitch JE. Comparative efficacy and incremental cost per responder of methotrexate versus apremilast for methotrexate-naive patients with psoriasis. J Am Acad Dermatol. 2016;75(4):740–6. https://doi.org/10.1016/j.jaad.2016.05.040.

31. Hinde S, Wade R, Palmer S, Woolacott N, Spackman E. Apremilast for the treatment of moderate to severe plaque psoriasis: a critique of the evidence. PharmacoEconomics. 2016;34(6):587–96. https://doi.org/10.1007/s40273-016-0382-3.

32. Sideris E, Corbett M, Palmer S, Woolacott N, Bojke L. The clinical and cost effectiveness of apremilast for treating active psoriatic arthritis: a critique of the evidence. PharmacoEconomics. 2016. https://doi.org/10.1007/s40273-016-0419-7.

33. Schlaak JF, Buslau M, Jochum W, Hermann E, Girndt M, Gallati H, et al. T cells involved in psoriasis vulgaris belong to the Th1 subset. J Invest Dermatol. 1994;102(2):145–9.

34. Lowes MA, Kikuchi T, Fuentes-Duculan J, Cardinale I, Zaba LC, Haider AS, et al. Psoriasis vulgaris lesions contain discrete populations of Th1 and Th17 T cells. J Invest Dermatol. 2008;128(5):1207–11. https://doi.org/10.1038/sj.jid.5701213.

35. Austin LM, Ozawa M, Kikuchi T, Walters IB, Krueger JG. The majority of epidermal T cells in psoriasis vulgaris lesions can produce type 1 cytokines, interferon-gamma, interleukin-2, and tumor necrosis factor-alpha, defining TC1 (cytotoxic T lymphocyte) and TH1 effector populations: a type 1 differentiation bias is also measured in circulating blood T cells in psoriatic patients. J Invest Dermatol. 1999;113(5):752–9. https://doi.org/10.1046/j.1523-1747.1999.00749.x.

36. Arican O, Aral M, Sasmaz S, Ciragil P. Serum levels of TNF-alpha, IFN-gamma, IL-6, IL-8, IL-12, IL-17, and IL-18 in patients with active psoriasis and correlation with disease severity. Mediat Inflamm. 2005;2005(5):273–9. https://doi.org/10.1155/MI.2005.273.

37. Nair RP, Duffin KC, Helms C, Ding J, Stuart PE, Goldgar D, et al. Genome-wide scan reveals association of psoriasis with IL-23 and NF-kappa B pathways. Nat Genet. 2009;41(2):199–204. https://doi.org/10.1038/ng.311.

38. Papp KA, Kaufmann R, Thaci D, Hu C, Sutherland D, Rohane P. Efficacy and safety of apremilast in subjects with moderate to severe plaque psoriasis: results from a phase II, multicenter, randomized, double-blind, placebo-controlled, parallel-group, dose-comparison study. J Eur Acad Dermatol Venereol. 2013;27(3):e376–83. https://doi.org/10.1111/j.1468-3083.2012.04716.x.

39. Papp K, Cather JC, Rosoph L, Sofen H, Langley RG, Matheson RT, et al. Efficacy of apremilast in the treatment of moderate to severe psoriasis: a randomised controlled trial. Lancet. 2012;380(9843):738–46. https://doi.org/10.1016/S0140-6736(12)60642-4.

40. Gottlieb AB, Strober B, Krueger JG, Rohane P, Zeldis JB, CC H, et al. An open-label, single-arm pilot study in patients with severe plaque-type psoriasis treated with an oral anti-inflammatory agent, apremilast. Curr Med Res Opin. 2008;24(5):1529–38. https://doi.org/10.1185/030079908X301866.

41. Gottlieb AB, Matheson RT, Menter A, Leonardi CL, Day RM, Hu C, et al. Efficacy, tolerability, and pharmacodynamics of apremilast in recalcitrant plaque psoriasis: a phase II open-label study. J Drugs Dermatol. 2013;12(8):888–97.

42. Paul C, Cather J, Gooderham M, Poulin Y, Mrowietz U, Ferrandiz C, et al. Efficacy and safety of apremilast, an oral phosphodiesterase 4 inhibitor, in patients with moderate-to-severe plaque psoriasis over 52 weeks: a phase III, randomized controlled trial (ESTEEM 2). Br J Dermatol. 2015;173(6):1387–99. https://doi.org/10.1111/bjd.14164.

43. AbuHilal M, Walsh S, Shear N. Use of Apremilast in combination with other therapies for treatment of chronic plaque psoriasis: a retrospective study. J Cutan Med Surg. 2016. https://doi.org/10.1177/1203475416631328.

44. Danesh MJ, Beroukhim K, Nguyen C, Levin E, Koo J. Apremilast and adalimumab: a novel combination therapy for recalcitrant psoriasis. Dermatol Online J. 2015;21(6)

45. Rothstein BE, McQuade B, Greb JE, Goldminz AM, Gottlieb AB. Apremilast and secukinumab combined therapy in a patient with recalcitrant plaque psoriasis. J Drugs Dermatol. 2016;15(5):648–9.

46. Bartos S, Hill D, Feldman SR. Review of maintenance of response to psoriasis treatments. J Dermatolog Treat. 2016;27(4):293–7. https://doi.org/10.1080/09546634.2016.1177158.

47. Reich K, Gooderham M, Green L, Bewley A, Zhang Z, Khanskaya I, et al. The efficacy and safety of apremilast, etanercept, and placebo, in patients with moderate to severe plaque psoriasis: 52-week results from a phase 3b, randomized, placebo-controlled trial (LIBERATE). J Eur Acad Dermatol Venereol. 2016. https://doi.org/10.1111/jdv.14015.

48. Smith RL. Pediatric psoriasis treated with apremilast. JAAD Case Rep. 2016;2(1):89–91. https://doi.org/10.1016/j.jdcr.2015.12.005.

49. Schett G, Wollenhaupt J, Papp K, Joos R, Rodrigues JF, Vessey AR, et al. Oral apremilast in the treatment of active psoriatic arthritis: results of a multicenter, randomized, double-blind, placebo-controlled study. Arthritis Rheum. 2012;64(10):3156–67. https://doi.org/10.1002/art.34627.

50. Kavanaugh A, Mease PJ, Gomez-Reino JJ, Adebajo AO, Wollenhaupt J, Gladman DD, et al. Longterm (52-week) results of a phase III randomized, controlled trial of apremilast in patients with psoriatic arthritis. J Rheumatol. 2015;42(3):479–88. https://doi.org/10.3899/jrheum.140647.

51. Cutolo M, Myerson GE, Fleischmann RM, Liote F, Diaz-Gonzalez F, Van den Bosch F, et al. A phase III, randomized, controlled trial of apremilast in patients with psoriatic arthritis: results of the PALACE 2 trial. J Rheumatol. 2016. https://doi.org/10.3899/jrheum.151376.

52. Wells A, Edwards C, Adebajo A, Kivitz A. Apremilast in the treatment of DMARD-Naïve psoriatic arthritis patients: results of a phase 3 randomized, controlled trial (PALACE 4). 2013. http://acrabstracts.org/abstract/apremilast-in-the-treatment-of-dmard-naive-psoriatic-arthritis-patients-results-of-a-phase-3-randomized-controlled-trial-palace-4/. Accessed 26 July 2016.

53. Kavanaugh A, Adebajo AO, Gladman DD, Gomez-Reino JJ, Hall S, Lespessailles E. Long-term (156-week) efficacy and safety profile of apremilast, an oral phosphodiesterase 4 inhibitor, in patients with psoriatic arthritis: results from a phase III, randomized, controlled trial and open-label extension (PALACE 1). American College of Rheumatology. 2015. http://acrabstracts.org/abstract/long-term-156-week-efficacy-and-safety-profile-of-apremilast-an-oral-phosphodiesterase-4-inhibitor-in-patients-with-psoriatic-arthritis-results-from-a-phase-iii-randomized-controlled-trial-and/. Accessed 29 July 2016.

54. Wells A, Edwards C, Adebajo A, Kivitz A. Long-term (104-week) safety and efficacy of monotherapy with apremilast in dmard-naïve patients with psoriatic arthritis: a phase 3, randomized, controlled trial and open-label extension (PALACE 4). American College of Rheumatology. 2014. http://acrabstracts.org/abstract/long-term-104-week-safety-and-efficacy-of-monotherapy-with-apremilast-in-dmard-naive-patients-with-psoriatic-arthritis-a-phase-3-randomized-controlled-trial-and-open-label-extension-palace-4/. Accessed 26 July 2016.

55. Farley E, Masrour S, McKey J, Menter A. Palmoplantar psoriasis: a phenotypical and clinical review with introduction of a new quality-of-life assessment tool. J Am Acad Dermatol. 2009;60(6):1024–31. https://doi.org/10.1016/j.jaad.2008.11.910.

56. Adisen E, Tekin O, Gulekon A, Gurer MA. A retrospective analysis of treatment responses of palmoplantar psoriasis in 114 patients. J Eur Acad Dermatol Venereol. 2009;23(7):814–9. https://doi.org/10.1111/j.1468-3083.2009.03197.x.

57. Bissonnette R, Pariser DM, Wasel NR, Goncalves J, Day RM, Chen R, et al. Apremilast, an oral phosphodiesterase-4 inhibitor, in the treatment of palmoplantar psoriasis: results of a pooled analysis from phase II PSOR-005 and phase III efficacy and safety trial evaluating the effects of apremilast in psoriasis (ESTEEM) clinical trials in patients with moderate to severe psoriasis. J Am Acad Dermatol. 2016;75(1):99–105. https://doi.org/10.1016/j.jaad.2016.02.1164.

58. Rich P, Gooderham M, Bachelez H, Goncalves J, Day RM, Chen R, et al. Apremilast, an oral phosphodiesterase 4 inhibitor, in patients with difficult-to-treat nail and scalp psoriasis: results of 2 phase III randomized, controlled trials (ESTEEM 1 and ESTEEM 2). J Am Acad Dermatol. 2016;74(1):134–42. https://doi.org/10.1016/j.jaad.2015.09.001.

59. Gittler JK, Shemer A, Suarez-Farinas M, Fuentes-Duculan J, Gulewicz KJ, Wang CQ, et al. Progressive activation of T(H)2/T(H)22 cytokines and selective epidermal proteins characterizes acute and chronic atopic dermatitis. J Allergy Clin Immunol. 2012;130(6):1344–54. https://doi.org/10.1016/j.jaci.2012.07.012.

60. Koga C, Kabashima K, Shiraishi N, Kobayashi M, Tokura Y. Possible pathogenic role of Th17 cells for atopic dermatitis. J Invest Dermatol. 2008;128(11):2625–30. https://doi.org/10.1038/jid.2008.111.

61. Volf EM, SC A, Dumont N, Scheinman P, Gottlieb ABA. Phase 2, open-label, investigator-initiated study to evaluate the safety and efficacy of apremilast in subjects with recalcitrant allergic contact or atopic dermatitis. J Drugs Dermatol. 2012;11(3):341–6.

62. Saporito RC, Cohen DJ. Apremilast use for moderate-to-severe atopic dermatitis in pediatric patients. Case Rep Dermatol. 2016;8(2):179–84. https://doi.org/10.1159/000446836.

63. Suarez-Farinas M, Ungar B, Noda S, Shroff A, Mansouri Y, Fuentes-Duculan J, et al. Alopecia areata profiling shows TH1, TH2, and IL-23 cytokine activation without parallel TH17/TH22 skewing. J Allergy Clin Immunol. 2015;136(5):1277–87. https://doi.org/10.1016/j.jaci.2015.06.032.

64. Huang KP, Mullangi S, Guo Y, Qureshi AA. Autoimmune, atopic, and mental health comorbid conditions associated with alopecia areata in the United States. JAMA Dermatol. 2013;149(7):789–94. https://doi.org/10.1001/jamadermatol.2013.3049.

65. Gilhar A, Keren A, Shemer A, d'Ovidio R, Ullmann Y, Paus R. Autoimmune disease induction in a healthy human organ: a humanized mouse model of alopecia areata. J Invest Dermatol. 2013;133(3):844–7. https://doi.org/10.1038/jid.2012.365.

66. Culp B, Scheinfeld N. Rosacea: a review. P T. 2009;34(1):38–45.

67. Thompson BJ, Furniss M, Zhao W, Chakraborty B, Mackay-Wiggan J. An oral phosphodiesterase inhibitor (apremilast) for inflammatory rosacea in adults: a pilot study. JAMA Dermatol. 2014;150(9):1013–4. https://doi.org/10.1001/jamadermatol.2013.10526.

68. Magro CM, Crowson AN. The clinical and histomorphological features of pityriasis rubra pilaris. A comparative analysis with psoriasis. J Cutan Pathol. 1997;24(7):416–24.

69. Adnot-Desanlis L, Antonicelli F, Tabary T, Bernard P, Reguiai Z. Effectiveness of Infliximab in pityriasis rubra pilaris is associated with pro-inflammatory cytokine inhibition. Dermatology. 2013;226(1):41–6. https://doi.org/10.1159/000346640.

70. Krase IZ, Cavanaugh K, Curiel-Lewandrowski C. Treatment of refractory pityriasis rubra pilaris with novel phosphodiesterase 4 (PDE4) inhibitor apremilast. JAMA Dermatol. 2016;152(3):348–50. https://doi.org/10.1001/jamadermatol.2015.3405.

71. Toro JR, Finlay D, Dou X, Zheng SC, LeBoit PE, Connolly MK. Detection of type 1 cytokines in discoid lupus erythematosus. Arch Dermatol. 2000;136(12):1497–501.

72. Albrecht J, Taylor L, Berlin JA, Dulay S, Ang G, Fakharzadeh S, et al. The CLASI (cutaneous lupus Erythematosus disease area and severity index): an outcome instrument for cutaneous lupus erythematosus. J Invest Dermatol. 2005;125(5):889–94. https://doi.org/10.1111/j.0022-202X.2005.23889.x.

73. Zierhut M, Mizuki N, Ohno S, Inoko H, Gul A, Onoe K, et al. Immunology and functional genomics of Behcet's disease. Cell Mol Life Sci. 2003;60(9):1903–22. https://doi.org/10.1007/s00018-003-2333-3.

74. Zhou ZY, Chen SL, Shen N, Lu Y. Cytokines and Behcet's disease. Autoimmun Rev. 2012;11(10):699–704. https://doi.org/10.1016/j.autrev.2011.12.005.

75. Mege JL, Dilsen N, Sanguedolce V, Gul A, Bongrand P, Roux H, et al. Overproduction of monocyte derived tumor necrosis factor alpha, interleukin (IL) 6, IL-8 and increased neutrophil superoxide generation in Behcet's disease. A comparative study with familial Mediterranean fever and healthy subjects. J Rheumatol. 1993;20(9):1544–9.

76. Hatemi G, Melikoglu M, Tunc R, Korkmaz C, Turgut Ozturk B, Mat C, et al. Apremilast for Behcet's syndrome—a phase 2, placebo-controlled study. N Engl J Med. 2015;372(16):1510–8. https://doi.org/10.1056/NEJMoa1408684.

77. Sugerman PB, Savage NW, Walsh LJ, Zhao ZZ, Zhou XJ, Khan A, et al. The pathogenesis of oral lichen planus. Crit Rev Oral Biol Med. 2002;13(4):350–65.

78. Khan A, Farah CS, Savage NW, Walsh LJ, Harbrow DJ, Sugerman PB. Th1 cytokines in oral lichen planus. J Oral Pathol Med. 2003;32(2):77–83.

79. Paul J, Foss CE, Hirano SA, Cunningham TD, Pariser DM. An open-label pilot study of apremilast for the treatment of moderate to severe lichen planus: a case series. J Am Acad Dermatol. 2013;68(2):255–61. https://doi.org/10.1016/j.jaad.2012.07.014.

80. Haimovic A, Sanchez M, Judson MA, Prystowsky S. Sarcoidosis: a comprehensive review and update for the dermatologist: part I. Cutaneous disease. J Am Acad Dermatol. 2012;66(5):699. e1–718.e1. https://doi.org/10.1016/j.jaad.2011.11.965; quiz 717–8.

81. Judson MA, Marchell RM, Mascelli M, Piantone A, Barnathan ES, Petty KJ, et al. Molecular profiling and gene expression analysis in cutaneous sarcoidosis: the role of interleukin-12, interleukin-23, and the T-helper 17 pathway. J Am Acad Dermatol. 2012;66(6):901–10. https://doi.org/10.1016/j.jaad.2011.06.017, 10.e1–2.

82. Baughman RP, Judson MA, Ingledue R, Craft NL, Lower EE. Efficacy and safety of apremilast in chronic cutaneous sarcoidosis. Arch Dermatol. 2012;148(2):262–4. https://doi.org/10.1001/archdermatol.2011.301.

83. Chapman RW, House A, Richard J, Prelusky D, Lamca J, Wang P, et al. Pharmacology of a potent and selective inhibitor of PDE4 for inhaled administration. Eur J Pharmacol. 2010;643(2–3):274–81. https://doi.org/10.1016/j.ejphar.2010.06.054.

84. Dong C, Virtucio C, Zemska O, Baltazar G, Zhou Y, Baia D, et al. Treatment of skin inflammation with benzoxaborole PDE inhibitors: selectivity, cellular activity, and effect on cytokines associated with skin inflammation and skin architecture changes. J Pharmacol Exp Ther. 2016. https://doi.org/10.1124/jpet.116.232819.

85. Andoh T, Yoshida T, Kuraishi Y. Topical E6005, a novel phosphodiesterase 4 inhibitor, attenuates spontaneous itch-related responses in mice with chronic atopy-like dermatitis. Exp Dermatol. 2014;23(5):359–61. https://doi.org/10.1111/exd.12377.

86. Nemoto O, Hayashi N, Kitahara Y, Furue M, Hojo S, Nomoto M, et al. Effect of topical phosphodiesterase 4 inhibitor E6005 on Japanese children with atopic dermatitis: results from a randomized, vehicle-controlled exploratory trial. J Dermatol. 2015. https://doi.org/10.1111/1346-8138.13231.

87. Zane LT, Kircik L, Call R, Tschen E, Draelos ZD, Chanda S, et al. Crisaborole topical ointment, 2% in patients ages 2 to 17 years with atopic dermatitis: a phase 1b, open-label, maximal-use systemic exposure study. Pediatr Dermatol. 2016. https://doi.org/10.1111/pde.12872.

88. Tom WL, Van Syoc M, Chanda S, Zane LT. Pharmacokinetic profile, safety, and tolerability of crisaborole topical ointment, 2% in adolescents with atopic dermatitis: an open-label phase 2a study. Pediatr Dermatol. 2016;33(2):150–9. https://doi.org/10.1111/pde.12780.

89. Paller AS, Tom WL, Lebwohl MG, Blumenthal RL, Boguniewicz M, Call RS, et al. Efficacy and safety of crisaborole ointment, a novel, nonsteroidal phosphodiesterase 4 (PDE4) inhibitor for the topical treatment of atopic dermatitis (AD) in children and adults. J Am Acad Dermatol. 2016. https://doi.org/10.1016/j.jaad.2016.05.046.

90. Armstrong AW, Robertson AD, Wu J, Schupp C, Lebwohl MG. Undertreatment, treatment trends, and treatment dissatisfaction among patients with psoriasis and psoriatic arthritis in the United States: findings from the National Psoriasis Foundation surveys, 2003–2011. JAMA Dermatol. 2013;149(10):1180–5. https://doi.org/10.1001/jamadermatol.2013.5264.

91. Lebwohl MG, Bachelez H, Barker J, Girolomoni G, Kavanaugh A, Langley RG, et al. Patient perspectives in the management of psoriasis: results from the population-based multinational assessment of psoriasis and psoriatic arthritis survey. J Am Acad Dermatol. 2014;70(5):871–881.e1–30. https://doi.org/10.1016/j.jaad.2013.12.018.

92. Lebwohl MG, Kavanaugh A, Armstrong AW, Van Voorhees AS. US perspectives in the management of psoriasis and psoriatic arthritis: patient and physician results from the population-based multinational assessment of psoriasis and psoriatic arthritis (MAPP) survey. Am J Clin Dermatol. 2016;17(1):87–97. https://doi.org/10.1007/s40257-015-0169-x.

Oral Retinoids in Dermatology

22

Mio Nakamura, Sahil Sekhon, Amanda Raymond,
and John Koo

Abbreviations

ALT	Alanine aminotransferase
AST	Aspartate aminotransferase
BB-UVD	Broadband ultraviolet B
CBC	Complete blood count
CD	Crohn's disease
FDA	Food and Drug Administration
Free T4	Free thyroxine
IBD	Inflammatory bowel disease
LFT	Liver function tests
PASI	Psoriasis Area and Severity Index
PUVA	Psoralen plus ultraviolet A
RAR	Retinoic acid receptor
RXR	Retinoid X receptor
TSH	Thyroid-stimulating hormone
UC	Ulcerative colitis
UVB	Ultraviolet B
WBC	White blood cells

Introduction

Retinoids have been used in dermatology since the 1940s when vitamin A was first used to treat acne vulgaris. Currently, three retinoids are approved for dermatologic indications in the United States: acitretin for moderate-to-severe psoriasis vulgaris, isotretinoin for severe recalcitrant nodular acne vulgaris, and bexarotene for cutaneous T-cell lymphoma. This chapter will focus on these three medications.

M. Nakamura, MD (✉) • S. Sekhon, MD
A. Raymond, MD • J. Koo, MD
Department of Dermatology, University of California San Francisco, San Francisco, CA, USA
e-mail: mionak24@gmail.com; John.Koo2@ucsf.edu

Acitretin

Acitretin (Soriatane) is an oral retinoid approved for the treatment of moderate-to-severe psoriasis [1]. It is thought to modulate epidermal proliferation and differentiation and to have immunomodulatory and anti-inflammatory activity. Acitretin has no direct immunosuppressive effects and can therefore be used in patients who are not candidates for systemic immunosuppressive therapy, such as those with active chronic infections (hepatitis B, hepatitis C, HIV, etc.), history of serious infection, malignancy, or the elderly. Acitretin is also used in combination with ultraviolet B (UVB) or psoralen plus ultraviolet A (PUVA) phototherapy for synergistic efficacy [2]. Off-label, acitretin is used for chemoprevention of cutaneous malignancies in high-risk patients [3], as well as other inflammatory and keratinization disorders such as pityriasis rubra pilaris, ichthyosis, and hyperkeratotic palmoplantar dermatitis [4].

Mechanism of Action

Vitamin A exhibits its biological effects through two members of the steroid/thyroid superfamily of nuclear hormone receptors: the retinoic acid receptors (RAR α, β, γ) and the retinoid X receptors (RXR α, β, γ). Acitretin is a second-generation vitamin A derivative that activates all three RAR subtypes (α, β, γ), which then bind to retinoid response elements in the promotor region of the target genes and alter gene transcription [5]. In psoriasis, acitretin appears to have direct effect on keratinocyte gene transcription to normalize proliferation and differentiation. Skin biopsies from psoriasis lesions of patients treated with acitretin show a reduction in the typical pathologic characteristics of psoriasis including epidermal/suprapapillary thickness ratio and a thickened basal cell layer [6]. Acitretin also appears to have anti-angiogenic and anti-inflammatory effects through modulation of T-cell responses and inhibition of neutrophil chemotaxis [4].

© Springer International Publishing AG 2018
P.S. Yamauchi (ed.), *Biologic and Systemic Agents in Dermatology*, https://doi.org/10.1007/978-3-319-66884-0_22

Pharmacokinetics and Metabolism

Acitretin is derived from its precursor drug etretinate, an ethyl ester second-generation retinoid. Etretinate was a widely used systemic retinoid for psoriasis until 1980 when it was replaced by acitretin. The efficacy of etretinate and acitretin is shown to be comparable [7]. The difference between etretinate and acitretin is that etretinate is extremely lipophilic and stored in fat; consequently, its half-life is 120 days [8]. Acitretin is more water soluble, and its half-life is approximately 60 h [1]. However, the concurrent use of alcohol and acitretin leads to reverse metabolism to etretinate [9, 10]. Although the exact amount of alcohol required to produce this effect is unknown, it is necessary to avoid the use of alcohol during acitretin therapy and for 3 years after discontinuation.

Acitretin is taken orally, and the absorption of the medication is enhanced two- to five-fold when taken with high-fat meals [11]. It has a bioavailability of approximately 60%, with 99% of the circulating drug bound to plasma proteins. The drug is metabolized in the liver and is excreted as bile or as water-soluble metabolites in the kidneys [12].

Use and Dosage

For the treatment of moderate-to-severe psoriasis, the typical dose of acitretin is 10–50 mg/day given as a single dose [13]. Although higher doses of acitretin lead to relatively faster onset of action and greater improvement of psoriasis, many patients are unable to tolerate the side effects of acitretin at high doses (see section Safety and Tolerability). After decades of use, most psoriasis experts in the United States are of the consensus that, for most patients, acitretin is best used at a "low dose" of 25 mg/day or less, taken with food. When higher than 25 mg/day is used (such as in the phase III pivotal trial for U.S. Food and Drug Administration (FDA) approval), annoying side effects such as dry skin, hair loss, and skin irritation become more noticeable than the therapeutic effect. Therefore, although the FDA approval involved high doses, low dose of 25 mg/day or less is recommended, especially for long-term use. Furthermore, in the authors' experience, the optimal dose in the elderly tends to be, on average, lower than the optimal dose for the non-elderly population.

Because both efficacy and side effects of acitretin can vary substantially among individual patients, proper dosing of acitretin requires careful titration to achieve a balance between optimizing response and minimizing toxicity. Optimal dosing may be achieved using a "dose-escalation strategy" involving initiation of therapy at low doses (10–25 mg/day) and, if necessary, gradually increasing the dose as tolerated until adequate response is achieved [14]. The "dose-escalation strategy" is derived from a study that compared three different dosing regimens of acitretin. The first group of patients received increasing doses of acitretin, starting with 10 mg/day for 2 weeks, then 30 mg/day for 2 weeks, and then 50 mg/day for 2 weeks (dose-escalation group). The second group was treated with a stable dose of acitretin 30 mg/day for 6 weeks (stable dose group). The third group received decreasing doses starting with 50 mg/day for 2 weeks, then 30 mg/day for 2 weeks, and then 10 mg/day for 2 weeks (dose-declining group). The three dosing regimens used in this study were shown to have comparable efficacy; however, the dose-escalation group experienced the lowest toxicity [15].

Acitretin is dosed similarly for other uses such as pityriasis rubra pilaris and other keratinization disorders [4]. For chemoprevention of malignancy in patients with solid organ transplantation, acitretin is typically used at 0.2–0.4 mg/kg/day [16–18]. Table 22.1 summarizes the use of acitretin in various dermatologic conditions, both on- and off-label.

Efficacy

Psoriasis

The efficacy of acitretin is dose dependent, with higher doses leading to faster and more effective improvement of psoriasis. In patients with moderate-to-severe chronic plaque psoriasis, various dosages have been used in clinical trials. When 50 mg/day is used, approximately 23% and 70% of patients

Table 22.1 The use of acitretin in dermatologic conditions

On-label use	Moderate-to-severe psoriasis
Reported off-label use	Non-melanoma skin cancer chemoprevention for high-risk patients • Solid-organ transplant recipients • Patients who have undergone long-term PUVA • Patients with extensive sun damage • Patients with xeroderma pigmentosum, nevoid basal cell carcinoma syndrome, Bazex syndrome, Rombo syndrome, and epidermodysplasia verruciformis Inherited keratinization disorders • Lamellar ichthyosis • Non-bullous and bullous ichthyosiform erythroderma • Pityriasis rubra pilaris • Inflammatory linear verrucous epidermal nevus • Darier's disease • Sjogren-Larsson syndrome Other keratinization disorders • Lichen sclerosus et atrophicus • Lichen planus • Palmoplantar pustulosis • Pityriasis rubra pilaris • Subcorneal pustular dermatosis Others • Cutaneous lupus erythematosus (in combination with hydroxychloroquine)

achieve 75% improvement or greater in the Psoriasis Area and Severity Index from baseline (PASI-75) at weeks 8 and 12, respectively [7, 19]. After 6 and 12 months of continuous treatment, 75% and 88% of patients, respectively, reach 50% improvement or greater in PASI from baseline (PASI-50) [20], indicating that acitretin is an effective maintenance therapy.

Acitretin has a quicker onset of action and is effective for treatment of pustular psoriasis. Patients with severe, generalized pustular disease will often require a more aggressive treatment with higher starting dose (50–75 mg/day). Lesions can begin to resolve in as little as 10 days after starting treatment [21], and acitretin is overall effective with one study showing improvement in 84% of patients with generalized pustular psoriasis [22]. Acitretin can also be used effectively to treat erythrodermic psoriasis [21].

Acitretin can be used as part of combination therapy for the treatment of recalcitrant moderate-to-severe psoriasis, especially in patients with thick, scaly plaques (Fig. 22.1). Many studies have shown that combination of acitretin with UVB and PUVA phototherapy is not only more effective but reduces the cumulative UV dose, as well as number and duration of treatment required, compared to phototherapy alone [23–28]. In a randomized, double-blind comparative study of 60 patients with severe, widespread psoriasis treated with PUVA, marked or complete clearing of psoriasis occurred in 80% of the patients without acitretin and in 96% of the patients with acitretin. The mean cumulative UVA dose given to patients in the acitretin-PUVA group was 42% less than that required for patients in the placebo-PUVA group [24]. Acitretin is also shown to enhance the efficacy of UVB phototherapy in an 8-week, randomized, comparator study, which found that more than double the number of patients in the combined broadband-UVB (BB-UVB) and acitretin cohort reached PASI-75 as compared to the BB-UVB-only cohort [28]. When adding acitretin to a treatment regimen in a patient who is already receiving phototherapy, the UV dose should be decreased by 50% and increased as tolerated at subsequent treatment sessions in order to avoid *delayed retinoid burn*. Delayed retinoid burn is a phenomenon in which lesional skin of psoriasis, but not normal skin, burns approximately 2–4 weeks after adding acitretin, if UVB dose is not appropriately decreased [29].

Acitretin can also be used safely in combination with topical corticosteroids and calcipotriene. It can also be used with cyclosporine as part of sequential therapy, in which cyclosporine can clear psoriasis rapidly and acitretin can be used to maintain its effects [21]. Acitretin should not be used in combination with methotrexate due to theoretical risk of hepatotoxicity, although not absolutely contraindicated [30]. In appropriately selected patients, the combination of acitretin and biologics may be an effective treatment option [31].

Chemoprevention

Acitretin can be used to prevent or delay the development of non-melanoma skin cancers, especially in solid organ transplant recipients [16, 32]. In a 5-year study, 12 of 16 renal transplant recipients on acitretin 0.3 mg/kg/day showed significant reduction in the number of new tumors excised during the treatment period compared to the pretreatment period [17]. Another study showed that acitretin 0.2 mg/kg/day decreased the thickness and number of actinic keratosis but did not affect the incidence of new skin malignancies [18]. Discontinuation of acitretin can cause rapid recurrence of actinic keratoses and squamous cell carcinomas [32, 33]. Since there is no proven cumulative side effect from long-term use of low-dose acitretin, the authors recommend that patients who are benefiting from skin cancer chemoprevention not be discontinued without good reason. Patients with xeroderma pigmentosum, nevoid basal cell carcinoma syndrome, Bazex syndrome, Rombo syndrome, and epidermodysplasia verruciformis may also be candidates for acitretin therapy for non-melanoma skin cancer prevention. Patients who have had PUVA or significant sun damage may also benefit from acitretin chemoprevention [34].

Other Dermatologic Conditions

Acitretin is considered a first-line agent for the treatment of hyperkeratotic palmoplantar dermatitis [35]. Acitretin can also be used to treat pediatric patients with inherited keratinization disorders such as lamellar ichthyosis, non-bullous and bullous ichthyosiform erythroderma, pityriasis rubra pilaris, inflammatory linear verrucous epidermal nevus, Darier's disease, and Sjogren-Larsson syndrome [36, 37]. Acitretin has also been used to treat lichen sclerosus et atrophicus, lichen planus, palmoplantar pustulosis, pityriasis rubra pilaris, and subcorneal pustular dermatosis [4]. Acitretin has been used in combination with hydroxychloroquine for treatment of cutaneous lupus erythematosus [38].

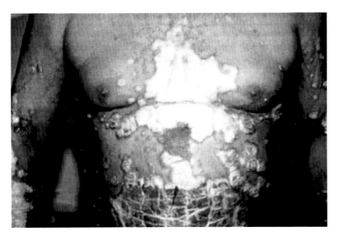

Fig. 22.1 Psoriasis patients with thick scale may benefit from combination treatment of acitretin and phototherapy

Table 22.2 Common side effects of acitretin which are dose dependent

Adverse event	Acitretin >25 mg/day (%)	≤25 mg/day (%)
Cheilitis	>75	70
Skin peeling	50–75	30
Alopecia	50–75	13
Pruritus	25–50	26
Dry skin	25–50	4
Nail disorder	25–50	0
Arthralgia	10–25	4
Headache	1–10	13
Myalgia	1–10	0
Depression	1–10	0

Safety and Tolerability

Many of the reported adverse effects of acitretin as discussed below are dose dependent [39] (Table 22.2). Clinical trials report much lower incidences of adverse effects in patients treated with low-dose acitretin (≤25 mg/day) versus high-dose acitretin (>25 mg/day) [21].

Teratogenicity
Acitretin, as with all systemic retinoids, is teratogenic and therefore labeled pregnancy category X by the FDA. Exposure to systemic retinoids during the first 6 weeks of gestation leads to abnormalities in cephalic neural crest development. Characteristic fetal irregularities involve craniofacial (high palate, anophthalmia), musculoskeletal (syndactyly, absence of terminal phalanges, hip malformations), and central nervous system (meningomyelocele, meningoencephalocele, and multiple synostosis) [1, 40]. Acitretin is generally avoided in female patients of reproductive potential, and patients are instructed to refrain from becoming pregnant and use appropriate contraception during and for 3 years following cessation of acitretin therapy. Patients should be advised to avoid alcohol consumption while taking acitretin because, as stated earlier, alcohol can convert acitretin to etretinate, which has an extremely long half-life.

Mucocutaneous Toxicity
The most common side effect of acitretin is cheilitis, which occurs in approximately 70% of patients regardless of the dose [21, 39]. Other common side effects, including skin peeling, pruritus, xerosis, and sticky sensation of the skin, are more likely to be observed on higher doses of acitretin [41]. Potential nail diseases include onychorrhexis and onychoschizia, as well as pyogenic granulomas when high-dose therapy is used long-term. Alopecia (46%) can occur a few weeks following initiation of acitretin but should be reversible with dose reduction or discontinuation of therapy [39]. All of the aforementioned side effects are dose dependent, except for cheilitis, and can be managed by reducing the dose as needed. Routine skin care such as use of emollients may help alleviate some of the associated discomfort.

Hepatotoxicity
Liver function test (LFT) abnormalities can occur 2–8 weeks after initiating acitretin in approximately 25–30% of patients, usually in association with high-dose therapy [42]. It has been the authors' experience that LFT abnormalities are very rare when low dose (25 mg/day or less) is used. The elevations are transient, and severe or persistent elevations are rare. Patients who present with transaminase elevations two to three times the upper limit of normal should decrease the acitretin dose by 50% and LFTs rechecked in 2 weeks. Alternatively, acitretin may be discontinued until labs normalize and then restarted at a lower dose with close laboratory monitoring [21]. Acitretin should be used with caution in patients with preexisting liver disease. Patients should be counseled about minimizing ethanol and acetaminophen consumption while taking acitretin to reduce the risk of hepatotoxicity. If LFT elevations persist, hepatology consultation may be warranted. Routine liver biopsy is not required for patients on long-term acitretin therapy.

Hyperlipidemia
Hypertriglyceridemia and hypercholesterolemia occur in 66 and 33% of patients on high-dose acitretin, respectively [42]. The risks are much less common with low-dose therapy. Most cases are mild, and fulminant pancreatitis secondary to severely elevated serum triglycerides is rare [1]. Most cases can be managed with lifestyle changes (decreasing dietary fat intake and increasing exercise) and medical management with lipid-lowering agents, if necessary. If triglycerides are >499 mg/dL, acitretin dose should be decreased by 50%. If triglycerides are >800 mg/dL, acitretin should be discontinued. Acitretin can be reinitiated once hypertriglyceridemia is under control [21].

Myalgias and Arthralgias
Myalgias can occur without creatinine phosphokinase (CPK) elevation. Arthralgias can also occur in a small proportion of patients and usually resolve on discontinuation of therapy [21].

Pseudotumor Cerebri
There have been a limited number of case reports of pseudotumor cerebri (idiopathic intracranial hypertension) during systemic retinoid therapy. However, the exact incidence is unclear, and there is no evidence-based data to support an association between acitretin and pseudotumor cerebri [43]. The use of tetracycline antibiotics should be avoided, as there may be an increased risk of pseudotumor cerebri with the combination of systemic retinoids and tetracyclines [44]. Patients should be counseled for signs and symptoms including severe headaches, nausea, emesis, and visual changes.

Ophthalmologic evaluation to rule out papilledema is warranted if pseudotumor cerebri is suspected.

Skeletal Abnormalities

Some retrospective studies evaluating the effects of etretinate and acitretin have suggested a possible association between systemic retinoid use and development of hyperostosis. However, all prospective studies using low-dose acitretin to date have not shown convincing evidence of this association. The development of hyperostosis previously reported in retrospective studies where all bone spurs were thought to be due to acitretin may, in retrospect, be a normal aging process rather than due to acitretin therapy [45]. Screening radiographs or follow-up X-rays are likely unnecessary for adults unless they report symptoms of bone pain or using high-dose acitretin [21].

Psychiatric Effects

There is a warning of depression on the package insert of acitretin; however, there is no convincing evidence that acitretin is associated with increased risk of depression, and the warning is likely to reflect a class label from the depression controversy surrounding isotretinoin [21].

Monitoring

Baseline labs, including a complete blood count (CBC), LFTs, and a fasting lipid panel, are recommended before initiating therapy with acitretin. Labs should be repeated monthly while dose adjustments are made. Once the patient is on a stable maintenance dose and demonstrates normal laboratory values, routine monitoring can be decreased to every 2–3 months (Table 22.3). Although acitretin therapy is not recommended for females of childbearing potential, two negative pregnancy tests are required before initiating acitretin therapy and monthly during treatment [1].

Isotretinoin

Isotretinoin is an oral first-generation retinoid initially approved in 1982 for the treatment of severe recalcitrant nodular acne [46]. It was originally marketed under the name Accutane but is now marketed under several brand and generic

Table 22.3 Laboratory monitoring during acitretin therapy

Laboratory tests	Frequency
Complete blood count, liver function tests, fasting lipid panel	Baseline, then monthly while dose adjustments are made, then every 2–3 months during stable dosing
Pregnancy tests (for females of reproductive age)	Two negative results at baseline, then monthly thereafter

names. Isotretinoin was originally developed and researched for treatment of ichthyosis and other keratinizing disorders in the United States [47] but was found to also have a significant effect on improving nodulocystic acne vulgaris in these clinical trial patients. Isotretinoin was then studied in clinical trials for the treatment of acne vulgaris and, soon thereafter, gained approval by the FDA for treatment of severe recalcitrant nodular acne [48], which is defined as multiple, inflammatory lesions greater than 5 mm in size that are unresponsive to conventional therapy including oral antibiotics [46].

Mechanism of Action

Isotretinoin, like other medications in the retinoid class, binds to RAR and RXR, both of which have three subtypes, α, β, γ. Isotretinoin binds to all six subtypes and does not have any known affinity for one receptor type or subtype. In general, RAR and RXR exist as heterodimers, with RAR always binding to RXR while RXR can form homodimers with other RXR as well as with thyroid hormone receptor, vitamin D_3, and others [5, 49]. It is thought that retinoids have two main effects: a direct effect on gene transcription that results in cellular differentiation and an indirect effect on gene transcription that results in reduced cellular proliferation and inflammation [49]. In acne, isotretinoin decreases sebum production, abnormal desquamation of follicular epithelial cells, inflammation, and *P. acnes* in areas prone to acne [50–54]. It is thought that the combination of all of these effects and the alteration of the biology of the skin result in the long-term remission of acne vulgaris seen in many patients.

Pharmacokinetics and Metabolism

Isotretinoin (13-*cis*-retinoic acid) is a first-generation retinoid, derived from manipulation of the polar end group and the polyene side group of vitamin A. Isotretinoin has bioavailability of 25%, which can be slightly enhanced with food intake, although this effect is not nearly as significant as with acitretin or bexarotene. In plasma, it is typically protein-bound to albumin and has a half-life of 10–20 h [55]. It is metabolized in the liver by the 3A4 isoform of cytochrome P-450 into 4-oxo-isotretinoin, which is then excreted in the bile and the urine. Given that it is more water soluble than other oral retinoids like etretinate, it is poorly stored in the liver and is undetectable in serum 1 month after therapy is stopped.

Use and Dosage

Isotretinoin is the only oral retinoid approved for the treatment of nodulocystic acne vulgaris. For the treatment of acne vulgaris, the standard range of dosing is 0.5–1 mg/kg/day, which is based on several studies that evaluated different dosing regimens [56]. One study evaluated the response to daily dosing at 0.1, 0.5, and 1 mg/kg over the course of 20 weeks and showed relatively similar clinical improvement. However, the 0.1 mg/kg daily group had a much higher relapse rate with 42% of patients requiring retreatment, while the clinical side effects and lab abnormalities experienced between the three groups were relatively similar [57]. In a study evaluating long-term success of isotretinoin treatment, it was found that the dose schedule, and especially the cumulative dose of isotretinoin, was important in determining relapse rate. Patients receiving 0.5 mg/kg/day or patients with a cumulative dose <120 mg/kg had a significantly higher rate of relapse compared to patients with cumulative dose >120 mg/kg [58]. Some studies have evaluated alternative cumulative dosing regimens; one study showed that patients treated with cumulative dose of 220 mg/kg had significantly lower rates of relapse of acne vulgaris while having very similar rates of adverse effects of the medication except for a higher incidence of retinoid dermatitis [59]. Other studies have evaluated the efficacy of low-dose regimens in mild-to-moderate acne and found that the low-cumulative dosing regimens had similar efficacy when compared to standard dosing regimens [60, 61]. The American Academy of Dermatology work group suggests the following regimen for isotretinoin therapy: starting therapy with a dose of 0.5 mg/kg/day and increasing to 1 mg/kg/day after 1 month as tolerated with a goal of cumulative dose of 120–150 mg/kg [62]. Absolute contraindications for isotretinoin use include active pregnancy, active nursing, women seeking to become pregnant, and inadequate contraceptive usage.

Efficacy

Isotretinoin has been shown to improve acne to clear or almost clear in at least 70% of patients [63, 64]. Typically, patients can initially expect to have some worsening of their acne in the first 2 months of treatment with near complete clearance by the end of their treatment, which can vary depending on how the medication is prescribed (as described above).

Safety and Tolerability

Isotretinoin is usually well tolerated with minimal and reversible adverse effects. The most common adverse effects include cheilitis, dryness in the nares, xerosis or exacerbation of xerosis (more common in atopic patients) [65], arthralgias, myalgias, and elevated serum triglycerides and/

or cholesterol. Triglyceride elevation rarely requires treatment or discontinuation of treatment and an increase to the range where pancreatitis due to hypertriglyceridemia is rare [66]. Similarly, LFT abnormalities are usually transient and reversible and do not warrant interruption of isotretinoin therapy [67]. Other relatively common adverse events include decreased night vision, bacterial conjunctivitis, blepharoconjunctivitis, and corneal opacities [68–71]. Of note, decreased night vision resolves with cessation of therapy, and corneal opacities are often found incidentally on ophthalmic exam and do not cause visual disturbances. Rare adverse events that have been seen in isotretinoin therapy in acne vulgaris patients include pyogenic granuloma-like lesions, acne fulminans, and pseudotumor cerebri [72–75]. Notably, pseudotumor cerebri risk is increased with concomitant usage of tetracyclines and isotretinoin. However, pseudotumor cerebri has a much stronger association with tetracycline exposure, and isotretinoin has been used safely in patients who have had pseudotumor cerebri due to minocycline [76, 77]. Given the link between tetracyclines and pseudotumor cerebri, it is best to avoid the combination of isotretinoin and tetracyclines for treatment of acne.

Isotretinoin usage has been linked to depression, suicidal ideation/attempts, completed suicide, and other psychiatric disturbances [46, 78]. A warning was added to the label in 1998; however, large-scale studies have not shown this association and causality [79, 80]. Some studies have posited that a small subset of isotretinoin patients may have a small risk of depression or suicide, but depression in these patients is quickly reversible with cessation of the medication, taking 2–7 days to resolve, which is likely prior to achievement of complete drug clearance [81]. It is likely that some patients with acne vulgaris have preexisting mild depression or increased risk of depression, and it is important for clinicians to be aware of a patient's risk factors and discontinue isotretinoin if depression in their patient becomes more profound and severe. Additionally, there is stronger evidence for the improvement of depression and anxiety in patients with acne treated with isotretinoin, suggesting that isotretinoin may do more good than harm psychiatrically [82–85]. Patients with untreated acne are at risk for psychiatric conditions such as suicide and depression, and therefore, it is important to inquire about them before initiating therapy and continue to monitor for these conditions during therapy. If a patient has a history of depression or exhibits depressive symptoms, clinicians should consider consultation with a psychiatrist and using a lower than standard dose of isotretinoin with close monitoring of depressive symptoms with a gradual dose increase as tolerated [86].

Isotretinoin may also be associated with inflammatory bowel disease (IBD), including both ulcerative colitis (UC) and Crohn's Disease (CD); however, the evidence for this is also mixed. Some studies have shown probable association between IBD and isotretinoin use, but even in these studies, it is difficult to declare that isotretinoin has caused IBD given that the age of patients at first diagnosis of IBD is similar to the age of patients being treated with isotretinoin [60]. One large case-control study found that isotretinoin use was associated with the development of UC but not with CD [87]. However, a large population-based cohort study conducted over 12 years evaluating 46,922 patients treated with isotretinoin in Canada found no association between isotretinoin and IBD [88]. This study did find some evidence of associations between IBD and isotretinoin and with topical acne medications, which could suggest an association between IBD and acne itself. A retrospective cohort study in the United Kingdom found that tetracyclines, particularly doxycycline, may be associated with the development of IBD [89]. Given the lack of a clear association between isotretinoin and IBD, it is best to be cautious in using isotretinoin in patients with a strong family history of IBD and consider co-managing with gastroenterology for patients with IBD who are deemed to be appropriate candidates for isotretinoin therapy.

Monitoring

Laboratory Tests

Monitoring during treatment with isotretinoin involves the following baseline and routine tests: CBC with platelets, fasting lipid profile, LFTs, and kidney function tests (Table 22.4). Currently, there is no consensus on guidelines for laboratory monitoring. Some recommend testing weekly or biweekly until stable response to medication is established [46]. Current recommended monitoring parameters include fasting lipid profile (including triglycerides) and transaminase collection at baseline and then repeated weekly or biweekly until a stable response is established. However, physician instruction regarding laboratory interpretation and associated treatment modification or discontinuation is limited, and modified monitoring schedules have been proposed to decrease superfluous testing and associated costs that may not provide higher quality of care [90, 91]. One regimen that has been suggested involves testing baseline values of the above parameters and then testing at 1 month after starting therapy as well as 2 months after therapy, with monthly lab testing thereafter if any significant laboratory test results are observed (triglycerides >300 mg/dL, alkaline phosphatase >200 U/L (female) and >350 U/L (male), ALT >45 U/L, AST >60 U/L, cholesterol >250 mg/dL, WBC <3000). Discontinuation of therapy should be considered if lab results are above these close monitoring values (triglycerides >400 mg/dL, alkaline phosphatase >264 U/L (female) and >500 U/L (male), ALT >62 U/L, AST >80 U/L, cholesterol >300 mg/dL, WBC <2500) [92]. Another monitoring regimen involves testing

Table 22.4 Monitoring during isotretinoin therapy

Monitoring	Frequency
Complete blood count, liver function tests, fasting lipid panel, kidney function tests	Current guideline: Baseline, then weekly or biweekly until stable response to medication is established [46]
	Alternative regimen: Baseline, then 1 and 2 months after initiating therapy. If significant elevations are observed, continue with monthly monitoring or consider discontinuation of isotretinoin [92]
Pregnancy testing (for females of reproductive age)	Two negative results at baseline, then monthly thereafter
iPledge	All patients, prescribers, and pharmacies must be enrolled in the iPledge program and complete all required steps monthly before the patient receives the medication

at baseline and then again after 2 months of therapy for most patients and more frequent testing based on baseline abnormalities and medical history [93].

Pregnancy

Given that teratogenicity is a very important adverse effect of retinoids and many patients using isotretinoin are of childbearing age, women of childbearing potential must adhere to strict pregnancy monitoring that includes two negative urine or serum pregnancy tests with sensitivity of at least 25 mIU/mL prior to receiving the first prescription for isotretinoin. The first test must occur at the time of initial decision to start isotretinoin and the second test during the first 5 days of the menstrual period immediately prior to beginning isotretinoin. Patients with amenorrhea should have the second test done at least 11 days after their last unprotected sexual intercourse, defined as intercourse without using two effective forms of contraception. Monthly urine or serum pregnancy tests should occur throughout isotretinoin therapy.

These guidelines were published in the original package insert for Accutane, but despite the strict guidelines, pregnancy during isotretinoin therapy continued to occur. As such, the FDA and pharmaceutical companies agreed to form a federal registry called the iPledge registry in order to try to decrease the number of pregnancies during isotretinoin therapy. Pharmacies, prescribers, and patients participate in the registry that outlines certain requirements prior to dispensing of medication to patients. Women of childbearing potential must have two forms of birth control that they must confirm each month to the iPledge registry. The only exceptions are women who are abstinent and women who have had a hysterectomy. Men are also enrolled in the iPledge registry. Physicians must also access the registry to confirm that they have provided counseling to the patient. Despite the iPledge registry being implemented, fetal exposure to isotretinoin has not decreased significantly [94]. As such, it is imperative that physicians prescribing isotretinoin provide in-depth counseling to their patients on contraception and the teratogenic risk of isotretinoin.

Bexarotene

Bexarotene was approved by the FDA in 1999 for treatment of cutaneous T-cell lymphoma after at least one systemic therapy has been tried without adequate response [95]. Bexarotene is a third-generation retinoid that selectively binds to the α, β, γ subtypes of RXR and is typically dosed at 300 mg/m^2/day. Response to treatment with bexarotene varies by stage: stage I–IIA has a response rate of 54% at 300 mg/m^2 and 67% at higher doses; stage IIIB–IVB has a response rate of 48% at 300 mg/m^2 and 55% at higher doses [96, 97].

Like all other retinoids, bexarotene is pregnancy category X and shares some of the same adverse events such as hypertriglyceridemia and hypercholesterolemia. Patients on bexarotene are much more likely to experience these effects compared to acitretin and isotretinoin and should be monitored closely. Dose adjustments or initiation of lipid-lowering agents may be necessary. Caution is advised on the selection of a lipid-lowering agent, as gemfibrozil can actually cause an increase in both the bexarotene and triglyceride levels [89]. Bexarotene also has some adverse effects that are unique. Nearly all patients taking bexarotene develop hypothyroidism that requires thyroid hormone supplementation [98]. Many patients can experience dose-related but reversible leukopenia that usually presents at 1–2 months of treatment [95, 96].

Monitoring while on bexarotene is quite similar to monitoring while on isotretinoin; however, it is important to note that there are additional laboratory tests that should be performed before and during bexarotene treatment. This includes thyroid-stimulating hormone (TSH) and free thyroxine (free T4); the free T4 level should dictate the need for thyroid hormone supplementation. Laboratory monitoring should be performed every 1–2 weeks for fasting lipid panel until lipid response to bexarotene is established; CBC with platelets and cell differential counts, LFTs, kidney function tests, TSH, free T4, and pregnancy tests (urine or serum) in females of childbearing potential should be performed monthly for the first 3–6 months and then every 3 months thereafter.

Case Report: Systemic Retinoids (Acitretin)
An 81-year-old male presents with long-standing history of plaque psoriasis. Over the past 5 years, his psoriasis had been well controlled on etanercept. However, he was recently diagnosed with invasive melanoma. Etanercept was stopped approximately 3 weeks ago, and his psoriasis has started to flare up on his scalp, trunk, arms, and legs. Topical medications

have not been able to control the flare. He complains of severe itching due to his psoriasis. There is no family history of psoriasis. He denies joint pain or joint swelling concerning for psoriatic arthritis.

Past Medical History
- Invasive melanoma
- Hypertension

Social History
- Denies alcohol or tobacco use
- Married
- Retired

Previous Therapies
- Topical steroids
- Narrowband UVB
- Etanercept

Physical Exam
- Psoriatic plaques on the scalp, trunk, upper, and lower extremities covering 15% of the body surface area
- No features of psoriatic arthritis (dactylitis, enthesitis, tender and swollen joints, etc.)

Management
The patient has severe, generalized psoriasis, which likely requires treatment with a systemic agent. Given his recent diagnosis of invasive melanoma and his advanced age, immunosuppressive agents are avoided. Acitretin is chosen given its lack of immunosuppressive effects, and it may also have chemopreventive benefits. Acitretin is also well tolerated in the elderly population. Acitretin is not effective for treating psoriatic arthritis, but this patient does not have any signs or symptoms concerning for arthritis. Screening labs including CBC, LFTs, and lipid panel are obtained and found to be within normal limits. He is started on a standard dose of acitretin 25 mg daily, taken with food to maximize absorption.

Over the next 6 weeks, induration and scale of his psoriasis improved significantly; however, erythema remained. The patient was reassured that redness takes longer to resolve. Only minor side effects of cheilitis, dry mouth, and xerosis were noted. The patient was reminded that laboratory tests are obtained every 2–3 months to monitor for the rare risks of hepatotoxicity and hypertriglyceridemia.

At follow-up 6 months later, the erythema was found to be much improved and his psoriasis was nearly clear. Hypertriglyceridemia to 350 mg/dL was observed; therefore, he was referred to his primary care physician and his triglycerides stabilized after appropriate medical therapy.

After 9 months of treatment, the patient came in for a follow-up appointment and complained of skin fragility. Given skin fragility is a dose-dependent side effect of acitretin, the acitretin was held until the skin was restored. The acitretin was then restarted at a lower dose of 17.5 mg daily. The patient was advised that the dose can be increased back up to 25 mg if he experiences a flare of his psoriasis. Alternatively, if he continues to experience side effects, which are typically dose dependent, the dose can be further decreased to 25 mg every other day (average of 12.5 mg daily) or to 10 mg daily. The patient tolerated acitretin 17.5 mg well without any side effects or further laboratory abnormalities. He was continued on acitretin long-term with good control of his psoriasis.

References

1. Soriatane. package insert. Research Triangle Park, NC: Stiefel; 2015.
2. Lebwohl M, Drake L, Menter A, et al. Consensus conference: acitretin in combination with UVB or PUVA in the treatment of psoriasis. J Am Acad Dermatol. 2001;45(4):544–53.
3. Khera P, Koo JYM. A review of the chemopreventive and chemotherapeutic effects of topical and oral retinoids for both cutaneous and internal neoplasms. J Drugs Dermatol. 2005;4(4):432–47.
4. Dunn LK, Garr LR, Yentzer BA, O'Neill JL, Feldman SR. Acitretin in dermatology: a review. J Drugs Dermatol. 2011;10(7):772–82.
5. Chandraratna RA. Rational design of receptor-selective retinoids. J Am Acad Dermatol. 1998;39(4 Pt 2):S124–8.
6. Werner B, Bresch M, Brenner FM, Lima HC. Comparative study of histopathological and immunohistochemical findings in skin biopsies from patients with psoriasis before and after treatment with acitretin. J Cutan Pathol. 2008;35(3):302–10.
7. Gollnick H, Bauer R, Brindley C, et al. Acitretin versus etretinate in psoriasis. Clinical and pharmacokinetic results of a German multicenter study. J Am Acad Dermatol. 1988;19(3):458–68.
8. Massarella J, Vane F, Buggé C, et al. Etretinate kinetics during chronic dosing in severe psoriasis. Clin Pharmacol Ther. 1985;37(4):439–46.
9. Grønhøj Larsen F, Steinkjer B, Jakobsen P, Hjorter A, Brockhoff PB, Nielsen-Kudsk F. Acitretin is converted to etretinate only during concomitant alcohol intake. Br J Dermatol. 2000;143(6):1164–9.
10. FG L, Jakobsen P, Knudsen J, Weismann K, Kragballe K, Nielsen-Kudsk F. Conversion of acitretin to etretinate in psoriatic patients is influenced by ethanol. J Invest Dermatol. 1993;100(5):623–7.
11. McNamara PJ, Jewell RC, Jensen BK, Brindley CJ. Food increases the bioavailability of acitretin. J Clin Pharmacol. 1988;28:1051–5.
12. Wolverton SE. Comprehensive dermatologic drug therapy. Philadelphia, PA: Saunders Elsevier; 2007.
13. Menter A, Korman NJ, Elmets CA, et al. Guidelines of care for the management of psoriasis and psoriatic arthritis. Section 4. Guidelines of care for the management and treatment of psoriasis with traditional systemic agents. J Am Acad Dermatol. 2009;61:451–85.
14. Ling MR. Acitretin: optimal dosing strategies. J Am Acad Dermatol. 1999;41:S13–7.
15. Berbis P, Geiger JM, Vaisse C, Rognin C, Privat Y. Benefit of progressively increasing doses during the initial treatment with acitretin in psoriasis. Dermatologica. 1989;178:88–92.
16. Bavinck JN, Tieben LM, Van der Woude FJ, et al. Prevention of skin cancer and reduction of keratotic skin lesions during acitretin therapy in renal transplant recipients: a double-blind, placebo-controlled study. J Clin Oncol. 1995;13(8):1933–8.
17. McKenna DB, Murphy GM. Skin cancer chemoprophylaxis in renal transplant recipients: 5 years of experience using low-dose acitretin. Br J Dermatol. 1999;140(4):656–60.
18. de Sévaux RG, Smit JV, de Jong EM, van de Kerkhof PC, Hoitsma AJ. Acitretin treatment of premalignant and malignant skin disorders in renal transplant recipients: clinical effects of a randomized trial comparing two doses of acitretin. J Am Acad Dermatol. 2003;49(3):407–12.
19. Kragballe K, Jansen CT, et al. A double-blind comparison of acitretin and etretinate in the treatment of severe psoriasis: results of a Nordic multi-center study. Acta Derm Venereol. 1989;69:35–40.
20. Geiger JM. Efficacy of acitretin in severe psoriasis. Skin Therapy Lett. 2003;8:1–3. 7
21. Pang ML, Murase JE, Koo J. An updated review of acitretin—a systemic retinoid for the treatment of psoriasis. Expert Opin Drug Metab Toxicol. 2008;4(7):953–64.
22. Ozawa A, Ohkido M, Haruki Y, et al. Treatments of generalized pustular psoriasis: a multicenter study in Japan. J Dermatol. 1999;26:141–9.
23. Lauharanta J, Geiger JM. A double-blind comparison of acitretin and etretinate in combination with bath PUVA in the treatment of extensive psoriasis. Br J Dermatol. 1989;121:107–12.
24. Tanew A, Guggenbichler A, Honigsmann H, et al. Photochemotherapy for severe psoriasis without or in combination with acitretin: a randomized, double-blind comparison study. J Am Acad Dermatol. 1991;26:682–4.
25. Saurat JH, Geiger JM, Amblard P, et al. Randomized double-blind multicenter study comparing acitretin-PUVA, etretinate-PUVA, and placebo-PUVA in the treatment of severe psoriasis. Dermatologica. 1988;177:218–24.
26. Iest J, Boer J. Combined treatment of psoriasis with acitretin and UVB phototherapy compared with acitretin alone and UVB alone. Br J Dermatol. 1989;120:665–70.
27. Lowe N, Prystowsky JH, Bourget T, et al. Acitretin plus UVB therapy for psoriasis: comparisons with placebo plus UVB and acitretin alone. J Am Acad Dermatol. 1991;24(4):591.
28. Ruzicka T, Sommerburg C, Braun-Falco O, et al. Efficiency of acitretin in combination with UV-B in the treatment of severe psoriasis. Arch Dermatol. 1990;126:482–6.
29. Busse K, Koo J. Introducing the delayed-retinoid burn: a case report and discussion of this potential risk of retinoid-phototherapy combination management. J Am Acad Dermatol. 2011;64:1011–2.
30. Lowenthal KE, Horn PJ, Kalb RE. Concurrent use of methotrexate and acitretin revisited. J Dermatol Treat. 2008;19:22–6.
31. Armstrong AW, Bagel J, Van Voorhees AS, Robertson AD, Yamauchi PS. Combining biologic therapies with other systemic treatments in psoriasis: evidence-based, best-practice recommendations from the medical Board of the National Psoriasis Foundation. JAMA Dermatol. 2015;151(4):432–8.
32. Smit JV, de Sevaux RG, Blokx WA, et al. Acitretin treatment in (pre)malignant skin disorders of renal transplant recipients: histologic and immunohistochemical effects. J Am Acad Dermatol. 2004;50(2):189–96.
33. George R, Weightman W, Russ GR, et al. Acitretin for chemoprevention of non-melanoma skin cancers in renal transplant recipients. Australas J Dermatol. 2002;43(4):269–73.
34. Bettoli V, Zauli S, Virgili A. Retinoids in the chemoprevention of non-melanoma skin cancers: why, when and how. J Dermatolog Treat. 2013;24(3):235–7.
35. Thestrup-Pedersen K, Andersen KE, Menne T, et al. Treatment of hyperkeratotic dermatitis of the palms (eczema keratoticum) with oral acitretin. A single-blind placebo-controlled study. Acta Derm Venereol. 2001;81(5):353–5.
36. Lacour M, Mehta-Nikhar B, Atherton DJ, et al. An appraisal of acitretin therapy in children with inherited disorders of keratinization. Br J Dermatol. 1996;134(6):1023–9.
37. Zhang XB, Luo Q, Li CX, et al. Clinical investigation of acitretin in children with severe inherited keratinization disorders in China. J Dermatol Treat. 2008;19(4):221–8.

38. Ruzicka T, Sommerburg C, Goerz G, et al. Treatment of cutaneous lupus erythematosus with acitretin and hydroxychloroquine. Br J Dermatol. 1992;127(5):513–8.

39. Pearce DJ, Klinger S, Ziel KK, Murad EJ, Rowell R, Feldman SR. Low-dose acitretin is associated with fewer adverse events than high-dose acitretin in the treatment of psoriasis. Arch Dermatol. 2006 Aug;142(8):1000–4.

40. Rowe A. Retinoids X receptors. Int J Biochem Cell Biol. 1997;29:276–8.

41. Goldfarb MT, Ellis CN, Gupta AK, Tincoff T, Hamilton TA, Voorhees JJ. Acitretin improves psoriasis in a dose-dependent fashion. J Am Acad Dermatol. 1988;18(4 Pt 1):655–62.

42. Otley CC, Stasko T, Tope WD, et al. Chemoprevention of nonmelanoma skin cancer with systemic retinoids: practical dosing and management of adverse effects. Dermatol Surg. 2006;32:562–8.

43. Starling J, Koo J. Evidence based or theoretical concern? Pseudotumor cerebri and depression as acitretin side effects. J Drugs Dermatol. 2005;4:690–6.

44. Stuart BH, Litt IF. Tetracycline-associated intracranial hypertension in an adolescent: a complication of systemic acne therapy. J Pediatr. 1978;92:679–80.

45. Lee E, Koo J. Single-center retrospective study of long-term use of low-dose acitretin (Soriatane) for psoriasis. J Dermatolog Treat. 2004;15(1):8–13.

46. Isotretinoin. (Accutane) package insert. Nutley, NJ: Roche Laboratories; 2002.

47. Peck GL, Yoder FW. Treatment of lamellar ichthyosis and other keratinising dermatoses with an oral synthetic retinoid. Lancet. 1976;2(7996):1172–4.

48. Peck GL, Olsen TG, Yoder FW, et al. Prolonged remissions of cystic and conglobate acne with 13-cis-retinoic acid. N Engl J Med. 1979;300(7):329–33.

49. Mangelsdorf DJ, Evans RM. The RXR heterodimers and orphan receptors. Cell. 1995;83(6):841–50.

50. King K, Jones DH, Daltrey DC, Cunliffe WJ. A double-blind study of the effects of 13-cis-retinoic acid on acne, sebum excretion rate and microbial population. Br J Dermatol. 1982;107(5):583–90.

51. Leyden JJ, Mcginley KJ, Foglia AN. Qualitative and quantitative changes in cutaneous bacteria associated with systemic isotretinoin therapy for acne conglobata. J Invest Dermatol. 1986;86(4):390–3.

52. Strauss JS, Stranieri AM. Changes in long-term sebum production from isotretinoin therapy. J Am Acad Dermatol. 1982;6(4 Pt 2 Suppl):751–6.

53. Farrell LN, Strauss JS, Stranieri AM. The treatment of severe cystic acne with 13-cis-retinoic acid. Evaluation of sebum production and the clinical response in a multiple-dose trial. J Am Acad Dermatol. 1980;3(6):602–11.

54. Landthaler M, Kummermehr J, Wagner A, Plewig G. Inhibitory effects of 13-cis-retinoic acid on human sebaceous glands. Arch Dermatol Res. 1980;269(3):297–309.

55. Wiegand UW, Chou RC. Pharmacokinetics of oral isotretinoin. J Am Acad Dermatol. 1998;39(2 Pt 3):S8–12.

56. Goldsmith LA, Bolognia JL, Callen JP, et al. American academy of dermatology consensus conference on the safe and optimal use of isotretinoin: summary and recommendations. J Am Acad Dermatol. 2004;50(6):900–6.

57. Strauss JS, et al. Isotretinoin therapy for acne: results of a multicenter dose-response study. J Am Acad Dermatol. 1984;10(3):490–6.

58. Layton AM, Knaggs H, Taylor J, Cunliffe WJ. Isotretinoin for acne vulgaris—10 years later: a safe and successful treatment. Br J Dermatol. 1993;129(3):292–6.

59. Blasiak RC, Stamey CR, Burkhart CN, Lugo-somolinos A, Morrell DS. High-dose isotretinoin treatment and the rate of retrial, relapse, and adverse effects in patients with acne vulgaris. JAMA Dermatol. 2013;149(12):1392–8.

60. Borghi A, Mantovani L, Minghetti S, Giari S, Virgili A, Bettoli V. Low-cumulative dose isotretinoin treatment in mild-to-moderate acne: efficacy in achieving stable remission. J Eur Acad Dermatol Venereol. 2011;25(9):1094–8.

61. Lee JW, Yoo KH, Park KY, et al. Effectiveness of conventional, low-dose and intermittent oral isotretinoin in the treatment of acne: a randomized, controlled comparative study. Br J Dermatol. 2011;164(6):1369–75.

62. Zaenglein AL, Pathy AL, Schlosser BJ, et al. Guidelines of care for the management of acne vulgaris. J Am Acad Dermatol. 2016;74(5):945–973.e33.

63. Webster GF, Leyden JJ, Gross JA. Results of a phase III, double-blind, randomized, parallel-group, non-inferiority study evaluating the safety and efficacy of isotretinoin-Lidose in patients with severe recalcitrant nodular acne. J Drugs Dermatol. 2014;13(6):665–70.

64. Tan J, Humphrey S, Vender R, et al. A treatment for severe nodular acne: a randomized investigator-blinded, controlled, noninferiority trial comparing fixed-dose adapalene/benzoyl peroxide plus doxycycline vs. oral isotretinoin. Br J Dermatol. 2014;171(6):1508–16.

65. Leyden JJ. The role of isotretinoin in the treatment of acne: personal observations. J Am Acad Dermatol. 1998;39(2 Pt 3):S45–9.

66. Alcalay J, Landau M, Zucker A. Analysis of laboratory data in acne patients treated with isotretinoin: is there really a need to perform routine laboratory tests? J Dermatolog Treat. 2001;12(1):9–12.

67. Zane LT, Leyden WA, Marqueling AL, Manos MMA. Population-based analysis of laboratory abnormalities during isotretinoin therapy for acne vulgaris. Arch Dermatol. 2006;142(8):1016–22.

68. Maclean H, Wright M, Choi D, Tidman MJ. Abnormal night vision with isotretinoin therapy for acne. Clin Exp Dermatol. 1995;20(1):86.

69. Sieving PA, Chaudhry P, Kondo M, et al. Inhibition of the visual cycle in vivo by 13-cis retinoic acid protects from light damage and provides a mechanism for night blindness in isotretinoin therapy. Proc Natl Acad Sci U S A. 2001;98(4):1835–40.

70. Egger SF, Huber-spitzy V, Böhler K, et al. Ocular side effects associated with 13-cis-retinoic acid therapy for acne vulgaris: clinical features, alterations of tearfilm and conjunctival flora. Acta Ophthalmol Scand. 1995;73(4):355–7.

71. Fraunfelder FT, Fraunfelder FW, Edwards R. Ocular side effects possibly associated with isotretinoin usage. Am J Ophthalmol. 2001;132(3):299–305.

72. Hagler J, Hodak E, David M, Sandbank M. Facial pyogenic granuloma-like lesions under isotretinoin therapy. Int J Dermatol. 1992;31(3):199–200.

73. Chivot M. Acne flare-up and deterioration with oral isotretinoin. Ann Dermatol Venereol. 2001;128(3 Pt 1):224–8.

74. Lee AG. Pseudotumor cerebri after treatment with tetracycline and isotretinoin for acne. Cutis. 1995;55(3):165–8.

75. Roytman M, Frumkin A, Bohn TG. Pseudotumor cerebri caused by isotretinoin. Cutis. 1988;42(5):399–400.

76. Friedman DI. Medication-induced intracranial hypertension in dermatology. Am J Clin Dermatol. 2005;6(1):29–37.

77. Bettoli V, Borghi A, Mantovani L, et al. Safe use of oral isotretinoin after pseudo-tumor cerebri due to minocycline. Eur J Dermatol. 2011;21(6):1024–5.

78. Scheinman PL, Peck GL, Rubinow DR, Digiovanna JJ, Abangan DL, Ravin PD. Acute depression from isotretinoin. J Am Acad Dermatol. 1990;22(6 Pt 1):1112–4.

79. Cohen J, Adams S, Patten S. No association found between patients receiving isotretinoin for acne and the development of depression in a Canadian prospective cohort. Can J Clin Pharmacol. 2007;14(2):e227–33.

80. Marqueling AL, Zane LT. Depression and suicidal behavior in acne patients treated with isotretinoin: a systematic review. Semin Cutan Med Surg. 2007;26(4):210–20.

81. Wolverton SE, Harper JC. Important controversies associated with isotretinoin therapy for acne. Am J Clin Dermatol. 2013;14(2):71–6.
82. Mcgrath EJ, Lovell CR, Gillison F, Darvay A, Hickey JR, Skevington SM. A prospective trial of the effects of isotretinoin on quality of life and depressive symptoms. Br J Dermatol. 2010;163(6):1323–9.
83. Kaymak Y, Taner E, Taner Y. Comparison of depression, anxiety and life quality in acne vulgaris patients who were treated with either isotretinoin or topical agents. Int J Dermatol. 2009;48(1):41–6.
84. Hahm BJ, Min SU, Yoon MY, et al. Changes of psychiatric parameters and their relationships by oral isotretinoin in acne patients. J Dermatol. 2009;36(5):255–61.
85. Ferahbas A, Turan MT, Esel E, Utas S, Kutlugun C, Kilic CG. A pilot study evaluating anxiety and depressive scores in acne patients treated with isotretinoin. J Dermatolog Treat. 2004;15(3):153–7.
86. Borovaya A, Olisova O, Ruzicka T, Sárdy M. Does isotretinoin therapy of acne cure or cause depression? Int J Dermatol. 2013;52(9):1040–52.
87. Crockett SD, Porter CQ, Martin CF, Sandler RS, Kappelman MD. Isotretinoin use and the risk of inflammatory bowel disease: a case-control study. Am J Gastroenterol. 2010;105(9):1986–93.
88. Alhusayen RO, Juurlink DN, Mamdani MM, et al. Isotretinoin use and the risk of inflammatory bowel disease: a population-based cohort study. J Invest Dermatol. 2013;133(4):907–12.
89. Margolis DJ, Fanelli M, Hoffstad O, Lewis JD. Potential association between the oral tetracycline class of antimicrobials used to treat acne and inflammatory bowel disease. Am J Gastroenterol. 2010;105(12):2610–6.
90. Barth JH, Macdonald-hull SP, Mark J, Jones RG, Cunliffe WJ. Isotretinoin therapy for acne vulgaris: a re-evaluation of the need for measurements of plasma lipids and liver function tests. Br J Dermatol. 1993;129(6):704–7.
91. Shinkai K, McMichael A, Linos E. Isotretinoin laboratory test monitoring—a call to decrease testing in an era of high-value, cost-conscious care. JAMA Dermatol. 2016;152(1):17–9.
92. Altman RS, Altman LJ, Altman JS. A proposed set of new guidelines for routine blood tests during isotretinoin therapy for acne vulgaris. Dermatology (Basel). 2002;204(3):232–5.
93. Lee YH, Scharnitz TP, Muscat J, Chen A, Gupta-Elera G, Kirby JS. Laboratory monitoring during isotretinoin therapy for Acne A systematic review and meta-analysis. JAMA Dermatol. 2016;152(1):35–44.
94. Shin J, Cheetham TC, Wong L, et al. The impact of the iPLEDGE program on isotretinoin fetal exposure in an integrated health care system. J Am Acad Dermatol. 2011;65(6):1117–25.
95. Bexarotene. (Targretin) package insert and product monograph. Ligand Pharmaceuticals: San Diego, CA; 2000.
96. Duvic M, Martin AG, Kim Y, et al. Phase 2 and 3 clinical trial of oral bexarotene (Targretin capsules) for the treatment of refractory or persistent early-stage cutaneous T-cell lymphoma. Arch Dermatol. 2001;137(5):581–93.
97. Duvic M, Hymes K, Heald P, et al. Bexarotene is effective and safe for treatment of refractory advanced-stage cutaneous T-cell lymphoma: multinational phase II-III trial results. J Clin Oncol. 2001;19(9):2456–71.
98. Sherman SI, Gopal J, Haugen BR, et al. Central hypothyroidism associated with retinoid X receptor-selective ligands. N Engl J Med. 1999;340(14):1075–9.

Combination Therapy with Biologics and Other Systemic Treatments in Psoriasis

Kaitlyn M. Yim and April W. Armstrong

Psoriasis is a chronic inflammatory disease with a prevalence ranging from 0.5 to 11.4% in various regions worldwide [1]. Psoriasis is associated with cardiovascular, hepatic, renal, rheumatologic, and psychiatric comorbidities [2, 3]. Traditionally, moderate-to-severe psoriasis was treated with phototherapy and systemic oral agents such as methotrexate, acitretin, and cyclosporine [4]. Biologic agents have significantly changed the treatment landscape for psoriasis and have become widely used since the early twenty-first century. The FDA-approved agents to date include etanercept, adalimumab, infliximab, ustekinumab, secukinumab, and ixekizumab.

Dermatologic research has led to an increased understanding of psoriatic disease mechanisms at a molecular level. Mediated by cytokines such as interleukin 12 (IL-12), IL-23, IL-17A, and TNF-α, the T-helper 1 and T-helper 17 pathways have been found to act synergistically in the dysregulation of inflammation, proliferation of keratinocytes, and formation of plaques in psoriasis [5–7]. By inhibiting various cytokines and their receptors in these inflammatory cascades, biologics provide a novel, precise, and effective treatment approach against psoriasis.

Biologics are not only useful as monotherapies for moderate-to-severe psoriasis, but they also have synergistic potential when used in combination therapies with systemic agents [8]. While many patients respond adequately to first-line systemic or biologic monotherapies, some patients are refractory to FDA-approved dosages [4]. Clinically, these patients with difficult-to-treat, unremitting psoriasis may require combination therapy.

The concept of combination therapy began before the introduction of biologics. One long-standing approach is the concomitant use of a retinoid agent, such as acitretin, and phototherapy. Previous investigators have found that the combined use of acitretin and psoralen ultraviolet A (PUVA) phototherapy is significantly more effective than either treatment alone [9–11]. Similarly, combining acitretin with TL-01 narrow-band ultraviolet B (NB-UVB) phototherapy has been shown to have comparable therapeutic efficacy as that with PUVA [12]. This was among the first demonstrations in psoriasis treatments that combining therapies may augment overall effectiveness.

In addition to enhancing efficacy, combination therapy may also minimize toxicity. For example, combining acitretin and PUVA reduces the PUVA dosage needed to achieve clinical remission [9–11]. Increasing monotherapy dosages is one method of treating aggressive psoriasis, but it also raises concerns about dose-related adverse effects, particularly that of systemic therapies. Specifically, both PUVA and UVB phototherapy induce acute erythema, itching, and dryness, and PUVA is also associated with blistering and GI distress [13]. With long-term use, particularly after 150 treatments, the most common adverse effect of high-dose PUVA therapy is an increased risk of squamous cell carcinoma [14, 15]. This is most evident in Caucasian populations, but it is not proven in patients of darker-skin ethnicities [16]. Some studies have also found that PUVA increases the lifetime risk of malignant melanoma, though the data is conflicting [15, 17–19]. High-dose acitretin is associated with mucocutaneous inflammation, dyslipidemias, skeletal abnormalities, and teratogenicity [20, 21]. Methotrexate use has a significant risk of hepatotoxicity, particularly in patients with type 2 diabetes mellitus, and, less commonly, fatal myelosuppression [22–25]. Prolonged use of high-dose cyclosporine is not recommended due to concerns for irreversible renal toxicity, hypertension, and non-melanoma skin cancer [21, 26–28]. In contrast, data on the approved anti-psoriatic biologic agents shows that they have acceptable short- and long-term safety profiles, especially for the TNF inhibitors and IL-12/23 inhibitor [29].

Despite high efficacy with biologic agents, combining biologics with other agents may be necessary in patients with

K.M. Yim, BA • A.W. Armstrong, MD, MPH (✉)
Department of Dermatology, University of Southern California, 1975 Zonal Avenue, KAM 510, MC 9034, Los Angeles, CA 90089, USA
e-mail: kaitlyny@usc.edu; april.armstrong@med.usc.edu

© Springer International Publishing AG 2018
P.S. Yamauchi (ed.), *Biologic and Systemic Agents in Dermatology*, https://doi.org/10.1007/978-3-319-66884-0_23

refractory psoriasis, and combination therapies may enable greater therapeutic effectiveness without additive toxicity. However, there is a paucity of robust clinical trials evaluating the safety and efficacy of combination approaches. The choice of co-medication approach may vary based on patient demographics, comorbidities, and psoriasis disease severity. The National Psoriasis Foundation has published evidence-based recommendations regarding combining biologic therapies with other treatment modalities [4]. This chapter will examine combining biologic agents with methotrexate, acitretin, cyclosporine, and phototherapy.

Biologics and Methotrexate

Of the available oral agents for moderate-to-severe psoriasis, methotrexate is the most well-documented systemic medication used in combination with biologics in clinical practice [30]. Methotrexate interferes with DNA synthesis, repair, and replication, modulating both immune function and epithelial proliferation in psoriasis. While the exact mechanism underlying the synergistic effects of combining methotrexate with biologics is still being explored, it is proposed that methotrexate may decrease the production of anti-drug antibodies that may contribute to the loss of response to biologics [31]. Biologics and methotrexate combination therapy is typically reserved for patients with refractory psoriasis who have responded inadequately to either biologic or methotrexate monotherapy [4, 32]. The biologic agents that have been investigated with methotrexate include etanercept, infliximab, adalimumab, and ustekinumab.

Etanercept and Methotrexate

Combination therapy with etanercept and methotrexate is most robustly studied [4]. Etanercept is a fusion protein that inhibits TNF, a major inflammatory cytokine in the development of psoriasis. Two randomized controlled trials, two retrospective analyses, and a cross-sectional study all demonstrate that this combination approach results in increased efficacy with adequate safety and tolerability [33–37]. For example, in a study conducted by Gottlieb et al., 478 patients with moderate-to-severe psoriasis were randomized to receive etanercept plus methotrexate or etanercept monotherapy [33]. Specifically, all patients received 12 weeks of 50 mg etanercept twice weekly and 12 weeks of 50 mg etanercept once weekly, while half of the patients also received 7–15 mg methotrexate once weekly for the full period of 24 weeks. These patients had a BSA of at least 10% at the start of the study. At the end of 24 weeks, based on the Psoriasis Area and Severity Index (PASI), 77% of those on combination therapy experienced a 75% reduction, also referred to as a PASI-75. This was in comparison to 60% of the etanercept monotherapy group. While those on combination therapy reported more adverse events (75% vs. 60%), these events were not severe.

Similarly, Zachariae et al. conducted a randomized trial of 59 psoriasis patients with a BSA of 10% or greater [34]. Prior to the study, these patients had shown an inadequate response to methotrexate monotherapy. Thirty-one patients received etanercept with methotrexate and 28 patients received etanercept with a 4-week methotrexate taper. The regimen of etanercept in this study was 50 mg twice weekly for 12 weeks, followed by 25 mg twice weekly for 12 weeks. At the end of 24 weeks, 67% of those on combination therapy had a Physician Global Assessment (PGA) rating of clear or almost clear, and this was significantly higher than the 37% on etanercept monotherapy achieving the same endpoint.

Furthermore, two retrospective studies showed that co-medication with etanercept and methotrexate is effective in treating patients who are refractory to either medication as monotherapy [35, 36]. This combination approach seldom resulted in serious adverse events causing treatment cessation. Altogether, these studies suggest that combined therapy with etanercept and methotrexate offers a viable treatment alternative for persistent cases of moderate-to-severe psoriasis.

Infliximab and Methotrexate

Several studies examine the efficacy of combination therapy with infliximab and methotrexate [4, 37–40]. Infliximab is a chimeric, monoclonal antibody that inhibits TNF-α. One study conducted by Goedkoop et al. analyzed the effect of concomitant infliximab and methotrexate on 11 patients with active psoriasis and psoriatic arthritis [38]. These patients were already taking 5–20 mg methotrexate and, in addition, were given 3 mg/kg intravenous infliximab at weeks 0, 2, 6, 14, and 22. Based on PASI score, these patients experienced a mean 85% reduction by week 16. Furthermore, consistent with the patients' clinical improvement, skin biopsies taken at week 4 of treatment showed decreased neoangiogenesis and cell infiltration on immunohistochemistry, which are both typically increased in psoriatic inflammation.

Kavanaugh et al. performed a similar study on 47 patients diagnosed with psoriatic arthritis and psoriasis with greater than 3% BSA involvement [39]. Clinically, these patients were already on a weekly regimen of methotrexate at the start of the study and were then started on 5 mg/kg infliximab. After 54 weeks, 53% had achieved a PASI-75, compared to 48% of those on infliximab monotherapy. While this difference was found to be statistically insignificant, it indicated a possible benefit and the need for further investigation.

In a third study conducted by Dalaker et al., 23 patients on infliximab combination therapy were examined retrospectively [40]. These patients received either infliximab and methotrexate or infliximab and azathioprine, with a majority (17 of 23) receiving methotrexate. By week 14, 70% achieved a PASI-75 and 39% achieved a PASI-90. These combination approaches were also well tolerated. While more robust clinical trials are needed to evaluate the safety and efficacy of infliximab and methotrexate combination therapy, these studies suggest it may be another valuable combination approach.

Adalimumab and Methotrexate

There is limited data on methotrexate combination therapy with adalimumab, a fully human monoclonal antibody against TNF-α. De Groot et al. found that 4 weeks of co-medication with adalimumab and methotrexate decreases the levels of CD3, CD68, CD161, elastase, BDCA-2, and TNF, all of which are inflammatory markers in psoriatic skin [41]. Clinically, in a cross-sectional study performed by Takeshita et al., compared to methotrexate alone, adalimumab-methotrexate combination therapy was 3.04 times more effective (95% CI: 2.12–4.36); the efficacy of adalimumab-methotrexate combination therapy also appears to be higher than etanercept-methotrexate and infliximab-methotrexate combinations [37]. These findings suggest that combination therapy with adalimumab can be highly beneficial and result in clinical improvement by reducing psoriatic inflammation.

However, depending on the dose of adalimumab and methotrexate, the magnitude of benefit for this combination therapy is variable [42]. Therefore, additional studies are needed to determine the clinical efficacy and safety of adalimumab and methotrexate combination therapy.

Ustekinumab and Methotrexate

Ustekinumab is a monoclonal antibody that blocks the inflammatory action of IL-12 and IL-23. Heinecke et al. retrospectively analyzed 22 patients on ustekinumab therapy who were later started on an additional systemic or biologic agent [43]. Methotrexate was the most frequent agent prescribed to a total of 12 patients. Eight patients switched to combination therapy for concurrent psoriatic arthritis, which resulted in a mean 81% reduction in BSA involvement. Four patients added methotrexate due to limited response to ustekinumab monotherapy, and this proved to be a more effective treatment approach with a mean 71% reduction in BSA involvement. Notably, two of the patients who had inadequate control of their psoriasis on monotherapy achieved almost complete remission (BSA 0–1%) on

combination therapy. Furthermore, among all patients who received combined treatment, adverse effects were mild and few in number. Concomitant ustekinumab and methotrexate may offer another viable treatment option for patients with challenging or refractory psoriasis.

Biologics and Acitretin

Following biologics and methotrexate, psoriasis specialists recommend combined treatment with biologics and acitretin. Acitretin, an oral retinoid, is thought to inhibit the expression of IL-6 and its downstream induction of the T-helper 17 cascade, which plays a large role in the development of psoriasis [44]. Robust evidence for combination therapy with biologics and acitretin is lacking. A few studies suggest that combining etanercept or ustekinumab with acitretin may be beneficial in patients who have failed other treatments [45–48]. By specifically targeting psoriatic inflammation and not causing overall immunosuppression, acitretin is also particularly useful because it may be used for infectious or cancer patients who cannot be immunosuppressed [44].

Etanercept and Acitretin

Gisondi et al. conducted a randomized trial in which 60 patients received etanercept monotherapy, acitretin monotherapy, or a combination of both agents [45]. The dosages prescribed were 25 mg etanercept twice weekly, 0.4 mg/kg acitretin daily, or a combination of 25 mg etanercept once weekly with 0.4 mg/kg acitretin daily. After 24 weeks of treatment, these investigators found that combination therapy and etanercept monotherapy were similar in effectiveness, but both were more effective than acitretin monotherapy. In terms of PASI score, 44% of those on combination therapy and 45% of those on etanercept monotherapy achieved a PASI-75, compared to 30% of those on acitretin monotherapy. The combination group and etanercept group also had similar rates of BSA improvement (78% and 80%, respectively), whereas the acitretin group only had 46% BSA improvement. These findings suggest that patients who are refractory to oral acitretin may still be susceptible to combination approaches with etanercept.

Likewise, Lee et al. came to a similar conclusion by performing an almost identical study in 60 Korean patients with moderate-to-severe psoriasis [46]. Though the dosages differed slightly, these patients were randomized to the same three treatment arms: etanercept, acitretin, or combination therapy with both agents. The combination group received 25 mg etanercept twice weekly with 10 mg acitretin twice daily for 24 weeks. At the end of the study, 52.4% of the etanercept group, 22.2% of the acitretin group, and 57.9% of the combination group achieved a PASI-75. Together, these studies demonstrate that etanercept and acitretin combination therapy may be a more effective option for patients who require a stronger treatment regimen.

Ustekinumab and Acitretin

In addition to etanercept, one small study reported on the clinical efficacy of ustekinumab and acitretin combination therapy. Arakawa et al. described three patients with persistent pustular psoriasis in whom concomitant ustekinumab and acitretin proved to be a saving treatment [48]. These patients had previously failed a variety of treatments, including methotrexate, cyclosporine, biologic agents, and even etanercept and acitretin combination therapy. However, they all achieved remission with ustekinumab and acitretin and had remained psoriasis-free for 17–24 months at the conclusion of the study. While randomized trials are needed to substantiate these anecdotal reports, these cases suggest that concomitant ustekinumab and acitretin may be another effective combination approach for the future.

Biologics and Cyclosporine

Several studies have shown that combination therapy with biologics and cyclosporine may be useful as a short-term *bridging* therapy to biologic monotherapy [43, 49]. This combination is particularly useful in patients with very severe psoriasis, including those with erythroderma and those experiencing exacerbation due to abrupt taper or withdrawal of cyclosporine [49].

Yamauchi et al. analyzed eight patients with severe psoriasis who were transitioned from cyclosporine monotherapy to etanercept monotherapy by a period of combination therapy with both agents [49]. After starting 50 mg etanercept weekly, combined treatment was administered for 2–4 weeks before cyclosporine was tapered. The patients started on a regimen of 400 mg cyclosporine per day and were tapered by 100 mg per day every 2–4 weeks. When the patients reached 100 mg per day, they were tapered further to 100 mg every other day for 2–4 weeks and then discontinued completely. During this period, no rebound, flares, or adverse events occurred, demonstrating that concomitant etanercept and cyclosporine is a viable transition therapy.

Gattu et al. published a case series of five patients who used adalimumab and cyclosporine combination therapy to transition from cyclosporine to adalimumab. The cyclosporine taper occurred over 6–11 weeks. During the duration of the taper, no intermediate psoriatic flares were observed, and the patients were switched to long-term adalimumab without complications. While larger studies are warranted, this supports the feasibility of using adalimumab and cyclosporine combination therapy to initiate long-term biologic monotherapy.

Lastly, in a retrospective study of 22 patients on ustekinumab combination therapy, Heinecke et al. found that six patients required cyclosporine as a transitional therapy to ustekinumab monotherapy [43]. The bridging period ranged from 4 to 28 weeks and was fairly well tolerated. The most common reported adverse event was hypertension, which resolved after cessation of cyclosporine.

Overall, these studies support the potential utility of combining biologics and cyclosporine as a bridging technique to biologic monotherapy. However, combination therapy with biologics and cyclosporine is not recommended for long-term treatment of moderate-to-severe psoriasis [4]. High-dose cyclosporine places psoriasis patients at significant risk for malignancy and irreversible renovascular toxicity [21, 26, 28].

Biologics and Phototherapy

Combination therapy with biologics and phototherapy is often reserved for patients with refractory psoriasis who have responded inadequately to biologic monotherapy and for whom further immunosuppression is not desired [4]. However, concomitant phototherapy is complicated by the known increased risk of non-melanoma skin cancer associated with certain types of ultraviolet light therapies. A number of studies suggest that clinical outcomes are improved when NB-UVB is used in conjunction with biologics, namely, etanercept, adalimumab, and ustekinumab.

Etanercept and NB-UVB

The most commonly studied combination approach is etanercept and NB-UVB. Three randomized trials, three single-arm studies, and a retrospective analysis all support its clinical efficacy and safety [50–56]. Specifically, Wolf et al. conducted a study on five patients in which etanercept and NB-UVB was administered to one half of the body, while the other half was treated with etanercept monotherapy [50]. These patients had failed to reach a PASI-75 on etanercept alone. After 6 weeks of combination treatment, the patients experienced a mean PASI reduction of 89%, compared to 68% with just etanercept. Analogously, Gambichler et al. compared the same treatment arms in two psoriatic lesions. These investigators found that plaques treated with combination therapy displayed greater improvement in regard to PASI score, histology, and immunoreactivity [51].

In another trial by Lynde et al., 75 patients who did not show a PASI-90 response with etanercept monotherapy were randomized to receive etanercept and NB-UVB combination therapy or remain on etanercept [52]. Initially, these investigators found that the two treatments had similar effectiveness. However, after adjusting for patient compliance, combination therapy was evidently more efficacious. While only 3.4% of patients on monotherapy achieved a PASI-90 after 4 months, 42.9% of those on combination therapy achieved the same outcome.

Additionally, multiple single-arm studies have also shown that combination therapy with etanercept and NB-UVB is effective in treating moderate-to-severe psoriasis [53–55]. For example, Kircik et al. studied this combination approach by evaluating the PASI score of 86 patients [53]. These patients received etanercept 50 mg twice weekly and NB-UVB three times weekly. At the end of 12 weeks, 84.9% of patients experienced at least a PASI-75, 58.1% experienced at least a PASI-90, and 26.0% experienced a PASI-100, all without significant adverse effects. In an almost identical study only differing by dosage, De Simone et al. found that 81.8%, 57.6%, and 24.2% achieved a PASI-75, PASI-90, and PASI-100, respectively [54]. Interestingly, Calzavara-Pinton et al. selectively evaluated eight patients who were refractory to both agents as monotherapies [55]. When switched to combination therapy, they all achieved a PASI-75 and three of the patients even achieved complete remission.

Altogether, these studies suggest that combination therapy with etanercept and NB-UVB has therapeutic potential in the treatment of persistent moderate-to-severe psoriasis. However, it is also important to recognize that this combination may not be equally effective across different patient populations. For example, Park et al. showed that etanercept and NB-UVB combination therapy resulted in statistically similar rates of psoriasis remission as etanercept monotherapy in 30 obese patients [57]. Specifically, 53% of the combination group and 47% of the monotherapy group achieved remission. Further studies are needed to identify the patients who may benefit most from etanercept and NB-UVB combination therapy and to establish more robust evidence for the safety and efficacy of this approach.

Adalimumab and NB-UVB

Investigators have also explored adalimumab in combination with NB-UVB. Though the evidence is not as abundant, a handful of studies have shown that this combination approach enhances the clearance of moderate-to-severe psoriasis. In a clinical trial by Wolf et al., four patients who were on adalimumab monotherapy were exposed to NB-UVB on a randomly selected half of their body [58]. The dosages administered were 80 mg of loading dose adalimumab followed by 40 mg every other week and NB-UVB thrice weekly. After 6 weeks of treatment, the halves treated with combination therapy experienced a mean PASI-86, while the non-irradiated halves experienced a mean PASI-53.

Another study conducted by Belinchon et al. found that combined treatment with adalimumab and NB-UVB was able to reestablish a clinical response in three of four patients who had stopped responding to adalimumab monotherapy [56]. In conjunction with 40 mg adalimumab every other week, these patients received increasing radiation dosages of NB-UVB starting at 200–300 mJ/cm^2. NB-UVB was administered three times weekly for a total of 22–30 treatments. As a result, one patient experienced a PASI-75 and two experienced a PASI-90.

In a single-arm investigation conducted by Bagel et al., 20 psoriasis patients were treated with a 12-week regimen of adalimumab every other week and NB-UVB thrice weekly [59]. As a result, the patients achieved an average of PASI-95, with 95% of patients achieving PASI-75, 75% achieving PASI-90, and 55% achieving PASI-100. While this data is encouraging, additional higher-quality trials are needed to validate this combination approach.

Ustekinumab and NB-UVB

In regard to ustekinumab, two small studies have shown that combined treatment with NB-UVB may accelerate or recover clearance of moderate-to-severe psoriasis [56, 60]. In a study conducted by Wolf et al., combination therapy with ustekinumab and NB-UVB resulted in a mean 82% PASI reduction in nine patients, whereas ustekinumab monotherapy resulted in a mean 54% reduction [60]. This occurred after 6 weeks of 45 or 90 mg ustekinumab (depending on body weight) and NB-UVB three times weekly.

In another study by Belinchon et al., three patients who had previously failed ustekinumab monotherapy all showed a renewed response to concomitant ustekinumab and NB-UVB [56]. After 16–18 phototherapy sessions, these patients achieved PASI reductions ranging from 79 to 93%. These two studies suggest that the addition of phototherapy to ustekinumab therapy may increase overall effectiveness and offer a safe treatment alternative for patients with refractory psoriasis.

Conclusion

Biologic agents have transformed the treatment of moderate-to-severe psoriasis. As monotherapies, biologic agents are generally effective and well-tolerated in many patients. However, biologic monotherapies do not adequately address refractory psoriasis in a proportion of patients. Therefore, using certain combination therapies in appropriately selected patients can afford synergistic effectiveness without additive toxicity. In clinical practice, combining biologics with oral systemic agents or phototherapy is often used for patients with refractory psoriasis. While the choice of oral agents may differ based on patient demographics, comorbidities, or previously attempted therapies, biologics with concomitant methotrexate has the most evidence, followed by concomitant acitretin and then NB-UVB. However, a therapy or a combination therapy that has "most evidence" does not necessarily mean it is "most effective." Therefore, considerations must be given on a case-to-case basis with regard to which therapies will afford the best benefit-risk ratio in an individual patient. Future studies are needed to better understand and validate combination therapy involving biologic agents and other systemic treatments for psoriasis.

Case Report
History of Present Illness

A 68-year-old White male was diagnosed with psoriasis about 1 year ago. He was started on adalimumab 80 mg initially and then maintained on 40 mg every other week, and he responded well to this therapy for a year. BSA involvement decreased from 18 to 2%. However, during the second year of treatment, psoriasis began to increase gradually in severity with worsening plaques on his elbows, knees, and lower back. BSA involvement increased from 2 to 8% during this period, and he also experienced persistent itching. Due to concerns about additive immunosuppression, he does not want to escalate his dose of adalimumab or start another therapy that could add to immunosuppression. His weight is 73 kg. He denies joint pain and swelling. He is currently retired and lives at home with his wife.

Past Medical History
– Hypertension
– Hyperlipidemia

Social History
– Lives at home with wife
– Retired professor
– Denies smoking or alcohol use

Previous Therapies
– Topical treatments

Physical Exam
– Thick, silver, scaly psoriatic plaques on bilateral elbows, knees, and lower back
– No tender or swollen joints

Management
Given that this patient has refractory psoriasis to adalimumab and he does not want to increase the dose or add another agent that may increase his risk of immunosuppression (i.e., methotrexate), this patient is an appropriate candidate for NB-UVB phototherapy, which, in general, does not afford significant immunosuppression.

He is also retired and has a more flexible schedule to be compliant with NB-UVB treatments. Along with his dose of 40 mg adalimumab every other week, NB-UVB was given three times per week for a total of 3 months. The patient responded well and BSA decreased to 3%. After the patient showed adequate improvement, NB-UVB was tapered down to twice a week for 2 months. He continued to do well with a BSA of 2%, so NB-UVB was again tapered to once a week and he was maintained at that dose.

References

1. Michalek IM, Loring B, John SM. A systematic review of worldwide epidemiology of psoriasis. J Eur Acad Dermatol Venereol. 2016. https://doi.org/10.1111/jdv.13854.
2. Yeung H, Takeshita J, Mehta NN, Kimmel SE, Ogdie A, Margolis DJ, Shin DB, Attor R, Troxel AB, Gelfand JM. Psoriasis severity and the prevalence of major medical comorbidity: a population-based study. JAMA Dermatol. 2013;149(10):1173–9. https://doi.org/10.1001/jamadermatol.2013.5015.
3. Dowlatshahi EA, Wakkee M, Arends LR, Nijsten T. The prevalence and odds of depressive symptoms and clinical depression in psoriasis patients: a systematic review and meta-analysis. J Invest Dermatol. 2014;134(6):1542–51. https://doi.org/10.1038/jid.2013.508.
4. Armstrong AW, Bagel J, Van Voorhees AS, Robertson AD, Yamauchi PS. Combining biologic therapies with other systemic treatments in psoriasis: evidence-based, best-practice recommendations from the medical Board of the National Psoriasis Foundation. JAMA Dermatol. 2015;151(4):432–8. https://doi.org/10.1001/jamadermatol.2014.3456.
5. Armstrong AW, Voyles SV, Armstrong EJ, Fuller EN, Rutledge JC. A tale of two plaques: convergent mechanisms of T-cell-mediated inflammation in psoriasis and atherosclerosis. Exp Dermatol. 2011;20(7):544–9. https://doi.org/10.1111/j.1600-0625.2011.01308.x.
6. Ward NL, Umetsu DT. A new player on the psoriasis block: IL-17A- and IL-22-producing innate lymphoid cells. J Invest Dermatol. 2014;134(9):2305–7. https://doi.org/10.1038/jid.2014.216.
7. Golden JB, Groft SG, Squeri MV, Debanne SM, Ward NL, McCormick TS, Cooper KD. Chronic psoriatic skin inflammation leads to increased monocyte adhesion and aggregation. J immunol (Baltimore, MD: 1950). 2015;195(5):2006–18. https://doi.org/10.4049/jimmunol.1402307.
8. Lebwohl M. Combining the new biologic agents with our current psoriasis armamentarium. J Am Acad Dermatol. 2003;49(2 Suppl):S118–24.
9. Tanew A, Guggenbichler A, Honigsmann H, Geiger JM, Fritsch P. Photochemotherapy for severe psoriasis without or in combination with acitretin: a randomized, double-blind comparison study. J Am Acad Dermatol. 1991;25(4):682–4.
10. Saurat JH, Geiger JM, Amblard P, Beani JC, Boulanger A, Claudy A, Frenk E, Guilhou JJ, Grosshans E, Merot Y, et al. Randomized double-blind multicenter study comparing acitretin-PUVA, etretinate-PUVA and placebo-PUVA in the treatment of severe psoriasis. Dermatologica. 1988;177(4):218–24.
11. Lauharanta J, Juvakoski T, Lassus A. A clinical evaluation of the effects of an aromatic retinoid (Tigason), combination of retinoid and PUVA, and PUVA alone in severe psoriasis. Br J Dermatol. 1981;104(3):325–32.
12. Ozdemir M, Engin B, Baysal I, Mevlitoglu I. A randomized comparison of acitretin-narrow-band TL-01 phototherapy and acitretin-

psoralen plus ultraviolet a for psoriasis. Acta Derm Venereol. 2008;88(6):589–93. https://doi.org/10.2340/00015555-0529.

13. Menter A, Korman NJ, Elmets CA, Feldman SR, Gelfand JM, Gordon KB, Gottlieb A, Koo JY, Lebwohl M, Lim HW, Van Voorhees AS, Beutner KR, Bhushan R. Guidelines of care for the management of psoriasis and psoriatic arthritis: section 5. Guidelines of care for the treatment of psoriasis with phototherapy and photochemotherapy. J Am Acad Dermatol. 2010;62(1):114–35. https://doi.org/10.1016/j.jaad.2009.08.026.

14. Stern RS. The risk of squamous cell and basal cell cancer associated with psoralen and ultraviolet a therapy: a 30-year prospective study. J Am Acad Dermatol. 2012;66(4):553–62. https://doi.org/10.1016/j.jaad.2011.04.004.

15. Archier E, Devaux S, Castela E, Gallini A, Aubin F, Le Maitre M, Aractingi S, Bachelez H, Cribier B, Joly P, Jullien D, Misery L, Paul C, Ortonne JP, Richard MA. Carcinogenic risks of psoralen UV-A therapy and narrowband UV-B therapy in chronic plaque psoriasis: a systematic literature review. J Eur Acad Dermatol Venereol. 2012;26(Suppl 3):22–31. https://doi.org/10.1111/j.1468-3083.2012.04520.x.

16. Murase JE, Lee EE, Koo J. Effect of ethnicity on the risk of developing nonmelanoma skin cancer following long-term PUVA therapy. Int J Dermatol. 2005;44(12):1016–21. https://doi.org/10.1111/j.1365-4632.2004.02322.x.

17. Stern RS. The risk of melanoma in association with long-term exposure to PUVA. J Am Acad Dermatol. 2001;44(5):755–61. https://doi.org/10.1067/mjd.2001.114576.

18. Stern RS, Nichols KT, Vakeva LH. Malignant melanoma in patients treated for psoriasis with methoxsalen (psoralen) and ultraviolet a radiation (PUVA). The PUVA follow-up study. N Engl J Med. 1997;336(15):1041–5. https://doi.org/10.1056/nejm199704103361501.

19. Lindelof B, Sigurgeirsson B, Tegner E, Larko O, Johannesson A, Berne B, Ljunggren B, Andersson T, Molin L, Nylander-Lundqvist E, Emtestam L. PUVA and cancer risk: the Swedish follow-up study. Br J Dermatol. 1999;141(1):108–12.

20. Gollnick HP. Oral retinoids--efficacy and toxicity in psoriasis. Br J Dermatol. 1996;135(Suppl 49):6–17.

21. Warren RB, Griffiths CE. Systemic therapies for psoriasis: methotrexate, retinoids, and cyclosporine. Clin Dermatol. 2008;26(5):438–47. https://doi.org/10.1016/j.clindermatol.2007.11.006.

22. Malatjalian DA, Ross JB, Williams CN, Colwell SJ, Eastwood BJ. Methotrexate hepatotoxicity in psoriatics: report of 104 patients from Nova Scotia, with analysis of risks from obesity, diabetes and alcohol consumption during long term follow-up. Can J Gastroenterol. 1996;10(6):369–75.

23. Conway R, Low C, Coughlan RJ, O'Donnell MJ, Carey JJ. Risk of liver injury among methotrexate users: a meta-analysis of randomised controlled trials. Semin Arthritis Rheum. 2015;45(2):156–62. https://doi.org/10.1016/j.semarthrit.2015.05.003.

24. Rosenberg P, Urwitz H, Johannesson A, Ros AM, Lindholm J, Kinnman N, Hultcrantz R. Psoriasis patients with diabetes type 2 are at high risk of developing liver fibrosis during methotrexate treatment. J Hepatol. 2007;46(6):1111–8. https://doi.org/10.1016/j.jhep.2007.01.024.

25. Jariwala P, Kumar V, Kothari K, Thakkar S, Umrigar DD. Acute methotrexate toxicity: a fatal condition in two cases of psoriasis. Case Rep Dermatol Med. 2014;2014:946716. https://doi.org/10.1155/2014/946716.

26. Griffiths CE, Dubertret L, Ellis CN, Finlay AY, Finzi AF, Ho VC, Johnston A, Katsambas A, Lison AE, Naeyaert JM, Nakagawa H, Paul C, Vanaclocha F. Ciclosporin in psoriasis clinical practice: an international consensus statement. Br J Dermatol. 2004;150(Suppl 67):11–23. https://doi.org/10.1111/j.0366-077X.2004.05949.x.

27. Menter A, Korman NJ, Elmets CA, Feldman SR, Gelfand JM, Gordon KB, Gottlieb AB, Koo JY, Lebwohl M, Lim HW, Van Voorhees AS, Beutner KR, Bhushan R. Guidelines of care for the management of psoriasis and psoriatic arthritis: section 4. Guidelines of care for the management and treatment of psoriasis with traditional systemic agents. J Am Acad Dermatol. 2009;61(3):451–85. https://doi.org/10.1016/j.jaad.2009.03.027.

28. Paul CF, Ho VC, McGeown C, Christophers E, Schmidtmann B, Guillaume JC, Lamarque V, Dubertret L. Risk of malignancies in psoriasis patients treated with cyclosporine: a 5 year cohort study. J Invest Dermatol. 2003;120(2):211–6. https://doi.org/10.1046/j.1523-1747.2003.12040.x.

29. Campanati A, Ganzetti G, Giuliodori K, Molinelli E, Offidani A. Biologic therapy in psoriasis: safety profile. Curr Drug Saf. 2016;11(1):4–11.

30. Iskandar IY, Ashcroft DM, Warren RB, Evans I, McElhone K, Owen CM, Burden AD, Smith CH, Reynolds NJ, Griffiths CE. Patterns of biologic therapy use in the management of psoriasis: cohort study from the British Association of Dermatologists biologic interventions register (BADBIR). Br J Dermatol. 2016. https://doi.org/10.1111/bjd.15027.

31. Farhangian ME, Feldman SR. Immunogenicity of biologic treatments for psoriasis: therapeutic consequences and the potential value of concomitant methotrexate. Am J Clin Dermatol. 2015;16(4):285–94. https://doi.org/10.1007/s40257-015-0131-y.

32. Callis Duffin K, Yeung H, Takeshita J, Krueger GG, Robertson AD, Troxel AB, Shin DB, Van Voorhees AS, Gelfand JM. Patient satisfaction with treatments for moderate-to-severe plaque psoriasis in clinical practice. Br J Dermatol. 2014;170(3):672–80. https://doi.org/10.1111/bjd.12745.

33. Gottlieb AB, Langley RG, Strober BE, Papp KA, Klekotka P, Creamer K, Thompson EH, Hooper M, Kricorian G. A randomized, double-blind, placebo-controlled study to evaluate the addition of methotrexate to etanercept in patients with moderate to severe plaque psoriasis. Br J Dermatol. 2012;167(3):649–57. https://doi.org/10.1111/j.1365-2133.2012.11015.x.

34. Zachariae C, Mork NJ, Reunala T, Lorentzen H, Falk E, Karvonen SL, Johannesson A, Clareus B, Skov L, Mork G, Walker S, Qvitzau S. The combination of etanercept and methotrexate increases the effectiveness of treatment in active psoriasis despite inadequate effect of methotrexate therapy. Acta Derm Venereol. 2008;88(5):495–501. https://doi.org/10.2340/00015555-0511.

35. Driessen RJ, van de Kerkhof PC, de Jong EM. Etanercept combined with methotrexate for high-need psoriasis. Br J Dermatol. 2008;159(2):460–3. https://doi.org/10.1111/j.1365-2133.2008.08669.x.

36. Babino G, Giunta A, Ruzzetti M, Sole Chimenti M, Chimenti S, Esposito M. Combination therapy with etanercept in psoriasis: retrospective analysis of efficacy and safety outcomes from real-life practice. J Int Med Res. 2016;44(1 suppl):100–5. https://doi.org/10.1177/0300060515593260.

37. Takeshita J, Wang S, Shin DB, Callis Duffin K, Krueger GG, Kalb RE, Weisman JD, Sperber BR, Stierstorfer MB, Brod BA, Schleicher SM, Robertson AD, Linn KA, Shinohara RT, Troxel AB, Van Voorhees AS, Gelfand JM. Comparative effectiveness of less commonly used systemic monotherapies and common combination therapies for moderate to severe psoriasis in the clinical setting. J Am Acad Dermatol. 2014;71(6):1167–75. https://doi.org/10.1016/j.jaad.2014.08.003.

38. Goedkoop AY, Kraan MC, Picavet DI, de Rie MA, Teunissen MB, Bos JD, Tak PP. Deactivation of endothelium and reduction in angiogenesis in psoriatic skin and synovium by low dose infliximab therapy in combination with stable methotrexate therapy: a prospective single-centre study. Arthritis Res Ther. 2004;6(4):R326–34. https://doi.org/10.1186/ar1182.

39. Kavanaugh A, Krueger GG, Beutler A, Guzzo C, Zhou B, Dooley LT, Mease PJ, Gladman DD, de Vlam K, Geusens PP, Birbara C, Halter DG, Antoni C. Infliximab maintains a high degree of clinical

response in patients with active psoriatic arthritis through 1 year of treatment: results from the IMPACT 2 trial. Ann Rheum Dis. 2007;66(4):498–505. https://doi.org/10.1136/ard.2006.058339.

40. Dalaker M, Bonesronning JH. Long-term maintenance treatment of moderate-to-severe plaque psoriasis with infliximab in combination with methotrexate or azathioprine in a retrospective cohort. J Eur Acad Dermatol Venereol. 2009;23(3):277–82. https://doi.org/10.1111/j.1468-3083.2008.03039.x.

41. de Groot MTM, Picavet DI, van Kuijk AW, Tak PP, de Rie MA, Bos JD. Adalimumab in combination with methotrexate more effectively reduces the numbers of different inflammatory cell types in lesional psoriatic skin than does single treatent with adalimumab or methotrexate. Br J Dermatol. 2008;158(6):1401.

42. Behrens F, Koehm M, Arndt U, Wittig BM, Greger G, Thaci D, Scharbatke E, Tony HP, Burkhardt H. Does concomitant methotrexate with adalimumab influence treatment outcomes in patients with psoriatic arthritis? Data from a large observational study. J Rheumatol. 2016;43(3):632–9. https://doi.org/10.3899/jrheum.141596.

43. Heinecke GM, Luber AJ, Levitt JO, Lebwohl MG. Combination use of ustekinumab with other systemic therapies: a retrospective study in a tertiary referral center. J Drugs Dermatol. 2013;12(10):1098–102.

44. Booij MT, Van De Kerkhof PC. Acitretin revisited in the era of biologics. J Dermatol Treat. 2011;22(2):86–9. https://doi.org/10.3109/09546630903578582.

45. Gisondi P, Del Giglio M, Cotena C, Girolomoni G. Combining etanercept and acitretin in the therapy of chronic plaque psoriasis: a 24-week, randomized, controlled, investigator-blinded pilot trial. Br J Dermatol. 2008;158(6):1345–9. https://doi.org/10.1111/j.1365-2133.2008.08564.x.

46. Lee JH, Youn JI, Kim TY, Choi JH, Park CJ, Choe YB, Song HJ, Kim NI, Kim KJ, Lee JH, Yoo HJ. A multicenter, randomized, open-label pilot trial assessing the efficacy and safety of etanercept 50 mg twice weekly followed by etanercept 25 mg twice weekly, the combination of etanercept 25 mg twice weekly and acitretin, and acitretin alone in patients with moderate to severe psoriasis. BMC Dermatol. 2016;16(1):11. https://doi.org/10.1186/s12895-016-0048-z.

47. Smith EC, Riddle C, Menter MA, Lebwohl M. Combining systemic retinoids with biologic agents for moderate to severe psoriasis. Int J Dermatol. 2008;47(5):514–8. https://doi.org/10.1111/j.1365-4632.2008.03470.x.

48. Arakawa A, Ruzicka T, Prinz JC. Therapeutic efficacy of interleukin 12/interleukin 23 blockade in generalized pustular psoriasis regardless of IL36RN mutation status. JAMA Dermatol. 2016;152(7):825–8. https://doi.org/10.1001/jamadermatol.2016.0751.

49. Yamauchi PS, Lowe NJ. Cessation of cyclosporine therapy by treatment with etanercept in patients with severe psoriasis. J Am Acad Dermatol. 2006;54(3 Suppl 2):S135–8. https://doi.org/10.1016/j.jaad.2005.11.1043.

50. Wolf P, Hofer A, Legat FJ, Bretterklieber A, Weger W, Salmhofer W, Kerl H. Treatment with 311-nm ultraviolet B accelerates and

improves the clearance of psoriatic lesions in patients treated with etanercept. Br J Dermatol. 2009;160(1):186–9. https://doi.org/10.1111/j.1365-2133.2008.08926.x.

51. Gambichler T, Tigges C, Scola N, Weber J, Skrygan M, Bechara FG, Altmeyer P, Kreuter A. Etanercept plus narrowband ultraviolet B phototherapy of psoriasis is more effective than etanercept monotherapy at 6 weeks. Br J Dermatol. 2011;164(6):1383–6. https://doi.org/10.1111/j.1365-2133.2011.10358.x.

52. Lynde CW, Gupta AK, Guenther L, Poulin Y, Levesque A, Bissonnette R. A randomized study comparing the combination of nbUVB and etanercept to etanercept monotherapy in patients with psoriasis who do not exhibit an excellent response after 12 weeks of etanercept. J Dermatol Treat. 2012;23(4):261–7. https://doi.org/10.3109/09546634.2011.607795.

53. Kircik L, Bagel J, Korman N, Menter A, Elmets CA, Koo J, Yang YC, Chiou CF, Dann F, Stevens SR. Utilization of narrow-band ultraviolet light B therapy and etanercept for the treatment of psoriasis (UNITE): efficacy, safety, and patient-reported outcomes. J Drugs Dermatol. 2008;7(3):245–53.

54. De Simone C, D'Agostino M, Capizzi R, Capponi A, Venier A, Caldarola G. Combined treatment with etanercept 50 mg once weekly and narrow-band ultraviolet B phototherapy in chronic plaque psoriasis. Eur J Dermatol. 2011;21(4):568–72. https://doi.org/10.1684/ejd.2011.1330.

55. Calzavara-Pinton PG, Sala R, Arisi M, Rossi MT, Venturini M, Ortel B. Synergism between narrowband ultraviolet B phototherapy and etanercept for the treatment of plaque-type psoriasis. Br J Dermatol. 2013;169(1):130–6. https://doi.org/10.1111/bjd.12277.

56. Belinchon I, Arribas MP, Soro P, Betlloch I. Recovery of the response to biological treatments using narrow band ultraviolet-B in patients with moderate to severe psoriasis: a retrospective study of 17 patients. Photodermatol Photoimmunol Photomed. 2014;30(6):316–22. https://doi.org/10.1111/phpp.12134.

57. Park KK, JJ W, Koo J. A randomized, 'head-to-head' pilot study comparing the effects of etanercept monotherapy vs. etanercept and narrowband ultraviolet B (NB-UVB) phototherapy in obese psoriasis patients. J Eur Acad Dermatol Venereol. 2013;27(7):899–906. https://doi.org/10.1111/j.1468-3083.2012.04611.x.

58. Wolf P, Hofer A, Weger W, Posch-Fabian T, Gruber-Wackernagel A, Legat FJ. 311 nm ultraviolet B-accelerated response of psoriatic lesions in adalimumab-treated patients. Photodermatol Photoimmunol Photomed. 2011;27(4):186–9. https://doi.org/10.1111/j.1600-0781.2011.00594.x.

59. Bagel J. Adalimumab plus narrowband ultraviolet B light phototherapy for the treatment of moderate to severe psoriasis. J Drugs Dermatol. 2011;10(4):366–71.

60. Wolf P, Weger W, Legat FJ, Posch-Fabian T, Gruber-Wackernagel A, Inzinger M, Salmhofer W, Hofer A. Treatment with 311-nm ultraviolet B enhanced response of psoriatic lesions in ustekinumab-treated patients: a randomized intraindividual trial. Br J Dermatol. 2012;166(1):147–53. https://doi.org/10.1111/j.1365-2133.2011.10616.x.

Jerry Bagel

The act of bridging from one biologic agent to another biologic agent is a therapeutic switch based on very little scientific data. In randomized, psoriatic clinical trials, subjects are required to wash out from systemic therapies for 4 weeks and biologic therapies for 12 weeks prior to randomizing. Hence, no clinical trial data is applicable to switching between biologic agents.

The first scenario to address is the patient who is on a biologic agent and although is not flaring is not responding effectively, i.e. not achieved at least a PASI 75 (primary failure) or after obtaining a PASI 75 has lost efficacy (secondary failure). Since the patient is not flaring, time is not of the essence. In this case the time between discontinuing the original treatment and starting a new treatment would "theoretically" be based on the half-life of the original agent. The half-lives for etanercept, adalimumab, infliximab, ustekinumab, secukinumab, and ixekizumab are 4.5, 14, 7, 21, 21, and 17 days, respectively. It takes five half-lives for complete elimination; however, at three half-lives, there is only 12.5% of the biologic agent remaining which one could assume does not have therapeutic efficacy or immunosuppression. Utilizing this metric, it would require a 2, 6, 3, 9.9, and 7 week washout before starting a new biologic agent after discontinuing etanercept, adalimumab, infliximab, ustekinumab, secukinumab, and ixekizumab, respectively.

In reality this is rarely done. Typically, it takes 2–3 weeks to get a biologic agent approved through the insurance process and another week for the patient to come to the office to be instructed how to administer the drug. In most cases, it would seem appropriate to not have the patient wait any longer than 4 weeks after discontinuing the previous agent. If the reason for switching biologics is for lack of efficacy, it would be appropriate to administer the next dose of the new biologic at the next dosing interval, i.e. for a new biologic

J. Bagel, MD, MS
Psoriasis Treatment Center of Central New Jersey,
University of Pisa, Pisa, Italy
e-mail: Dreamacres1@aol.com

after etanercept in week and for adalimumab in 2 weeks. The new biologic should be administered in the approved dosing regimen. Similarly, if non-medical switching is required (switching because insurance mandates), the time frame to start the approved agent should not have to wait more than the normal interval of dosing [1].

On the other hand, if a biologic agent was discontinued because of safety reasons (adverse event), then one must be prudent in the time frame before initiating the next biologic agent. It would be necessary to evaluate clinical and lab parameters prior to resuming biologic therapy independent on the half-life of the preceding biologic agent. Another aspect of washout that needs to be considered are the co-morbidities of the individual, i.e. diabetes, kidney failure, obesity, advanced age where increased risks of infection occur. In these cases even when biologics are switched, even for efficacy purposes, the "theoretical" washout would be prudent.

With more efficacious biologic agents in our tool box, and with PASI 100 in the FDA label for ixekizumab, the physician-patient dialogue continues to press the envelope to the point where 3% body surface area may no longer be acceptable and switching to more efficacious biologics becomes more commonplace. Not only is complete clearing at 12 weeks a reality, but a maintenance of response is becoming an expectation. Therefore, switching from "older" biologics to more efficacious biologics could be a common occurrence. Ganzetti et al. reviewed switching from one biological therapy to another biological therapy: the experience of the PsOMarche group, which evaluated 38 subjects, with an average PASI of 22.6, of which 9 switched for primary failure and 73% for secondary failure (loss efficacy after obtaining a PASI 75). The average time for treatment with the first biologic was 1 year. The theoretical washout periods utilized were 2 weeks for adalimumab, 1 week for etanercept, 2–4 weeks for infliximab, and 8–12 weeks for ustekinumab [2]. However, in practice, switching from one biologic to next directly occurred 56% of the time whereas a washout period was utilized 44%. PASI 75 was achieved in 53% and 89.4% of subjects after 8 and 16 weeks of switching to the second biologic agent. Subjects were

P.S. Yamauchi (ed.), *Biologic and Systemic Agents in Dermatology*, https://doi.org/10.1007/978-3-319-66884-0_24

switched primarily to adalimumab followed by ustekinumab and were well tolerated with no safety concerns occurring during the observation period. Mrowietz et al. does not recommend a "theoretical" washout in cases of lack of efficacy and states the washout after discontinuing ustekinumab to be as early as 2–4 weeks [3].

Another scenario is transitioning to a biologic agent after a patient has been on methotrexate for an extended period of time to decrease the potential of hepatotoxicity in the psoriatic population with a high incidence of fatty liver secondary to obesity, diabetes, hyperlipidaemia, and alcoholism, similarly transitioning to a biologic agent if someone was on cyclosporine and the desire to discontinue to avoid nephrotoxicity or discontinue acitretin to avoid persistent hyperlipidaemia.

Ganzetti et al. evaluated 47 subjects on conventional systemic agents over a 6-month period. Transitioning from a conventional systemic to a biologic agent occurred in 66% for lack of efficacy whereas 25% for safety reasons, i.e. hypertension and increased creatinine related to cyclosporine treatment and hyperlipidemia due to acitretin. Transitioning to a biologic agent occurred without washout in 37%, with washout in 51%, and with overlapping the previous systemic and the new biologic in 12% of the cases [4].

There are acute circumstances when patients are flaring widespread, or possibly palmar plantar or intertriginous areas, where their psoriasis is disabling. In these cases the two options would be to start the second biologic agent immediately after discontinuing the first. This may work with IL-17 inhibitors partially due to their high loading dose results in quick and effective results.

The question that is asked and only answered from an empirical perspective is when overlapping a conventional systemic and a biologic: How to taper the systemic therapy while adding the biologic agent. In patients with rapidly flaring psoriasis, adding a bridge such as cyclosporine is very useful. A practical approach is to initiate cyclosporine 3.5–5 mg/kg/day until a PASI 50 improvement is obtained. At that time a biologic agent could be administered. Monitoring should be at the level of the riskiest medication, in this case it would be cyclosporine. The combination data of cyclosporine with adalimumab and etanercept have been studied in small numbers. The tapering of cyclosporine reported varies but it is important not to taper too quickly nor keep it on board too long hence a taper of 0.5 mg/kg/week once the patient has added the biologic agent for a few weeks.

The fact that most of the biologic agents approved for psoriasis are also approved for psoriatic arthritis, and the fact that methotrexate is not discontinued in the psoriatic arthritis trials allows us to have a better handle on the safety of methotrexate in combination with biologic agents. If methotrexate needs to be discontinued because of a safety event, then one needs to make sure all aspects of the adverse event are resolved prior to initiating a biologic agent. On the other hand, if methotrexate is being discontinued because of lack of efficacy or to prevent future toxicity, overlapping with a biologic agent would be helpful to prevent flare. The question again is for how long to you keep methotrexate onboard. In view of no known toxicity going with a slow taper would be prudent, i.e. as slowly as 2.5 mg decrease per month.

With more efficacious biologics available, i.e. secukinumab and ixekizumab, with the latter's phase 3 data revealing 40% of patients obtaining PASI 100 at week 12. In addition ixekizumab shows the same efficacy in bio-naive and patients who have received numerous biologics in the past; it is reasonable if you can get these medications approved expeditiously to start them as soon as possible. The high loading doses with these two agents assists in the rapid onset of efficacy which would be helpful in the control of a flaring patient.

Yamauchi and Lowe evaluated patients who were placed on cyclosporine until they were 50% better. They then added etanercept as cyclosporine was discontinued. The eight patients in this study remained clear on etanercept 12 weeks after cyclosporine was discontinued [5].

Another small study looked at five patients on cyclosporine and adalimumab as a cyclosporine-tapering regimen that ranged from 6 to 11 weeks. All patients were able to transition to adalimumab as a monotherapy without flare [6].

Unfortunately, there is very limited data in regard to risks of malignancy and infection when combining cyclosporine and biologic agents. As data has shown when combination anti-suppressants are added to the mix the risk of infections and malignancies increase. Hence it would be prudent to overlap with caution. Nonetheless when you do overlap, do not taper too quickly as your patient may flare. This is truly the art of medicine.

Case Report

A 44-year-old Indian male with psoriatic plaques on scalp, elbows, and knees presents to his internist after gardening with extensive poison ivy and was given 40 mg IM Kenalog.

Past Medical History:
Bell's palsy, GERD
Medications: Prilosec

Social History:
Drinks occasionally
Married
Electrical Engineer

Previous Treatments:
Topical Steroids
Narrow band UVB

Physical Exam:
Exfoliative erythroderma
Blood pressure = 126/88

Fasting glucose = 106

Creatinine = 1.0

Magnesium = within normal limits

QuantiFERON Gold = negative

Hepatitis B and C profile = within normal limits

Management:

Cyclosporine 4 mg/kg in split doses

Prescribed adalimumab

After 3 weeks patient is 50% improved

Initiated adalimumab week 0, 80 mg SQ; week 1, 40 mg SQ, subsequently 40 mg SQ, QO week

After 2 weeks on adalimumab, began taper of cyclosporine by 0.5 mg QO week

After 10 weeks on adalimumab, cyclosporine was discontinued and patient continued to do well

References

1. Woo WA. Switching biological agents for psoriasis in secondary care: a single-center, retrospective, open-label study. Br J Derm. 2014;170(4):989–90.
2. Ganzietti G, et al. The transitioning from conventional therapy to biological treatment in psoriatic patients: STRATOS, a project of Marche region. G Ital Dermatol Venereol. 2016;151(4):340–6.
3. Mrowietz U, et al. A consensus report on appropriate treatment optimization and transitioning in the management of moderate-to-severe plaque psoriasis. JEADV. 2014;28(4):439–53.
4. Ganzietti G, et al. The switching from a biological therapy to another biologic agent in psoriatic patients: the experience of PsOMarche group. G Ital Dermatol Venereol. 2016.; {Epub ahead of print}
5. Yamauchi PS, Lowe NJ. Cessation of cyclosporine therapy by treatment with etanercept in patients with severe psoriasis. Am Acad Dermatol. 2006;54(3 Suppl 2):S135–8.
6. Armstrong AW, et al. Combining biologic therapies with other systemic treatments in psoriasis. JAMA Dermatol. 2015;151(4):432–8.

Paul S. Yamauchi

Case Study #1: Severe Flare During Therapy

Psoriasis Medical History

1. 45-year-old male with a history of psoriasis for 3 years.
2. Started as guttate psoriasis after documented strep throat infection.
3. Despite topical and phototherapy, guttate psoriasis evolved into plaque psoriasis.
4. Maximum psoriasis severity—35%.
5. No family history of psoriasis.
6. No psoriatic arthritis symptoms.

Past Medical History

1. Hypercholesterolemia
2. Obesity (weight 230 lbs., BMI—30.1)
3. Hypertension
4. Smokes 1 ppd
5. Alcohol intake: one to two beers every night

Therapeutic History for Psoriasis

1. NB-UVB—did not improve his guttate psoriasis or plaque psoriasis
2. Topical agents.
3. Initiated on ustekinumab at 90 mg dose when his BSA was 35%.
4. Psoriasis improved down to 1% BSA after 3 months.

P.S. Yamauchi, MD, PhD
David Geffen School of Medicine at UCLA, Dermatology Institute and Skin Care Center, 2001 Santa Monica Blvd Suite 1160W, Santa Monica, CA 90404, USA
e-mail: paulyamauchi@yahoo.com

5. Patient has been on ustekinumab for 2 years with stable maintenance of response.
6. His next shot of ustekinumab is due in 1 month.

Complication

1. Patient was hiking in woods and developed severe contact dermatitis from poison oak.
2. He presented to the ER and was given intramuscular and oral systemic steroids.
3. The contact dermatitis resolved after 1 week.
4. 2 weeks after systemic steroid administration, the patient developed erythrodermic psoriasis.

Clinical Course Options

1. The laboratories that were measured at the ER showed normal CBC and chemistry panel (including LFTs and renal function test)
2. Despite being on ustekinumab, the patient developed erythrodermic psoriasis, presumably from steroid withdrawal. What would be an appropriate next step?
   (a) Administer an immediate dose of ustekinumab at 90 mg.
   (b) Administer another biologic agent.
   (c) Add phototherapy.
   (d) Add cyclosporine.
   (e) Add acitretin.
   (f) Add methotrexate.
   (g) Add apremilast.

Management and Response

1. Cyclosporine was administered at a starting dose of 5 mg/kg.
2. After 10 days, the patient was 90% improved.
3. The dose cyclosporine was tapered down 100 mg per week and then discontinued.
4. During the taper, another 90 mg dose of ustekinumab was administered at the normal 3-month dosing interval.

P.S. Yamauchi (ed.), *Biologic and Systemic Agents in Dermatology*, https://doi.org/10.1007/978-3-319-66884-0_25

Discussion

1. Retrospective analysis using cyclosporine as rescue therapy to control psoriasis flare-ups in 10 patients who had received continuous efalizumab therapy (a biologic agent for psoriasis that was discontinued in 2009) has been reported [1, 2].
2. Combination therapy with cyclosporine and efalizumab was generally well tolerated and controlled the relapse effectively.
3. The data on managing flare-ups during biologic therapy with systemic agents (including cyclosporine) is limited.
4. There are several case reports on combination therapy with biologic agents [1, 2].

Case Study #2: Loss of Response During Therapy

Psoriasis Medical History

1. 32-year-old female.
2. History of psoriasis for 10 years.
3. Family history of psoriasis in mother.
4. No psoriatic arthritis symptoms.
5. Initially mild psoriasis limited to scalp, knees, and elbows that was controlled with topical agents.
6. 2 years ago, the psoriasis worsened to a maximum severity of 15% BSA.

Past Medical History

1. Has two children
2. Does not plan on becoming pregnant and is on birth control
3. Nonsmoker
4. Alcohol intake—one glass of wine every night

Therapeutic History for Psoriasis

1. Topical agents.
2. Phototherapy—good initial response after 4 months of treatment but relapsed soon after discontinuing.
3. The BSA was 15%.
4. The patient was then treated with etanercept at 50 mg BIW for 12 weeks and then 50 mg weekly for maintenance.
5. For 9 months, the BSA was reduced a stable level at 2%.

Complication

1. Despite being compliant on etanercept therapy, the psoriasis relapsed after 9 months of stable clearance.
2. The BSA increased to 11% within 1 month
3. Topical therapy did not control the relapse.

Clinical Course Options

1. The patient's psoriasis is worsening despite being on etanercept.
2. Assuming all laboratory values are normal, what would be an appropriate next step?
    (a) Increase etanercept to 50 mg BIW.
    (b) Add methotrexate.
    (c) Add cyclosporine.
    (d) Add acitretin.
    (e) Add apremilast.
    (f) Switch to a biologic agent that is not a TNF inhibitor.
    (g) Switch to a different biologic agent that is a TNF inhibitor.
    (h) Others.

Management and Response

1. The dosage of etanercept was increased to 50 mg BIW.
2. No improvement of the psoriasis was evident after 6 weeks.
3. What would be the next step?
    (a) Add methotrexate.
    (b) Add cyclosporine.
    (c) Add acitretin.
    (d) Add apremilast.
    (e) Switch to a biologic agent that is not a TNF inhibitor.
    (f) Switch to a different biologic agent that is a TNF inhibitor.
    (g) Others.

Management and Response (continued)

1. Etanercept was discontinued, and adalimumab was initiated at a dose of 80 mg at week 0, 40 mg at week 1, and then 40 mg every other week.
2. Within 2 weeks, the psoriasis had begun to improve.
3. After 3 months, the BSA decreased to 1%.
4. The patient continues to treat her psoriasis with adalimumab.

Discussion

1. A primary nonresponse occurs where there is no or minimal response to the therapy (e.g., less than a PASI 50 response).
2. A secondary nonresponse occurs where the drug is starting to lose efficacy after attaining the desired response (e.g., losing 50% of a PASI 75 response).
3. Although there are no specific guidelines on switching biologic agents, the usual route is to transition from one biologic to another without any washout period. In formal clinical trials, a typical washout period is 3 months. This is not necessary and the switch can occur once a patient is

approved for the new biologic agent. It is not necessary to base the switch on the half-life of the original biologic.

4. When transitioning biologics, the switch may be within the same class (e.g., one TNF inhibitor to a different TNF inhibitor) or a different class (e.g., TNF inhibitor to IL-12/IL-23 or IL-17 inhibitor). For a primary nonresponse, the recommendation is to switch to a different class. For a secondary nonresponse, switching can occur within the same class [3] or to a different mechanism of action.

Case Study #3: Managing Recalcitrant Psoriasis and Psoriatic Arthritis

Psoriasis Medical History

1. 41-year-old male
2. History of psoriasis for 11 years.
3. Family history of psoriasis and psoriatic arthritis (mother).
4. Psoriasis mild (1–2% BSA) for the first 10 years.
5. Patient started to develop morning stiffness that lasted 30 min and lower back pain that he attributed to getting older.
6. Pain and swelling in two fingers in his left hand.
7. Pitting and onycholysis of his nails.
8. Feeing more fatigued.

Past Medical History

1. Hyperlipidemia
2. Obesity (weight 230 lbs., BMI—30.1)
3. Hypertension
4. Smokes 1 ppd
5. Alcohol intake: one to two beers every night

Therapeutic History for Psoriasis

1. For the first 10 years, his mild psoriasis was controlled with topical steroids by his primary care physician.
2. When the patient developed arthritic symptoms, his primary care physician attributed this to osteoarthritis and prescribed NSAIDs with moderate improvement
3. However the psoriasis began to worsen and affected his scalp, trunk, and extremities (15% BSA).
4. The patient was then referred to a dermatologist for further management.

Management and Response

1. The dermatologist diagnosed the patient with psoriasis and psoriatic arthritis based on morning stiffness, asymmetric oligoarthritis, and nail changes.

2. Before checking labs, which course of therapy would you consider?
   (a) Methotrexate
   (b) TNF inhibitor (etanercept, adalimumab, infliximab, certolizumab)
   (c) Ustekinumab
   (d) Apremilast
   (e) IL-17 inhibitor (secukinumab, ixekizumab, brodalumab)
   (f) Others.
3. The QuantiFERON Gold assay test was negative, and all laboratory parameters were normal including negative a hepatitis B panel.
4. Adalimumab was initiated at a dose of 80 mg at week 0, 40 mg at week 1, and then 40 mg every other week.
5. Within 1 month, the morning stiffness and oligoarthritis improved and the patient felt less fatigued and more functional.
6. After 3 months, the psoriatic arthritis was not bothering the patient. However, there was minimal improvement in his psoriasis (15% BSA) and the patient desired clearer skin.
7. The psoriatic arthritis is stable but the psoriasis has remained unchanged
8. What would you consider next?
   (a) Continue adalimumab and wait and see.
   (b) Add methotrexate.
   (c) Add apremilast.
   (d) Switch to apremilast.
   (e) Switch to etanercept.
   (f) Switch to infliximab.
   (g) Switch to ustekinumab.
   (h) Switch to IL-17 inhibitor.
   (i) Others.
9. The patient was switched from adalimumab to ustekinumab at 90 mg at weeks 0 and 4 and at every 3 months of dosing.
10. Within 2 months, the BSA decreased to 2%.
11. However, he developed a small effusion in his left knee with pain and swelling, and his oligoarthritis redeveloped in his hands.
12. At month 4 after 3 doses of ustekinumab, the psoriasis was 100% clear, but his psoriatic arthritis continued to worsen.
13. The psoriasis is clear but the psoriatic arthritis has worsened during ustekinumab therapy
14. At this point, what would you consider?
    (a) Remain on ustekinumab and wait and see.
    (b) Add methotrexate.
    (c) Add apremilast.
    (d) Switch to apremilast.
    (e) Switch to etanercept.
    (f) Switch to infliximab.
    (g) Switch to IL-17 inhibitor.
    (h) Others.

15. Apremilast was added in combination with ustekinumab.
16. Within 1 month, the psoriatic arthritis improved with a reduction of morning stiffness and less pain and swelling in his fingers.
17. After 2 months, his psoriasis remained 100% clear, and the psoriatic arthritis was stable and under control.

Discussion

1. Another option would have been to switch to an IL-17 inhibitor such as secukinumab which has the indication for both psoriasis and psoriatic arthritis.
2. It is generally not recommended to combine two biologic agents together due to potential risk of adverse events such as serious infections.
3. Point to consider—if the patient requested that ustekinumab be discontinued and only remain on apremilast as monotherapy, would you consider this?
    (a) Yes
    (b) No
    (c) Not sure

Case Study #4: Malignancy During Therapy

Psoriasis Medical History

1. 52-year-old male
2. History of psoriasis for 25 years
3. No family history of psoriasis
4. No psoriatic arthritis symptoms
5. Maximal psoriasis severity in his lifetime—30% BSA:
    (a) Scalp
    (b) Trunk
    (c) Extremities

Past Medical History

1. Hypertension
2. Type 2 diabetes mellitus
3. BMI—27
4. Nonsmoker
5. Alcohol intake—one glass of wine every night

Therapeutic History for Psoriasis

1. Topical agents.
2. Phototherapy—tried for 4 weeks but unable to continue due to busy schedule.
3. Methotrexate—minimal response and could not tolerate.
4. Etanercept—50 mg weekly for 10 years.
5. Psoriasis is stable and controlled. BSA is 1–2%.

Complication

1. The patient was diagnosed with colon cancer during a colonoscopy screening exam.
2. Etanercept was discontinued following the diagnosis.
3. Surgery and chemotherapy was performed and the colon cancer was in remission.
4. At this point, the psoriasis has relapsed and the BSA is 20%.
5. The patient inquires if he can go back on etanercept.

Clinical Course Options

1. The colon cancer is in remission, but the psoriasis has relapsed (20% BSA). The patient requests that etanercept be restarted.
2. What would be your next step?
    (a) Resume etanercept.
    (b) Initiate another biologic.
    (c) Phototherapy.
    (d) Apremilast.
    (e) Methotrexate.
    (f) Cyclosporine.
    (g) Acitretin (with or without phototherapy).
    (h) Others.

Management and Response

1. The case was discussed with the patient's oncologist.
2. The oncologist stated he had no reservations about restarting the patient back on etanercept.
3. The patient was restarted on etanercept after the risks and benefits were discussed.
4. The same degree of efficacy as before was recaptured.
5. The patient continues to be closely monitored by both the dermatologist and oncologist.

Discussion

1. Several studies do support the favorability of the safety profile of biologics in patients with psoriasis in terms of the risk of developing malignancy [4].
2. A few studies in patients with a previous history of cancer show no increased risk of recurrence in those treated with biologics compared to nonbiologic therapy.
3. Recent studies do not show an increased risk of new or recurrent malignancy in patients with psoriasis treated with biologic agents.
4. Coordinating the management of patients that develop or have a history of previous malignancy with an oncology team is crucial for patient-centered care until clear evidence-based guidelines are developed

Case Study #5: Paradoxical Anti-TNF Pustular-Induced Psoriasis

Past Medical History

1. 28-year-old female
2. History of Crohn's for 3 years
3. Currently on infliximab for 1½ years with good control
4. BMI—22
5. Nonsmoker
6. No alcohol consumption
7. No history or FH of psoriasis

Complication

1. The patient developed an intensely pruritic rash on her distal extremities.
2. Her internist prescribed a high potency steroid which did not improve the rash.
3. She was then referred to a dermatologist for further evaluation and treatment.
4. On physical examination, erythematous, scaly patches with overlying 2 mm pustules were present on the distal extremities.
5. A punch biopsy was performed which parakeratosis, acanthosis with intraepidermal neutrophils, and a perivascular lymphocytic infiltrate in the dermis with neutrophil accumulation at the dermal papillae.

Clinical Course Options

1. The presumed diagnosis of paradoxical anti-TNF pustular-induced psoriasis was made in this patient with Crohn's disease.
2. What would be your next step?
   (a) Phototherapy.
   (b) Add apremilast.
   (c) Add cyclosporine.
   (d) Add methotrexate.
   (e) Switch to another TNF inhibitor.
   (f) Switch to ustekinumab.
   (g) Others.

Management and Response

1. The infliximab was not withheld and apremilast was added.
2. The patient developed nausea and diarrhea soon afterward and was not able to tolerate apremilast.
3. In discussion with the gastroenterologist, the decision was made to switch to ustekinumab to treat the psoriasis and to control her Crohn's disease.
4. The psoriasis dosing was used at 45 mg at weeks 0 and 4 and every 3 months.

5. The patient's psoriasis resolved within 2 months and her Crohn's disease remained stable on ustekinumab.

Discussion

1. A case review report examined the incidence of paradoxical anti-TNF pustular-induced psoriasis [5]:
   (a) 127 cases in patients with rheumatoid arthritis, ankylosing spondylitis, and Crohn's disease.
   (b) Infliximab (55.1%), etanercept (27.6%), adalimumab (17.3%).
   (c) Palmoplantar pustular psoriasis 40.5% of the cases, with plaque-type psoriasis in 33.1%, and other types comprising the remainder.
   (d) Topical corticosteroids were the most commonly employed treatment modality but led to resolution in only 26.8% of cases.
   (e) Switching to a different anti-TNF agent led to resolution in 15.4% of cases.
   (f) Cessation of anti-TNF therapy with systemic therapy led to resolution in 64.3% of cases.
2. Almost two-thirds of patients with Crohn's disease refractory to at least one anti-TNF agent receive clinical benefit from ustekinumab therapy, not requiring steroids for up to 12 months afterward [6].
3. Anti-IL-17 inhibitors have a class warning about a very small but potential risk of exacerbation of inflammatory bowel disease. Utilization of using these agents in situations of paradoxical anti-TNF pustular-induced psoriasis in patients with inflammatory bowel disease can be considered if there is lack of response from ustekinumab.
4. Oral systemic agents such as acitretin, apremilast, methotrexate, or cyclosporine may be considered as well.
5. Phototherapy may also be considered as well.

Pregnancy
Scenario

1. 28-year-old female with a 5-year history of psoriasis.
2. Initiated on ustekinumab when her baseline BSA was 35%.
3. Psoriasis 100% improved with ixekizumab after 6 months.
4. Patient informs you she is pregnant with her first child and wants to discuss whether to continue or stop the ixekizumab.
5. What would you do?
   (a) Stop ixekizumab.
   (b) Continue ixekizumab.

Discussion

1. There are no specific guidelines in the management of women who become pregnant while on a biologic agent. Each case is individualized and handled accordingly [7].

Table 25.1 Prevalence and risk ratios of pregnancy outcomes in psoriasis

Pregnancy outcome (ICD-9 code)	Psoriasis $N = 358$ (%)	Non-psoriasis $N = 131,424$ (%)	Risk ratio	95% CI
Spontaneous abortion (634)	28.1	7.2	3.90	3.33, 4.56
Preterm birth (644)	21.7	7.4	2.92	2.41, 3.54
Severe pre-eclampsia and eclampsia (642.5 and 642.6)	14.2	2.9	4.92	3.79, 6.39
Placenta previa without and with hemorrhage (641.0 and 641.1)	18.6	5.3	3.49	2.81, 4.33
Ectopic pregnancy (633)	13.6	3.0	4.56	3.48, 5.97
Cesarean section (669.7)	7.3	20.5	0.35	0.24, 0.53

Lima X, et al. Presented at: American Academy of Dermatology 68th Annual Meeting; March 5–9, 2010; Miami Beach, Florida. Poster P3308

2. For moderate-to-severe psoriasis, ultraviolet B phototherapy is preferred [8].
3. Despite regulated safety data, biologics are favored over other systemic medications when needed.
4. All biologics for psoriasis are pregnancy category B.
5. Certolizumab does not cross the placenta.
6. Limited data for TNF inhibitor indicate numerous cases of safe use during pregnancy and no clear pattern of malformations.
7. Increased rate of spontaneous abortion if etanercept is used during the first trimester.
8. Data limited for ustekinumab but no maternal, fetal, or infantile toxicities in animal studies.
9. Table 25.1 shows the prevalence and risk ratios of pregnancy outcomes in psoriasis.

Hepatitis B and C Case Reports [9]

1. Hepatitis B and hepatitis C
2. Five patients with concurrent viral hepatitis had plaque psoriasis with two having psoriatic arthritis (PsA) (2 M, 3F, mean age 54.5 years, average duration 8.8 years).
3. Three patients had HBV and two had HCV.
4. All the patients had received at least one biologic agent: four treatments of etanercept and one treatment of adalimumab.
5. Patients were evaluated by a hepatologist and were cleared to use the biologics with regular monitoring.
6. Psoriasis improved in all patients and no worsening of HBV or HCV.
7. Close monitoring required.

Table 25.2 Interpretation of Hepatitis B serologies

HBsAg	Negative	Susceptible
Anti-HBc	Negative	
Anti-HBs	Negative	
HBsAg	Negative	Immune due to natural infection
Anti-HBc	Positive	
Anti-HBs	Positive	
HBsAg	Negative	Immune due to hepatitis B vaccination
Anti-HBc	Negative	
Anti-HBs	Positive	
HBsAg	Positive	Acutely infected
Anti-HBc	Positive	
IgM anti-HBc	Positive	
Anti-HBs	Negative	
HBsAg	Positive	Chronically infected
Anti-HBc	Positive	
IgM anti-HBc	Negative	
Anti-HBs	Negative	
HBsAg	Negative	Interpretation unclear; four possibilities:
Anti-HBc	Positive	1. Resolved infection (most common)
Anti-HBs	Negative	2. False-positive anti-HBc, thus susceptible
		3. "Low level" chronic infection
		4. Resolving acute infection

Reprinted with permission from https://www.cdc.gov/hepatitis/hbv/hbvfaq.htm

8. Table 25.2 lists the interpretation of hepatitis B serologic test results:
   (a) When clinical trials are conducted for psoriasis, patients are excluded if the HbsAg is positive indicating infection (acute or chronic) or anti-HBc is positive and the HbsAg and anti-HBs are both negative indicating the interpretation is unclear with four possibilities:
      Resolved infection (most common)
      False-positive anti-HBc and thus susceptible
      "Low level" chronic infection
      Resolving acute infection

HIV Reports

1. Three HIV-positive patients all had plaque psoriasis with two having psoriatic arthritis (3 males, mean age 54.6 years, average duration 12.3 years) [9].
2. All were receiving HAART therapy under the care of infectious diseases physicians.
3. Two received etanercept and one adalimumab treatments and were followed up closely by the dermatologist and infectious disease physicians.
4. Psoriasis improved in all patients and no worsening of HIV.

5. Close monitoring required.
6. HIV and tumor necrosis factor (TNF) inhibitors [10]:
   (a) 27 published cases of patients with HIV being treated with TNF inhibitors.
   (b) Patients with HIV may have recalcitrant inflammatory disorders.
   (c) Clinical trials and case series demonstrate that tumor necrosis factor-alpha inhibitors can provide improvement in patients with HIV/AIDS with few complications.
   (d) Physicians may consider TNF inhibitors in motivated patients with HIV/AIDS, who are monitored for their CD4 count.

Vaccinations
Scenario

1. A 55-year-old male with a 20-year history of psoriasis.
2. He developed psoriatic arthritis 12 years after the onset of psoriasis.
3. His psoriatic arthritis and psoriasis has been well controlled on a 50 mg weekly dosing etanercept for 8 years.
4. The patient informs the dermatologist he wants to receive the live zoster vaccine.
5. How would you handle this?

Discussion

1. The package insert for biologics generally state that live vaccines should not be given while on therapy.
2. The general recommendation is for patients to be vaccinated first (on vaccines they wish to receive) and wait 1 month before the first dose of the biologic agent.
3. There are no specific guidelines for how long to withhold the biologic therapy prior to administering a live vaccine. The author's strategy is to withhold the biologic agent at the time when patient is due for their next dose, wait 1 month, have the live vaccine administered, wait another month, and then resume therapy. Another strategy is to withhold the biologic agent for five half-lives prior after the last dose prior to administering the live vaccine.
4. An analysis that included nearly 20,000 vaccinated Medicare patients reported that the administration of the live zoster vaccine was not associated with an increased risk of zoster shortly when concurrent biologics were not withheld. The study also showed a reduced longer-term risk of zoster in patients with an immune-mediated disease [11].
5. For heat-killed vaccines, the author does not generally withhold the biologic agent although the package insert for some biologics states that non-live vaccinations received during a course of biologic therapy may not elicit an immune response sufficient to prevent disease while studies performed on other biologics have demonstrated that antibody responses were elicited to certain non-live vaccines.

Surgery
Scenario

1. A 40-year-old woman with a 6 year history of severe psoriasis.
2. Her BMI at baseline was 32 and her weight was 250 lbs.
3. She has been on ustekinumab 3 years for and she is 100% clear.
4. Through diet and exercising, she lost 50 lbs. and her BMI is down to 25.
5. She wishes to undergo abdominoplasty to improve her appearance.
6. When would be an optimal time to schedule her surgery since she is on a biologic agent?

Discussion

1. A literature review reported that biologic and systemic agents can be safely continued through low-risk operations (e.g., simple excisions and Mohs surgery) in patients with psoriasis and psoriatic arthritis without increased incidence of delayed wound healing and prolonged infections. For moderate- and high-risk surgeries such as total joint replacement, a case-by-case approach should be taken based on the patient's individual risk factors and comorbidities [12].
2. The author generally recommends withholding the biologic agent 1–2 weeks prior to major surgery and resuming therapy 1 week after surgery.

Latent Tuberculosis
Scenario

1. A 40-year-old male from the Philippines has severe psoriasis for 10 years.
2. Topical agents and phototherapy have not been adequate.
3. He wishes to be treated with secukinumab after a female coworker told him this drug cleared her psoriasis.
4. His BSA at baseline is 40% with no symptoms or signs of psoriatic arthritis.
5. He has no history or family history of inflammatory bowel disease.
6. You decide that secukinumab would be appropriate for this patient.
7. The patient informs you he received the BCG vaccine.
8. Would you still test for tuberculosis?
   (a) Yes
   (b) No
9. Checking for tuberculosis should always be performed even if the patient has received the BCG vaccine before.
10. A QuantiFERON Gold assay test was performed and was positive.
11. What is your next step?
    (a) Because the patient has a positive QuantiFERON Gold assay, he should not be on any biologic agent.
    (b) Initiate isoniazid therapy.
    (c) Check a chest X-ray.

12. A chest X-ray was ordered and no signs of active tuberculosis were seen.
13. Isoniazid was prescribed for 9 months. One month into therapy with isoniazid, the patient was initiated on secukinumab.

Discussion

1. People with latent tuberculosis are not infectious and cannot transmit tuberculosis to other people.
2. Overall, without treatment, about 5–10% of people with latent tuberculosis will develop active tuberculosis disease at some time in their lives. About half of those people who develop tuberculosis will do so within the first 2 years of infection.
3. The BCG vaccination may cause the PPD test to be positive even though there was no exposure. The QuantiFERON Gold assay test is not likely to be positive in individuals who have received the BCG vaccination. In the event the assay is positive, then prophylactic therapy should be instituted because the vaccine may have worn off.
4. The biologic therapy can be initiated following 1 month of prophylactic treatment for latent tuberculosis.
5. Tuberculosis screening is usually done annually while patients are on biologics or whenever there has been an exposure.

References

1. Armstrong AW, Bagel J, van Voorhees AS, Robertson AD, Yamauchi PS. Combining biologic therapies with other systemic treatments in psoriasis: evidence-based, best-practice recommendations from the Medical Board of the National Psoriasis Foundation. JAMA Dermatol. 2015;151:432–8.
2. Costanzo A, Talamonti M, Botti E, Spallone G, Papoutsaki M, Chimenti S. Efficacy of efalizumab in psoriasis patients previously treated with tumour necrosis factor blockers. Dermatology. 2009;219:48–53.
3. Yamauchi PS, Bissonnette R, Teixeira HD, Valdecantos WC. Systematic review of efficacy of anti-tumor necrosis factor (TNF) therapy in patients with psoriasis previously treated with a different anti-TNF agent. J Am Acad Dermatol. 2016;75:612–8.
4. Patel S, Patel T, Kerdel FA. The risk of malignancy or progression of existing malignancy in patients with psoriasis treated with biologics: case report and review of the literature. Int J Dermatol. 2016;55:487–93.
5. Ko JM, Gottlieb AB, Kerbleski JF. Induction and exacerbation of psoriasis with TNF-blockade therapy: a review and analysis of 127 cases. J Dermatol Treat. 2009;20:100–8.
6. Wils P, Bouhnik Y, Michetti P, Flourie B, Brixi H, Bourrier A, Allez M, Duclos B, Grimaud JC, Buisson A, Amiot A, Fumery M, Roblin X, Peyrin-Biroulet L, Filippi J, Bouguen G, Abitbol V, Coffin B, Simon M, Laharie D, Pariente B; Groupe d'Etude des affections Inflammatoires du tube Digestif. Subcutaneous Ustekinumab provides clinical benefit for two-thirds of patients with Crohn's disease refractory to anti-tumor necrosis factor agents. Clin Gastroenterol Hepatol. 14:242–50.
7. Murase JE, Heller MM, Butler DC. Safety of dermatologic medications in pregnancy and lactation: Part I. Pregnancy. J Am Acad Dermatol. 2014;70:401.e1–14.
8. Hoffman MB, Farhangian M, Feldman SR. Psoriasis during pregnancy: characteristics and important management recommendations. Expert Rev Clin Immunol. 2015;11:709–20.
9. Zarei M, Villada G, Romanelli R. Biologics therapy in psoriasis patients with viral hepatitis, HIV, and cardiovascular diseases. J Am Acad Dermatol Suppl. 2016;74:3532.
10. Gallitano SM, McDermott L, Brar K, Lowenstein E. Use of tumor necrosis factor (TNF) inhibitors in patients with HIV/AIDS. J Am Acad Dermatol. 2016;74:974–80.
11. Zhang J, Xie F, Delzell E, Chen L, Winthrop KL, Lewis JD, Saag KG, Baddley JW, Curtis JR. Association between vaccination for herpes zoster and risk of herpes zoster infection among older patients with selected immune-mediated diseases. JAMA. 2012;308:43–9.
12. Choi YM, Debbaneh M, Weinberg JM, Yamauchi PS, Van Voorhees AS, Armstrong AW, Siegel M, JJ W. From the Medical Board of the National Psoriasis Foundation: perioperative management of systemic immunomodulatory agents in patients with psoriasis and psoriatic arthritis. J Am Acad Dermatol. 2016;75:798–805.

Biosimilars in Dermatology

26

Paul S. Yamauchi

Introduction

Biologics are complex, high molecular weight molecules manufactured through recombinant DNA technology in living system host cells such as bacteria, yeast insect, plant, or mammalian cells grown in culture [1]. Biologics comprise an array of proteins that include monoclonal antibodies, receptor fusions proteins, blood and plasma products, recombinant proteins, and vaccines [2]. They play a critical role in clinical care by eliciting a therapeutic response through the binding of specific targets and antigens in the body.

Biosimilars are copies or imitations of original biologics (reference product) that are structurally similar and have the same pharmacologic mechanism of action [3, 4]. In the United States, the Federal Drug Agency (FDA) defines a biosimilar as "a biologic product that is highly similar to a US licensed reference biological product notwithstanding minor differences in clinically inactive components, and for which there are no clinically meaningful differences between the biological product and the reference product in terms of the safety, purity, and potency of the product" [5]. The European Medicines Agency (EMA) defines a biosimilar as a biological medicinal product that contains a version of the active substance of an already authorized original biological medicinal product, referred to as the reference medicinal product, or simply "reference product" [6]. A biosimilar demonstrates similarity to the reference product in terms of quality characteristics, biological activity, safety, and efficacy based on a comprehensive comparability exercise [7]. The World Health Organization (WHO) refers to a biosimilar as a similar biotherapeutic product (SBP), defined as "a biotherapeutic product which is similar in terms of quality, safety and efficacy to an already licensed reference biotherapeutic product" [8]. Unlike generic medications, biosimilars are not identical to the reference biologic or to other biosimilars of the same reference biologic.

With patent expiration dates of important biologic drugs having already occurred or are on the horizon (Table 26.1), focus on developing biosimilars have heavily intensified [9]. The foremost intention of biosimilar availability is to improve patient access to biologic therapies by reducing clinical developmental expenses and offering an economic advantage through substantial reduction of cost. However, the introduction of these agents into the US health care marketplace has elicited concern and debate because biosimilars are not identical copies of their originator drugs and pharmacovigilance studies are limited. Nonetheless, several biosimilar are approved globally and as more enter the market, it is important that health care providers understand their role and characteristics.

This review aims to provide a comprehensive treatise of biosimilars and its relevance in dermatology with emphasis on the current landscape in this continuous evolving area.

Table 26.1 Anticipated United States and European Union patent expiration years for innovator biologics

Biologic name	Brand name	Anticipated expiration year	
		US	EU
Adalimumab	Humira®	2016	2018
Certolizumab pegol	Cimzia®	2024	2021
Etanercept	Enbrel®	2028	2015
Golimumab	Simponi®	2024	2024
Infliximab	Remicade®	2018	2015
Ustekinumab	Stelara®	2023	2024

P.S. Yamauchi, MD, PhD
David Geffen School of Medicine at UCLA, Dermatology Institute and Skin Care Center, 2001 Santa Monica Blvd Suite 1160W, Santa Monica, CA 90404, USA
e-mail: paulyamauchi@yahoo.com

© Springer International Publishing AG 2018
P.S. Yamauchi (ed.), *Biologic and Systemic Agents in Dermatology*, https://doi.org/10.1007/978-3-319-66884-0_26

Manufacturing and Structure of Biologics and Biosimilars

Biosimilars differ from generic drugs in numerous important ways and are not synonymous with each other (biosimilar ≠ generic) (Fig. 26.1). Unlike generic drugs, which are identical to the reference drug in dosage, safety, strength, route of administration, quality, and intended use, biosimilars are not exact copies of their reference product. The molecular weight of the biosimilar is typically in the thousands of daltons while the size of a generic in the hundreds of daltons [12]. The structure of the biosimilar is complex and heterogenous while generics have a simple and defined structure [12, 13]. While generics are small molecules that can be fully characterized, biosimilars are dynamic structures that cannot be fully characterized 100% in the laboratory. Biosimilars can be sensitive to slight changes in physical conditions such as temperature, storage, and handling while generics are relatively stable under similar conditions. Biosimilars have intrinsic potential for immunogenicity while generics have a low potential. Generics are synthesized from predictable chemical reactions and identical copies can be produced.

Because biologics and biosimilars are produced in living systems (Fig. 26.2), they are more complicated to develop and manufacture than small molecules (Fig. 26.3). Small molecule drugs are synthesized through a series of chemical reactions and are readily reproducible in laboratories and highly equivalent due to their simple structure [10]. One of the initial steps in the development of a biologic is to isolate the gene that encodes the protein of interest [11]. The isolated gene is expressed on a DNA vector which is then transfected into a cell line. A unique cell clone is subsequently identified and expanded into a master cell bank that produces vast quantities of the desired protein. The protein is subsequently extracted and purified through a series of manufacturing processing steps that leads to the final dispensed product. Quality control and quality assurance are monitored at all stages of the manufacturing process to ensure that product attributes meet the stringent requirements for identity, purity, potency, and stability. Adding to another level of variable complexity with biologics and biosimilars, the manufacturing processes may be similar but not identical between different manufacturers (Fig. 26.4). Each step during manufacturing can potentially introduce variability between a biosimilar and its reference drug. Such differences may lead to

Biologics and Biosimilars Are Made by Living Cells Through Well-Controlled Processes

A typical biotechnology manufacturing process includes multiple stages

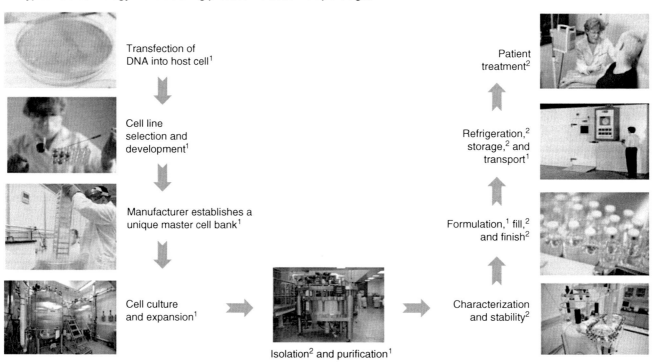

Transfection of DNA into host cell[1]

Cell line selection and development[1]

Manufacturer establishes a unique master cell bank[1]

Cell culture and expansion[1]

Isolation[2] and purification[1]

Characterization and stability[2]

Formulation,[1] fill,[2] and finish[2]

Refrigeration,[2] storage,[2] and transport[1]

Patient treatment[2]

DNA = deoxyribonucleic acid.
1. Kresse GB. *Eur J Pharm Biopharm.* 2009;72:479-486. 2. Sharma BG. EJHP Pract. 2007;13:54-56.

Fig. 26.1 Biosimilars are different from generics (reprinted with permission from Amgen)

Biologics Are Larger and Structurally More Complex Than Chemically Synthesized Drugs

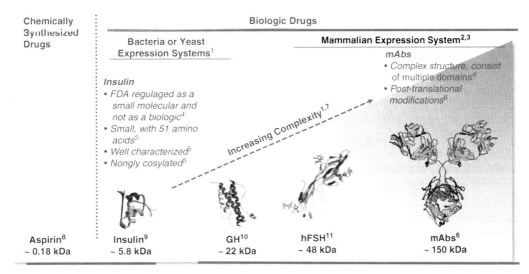

Images are not shown to relative scale.
FDA =Food and Drug Administration; mAbs =monoclonal antibodies; GH1 =human growth hormone 1; hFSH = human follicle-stimulating hormone.
1. EMA. Biosimilar Medicines. www.ema.europa.eu/ema/index.jsp?curf=pages/special_topics/document_listing/document_listing_000318.jsp. Accessed March 5, 2015. 2. Rosser MP, et al. *Protein Express Pur.* 2005;40:237-243. 3. Lackner A, et al. *Anal Biochem.* 2008;380:146-148. 4. Johnson JA; Congressional Research Service *FDA Regulation of Follow-On Biologics.* CRS Report for Congress. Published April26, 2010. 5. EMA. *Guideline on Non-Clinical and Clinical Development of Similar Biological Medicinal Products Containing Recombinant Human Insulin and Insulin Analogues.* Published February 26, 2015. 6. Schneider C, et al. Nat *Biotechnol.* 2008;26: 985-990. 7. Berkowitz S, et al. *Nat Rev Drug Discov.* 2012; 11 :527-540. 8. Aspirin (acetylsalicylic acid) prescribing information, www. fda.gov/ohrms/DOCKETS/ac/03/briefing/4012B1_03_Appd%201-Professionai%20Labeling.pdf. Accessed October 19, 2016. 9. Sigma Aldrich. Product Information: Insulin. http://www.sigmaaldrich.com/content/dam/sigmaaldrich/docs/Sigma/Produd_Information_Sheet/2/i6634pis.pdf.Accessed October 23, 2016.10. OMIM. Growth Hormone. www.omim.org/entry/139250?search=human%20growth%20hormone&highlight= hormone%20growth%20human. Accessed October 19, 2016.11. Na KH, et al. *J Microbial Biotechnol.* 2005; 15:395-402.

Fig. 26.2 Biologics and biosimilars are made by living cells through well-controlled processes (reprinted with permission from Amgen)

Each Biosimilar Is Unique Because of Differences in Manufacturing

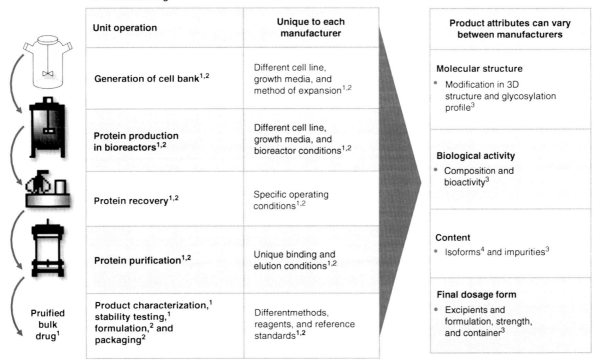

1. Mellstedt H, et al. *Ann Oncol.* 2008:411-419. 2. Roger SD. *Nephrology (Carlton).* 2006; 11:341-346. 3. FDA. *Scientific Considerations in Demonstrating Biosimilarity to a Reference Product. Guidance for Industry.* Published April 2015. 4. FDA. *]Quality Considerations in Demonstrating Biosimilarity to a Reference Protein Product. Guidance for Industry* Published April 2015.

Fig. 26.3 Biologics are larger and structurally more complex than chemically synthesized drugs (reprinted with permission from Amgen)

Biosimilars Are Different From Generics

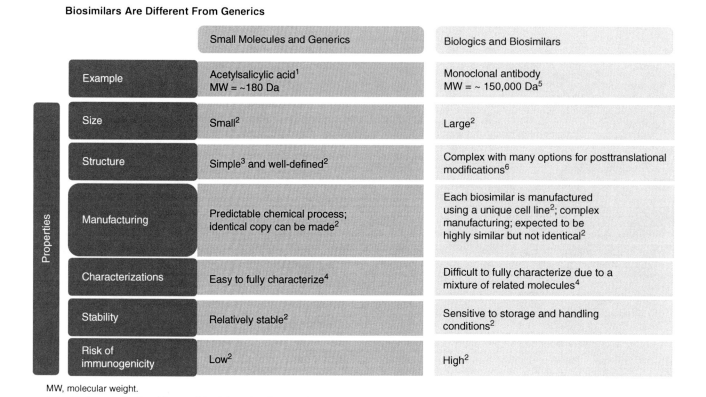

Properties		Small Molecules and Generics	Biologics and Biosimilars
	Example	Acetylsalicylic acid[1] MW = ~180 Da	Monoclonal antibody MW = ~ 150,000 Da[5]
	Size	Small[2]	Large[2]
	Structure	Simple[3] and well-defined[2]	Complex with many options for posttranslational modifications[6]
	Manufacturing	Predictable chemical process; identical copy can be made[2]	Each biosimilar is manufactured using a unique cell line[2]; complex manufacturing; expected to be highly similar but not identical[2]
	Characterizations	Easy to fully characterize[4]	Difficult to fully characterize due to a mixture of related molecules[4]
	Stability	Relatively stable[2]	Sensitive to storage and handling conditions[2]
	Risk of immunogenicity	Low[2]	High[2]

MW, molecular weight.

1. Aspirin (acetylsalicylic acid) prescribing information, Bayer. 2. Genazzani AA, et al. *BioDrugs.* 2007;21:351-356. 3. Prugnaud JL. *Br J Clin Pharmacal.* 2008;65:619-620. 4. GottliebS. *AmJ Health Syst Pharm.* 2008;65(14 supp 6):S2-S8. 5. Lipman NS, et ai. *ILAR J.* 2005;46:258-268. 6. Roger SD. *Nephrology (Carlton).* 2006;11:341-346.

Fig. 26.4 Each biosimilars is unique because of differences in manufacturing (reprinted with permission from Amgen)

structural variances in the resulting biologic protein which could alter the safety or efficacy of the product.

It is important to note that biosimilars are derived from a cell line that is different from the reference biologic due to proprietary rights of the original sponsor. As a result, biosimilars are not exact copies to their reference products but are similar to each other with some minor variations. The development of a biosimilar first starts with the identification of the primary acid sequence of the reference product followed by the construction of the corresponding recombinant DNA gene which is then transfected and expressed in a different cell line through reverse engineering. Analytical characterization is conducted to demonstrate similarity to the reference product followed by comparative clinical studies in safety, efficacy, and immunogenicity to confirm biosimilarity.

The environment in the cell dictates the structural properties of the protein and its function. The primary structure of the protein establishes the amino acid sequence chain and the secondary and tertiary structure determine the folding and three-dimensional shape of the protein (Fig. 26.5). Any small changes in the conformation of the protein can alter its function and cause clinically meaningful differences in efficacy and safety [14]. In addition, proteins undergo posttranslational modifications that further contribute to the function,

diversity, and complexity [15] (Fig. 26.5). There are more than 300 types of posttranslational modifications that have been identified including glycosylation, phosphorylation, methylation, amidation, and acetylation. While a biosimilar may have the same primary amino acid sequence as the reference product, differences in posttranslational modifications may potentially result in low level sequence variants that can change biological function or stability. Some of these variability in posttranslational modifications can be attributed to the actual cell line itself or the bioreactor conditions in which the biosimilar is produced. Ongoing inherent mutations with each passing generation of the cell line or even batch-to-batch within the same production line may also contribute to minor posttranslational variants [16]. These minor differences between the proposed biosimilar and the reference product can influence the pharmacokinetics, pharmacodynamics, efficacy, safety, and immunogenicity, and careful identification and quantification from the onset must be determined to ensure these differences are clinically non-meaningful [17–19].

Manufacturing processes periodically undergo changes to improve certain aspects of development such as increased scale production, enhanced product stability, or to comply with regulatory requirement changes. There may

Fig. 26.5 Protein folding and posttranslational modifications affect clinical characteristics (reprinted with permission from Amgen)

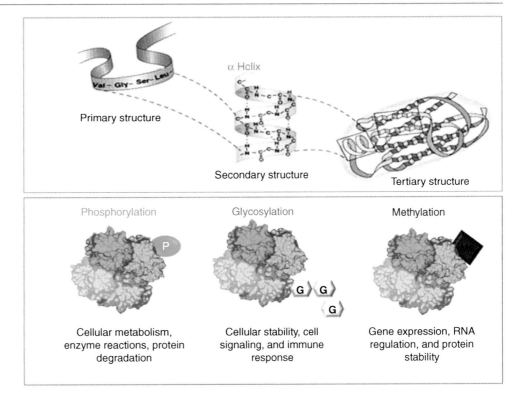

Primary structure

α Helix

Secondary structure

Tertiary structure

Phosphorylation

Cellular metabolism, enzyme reactions, protein degradation

Glycosylation

Cellular stability, cell signaling, and immune response

Methylation

Gene expression, RNA regulation, and protein stability

be occasional small shifts in product attributes because of these manufacturing changes that need to be justified by analytic tests so there is no adverse effect on safety, efficacy, and immunogenicity. The phenomena called process drift is an unexpected trend or shift in the quality attribute of a product over time such as changes in glycosylation. Some potential sources of drift away from the intended target value are changes in raw materials, operator practices, facilities, equipment, etc. [20]. For example, chemical characterization of different commercial lots etanercept produced between 2007 and 2011 revealed variations in both C-terminal lysine content and glycosylation [21]. Despite these substantial differences from drifting presumably due to changes in the manufacturing process, etanercept was continuously marketed throughout this time frame without any change in label indicating the observed changes were predicted not to alter the clinical profile of the drug and were considered not clinically meaningful by the health authorities. The FDA has stated that assessing the differences arising from drifting due to a manufacturing change is not comparable to demonstrating biosimilarity between the proposed biosimilar and reference product for any posttranslational modifications. Drifting does not result in an original product becoming a biosimilar because it was not reversed engineered in its development and the original company has proprietary and historical information of its manufacturing process. Although some of the determinants used to measure drifting may also be applicable to demonstrate

biosimilarity, further data are needed to determine biosimilarity because of uncertainties and lack of long-term experience.

Development of Biosimilars

In the US, the FDA gained authority to approve biosimilars as part of the Patient Protection and Affordable Care Act in 2010, which created an abbreviated approval pathway for biological products shown to be biosimilar or interchangeable with an FDA licensed reference biologic drug. This is under Section 7002 of H.R. 3590 referred to as the Biologic Price Competition and Innovation (BPCI) Act of 2009, an amendment of Section 351 of the PHS Act intended to improved patient access to expensive biologic therapies. The proposed biosimilar and reference product must have the same presumed mechanism of action, administration route, dosage, and potency to be considered for an abbreviated Biological License Application (BLA).

The regulatory pathway for the development and approval of biosimilars differs from reference biologics and generics (Table 26.2). Given the complex nature of biologics, the FDA developed a biosimilar development program to issue recommendations that focused on the "totality of evidence" to evaluate biosimilarity through a stepwise investigational approach (Fig. 26.6) [22]. The purpose of the program was to support a demonstration of biosimilarity between the proposed biosimilar and reference product that included an

Table 26.2 Differences in regulatory requirements for reference biologics, biosimilars, and generics

	Reference Biologics	Biosimilars	Generic
Quality	Comprehensive product analysis	Comprehensive product analysis Comparison with reference biologic	Comprehensive product analysis Comparison with reference small drug
Preclinical	Full preclinical program	Abbreviated program based on complexity	Not required
Clinical	Phase 1	PK equivalence PD equivalence	Bioequivalence only
	Phase 2	Phase 2 not required	Phase 2 not required
	Phase 3 in all indications	Phase 3 in at least one representative indication. Extrapolation to other indications allowed if the mechanism of action is the same	Phase 3 not required
	Pharmacovigilance program	Yes	Yes

PK pharmacokinetics, *PD* pharmacodynamics

Fig. 26.6 Regulatory approval pathway for biosimilars development differs from that of innovator products. (Reprinted with permission from Kozlowski,S. Presented at Biotechnology Summit; June 13, 2014; Rockville, MD. https://www.ibbr.umd.edu/sites/default/files/public_page/Kozlowski%20-%20 Biomanufacturing%20 Summit.pdf)

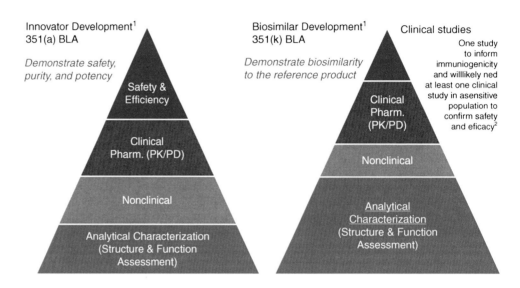

Structural Analyses

The FDA expects that the expression construct for the proposed biosimilar encodes the same primary amino acid sequence as its reference product. However, minor modifications such as N- or C- terminal truncations that are not expected to change the product performance are acceptable. All physical characteristics of the biosimilar (primary, secondary, tertiary, quaternary structure; posttranslational modifications; and biological activities) be highly similar to the reference product notwithstanding minor differences in its clinically inactive components.

Functional Assays

The pharmacologic activity of biosimilars is compared to the reference product through several vitro and/or in vivo functional

assessment of the effects of any observed differences between the products, but not to independently establish the safety and efficacy of the biosimilar itself [23].

assays. In vitro assays include biological assays, binding assays, and enzyme kinetics to compare the mechanism of action of both products. In vivo assays may include the use of animal models of disease to evaluate functional effects on pharmacodynamics markers and efficacy measures. Functional assessment of monoclonal antibody biosimilars focuses on biological activity associated with antigen binding at the Fab region and complement interactions on the Fc region. Functional assessment also includes measuring the inhibition of proliferation in an appropriate cell line such as antibody-dependent cell-mediated cytotoxicity.

Animal Data (Nonclinical Studies)

Animal studies may be utilized to demonstrate safety evaluation and support biosimilarity between the biosimilar and the reference product. However, toxicity data for biosimilars from animal studies may not be necessary or expected if structural and functional data provide strong evidence supporting analytic similarity to the reference product based on the pharmacokinetics (PK) and pharmacodynamics (PD) profiles of the proposed product and the reference product. It is important to note that PK and PD assessments from animal data will not replace the requirement for human PK and PD studies. Animal immunogenicity assessments may be conducted to assist in the interpretation of the animal study results but generally do not reflect potential immune responses in humans.

Clinical Pharmacology

Human PK studies comparing the proposed biosimilar product to the reference product are required and considered the foundation to demonstrate pharmacologic bioequivalence. Human PD studies may or may not be required but are often conducted to supplement PK studies if sensitive PD markers and clinical endpoints are available. Human PK studies that have demonstrated similar exposure measurements such as serum concentration over time between the proposed biosimilar product and the reference product provide evidence of biosimilarity that can be correlated with clinical safety and efficacy. Likewise, human PD studies that exert a similar effect on PD outcomes relevant to defined efficacy measurements such as a dose response curve or specific safety events represent further support for biosimilarity determination.

Immunogenicity assessment is required to evaluate potential differences between the proposed biosimilar and the reference product and serves to establish there are no clinically meaningful differences [24–27]. Any difference in immune responses may potentially promote the development of neutralizing antibodies and induce changes in PK and PD responses. The FDA expects at least one clinical assay study to compare the immunogenicity of the biosimilar to the reference product that considers antibody parameters such as titer changes, specificity, time course of development, impact on PK responses, and neutralizing of product activity.

Safety and Efficacy Studies

All clinical studies need to demonstrate that the proposed biosimilar product is neither inferior to the reference product by a specified margin nor superior to the reference product by a specified margin. The pyramid scheme in Fig. 26.6 shows almost equal partitioning of the four segments comprising the clinical development of the reference product for analytical characterization, nonclinical studies, clinical pharmacology, and safety plus efficacy. Conversely, there is greater emphasis on analytical characterization and clinical pharmacology over nonclinical studies and safety plus efficacy for the development of the biosimilar counterpart. Whereas clinical trials are required and conducted for all indications for the reference (innovator) product, at least one clinical trial for a specific indication is recommended for the biosimilar product that is compared head-to-head to the reference product. The clinical trial protocol for the biosimilar matches and parallels the phase 3 trial of the innovator that was previously conducted for that indication. It is up to the sponsor that is developing the biosimilar product to choose the indication for testing in the clinical trial. Results for the safety and efficacy endpoints should closely match between the reference product and biosimilar within specified parameters. Hypothetically, even if the biosimilar demonstrates superior efficacy outside the specified margins over the reference product which might be interpreted as being favorable for the biosimilar, biosimilarity is not established because the two products are not equivalent since clinical meaningful differences are evident.

Extrapolation

The term extrapolation refers to a biosimilar product obtaining approval in one or more indications that the reference product is licensed for in the absence of performing clinical trials for that particular indication [22]. Extrapolation is allowable provided that analytical characterization, PK/PD activities, and immunogenicity profiles for the biosimilar closely matche the reference product without clinically meaningful differences. Usually at least one clinical trial is chosen for a therapeutic indication at the sponsor's discretion to demonstrate similar efficacy and safety. For example, if the efficacy endpoints and safety measurements in a psoriasis comparator trial between an antitumor necrosis factor (TNF) inhibitor biosimilar and the reference product revealed no clinically relevant differences between the two agents, then extrapolation would be allowed for other indications such as rheumatoid arthritis or inflammatory bowel disease even though they were not tested in clinical trials. Because clinical trials in psoriasis have lower placebo rates with higher efficacy changes from baseline and concomitant systemic agents are not used (unlike rheumatoid arthritis or Crohn's disease trials where combination therapy is allowed), extrapolation from psoriasis trials could be a preferable benchmark in comparison to other approved indications such rheumatoid arthritis, Crohn's disease, or ankylosing spondylitis [10]. In certain instances, exclusivity may be granted for an indication that the reference product had recently been approved for and extrapolation would be denied. For example, the reference product for adalimumab recently had approvals in adults for moderate to severe hidradenitis suppurativa and noninfectious intermediate, posterior, and panuveitis that the currently approved biosimilar for adalimumab does not have.

On April 5, 2016, the FDA approved the first monoclonal antibody biosimilar in the United States called Inflectra® (designated as CT-P13 in clinical trials) which demonstrated biosimilarity to Remicade® (infliximab). Based on analytic characterization, clinical pharmacology, and the phase 3 trials for rheumatoid arthritis [28] and ankylosing spondylitis [29] in comparison to Remicade®, Inflectra® was approved for rheumatoid arthritis and ankylosing spondylitis and extrapolation was allowed for Crohn's disease, ulcerative colitis, psoriatic arthritis, and plaque psoriasis but not for the pediatric indications. Prior to FDA approval, the European Commission had already approved Inflectra® and allowed extrapolation for all infliximab indications including pediatric indications. In addition, an independent small psoriasis trial demonstrated clinical responses in infliximab naïve patients who were treated with CT-P13 [30]. Furthermore, patients were able to maintain responses initially attained by Remicade® and then switched over to CT-P13.

Interchangeability

The BPCI Act defines interchangeability as a biosimilar product that is expected to have the same clinical result as the reference product in any given patient without the safety and efficacy being compromised as a result of switching when compared to using the reference product alone. The BPCI Act states that an interchangeable biologic may be substituted for the reference product without the intervention of the health care provider who originally prescribed the reference product. Currently none of the approved biosimilars in the US have a designation for interchangeability at the time of preparation of this manuscript.

In early 2017, the FDA drafted and issued initial guidelines detailing the agency's expectations for demonstrating biosimilar interchangeability [31]. The sponsors have 90 days to respond to the proposed guidelines before the FDA finalizes its recommendations which may be announced later in 2017. For biological products that are intended to be administered to an individual more than once, the sponsors generally will be expected to conduct a switching study or studies to address the provision "for a biological product that is administered more than once to an individual, the risk in terms of safety or diminished efficacy of alternating or switching between use of the biological product and the reference product is not greater than the risk of using the reference without such alternation or switch" set forth in section 351(k)(4)(B) of the PHS Act. The switch study should evaluate changes in treatment that result in at least two separate exposure periods to each of the two products (i.e., at least three switches with each switch crossing over to the alternate product). The recommendations for primary analysis in a multi-switch study are PK endpoints and secondary endpoints include safety, immunogenicity, and efficacy. However, for biosimilars that are not intended to be interchangeable multi-switch studies would not be needed. The FDA also recommends that clinical PK and PD studies be utilized to assess the impact of switching since changes in immunogenicity and exposure may potentially arise as a result of alternating therapies. If apparent differences in the immune responses or adverse events are noticed in the switch arms of the study, there would be concerns whether the proposed biosimilar would be interchangeable irrespective of whether the biosimilar or the reference product caused the event.

Switch studies could be designed with a lead-in period of the reference product followed by a randomized two-cohort period with one arm incorporating the switch to the biosimilar and the other arm remaining as a non-switch arm with the reference product only. The switch arm is expected to undergo at least three switches: reference product → biosimilar → reference product → biosimilar. If the biosimilar is deemed to be interchangeable based on a study in a specific indication or more, then the sponsor may seek designation for interchangeability to be extrapolated to other indications for which the reference product is licensed. In addition, if the reference product is only marketed in a vial or prefilled syringe, the sponsor may not seek licensure for the biosimilar to be dispensed in a different presentation such as an auto-injector.

Labeling of Biosimilars

The FDA has issued a statement that the labeling of biosimilars includes a description of the clinical data that supports safety and efficacy of the reference product as described in the package information [32]. This mechanism follows the same labeling procedures similar to generic small molecule drugs. However, the labeling of biosimilars should not include a description of clinical studies that supports a demonstration that there are no clinically meaningful differences between the proposed biosimilar and the reference product. Basically, the package information for the biosimilar will be composed of the same information that is found in the reference product with regard to safety, efficacy, warnings, etc. and have no mention of clinical trial outcomes and any differences in PK/PD or immunogenicity assays. The reasoning for this by the FDA is that data from clinical studies designed to support a demonstration of biosimilarity are not likely to be relevant to health care provider's considerations with regard to safety and efficacy and potentially may cause confusion that could result in an inaccurate understanding of the risk-benefit profile of the biosimilar. One difference in the labeling is in circumstances where the biosimilar does not have all the indications that the reference product is approved and licensed (exclusions for extrapolation or an exclusive indication for the reference product).

Nonproprietary Naming of Biosimilars

The FDA issued guidance for nonproprietary naming of biosimilars that comprises a combination of the core name and a distinguishable suffix that is devoid of meaning and composed of four lower case letters [33]. An example of this is Erelzi® (designated as GP2015 in clinical trials) which is the biosimilar to Enbrel® that received FDA approval on August 30, 2016. The approval was based on clinical trials in psoriasis that demonstrated equivalent efficacy, safety, and immunogenicity results in comparison to Enbrel® [34].

The nonproprietary naming of Erelzi® is etanercept-szzs. The role of nonproprietary naming is to assist in the facilitation of correct identification of biosimilars from the reference product and other biosimilars for health care professionals, pharmacists, and patients. The unique suffixes are designed to prevent inadvertent substitution of biosimilars that have not been deemed to be interchangeable.

The FDA is strongly committed to the development of safe and optimal pharmacovigilance programs for biosimilars. One item in the framework would be the use of nonproprietary names with distinguishing suffixes that can serve as a key component to identify specific biosimilars in adverse event reporting and to reinforce accurate product identification in billing and claims records used for active pharmacovigilance [33].

Adalimumab-atto (Amjevita®, ABP-501): An Example of Demonstrating Biosimilarity

Adalimumab-atto (Amjevita®; also designated as ABP-501 in clinical trials) is a biosimilar to Humira® (adalimumab) that received FDA approval on September 23, 2016, based on analytic characterization, clinical pharmacology, and two phase 3 trials for plaque psoriasis [35, 36] and rheumatoid arthritis

[36]. Extrapolation was allowed for psoriatic arthritis, ankylosing spondylitis, juvenile idiopathic arthritis, adult Crohn's disease, and adult ulcerative colitis and excluded other approved indications for Humira®. Adalimumab-atto exhibited similar PK serum concentration profiles and immunogenicity antibody results when compared to US and European derived Humira® (Fig. 26.7a, b). The mean Psoriasis Area Severity Index (PASI) improvement was similar between adalimumab-atto and Humira® up to week 16. In addition, switching from Humira® to adalimumab-atto at week 16 showed similar maintenance of PASI response up to week 52 when compared to continuing Humira® during the same time frame (Fig. 26.7c). In a comparator trial for rheumatoid arthritis where the American College of Rheumatology (ACR) response was used as the endpoint, the ACR 20, 50, and 70 scores were similar between adalimumab-atto and Humira® up to week 24 (Fig. 26.7d). Table 26.3 shows that the incidence of adverse events was generally similar in the 24-week rheumatoid arthritis trial and for the first 16 weeks in the psoriasis trial. Based on the collective data, the FDA determined there were no meaningful clinical differences between the products and the requirements for establishing biosimilarity were fulfilled. It is important to note that the single switch period in the psoriasis trial was not designed for

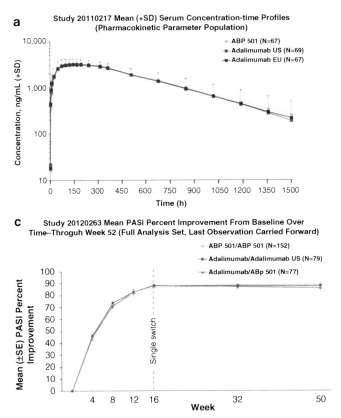

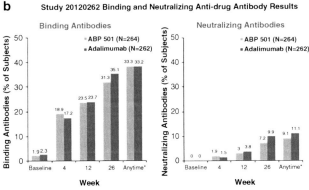

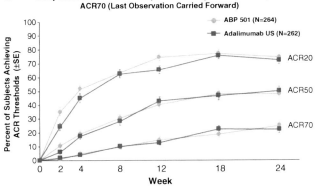

Fig. 26.7 Establishing biosimilarity of ABP-501 when compared to reference adalimumab (Reprinted with permission from FDA Briefing Document Arthritis Advisory Committee Meeting July 12, 2016 BLA 761024 ABP 501, a proposed biosimilar to Humira (adalimumab) Amgen).

https://www.fda.gov/downloads/AdvisoryCommittees/ CommitteesMeetingMaterials/Drugs/ArthritisAdvisoryCommittee/ UCM510293.pdf)

Table 26.3 Adverse events of interest in rheumatoid arthritis and plaque psoriasis studies

Event of interest category	Rheumatoid Arthritis Study 20120262		Plaque Psoriasis Study 20120263				
			Through week 16		Weeks 16–52 (re-randomized)		
	ABP 501	Adalimumab	ABP 501	Adalimumab	ABP 501/ABP 501	Adalimumab/Adalimumab	Adalimumab/ABP 501
	$N = 264$	$N = 262$	$N = 174$	$N = 173$	$N = 152$	$N = 79$	$N = 77$
	n (%)	n (%)	n (%)	n (%)	n (%)	n (%)	n (%)
Any adverse event of interest	80 (30.3)	94 (35.9)	68 (39.1)	69 (39.9)	75 (49.3)	31 (39.2)	39 (50.6)
Infections and infestations	61 (23.1)	68 (26.0)	59 (33.9)	58 (33.5)	67 (44.1)	29 (36.7)	37 (48.1)
Hypersensitivity	14 (5.3)	10 (3.8)	8 (4.6)	7 (4.0)	8 (5.3)	2 (2.5)	3 (3.9)
Liver enzyme elevations	13 (4.9)	10 (3.8)	4 (2.3)	2 (1.2)	9 (5.9)	2 (2.5)	2 (2.6)
Injection site reactions	6 (2.3)	13 (5.0)	3 (1.7)	9 (5.2)	2 (1.3)	3 (3.8)	0 (0.0)
Hematological reactions	5 (1.9)	5 (1.9)	0 (0.0)	3 (1.7)	0 (0.0)	1 (1.3)	1 (1.3)
Malignancies	1 (0.4)	1 (0.4)	1 (0.6)	1 (0.6)	1 (0.7)	0 (0.0)	0 (0.0)
Heart failure	1 (0.4)	2 (0.8)	0 (0.0)	0 (0.0)	0 (0.0)	0 (0.0)	0 (0.0)
Demyelinating diseases	0 (0.0)	0 (0.0)	0 (0.0)	0 (0.0)	0 (0.0)	0 (0.0)	0 (0.0)
Lupus-like syndromes	0 (0.0)	0 (0.0)	0 (0.0)	0 (0.0)	0 (0.0)	0 (0.0)	0 (0.0)

(Reprinted with permission from FDA Briefing Document Arthritis Advisory Committee Meeting July 12, 2016 BLA 761024 ABP 501, a proposed biosimilar to Humira (adalimumab) Amgen https://www.fda.gov/downloads/AdvisoryCommittees/CommitteesMeetingMaterials/Drugs/ArthritisAdvisoryCommittee/UCM510293.pdf)

winterchangeability and none of the biosimilars, including adalimumab-atto, are currently designated for interchangeability by the FDA at the time of preparation of this manuscript.

State Laws Regarding Biosimilar Substitution

For the past several years a total of at least 37 states have deliberated on legislature to establish state standards for the substitution of a biosimilar to replace the original reference prescription biologic [37]. As of 3/16/2017, 27 states and Puerto Rico have enacted laws regulating the substitution of biosimilars while other states have filed but not passed any laws (Fig. 26.8) [37]. The provisions of state legislation vary state by state but there are several features and requirements that have commonality.

- Any biosimilar under consideration for substitution must first be designated as interchangeable by FDA.
- The prescriber health care provider would be able to prevent substitution by stating "dispense as written" or "brand medically necessary."
- The prescriber must be notified of the substitution by the pharmacist.
- The patient must be notified that a substitution will be made and in some states patient consent would be required before any such switch is made.
- The pharmacist and the physician must retain records of substituted biosimilars.
- Some state laws provide immunity for pharmacists who make a substitution that is in compliance with the state law.
- Some state legislation requires the pharmacist to explain the price difference between the reference product and the biosimilar and that the substituted product must have a lower cost.

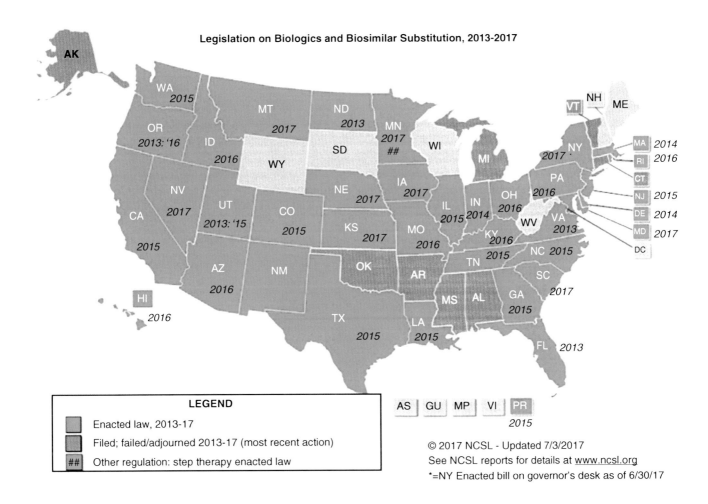

Fig. 26.8 Legislation on Biologics and Biosimilar Substitution, 2013–2017 (Reprinted with permission from National Conference of State Legislatures. State laws and legislation related to biologic medications and substitution of biosimilars. 10/12/2017. http://www.ncsl.org/research/health/state-laws-and-legislation-related-to-biologic-medications-and-substitution-of-biosimilars.aspx)

Pharmacoeconomics of Biosimilars

Estimated cost savings of biosimilars in the US have varied widely in several independent analysis studies. Despite recent approval of biosimilars in the US, there has been delayed entry into the market for various reasons including ongoing patent disputes and litigation processes between sponsors of the reference product and biosimilar and none of the currently approved biosimilars have been designated to be interchangeable. As a result, some of the predictions in cost savings have lagged. Nonetheless, many evaluations have projected billions of dollars worth of savings in the US for the future.

The US market is predicted to be the biggest market for biosimilars internationally by the 2015 Global & USA Biosimilar Market Analysis and biosimilars will account for 4–10% of all marketed biologics globally [38]. When the BPCI act was passed 2009, the Congressional Budget Office had already estimated one year before that total expenditures on biologics would decrease by $25 billion between 2009 and 2018 with savings of $5.9 billion for the federal government alone [38]. Analysis from Rand Corporation predicted that biosimilars will lead to a $44.2 billion reduction in direct spending on biologic drugs from 2014 to 2024, or about 4% of total biologic spending over that same period, with a range of $13 billion to $66 billion [39].

Biosimilars have never been projected to equal the 70–80% cost savings that generics are associated with. In Europe which has approved 23 biosimilars since 2006 and other countries, the average reduction in price for biosimilars is 20–30% lower than reference biologics [38]. The price reductions are highly variable from country to country and product to product in each country. For example, the biosimilar to etanercept is 10–15% cheaper in Denmark but the biosimilar to infliximab is 60% lower relative to their reference products. For the US, payers have aligned their expectations that cost reductions for biosimilars will be in the 10–35% range [38].

Clinical Considerations for Dermatologists

Biosimilars represent a new category of drugs that are intended to increase access to patients by making them more affordable. However, cost savings will be evident only to the extent they are utilized by prescribers, pharmacists, and payers. Reluctance and uncertainty about unprecedented landmarks established during the drug development of biosimilars such as extrapolation may result in initial slow adoption of biosimilars by clinicians. But over time the uptake may gradually escalate, either through greater comfort and acceptance by health care professionals as more data is accumulated from pharmacovigilance programs, or the enforcement of mandates by payers to increase accessibility to biologic agents in the form of biosimilars. The utilization of marketed biosimilars in Europe where there has been more experience has steadfastly risen in the past several years. In fact, the acceptance of generics in the US took many years to attain but today greater than 85% of dispensed prescriptions are generic in nature [40].

The regulatory approval of biosimilars is based on the "totality of evidence" through comprehensive analytical, functional, and clinical assessments by the sponsors to ensure there are no clinically meaningful differences between the reference product and biosimilars. The working principle of this embodiment leads to the conceptualization of extrapolation. This differs from the paradigm of well-controlled placebo controlled trials where each new indication is clinically tested. The FDA considers the types of analysis to support a finding of biosimilarity based on the "totality of evidence" are generally more sensitive to product differences than in noninferiority-controlled trials [22, 23].

To date three anti-TNF inhibitor biosimilars have been approved by the FDA and a plethora of biosimilars are under clinical investigation globally (Table 26.4). The next decade will see several more biosimilars receiving approval as the market intensifies. Currently none of the approved biosimilars in the US have been authorized to be

Table 26.4 Biosimilars that target antitumor necrosis factor[a]

Reference product	Biosimilar	Maker and distributor
Infliximab	Remsima®/Inflectra® (CT-P13)	Celltrion/Hospira/Pfizer
Infliximab	BS	Nippon Kayaku
Infliximab	Flixabi®/Renflexis® (SB2)	Samsung Bioepis/Biogen/Merck
Infliximab	ABP-710	Amgen
Infliximab	GP1111	Sandoz
Adalimumab	Amjevita®/adalimumab-atto (ABP-501)	Amgen
Adalimumab	SB5	Samsung Bioepis/Biogen/Merck
Adalimumab	GP2017	Sandoz
Adalimumab	BI695501	Boehringer Ingelheim
Adalimumab	CHS-1420	Coherus Biosciences
Etanercept	Erelzi®/etanercept-szzs (GP2015)	Sandoz
Etanercept	Benepali® (SB4)	Samsung Bioepis/Biogen/Merck
Etanercept	CHS-2014	Coherus Biosciences

[a]This list is not all-inclusive

interchangeable. Interchangeability is an area that remains indeterminate as sponsors negotiate with the FDA to issue finalized guidelines. Until such time substitution may not occur until a biosimilar is deemed to be interchangeable with the reference product.

With any innovation comes uncertainty and hesitancy. The potential development of robust pharmacovigilance programs for biosimilars which is a recommendation in the FDA regulatory guidelines [22] may assuage concerns amongst health care providers in the US. If indeed the availability of biosimilars results in cost savings and increased access to patients overall, then biosimilars may one day gain acceptance analogous to generic drugs.

References

1. National Cancer Institute Dictionary of Cancer Terms. Biologic drug. Available at http://www.cancer.gov/dictionary?cdrid=426407.
2. Strober BE, Armour K, Romiti R, Smith C, Tebbey PW, Menter A, Leonardi C. Biopharmaceuticals and biosimilars in psoriasis: what the dermatologist needs to know. J Am Acad Dermatol. 2012;66:317–22.
3. Mellstedt H, Niederwieser D, Ludwig H. The challenge of biosimilars. Ann Oncol. 2008;19:411–9.
4. Schneider CK, Vleminckx C, Gravanis I, Ehmann F, Trouvin JH, Weise M, Thirstrup S. Setting the state for biosimilar monoclonal antibodies. Nat Biotechnol. 2012;30:1179–85.
5. Food and Drug Administration. Patient Protection and Affordable Care Act. Available at https://www.gpo.gov/fdsys/pkg/BILLS-111hr3590pp/pdf/BILLS-111hr3590pp.pdf.
6. Guideline on similar biological medicinal products containing biotechnology-derived proteins as active substance: nonclinical and clinical issues. Available at http://www.ema.europa.eu/docs/en_GB/document_library/Scientific_guideline/2013/06/WC500144124.pdf.
7. European Medicines Agency. Guideline on similar biological medicinal products, 2014. Available at http://www.ema.europa.eu/docs/en_GB/document_library/Scientific_guideline/2014/10/WC500176768.pdf.
8. Guidelines on evaluation of Similar Biotherapeutic Products (SBPs). World Health Organization. Available at http://www.who.int/biologicals/areas/biological_therapeutics/BIOTHERAPEUTICS_FOR_WEB_22APRIL2010.pdf.
9. US$54 billion worth of biosimilar patents expiring before 2020. GABA Online. September 30, 2011. Available at http://gabionline.net/Biosimilars/Research/US-54-billion-worth-of-biosimilar-patents-expiring-before-2020.
10. Blauvelt A, Cohen AD, Puig L, Vender R, van der Walt J, Wu JJ. Biosimilars for psoriasis: preclinical analytical assessment to determine similarity. Br J Dermatol. 2016;174:282–6.
11. Gottlieb S. Biosimilars: policy, clinical, and regulatory considerations. Am J Health Syst Pharm. 2008;65:S2–8.
12. Roger SD. Biosimilars: how similar or dissimilar are they? Nephrology (Carlton). 2006;11:341–6.
13. Prugnaud JL. Similarity of biotechnology-derived medicinal products: specific problems and new regulatory framework. Br J Clin Pharmacol. 2008;65:619–20.
14. Crommelin DJ, Storm G, Verrijk R, de Leede L, Jiskoot W, Hennink WE. Shifting paradigms: biopharmaceuticals versus low molecular weight drugs. Int J Pharm. 2003;266:3–16.
15. Walsh CT, Garneau-Tsodikova S, Gatto GJ Jr. Protein posttranslational modifications: the chemistry of proteome diversifications. Angew Chem Int Ed Engl. 2005;44:7342–72.
16. Fleischmann C, Bevan S, Neil JC, Terry A, Houlston RS. Mutations in the candidate tumour suppressor gene FLJ12973 on chromosome 15q15 are rare in colorectal cancer. Cancer Lett. 2003;196:65–7.
17. Barnes HJ, Ragnarrson G, Alvan G. Quality and safety considerations for recombinant biological medicines: a regulatory perspective. Int J Risk Saf Med. 2009;21:13–22.
18. Colbert RA, Cronstein BN. Biosimilars: the debate continues. Arthritis Rheum. 2011;63:2848–50.
19. Kuhlmann M, Covic A. The protein science of biosimilars. Nephrol Dial Transplant. 2006;21
20. PQRI-FDA Workshop on Process Drift: Detection, Measurement, and Control in the Manufacture of Pharmaceuticals. Available at http://pqri.org/wpcontent/uploads/2015/08/pdf/processdrift_final-program.pdf.
21. Schiestl M, Stangler T, Torella C, Cepeljnik T, Toll H, Grau R. Acceptable changes in quality attributes of glycosylated biopharmaceuticals. Nat Biotechnol. 2011;29:310–2.
22. USFDA. Guidance for industry: scientific considerations in demonstrating biosimilarity to a reference product; 2015. Available at http://www.fda.gov/downloads/DrugsGuidanceComplianceRegulatoryInformation/Guidances/UCM291128.pdf.
23. USFDA. Guidance for industry: quality considerations in demonstrating biosimilarity of a therapeutic protein product to a reference product; 2015. Available at http://www.fda.gov/downloads/drugs/guidancecomplianceregulatoryinformation/guidances/ucm291134.pdf.
24. USFDA.2014. Guidance for industry: immunogenicity assessment for therapeutic protein products. Available at: http://www.fda.gov/downloads/drugs/guidancecomplianceregulatoryinformation/guidances/ucm338856.pdf
25. Shankar G, Arkin S, Cocea L, et al. Assessment and reporting of the clinical immunogenicity of therapeutic proteins and peptides—harmonized terminology and tactical recommendations. AAPS J. 2014;16:658–73.
26. Kirshner SL. Mechanisms underlying the immunogenicity of therapeutic proteins: risk assessment and management strategies. J Interferon Cytokine Res. 2014;34:923–30.
27. Rosenberg AS. Effects of protein aggregates: an immunologic perspective. AAPS J. 2006;8:E501–7.
28. Yoo DH, Hrycaj P, Miranda P, Ramiterre E, Piotrowski M, Shevchuk S, Kovalenko V, Prodanovic N, Abello-Banfi M, Gutierrez-Ureña S, Morales-Olazabal L, Tee M, Jimenez R, Zamani O, Lee SJ, Kim H, Park W, Müller-Ladner U. A randomised, double-blind, parallel-group study to demonstrate equivalence in efficacy and safety of CT-P13 compared with innovator infliximab when coadministered with methotrexate in patients with active rheumatoid arthritis: the PLANETRA Study. Ann Rheum Dis. 2013;72:1613–20.
29. Park W, Hrycaj P, Jeka S, Kovalenko V, Lysenko G, Miranda P, Mikazane H, Gutierrez Ureña S, Lim M, Lee YA, Lee SJ, Kim H, Yoo DH, Braun J. A randomised, double-blind, multicentre, parallel-group, prospective study comparing the pharmacokinetics, safety, and efficacy of CT-P13 and innovator infliximab in patients with ankylosing spondylitis: the PLANETAS Study. Ann Rheum Dis. 2013;72:1605–12.
30. Dapavo P, Vujic I, Fierro MT, Quaglino P, Sanlorenzo M. The infliximab biosimilar in the treatment of moderate to severe plaque psoriasis. J Am Acad Dermatol. 2016;75:736–9.
31. USFDA. Guidance for industry: considerations in demonstrating interchangeability with a reference product; 2017. Available at http://www.fda.gov/downloads/Drugs/GuidanceComplianceRegulatoryInformation/Guidances/UCM537135.pdf.
32. USFDA. Guidance for industry: labeling for biosimilar products; 2016. http://www.fda.gov/downloads/Drugs/GuidanceComplianceRegulatoryInformation/Guidances/UCM493439.pdf.
33. USFDA. 2017. Guidance for Industry: Nonproprietary Naming of Biological Products www.fda.gov/downloads/Drugs/GuidanceComplianceRegulatoryInformation/Guidances/UCM459987.pdf.

34. Griffiths CE, Thaçi D, Gerdes S, Arenberger P, Pulka G, Kingo K, Weglowska J, EGALITY study group, Hattebuhr N, Poetzl J, Woehling H, Wuerth G, Afonso M. The EGALITY study: a confirmatory, randomized, double-blind study comparing the efficacy, safety and immunogenicity of GP2015, a proposed etanercept biosimilar, vs. the originator product in patients with moderate-to-severe chronic plaque-type psoriasis. Br J Dermatol. 2016:27.

35. Papp K, Bachelez H, Costanzo A, Foley P, Gooderham M, Kaur P, Narbutt J, Philipp S, Spelman L, Weglowska J, Zhang N, Strober B. Clinical similarity of biosimilar ABP 501 to adalimumab in the treatment of patients with moderate to severe plaque psoriasis: a randomized, double-blind, multicenter, phase III study. J Am Acad Dermatol. 2017;10

36. FDA Briefing Document Arthritis Advisory Committee Meeting July 12, 2016 BLA 761024 ABP 501, a proposed biosimilar to Humira (adalimumab) Amgen. Available on https://www.fda.gov/downloads/AdvisoryCommittees/CommitteesMeetingMaterials/Drugs/ArthritisAdvisoryCommittee/UCM510293.pdf.

37. State Laws and Legislation Related to Biologic Medications and Substitution of Biosimilars. Available on http://www.ncsl.org/research/health/state-laws-and-legislation-related-to-biologic-medications-and-substitution-of-biosimilars.aspx.

38. Singh SC, Bagnato KM. The economic implications of biosimilars. Am J Manag Care. 2015;21:s331–40.

39. The Cost Savings Potential of Biosimilar Drugs in the United States. Available on http://www.rand.org/content/dam/rand/pubs/perspectives/PE100/PE127/RAND_PE127.pdf.

40. Christl LA, Woodcock J, Kozlowski S. Biosimilars: the US Regulatory Framework. Annu Rev Med. 2017;68:243–54.

Biological Agents in Pediatric Dermatology

27

Emily B. Lund and Amy S. Paller

Introduction

Biological agents ("biologics") include a broad group of often complex products, such as antibodies, blood components, vaccines, gene therapy, and recombinant proteins. They may be isolated from natural sources, whether microorganism, animal, or human, or produced using biotechnology methods. They can be designed to specifically target disease pathogenesis.

Structurally, biologics used for psoriasis fall into two classes: antibodies and fusion proteins. Functionally, biologics modulate the immune system by interfering with cytokine production, inhibiting T-cell activation, or depleting B-cells. While used widely in adult dermatology and for many years in pediatric patients with rheumatologic and gastrointestinal disorders, biologics have only recently been approved for pediatric psoriasis in Europe and the United States. To date, three biologics have been tested in double-blinded, randomized controlled trials for pediatric psoriasis: etanercept, adalimumab, and ustekinumab (1, 2, 3; Table 27.1). All of these are anti-cytokine agents, with etanercept and adalimumab targeting tumor necrosis factor alpha (TNF-α), and ustekinumab targeting the shared p40 component of interleukin (IL) -12 and 23. Etanercept and ustekinumab are now approved by the Food and Drug Administration (FDA) for treatment of moderate-to-severe chronic plaque psoriasis in children, for ages 4–17 years and 12–17 years respectively. Adalimumab is approved in Europe for the treatment of severe plaque psoriasis in children starting at age 4 etanercept at age 6, and ustekinumab is approved for the treatment of moderate-to-severe plaque psoriasis starting at age 12. Although infliximab has occasionally been used in severe cases that require rapid-acting intravenous administration, it is not approved and rarely considered for plaque psoriasis in children.

Approximately one-third of individuals with psoriasis experience disease onset prior to 16 years of age, with the prevalence increasing linearly throughout childhood [1, 2]. The most common predisposing genetic risk factor is the human leukocyte antigen (HLA) type Cw6 (*PSOR1*). Having a pathogenic mutation in *CARD14* (caspase recruitment domain family 14; *PSOR2*) causes a rare familial form, which may manifest as pityriasis rubra pilaris or psoriasis [3, 4]. Triggering environmental factors are skin trauma (Koebner phenomenon), infections (most notably streptococcal, but also staphylococcal and varicella), Kawasaki disease, certain medications, as well as psychological and physical stress [5–10].

The role of the immune system in the pathophysiology of psoriasis accounts for the responsiveness of this disease to the targeted immunomodulatory effects of biologics. Although our understanding of psoriasis is based strictly on studies in adults, it is thought that TNF-α and IL-17A synergistically upregulate the production of other cytokines, chemokines, and antimicrobial peptides from keratinocytes and regional immune cells, initiating and perpetuating the immune activation of psoriasis [11]. Most pediatric psoriasis can be managed topically; however, approximately 10% are either recalcitrant to topical therapy, associated with juvenile psoriatic arthritis, or significantly severe and diffuse enough to require systemic medications or phototherapy, most often narrow-band ultraviolet light. Methotrexate is the most commonly prescribed systemic medication (69% of pediatric patients prescribed a systemic medication), but cyclosporine, retinoids, and fumaric acid are non-biologic alternatives [12]. Recent studies suggest that the more targeted biologics have superior efficacy and side-effect profiles compared to these more nonspecific systemic therapies [12, 13].

E.B. Lund, MD • A.S. Paller, MS, MD (✉)
Departments of Dermatology and Pediatrics, Feinberg School of Medicine, Northwestern University, 676 N St. Clair St., Suite 1600, Chicago, IL, USA
e-mail: apaller@northwestern.edu

© Springer International Publishing AG 2018
P.S. Yamauchi (ed.), *Biologic and Systemic Agents in Dermatology*, https://doi.org/10.1007/978-3-319-66884-0_27

267

Table 27.1 Biologics for pediatric psoriasis

Biologic	Target	Type	Dosing	Frequency
Etanercept	TNF-α	Fusion protein	0.8 mg/kg (maximum 50 mg)	Administered subcutaneously every week
Adalimumab	TNF-α	Human monoclonal antibody	0.8 mg/kg (maximum 40 mg) A loading dose of twice the calculated dose can be given the initial week	Administered subcutaneously every other week
Ustekinumab	Common p40 subunit of IL-12 and IL-23	Human monoclonal antibody	<60 kg: 0.75 mg/kg 60–100 kg: 45 mg >100 kg: 90 mg	Administered subcutaneously every 12 weeks, with an additional loading dose given 4 weeks after the initial injection.

Tumor Necrosis Factor Inhibitors

Among the biologics, TNF inhibitors are most often used. In an international study of 390 children using systemic medications for pediatric psoriasis, 27% were treated with a TNF inhibitor, second only to methotrexate in frequency; the majority of these children were treated with etanercept [12].

All TNF inhibitors carry a boxed warning about serious infections and malignancies, although to-date an increased risk of malignancy has not been documented in children treated with TNF inhibitors for psoriasis. In the end, these risks must be balanced with the risks of conventional therapies for these diseases, as well as the inherent risks of immune-mediated disease (i.e., the known increased risk of lymphoma in individuals with severe psoriasis itself) [14]. The decision to treat with a TNF blocker must weigh the potential benefits of treatment with the specific risk profile of individual patients in order to maximize the therapeutic effect of these medications.

Etanercept

Etanercept is a soluble TNF-α receptor fusion protein, consisting of two p75 TNF receptors bound to the Fc portion of immunoglobulin G, which can reversibly bind two TNF-α molecules. As the longest used and best studied biologic for pediatric psoriasis, it is currently the only TNF inhibitor FDA-approved for this indication. It is also FDA-approved for adults with psoriasis, rheumatoid arthritis, psoriatic arthritis, and ankylosing spondylitis, and for children with polyarticular juvenile idiopathic arthritis (JIA). It has been approved in Europe for pediatric psoriasis since 2008.

Etanercept was first investigated as a treatment for pediatric psoriasis in a phase III, double-blinded, placebo-controlled trial published by Paller et al. in 2008. Children ages 4 to 17 with moderate-to-severe plaque psoriasis, defined as a Psoriasis Area and Severity Index (PASI) score of at least 12, a static Physician's Global Assessment (PGA) of at least 3, and involvement of at least 10% of the body surface area (BSA), were enrolled. Subjects were then randomized to either placebo or etanercept 0.8 mg/kg (max 50 mg) weekly for 12 weeks. After 12 weeks, subjects entered 24 weeks of open-label treatment with etanercept. Those who achieved PASI 75 entered a 12-week blinded withdrawal-retreatment period, during which they were randomized to either placebo or weekly etanercept. Efficacy endpoints were PASI 50, PASI 75, PASI 90, and PGA 0/1 at week 12, as well as the Children's Dermatology Life Quality Index (CDLQI) score. Safety endpoints were adverse events, serious adverse events, laboratory values, serum concentrations of etanercept, and disease rebound during the withdrawal period.

The study enrolled 211 children, aged 4–17. At week 12, significantly more subjects in the etanercept group reached a PASI 75 response compared to those receiving placebo (57% vs. 11%, $p < 0.001$). Similar trends were observed for PASI 50 (75% vs. 23%, $p < 0.001$) and PASI 90 (27% vs 7%, $p < 0.001$) responses. These results were sustained throughout the 24-week open-label treatment phase. Both the original placebo group and the etanercept group experienced mean percentage improvement in their PASI scores that were greater than 70% [15]. These efficacy findings were unchanged in subgroup analysis [16]. Quality of life, as measured by the CDLQI, also improved significantly more in the etanercept group than in the placebo group (52.3% versus 17.5%, $p = 0.0001$; [17]).

During the withdrawal-retreatment phase, 42% of those assigned to placebo lost their PASI 75 response and were retreated with etanercept. These subjects were retreated with etanercept and achieved response rates similar to those seen in the initial double-blind treatment phase. Nearly half of the subjects on placebo maintained their PASI 75 response through the end of the study (week 48). No rebound of psoriasis was observed during this period [15]. In a 5-year, open-label extension of the double-blinded trial for patients who had achieved at least PASI 50 completed by 69 subjects, the percentage of patients achieving PASI 75 or PASI 90 responses remained constant [18]. Regarding safety, similar rates of infectious and noninfectious adverse events were observed between the two groups [15, 18]. In the 5-year, open-label extension, the most common adverse events reported were upper respiratory tract infection, nasopharyngitis, and headache. No malignancies or opportunistic infections were observed [18].

Etanercept is administered subcutaneously at a dose of 0.8 mg/kg (maximum 50 mg) every week. Although the American College of Rheumatology recommends baseline complete blood counts (CBC), liver function tests, and serum creatinine and every 3–6 months thereafter for individuals with JIA who are starting a TNF-α inhibitor, this recommendation is based on consensus (level D evidence); there is no recommendation in the current dermatologic literature [19]. At a minimum, however, providers should perform a baseline history and physical examination and obtain annual TB testing. Patients administered etanercept and other TNF inhibitors should avoid live vaccines while on these medications, as infection transmission from these vaccines has not been characterized in individuals on these medications [20].

Adalimumab

Adalimumab is a recombinant, fully human monoclonal antibody to TNF-α. It binds specifically to TNF-α, preventing its interactions with the p55 and p75 cell surface receptors. In adults, it is currently FDA-approved for the treatment of psoriasis and psoriatic arthritis, rheumatoid arthritis, arthritis, ankylosis spondylitis, Crohn's disease, ulcerative colitis, hidradenitis suppurativa, and uveitis. In children, adalimumab is approved for the treatment of JIA and Crohn's disease [21]. In 2015, it was approved by the European Commission for severe plaque psoriasis in children as young as 4 years. It was studied for this indication in an international multicenter double-blinded, randomized controlled trial comparing the efficacy and safety of adalimumab to methotrexate in pediatric patients [22]. A similar study conducted in adults several years prior demonstrated the superior efficacy and comparable safety of adalimumab vs. methotrexate [23].

The pediatric trial conducted by Papp et al. enrolled 114 children ages 5 to 18. Subjects had moderate-to-severe plaque psoriasis, defined as PGA ≥ 4, BSA involved >20%, PASI >20, or PASI >10 with psoriatic arthritis unresponsive to nonsteroidal anti-inflammatory drugs, clinically relevant facial, genital, or hand/foot involvement, or Children's Dermatology Life Quality Index >10. They were randomized to either adalimumab 0.8 mg/kg up to 40 mg every other week, adalimumab 0.4 mg/kg up to 20 mg every other week, or methotrexate 0.1–0.4 mg/kg up to 25 mg every week. After 16 weeks of double-blind treatment, treatment responders (those who had achieved at least a PASI 75 response and PGA of 0/1) proceeded to the next phase, during which treatment was withdrawn until loss of disease control. Subjects

completing the second phase were then retreated with adalimumab (0.8 mg/kg for patients who previously received adalimumab 0.8 mg/kg or methotrexate, and 0.4 mg/kg for patients who previously received adalimumab 0.4 mg/kg) for 16 weeks. After this blinded retreatment stage, patients were treated and followed for 52 weeks.

After 16 weeks of treatment, significantly more subjects treated with adalimumab 0.8 mg/kg reached a PASI 75 response than those treated with adalimumab 0.4 mg/kg or methotrexate (57.9% versus 43.6 and 32.4%, respectively). Similarly, 60.5% of patients treated with standard-dose adalimumab achieved PGA 0/1 vs. 40.5% with low-dose adalimumab and 41.0% with methotrexate. PASI 100 was achieved in 18.4% of patients treated with standard-dose adalimumab vs. 10.4% with low-dose adalimumab and 2.7% with methotrexate. Adverse events were similar among the three treatment groups, and there were no serious adverse events reported in the adalimumab 0.8 mg/kg treatment group [22].

Adalimumab is administered via subcutaneous injection at a dose of 0.8 mg/kg (maximum 40 mg) every other week. A loading dose of 80 mg can be given the initial week. Prior to starting the medication, as with etanercept, TB testing should be performed and repeated annually. Immunizations should also be updated, and live vaccines withheld during treatment.

Ustekinumab

Ustekinumab is a human immunoglobulin G1 kappa monoclonal antibody targeting the common p40 subunit of IL-12 and IL-23. It prevents these cytokines from binding to the IL-12 receptor, found on the surface of immune cells. Canada approved it in 2008 for the treatment of moderate-to-severe plaque psoriasis in adults following the two global phase 3 trials (PHOENIX 1 and PHOENIX 2), which demonstrated the efficacy and safety of ustekinumab for this indication [24, 25]. FDA approval for psoriasis and psoriatic arthritis followed in 2009. It is also approved for adults with Crohn's disease [26] and, in Canada and the European Union, for adolescents 12 and older [27]. It was approved by the FDA in 2017 for treating pediatric psoriasis (12 years and older). Anecdotally, it appears to be the current treatment of choice for pediatric patients with *CARD14* mutations, with a better reported efficacy than non-biologics and TNF inhibitors.

Ustekinumab was evaluated in adolescents with moderate-to-severe plaque psoriasis in the CADMUS trial, which ultimately led to its approval in Canada and the European Union. This multicenter, double-blinded, placebo-controlled trial enrolled children ages 12 through 17 with chronic (diagnosed at least 6 months prior to screening) moderate-to-severe plaque psoriasis (PASI ≥12, PGA ≥ 3, and ≥10% BSA involved). These subjects were randomized to receive either standard (0.75 mg/kg for ≤60 kg, 45 mg for 60 kg–100 kg, or 90 mg for >100 kg) or half-standard ustekinumab dosing (0.375 mg/kg, for ≤60 kg, 22.5 mg for 60 kg–100 kg, or 45 mg for >100 kg) or to placebo with crossover to standard to half-standard ustekinumab at week 12. Open-label treatment was continued through week 40, with adverse events collected through week 60.

Overall, 110 patients were enrolled. Ustekinumab resulted in significant clinical improvement, which was quite rapid in some cases. At week 12, 67.6% of patients on half-standard dosing and 69.4% of patients on standard dosing had a PGA of 0/1, compared to 5.4% of the placebo group ($p < 0.001$). One-third of each ustekinumab group achieved this effect by week 4. Furthermore, more than two-thirds of subjects on ustekinumab reached PASI 75 (half-standard 78.4%, standard 80.4%) and more than half attained PASI 90 (half-standard 54.1% and 61.1%) compared to placebo (10.8% and 5.4%, respectively; $p < 0.001$).

Therapeutic response was sustained during the course of the study period, with little change in the proportions of patients who achieved PGA0/1, PASI 75, or PASI 90 from week 12 to week 52. Beyond week 12, the clinical response in the standard dosing group was sustained better than in the half-standard dosing group.

Nine subjects (8.2%) discontinued study treatment because of poor clinical response ($n = 5$), adverse events ($n = 3$), or death ($n = 1$, car accident). There was no significant difference between the groups in the number or types of adverse events, which were reported. Most were mild or moderate, with only six serious adverse events reported throughout the course of the study. The most common adverse events were infections, specifically nasopharyngitis. There were no malignancies or active TB infections reported [28].

Like other biologics, the immunogenicity of ustekinumab may decrease its effectiveness with time. In the Landells et al. study, 8.2% of subjects tested positive for antibodies to ustekinumab at week 60. Most of these patients had minimal disease at this time point, further confirming that these are not neutralizing antibodies [28]. Studies in adults suggest that the durability of ustekinumab may be superior to that of the TNF inhibitors [29].

Ustekinumab is typically administered by subcutaneous injection. Dosing is weight-based. Individuals weighing less than 60 kilograms should be given 0.75 mg/kg, 60–100 kilograms should be given 45 mg, and those weighing more than 100 kilograms given 90 mg. Injections are given every 12 weeks, with an additional loading dose given 4 weeks after the initial injection. As with the TNF inhibitors, there are currently no formal recommendations for baseline or monitoring laboratory testing. However, taking a baseline history, including of immunization history, performing a physical examination, and testing for tuberculosis are a minimal expectation to identify those at increased risk for a serious infection on an immunomodulatory drug. TB testing should be repeated on an annual basis. Furthermore, as there is no data available on the transmission of infection from live vaccines while on ustekinumab, it is currently recommended that patients on ustekinumab avoid live vaccines. Vaccines should be updated prior to starting ustekinumab, and if a live vaccine needs to be administered, ustekinumab should be discontinued for 15 weeks prior to the vaccination. It can be restarted 2 weeks after the vaccine is given [27].

Conclusions

While biologics are highly effective for treatment of psoriasis and well tolerated, access is limited by cost, lack of guidelines for pediatric use, and limited long-term safety data. The cost of 1 year of induction and maintenance treatment can exceed $50,000, with out-of-pocket costs for patients between $250 and $350 each month. Because of these high costs, obtaining insurance coverage for these medications can be difficult, particularly in children, and treatment abandonment by patients is high [30]. Furthermore, there is no published consensus on the dosing and course length, or the baseline evaluation and optimal monitoring required by these medications in pediatric psoriasis. As a result, treatment paradigms are extrapolated from experiences in adult dermatology or other pediatric disciplines. Also complicating the use of the medications is the theoretical decrease in therapeutic effect of biologics with time, which is problematic for children with a chronic disease that may require lifelong therapy. In one report in adults, the 1-year drug survival rates for ustekinumab, adalimumab, and etanercept were 85%, 74%, and 68%, respectively, with overall 79% showing good quality of life [31]. Regarding safety, in addition to concerns about increased risk for malignancies and opportunistic infections, the effect of these immunomodulatory medications on the developing immune system is unknown. As these and other biological agents will increasingly be used to treat children with psoriasis and other immune-mediated dermatologic conditions, collaborative research is important to optimize efficacy, safety, and access to these medications for children with psoriasis.

Case

KK is a 16-year-old girl with moderate plaque psoriasis whose course began at age 7 years when she developed guttate psoriasis after streptococcal pharyngitis. During the subsequent years, her guttate psoriasis evolved into plaque psoriasis. She was initially managed with topical corticosteroids and a topical vitamin D analog, but advanced to narrowband UVB therapy because of suboptimal control, with subsequent improvement. However, due to continued flares, she initiated weekly oral methotrexate and 6 days per week of folate (skipping on the day of the methotrexate). Although showing signs of improvement within the first 2 months of use, she was unable to tolerate the nausea, leading to discontinuation. Physical examination showed psoriatic plaques on the scalp, trunk, upper and lower extremities, covering approximately 15% of the body surface area. She underwent tuberculosis testing (negative) and transitioned to adalimumab 40 mg administered subcutaneously every other week. She experienced excellent improvement within two months after initiation of the adalimumab. Other than discomfort at her injection site, she tolerates adalimumab well and continues to maintain control.

References

1. Michalek IM, Loring B, John SM. A systematic review of worldwide epidemiology of psoriasis. J Eur Acad Dermatol Venereol. 2016. https://doi.org/10.1111/jdv.13854.
2. Raychaudhuri SP, Gross J. A comparative study of pediatric onset psoriasis with adult onset psoriasis. Pediatr Dermatol. 2000;17:174–8.
3. Jordan CT, Cao L, Roberson ED, Pierson KC, Yang CF, Joyce CE, et al. PSORS2 is due to mutations in CARD14. Am J Hum Genet. 2012;90:784–95.
4. Eytan O, Sarig O, Sprecher E, van Steensel MA. Clinical response to ustekinumab in familial pityriasis rubra pilaris caused by a novel mutation in CARD14. Br J Dermatol. 2014;171:420–2.
5. Shah KN. Diagnosis and treatment of pediatric psoriasis: current and future. Am J Clin Dermatol. 2013;14:195–213.
6. Nyfors A, Lemholt K. Psoriasis in children. A short review and a survey of 245 cases. Br J Dermatol. 1975;92:437–42.
7. Pouessel G, Ythier H, Carpentier O, Vachée A, Etienne J, Catteau B. Childhood pustular psoriasis associated with Panton-valentine leukocidin-producing Staphylococcus Aureus. Pediatr Dermatol. 2007;24:401–4.
8. Ito T, Furukawa F. Psoriasis guttate acuta triggered by varicella zoster virus infection. Eur J Dermatol. 2000;10:226–7.
9. Ergin S, Karaduman A, Demirkaya E, Bakkaloğlu A, Ozkaya O. Plaque psoriasis induced after Kawasaki disease. Turk J Pediatr. 2009;51:375–7.
10. Nestle FO, Kaplan DH, Barker J. Psoriasis. N Engl J Med. 2009;361:496–509.
11. Guttman-Yassky E, Nograles KE, Krueger JG. Contrasting pathogenesis of atopic dermatitis and psoriasisDOUBLEHYPHENpart II: immune cell subsets and therapeutic concepts. J All Clin Immunol. 2011;127(6):1420–32.
12. Bronckers IM, Seyger MM, West D, Lara-Corrales I, Tollefson M, Tom W, et al. Safety of systemic agents in pediatric psoriasis: an international multicenter study. JAMA Dermatol. 2017; 153(11):1147–1157. https://doi.org/10.1001/jamadermatol.2017.3029. [Epub ahead of print]
13. Garber C, Creighton-Smith M, Sorensen EP, Dumont N, Gottlieb AB. Systemic treatment of recalcitrant pediatric psoriasis: a case series and literature review. J Drugs Dermatol. 2015;14:881–6.
14. Chiesa Fuxench ZC, Shin DB, Ogdie Beatty A, Gelfand JM. The risk of cancer in patients with psoriasis: a population-based cohort study in the health improvement network. JAMA Dermatol. 2016;152:282–90.
15. Paller AS, Siegfried EC, Langley RG, Gottlieb AB, Pariser D, Landells I, et al. Etanercept treatment for children and adolescents with plaque psoriasis. N Engl J Med. 2008;358:241–51.
16. Paller AS, Eichenfield LF, Langley RG, Leonardi CL, Siegfried EC, Creamer K, et al. Subgroup analyses of etanercept in pediatric patients with psoriasis. J Am Acad Dermatol. 2010;63:e38–41.
17. Langley RG, Paller AS, Hebert AA, Creamer K, Weng HH, Jahreis A, et al. Patient-reported outcomes in pediatric patients with psoriasis undergoing etanercept treatment: 12-week results from a phase III randomized controlled trial. J Am Acad Dermatol. 2011;64:64–70.
18. Paller AS, Siegfried EC, Pariser DM, Rice KC, Trivedi M, Iles J, et al. Long-term safety and efficacy of etanercept in children and adolescents with plaque psoriasis. J Am Acad Dermatol. 2016;74:280–7.
19. Beukelman T, Patkar NM, Saag KG, Tolleson-Rinehart S, Cron RQ, DeWitt EM, et al. American College of Rheumatology recommendations for the treatment of juvenile idiopathic arthritis: initiation and safety monitoring of therapeutic agents for the treatment of arthritis and systemic features. Arthritis care res. 2011. 2011;63:465–82.
20. Enbrel [Full prescribing information]. [Internet]. 2016 [cited 5 January 2017]. Available from: http://pi.amgen.com/~/media/amgen/repositorysites/pi-amgen-com/enbrel/enbrel_pi.ashx.
21. Humira [Full prescribing information] [Internet]. 2016 [cited 5 January 2017]. Available from: http://www.rxabbvie.com/pdf/humira.pdf
22. Papp K, Thaçi D, Marcoux D, Weibel L, Philipp S, Ghislain PD, et al. Efficacy and safety of adalimumab every other week versus methotrexate once weekly in children and adolescents with severe chronic plaque psoriasis: a randomised, double-blind, phase 3 trial. Lancet. 2017;390:40–9.
23. Saurat JH, Stingl G, Dubertret L, Papp K, Langley RG, Ortonne JP, et al. Efficacy and safety results from the randomized controlled comparative study of adalimumab vs. methotrexate vs. placebo in patients with psoriasis (CHAMPION). Br J Dermatol. 2008;158:558–66.
24. Leonardi CL, Kimball AB, Papp KA, Yeilding N, Guzzo C, Wang Y, et al. Efficacy and safety of ustekinumab, a human interleukin-12/23 monoclonal antibody, in patients with psoriasis: 76-week results from a randomised, double-blind, placebo-controlled trial (PHOENIX 1). Lancet. 2008;371:1665–74.
25. Papp KA, Langley RG, Lebwohl M, Krueger GG, Szapary P, Yeilding N, et al. Efficacy and safety of ustekinumab, a human interleukin-12/23 monoclonal antibody, in patients with psoriasis: 52-week results from a randomised, double-blind, placebo-controlled trial (PHOENIX 2). Lancet. 2008;371:1675–84.
26. Stelara [Full prescribing information]. [Internet]. 2016 [cited 5 January 2017]. Available from: https://www.stelarainfo.com/pdf/prescribinginformation.pdf
27. Ustekinumab [summary of product characteristics]. [Internet]. Cited, vol. 5. Available from: January; 2017. http://www.ema.europa.eu/docs/en_GB/document_library/EPAR_-_Product_Information/human/000958/WC500058513.pdf
28. Landells I, Marano C, Hsu MC, Li S, Zhu Y, Eichenfield LF, et al. Ustekinumab in adolescent patients age 12 to 17 years with moderate-to-severe plaque psoriasis: results of the randomized phase 3 CADMUS study. J Am Acad Dermatol. 2015;73:594–603.
29. Menter A, Papp KA, Gooderham M, Pariser DM, Augustin M, Kerdel FA, et al. Drug survival of biologic therapy in a large, disease-based registry of patients with psoriasis: results from the psoriasis longitudinal assessment and registry (PSOLAR). J Eur Acad Dermatol Venereol. 2016;30:1148–58.
30. Albrecht J, Lebwohl M, Asgari MM, Bennett DD, Cook A, Evans CC, et al. The state and consequences of dermatology drug prices in the United States. J Am Acad Dermatol. 2016;75:603–5.
31. Van den Reek JM, Zweegers J. Kievit W, et al. 'happy' drug survival of adalimumab, etanercept and usteinumab in psoriasis in daily practice care: results from the BIOCAPTURE network. Br J Dermatol. 2014;171:1189–96.

Oral Systemic Agents in Pediatric Dermatology

Nancy Cheng and Wynnis L. Tom

Oral systemic agents are used in pediatric dermatology for a broad range of conditions including inflammatory disorders, vascular tumors and malformations, connective tissue diseases, and immunobullous diseases, among others. They represent a vital component of the treatment spectrum and their utilization may be indicated after failure of standard non-systemic therapies or in the setting of certain indicators of greater disease impact or severity. However, in contrast to their use in adults, the use of systemic agents in children remains limited in the United States due to the relative paucity of indications approved by the Food and Drug Administration (FDA). Availability of data informing their appropriate use remains subject to the inherent obstacles of conducting large-scale studies in pediatric patients including randomized controlled trials. As such the choice of agent, determination of optimal dosing and duration, and selection of monitoring parameters often rely heavily on well-informed clinical judgement that reconciles broader literature-based strategies with individual patient considerations and provider experience.

Atopic Dermatitis

The chronic, pruritic, and multifactorial nature of atopic dermatitis (AD) can pose a challenging therapeutic conundrum. Systemic treatment is generally warranted in cases that are severe, not responsive to topical therapies and/or phototherapy, and/or which carry a significant burden in quality of life for the patient or family. Various systemic agents have been used with success, though mainly off-label.

Systemic corticosteroids inhibit T-cell proliferation, cytokine production (e.g., interleukin (IL)-1, IL-2, interferon-

gamma), eosinophil activity, and mast cell mediator release, which can help alleviate the symptoms and signs of AD. Although short courses are effective in the immediate period, the potential benefits must be weighed against the well-known adverse effects that include hypertension, mood changes, sleep disturbance, and weight gain. Chronic treatment can adversely affect linear growth in children and bone density, and may lead to cataract formation [1, 2]. A significant rebound flare upon discontinuation of therapy is another major concern. Thus, in general, systemic corticosteroids should be reserved only for severe "crises" with intent to bridge to another systemic agent or to phototherapy for long-term control. The other main oral agents used for refractory atopic dermatitis in children are cyclosporine, methotrexate, azathioprine, and mycophenolate mofetil.

Cyclosporine

Since its introduction as an anti-rejection immunosuppressant for solid organ transplant recipients, the calcineurin inhibitor cyclosporine has seen its role greatly expanded to treat many dermatologic conditions. Its use for atopic dermatitis is currently off-label in the US, although it is approved for this purpose in many other countries. In addition to the original formulation, a newer microemulsion offers more complete and more predictable bioavailability. Both are available as oral solutions and capsules.

In a recent survey of pediatric dermatologists, cyclosporine was the most frequently chosen first-line systemic therapy for atopic dermatitis [3]. The relatively rapid onset of action makes cyclosporine a favorable choice when acute control of disease is desired, with improvement reported as early as 2 weeks into treatment. This is especially seen in the microemulsion formulation, which has shown faster onset of improvement and greater initial efficacy [4]. Doses of 3–6 mg/kg/day have been used with success (notably slightly higher than the standard adult dosing of 2.5–5 mg/kg/day), with some suggestion that higher doses can afford more

N. Cheng, MD • W.L. Tom, MD (✉)
Pediatric and Adolescent Dermatology, University of California, San Diego/Rady Children's Hospital, 8010 Frost Street, Suite 602, San Diego, CA 92123, USA
e-mail: wtom@rchsd.org

© Springer International Publishing AG 2018
P.S. Yamauchi (ed.), *Biologic and Systemic Agents in Dermatology*, https://doi.org/10.1007/978-3-319-66884-0_28

rapid control of symptoms. Cyclosporine may be used as a short-term intermittent therapy for 3–6 months or as a longer-term therapy for up to 12 months. As expected, more adverse effects are seen with longer durations of therapy.

The use of cyclosporine comes with a well-recognized set of potential adverse effects, most notably nephrotoxicity and hypertension, both of which are thought to be dose- and duration-dependent and generally reversible upon discontinuation. Other characteristic side effects, including hyperlipidemia, hyperkalemia, gingival hyperplasia, and hypertrichosis, are relatively rare in children but should be monitored as well. Medication interactions are a significant concern with cyclosporine, which is a well-known substrate of cytochrome (CYP) 3A4. Careful consideration should be given to any concurrent medications sharing this metabolic pathway, as they can affect serum levels of cyclosporine, increase renal toxicity, or themselves be affected by co-administration with cyclosporine.

Methotrexate

Methotrexate is a versatile medication used off-label for numerous conditions in dermatology, including atopic dermatitis. Its action as a folic acid antagonist is mediated by inhibition of dihydrofolate reductase, essentially blocking the pathway needed to synthesize key nucleotides for DNA and RNA. It also has anti-inflammatory effects via induction of adenosine production.

Even though data is limited on the effectiveness of methotrexate for atopic dermatitis, it is a commonly chosen first-line systemic treatment, second to cyclosporine in popularity according to one study [3]. Studies have shown it to be safe and well tolerated [5]. While oral administration is most common, some physicians prefer the subcutaneous formulation, which provides more predictable absorption at doses greater than 15 mg and decreases the risk for gastrointestinal discomfort [6, 7]. Dosing is generally within the range of 7.5–25 mg weekly, with most regimens starting on the lower end and increasing as needed for effect.

The most notable adverse effects tend to be hepatotoxicity, gastrointestinal upset, stomatitis, teratogenicity, and uncommon but potentially serious pancytopenia. Most appear to be reversible upon discontinuation of the medication. The utility of folic acid supplementation is debated by some, given some reports showing reduced risk of pancytopenia and gastrointestinal symptoms but others suggesting decreased effectiveness of methotrexate. It remains generally accepted that folic acid should be recommended for all children being treated with methotrexate for atopic dermatitis. This recommendation is supported by a systematic review and meta-analysis of adult patients showing that folic acid significantly reduced risk of any reported adverse events

from methotrexate [7]. The review further showed that adverse events did not seem to be methotrexate dose- or duration-dependent, highlighting the need for careful monitoring across all patients [7]. Due to its action on the folate pathway, methotrexate should never be combined with the antibiotic trimethoprim-sulfamethoxazole, a highly noted drug interaction.

A 2009 consensus conference on the long-term use of methotrexate in psoriasis suggested liver biopsy to assess for hepatotoxicity may be done less frequently or avoided altogether in patients deemed low risk [8]. Although there is a lack of specific data for atopic dermatitis, the risk would appear lower given decreased prevalence of fatty liver disease, obesity, and other relevant comorbidities compared to patients with psoriasis.

Azathioprine

Azathioprine is purine analog that was originally synthesized from 6-mercaptopurine. It is thought to inhibit purine metabolism, cell division, and the function of T-cells, B-cells, and antigen-presenting cells [9]. Its use in atopic dermatitis is off-label, but it has been demonstrated to be effective for refractory atopic dermatitis. One systematic review suggested it may be less effective than cyclosporine for adult atopic dermatitis, although no direct comparative studies have been conducted [9]. Onset of effect is slower (8–12 weeks), but it can be used for longer durations than cyclosporine. Currently, the only available formulation of azathioprine in the United States is a tablet, requiring compounding should a liquid suspension be necessary in the case of young children.

In children, azathioprine is often started at 2.5 mg/kg/day and increased as needed to a higher possible maximum of 4 mg/kg/day [10], compared to 1–3 mg/kg/day in adults. A baseline level of the catabolic enzyme thiopurine-S-methyltransferase (TPMT) should be checked, as abnormally low levels may require lower dosing to avoid toxic accumulation of the precursor metabolite. Interestingly, TPMT levels have been inversely correlated with response to therapy, with some patients showing inducible levels over the course of azathioprine treatment that corresponded to evolving effectiveness of the medication [11]. As always, the minimum effective dose should be used, and systemic therapy should be tapered or discontinued once clearance is achieved.

Studies have found relatively mild adverse effects, with gastrointestinal upset being the most common. Other negative effects, such as hepatotoxicity and hematologic abnormalities, may vary in severity and uncommonly lead to discontinuation of azathioprine [12]. The associations with malignancy, infection, and myelosuppression have not been well established in children with atopic dermatitis

Table 28.1 Typical pediatric dosing ranges and monitoring considerations for oral systemic agents for atopic dermatitis and psoriasis

Medication	Dosing: atopic dermatitis	Dosing: psoriasis	Special considerations in monitoring	Pregnancy category[a]
Cyclosporine	3–6 mg/kg/day	2.5–5 mg/kg/day	Blood pressure, CBC, K, Cr, Mg, uric acid, LFTs, cytochrome p450 drug interactions	C
Methotrexate	7.5–25 mg qweek	7.5–25 mg qweek	CBC, Cr, LFTs, cumulative dose, drugs acting on folate pathway	X
Azathioprine	2.5–4 mg/kg/day (half dose for those with intermediate TPMT activity)		TPMT activity, CBC, LFTs, drugs acting on xanthine oxidase pathway	D
Mycophenolate mofetil	600–1200 mg/m² (body surface area)		CBC, gastrointestinal discomfort	D
Acitretin		0.5–1 mg/kg/day	LFTs, fasting lipids, mucocutaneous dryness	X

CBC cell blood count, *K* potassium, *Cr* creatinine, *Mg* magnesium, *LFTs* liver function tests, *TPMT* thiopurine methyltransferase
[a]Negative baseline testing, proper counseling and initiation of contraception is necessary in females of childbearing age. Drugs in pregnancy categories D and X can cause birth defects or fetal death if taken during pregnancy

but should be noted and watched for during treatment. Of the relatively few drug interactions with azathioprine, caution should be used with concurrent administration of allopurinol, angiotension-converting enzyme inhibitors, and sulfasalazine, which all act on the same metabolic pathway and can increase the risk of various forms of toxicity.

Mycophenolate Mofetil

Mycophenolate mofetil (MMF) is an immunosuppressant whose active metabolite blocks inosine monophosphate dehydrogenase, the key enzyme in *de novo* purine synthesis, which in turn inhibits the major pathway for production of B- and T-cells. Its efficacy is variable compared to other systemic medications discussed above, leading to its classification as an alternative therapy for recalcitrant atopic dermatitis. However, in some cases, MMF can be a desirable first choice for its favorable side effect profile. Interestingly, when compared to cyclosporine, its delayed effect but prolonged response after discontinuation suggests the utility of treating with faster-acting cyclosporine followed by longer-acting MMF [13]. Dosing is recommended to be based on body surface area, 600–1200 mg/m². It is available as a capsule, tablet, and oral solution.

Gastrointestinal discomfort is common but usually mild, and tolerability can be improved using the enteric-coated formulation. Increased risk of infections has been observed in solid organ transplant patients, but the relevance for children with atopic dermatitis remains unknown. Other adverse effects, such as hematologic abnormalities, are generally mild, dose-dependent, and reversible upon discontinuation of the medication. The advantageous safety profile may facilitate longer durations of therapy, and cases

of successful continued use for 24 months have been reported [10].

Dosing and considerations in monitoring for these agents is summarized in Table 28.1. Additional guidelines detailing their use in the management of atopic dermatitis has been published by a working group of the American Academy of Dermatology [10]. They note that the limited data precludes any definitive recommendations for a therapeutic ladder among these agents. Head-to-head pediatric data is limited to one single study comparing 12 weeks of treatment with low-dose cyclosporine compared to low-dose methotrexate, with cyclosporine having faster effect but also faster relapse during the 12 week follow-up period [14]. An international initiative is underway to develop a uniform core set of items to be captured in patient registries, to improve the ability to compare efficacy, safety, and cost-effectiveness of treatment options with time [15].

Case Study
An 11-year-old female has had atopic dermatitis since infancy. Her mother is concerned as the disease is not improving with time, as she had been told, and it is not responding well to even high potency topical steroids. Many products sting on her skin, so she mainly applies petrolatum ointment as her emollient. The patient is distraught over her condition and it is affecting her social interactions at school. Her medical history is significant for asthma and she is allergic to peanut, shellfish, and wheat. She has not yet had menarche. On exam, she has multiple pink, lichenified and crusted plaques scattered diffusely on the trunk and extremities (Fig. 28.1a), with some scaling on the scalp as well. Over 60% of her body surface area is affected, and they report that many times her skin condition is even worse. The lesions do not appear to be infected.

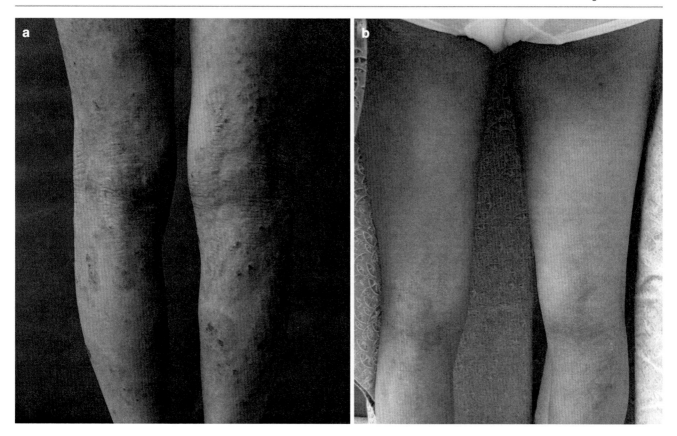

Fig. 28.1 (a) 11-year-old female with long-standing severe atopic dermatitis, including the lower extremities. (b) Significant improvement in her lesions after 11 months of treatment with mycophenolate mofetil

Management

Given the prolonged course and severity of her atopic dermatitis, escalation of therapy is appropriate. Narrow-band phototherapy was discussed, but the mother's work schedule precluded bringing the patient in three times weekly. The main systemic treatment options considered were azathioprine, mycophenolate mofetil, and methotrexate, as it was not felt that cyclosporine would likely provide a sufficient course given her long-standing disease. Mycophenolate was started at 500 mg twice daily (860 mg/m²) and increased to 750 mg twice daily after 4 months (1200 mg/m²), while topical corticosteroids were continued. She had mild diarrhea the first few weeks that self-resolved and no major laboratory abnormalities during her treatment. Her atopic dermatitis significantly improved (Fig. 28.1b is after 11 months of mycophenolate therapy) and the drug was tapered off for a total course of 23 months. She now has mild disease with only occasional need for low and mid potency topical steroids.

Psoriasis

Similar to their use in atopic dermatitis, oral systemic agents in psoriasis are commonly used off-label. Candidates for systemic therapy have typically failed topical steroids, with

or without topical vitamin D derivatives, and/or phototherapy. While access to biologic agents is increasing for affected children, this chapter will focus only on oral systemic agents including methotrexate, cyclosporine, and acitretin. All are considered appropriate first-line agents with reasonable safety and efficacy profiles. Literature suggests some subtypes of psoriasis may respond better to certain agents (discussed below). It should be noted that generalized pustular psoriasis and erythrodermic psoriasis typically warrant direct-to-systemic treatment regardless of prior topical or phototherapy.

Methotrexate

In terms of oral agents, methotrexate is considered the drug of choice for moderate to severe plaque psoriasis in children and has been found to be safe and effective for other types of psoriasis as well. Studies have shown an effect as early as 5 weeks, with clinical remission of disease lasting up to 3 years. The Child-CAPTURE study followed 25 children with plaque psoriasis treated with methotrexate over 48 weeks and found significant improvement in their Psoriasis Area and Severity Index (PASI) scores and quality of life, with relatively few and mild adverse effects [16, 17]. Dosing varies widely and has been generally based on adult dosing for psoriasis, ranging from 7.5 to 25 mg weekly, aiming to use the lowest effective dose. Treatment duration may be limited by cumulative dose, although expert consensus in pediatric psoriasis suggests liver biopsy at 1.5 grams of intake may not necessarily be required in children at relatively low risk of hepatotoxicity [8]. Although a more in-depth discussion of biologics is in Chap. 27, biologics have been found to be effective in combination with methotrexate. Limited data suggests biologic agents can be a useful adjunct therapy when insufficient improvement is seen with methotrexate alone [18]. Etanercept is a common first biologic in these situations, with FDA approval based on the positive results of short- and long-term pediatric trials [19], followed by adalimumab and ustekinumab.

Cyclosporine

Cyclosporine has been well established as a treatment for psoriasis in adults, and recent studies have shown it to be safe and effective in children as well. The relatively quick onset of improvement, with total clearance reported even at 4 weeks, allows for a potentially shorter duration of treatment [20]. Dosing commonly ranges from 2.5 to 5 mg/kg/day. It is notable that the maximum recommended dose for psoriasis in adults is 4 mg/kg/day; however, children have been proposed to require higher doses due to their greater surface area to weight ratio and age-dependent differences in pharmacokinetics [21]. For this reason, in children with quite severe disease, one may consider starting more aggressively at 5 mg/kg/day and decreasing the dose once improved [22]. Recurrence of disease may be seen in some patients during the taper, when the dose is decreased to about 1 mg/kg/day, or in the several months after discontinuation. Some cases have been reported to improve again with resuming the original dose, while others have required switching to another systemic agent such as methotrexate [20]. Infrequently, patients have had to discontinue treatment due to laboratory abnormalities or mild adverse effects such as hypertrichosis or flu-like symptoms [20, 23]. In total, treatment may continue for several months or longer but it is recommended not to exceed 1–2 years in order to avoid nephrotoxicity [22].

Acitretin

Oral retinoids offer a non-immunosuppressive treatment option for children with psoriasis. Acitretin is thought to be most effective in guttate and pustular psoriasis and is a first-line choice for generalized pustular psoriasis. It is recommended not to exceed a dosing of 0.5 to 1 mg/kg/day to minimize the risk of toxicities, including mucocutaneous effects, which are dose-dependent and generally reversible [22]. Patients may note dryness of the skin and lips, thinning of the hair and nails,

or epistaxis. Lower doses can lessen these adverse effects; however, in some patients doses low enough to render tolerability may not be sufficient to produce adequate improvement in the skin. Elevated lipids and liver enzymes are not uncommon, and it is advisable to check these at baseline and during treatment. One multicenter retrospective study found a mean duration of treatment of nearly two years to achieve satisfactory and sustained improvement in PASI scores, and mucocutaneous effects in all patients were mild enough not to affect therapy [24]. As is the case with most literature in pediatric psoriasis, the sample sizes are too small to allow broader generalizability of data. Long-term use of acitretin is limited by the potential for skeletal anomalies (e.g., periosteal thickening, premature closure of the epiphyses, and ossification similar to that seen in diffuse idiopathic skeletal hyperostosis) and continuous administration, particularly at higher doses, is not advised. The known teratogenic effects can also limit its use in females of childbearing potential.

Other Agents

Oral apremilast is a small molecule inhibitor of the phosphodiesterase 4 enzyme, leading to increased cyclic adenosine monophosphate (cAMP) levels and decreased production of pro-inflammatory mediators like tumor necrosis factor (TNF)-α, interferon (IFN)-γ, IL-12/23p40, IL-23p19, and IL-22. It is approved for the treatment of moderate to severe plaque psoriasis in adults. The most commonly reported side effects are diarrhea, nausea, and headache, and some experience weight loss during treatment. Gradual titration of dose appears to lessen the risk of gastrointestinal symptoms. Pediatric trials are currently underway.

Hemangiomas of Infancy

The use of oral beta-blockershas revolutionized the treatment of complicated infantile hemangiomas. Whereas prior regimens resorted to medications with considerably greater risk, such as systemic corticosteroids or chemotherapy agents, the discovery of propranolol's effectiveness in treatment of this vascular tumor has truly transformed the landscape of available treatments. This chapter will focus on oral agents, but it should be noted that topical timolol offers a safe and effective topical alternative for suitable hemangiomas, typically those that are small, superficial, and without clinically concerning features.

Propranolol

Infantile hemangiomas are vascular tumors that may require specialty evaluation for clinically concerning features or questions of management, particularly during the rapid growth phase. Multiple studies have attested to propranolol's excellent safety profile and demonstrated effectiveness for this particular lesion, and it is an exception to the rule with a large randomized, double-blind, placebo-controlled pediatric study having been performed and published [25]. Propranolol is a nonselective beta-blocker widely used for hemangiomas that pose a risk of disfigurement, ulceration, bleeding, functional impairment (including visual impairment), airway obstruction, or cardiovascular compromise. With few exceptions that will be described below, it is the first-line agent for hemangiomas requiring systemic treatment. Adverse effects are uncommon and are most notable for hypotension and hypoglycemia. As such, routine monitoring includes baseline blood pressure and heart rate, which should be rechecked with each dosage increase, and propranolol should always be given with food and held during periods of decreased oral intake. Beta-blockade could exacerbate existing reactive airway disease, although a recent review of 683 children found no increased risk of wheezing or respiratory episodes between cases and controls [26]. However, cases of congenital or persistent stridor including laryngomalacia were not included in this study. The utility of routine screening with a baseline electrocardiogram remains debatable, as very few cardiac conditions would preclude the use of propranolol. Expert consensus suggests screening be reserved for patients with a history of arrhythmia, below-normal heart rate for their age, or family history of arrhythmias, congenital heart conditions, or connective tissue disease in the mother [27]. Dosing is typically started at 1 mg/kg/day divided twice daily, with increase to 2 mg/kg/day divided twice daily after the first week if vitals remain stable. Dosing can be increased to 3 mg/kg/day as needed.

Importantly, in lesions concerning for PHACE syndrome (Posterior fossa abnormalities, Hemangioma, Arterial lesions, Cardiac abnormalities, Eye abnormalities), propranolol should be avoided until workup is complete, as risk stratification of any cerebral vascular or cardiac anomalies is crucial in determining whether to use propranolol and at what dose. A 2014 consensus conference categorized high risk abnormalities as generally representing those involving significant (>25%) stenosis and located distal to the circle of Willis, while intermediate risk abnormalities generally represent those located proximal to the circle of Willis with no perceived hemodynamic risk [28]. It is recommended that any intermediate risk lesions be discussed with neurology or neurosurgery for consideration of treatment options. In some cases, it may be appropriate to start low-dose propranolol at around 0.5 mg/kg/day divided three times a day. The use of propranolol in high risk lesions remains controversial, in part due to the risk of stroke from cardiac steal; a drop in blood pressure could attenuate flow through narrowed or absent vessels. The risk remains very real even when propranolol is used in combination with systemic steroids, and acute ischemic stroke was reported in two patients with PHACE syndrome on this dual treatment regimen [28]. As such, careful weighing of risks and benefits remains essential in this scenario.

Other Beta-Blockers

Other oral beta-blockers have been utilized for infantile hemangiomas. While acebutolol and atenolol are limited to only a few reported cases, oral nadolol has been used in over 50 infants in the published literature [29, 30]. Head to head studies in comparison with propranolol remain to be performed, but oral nadolol does not cross the blood brain barrier and has been an effective alternative in some cases of sleep disturbance (e.g., agitation and nightmares) with propranolol administration [29].

Case Study

A 7-week-old female is brought into clinic for a lesion on the right side of the head that was becoming more red and "a little more bumpy" since it was first noticed at 2 weeks of age (Fig. 28.2a). No treatments have been tried. The infant is otherwise healthy, with no history of heart murmur or wheezing. Physical exam is notable for a large 12 × 7 cm reddish-blue plaque extending from the right temporal scalp down to the ear, lateral cheek, and neck, within which are some scattered more palpable areas. There is no ulceration.

Management

Given the growth of a large facial hemangioma that could cause significant deformity, systemic treatment was indicated. However, the segmental distribution indicated the possibility for the lesion to be a part of PHACE syndrome and airway hemangiomas have also been found in association with cutaneous hemangiomas located at the "beard area." A workup was first initiated with magnetic resonance (MR) imaging and MR angiography of the head and neck, electrocardiogram, echocardiogram, bronchoscopy, and eye examination being performed. Absence of the A1 component of the right anterior cerebral artery and reconstitution of the A2 component, likely from the left anterior cerebral artery, with a patent anterior communicating artery was noted on the MRA, with the remaining studies being negative for significant findings. After conferring with neurology and neurosurgery, the child was deemed to have PHACE syndrome with low to moderate risk congenital vascular anomalies. Oral propranolol was started at 1 mg/kg/day and more conservatively divided three times daily, with careful monitoring. No adverse effects were noted and over the following 8 weeks,

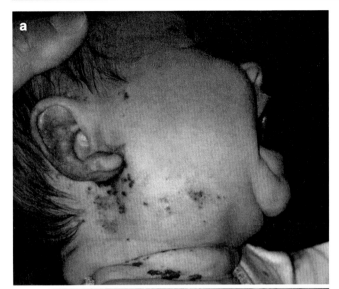

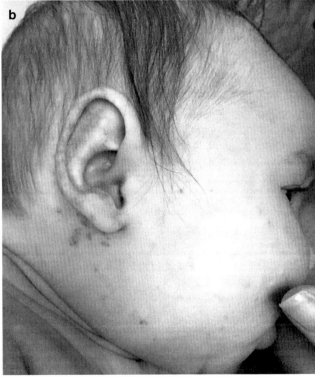

Fig. 28.2 (**a**) Large segmental hemangioma involving the right temporal scalp down to the lateral neck. (**b**) The hemangioma is less red and thick after oral propranolol treatment for 3 months

propranolol was increased in several steps to 2 mg/kg/day. The lesion became less red and thick over the next few months, with fewer palpable areas (Fig. 28.2b). Starting at 11 months of age, propranolol was slowly weaned and no rebound growth was noted. The child continues to be followed by neurology, and to date, no developmental anomalies have been noted.

References

1. Daley-Yates PT, Richards DH. Relationship between systemic corticosteroid exposure and growth velocity: development and validation of a pharmacokinetic/pharmacodynamic model. Clin Ther. 2004;26(11):1905–19.
2. Bair B, Dodd J, Heidelberg K, Krach K. Cataracts in atopic dermatitis: a case presentation and review of the literature. Arch Dermatol Am Med Assoc. 2011;147(5):585–8.
3. Totri CR, Eichenfield LF, Logan K, Proudfoot L, Schmitt J, Lara-Corrales I, et al. Prescribing practices for systemic agents in the treatment of severe pediatric atopic dermatitis in the US and Canada: the PeDRA TREAT survey. J Am Acad Dermatol. 2017;76(2):281–5.
4. Zurbriggen B, Wüthrich B, Cachelin AB, Wili PB, Kägi MK. Comparison of two formulations of Cyclosporin A in the treatment of severe atopic dermatitis. Dermatology (Basel). 1999;198(1):56–60.
5. Dadlani C, Orlow SJ. Treatment of children and adolescents with methotrexate, cyclosporine, and etanercept: review of the dermatologic and rheumatologic literature. J Am Acad Dermatol. 2005;52(2):316–40.
6. van Roon EN, van de Laar MAFJ. Methotrexate bioavailability. Clin Exp Rheumatol. 2010;28(5 Suppl 61):S27–32.
7. Mazaud C, Fardet L. Relative risk of and determinants for adverse events of methotrexate prescribed at a low dose: a systematic review and meta-analysis of randomized. Placebo-Controlled Trials Br J Dermatol. 2017;9
8. Kalb RE, Strober B, Weinstein G, Lebwohl M. Methotrexate and psoriasis: 2009 National Psoriasis Foundation Consensus Conference. 2009. pp. 824–37.
9. Schmitt J, Abraham S, Trautmann F, Stephan V, Fölster-Holst R, Homey B, et al. Usage and effectiveness of systemic treatments in adults with severe atopic eczema: first results of the German Atopic eczema registry TREAT Germany. J Dtsch Dermatol Ges. 2017;15(1):49–59.
10. Sidbury R, Davis DM, Cohen DE, Cordoro KM, Berger TG, Bergman JN, et al. Guidelines of care for the management of atopic dermatitis: section 3. Management and treatment with phototherapy and systemic agents. J Am Acad Dermatol. 2014;71:327–49.
11. Caufield M, Tom WL. Oral azathioprine for recalcitrant pediatric atopic dermatitis: clinical response and thiopurine monitoring. J Am Acad Dermatol. 2013;68(1):29–35.
12. Fuggle NR, Bragoli W, Mahto A, Glover M, Martinez AE, Kinsler VA. The adverse effect profile of oral azathioprine in pediatric atopic dermatitis, and recommendations for monitoring. J Am Acad Dermatol. 2015;72(1):108–14.
13. Haeck IM, Knol MJ, Berge Ten O, van Velsen SGA, de Bruin-Weller MS, Bruijnzeel-Koomen CAFM. Enteric-coated mycophenolate sodium versus cyclosporin a as long-term treatment in adult patients with severe atopic dermatitis: a randomized controlled trial. J Am Acad Dermatol. 2011;64(6):1074–84.
14. El-Khalawany MA, Hassan H, Shaaban D, Ghonaim N, Eassa B. Methotrexate versus cyclosporine in the treatment of severe atopic dermatitis in children: a multicenter experience from Egypt. Eur J Pediatr. 2013;172(3):351–6.
15. Gerbens LAA, Boyce AE, Wall D, Barbarot S, de Booij RJ, Deleuran M, et al. TREatment of ATopic eczema (TREAT) registry taskforce: protocol for an international Delphi exercise to identify a core set of domains and domain items for national atopic eczema registries. Trials BioMed Central. 2017;18(1):87.
16. van Geel MJ, Oostveen AM, Hoppenreijs EPAH, Hendriks JCM, van de Kerkhof PCM, de Jong EMGJ, et al. Methotrexate in pediatric plaque-type psoriasis: long-term daily clinical practice

results from the child-CAPTURE registry. J Dermatolog Treat. 2015;26(5):406–12.

17. Oostveen AM, de Jager MEA, van de Kerkhof PCM, Donders ART, de Jong EMGJ, Seyger MMB. The influence of treatments in daily clinical practice on the Children's dermatology life quality index in juvenile psoriasis: a longitudinal study from the child-CAPTURE patient registry. Br J Dermatol. 2012;167(1):145–9.

18. Klufas DM, Wald JM, Strober BE. Treatment of moderate to severe pediatric psoriasis: a retrospective case series. Pediatr Dermatol. 2016;33(2):142–9.

19. Sanclemente G, Murphy R, Contreras J, García H, Bonfill CX. Anti-TNF agents for paediatric psoriasis. Cochrane database syst rev. 2015;(11):CD010017.

20. Bulbul Baskan E, Yazici S, Tunali S, Saricaoglu H. Clinical experience with systemic cyclosporine a treatment in severe childhood psoriasis. J Dermatol Treat. 2016;27(4):328–31.

21. Perrett CM, Ilchyshyn A, Berth-Jones J. Cyclosporin in childhood psoriasis. J Dermatol Treat. 2003;14(2):113–8.

22. Marqueling AL, Cordoro KM. Systemic treatments for severe pediatric psoriasis: a practical approach. Dermatol Clin. 2013; 31(2):267–88.

23. Di Lernia V, Stingeni L, Boccaletti V, Calzavara Pinton PG, Guarneri C, Belloni Fortina A, et al. Effectiveness and safety of cyclosporine in pediatric plaque psoriasis: a multicentric retrospective analysis. J Dermatol Treat. 2016;27(5):395–8.

24. Di Lernia V, Bonamonte D, Lasagni C, Belloni Fortina A, Cambiaghi S, Corazza M, et al. Effectiveness and safety of Acitretin in children with plaque psoriasis: a multicenter retrospective analysis. Pediatr Dermatol. 2016;33(5):530–5.

25. Léauté-Labrèze C, Voisard J-J, Moore N. Oral propranolol for infantile hemangioma. N Engl J Med. 2015;373(3):284–5.

26. Mei-Zahav M, Blau H, Hoshen M, Zvulunov A, Mussaffi H, Prais D, et al. Propranolol treatment for infantile hemangioma does not increase risk of childhood wheezing. Pediatr Pulmonol. 2017;25:168.

27. Drolet BA, Frommelt PC, Chamlin SL, Haggstrom A, Bauman NM, Chiu YE, et al. Initiation and use of propranolol for infantile hemangioma: report of a consensus conference. Pediatrics. 2013;131(1):128–40.

28. Garzon MC, Epstein LG, Heyer GL, Frommelt PC, Orbach DB, Baylis AL, et al. PHACE syndrome: consensus-derived diagnosis and care recommendations. J Pediatr. 2016;178:24–33.e2

29. Bernabeu-Wittel J, Narváez-Moreno B, de la Torre-García JM, Fernández-Pineda I, Domínguez-Cruz JJ, Coserría-Sánchez F, et al. Oral propranolol for children with infantile hemangiomas and sleep disturbances with oral propranolol. Pediatr Dermatol. 2015;32(6):853–7.

30. Randhawa HK, Sibbald C, Garcia Romero MT, Pope E. Oral Nadolol for the treatment of infantile hemangiomas: a single-institution retrospective cohort study. Pediatr Dermatol. 2015; 32(5):690–5.

Utilization of Biologic and Systemic Agents in the Elderly

Alexander S. Hoy, Kristyn D. Beck, and Abby S. Van Voorhees

Conventional Systemic Agents

Acitretin

Acitretin is a systemic retinoid that is commonly used in dermatology for the treatment of psoriasis as well as various other diseases keratinization. It modulates the immune system and lowers keratinocyte proliferation [1]. One of the largest advantages of acitretin when compared to other systemic psoriasis treatments is that it is not immunosuppressive. Acitretin's largest drawback, its teratogenicity, is fortunately not an issue for elderly patients [2]. However, acitretin can take several weeks in order to reach peak effectiveness and is often less effective than other systemic medications in reaching PASI 75 for plaque psoriasis [3, 4]. Response is generally considered dose dependent, however there have been some studies where this has not been seen [3, 5]. In a double-blinded, randomized study that looked at dosing, patients treated with 25, 35, and 50 mg per day saw 54, 76, and 54% PASI score reductions after 12 weeks of therapy [3]. In another study that initially treated patients with 10–25 mg/day before increasing it to 20–50 mg/day, after 3 months the median PASI score was reduced from 19.25 to 5.75 [6]. In a 12 week study that looked at psoriasis treatments in the elderly, only 27% reached a PASI 75 when treated with a mean dose of 0.38 mg/kg [4]. The conclusion from these studies is that dosing will need to be tailored to the patient and individuals should be counseled to expect a relatively longer period of time before the maximum response to treatment is achieved.

The side effects from acitretin include a number of mucocutaneous irritations, increased serum triglycerides, and increased liver enzymes [4, 7]. The most common adverse effects include cheilitis, skin peeling, pruritus, rhinitis, dry skin, and alopecia [7]. All of these were found to be dose dependent, barring pruritus. A retrospective analysis of two 24 week randomized double-blinded studies found that cheilitis was present in 57% of patients at 25 mg/day which increased to 77% in patients on a 50 mg/day dose. Skin peeling was the second most common side effect and was seen in 25% of lower dose patients and 47% in higher dose patients. In total, 77 and 95% of patients on 25 mg/day and 50 mg/day, respectively, developed adverse effects compared to 48% that were on a placebo [7]. In a study of psoriasis in the elderly, of 62 patients treated with a mean dose of 0.38 mg/kg, only four patients had skin xerosis and one developed alopecia [4]. However, this study duration was limited to only 12 weeks. Conjunctival inflammation is also common and patients with contact lenses should be encouraged to use glasses instead [8].

Hyperlipidemia that can develop as a result of acitretin treatment may put older persons with a history of elevated lipids at additional risk. During acitretin clinical trials, 66% of patients had an increase in their triglyceride levels of greater than 20 mg/dL when treated with 10–75 mg/day [2]. 33% of patients had their cholesterol increase by more than 100%. In a study of acitretin usage in the elderly, after 12 week of treatment with 0.38 mg/kg, 6 of 62 patients had increased serum triglycerides [4]. Should a patient develop hypertriglyceridemia, terminating treatment is not always necessary and the European S3 guidelines recommend attempting dietary and lifestyle modifications before using lipid-modifying drugs should triglyceride become greater than 5 mmol/L [8].

Acitretin has also been associated with increases in serum liver enzyme levels in about one-third of patients [2]. These changes can be temporary and will often return to normal by reducing or removing treatment. Acitretin's effects on the liver do not appear to be significant [9]. A study of 128 patients who took acitretin for 2 years found that increases in serum liver enzyme levels did not result in significant changes in the patient's liver biopsies. However, it is still recommended that physicians monitor serum liver enzyme

A.S. Hoy, BS • K.D. Beck, MD • A.S. Van Voorhees, MD (✉)
EVMS Dermatology, 721 Fairfax Avenue Suite 200, Norfolk, VA 23507-2007, USA
e-mail: vanvooas@evms.edu

© Springer International Publishing AG 2018
P.S. Yamauchi (ed.), *Biologic and Systemic Agents in Dermatology*, https://doi.org/10.1007/978-3-319-66884-0_29

levels for significant changes, particularly for patients already at risk for liver damage [8]. Additionally during treatment, alcohol use should be prohibited, as it can cause conversion of acitretin to etretinate, which has been reported in association with chronic active hepatitis [2, 10, 11]. As a result of this side effect, elderly patients with hepatic dysfunction or alcoholism should be treated with caution when using acitretin [8].

Acitretin has fewer reported drug interactions than many of the other conventional, systematic treatments for psoriasis. Despite this, it is imperative to ensure elderly patients taking acitretin avoid overconsuming vitamin A through diet and supplements to prevent hypervitaminosis [12]. Tetracycline also needs to be avoided as it can cause an increase in photosensitivity and an increased risk of developing pseudotumor cerebri [2]. Combination therapy with methotrexate is discouraged due to an increased risk of hepatotoxicity. In addition, acitretin is strongly contraindicated in individuals with severe renal dysfunction [8].

Acitretin's role as a non-immunosuppressant systemic psoriasis treatment uniquely positions it among other treatments for the elderly who may already be immunosuppressed [13]. Lastly, acitretin may serve as chemoprevention for nonmelanoma skin cancer and therefore may be helpful in elderly patients with a history of numerous nonmelanoma skin cancers as a dual purpose when treating comorbid psoriasis [14]. While its efficacy in achieving PASI 75 may be lacking when compared to other systemic and newer biologic agents, it may provide relief to some patients who may otherwise go untreated due to drug interactions or comorbidities.

Methotrexate

Methotrexate is a folate antagonist that acts as an immunomodulator [15, 16]. Its efficacy in reducing PASI scores, its relative safety, and its low cost have made it a mainstay of psoriasis treatment. It can be used for both induction and long-term treatment [8]. Methotrexate's efficacy is roughly comparable to cyclosporine, with a study comparing the two finding that 26 of 43 and 30 of 42 reaching PASI 75 respectively after 16 weeks [17]. Another study that looked at its use in 74 elderly patients found that after 12 weeks, 49% of patients had reached a PASI 75 on a mean dose of 11.7 mg/week [4]. In addition, the rate of adverse effects was only 0.12/patient year compared to 1.4/patient year with cyclosporine. For the elderly, however, special consideration for dosing and for side effects must be considered before selecting it as a treatment.

Older patients may require a smaller dose of methotrexate in order to see the desired results [18]. This has been correlated with decreasing creatinine excretion rates and increasing age in patients over 50. The decline in renal function, often seen with age, is thought to be responsible for the need for dose reduction [19]. Renal impairment has also been associated with increased adverse effects [20]. As a result of these factors, it has been recommended that renal function is assessed before initiating and monitored throughout treatment and that patients with kidney disease may need an alternative regimen [8, 19]. In addition, lower dosing is usually appropriate [8].

Two of the most significant adverse effects that can result from methotrexate are myelosuppression and hepatotoxicity. In addition to these side effects, methotrexate can also more commonly cause nasopharyngitis, nausea, and headache [17, 21]. Changes in blood count can be a relatively common adverse effect, with one study reporting that these abnormalities account for up to 27% of all adverse events seen within the first 90 days of beginning treatment with 7.5–40 mg methotrexate/week and 15 mg folate/week [22]. Of these hematologic changes, anemia was the most common, followed by thrombocytopenia and leukopenia. Stemming from this, infections can pose a problem, particularly for the elderly who may already be immunosuppressed [23]. A clinical trial comparing adalimumab with methotrexate found that 46 of 110 patients treated with 15–25 mg methotrexate/week and 5 mg folate/week developed infections during the 16 weeks they were treated [24]. Patients that are on methotrexate for longer have been observed to be at a greater risk for infections as they were significantly more frequent in a population of patients that had cumulatively received more than 2 g of methotrexate [22]. In order to monitor the myelosuppression, it is recommended that a blood count is done before treatment, after the first week, every 2 weeks for the first 2 months, and every 2–3 months subsequently [8]. As a result of these side effects, methotrexate is contraindicated for patients with severe infections, who are immunocompromised, or who have baseline hematologic abnormalities.

The hepatotoxicity caused by methotrexate can be problematic for older patients who may have a reduced drug metabolism and decreased self-healing ability [19]. One study of 110 patients found that 1% of individuals had elevated liver enzymes when treated with 15–25 mg methotrexate/week for 4 weeks [24]. However another study observed 45 cases of increased serum liver enzymes in 103 patients after 90 days when treated with doses ranging from 7.5 to 40 mg/week methotrexate and 15 mg/week folate [22]. The implication of this is that individuals on methotrexate should have their serum liver enzymes monitored and those with potential risk factors for liver damage should utilize another medication. These include strong contraindications for patients with alcohol abuse and careful consideration before prescribing it for patients with a history of hepatitis [8].

For patients that have been on methotrexate for extended periods of time, there is still much debate as to the effects of chronic methotrexate exposure. A study that compared patients who had been treated with greater than 2 g or less than 2 g total did not find a significant difference in the number of adverse effects over the same period of time [22]. There were also a comparable number of severe adverse effects. Another study looked at liver biopsies before treatment and after cumulative doses ranging from 1 to 4 g among 28 enrolled patients [25]. This study found that patients who had received 3–4 g of methotrexate tended to have "fibrosis formation, inflammation enhancement in the portal area, and fibrous septa." They recommended doing liver biopsies every time a 1 g total had been administered in patients with no risk factors. Although due to the invasive nature of this test, these recommendations have been subject to a large amount of controversy in the field of dermatology and are not widely performed [26].

Given the efficacy and potential adverse effects, methotrexate is a viable treatment plan for many elderly patients once potential contraindications have been accounted for. However, liver and kidney function will need to be carefully followed to avoid hazardous side effects that older individuals may be particularly susceptible to. Drug interactions need to be taken into consideration to prevent amplification of side effects. NSAIDS, estimated to be the single most used drug in older adults, may lower methotrexate clearance rates in the kidney and increase the risk of bone marrow toxicity as well as the risk for gastrointestinal side effects [8, 19, 27]. Some antibiotics including penicillin and tetracycline should be avoided while concurrently on methotrexate [8, 28]. As previously mentioned, patients should be advised not to drink alcohol [8]. Ultimately, methotrexate should be considered as an oral agent for a subset of older psoriasis patients with special attention to coexistent risk factors for hepatic and hematologic toxicity.

Cyclosporine

Cyclosporine is an immunosuppressive agent that works by decreasing active T-cell populations [29]. In dermatology, it is most notably used to treat severe psoriasis in the acute setting of a flare. It can be administered rarely as a long-term treatment, but is most strongly recommended as a short course and often used as a bridge to safer maintenance therapies [30]. A major benefit of its use is the ability to allow for reductions in PASI relatively quickly. Reduction in PASI is dose dependent and treatment with 5 mg/kg/day has been reported to reduce PASI scores by 50% in 72% of patients after 10–12 weeks while a 50% reduction in PASI was reported in 66% of patients taking 2.5 mg/kg/day [29]. In a study focusing on treatment of psoriasis in the elderly, 46% of patients reached a 75% reduction in PASI by week 12 [4]. Although dosage varied in this study, the mean dose was 3.5 mg/kg. In another study, patients saw a mean decrease in

PASI score from 14.0 ± 6.6 to 3.8 ± 0.5 after 16 weeks on 3 mg/kg cyclosporine for the first 4 weeks, followed by 5 mg/kg cyclosporine [17]. These benefits must of course be weighed against the risk of serious adverse effects that can be seen in treatment with cyclosporine and may be of higher consequence in the elderly population.

Cyclosporine's potential adverse effects are most notable for an increased risk of hypertension, renal insufficiency, malignancy, and infection. A 2001 meta-analysis of 3 randomized, controlled trials found that systolic blood pressures increased to or above 160 mmHg in 1.9% of patients on 1.25 mg/kg/day of cyclosporine, 1.1% of patients on 2.5 mg/kg/day, and 3.4% of patients on 5 mg/kg/day [29]. Diastolic blood pressure was also affected with risk of developing a diastolic pressure of 95 mmHg or higher being 4.9%, 13.7%, and 8.6% for 1.25 mg/kg/day, 2.5 mg/kg/day, and 5 mg/kg/day doses, respectively. Another study that looked at the safety of systemic treatments for psoriasis in the elderly reported that 11 of the 32 patients taking cyclosporine developed hypertension [4]. Demographic data was not given for individual treatment plans, but comorbidities were common (more than 90% of enrolled patients), with cardiovascular disease reported most frequently. The implication of these studies is to exercise extreme caution when using cyclosporine in patients with preexisting hypertension, which is widespread in the elderly and reported in up to 65% of the US population over the age of 60 [31]. Patients with poorly controlled hypertension should not take cyclosporine [8]. This adverse effect should be monitored with regular blood pressure checks.

Patients taking cyclosporine are also at risk for developing nephrotoxicity [32]. One meta-analysis found that serum creatinine increased more than 30% in 4.4% of patients ($n = 756$) receiving doses of 1.5–5 mg/kg/day for 10–12 weeks [29]. Serum creatinine elevations were also dose related with elevations of 1.9, 6.8, and 11.4% in patients taking 1.5, 2.5, and 5 mg/kg/day. Treatment with cyclosporine is thought to put elderly patients at an increased risk for nephrotoxicity due to age-related decreases in drug excretion rates [8, 19, 33]. The European S3 guidelines advise adhering closely to lab monitoring recommendations for the elderly and generally recommend testing for several renal function markers throughout treatment for all patients [8]. These lab values include frequent serum creatinine levels, which should be tested before treatment and at weeks 2, 4, 8, 12, and 16 weeks. Full blood counts, liver function tests, and electrolytes can be evaluated at the same intervals to monitor for hematological alterations, hepatotoxicity, and blood potassium abnormalities, respectively. Uric acid should be tested at least at baseline to monitor kidney function. They also recommend checking urine status, magnesium, cholesterol, and triglycerides before treatment and at weeks 4 and 16 for further observation of kidney function and alterations in lipid profile.

In addition to monitoring, the guidelines recommend a nephrology consult for extended periods of treatments. In a small study of elderly patients treated with cyclosporine, 5 of 36 patients developed renal insufficiency [4]. They found the risk of developing renal insufficiency to be 0.35/patient year. Given the risk of renal toxicity, cyclosporine should be avoided if feasible in patients with baseline impaired renal function [8].

Cyclosporine also puts patients at an increased risk for skin malignancies, particularly if the individual has had UV treatment in the past [34]. Patients treated with cyclosporine had an increased relative risk of developing nonmelanoma skin cancer. Individuals that have received past PUVA treatment or other immunosuppressants were reported to have a higher incidence of developing any type of malignancy. In addition to the development of skin malignancies, cyclosporine may also put patients at an increased risk for infection [8]. As a result of immunosuppression, live vaccines are contraindicated during treatment [35]. Administration of inactivated vaccines during treatment may lead to a reduced immune response that may lower efficacy. As a result of this immunosuppression, cyclosporine should be avoided in elderly patients with a history of or current malignancy, who are undergoing PUVA therapy, or who have a serious infectious disease [8]. Individuals taking cyclosporine should also be carefully watched for the development of skin malignancies.

Comorbidities should be carefully accounted for and evaluated prior to administration of cyclosporine. Due to the potential for drug interactions, it is also important to evaluate for medication interactions, particularly in regard to their effect on renal function. In the context of other available medications, the clinical use of cyclosporine must be carefully weighed against other traditional and biologic systemic treatments, particularly in the elderly population. Statins are one of the most commonly prescribed drugs for the elderly, but most are heavily contraindicated [27, 36, 37]. Potassium-sparing diuretics and ACE inhibitors are also highly prescribed but contraindicated medications [27, 37, 38]. Cyclosporine metabolism can be lowered by grapefruit juice so patients should be advised to avoid consuming it while on cyclosporine [39]. In summary, in light of these side effects, despite the relatively quick efficacy of cyclosporine, its use in the elderly should only be considered in severe cases of psoriasis that have been unsuccessfully treated with other first-line medications.

Mycophenolate Mofetil

Mycophenolate Mofetil (MMF) is often used in dermatology as a corticosteroid-sparing immunosuppressive agent in the treatment of numerous inflammatory skin conditions, especially immunobullous and connective tissue diseases. It functions as a pro-drug, which is converted in the plasma,

liver, and kidneys to the active antimetabolite mycophenolate acid (MPA) [40]. This metabolite then inhibits the enzyme, inosine monophosphate dehydrogenase, involved in "de novo" purine nucleotide synthesis in activated lymphocytes. MPA is inactivated in the liver by enzymatic alteration to form a phenolic glucoronide of MPA (MPAG), which is excreted into bile. Subsequent enterohepatic circulation is important for maintaining serum concentrations at therapeutic levels. The inactive MPAG is converted back to the active MPA by the enzyme beta-glucoronidase, which is found in high concentrations in both the skin and the gastrointestinal tract. This explains both the therapeutic effects in the skin as well as the commonly reported adverse side effects of diarrhea and abdominal pain [41]. It is important to note that although the kidneys excrete up to 90% of MPAG, MPA levels are not significantly affected by renal disease and therefore no dose adjustment is required for renal impairment [42]. MPA and MPAG are mostly bound in the serum to albumin and therefore dose adjustments may be required in patients with low albumin and in those patients taking other medications that compete with protein binding sites.

As discussed above, the use of MMF in the elderly is often limited by abdominal symptoms such as diarrhea, vomiting, and abdominal pain. However, the elderly population is at a significantly higher risk for serious complications of diarrhea, specifically dehydration and electrolytes abnormalities and should be monitored more closely for these symptoms to avoid adverse sequela. In general, the risk for hypoalbuminemia is higher in the elderly and can be secondary to various etiologies including malnutrition, gastrointestinal loss, liver dysfunction, and kidney disease. This can result in increased levels of free MPA in the serum and a theoretically higher risk for hematologic toxicity and infection [43]. Hematologic toxicity is a serious adverse effect, especially in the elderly population, and should be monitored for along with liver function tests and serum creatinine every 2–4 weeks after a dose escalation and every 2–3 months once the dose has stabilized [44]. As with all patients being treated with MMF, elderly patients should be monitored for development of side effects and may actually require modifications to their dose or regimen more frequently compared to younger patients. Unfortunately data is limited on the relative risk of these side effects in elderly patients being treated for dermatologic conditions; however, in one report, up to 60% of organ transplant recipients over 60 years of age being treated with MMF will eventually require an alternative antimetabolite-sparing regimen [45].

Also, the elderly population as a whole is at a higher risk for medication interactions, which can alter levels of the active metabolite MPA. Sub-therapeutic levels of MPA can develop in patients on a medication that interferes with enterohepatic circulation such as cholestyramine or a variety of systemic antibiotics including cephalosporins, penicillin, macrolides, sulfonamides, and flouroquinolones. Also, many elderly patients who are on daily salicylates can develop increased free levels of MPA due to competition for protein binding sites in the serum. Phenytoin has been reported to have a similar effect and can also elevate free MPA levels. Caution should be using when co-prescribing antiviral medications such as acyclovir, valacyclovir, ganciclovir, valganciclovir with MMF as elevated levels of MPA may result and increased risk for neutropenia has been reported with valacyclovir [44]. Fortunately, phase 2 metabolism such as occurs in the activation of MMF to MPA does not appear to be inherently affected by the normal aging process.

A recent study of 69 patients with various dermatologic conditions who were treated with an average dose of 2 g daily of MMF revealed a complete response in 56, 53, 46, and 0% of patients with atopic dermatitis, immunobullous diseases, neutrophillic dermatoses, and psoriasis, respectively [46]. The use of MMF in the treatment of psoriasis is usually considered a last resort given the overall lower efficacy and higher risk of adverse side effects. However, its use may be attempted in patients with severe refractory psoriasis who may otherwise have contraindications to or who have not responded to multiple other first-line agents. When compared to other conventional agents in a multicenter randomized open-label clinical trial evaluating mycophenolate mofetil and cyclosporine in 54 patients with plaque psoriasis, cyclosporine was found to have significantly superior efficacy and along with methotrexate would be the preferred first-line conventional systemic agents in elderly patients with moderate to severe plaque psoriasis [47]. In summary, mycophenolate mofetil's use as a systemic agent for the treatment of psoriasis in the elderly is limited by its relatively lower efficacy weighed with the concern for immunosuppression and medication interactions but can be considered in patients with contraindications to other systemic agents or in patients with comorbidities that could be simultaneously targeted with this agent.

Biologic Agents

Tumor Necrosis Factor: Alpha Inhibitors

Etanercept
Etanercept isafullyhuman, dimeric fusion protein that binds to both soluble and membrane bound TNF-α and TNF-β, preventing further binding to cell membrane receptors [48]. When active, TNF-α not only stimulates the Th1 response but also plays a complex role in cross-activation of multiple other inflammatory mediators leading to enhanced production of IL-23 by dendritic cells which is a well known activator of the Th17 response [49, 50]. IL-17 then acts synergistically with IL-22 to increase keratinocyte proliferation up to fivefold [51]. TNF-α can also act directly to stimulate neutrophils, which are important in the pathogenesis of psoriasis. Although etanercept has a much higher affinity for TNF-α than the other monoclonal antibodies, it releases the cytokine quickly with 90% released within 2–3 h. The molecule is absorbed slowly reaching peak levels at about 2 days with an absolute bioavailability of 58% [52]. The complex is thought to then be metabolized by proteolysis and excreted in urine, bile, or both [53].

Etanercept has long been a first-line biologic agent in the treatment of moderate to severe plaque psoriasis and appears to have equal efficacy in the elderly population. One recent study compared 1158 patients <65 years of age to 77 patients >65 years of age and found no statistically significant difference in the number of patients reaching at least a PASI 50 or 75 between the two age groups. The same study also demonstrated improved quality of life index scores in the elderly population with no significant difference between the two age groups studied [54].

Lastly, etanercept has not been shown to have an age-related increase in toxicity when used to treat psoriasis in the elderly. One study comparing the rate of adverse events in 187 psoriasis patients >65 years of age reported etanercept to have the lowest rate (0.11) when compared to numerous other conventional and biologic agents such as methotrexate (0.12), acitretin (0.32), cyclosporine (1.4), PUVA (0.5), adalimumab (0.35), infliximab (0.19), efalizumab (0.3), and ustekinumab (0.26) [4]. An analysis of 4322 patients >65 years of age who were treated with etanercept for various rheumatologic diseases did not reveal any statistically significant increased risk for serious adverse events including infection and malignancy when compared to the population <65 years of age. Of note, demyelinating disease only occurred in patients <65 years of age [55]. Another important factor for the elderly population is the concern for medication interactions. Due to the presumed proteolytic metabolism, etanercept is unlikely to interfere with the metabolism or excretion of most drugs but has been shown to increase the risk for serious infections when given simultaneously with anakinra [56].

Infliximab
Infliximab is a chimeric IgG (25% mouse and 75% human) monoclonal antibody that binds soluble and membrane bound TNF-α [57]. The proposed mechanism of action in the treatment of psoriasis is therefore similar to that of other TNF-α inhibitors. It is uniquely administered by infusion and concentrations in the serum are directly correlated with dosing but do not appear to be affected by the normal aging process [58]. Infliximab is assumed to be metabolized by proteolysis and therefore metabolism is also not significantly affected by liver or kidney disease [59, 60].

Several major trials have been performed to evaluate the efficacy of infliximab in the treatment of plaque psoriasis, which have all shown promising results. One study of 249 patients with moderate to severe plaque psoriasis showed a

PASI 75 of close to 80%, which was maintained for 3–4 months after the last infusion [61]. Other studies have reported a PASI 75 as high as 93% at week 12 of treatment [4]. A retrospective, cohort study by Garber et al. [62] compared 48 elderly (>65 years of age) psoriasis patients to 146 adult (18–64 years of age) psoriasis patients and documented no statistically significant difference in simple-measure for assessing psoriasis activity (S-MAPA) between several biologic agents including infliximab [62]. Infliximab's efficacy in the treatment of psoriasis and rheumatoid arthritis was not significantly different between elderly patient and younger patients, according to infliximab's package insert [63].

• The original sentence may be too similar to a sentence in Grozdev IS, Van Voorhees AS, Gottlieb AB, Hsu S, Lebwohl MG, Bebo BF Jr, et al. Psoriasis in the elderly: from the Medical Board of the National Psoriasis Foundation. J Am Acad Dermatol. 2011;65:537–45.
• No difference in the efficacy of infliximab has been seen in elderly patients compared with younger patients [63].

High dose infliximab is contraindicated in patients with congestive heart failure (CHF)as a significant increase in mortality and hospitalizations was seen in patients receiving doses of 10 mg/kg. However, these side effects were not seen at the lower psoriasis dosing of ≤5 mg/kg. Therefore, smaller doses as are given in the treatment of psoriasis (3–5 mg/kg) may be considered in patients with CHF if indicated after cardiologic evaluation [64]. Overall, the incidence of total adverse events in the elderly population after a 1-year treatment with infliximab has been reported to be 0.19 per patient year. This same retrospective, observational study reported a 1-year infection rate of 0.05 for elderly patients being treated with infliximab for psoriasis with only one serious infection requiring hospitalization [4]. A retrospective study also found no statistically significant difference in adverse events or infection rates between elderly and adult psoriasis patients treated with several biologic agents including infliximab. Furthermore, they found data to suggest that several biologic agents, including infliximab, may be safer options for elderly psoriasis patients when compared to conventional systemic agents such as acitretin, methotrexate, and cyclosporine [62]. Unfortunately, no prospective studies currently exist to evaluate the safety of infliximabInfliximabsafety of for the treatment of psoriasis in the elderly.

Adalimumab

Adalimumab is a recombinant antibody to TNF-α that is fully human and works similarly to the other TNF-α inhibitors in its class by preventing binding to the TNFR. Like infliximab, it is also capable of lysing cells that express TNF-α. Unlike infliximab, it is administered subcutaneously and reaches peak concentrations at 131 h with a bioavailability of 64% [65]. It is most likely metabolized by proteolysis and clearance does not seem to be effected by liver or renal disease.

Adalimumab has been used to treat moderate to severe plaque psoriasis and in phase III clinical trials, 71% of patients have been reported to achieve a PASI-75 at 16 weeks of treatment [66]. However, in one recent study, 65% of patients over the age of 65 were reported to achieve a PASI-75. The overall adverse event rate in the elderly population (age 65 and older) has been reported at 0.35, which trended slightly higher than the adverse event rates reported for other biologic agents including etanercept, infliximab, and ustekinumab. However, this difference was only found to be statistically significant when compared to etanercept, which had an adverse event rate of 0.11 in this same population. When compared to methotrexate in this same study, adalimumab was also noted to have a statistically higher increased risk for infection in the elderly population [4].

Due to the presumed proteolytic metabolism, adalimumab is unlikely to interfere with the metabolism or excretion of most drugs. In general, medication interactions in the elderly population are rarely reported, although adalimumab, like etanercept, should also not be given to patients on anakinra due to the increased risk for infection. Also, methotrexate has been reported to reduce clearance of adalimumab by up to 44% although this does not appear to clinically alter efficacy [67]. Further discussion of the TNF-inhibitors as a group will be addressed below.

TNF-α Inhibitors

Concern for increased risk of malignancy in the elderly population is often cited as a reason for avoiding systemic treatments with hematologic malignancy being the most common concern. Unfortunately, data is limited with regard to lymphoma risk associated with TNF-α inhibitors as a class. Several clinical trials have suggested a slight increased risk of lymphoma compared to control patients; however, these studies were all limited by small sample size and short-term follow-up [68]. To confound the issue further, psoriasis patients have an estimated baseline increased relative risk of 2.95 for lymphoma when compared to the general population [69]. Unfortunately, the majority of observational studies in the current literature have evaluated patients with rheumatoid arthritis (RA). These studies have questionable applicability to psoriasis patients, especially given the higher likelihood for RA patients to be treated with higher dose immunosuppressants and simultaneously with more than one agent. In general, most studies suggest that all but very small increases in the risk for lymphoma in patients treated with monotherapy TNF-α inhibitors can be ruled out. However, an extremely rare and often fatal hepatosplenic T cell lymphoma has been reported in 18 patients receiving combination therapy with TNF-α inhibitors and either azathioprine or 6-mercaptopurine [70]. TNF-α inhibitors as a whole have been reported in some studies to carry an increased risk for nonmelanoma skin cancer and a trend has been reported in two large registries toward an increased risk for malignant melanoma in RA patients specifically [71].

Although a causal relationship has not been firmly established, worsening neurologic disease has been reported in three case series in association with all three TNF-α inhibitors. This risk should be considered and a different medication selected, if feasible, when treating elderly psoriasis patients with comorbid multiple sclerosis, optic neuritis, Guillain-Barre syndrome, and other demyelinating disorders [72]. Current literature is lacking with regard to specific risks for demyelinating disorders in the elderly population specifically.

Another common concern of clinicians when prescribing TNF-α inhibitors to the elderly population is an increased risk for infection. Clinical trials have suggested a trend toward increased rates of serious infections in patients treated with both infliximab and adalimumab. In general, it is prudent to screen elderly patients for signs of infection and to temporarily withdraw treatment with all TNF-α inhibitors during an active infection. The increased risk for primary infection and possible reactivation of latent tuberculosis is a concern in any age and should be screened for annually. Overall, the risk of tuberculosis has been reported to be higher in patients treated with infliximab and adalimumab compared to etanercept [73]. Invasive fungal infections have been reported more commonly in patients treated for RA with infliximab and etanercept although 98% of these cases were seen in patients on at least one other immunosuppressive agent [74]. Reactivation of hepatitis B has been reported in association with all three TNF-α inhibitors and should be screened for prior to consideration for therapy [75]. Lastly, a recent study evaluating a cohort of patients treated for RA, psoriatic arthritis and inflammatory bowel disease, 20% of whom were 65 years or older, found no significant increased risk of herpes zoster infection associated with TNF-α inhibitor therapy [76].

Congestive heart failure (CHF) is a common comorbidity in the elderly population and should be screened for in all psoriasis patients considering biologic therapy. Two large studies evaluating etanercept for the treatment of congestive heart failure were stopped prematurely due to failure to show any improvement compared to placebo and there is some evidence for a trend toward increased mortality in CHF patients treated with either etanercept or infliximab [64]. However, there is no good evidence that this class of medications increases the risk for new onset CHF [77]. It is the opinion of the authors that with careful patient selection as well as appropriate counseling and monitoring, TNF-α inhibitors can be an appropriate option for moderate to severe plaque psoriasis in the elderly with special consideration and avoidance when feasible in patients with comorbid CHF and/or demyelinating neurologic disease.

Ustekinumab

Ustekinumab is a veryefficacious human monoclonal antibody against interleukin-12 and interleukin-23 and is used in the treatment of moderate to severe plaque psoriasis. Maintenance doses of ustekinumab are uniquely administered every 12 weeks after completion of the loading dose, which may present a distinct advantage for a subset of elderly patients in which frequent self-injections are difficult or impractical. Furthermore, it benefits from a low rate of adverse effects, particularly in comparison with many of the conventional systemic treatments for psoriasis. In a meta-analysis of five studies exploring the efficacy of ustekinumab, after 24–28 weeks of 45 mg, patients were 10.92 times more likely to reach a PASI 75 than in those not treated with ustekinumab [30]. Those on the 90 mg dose were 11.60 times more likely to reach a PASI 75 when compared to the placebo group. One of the phase III clinical trials within this meta-analysis found that after 12 weeks, 273/409 (66.7%) patients on 45 mg and 311/411 (75.7%) on 90 mg reached a PASI 75 compared with only 15/410 (3.7%) of the placebo group [78]. Another clinical trial that looked at responses over 5 years found that by week 52, 71.4% of patients on 45 mg reached a PASI 75 compared with 78.9% of patients treated with the 90 mg dose [79]. This study was placebo controlled for 12 weeks and patients withdrawn secondary to adverse effects, usage of prohibited medications, or insufficient response were considered to be nonresponders for the remainder of the study. Additionally, after 12 weeks, patients who were previously on placebo were randomly assigned to either 45 mg or 90 mg per week. Of the 1212 patients on either dose initially enrolled, 7.31% had serious adverse events and 2.43% of patients had adverse events leading to discontinuation during the 264 weeks.

The most notable potential adverse effect associated with ustekinumab treatment is infection. In a study of 606 patients on 45 mg and 809 patients on 90 mg, 26.0% and 23.6% of patients developed infections requiring treatment after 5 years of therapy [79]. Fortunately, only 1.08 and 0.88% of patients, respectively, developed serious infections. It should be noted that the age range in this study was relatively young, with the mean age being 46.2 ± 12.2 years. The literature regarding the extent of immunosuppression in elderly patients treated with ustekinumab is currently sparse. A small retrospective study of 22 elderly patients with a mean age of 70.3 had no reported serious infections after 2 years of treatment, suggesting ustekinumab's immunosuppression may not be significantly worsened by immunosenescence [80]. A confirmatory observational study looking at 3474 patients on ustekinumab from the PSOLAR registry did not find an increased risk of serious infection in patients treated with ustekinumab when compared with psoriasis patients treated with non-biologic therapies [81]. Conversely, another study did suggest that age, diabetes mellitus, and a history of significant infections were associated with an increased risk of serious infection. As with all biologics, it is therefore recommended that patients be prescreened for tuberculosis, current infection, and a history of frequent infections [8]. It would be prudent to check a complete blood count prior to initiating treatment and every 3–6 months thereafter. It is also recommended that patients do not receive live vaccinations during treatment or for 12 weeks following discontinuation of treatment [8]. Interestingly, one study exploring the efficacy of 23-valent pneumococcal and tetanus toxoid vaccines in patients taking ustekinumab found that both had responses similar to control patients [82].

In addition to an increased risk of infection, ustekinumab has also been associated with an increased risk for malignancy. In a 5-year study of 606 patients on 45 mg and 809 patients on 90 mg, 1.08% of patients on 45 mg and 1.07% on 90 mg developed any form of malignancy [79]. However, this study was not placebo controlled and there was not a trend toward an increased rate of any specific form of malignancy. The same study also saw a small number of major adverse cardiac events (MACE) in the patient population. This study found that 0.56% of patients on 45 mg and 0.42% of patients on 90 mg experienced one cardiac event after 5 years of treatment [79]. However, an analysis of data from 3308 patients enrolled in the PSOLAR trial from 2007 to 2013 did not find an association between ustekinumab use and an increased risk of MACE [83]. Other side effects of treatment include nasopharyngitis, upper respiratory infections, headache, arthralgia, diarrhea, back pain, injection-site erythema, and fatigue [84]. It is recommended that patients be screened for nonmelanoma skin cancer, lymphadenopathy, and cardiovascular risk factors prior to starting treatment to assess if they may be at higher risk for developing these adverse events [8]. Although data is currently limited in the elderly population, it is the opinion of the authors that with careful patient selection, counseling, and monitoring, ustekinumab can be an appropriate option for moderate to severe plaque psoriasis in the elderly with special consideration that advanced age may be associated with an increased risk for infection.

Interleukin-17 Inhibitors

Secukinumab

Secukinumab is one Interleukin-17 inhibitors secukinumab Secukinumab biologic agents of the newest biologic agents in the management of plaque psoriasis and is a human monoclonal antibody against interleukin-17A [85]. A phase III double-blinded, randomized clinical trial of 177 patients receiving 150, 300 mg, or a placebo found that by week 12, 69.5%, 75.9%, and 0% had reached a PASI 75, respectively. However, the average age of each group in this study was 45.1, 46.0, and 46.5, respectively, with no patients older than 62 [86]. Although

current data does not indicate an increased risk for adverse events specific to the elderly population, this conclusion is limited by the lack of time for post-marketing safety studies and a lack of investigation into its use in the elderly population.

The safety profile of secukinumab has been investigated in several clinical trials. One double-blinded, randomized clinical trial of 177 patients receiving 150, 300 mg, or a placebo found that during the 12 weeks of treatment, 57.6, 50.8, and 47.5% of patients, respectively, experienced an adverse event [86]. There were no serious adverse events in the 150 mg arm, 3 in the 300 mg arm, and only 1 in the placebo arm. All arms of the study had 59 patients each. These events included acute myocardial infarction, cerebrovascular accident, and sciatica for the three patients taking 300 mg and exfoliative dermatitis in the patient taking the placebo. The study reported that the patients who had experienced MACE had multiple cardiovascular risk factors. Diarrhea, nasopharyngitis, headache, pyrexia, back pain, bursitis, cough, depression, nausea, oropharyngeal pain, and rhinitis were also reported. Another double-blinded, randomized clinical trial including 61 patients receiving 150 mg, 60 patients on 300 mg, and 61 patients receiving placebo found that after 12 weeks, 63.9, 70.0, and 54.1%, respectively, experienced an adverse event [87]. One patient that received the 150 mg secukinumab dose developed malignant melanoma in situ, although researchers did not consider it to be related to the treatment [85].

Immunosuppression leading to an increased risk of infection and infestation is a concern for secukinumab, as with many biologics. A double blind, randomized clinical trial of secukinumab at 300 and 150 mg compared to 50 mg etanercept or placebo found that after 12 weeks, 26.7% of patients on 300 mg of secukinumab, 30.9% of patients on 150 mg secukinumab, 24.5% of patients on etanercept, and 19.3% of patients on placebo had an infection or infestation [85]. Unfortunately, the degree to which this holds true in the elderly has yet to be investigated [23]. Phase III trials also found a dose dependent increased risk of mild to moderate candida infections with one study reporting 4.7% of patients on 300 mg developed an infection after 52 weeks, compared with 2.3% on 150 mg. Fortunately, these were all effectively managed with standard therapy and did not significantly impact the course of treatment or cause discontinuation of the study drug [85]. Although data is currently limited, it is the opinion of the authors that with careful patient selection as well as appropriate counseling and monitoring, secukinumab can be an appropriate option for moderate to severe plaque psoriasis in the elderly with special consideration for patients with concurrent inflammatory bowel disease.

Ixekizumab

Ixekizumab is another recently FDA approved Il-17A monoclonal antibody used in the treatment of moderate to severe plaque psoriasis. Ixekizumab's efficacy during induction and during maintenance was explored during the UNCOVER phase 3 clinical trials. The trial consisted of 3 groups and the patient's mean ages were 46 ± 13, 45 ± 12, and 46 ± 13 years old, respectively. After 12 weeks of treatment, 89.1% achieved a PASI 75, 70.9% achieved a PASI 90, and 35.3% achieved a PASI 100 [88]. Furthermore, UNCOVER-3 observed continued treatment through 60 weeks. These studies show a drug that is highly efficacious in the treatment of plaque psoriasis. A stratification of this population to specify those age 65 or older was not performed and therefore it is not known if there is a difference in the efficacy for this age group specifically.

The serious adverse events reported include neutropenia, candida infections, and inflammatory bowel disease [88]. Other more common adverse events included upper respiratory tract infections, nasopharyngitis, headache, and injection site reactions [88]. Infections were most often reported as nonserious, mild, or moderate upper respiratory infections. Candida infections were frequently diagnosed as vulvovaginal or oral candidiasis, which is consistent with the proposed role of IL-17 in host defense against extracellular organisms such as yeast. Cellulitis was the most commonly reported serious adverse event in patients treated with ixekizumab. Importantly, there were no cases of active or clinically reactivated tuberculosis reported. Furthermore, Ixekizumab use was not associated with an increased risk for major adverse cardiovascular events of cerebrovascular events (MACE) [89].

Excluding the risk for nonmelanoma skin cancer, the risk for malignancy was similar in comparison to etanercept treated patients. Unfortunately, this data is limited by the lack of long-term follow-up for these patients and will need to be further monitored for in ongoing safety trials. Moreover, the rates of nonmelanoma skin cancer as well as other malignancies were comparable with the rates expected in patients with a history of psoriasis.

Current research suggests that ixekizumab is a relatively safe and highly efficacious systemic agent for the treatment of moderate to severe plaque psoriasis. Unfortunately, data specific to the elderly population is currently lacking and further research needs to be done to determine if the current data can be extrapolated to the elderly population. Although data is currently limited, it is the opinion of the authors that with careful patient selection and appropriate counseling and monitoring, ixekizumab can be an appropriate option for moderate to severe plaque psoriasis in the elderly with special consideration for patients with comorbid inflammatory bowel disease.

Small Molecule, Oral Agents

Apremilast

Apremilast is an oral agent that acts as an inhibitor of PDE4 and has recently been approved for the treatment of moderate to severe plaque psoriasis. It is the first small molecule inhibitor of its kind to be used in the treatment of patients with psoriasis and works by decreasing chronic inflammatory pathways in macrophages, monocytes, mast cells, dendritic cells, eosinophils, and T cells. The mechanism of action involves blocking degradation of cAMP and stimulating downstream production of anti-inflammatory cytokines such as IL-6 and IL-10 [90].

In the phase III ESTEEM trial, 28.8% of patients treated with apremilast achieved a PASI 75 and 55.5% of patients achieved a PASI 50 after 16 weeks of treatment [91]. In addition, it appears to be efficacious in the treatment of both nail and scalp psoriasis and therefore may serve a unique role in the management of significant but localized disease at these sites [92]. The oral administration is a unique advantage for apremilast and is desirable for a subset of patients as an alternative to injections. Of note, renal dose adjustment suggests a modified regimen for patients with a creatinine clearance <30 and therefore baseline renal function should be evaluated before starting therapy [91]. This is especially pertinent for elderly patients with a history of renal disease. Although drug interactions are rare, avoidance of concomitant use of potent cytochrome 450 enzyme inducers is recommended as administration with rifampin has been shown to decrease systemic exposure to apremilast [93].

Furthermore, apremilast thus far does not appear to be associated with an increased risk for infection other than nasopharyngitis and upper respiratory tract infections and large studies have reported no increased risk for reactivation of tuberculosis. This may be a distinct advantage when selecting an agent for elderly patients with psoriasis. The decrease in required laboratory monitoring may also be helpful for elderly patients who find frequent visits to be challenging. The most commonly reported side effects include diarrhea and headache and these were most often reported as mild to moderate in severity. Weight loss was reported in patients on apremilast more frequently than placebo which although may be advantageous for some, could be considered undesirable in a subset of elderly patients with difficulty maintaining an optimal weight [87]. According to the manufacturer, geriatric patients ≥65 years of age experienced no overall difference in the safety or efficacy profile compared to younger adult patients <65 years of age in the clinical studies. However, due to the limited data available in very elderly patients (≥75 years of age), apremilast should be used with caution in this patient population [94]. In summary, apremilast's favorable overall safety profile and adequate efficacy making it an appropriate oral treatment option for a subset of elderly patients with moderate to severe plaque psoriasis with special consideration for renal status, medication interactions, and risk factors for depression [90] (Table 29.1).

Table 29.1 Advantages and disadvantages of systemic agents for the treatment of psoriasis in the elderly population

Medications	Advantages	Disadvantages
Acitretin	Lack of immunosuppression or increased malignancy risk, decreased risk of nonmelanoma skin cancer, oral option	Delay in onset by several weeks, mucocutaneous irritation/xerosis, hyperlipidemia, transaminitis (especially in the setting of alcohol intake), contraindicated in severe renal or hepatic dysfunction
Methotrexate	Low cost, oral/intramuscular/subcutaneous options	Dose modification with decreased renal function, nausea, myelosuppression, hepatotoxicity (increased in the setting of alcohol intake), medication interactions (e.g., NSAIDs, antibiotics)
Cyclosporine	Rapid onset, oral option	Immunosuppression, hypertension, renal insufficiency, electrolyte abnormalities, increased risk for skin malignancies, medication interactions (e.g., statins, ACE inhibitors, and potassium-sparing diuretics)
Mycophenolate Mofetil	No dose adjustment in renal disease, oral option	Hematologic toxicity, diarrhea/abdominal pain, dose adjustment in hypoalbuminemia, medication interactions (e.g., phenytoin, salicylates, antiviral medications)
Etanercept	No age-dependent increase in adverse events, minimal medication interactions, good long-term safety data	Worsened CHF, immunosuppression, reactivation of tuberculosis and hepatitis B, possible increase in lymphoproliferative diseases, demyelinating disorders
Infliximab	Minimal medication interactions	Worsened CHF, immunosuppression, reactivation of tuberculosis and hepatitis B, possible increase in lymphoproliferative diseases, demyelinating disorders, infusion reactions, logistics of infusions
Adalimumab	Minimal medication interactions	Worsened CHF, immunosuppression, reactivation of tuberculosis and hepatitis B, possible increase in lymphoproliferative diseases, demyelinating disorders
Ustekinumab	Minimal medication interactions, decreased frequency of injections	Less long-term safety data than TNF-inhibitors, immunosuppression, rate of serious infections directly related to age and diabetes, controversial trend toward increased risk for MACE
Secukinumab	Minimal medication interactions	Limited long-term safety data, immunosuppression, increased risk for candida infections, worsened IBD
Ixekizumab	Minimal medication interactions	Limited long-term safety data, immunosuppression, myelosuppression, increased risk for candida infections, worsened IBD
Apremilast	Lower infection risk, no lab monitoring except if baseline renal status unknown, weight loss, oral option	Limited long-term safety data, dose adjustments for creatinine clearance, possible drug interactions with C450 enzyme inducers (e.g., Rifampin), diarrhea, weight loss, depression/suicidal ideation

Cases

Case 1

A 72-year-old white male developed psoriatic plaques on his elbows and knees 4 years ago, which was originally managed successfully with topical corticosteroids, but now reports decreased efficacy. His psoriasis acutely worsened 6 months ago after his wife passed away. The patient had undergone phototherapy for a few months but had minimal response. He also had difficulty arranging frequent transportation for treatments, as he is unable to drive his car due to macular degeneration. He complains of severe itching and burning due to his psoriasis. There is no family history of psoriasis. He does not endorse symptoms of psoriatic arthritis although does have a history of osteoarthritis in his hands and does not feel comfortable with self-injections at home.

Past Medical History
- Obesity (BMI – 35)
- Macular Degeneration
- Osteoarthritis

Social History
- Drinks a few glasses of wine each night
- Smokes 1 pack per day
- Retired engineer

Previous Therapies
- Topical steroids
- Narrow band UVB

Physical Exam
- Psoriatic plaques on the scalp, trunk, upper, and lower extremities covering 18% of the body surface area
- No features of psoriatic arthritis (dactylitis, enthesitis, tender and swollen joints, etc.)

Management

Because of the severity of his psoriasis, the biologic agent ustekinumab was chosen. Methotrexate was not considered because he was a drinker and obese which are both risk factors for liver toxicity. The quantiferon gold assay test was negative and he had negative hepatitis B serologies. Other baseline laboratory monitoring was normal including compete blood count, liver function tests, and his HIV status was negative. Due to anticipated difficulty with self-injections and transportation concerns, ustekinumab was chosen as injections could be administered in the office every 12 weeks after the loading dose was complete. The higher weight-based dose of ustekinumab was used starting at 90 mg on week 0 and 4 and then every 12 weeks after that. Within 3 months, his body surface area decreased to 1% and his itching and burn-ing had disappeared. The patient has remained on ustekinumab for 2 years and is satisfied with the treatment.

Case 2

A 65-year-old white female with history of mild psoriasis Mild psoriasis developed widespread psoriatic plaques on her scalp, trunk and extremities after a recent hospitalization for pneumonia. She reports that this was her third hospitalization for pneumonia this year. She is a current smoker and also has a history of numerous nonmelanoma skin cancers. She has previously been responsive to topical corticosteroids but now reports difficulty with application to widespread plaques. She complains of significant itching due to her psoriasis. She reports her father also had psoriasis. She does not endorse symptoms of psoriatic arthritis.

Past Medical History
- Basal Cell Carcinoma
- Squamous Cell Carcinoma
- Recurrent Pneumonia

Social History
- Does not drink alcohol
- Smokes 2 packs per day
- Retired teacher

Previous Therapies
- Topical steroids

Physical Exam
- Psoriatic plaques on the scalp, trunk, upper, and lower extremities covering 10% of the body surface area
- No features of psoriatic arthritis (dactylitis, enthesitis, tender and swollen joints, etc.)

Management

Because of the widespread involvement of her psoriasis, a systemic agent was chosen and the patient was started on acitretin. Several of the other systemic agents were not chosen due to the concern for immunosuppression in the setting of recurrent pneumonia. AcitretinAcitretinbiologic agents also has the added benefit of decreasing her risk for future nonmelanoma skin cancers. Her baseline labs included creatinine, liver function tests and a fasting lipid panel that were within normal limits. She was originally started on 10 mg acitretin daily in biologic agents conjunction with higher potency topical corticosteroids for the thickest plaques. Within 3 months, her body surface area decreased to 2% and her itching had significantly improved. The patient has remained on acitretin for 3 years and has had a decreased burden of skin cancer over this time as well.

References

1. Kelly J, Foley P, Strober B. Current and future oral systemic therapies for psoriasis. Dermatol Clin. 2015;33:91–109.
2. Katz HI, Waalen J, Leach E. Acitretin in psoriasis: an overview of adverse effects. J Am Acad Dermatol. 1999;41:S7–S12.
3. Dogra S, Jain A, Kanwar A. Efficacy and safety of acitretin in three fixed doses of 25, 35 and 50 mg in adult patients with severe plaque type psoriasis: a randomized, double blind, parallel group, dose ranging study. J Eur Acad Dermatol Venereol. 2012;27:e305–11.
4. Piaserico S, Conti A, Lo Console F, De Simone C, Prestinari F, Mazzotta A, et al. Efficacy and safety of systemic treatments for psoriasis in elderly patients. Acta Derm Venereol. 2014;94:293–7.
5. Goldfarb M, Ellis C, Tincoff T, Hamilton T, Voorhees J. Acitretin improves psoriasis in a dose-dependent fashion. J Am Acad Dermatol. 1988;18:655–62.
6. Karadag AS, Ertugrul DT, Kalkan G, Bilgili SG, Celik HT, et al. The effect of acitretin treatment on insulin resistance, retinol-binding protein-4, leptin, and adiponectin in psoriasis vulgaris: a non-controlled study. Dermatology. 2013;227:103–8.
7. Pearce D, Klinger S, Ziel K, Murad E, Rowell R, Feldman S. Low-dose acitretin is associated with fewer adverse events than high-dose acitretin in the treatment of psoriasis. Arch Dermatol. 2006;142:1000–4.
8. Nast A, Gisondi P, Ormerod AD, Saiag P, Smith C, Spuls PI, et al. European S3-Guidelines on the systemic treatment of psoriasis vulgaris. J Eur Acad Dermatol Venereol. 2015a;29:2277–94.
9. Roenigk H, Callen J, Guzzo C, Katz H, Lowe N, Madison K, Nigra T, Fiedler V, Armstrong R. Effects of acitretin on the liver. J Am Acad Dermatol. 1999;41:584–8.
10. Sanchez MR, Ross B, Rotterdam H, Salik J, Brodie R, Freedberg IM. Retinoid hepatitis. J Am Acad Dermatol. 1993;28:853–8.
11. Weiss VC, Layden T, Spinowitz A, Buys CM, Nemchausky BA, West DP, Emmons KM. Chronic active hepatitis associated with etretinate therapy. Br J Dermatol. 1985;112:591–7.
12. Carretero G, Ribera M, Belinchón I, Carrascosa JM, Puig L, Ferrandiz C, et al. Guidelines for the use of acitretin in psoriasis. Psoriasis Group of the Spanish Academy of Dermatology and Venereology. Actas Dermosifiliogr. 2013;104:598–616.
13. Grozdev IS, Van Voorhees AS, Gottlieb AB, Hsu S, Lebwohl MG, Bebo BF Jr, et al. Psoriasis in the elderly: from the Medical Board of the National Psoriasis Foundation. J Am Acad Dermatol. 2011;65:537–45.
14. Zwald FO, Brown M. Skin cancer in solid organ transplant recipients: advances in therapy and management. J Am Acad Dermatol. 2011;65:263–79.
15. Nesher G, Moore T, Dorner R. In vitro effects of methotrexate on peripheral blood monocytes: modulation by folinic acid and S-adenosylmethionine. Ann Rheum Dis. 1991;50:637–41.
16. Shen S, O'Brien T, Yap LM, Prince HM, McCormack CJ. The use of methotrexate in dermatology: a review. Australas J Dermatol. 2012;53:1–18.
17. Heydendael V, Spuls P, Opmeer B, de Borgie C, Reitsma J, Goldschmidt W, et al. Methotrexate versus cyclosporine in moderate-to-severe chronic plaque psoriasis. N Engl J Med. 2003;349:658–65.
18. Fairris GM, Dewhurst AG, White JE, Campbell MJ. Methotrexate dosage in patients aged over 50 with psoriasis. BMJ. 1989;298:801–2.
19. Flammiger A, Maibach H. Drug dosage in the elderly. Drug Aging. 2006;23:203–15.
20. Felson D, Chernoff M, Anderson JJ, Weinblatt M, Furst D, Schmid F, et al. The effect of age and renal function on the efficacy and toxicity of methotrexate in rheumatoid arthritis. J Rheumatol. 1995;22:218–23.
21. Saurat JH, Langley RG, Reich K, Unnebrink K, Sasso EH, Kampman W. Relationship between methotrexate dosing and clinical response in patients with moderate to severe psoriasis: subanalysis of the CHAMPION study. Br J Dermatol. 2011;165:399–406.
22. Wollina U, Ständer K, Barta U. Toxicity of methotrexate treatment in psoriasis and psoriatic arthritis – short- and long-term toxicity in 104 patients. Clin Rheumatol. 2001;20:406–10.
23. Wick G, Jansen-Dürr P, Berger P, Blasko I, Grubeck-Loebenstein B. Diseases of aging. Vaccine. 2000;18:1567–83.
24. Saurat JH, Stingl G, Dubertret L, Papp K, Langley R, Ortonne JP, et al. Efficacy and safety results from the randomized controlled comparative study of adalimumab vs. methotrexate vs. placebo in patients with psoriasis (CHAMPION). Br J Dermatol. 2008;158:558–66.
25. Carneiro C, Lamy CV, Ramos-e-Silva M. Methotrexate and liver function: a study of 13 psoriasis cases treated with different cumulative dosages. J Eur Acad Dermatol Venereol. 2008;22:25–9.
26. Kalb RE, Strober B, Weinstein G, Lebwohl M. Methotrexate and psoriasis: 2009 National Psoriasis Foundation Consensus Conference. J Am Acad Dermatol. 2009;60(5):824–37.
27. Qato D, Wilder J, Schumm P, Gillet V, Alexander C. Changes in prescription and over-the-counter medication and dietary supplement use among older adults in the United States, 2005 vs 2011. JAMA Internal Med. 2016;176:473.
28. Williams WM, Chen TS, Huang KC. Effect of penicillin on the renal tubular secretion of methotrexate in the monkey. Cancer Res. 1984;44:1913–7.
29. Faerber L, Braeutigam M, Weidinger G, Mrowietz U, Christophers E, Schulze HJ, et al. Cyclosporine in severe psoriasis. Results of a meta-analysis in 579 patients. Am J Clin Dermatol. 2001;2:41–7.
30. Nast A, Jacobs A, Rosumeck S, Werner R. Efficacy and safety of systemic long-term treatments for moderate-to-severe psoriasis: a systematic review and meta-analysis. J Invest Dermatol. 2015b;135:2641–8.
31. Nwankwo T, Yoon SS, Burt V, Gu Q. Hypertension among adults in the United States: National Health and nutrition examination survey, 2011-2012. NCHS Data Brief. 2013:1–8.
32. Lowe N, Wieder J, Rosenbach A, et al. Long-term low-dose cyclosporine therapy for severe psoriasis: effects on renal function and structure. J Am Acad Dermatol. 1996;35:710–9.
33. Balato N, Patruno C, Napolitano M, Patrì A, Ayala F, Scarpa R. Managing moderate-to-severe psoriasis in the elderly. Drug Aging. 2014;31:233–8.
34. Paul CF, Ho VC, McGeown C, Christophers E, Schmidtmann B, Guillaume JC, et al. Risk of malignancies in psoriasis patients treated with cyclosporine: a 5 y cohort study. J Invest Dermatol. 2003;120:211–216.
35. Arvas A. Vaccination in patients with immunosuppression. Türk Pediatri Arşivi. 2014;49:181–5.
36. Launay-Vacher V, Izzedine H, Deray G. Statins' dosage in patients with renal failure and cyclosporine drug–drug interactions in transplant recipient patients. Int J Cardiol. 2005;101:9–17.
37. Neuvonen P, Niemi M, Backman J. Drug interactions with lipid-lowering drugs: mechanisms and clinical relevance. Clin Pharmacol Ther. 2006;80:565–81.
38. Salem C, Badreddine A, Fathallah N, Slim R, Hmouda H. Drug-induced hyperkalemia. Drug Saf. 2014;37:677–92.
39. Sridharan K, Sivaramakrishnan G. Interaction of citrus juices with cyclosporine: systematic review and meta-analysis. Eur J Drug Metab Pharmacokinet. 2016;41(6):665–73.
40. Barraclough KA, Lee KJ, Staatz CE. Pharmacogenetic influences of mycophenolate therapy. Pharmacogenomics. 2010;11(3):369–90.
41. Gomez ED, Michaelover J, Frost P. Cutaneous beta-glucuronidase: cleavage of mycophenolic acid by preparations in mouse skin. Br J Dermatol. 1977;97(3):303–6.
42. Bullingham RE, Nicholls AJ, Kamm BR. Clinical pharmacokinetics of mycophenolate mofetil. Clin Pharmacokinet. 1998;34(6):429–55.

43. Atcheson BA, Taylor PJ, Mudge DW, Johnson DW, Hawley DM, Campbell SB, Isbel NM, Pillans PI, Tett SE. Mycophenolic acid pharmacokinetics and related outcomes early after renal transplant. Br J Clin Pharmacol. 2005;59(3):271–80.

44. Wolverton SE, et al. Comprehensive dermatologic drug therapy. Mycophenolate Mofetil. 3rd ed. Philadelphia: Elsevier; 2013. p. 190–1.

45. Brennan DC, Ramos E. Renal transplantation and the older adult patient. UpToDate. 2016.; (Accessed on May 27, 2016)

46. George L, Hamann I, Chen K, Choi J, Fernandez-Penas P. An analysis of the dermatological uses of Mycophenolate Mofetil in a tertiary hospital. J Dermatolog Treat. 2015;26(1):63–6.

47. Beissert S, Pauser S, Sticherling M, Frieling U, Loske KD, Frosch PJ, Haase I, Luger TA. A comparison of mycophenolate mofetil with cyclosporine for the treatment of chronic plaque-type psoriasis. Dermatology. 2009;219(2):126–32.

48. Moreland LW, Margolies G, Heck LW, Saway A, Blosch C, Hanna R, et al. Recombinant soluble tumor necrosis factor receptor (p80) fusion protein: toxicity and dose finding trial in refractory rheumatoid arthritis. J Rheumatol. 1996;23(11): 1849–55.

49. Lee E, Trepicchio WL, Oestreicher JL, Pittman D, Wang F, Chamian F, et al. Increased expression of interleukin 23 p19 and p40 in lesional skin of patients with psoriasis vulgaris. J Exp Med. 2004;199(1):125–30.

50. Zaba LC, Cardinale I, Gilleaudeau P, Sullivan-Whalen M, Suárez-Fariñas M, Fuentes-Duculan J, et al. Amelioration of epidermal hyperplasia by TNF inhibition is associated with reduced Th17 responses. J Exp Med. 2007;204(13):3183–94.

51. Eyerich S, Eyerich K, Pennino D, Carbone T, Nasorri F, Pallotta S, et al. Th22 cells represent a distinct human T cell subset involved in epidermal immunity and remodeling. J Clin Invest. 2009;119(12):3573–85.

52. Scallon B, Cai A, Solowski N, Rosenberg A, Song XY, Shealy D, et al. Binding and functional comparisons of two types of tumor necrosis factor antagonists. J Pharmacol Exp Ther. 2002;301(2):418–26.

53. Zhou H, Patat A, Parks V, Buckwalter M, Metzger D, Korth-Bradley J. Absence of a pharmacokinetic interaction between etanercept and warfarin. J Clin Pharmacol. 2004;44(5):543–50.

54. Militello G, Zia A, Stevens SR, Van Voorhees AS. Etanercept for the treatment of psoriasis in the elderly. J Am Acad Dermatol. 2006;55:517–9.

55. Fleischmann R, Baumgartner SW, Weisman MH, Liu T, White B, Peloso P. Long term safety of etanercept in elderly subjects with rheumatic diseases. Ann Rheum Dis. 2006;65:379–84.

56. Burls A, Jobanputra P. The trials of anakinra. Lancet. 2004;364(9437):827–8.

57. Mamula P, Mascarenhas MR, Baldassano RN. Biological and novel therapies for inflammatory bowel disease in children. Pediatr Clin North Am. 2002;49(1):1–25.

58. Gottlieb AB, Masud S, Ramamurthi R, Abdulghani A, Romano P, Chaudhari U, et al. Pharmacodynamic and pharmacokinetic response to anti-tumor necrosis factor-alpha monoclonal antibody (infliximab) treatment of moderate to severe psoriasis vulgaris. J Am Acad Dermatol. 2003;48(1):68–75.

59. Singh R, Cuchacovich R, Huang W, Espinoza LR. Infliximab treatment in a patient with rheumatoid arthritis on hemodialysis. J Rheumatol. 2002;29(3):636–7.

60. Zeltser R, Valle L, Tanck C, Holyst MM, Ritchlin C, Gaspari AA. Clinical, histological, and immunophenotypic characteristics of injection site reactions associated with etanercept: a recombinant tumor necrosis factor alpha receptor: Fc fusion protein. Arch Dermatol. 2001;137(7):893–9.

61. Gottlieb AB, Evans R, Li S, Dooley LT, Guzzo CA, Baker D, et al. Infliximab induction therapy for patients with severe plaque-type psoriasis: a randomized, double-blind, placebo-controlled trial. J Am Acad Dermatol. 2004;51(4):534–42.

62. Garber C, Plotnikova N, SC A, Sorensen EP, Gottlieb A. Biologic and conventional systemic therapies show similar safety and efficacy in elderly and adult patients with moderate to severe psoriasis. J Drugs Dermatol. 2015;14(8):846–52.

63. Infliximab [package insert] Available from: URL: http://www.remicade.com/remicade/assets/HCP_PPI.pdf. Accessed April 1, 2010.

64. Khanna D, McMahon M, therapy FDE A-t n f a, failure h. What have we learned and where do we go from here? Arthritis Rheum. 2004;50(4):1040–50.

65. Gordon KB, Langley RG, Leonardi C, Toth D, Menter MA, Kang S, et al. Clinical response to adalimumab treatment in patients with moderate to severe psoriasis: double-blind, randomized controlled trial and open-label extension study. J Am Acad Dermatol. 2006;55(4):598–606.

66. Menter A, Tyring SK, Gordon K, Kimball AB, Leonardi CL, Langley RB, et al. Adalimumab therapy for moderate to severe psoriasis: a randomized, controlled phase III trial. J Am Acad Dermatol. 2008;58(1):106–15.

67. Weisman MH, Moreland LW, Furst DE, Weinblatt ME, Keystone EC, Paulus HE, et al. Efficacy, pharmacokinetic, and safety assessment of adalimumab, a fully human anti-tumor necrosis factor-alpha monoclonal antibody, in adults with rheumatoid arthritis receiving concomitant methotrexate: a pilot study. Clin Ther. 2003;25(6):1700–21.

68. Baecklund E, Iliadou A, Askling J, Ekbom A, Backlin C, Granath F, et al. Association of chronic inflammation, not its treatment, with increased lymphoma risk in rheumatoid arthritis. Arthritis Rheum. 2006;54(3):692–701.

69. Gelfand JM, Berlin J, Van Voorhees A, Margolis DJ. Lymphoma rates are low but increased in patients with psoriasis: results from a population-based cohort study in the United Kingdom. Arch Dermatol. 2003;139(11):1425–9.

70. Dommasch E, Gelfand JM. Is there truly a risk of lymphoma from biologic therapies? Dermatol Ther. 2009;22(5):418–30.

71. Krathen MS, Gottlieb AB, Mease PJ. Pharmacologic immunomodulation and cutaneous malignancy in rheumatoid arthritis, psoriasis, and psoriatic arthritis. J Rheumatol. 2010;37(11):2205–15.

72. Bechtel M, Sanders C, Bechtel A. Neurological complications of biologic therapy in psoriasis: a review. J Clin Aesthet Dermatol. 2009;2(11):27–32.

73. Wallis RS. Tumor necrosis factor antagonists: structure, function, and tuberculosis risks. Lancet Infect Dis. 2008;8(10):601–11.

74. Tsiodras S, Samonis G, Boumpas DT, Kontoyiannis DP. Fungal infections complicating tumor necrosis factor alpha blockade therapy. Mayo Clin Proc. 2008;83(2):181–94.

75. Carroll MB, Forgione MA. Use of tumor necrosis factor alpha inhibitors in hepatitis B surface antigen-positive patients: a literature review and potential mechanisms of action. Clin Rheumatol. 2010;29(9):1021–9.

76. Winthrop KL, Baddley JW, Chen L, Liu L, Grijalva CG, Delzell E, et al. Association between the initiation of anti-tumor necrosis factor therapy and the risk of Herpes Zoster. JAMA Dermatol. 2013;309(9):887–95.

77. Listing J, Strangfeld A, Kekow J, Schneider M, Kapelle A, Wassenberg S, et al. Does tumor necrosis factor alpha inhibition promote or prevent heart failure in patients with rheumatoid arthritis? Arthritis Rheum. 2008;58(3):667–77.

78. Papp K, Langley R, Lebwohl M, Krueger GG, Szapary P, Yeilding N, et al. Efficacy and safety of ustekinumab, a human interleukin-12/23 monoclonal antibody, in patients with psoriasis: 52-week results from a randomized, double-blind, placebo-controlled trial (PHOENIX 2). Lancet. 2008;371:1675–84.

79. Langley R, Lebwohl M, Krueger G, Szapary PO, Wasfi Y, Chan D, et al. Long-term efficacy and safety of ustekinumab, with and without dosing adjustment, in patients with moderate-to-severe

psoriasis: results from the PHOENIX 2 study through 5 years of follow-up. Br J Dermatol. 2015;172:1371–83.

80. Megna M, Napolitano M, Balato N, Monfrecola G, Villani A, Ayala F, et al. Efficacy and safety of ustekinumab in a group of 22 elderly patients with psoriasis over a 2-year period. Clin Exp Dermatol. 2016;41:564–6.

81. Kalb RE, Fiorentino DF, Lebwohl MG, Toole J, Poulin Y, Cohen AD, et al. Risk of serious infection with biologic and systemic treatment of psoriasis: results from the Psoriasis Longitudinal Assessment and Registry (PSOLAR). JAMA Dermatol. 2015;151:961–9.

82. Brodmerkel C, Wadman E, Langley RG, Papp KA, Bourcier M, Poulin Y, et al. Immune response to pneumococcus and tetanus toxoid in patients with moderate-to-severe psoriasis following long-term ustekinumab use. J Drugs Dermatol. 2013;12: 1122–9.

83. Gottlieb AB, Kalb RE, Langley RG, Krueger GG, de Jong EM, Guenther L, et al. Safety observations in 12095 patients with psoriasis enrolled in an international registry (PSOLAR): experience with infliximab and other systemic and biologic therapies. J Drugs Dermatol. 2014;13:1441–8.

84. Papp K, Griffiths C, Gordon K, Lebwohl M, Szapary P, Wasfi Y, et al. Long-term safety of ustekinumab in patients with moderate-to-severe psoriasis: final results from 5 years of follow-up. Br J Dermatol. 2013;168:844–54.

85. Langley R, Elewski B, Lebwohl M, Reich K, Griffith CE, Papp K, et al. Secukinumab in plaque psoriasis—results of two phase 3 trials. N Engl J Med. 2014;371:326–38.

86. Blauvelt A, Prinz J, Gottlieb A, Kingo K, Sofen H, Ruer-Mulard M, et al. Secukinumab administration by pre-filled syringe: efficacy, safety and usability results from a randomized controlled trial in psoriasis (FEATURE). Br J Dermatol. 2014;172:484–93.

87. Paul C, Lacour JP, Tedremets L, Kreutzer K, Jazayeri S, Adams S, et al. Efficacy, safety and usability of secukinumab administration by autoinjector/pen in psoriasis: a randomized, controlled trial (JUNCTURE). J Eur Acad Dermatol. 2015b;29:1082–90.

88. Gordon KB, Blauvelt A, Papp KA, Langley RG, Luger T, Ohtsuki M, et al. Phase 3 trials of Ixekizumab in moderate-to-severe plaque psoriasis. N Engl J Med. 2016;375:345–56.

89. Strober B, Leonardi C, Papp K, Mrowietz U, Ohtsuki M, Bissonnette R, et al. Short and long-term safety outcomes with ixekizumab from 7 clinical trials in psoriasis: Etanercept comparisons and integrated data. J Am Acad Dermatol. 2016. https://doi.org/10.1016/j.jaad.2016.09.026.

90. Gisondi P, Girolomoni G. Apremilast in the therapy of moderate to sever chronic plaque psoriasis. Drug Des Devel Ther. 2016;10:1763–70.

91. Paul C, Cather J, Gooderham M, Poulin Y, Mrowietz U, Ferrandiz C, et al. Efficacy and safety of apremilast, an oral phosphodiesterase 4 inhibitor, in patients with moderate-to-severe plaque psoriasis over 52 weeks: a phase III, randomized controlled trial (ESTEEM 2). Br J Dermatol. 2015a;173(6):1387–99.

92. Rich R, Gooderham M, Bachelez H, Goncalves J, Day R, Chen R, et al. Apremilast, an oral phosphodiesterase 4 inhibitor, in patients with difficult to treat nail and scalp psoriasis: results of 2 phase III randomized, controlled trials (ESTEEM 1 and ESTEEM 2). J Am Acad Dermatol. 2016;74(1):134–42.

93. Gooderham M, Papp K. Selective Phosphodiesterase inhibitors for psoriasis: focus on Apremilast. BioDrugs. 2015;29(5):327–39.

94. Otezla® [package insert]. Celgene, Inc. Mississauga, ON. 2015. http://www.celgenecanada.net/pdfs/Otezla_Product_Monograph_English_Version.pdf.

Miscellaneous Uses of Biologic and Systemic Agents in Other Dermatologic Conditions

Grace W. Kimmel, John K. Nia, Peter W. Hashim, and Mark G. Lebwohl

Introduction

Biologics and related systemic agents were originally developed for use in a variety of rheumatologic and dermatologic conditions, including plaque psoriasis, psoriatic arthritis, and rheumatoid arthritis. These medications have dramatically changed the treatment and course of such diseases. Given their remarkable success in the treatment of the diseases for which they were originally tested, many have been used off-label in other conditions also thought to be characterized by autoimmune and inflammatory pathways. There are many reports of off-label uses of these drugs in the treatment of a range of dermatologic diseases, which we will explore here.

Erythrodermic Psoriasis

Erythrodermic psoriasis (EP) is a severe variation of psoriasis characterized by the presence of diffuse erythema, desquamation, and possible systemic symptoms. It often occurs in patients with preexisting plaque psoriasis, with potential triggers including infections, trauma to the skin, emotional stress, and withdrawal of anti-psoriatic treatment. In acute and rapidly progressing forms, EP can be life-threatening; such patients may present in septic shock. Treatment of this condition can be difficult, as there is little high-quality, evidence-based data to support the use of one specific medication over another [1]. The Medical Board of the National Psoriasis Foundation consensus guidelines published in 2010 recommend the use of cyclosporine or infliximab for severe, acute cases, as these are typically the most rapidly acting agents. Acitretin and methotrexate are also recommended as first-line therapies, although these are less rapidly acting. Etanercept or combination therapies are often second-line treatment options [2].

Notably, the traditional agents used in EP treatment, including acitretin, cyclosporine, and methotrexate, can be limited by treatment failure, inconvenience, or the occurrence of complications [1, 3, 4]. In recent years, as reflected in the treatment guidelines mentioned above, the biologics have shown promise as possible treatment alternatives. Although no large, randomized controlled trials have been performed in EP, as such patients are often excluded from the clinical trials for psoriasis, several case reports and small case studies have been published.

Infliximab, a chimeric mouse-human antitumor necrosis factor alpha (TNF-α) monoclonal antibody, is the most frequently reported biologic agent used in the treatment of EP [1]. Several case studies/small case series have been reported in the literature citing successful treatment with infliximab [5, 6]. In additional to these case reports, Poulalhon et al. [7] reported an open-label, uncontrolled clinical trial of five cases of EP treated with infliximab; after 14 weeks of treatment, results of Psoriasis Area and Severity Index (PASI) 90, PASI 75, and PASI 50 were seen in 40%, 60%, and 60% of cases, respectively.

Etanercept, a fully human recombinant fusion protein that binds to and inhibits TNF, has also been reported in the treatment of EP. Esposito et al. [4] published a 24-week open-label, uncontrolled clinical trial of 10 EP patients treated with etanercept; week 12 results of PASI 50 and PASI 75 were seen in 80% and 50% of cases, respectively. At week 24, all of the responders showed maintenance of at least PASI 50 response, with 75% remaining at or achieving PASI 75. Treatment was well tolerated. In addition, one case report of refractory EP in a pediatric patient treated with etanercept demonstrated an excellent treatment response without note of adverse effects [8].

Adalimumab is a fully human IgG1 monoclonal antibody against TNF-α used in the treatment of plaque psoriasis, among other conditions. Richetta et al. [9] reported a hepatitis

G.W. Kimmel, MD (✉) • J.K. Nia, MD
P.W. Hashim, MD, MHS • M.G. Lebwohl, MD
Department of Dermatology, Icahn School of Medicine at Mount Sinai, 5 East 98th Street, 5th Floor, New York, NY 10029, USA
e-mail: grace.kimmel@mssm.edu; john.nia@mssm.edu; peter.hashim@mssm.edu; Lebwohl@aol.com

© Springer International Publishing AG 2018
P.S. Yamauchi (ed.), *Biologic and Systemic Agents in Dermatology*, https://doi.org/10.1007/978-3-319-66884-0_30

C virus (HCV)-positive patient who developed resistant EP after anti-HCV therapy; treatment with adalimumab resulted in remission by week 3 of treatment with no reported adverse effects.

Ustekinumab is a fully human monoclonal antibody against the p40 subunit of interleukin (IL)-12 and IL-23, used in the treatment of plaque psoriasis. Several case studies and small case series have supported its use in the treatment of EP. One case series by Wang et al. [10] of 8 Chinese patients with EP treated with ustekinumab showed week 12 responses of PASI 50, PASI 75, and PASI 90 of 62.5%, 50%, and 12.5%, respectively. Week 28 results were even more impressive, with PASI 50, PASI 75, and PASI 90 responses of 75%, 50%, and 37.5%, respectively. A multicenter, retrospective study performed in Italy by Pescitelli et al. [11] evaluated 22 patients with EP treated with ustekinumab. At week 4, >50% of patients had at least a PASI 50 response, and at week 16, about two-thirds of patients achieved PASI 75. By week 28, 68.2% reached PASI 90, and 90.9% of patients achieved PASI 50. Long-term treatment success up to week 60 was observed, with only two patients withdrawing due to treatment failure. Additionally, there are reports of refractory EP patients who have failed treatment with TNF inhibitors who have responded successfully to ustekinumab [12, 13].

Although there has been little comparison between the difference biologic agents in the treatment of EP, one multicenter, retrospective study performed in France by Viguier et al. [14] evaluated 28 EP patients with a total of 42 flares who were treated with either infliximab ($n = 24$), adalimumab ($n = 7$), etanercept ($n = 6$), ustekinumab ($n = 3$), or efalizumab ($n = 2$). A successful result, defined by ≥75% improvement in body surface area (BSA) or Psoriasis Area and Severity Index (PASI) after 12–14 weeks of treatment, was found in 48% of flares treated with infliximab, 50% of flares treated with adalimumab, and 40% of flares treated with etanercept. Efalizumab showed no clinical benefit. Of the three patients treated with ustekinumab, one patient showed 50% improvement. Notably, despite this short-term efficacy, only one-third of patients remained on the same treatment at the 1-year time mark, as treatment switches due to treatment failure or side effects were common. The most significant safety concern was for serious infections. This study highlights the need for larger, long-term studies to further evaluate long-term efficacy and side effect profiles of biologic agents in the treatment of EP.

Pustular Psoriasis

Pustular psoriasis is another rare variation of psoriasis that may also be challenging to treat. Presenting clinically with many small pustules on a background of erythema, pustular psoriasis can be localized or generalized. Generalized forms may be severe and even life-threatening. In similarity with erythrodermic psoriasis, there are few high-quality, evidence-based studies on which to base management. Conventional agents including acitretin, methotrexate, and cyclosporine have been used in treatment of this condition; but again side effects and lack of efficacy may limit their usage. Biologic agents have been used in the treatment of pustular psoriasis patients in recent years, although to date no large clinical trials have been performed [15].

There are multiple reports of successful treatment of generalized pustular psoriasis (GPP) with infliximab (3–5 mg/kg^2) [16–18]. In one, patients had resolution of lesions as soon as within 48–72 h of infliximab infusion. No serious adverse effects were noted [16]. Given its fast onset of action, it was proposed as a first-line treatment for severe, acute cases of GPP by the Medical Board of the National Psoriasis Foundation in 2012 [15].

Adalimumab has also been reported in the treatment of pustular psoriasis. Adalimumab has been used successfully after secondary failure of infliximab therapy in several GPP patients [19]. It has also has been used in the treatment of pediatric GPP patients, including those who have failed treatment with conventional therapies and other biologics, with good efficacy [20, 21].

Case reports of successful treatment of generalized pustular psoriasis with ustekinumab have additionally been reported in recent years. In one, an elderly female who failed or could not tolerate methotrexate, acitretin, cyclosporine, and adalimumab had rapid clearing of her pustular psoriasis with ustekinumab, and maintained clear skin on maintenance dosing of the drug [22]. Another case report also detailed a recalcitrant GPP patient who had both short- and long-term success with ustekinumab treatment [22]. Localized palmoplantar pustular psoriasis has additionally been treated successfully with ustekinumab; one small case series of nine patients showed an average improvement in palmoplantar PASI scores of 71.6% after 24 weeks of treatment, with no major adverse effects [23].

Etanercept is another biologic that has shown utility in pustular psoriasis treatment. In one case of generalized annular pustular psoriasis, reported by Lo Shiavo et al. [24], the patient experienced complete clearance of pustular lesions within the first week of therapy with etanercept. Maintenance therapy was continued successfully. Fialova et al. [25] also described successful treatment of a pediatric GPP patient with etanercept, resulting in complete skin clearance at 6 months of therapy. In addition, etanercept showed good long-term efficacy in the treatment of a pediatric patient with palmoplantar pustular psoriasis. Although the response to treatment in this case was somewhat slow, it was progressive, with significant and sustained improvement over the course of months [26].

Secukinumab, an anti-IL-17A human monoclonal antibody approved for the treatment of plaque psoriasis, has been reported in the successful treatment of pustular psoriasis in a few cases [27, 28]. Polesie et al. [27] reported a patient with refractory disease who had clearing of lesions within 3 weeks of treatment initiation, and experienced maintained remission with continued dosing.

Despite the success of biologic agents in treating pustular psoriasis as reported in these case reports, it is notable that there are also multiple reports in the literature of pustular psoriasis being triggered by biologic agents. New-onset psoriasis, particularly pustular psoriasis, has been described as a paradoxical phenomenon in some patients started on TNF-α inhibitors including infliximab, etanercept, and adalimumab [29]. Ustekinumab has also been reported in some cases to induce flares of pustular psoriasis [30, 31]. The etiology of these responses remains unclear.

Hidradenitis Suppurativa

Hidradenitis supportive (HS) is a chronic, relapsing, inflammatory skin disease affecting the hair follicles. It is characterized by inflammatory skin nodules and abscesses in the apocrine gland-bearing areas of skin. Rupture of these lesions is common, leading to scarring and sinus tract formation. HS is notoriously difficult to treat. Adalimumab is currently the only approved treatment for moderate-to-severe HS. In the phase III trials (PIONEER I and II), patients receiving adalimumab had significantly better clinical response rates (defines as ≥50% reduction in abscess and inflammatory nodule count, and no increase in abscess and draining fistula count) at week 12 than those on placebo; 41.8% vs. 26% in PIONEER I and 58.9% vs. 27.6% in PIONEER II. Treatment was well tolerated, with adverse event rates similar to the placebo groups [32]. However, it is notable that there have also been case reports of HS paradoxically induced by adalimumab. Delobeau et al. [33] published a case series consisting of 4 patients with adalimumab paradoxically induced HS; time from adalimumab initiation to HS onset or exacerbation ranged from weeks to years. The pathogenesis behind such responses is unknown.

Other biologics have also been tried off-label in the treatment of HS. Successful use of infliximab has been described in case studies [34, 35]. In addition, a randomized, double-blind, placebo-controlled trial of infliximab in 38 moderate-to-severe HS patients was performed by Grant et al. [36]; 26% of patients in the treatment group experienced a ≥ 50% improvement in disease severity, as compared to only 5% of patients in the placebo group.

A systematic review by van Rappard et al. [37] reviewed 65 studies including 459 HS patients; four studies were randomized controlled trials whereas the rest were case reports or series. Overall, moderate-to-good responses were seen with infliximab (82%), adalimumab (76%), and etanercept (68%). Based on this evidence, the authors suggested that TNF-α inhibitors be tried in cases where conventional therapies have failed, with a preference for infliximab given that it has shown the most promising results thus far. Conversely, etanercept use was discouraged. Similarly, a randomized, double-blind, placebo-controlled clinical trial consisting of 20 moderate-to-severe HS patients failed to show benefit for treatment with etanercept 50 mg SC twice weekly, when compared to placebo at week 12 [38]. Another review by Haslund et al. [39] reported a positive treatment outcome for many patients treated with TNF-α inhibitors, but few patients (15/105) had long-term remission (≥3 months) after end of treatment. This again highlights the need for longer-term larger studies of these agents for use in HS.

In addition to TNF-α inhibitors, ustekinumab has also been used in a small number of cases for the treatment of HS. Gulliver et al. [40] described a case series of three patients with moderate-to-severe HS treated with 3–45 mg subcutaneous injections of ustekinumab at months 0, 1, and 4. One patient experienced complete disease remission; one patient saw some improvement (25–49%); and the third patient had no improvement. There are a few additional case reports in the literature citing successful treatment of HS with ustekinumab; however, improvement has been noted to take place slowly, over the period of several months [41–43].

Toxic Epidermal Necrolysis

Toxic epidermal necrolysis (TEN) is a severe adverse drug reaction resulting in full thickness epidermal necrosis with blistering and sloughing of the skin. TEN can be life-threatening. Treatment of this condition is often challenging, as there is no standardized treatment regimen, and little data is available to recommend one therapy over another. Although the pathogenesis underlying TEN remains unclear, high levels of TNF have been found in TEN-affected skin [44]. Therefore, biologic agents, particularly TNF-α inhibitors, have been tried off-label in the treatment of TEN.

Paradisi et al. [45] described a case series of 10 TEN patients treated with a single 50 mg subcutaneous dose of etanercept. All patients in this series responded quickly to treatment, and had complete reepithelialization with a mean healing time of 8.5 days. No adverse reactions were reported. Another case report of a patient who developed TEN after rituximab infusion also describes disease improvement and eventual clearance following etanercept treatment [46].

The similarly appearing condition toxic epidermal necrolysis-like acute cutaneous lupus erythematosus, which does not occur due to a drug exposure but rather to underlying autoimmune disease, has also been treated successfully with etanercept in a case series of three patients. Rapid clearance of the skin was seen following a single dose [47].

Successful use of infliximab in the treatment of TEN has also been described. Fischer et al. [48] reported a case of TEN in an adult patient following antibiotic exposure, which was treated with a single dose of infliximab. The progression of disease ceased after injection, and blisters/erythema resolved completely with only residual post-inflammatory pigmentary changes. A case series of four adult patients with TEN and extensive skin detachment also showed success with single dose infliximab treatment (300 mg); all four patients had complete reepithelialization. Although three patients developed bacteremia, none progressed to sepsis or septic shock, and mortality rate was 0% [49]. Infliximab has also been used with good results in a pediatric patient; Scott-Lang et al. [50] successfully treated a 7-year-old patient with TEN refractory to intravenous immunoglobulin therapy with infliximab. Rapid and marked improvement was also noted in this case.

Alopecia Areata

Alopecia areata (AA) is a relatively common immune-mediated disease, characterized by damage to the hair follicles resulting in hair loss. Some AA patients may have spontaneous regrowth, but others have rapidly progressive and severe disease. AA can progress to cause complete hair loss on the scalp (alopecia totalis, AT) or the entire body (alopecia universalis, AU). No FDA-approved treatment exists; common treatment options include topical, injected, or oral steroids, topical immunotherapy, phototherapy, and laser treatments [51]. However, AA may be refractory to these therapies and therefore biologic and other systemic agents have been tried as potential novel therapy options.

Janus kinase (JAK) inhibitors block numerous cytokine signaling pathways related to inflammation and have been trialed in the treatment of a variety of dermatologic conditions, including AA. In one case series, three patients with moderate-to-severe AA were treated with oral ruxolitinib (20 mg PO BID), which inhibits JAK1 and JAK2. All three experienced almost full hair regrowth within 3–5 months of treatment [52]. An open-label clinical trial of 12 patients treated with ruxolitinib for 3–6 months also showed success, with 9/12 patients showing significant (≥50%) improvement [53]. Tofacitinib, an inhibitor of JAK1 and JAK3, has also shown promising results. A patient coexisting alopecia universalis and psoriasis treated with tofacitinib experienced complete regrowth of scalp hair at 5 months, with significant regrowth noted in other areas. No adverse effects were noted [54]. A retrospective case study of adult patients with at least 40% scalp hair loss treated with tofacitinib was recently performed by Liu et al. [55], and found that of 65 potential responders, 77% had a clinical response to treatment and

58% had ≥50% improvement over 4–18 months of treatment. AA patients were noted to have greater improvement than AT/AU patients (81.8% vs. 59%). No serious adverse effects were reported. Additionally, the JAK1 and JAK2 inhibitor baricitinib has also been used successfully in AA; a 17-year-old patient described by Jabbari et al. [56] had complete hair regrowth on the scalp within 9 months of treatment initiation. These and other small studies show the promise of JAK inhibitors that will hopefully become even more apparent in future larger scale trials.

Ustekinumab has also been studied in the treatment of a small number of AA patients. Guttman-Yassky et al. [57] reported a case series consisting of 3 AA patients treated with ustekinumab 90 mg subcutaneously at weeks 0, 4, and 16. All three patients had hair regrowth at week 20, to varying degrees. At week 20, one patient with a 2-year history of alopecia universalis experienced regrowth of all eyebrows and body hair and 85% of scalp hair; full scalp regrowth was noted by week 49. The other two patients, who each presented with ~40% scalp involvement, also had improvement but to a somewhat lesser degree than the AU patient. Of these two, the patient with the shorter disease history had superior results. No adverse effects were reported.

It is also notable that AA may be triggered by treatment with some biologic agents. Alopecia has been described to occur as a rare adverse event in some patients treated with TNF-α inhibitors, particularly infliximab [58, 59]. One patient with psoriasis who developed alopecia after infliximab was then successfully treated for both conditions with ustekinumab [60].

Multicentric Reticulohistiocytosis

Multicentric reticulohistiocytosis (MRH) is a rare systemic disease characterized by tissue infiltration with histiocytes and multicentric giant cells. Patients frequently present with skin and joint involvement, and malignancies are also common in these patients. Skin findings frequently include widespread red-brown papulo-nodules that may coalesce into plaques. Although the disease often has spontaneous resolution after several years, early treatment is important, especially in preventing bone deformities. However, no treatment guidelines for MRH exist [61].

Given that histiocytes and TNF-α are found in the inflammatory infiltrate seen in MRH, TNF-α inhibitors have been tried in the treatment of MRH [61]. Infliximab is the most commonly used TNF inhibitor in MRH, typically dosed at 3 or 5 mg/kg at weeks 0, 2, 6 then every 8 weeks [61]. Reported treatment results vary. In one case report, the patient's joint symptoms significantly improved, without much change in skin lesions [62]. In other cases, skin disease improves, without effect on joint symptoms [63]. Other patients had improvement in skin disease and arthritis, but persistence of joint deformities and intermittent arthralgias [61, 64]. Adalimumab, dosed at 40 mg every other week, has also been used in the treatment of MRH. Again, results are variable. In one case, joint symptoms improved, but skin disease remained [65]. In another, skin disease was improved, but arthalgias persisted [66]. Etanercept 25 mg twice weekly has shown good results for both skin and joint manifestations in some patients [67, 68]. However, there are also reports of patients who failed treatment with etanercept [63, 64].

Cicatricial Pemphigoid

Cicatricial pemphigoid (mucus membrane pemphigoid) is a group of diseases characterized by chronic, relapsing blistering of the mucous membranes. Disease may be severe and result in scarring. Treatment of this condition can be difficult, as some patients fail or cannot tolerate conventional therapies such as steroids or other systemic anti-inflammatory or immunosuppressive medications.

Etanercept has been studied for use in the treatment of cicatricial pemphigoid. Canizares et al. [69] described a case series of three patients, all of whom had mucous membrane involvement and one of whom also had ocular involvement, treated with etanercept 25 mg subcutaneously twice weekly. All patients had improvement in oral lesions, and the patient with ocular disease experienced stabilization of disease. Other case reports also cite similar success with etanercept, including long-term remission, up to 18 months in one case [70, 71]. Rituxumab, a monoclonal antibody against the CD20 antigen of B-cells, has also been reported to have utility in treatment of cicatricial pemphigoid. One trial of 49 patients comparing the addition of rituximab to conventional immunosuppression versus conventional immunosuppression alone found that more patients who had the addition of rituximab achieved disease control (100% vs. 40%, respectively) [72].

Vitiligo

Vitiligo is a condition characterized by depigmented patches of skin, occurring secondary to destruction of melanocytes. The exact pathophysiology underlying the disease is unclear, but is thought to involve the immune system and inflammatory cytokines. It has been found that levels of TNF are increased in areas of skin affected by vitiligo, and directly associate with progressive depigmentation [73]. Therefore, TNF-α inhibitors have been tried as possible treatment for this disease, which can be difficult to treat and/or refractory to currently available therapies.

One clinical pilot study by Alghamdi et al. [74] evaluated six patients with widespread vitiligo treated with TNF-α inhibitors including infliximab, etanercept, and adalimumab,

administered according to the psoriasis treatment guidelines. One patient had disease progression, but 83% of the patients experienced stabilization of disease without progression for 6 months after completion of treatment. Other small case series have reported similar results of disease stabilization. Notably, this is not always followed by repigmentation [75].

Despite the reports of success in disease stabilization, there are also case reports documenting the paradoxical reaction of induction of vitiligo with TNF-α inhibitors. One case series of 10 patients reported new-onset nonsegmental vitiligo occurring in patients undergoing treatment with adalimumab (7 patients), infliximab (1 patient), ustekinumab (1 patient), and secukinumab (1 patient) for non-vitiligo indications. Mean time from medication initiation to onset of vitiligo lesions was quite long, at 17.4 ± 15.8 months [76]. A 2015 review by Webb et al. [75] found that of the 5928 patients reported in several case reports and observational studies of patients treated with TNF-α inhibitors for non-vitiligo conditions, only 18 developed de novo vitiligo while on therapy. Despite this reaction being relatively rare, these reports may limit more frequent use of TNF-α inhibitors in the treatment of vitiligo until more data is available.

Systemic Autoimmune Diseases

Biologic and systemic agents have been trialed off-label as treatment options in a number of systemic autoimmune diseases with dermatologic manifestations, including Behçet's disease, sarcoidosis, and others.

Behçet's disease (BD) is a systemic inflammatory vasculitis characterized clinically by recurrent oral and genital ulcers, cutaneous lesions, and uveitis. The presence of uveitis and/or central nervous system (CNS) involvement can lead to high morbidity, and overall mortality in this condition has been reported at 5% over a median of 7.7 years [77]. Treatment may involve colchicine, NSAIDs, topical agents, and immunosuppression for more severe manifestations. However, some patients may be refractory to these treatments and risk the development of irreversible organ damage [78]. TNF-α inhibitors have been used off-label successfully in the treatment of BD. A multicenter study performed by Vallet et al. [78] evaluated the outcomes of TNF-α inhibitors in 124 BD patients with severe and/or refractory disease manifestations. Treatment mainly consisted of infliximab (62%) and adalimumab (30%). Complete or partial response to treatment was seen in 90.4% of patients. Response rates for severe and/or refractory ocular, mucocutaneous, joint, gastrointestinal, CNS, and cardiovascular manifestations were reported at 96.3%, 88%, 70%, 77.8%, 92.3%, and 66.7%, respectively. Number of flares per year was also significantly lower during the TNF-α inhibitor treatment period than before, and patients were also able to significantly lower their prednisone dosages.

Arida et al. [79] reviewed available data on a total of 369 patients treated with TNF-α inhibitors for BD. In terms of the mucocutaneous manifestations of BD, the majority of patients treated with infliximab, etanercept, or adalimumab experienced improvement. Infliximab was the most commonly used agent. Rapid remission was induced in 91% of cases of oral ulcers, 96% of genital ulcers, 81% of erythema nodosum lesions, and 77% of other skin lesions. Twenty-one percent of patients in prospective studies evaluating repeated infliximab injections had sustained remission of mucocutaneous lesion at a median follow-up of 12.9 months, and 69% had partial response. Although the majority of data thus far has come from case reports or uncontrolled studies, these results suggest that TNF-α inhibitors may have a promising role in the treatment of BD.

Sarcoidosis is another systemic disease in which biologic agents have been used off-label. Sarcoidosis is characterized by noncaseating granulomas which may occur in a variety of tissues, particularly the lungs, lymph nodes, skin, and eyes. The etiology is unknown. Steroids and other immunosuppressants are often used in treatment, but some patients may be refractory or intolerant to such therapies. Biologic agents, in particular TNF-α inhibitors, have shown promise in sarcoidosis treatment. TNF-targeted treatments were the first biologics to be used in sarcoidosis, given that TNF-α is an important mediator in the development of sarcoid granulomas, and is secreted by macrophages in active sarcoidosis patients [80, 81]. Thielen et al. [82] reported a case of refractory chronic cutaneous sarcoidosis that was unresponsive to standard dosages of TNF-α inhibitors, but became responsive with dose escalation. High-dose infliximab (at 7.5 mg/kg every other month) and high-dose adalimumab (at 80 mg every other week) showed greater efficacy in this case than high-dose etanercept. Other studies have also found etanercept to be less efficacious in the treatment of sarcoid, possibly because it is a TNF-receptor antagonist and may be less effective than the monoclonal anti-TNF antibodies in preventing the formation of granulomas [81]. Baughman et al. [83] performed a double-blind randomized clinical trial of infliximab for chronic pulmonary sarcoidosis, which included a subset analysis of 26 patients with cutaneous sarcoidosis. They found a significant improvement with infliximab versus placebo for desquamation and induration at week 24, but no significant change in erythema, percentage of area involved, or evaluation of paired photographs. Infliximab has also improved lung function in studies of pulmonary sarcoidosis, with improvement in vital capacity in patients refractory to steroid therapy [84]. A systematic review published in 2008 by Ramos-Casals et al. [85] of biologic use in systemic autoimmune diseases reported that overall, 99% of sarcoid patients improved on infliximab therapy. Another TNF-α inhibitor, adalimumab, has also been used successfully in the treatment of sarcoidosis patients with refractory chronic uveitis and refractory pulmonary sarcoidosis [86, 87]. A double-blind, randomized, placebo-controlled trial of adalimumab in the treatment of 16 patients with cutaneous sarcoidosis found that there was significant improvement in target lesion area, target lesion volume, and Dermatology Life Quality Index score with adalimumab treatment. However, at 8 weeks after treatment cessation, there was some disease regression [88].

Notably, there are also case reports of paradoxical sarcoidosis development during treatment with TNF-α inhibitors for non-sarcoid conditions. Burns et al. [89] reported a case of cutaneous and pulmonary sarcoidosis development during etanercept therapy for rheumatoid arthritis, both of which were successfully treated with a switch to adalimumab. Cathcart et al. [90] described a case of sarcoidosis development in a patient on etanercept therapy, and also performed a literature review of similar cases, published in 2012. They found a total of 34 described cases, including their own. The lung and nearby lymph nodes were the most common site of sarcoidosis, and symptoms started an average of 22 months after initiation TNF-α inhibitors. With the exception of one patient, all had resolution of sarcoidosis symptoms upon cessation of TNF-α inhibitor treatment, at an average of 5.2 months.

The systematic review mentioned above by Ramos-Casals et al. [85] also reported high therapeutic response rates with biologic agents in other autoimmune conditions, including rituximab for systemic lupus erythematosus (SLE; 90% improvement), Sjogren syndrome (91% improvement), antiphospholipid syndrome (92%), and cryoglobulinemia (87%). Infliximab had high reported success in sarcoid (99%), adult-onset Still disease (90%), and polychondritis (86%). Etanercept also had high success rates in the treatment of Behçet's disease, with 96% of patients experiencing a therapeutic response, but did not show efficacy for sarcoidosis. Most of this data came from uncontrolled, observational studies.

Pityriasis Rubra Pilaris

Pityriasis rubra pilaris (PRP) is a chronic papulosquamous disease characterized by orange-pink, scaly plaques with islands of sparing, follicular hyperkeratosis, and palmoplantar keratoderma. There are six types of PRP, with type 1 (classical, adult form) being the most common [91]. Topical agents, retinoids, methotrexate, and UV light therapy may be used in treatment, but patients can be refractory to these therapies. Upregulation of TNF has been found to occur in lesional PRP skin [92]. Therefore, TNF blockade has been trialed in the condition, and there are case reports of successful treatment of PRP with adalimumab, infliximab, and etanercept [93–96]. Petrof et al. [91] performed a systematic review of TNF-α inhibitors in the treatment of PRP type 1, including 15 evaluable cases. They found that 12 of these cases showed a complete response (defined as ≥80%), with a mean time of 5 months to maximal response.

Balanitis Xerotica Obliterans

Balanitis xerotica obliterans is a variant of lichen planus affecting the penis. Scarring as well as urinary and sexual morbidities can occur and often have significant impact on patients' quality of life. The pathogenesis is not fully understood, but is thought to involve autoimmune and inflammatory pathways. Treatment of balanitis xerotica obliterans is difficult. Topical steroids are often used a first-line treatment, but may not be effective, especially in preventing scarring [97]. Lowenstein et al. [98] described a case of balanitis xerotica obliterans treated with intralesional adalimumab at 40 mg every other week. Dramatic improvement was noted by week 2, with near-clearing of disease by week 4. Treatment was continued, biweekly for 3 months and every 6 weeks thereafter. He remained nearly clear for 8 months, at which point he had a relapse that occurred after he did not receive an injection for 10 weeks. However, this relapse was successfully treated with resumed adalimumab.

Cutaneous Crohn's Disease

Cutaneous Crohn's disease (CDC) is a rare variant of Crohn's disease, in which patients have mucocutaneous noncaseating granulomatous lesions without gastrointestinal involvement. Patients may present with ulcers, nodules, or erosions in flexural areas. Stingeni et al. [99] described a case of CDC resistant to steroid therapy that was successfully treated with adalimumab, which is often used in cases of gastrointestinal Crohn's disease. The patient had noted improvement after 2 weeks and near complete clearing of lesions by week 4. Remission was sustained with continued treatment. There are additional reports of successful treatment of vulvar Crohn's disease with TNF-α inhibitors [100].

Dissecting Cellulitis of the Scalp

Dissecting cellulitis of the scalp is a chronic inflammatory disease characterized clinically by nodules and abscesses on the scalp, often with sinus tract formation. Disease may progress to cause scarring alopecia. Treatment of dissecting cellulitis is notoriously difficult. There are case reports of successful treatment of the condition with adalimumab, including a case series of three patients who had rapid improvement of disease along with histopathologic improvement in inflammation. Notably, disease did relapse upon cessation of treatment [101].

Atopic Dermatitis

At present, the treatment for moderate-to-severe atopic dermatitis (AD) centers on systemic immunosuppressive agents, such as cyclosporine, methotrexate, mycophenolate mofetil, or prednisone. Given the unfavorable side effect profile of these therapies, research continues into biologics as a means to provide safe and effective treatment options.

Several case reports have reported successful use of ustekinumab in patients with severe AD [102–104]. Only a single randomized, placebo-controlled trial has been conducted to date. Khattri et al. [105] randomized 33 patients to receive either placebo or ustekinumab at weeks 0, 4, and 16 (according to psoriasis dosing protocol). Results showed higher SCORAD50 responses (a marker of 50% clinical improvement) in the ustekinumab group at weeks 12, 16, and 20 versus placebo, but the difference between groups was not statistically significant.

Aphthous Stomatitis

Severe recurrent aphthous stomatitis is associated with odynophagia and significant eating difficulties. Although effective treatment options are limited, growing evidence has emerged for the use of TNF-α inhibitors.

In a case series by Sand et al. [106], 18 patients were treated with either adalimumab, etanercept, infliximab, or golimumab. All patients had previously failed systemic therapies, such as colchicine, thalidomide, prednisone, azathioprine, or dapsone. Overall, 89% of patients treated with TNF-α inhibitors achieved complete or almost complete clearance, with 50% requiring transition to another TNF-α inhibitor before obtaining adequate response.

O'Neill [107] reviewed 16 cases, gathered from individual reports or small series, that showed successful treatment with TNF-α inhibitors. Previously failed therapies included colchicine, thalidomide, dapsone, or methotrexate. Three of the 16 patients were affected by isolated recurrent aphthous stomatitis, while the remainder exhibited aphthous stomatitis as a feature of Behçet's disease or Crohn's disease. The majority of patients obtained complete or almost complete clearance within four weeks. Notably, 5 of the 16 patients remained on adjunctive systemic treatment, most commonly methotrexate.

Granuloma Annulare

Whereas localized granuloma annulare (GA) is often self-resolving in nature, generalized GA is typically a chronic condition. Systemic therapy can be considered in generalized GA, although patients classically show poor responses.

Recently, off-label use of TNF-α inhibitors has gained popularity in the treatment of generalized GA. The majority of evidence lies with adalimumab, though select authors have reported success with infliximab or etanercept [108–111].

In the largest series to date, Min and Lebwohl [112] performed a single-center observational study of seven patients with generalized GA. All patients had previously failed topical or intralesional corticosteroids, with 57% having also failed phototherapy. Patients were treated with adalimumab 80 mg, followed by 40 mg 1 week later, and 40 mg every other week thereafter. Patients demonstrated significant improvements in erythema (average reduction of 88%), induration (average reduction of 95%), and affected body surface area (average reduction of 87%). Notably, two patients required an increase to weekly dosing, which lead to enhanced results. Additional case reports have supported the successful use of adalimumab in generalized GA [113–116].

Systemic Sclerosis/Morphea

Systemic sclerosis is characterized by progressive fibrosis of the skin as well as the internal organs. Given the limited number of effective treatment options, clinicians have recently investigated the possible utility of TNF-α inhibitors in this patient population.

Omair et al. [117] performed a longitudinal cohort study of 10 patients with systemic sclerosis and inflammatory arthritis who were treated with a TNF-α inhibitor (infliximab, etanercept, or adalimumab). Subjects were monitored for improvements in arthritis, skin fibrosis, and lung function (if interstitial lung disease was present). At 6 months, no improvements were found in the subjects' skin scores or pulmonary function tests, although arthritis symptoms did improve over 12 months of treatment. A systematic review similarly found efficacy with the use of TNF-α inhibitors in systemic sclerosis-related inflammatory arthritis, but there were no clear benefits identified in skin disease [118].

Rarely, morphea has been reported as an adverse event of TNF-α inhibitors [119–121]. Ramirez et al. [121] described the development of morphea in a patient treated with adalimumab for ankylosing spondylitis. The patient's lesions manifested 12 months after the initiation of therapy and resolved within 18 months of treatment discontinuation.

Pyoderma Gangrenosum

Pyoderma gangrenosum (PG) is a neutrophilic dermatosis characterized by painful cutaneous ulcers with a necrotic base [122]. Local and systemic corticosteroids, antibiotics, colchicine, methotrexate, and other agents are often used in treatment; however biologics have recently proven to be a useful tool in the treatment of PG [123].

In multiple case reports, infliximab has been shown to be efficacious in treating PG [123–129]. Tan et al. [123] reported two patients with Crohn's disease and concurrent PG refractory to standard treatments. Both patients saw rapid, dramatic improvement after receiving 5 mg/kg infusion of infliximab. Of note, the signs of PG returned several months after cessation of infliximab, with similar resolution after reinitiating infliximab therapy. In 2006, Regueiro et al. [129] found infliximab to be safe and effective for the treatment of PG by examining thirteen patients with moderate-to-severe PG refractory to medical therapy. All patients demonstrated complete healing of the skin lesions; three patients responded to induction infliximab therapy only, while the remaining 10 patients maintained clearance with infusions every 4–12 weeks. The dose of infliximab for PG varies across the different case reports. While some clinicians choose to use infliximab as a bridge to another therapy, many use infliximab as maintenance therapy. One study supports using infliximab at the same dose and schedule as the one approved for plaque psoriasis—an induction dose of 5 mg/kg at weeks 0, 2, 6 and a maintenance dose of 5 mg/kg every 8 weeks thereafter [124].

Adalimumab has demonstrated effectiveness in treating PG. Fonder et al. [130] described a patient with PG and inflammatory bowel disease refractory to azathioprine and infliximab that responded completely to adalimumab 80 mg every other week. There are other reports of the effectiveness of adalimumab monotherapy as well as in combination with other systemic immunosuppressant medications for PG. [130–132]

Etanercept has also shown to be efficacious for PG [133, 134]. Further, there are reports of certolizumab in combination with systemic steroids for treating PG. [135, 136]

Ustekinumab has been used to treat PG. Guenova et al. [137] were able to identify significant expression of IL23 A in a PG lesion. In an effort to suppress IL 23 expression, investigators initiated treatment with ustekinumab, a monoclonal antibody against the p40 subunit of IL 12 and 23. The patient saw complete clearance of her PG lesion fourteen weeks after commencing ustekinumab and maintained clearance 6 months after her final dose of ustekinumab.

Lichen Planus

Lichen planus (LP) has often been associated with medications, viruses, infections, and contact allergens [122]. While approximately 66% of patients see spontaneous resolution of their symptoms, many require treatment. Identifying and removing a potential causative agent is paramount. Topical, intralesional, and systemic corticosteroids are widely used in treatment, as well as phototherapy and systemic agents in more widespread disease. While there are reports that describe the efficacy of adalimumab in treating lichen planus [138, 139], there are reports that point to adalimumab as causing lichen planus [140, 141]. Infliximab has also been associated with inducing lichen planus in some cases [142, 143].

Sweet's Syndrome

Sweet's syndrome, also known as acute febrile neutrophilic dermatosis, is characterized by painful erythematous papules or plaques, fever, and leukocytosis. While the exact cause is unknown, many cases are associated with an underlying inflammatory process or malignancy [122]. Typically, lesions resolve on their own, however they return in roughly 30% of patients. Treatment is targeted at identifying and treating a potential causative agent. Prednisone has long been the standard of care in treating Sweet's syndrome. Subcutaneous Sweet's syndrome (SSS), a rare variant of Sweet's syndrome characterized by subcutaneous neutrophilic lesions, is notoriously difficult to treat. One case reported a patient with SSS refractory to treatment with oral prednisone that resolved completely with adalimumab monotherapy [144]. However, adalimumab has also been implicated in triggering Sweet's syndrome [145].

Necrobiosis Lipoidica

Necrobiosis lipoidica (NL) is characterized by an atrophic plaque typically found on the anterior surface of lower extremities, and is commonly associated with diabetes mellitus. Lesions generally begin as painful yellow patches that can progress to form an atrophic plaque with telangiectasias [122]. In addition to glycemic control, topical, systemic, and intralesional corticosteroids have been effective in treating NL. Zeichner et al. [146] described one case in which a 35-year-old female with NL, refractory to topical steroid and pulsed dye laser, responded to intralesional etanercept. Once weekly injections of etanercept 25 mg were given into the dermis at 1-cm intervals throughout the surface area of the lesion. Improvement was seen after the first month of treatment and continued over the next 8 months. In addition to intralesional etanercept, subcutaneous etanercept and adalimumab have been reported to improve NL lesions [147].

Dermatomyositis/Polymyositis

Dermatomyositis frequently occurs with other immune-mediated connective tissue disorders and, in adults, is often associated with an occult malignancy [122]. Long-term prednisone tapers have been an effective treatment for dermatomyositis, but some patients may be refractory or intolerant to this treatment. Riley et al. [148] treated five patients with juvenile dermatomyositis with infliximab. All five patients saw improvement in their symptoms. In one case of dermatomyositis refractory to conventional treatment as well as etanercept and infliximab, adalimumab was found to be successful [149]. However, there also have been case reports that associate TNF inhibitor use with the development or exacerbation of dermatomyositis and polymyositis [150, 151].

SAPHO Syndrome

Synovitis, acne, pustulosis, hyperostosis, and osteitis syndrome (SAPHO) is a neutrophilic dermatosis associated with osteoarticular lesions [122]. The increased expression of TNF-α in samples taken from bone led investigators to explore TNF inhibitors as a treatment option [152]. In multiple case reports, infliximab was shown to improve bone, joint, and cutaneous manifestations of SAPHO [152–155]. In a case series of six patients treated with different TNF inhibitors, Abdelghani et al. [156] found TNF inhibitors to be a viable treatment option for refractory cases of SAPHO; however 2 of the 3 patients treated with infliximab saw worsening cutaneous lesions after a promising initial response. Etanercept has also been found to provide rapid and lasting responses in patients with SAPHO, with symptoms returning after discontinuing therapy [156, 157]. Adalimumab has demonstrated efficacy in several case reports [156, 158–161]. Palmoplantar pustulosis and hidradenitis suppurativa were reported to occur in patients treated with different TNF inhibitors, although they have also been associated with SAPHO syndrome [156, 158, 160].

Conclusion

Biologic agents show great promise for the treatment of a variety of dermatologic conditions which to date have been difficult to treat. However, the majority of the data thus far has come from small numbers of case reports and case series, as highlighted in the above sections. The need for further studies, especially in the form of randomized, controlled clinical trials, will be of key importance to fully evaluate their efficacy and side effect profiles in these conditions. Hopefully, future research will continue to reveal success with novel treatment options for affected patients.

Case Report: Granuloma Annulare

A 67-year-old female was referred to our dermatology clinic in January 2014 with a 6–8 month history of generalized granuloma annulare, which had been refractory to intralesional and topical corticosteroid treatments. At initial presentation, she had extensive disease, with numerous skin-colored and erythematous papules and plaques present on the trunk, upper extremities, and lower extremities (Fig. 30.1). Biopsy findings were consistent with the diagnosis of granuloma annulare. Treatment with adalimumab was initiated with 80 mg subcutaneously, followed by 40 mg every other week starting 1 week after initiation. After 2 months of therapy, she saw >90% improvement, with only a few isolated papules remaining on the elbows. After 6 months of therapy, she had complete clearance, and adalimumab was then discontinued (Fig. 30.2). The patient had relapse of disease 3 months after treatment discontinuation, at which point she was restarted on adalimumab. She again had disease improvement, with nearly complete clearance after 6 months of therapy. She continued treatment for 1 year with sustained disease remission, at which point adalimumab was discontinued. Lesions recurred within 3 months of treatment discontinuation, and the patient was again restarted on adalimumab. At 6 month follow-up in November 2016, the patient was completely clear. She has continued treatment with adaliumumab 40 mg every other week since that time, with no adverse events or disease relapse noted.

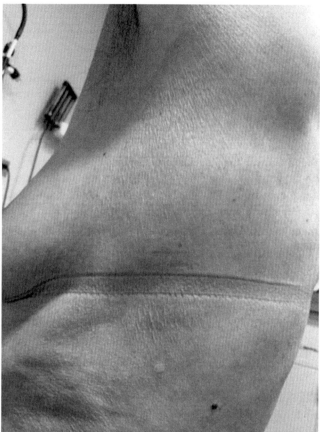

Fig. 30.2 Patient's trunk following treatment with adalimumab, showing clearance of granuloma annulare lesions

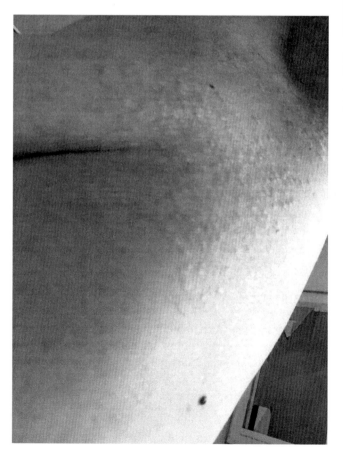

Fig. 30.1 Granuloma annulare lesions on the trunk, prior to treatment with adalimumab

References

1. Stinco G, Errichetti E. Erythrodermic psoriasis: current and future role of biologicals. BioDrugs. 2015;29(2):91–101.
2. Rosenbach M, et al. Treatment of erythrodermic psoriasis: from the medical board of the National Psoriasis Foundation. J Am Acad Dermatol. 2010;62(4):655–62.
3. Gottlieb AB. Novel immunotherapies for psoriasis: clinical research delivers new hope for patients and scientific advances. J Investig Dermatol Symp Proc. 2004;9(1):79–83.
4. Esposito M, et al. Treatment of erythrodermic psoriasis with etanercept. Br J Dermatol. 2006;155(1):156–9.
5. Lewis TG, et al. Life-threatening pustular and erythrodermic psoriasis responding to infliximab. J Drugs Dermatol. 2006;5(6):546–8.
6. Takahashi MD, Castro LG, Romiti R. Infliximab, as sole or combined therapy, induces rapid clearing of erythrodermic psoriasis. Br J Dermatol. 2007;157(4):828–31.
7. Poulalhon N, et al. A follow-up study in 28 patients treated with infliximab for severe recalcitrant psoriasis: evidence for efficacy and high incidence of biological autoimmunity. Br J Dermatol. 2007;156(2):329–36.
8. Fraga NA, et al. Refractory erythrodermic psoriasis in a child with an excellent outcome by using etanercept. An Bras Dermatol. 2011;86(4 Suppl 1):S144–7. (1806-4841 (Electronic))
9. Richetta AG, et al. Treatment of erythrodermic psoriasis in HCV+ patient with adalimumab. Dermatol Ther. 2009;22:S16–8.
10. Wang T-S, Tsai T-F. Clinical experience of ustekinumab in the treatment of erythrodermic psoriasis: a case series. J Dermatol. 2011;38(11):1096–9.

11. Pescitelli L, et al. Erythrodermic psoriasis treated with ustekinumab: an Italian multicenter retrospective analysis. J Dermatol Sci. 2015;78(2):149–51.

12. Santos-Juanes J, Coto-Segura P, et al. Ustekinumab induces rapid clearing of erythrodermic psoriasis after failure of antitumour necrosis factor therapies. Br J Dermatol. 2010;162(5):1144–6. https://doi.org/10.1111/j.1365-2133.2010.09669.x. (1365-2133 (Electronic))

13. CastiÑEiras I, et al. Sustained efficacy of ustekinumab in refractory erythrodermic psoriasis after failure of antitumor necrosis factor therapies. J Dermatol. 2012;39(8):730–1.

14. Viguier M, et al. Efficacy and safety of biologics in erythrodermic psoriasis: a multicentre, retrospective study. Br J Dermatol. 2012;167(2):417–23.

15. Robinson A, et al. Treatment of pustular psoriasis: from the medical Board of the National Psoriasis Foundation. J Am Acad Dermatol. 2012;67(2):279–88.

16. Kim H-S, et al. Two cases of generalized pustular psoriasis: successful treatment with infliximab. Ann Dermatol. 2014;26(6):787–8.

17. Chandran NS, Chong W-S. A dramatic response to a single dose of infliximab as rescue therapy in acute generalized pustular psoriasis of von Zumbusch associated with a neutrophilic cholangitis. Australas J Dermatol. 2010;51(1):29–31.

18. Trent JT, Kerdel FA. Successful treatment of von Zumbusch Pustular psoriasis with infliximab. J Cutan Med Surg. 2004;8(4):224–8.

19. Matsumoto A, et al. Adalimumab administration after infliximab therapy is a successful treatment strategy for generalized pustular psoriasis. J Dermatol. 2017;44(2):202–4. https://doi.org/10.1111/1346-8138.13632. (1346-8138 (Electronic))

20. Alvarez AC, et al. Recalcitrant pustular psoriasis successfully treated with adalimumab. Pediatr Dermatol. 2011;28(2):195–7. https://doi.org/10.1111/j.1525-1470.2010.01219.x. (1525-1470 (Electronic))

21. Callen JP, Jackson JH. Adalimumab effectively controlled recalcitrant generalized pustular psoriasis in an adolescent. J Dermatol Treat. 2005;16(5–6):350–2.

22. Storan ER, O'Gorman SM, Markham T. Generalized pustular psoriasis treated with ustekinumab. Clin Exp Dermatol. 2016;41(6):689–90.

23. Buder V, et al. Ustekinumab in the treatment of palmoplantar pustular psoriasis—a case series of nine patients. J Deutschen Dermatol Gesellschaft. 2016;14(11):1108–13.

24. Lo Schiavo A, et al. Etanercept in the treatment of generalized annular Pustular psoriasis. Ann Dermatol. 2012;24(2):233–4.

25. Fialová J, et al. Juvenile generalized pustular psoriasis treated with etanercept. Dermatol Ther. 2014;27(2):105–8.

26. Floristan U, et al. Recalcitrant palmoplantar pustular psoriasis treated with etanercept. Pediatr Dermatol. 2011;28(3):349–50.

27. Polesie S, Lidholm AG. Secukinumab in the treatment of generalized Pustular psoriasis: a case report. Acta Derm Venereol. 2017;96(7):124–5.

28. Bohner A, et al. Acute generalized Pustular psoriasis treated with the IL-17A antibody Secukinumab. JAMA Dermatol. 2016;152(4):482–4.

29. de Gannes GC, et al. Psoriasis and pustular dermatitis triggered by tnf-α inhibitors in patients with rheumatologic conditions. Arch Dermatol. 2007;143(2):223–31.

30. Langley RG, et al. Long-term efficacy and safety of ustekinumab, with and without dosing adjustment, in patients with moderate-to-severe psoriasis: results from the PHOENIX 2 study through 5 years of follow-up. Br J Dermatol. 2015;172(5):1371–83.

31. Wenk KS, Claros JM, Ehrlich A. Flare of pustular psoriasis after initiating ustekinumab therapy. J Dermatol Treat. 2012;23(3):212–4.

32. Kimball AB, et al. Two Phase 3 Trials of Adalimumab for Hidradenitis Suppurativa. N Engl J Med. 2016;375(5):422–34. https://doi.org/10.1056/NEJMoa1504370. (1533-4406 (Electronic))

33. Delobeau M, et al. Observational case series on adalimumab-induced paradoxical hidradenitis suppurativa. J Dermatolog Treat. 2016;27(3):251–3. https://doi.org/10.3109/09546634.2015. (1471-1753 (Electronic))

34. Lebwohl B, Sapadin AN. Infliximab for the treatment of hidradenitis suppurativa. J Am Acad Dermatol. 2003;49(5 Suppl):275–6.

35. Martinez F, et al. Hidradenitis suppurativa and Crohn's disease: response to treatment with infliximab. Inflamm Bowel Dis. 2001;7(4):323–6. (1078-0998 (Print))

36. Grant A, et al. Infliximab therapy for patients with moderate to severe hidradenitis suppurativa: a randomized, double-blind, placebo-controlled crossover trial. J Am Acad Dermatol. 2010;62(2):205–17.

37. van Rappard DC, Limpens J, Mekkes JR. The off-label treatment of severe hidradenitis suppurativa with TNF-alpha inhibitors: a systematic review. J Dermatolog Treat. 2013;24(5):392–404. https://doi.org/10.3109/09546634.2012.674193. (1471-1753 (Electronic))

38. Adams DR, et al. Treatment of hidradenitis suppurativa with etanercept injection. Arch Dermatol. 2010;146(5):501–4. https://doi.org/10.1001/archdermatol.2010.72. (1538-3652 (Electronic))

39. Haslund P, Lee RA, Jemec GB. Treatment of hidradenitis suppurativa with tumour necrosis factor-alpha inhibitors. Acta Derm Venereol. 2009;89(6):595–600. https://doi.org/10.2340/00015555-0747. (1651-2057 (Electronic))

40. Gulliver WP, Jemec GB, Baker KA. Experience with ustekinumab for the treatment of moderate to severe hidradenitis suppurativa. J Eur Acad Dermatol Venereol. 2012;26(7):911–4. https://doi.org/10.1111/j.1468-3083.2011.04123.x. (1468-3083 (Electronic))

41. Martin-Ezquerra G, et al. Use of biological treatments in patients with hidradenitis suppurativa. J Eur Acad Dermatol Venereol. 2015;29(1):56–60.

42. Sharon VR, et al. Management of recalcitrant hidradenitis suppurativa with ustekinumab. Acta Derm Venereol. 2012;92(3):320–1.

43. Lee RA, Eisen DB. Treatment of hidradenitis suppurativa with biologic medications. J Am Acad Dermatol. 2015;73(5 Suppl. 1):S82–8.

44. Paquet P, et al. Macrophages and tumor necrosis factor a in toxic epidermal necrolysis. Arch Dermatol. 1994;130(5):605–8.

45. Paradisi A, et al. Etanercept therapy for toxic epidermal necrolysis. J Am Acad Dermatol. 2014;71(2):278–83. https://doi.org/10.1016/j.jaad.2014.04.044. (1097-6787 (Electronic))

46. Didona D, et al. Successful use of etanercept in a case of toxic epidermal necrolysis induced by rituximab. J Eur Acad Dermatol Venereol. 2016;30(10):e83–4.

47. Napolitano M, et al. Toxic epidermal necrolysis-like acute cutaneous lupus erythematosus successfully treated with a single dose of etanercept: report of three cases. J Am Acad Dermatol. 2013;69(6):e303–5.

48. Fischer M, et al. Antitumour necrosis factor-α antibodies (infliximab) in the treatment of a patient with toxic epidermal necrolysis. Br J Dermatol. 2002;146(4):707–9.

49. Zarate-Correa LC, et al. Toxic epidermal necrolysis successfully treated with infliximab. J Invest Allergol Clin Immunol. 2013;23(1):61–3. (1018-9068 (Print))

50. Scott-Lang V, Tidman M, McKay D. Toxic epidermal necrolysis in a child successfully treated with infliximab. Pediatr Dermatol. 2014;31(4):532–4. https://doi.org/10.1111/pde.12029. (1525-1470 (Electronic))

51. Dainichi T, Kabashima K. Alopecia areata: what's new in epidemiology, pathogenesis, diagnosis, and therapeutic options? J Dermatol Sci. 2017;86(1):3–12. https://doi.org/10.1016/j.jdermsci.2016.10.004.

52. Xing L, et al. Alopecia areata is driven by cytotoxic T lymphocytes and is reversed by JAK inhibition. Nat Med. 2014;20(9):1043–9.

53. Mackay-Wiggan J, Jabbari A. Oral ruxolitinib induces hair regrowth in patients with moderate-to-severe alopecia areata. JCI Insight. 2016;1(15):e89790.

54. Craiglow BG, King BA. Killing two birds with one stone: oral Tofacitinib reverses alopecia Universalis in a patient with plaque psoriasis. J Invest Dermatol. 2014;134(12):2988–90.

55. Liu LY, et al. Tofacitinib for the treatment of severe alopecia areata and variants: a study of 90 patients. J Am Acad Dermatol. 2017;76(1):22–8.

56. Jabbari A, et al. Reversal of alopecia Areata following treatment with the JAK1/2 inhibitor Baricitinib. EBioMedicine. 2015;2(4):351–5.

57. Guttman-Yassky E, et al. Extensive alopecia areata is reversed by IL-12/IL-23p40 cytokine antagonism. J Allergy Clin Immunol. 2016;137(1):301–4.

58. Ribeiro LB, et al. Alopecia secondary to anti-tumor necrosis factor-alpha therapy. An Bras Dermatol. 2015;90(2):232–5.

59. Doyle LA, et al. Psoriatic alopecia/alopecia areata-like reactions secondary to anti-tumor necrosis factor-alpha therapy: a novel cause of noncicatricial alopecia. Am J Dermatopathol. 2011;33(2):161–6.

60. Andrisani G, et al. Development of psoriasis scalp with alopecia during treatment of Crohn's disease with infliximab and rapid response to both diseases to ustekinumab. Eur Rev Med Pharmacol Sci. 2013;17(20):2831–6.

61. Macía-Villa CC, Zea-Mendoza A. Multicentric reticulohistiocytosis: case report with response to infliximab and review of treatment options. Clin Rheumatol. 2016;35(2):527–34.

62. De Knop KJ, et al. Multicentric reticulohistiocytosis associated arthritis responding to anti-TNF and methotrexate. Acta Clin Belg. 2011;66(1):66–9.

63. Sellam J, et al. Refractory multicentric reticulohistiocytosis treated by infliximab: two cases. Clin Exp Rheumatol. 2005;23(1):97–9.

64. Kalajian AH, Callen JP. Multicentric reticulohistiocytosis successfully treated with infliximab: an illustrative case and evaluation of cytokine expression supporting anti–tumor necrosis factor therapy. Arch Dermatol. 2008;144(10):1360–6.

65. Shannon SE, et al. Multicentric reticulohistiocytosis responding to tumor necrosis factor-alpha inhibition in a renal transplant patient. J Rheumatol. 2005;32(3):565–7.

66. Yeter KC, Arkfeld DG. Treatment of multicentric reticulohistiocytosis with adalimumab, minocycline, methotrexate. Int J Rheum Dis. 2013;16(1):105–6.

67. Kovach BT, et al. Treatment of multicentric reticulohistiocytosis with etanercept. Arch Dermatol. 2004;140(8):919–21.

68. Matejicka C, Morgan GJ, Schlegelmilch JG. Multicentric reticulohistiocytosis treated successfully with an anti–tumor necrosis factor agent: comment on the article by Gorman et al. Arthritis Rheum. 2003;48(3):864–6.

69. Canizares MJ, et al. Successful treatment of mucous membrane pemphigoid with etanercept in 3 patients. Arch Dermatol. 2006;142(11):1457–61.

70. Kennedy JS, Devillez RL, Henning JS. Recalcitrant cicatricial pemphigoid treated with the anti-TNF-alpha agent etanercept. J Drugs Dermatol. 2010;9(1):68–70.

71. John H, Whallett A, Quinlan M. Successful biologic treatment of ocular mucous membrane pemphigoid with anti-TNF-alpha. Eye (Lond). 2007;21(11):1434–5.

72. Maley A, et al. Rituximab combined with conventional therapy versus conventional therapy alone for the treatment of mucous membrane pemphigoid (MMP). J Am Acad Dermatol. 2016;74(5):835–40.

73. Kim NH, et al. Tumor necrosis factor-α in vitiligo: direct correlation between tissue levels and clinical parameters. Cutan Ocul Toxicol. 2011;30(3):225–7.

74. Alghamdi KM, et al. Treatment of generalized vitiligo with anti-TNF-alpha agents. J Drugs Dermatol. 2012;11(4):534–9.

75. Webb KC, et al. Tumour necrosis factor-alpha inhibition can stabilize disease in progressive vitiligo. Br J Dermatol. 2015;173(3):641–50.

76. Mery-Bossard L, et al. THU0165 new onset Vitiligo under biological agents: a CASE series. Ann Rheum Dis. 2014;73(Suppl 2):237.

77. Saadoun D, et al. Mortality in Behçet's disease. Arthritis Rheum. 2010;62(9):2806–12.

78. Vallet H, et al. Efficacy of anti-TNF alpha in severe and/or refractory Behçet's disease: multicenter study of 124 patients. J Autoimmun. 2015;62:67–74.

79. Arida A, et al. Anti-TNF agents for Behcet's disease: analysis of published data on 369 patients. Semin Arthritis Rheum. 2011;41(1):61–70.

80. Beegle SH, et al. Current and emerging pharmacological treatments for sarcoidosis: a review. Drug Des Devel Ther. 2013;7:325–38.

81. Brito-Zeron P, et al. Sarcoidosis: an update on current pharmacotherapy options and future directions. Expert Opin Pharmacother. 2016;17(18):2431–48.

82. Thielen AM, et al. Refractory chronic cutaneous sarcoidosis responsive to dose escalation of TNF-alpha antagonists. Dermatology. 2009;219(1):59–62.

83. Baughman RP, et al. Infliximab for chronic cutaneous sarcoidosis: a subset analysis from a double-blind randomized clinical trial. Sarcoidosis Vasc Diffuse Lung Dis. 2016;32(4):289–95.

84. Rossman MD, et al. A double-blinded, randomized, placebo-controlled trial of infliximab in subjects with active pulmonary sarcoidosis. Sarcoidosis Vasc Diffuse Lung Dis. 2006;23(3):201–8.

85. Ramos-Casals M, et al. A systematic review of the off-label use of biological therapies in systemic autoimmune diseases. Medicine (Baltimore). 2008;87(6):345–64.

86. Erckens RJ, et al. Adalimumab successful in sarcoidosis patients with refractory chronic non-infectious uveitis. Graefes Arch Clin Exp Ophthalmol. 2012;250(5):713–20.

87. Baughman RP. Tumor necrosis factor inhibition in treating sarcoidosis: the American experience. Rev Port Pneumol. 2007;13:S47–50.

88. Pariser RJ, et al. A double-blind, randomized, placebo-controlled trial of adalimumab in the treatment of cutaneous sarcoidosis. J Am Acad Dermatol. 2013;68(5):765–73.

89. Burns AM, Green PJ, Pasternak S. Etanercept-induced cutaneous and pulmonary sarcoid-like granulomas resolving with adalimumab. J Cutan Pathol. 2012;39(2):289–93.

90. Cathcart S, Sami N, Elewski B. Sarcoidosis as an adverse effect of tumor necrosis factor inhibitors. J Drugs Dermatol. 2012;11(5):609–12.

91. Petrof G, et al. A systematic review of the literature on the treatment of pityriasis rubra pilaris type 1 with TNF-antagonists. J Eur Acad Dermatol Venereol. 2013;27(1):e131–5.

92. Zhang YH, et al. Type I pityriasis rubra pilaris: upregulation of tumor necrosis factor alpha and response to adalimumab therapy. J Cutan Med Surg. 2010;14(4):185–8.

93. Wassef C, Lombardi A, Rao BK. Adalimumab for the treatment of pityriasis rubra pilaris: a case report. Cutis. 2012;90(5):244–7.

94. Chiu HY, Tsai TF. Pityriasis Rubra Pilaris with polyarthritis treated with adalimumab. J Am Acad Dermatol. 2013;68(1):187–8.

95. Manoharan S, White S, Gumparthy K. Successful treatment of type I adult-onset pityriasis rubra pilaris with infliximab. Australas J Dermatol. 2006;47(2):124–9.

96. Seckin D, Tula E, Ergun T. Successful use of etanercept in type I pityriasis rubra pilaris [13]. Br J Dermatol. 2008;158(3):642–4.

97. Neill SM, et al. British Association of Dermatologists' guidelines for the management of lichen sclerosus 2010. Br J Dermatol. 2010;163(4):672–82.

98. Lowenstein EB, Zeichner JA. Intralesional adalimumab for the treatment of refractory balanitis xerotica obliterans. JAMA Dermatol. 2013;149(1):23–4.

99. Stingeni L, et al. Cutaneous Crohn's disease successfully treated with adalimumab. J Eur Acad Dermatol Venereol. 2016;30(10):e72–4.

100. Laftah Z, et al. Vulval Crohn's disease: a clinical study of 22 patients. J Crohns Colitis. 2015;9(4):318–25.

101. Navarini AA, Trueb RM. 3 cases of dissecting cellulitis of the scalp treated with adalimumab: control of inflammation within residual structural disease. Arch Dermatol. 2010;146(5):517–20.

102. Shroff A, Guttman-Yassky E. Successful use of ustekinumab therapy in refractory severe atopic dermatitis. JAAD Case Rep. 2015;1(1):25–6.

103. Wlodek C, Hewitt H, Kennedy CT. Use of ustekinumab for severe refractory atopic dermatitis in a young teenager. Clin Exp Dermatol. 2016;41(6):625–7.

104. Puya R, et al. Treatment of severe refractory adult atopic dermatitis with ustekinumab. Int J Dermatol. 2012;51(1):115–6.

105. Khattri S, et al. Efficacy and safety of ustekinumab treatment in adults with moderate-to-severe atopic dermatitis. Exp Dermatol. 2017;26(1):28–35.

106. Sand FL, Thomsen SF. Efficacy and safety of TNF-alpha inhibitors in refractory primary complex aphthosis: a patient series and overview of the literature. J Dermatolog Treat. 2013;24(6):444–6.

107. O'Neill ID. Efficacy of tumour necrosis factor-alpha antagonists in aphthous ulceration: review of published individual patient data. J Eur Acad Dermatol Venereol. 2012;26(2):231–5.

108. Hertl MS, et al. Rapid improvement of recalcitrant disseminated granuloma annulare upon treatment with the tumour necrosis factor-alpha inhibitor, infliximab. Br J Dermatol. 2005;152(3):552–5.

109. Murdaca G, et al. Anti-tumor necrosis factor-alpha treatment with infliximab for disseminated granuloma annulare. Am J Clin Dermatol. 2010;11(6):437–9.

110. Shupack J, Siu K. Resolving granuloma annulare with etanercept. Arch Dermatol. 2006;142(3):394–5.

111. Kreuter A, Altmeyer P, Gambichler T. Failure of etanercept therapy in disseminated granuloma annulare. Arch Dermatol. 2006;142(9):1236–7. author reply 1237

112. Min MS, Lebwohl M. Treatment of recalcitrant granuloma annulare (GA) with adalimumab: a single-center, observational study. J Am Acad Dermatol. 2016;74(1):127–33.

113. Rosmarin D, et al. Successful treatment of disseminated granuloma annulare with adalimumab. J Drugs Dermatol. 2009;8(2):169–71.

114. Werchau S, Enk A, Hartmann M. Generalized interstitial granuloma annulare--response to adalimumab. Int J Dermatol. 2010;49(4):457–60.

115. Kozic H, Webster GF. Treatment of widespread granuloma annulare with adalimumab: a case report. J Clin Aesthet Dermatol. 2011;4(11):42–3.

116. Knoell KA. Efficacy of adalimumab in the treatment of generalized granuloma annulare in monozygotic twins carrying the 8.1 ancestral haplotype. Arch Dermatol. 2009;145(5):610–1.

117. Omair MA, Phumethum V, Johnson SR. Long-term safety and effectiveness of tumour necrosis factor inhibitors in systemic sclerosis patients with inflammatory arthritis. Clin Exp Rheumatol. 2012;30(2):S55–9.

118. Phumethum V, Jamal S, Johnson SR. Biologic therapy for systemic sclerosis: a systematic review. J Rheumatol. 2011;38(2):289–96.

119. Mattozzi C, et al. Morphea, an unusual side effect of anti-TNF-alpha treatment. Eur J Dermatol. 2010;20(3):400–1.

120. Stewart FA, Gavino AC, Elewski BE. New side effect of TNF-alpha inhibitors: morphea. Skinmed. 2013;11(1):59–60.

121. Ramirez J, et al. Morphea associated with the use of adalimumab: a case report and review of the literature. Mod Rheumatol. 2012;22(4):602–4.

122. Bolognia J, Jorizzo JL, Schaffer JV. Dermatology. 3rd ed. Philadelphia: Elsevier Saunders; 2012.

123. Tan M, et al. Improvement of pyoderma gangrenosum and psoriasis associated with crohndisease with anti–tumor necrosis factor α monoclonal antibody. Arch Dermatol. 2001;137(7):930–3.

124. Adışen E, Öztaş M, Gürer MA. Treatment of idiopathic Pyoderma Gangrenosum with infliximab: induction dosing regimen or on-demand therapy? Dermatology. 2008;216(2):163–5.

125. Cocco A, et al. Successful treatment with infliximab of refractory pyoderma gangrenosum in 2 patients with inflammatory bowel diseases. Inflamm Bowel Dis. 2007;13(10):1317–9.

126. De la Morena F, et al. Refractory and infected pyoderma gangrenosum in a patient with ulcerative colitis: response to infliximab. Inflamm Bowel Dis. 2007;13(4):509–10.

127. Hewitt D, Tait C. Use of infliximab in pyoderma gangrenosum. Australas J Dermatol. 2007;48(2):95–8.

128. Juillerat P, et al. Infliximab for the treatment of disseminated pyoderma gangrenosum associated with ulcerative colitis. Case report and literature review. Dermatology. 2007;215(3):245–51.

129. Regueiro M, et al. Infliximab for treatment of pyoderma gangrenosum associated with inflammatory bowel disease. Am J Gastroenterol. 2003;98(8):1821–6.

130. Fonder MA, et al. Adalimumab therapy for recalcitrant pyoderma gangrenosum. J Burns Wounds. 2006;5:e8.

131. Heffernan MP, Anadkat MJ, Smith DI. Adalimumab treatment for pyoderma gangrenosum. Arch Dermatol. 2007;143(3):306–8.

132. Sagami S, et al. Successful use of Adalimumab for treating Pyoderma Gangrenosum with ulcerative colitis under corticosteroid-tapering conditions. Intern Med. 2015;54(17):2167–72.

133. Disla E, et al. Successful use of etanercept in a patient with pyoderma gangrenosum complicating rheumatoid arthritis. J Clin Rheumatol. 2004;10(1):50–2.

134. Rogge FJ, Pacifico M, Kang N. Treatment of pyoderma gangrenosum with the anti-TNFα drug – Etanercept. J Plast Reconstr Aesthet Surg. 2008;61(4):431–3.

135. Cinotti E, et al. Certolizumab for the treatment of refractory disseminated pyoderma gangrenosum associated with rheumatoid arthritis. Clin Exp Dermatol. 2014;39(6):750–1.

136. Hurabielle C, et al. Certolizumab pegol - A new therapeutic option for refractory disseminated pyoderma gangrenosum associated with Crohn's disease. J Dermatolog Treat. 2016;27(1):67–9.

137. Guenova E, et al. Interleukin 23 expression in pyoderma gangrenosum and targeted therapy with ustekinumab. Arch Dermatol. 2011;147(10):1203–5.

138. Chao TJ. Adalimumab in the management of cutaneous and oral lichen planus. Cutis. 2009;84(6):325–8.

139. Hollo P, et al. Successful treatment of lichen planus with adalimumab. Acta Derm Venereol. 2012;92(4):385–6.

140. Asarch A, et al. Lichen planus-like eruptions: an emerging side effect of tumor necrosis factor-alpha antagonists. J Am Acad Dermatol. 2009;61(1):104–11.

141. Au S, Hernandez C. Paradoxical induction of psoriasis and lichen Planus by tumor necrosis factor-alpha inhibitors. Skinmed. 2015;13(5):403–5.

142. Fernandez-Torres R, et al. Infliximab-induced lichen planopilaris. Ann Pharmacother. 2010;44(9):1501–3.

143. Worsnop F, et al. Reaction to biological drugs: infliximab for the treatment of toxic epidermal necrolysis subsequently triggering erosive lichen planus. Clin Exp Dermatol. 2012;37(8):879–81.

144. Agarwal A, et al. Refractory subcutaneous sweet syndrome treated with adalimumab. JAMA Dermatol. 2016;152(7):842–4.

145. Banse C, et al. Occurrence of sweet syndrome under anti-TNF. Clin Rheumatol. 2015;34(11):1993–4.

146. Zeichner JA, Stern DWK, Lebwohl M. Treatment of necrobiosis lipoidica with the tumor necrosis factor antagonist etanercept. J Am Acad Dermatol. 2006;54(3 Suppl. 2):S120–1.

147. Zhang KS, Quan LT, Hsu S. Treatment of necrobiosis lipoidica with etanercept and adalimumab. Dermatol Online J. 2009;15(12)

148. Riley P, et al. Effectiveness of infliximab in the treatment of refractory juvenile dermatomyositis with calcinosis. Rheumatology (Oxford). 2008;47(6):877–80.

149. Park JK, et al. Successful treatment for conventional treatment-resistant dermatomyositis-associated interstitial lung disease with adalimumab. Rheumatol Int. 2012;32(11):3587–90.

150. Klein R, et al. Tumor necrosis factor inhibitor-associated dermatomyositis. Arch Dermatol. 2010;146(7):780–4.

151. Ishikawa Y, et al. Etanercept-induced anti-Jo-1-antibody-positive polymyositis in a patient with rheumatoid arthritis: a case report and review of the literature. Clin Rheumatol. 2010;29(5):563–6.

152. Wagner AD, et al. Sustained response to tumor necrosis factor α–blocking agents in two patients with SAPHO syndrome. Arthritis Rheum. 2002;46(7):1965–8.

153. De Souza A, Solomon GE, Strober BE. SAPHO syndrome associated with hidradenitis suppurativa successfully treated with infliximab and methotrexate. Bull NYU Hosp Jt Dis. 2011;69(2):185–7.

154. Moll C, et al. Ilium osteitis as the main manifestation of the SAPHO syndrome: response to infliximab therapy and review of the literature. Semin Arthritis Rheum. 2008;37(5):299–306.

155. Sabugo F, et al. Infliximab can induce a prolonged clinical remission and a decrease in thyroid hormonal requirements in a patient with SAPHO syndrome and hypothyroidism. Clin Rheumatol. 2008;27(4):533–5.

156. Ben Abdelghani K, et al. Tumor necrosis factor-α blockers in SAPHO syndrome. J Rheumatol. 2010;37(8):1699–704.

157. Wolber C, et al. Successful therapy of sacroiliitis in SAPHO syndrome by etanercept. Wien Med Wochenschr. 2011;161(7):204–8.

158. Arias-Santiago S, et al. Adalimumab treatment for SAPHO syndrome. Acta Derm Venereol. 2010;90(3):301–2.

159. Castellvi I, et al. Successful treatment of SAPHO syndrome with adalimumab: a case report. Clin Rheumatol. 2010;29(10):1205–7.

160. Firinu D, et al. SAPHO syndrome: current developments and approaches to clinical treatment. Curr Rheumatol Rep. 2016;18(6):35.

161. Garcovich S, et al. *Long-term treatment of severe SAPHO syndrome with adalimumab: case report and a review of the literature*. Am J Clin Dermatol. 2012;13(1):55–9.

Biologics for the Treatment of Atopic Dermatitis

31

Tamar Hajar, Emma Hill, and Eric Simpson

Introduction

Atopic dermatitis (AD) is a chronic inflammatory skin condition affecting up to 20% of children and 10% of adults in industrialized countries [1, 2]. Clinical features of AD include xerosis, erythema, oozing, crusting, and lichenification. Pruritus is the hallmark symptom of the disease and is responsible for much of the well-documented disease burden for patients and their families [3].

AD pathogenesis has not been clearly elucidated; however, skin barrier dysfunction and dysregulated immune responses are two known key drivers of the disease [4]. Both genetic and environmental factors influence the risk of developing the disease and the prevalence of AD appears to be increasing in many parts of the globe, especially in urban areas [5].

As a result of various genetic and environmental factors, AD displays significant heterogeneity in regard to age of onset, remission rates, disease phenotype, comorbidity profile, disease severity, and response to treatment. Several phenotypes and corresponding endotypes have been proposed for the disease [6]. Despite our improved understanding of the molecular pathways in AD, most traditional therapies are not based on scientific mechanistic understanding.

Severity-Based Therapy Overview

The treatment strategy of AD relies heavily on the underlying disease severity. The skin barrier appears to play an important role in disease initiation. Emollient therapy has been studied for preventing the onset of AD (primary prevention) and can treat mild disease when combined with gentle skin care and reduction in disease triggers [7–9]. More moderate disease requires topical anti-inflammatory therapy with

either intermittent topical corticosteroids (TCS) or topical calcineurin inhibitors (TCI). As the disease becomes more severe, skin barrier approaches or topical therapy alone provide only limited benefit. Targeting inflammation with systemic immunomodulating therapy or phototherapy becomes necessary.

No one parameter or scoring system determines the need for systemic therapy in AD. Choosing whether a patient should start systemic treatment requires integrating several factors and balancing the patient's quality of life, patient preferences, skin severity, disease extent and location, adherence, and comorbidities with the benefits and risks of available systemic therapy.

Current guidelines recommend the use of traditional immunosuppressant medications including cyclosporine, methotrexate (MTX), mycophenolate mofetil (MMF), and azathioprine (AZA) in patients who fail conventional topical therapy or phototherapy [10]. The management of AD with systemic corticosteroids, although used frequently and shown to temporarily suppress disease activity, should generally be avoided because of an overall unfavorable risk-benefit profile. Additionally, short courses of oral corticosteroids may actually worsen the disease after discontinuation due to atopic flares [10]. A study by Schmitt and colleagues was terminated prematurely due to excessive AD flares in the corticosteroid group as compared to the continuous cyclosporine-treated group [11].

While traditional immunosuppressive therapies show some effectiveness in AD, their routine use is limited by inadequate disease responses (<50% improvement in most studies) and by end-organ toxicity [12, 13]. Thus treatment of moderate-to-severe atopic dermatitis is often frustrating in clinical practice for both patients and providers [14].

Biologic therapy holds promise for providing patients with moderate-to-severe AD a long-term effective option for disease control by virtue of their targeted effects on the dysregulated immune responses that underpin moderate-to-severe disease. As our specific understanding of the complex pathogenesis of AD improves, including immune and

T. Hajar, MD • E. Hill, BA • E. Simpson, MD, MCR (✉)
Oregon Health and Science University, Portland, OR, USA
e-mail: hajar@ohsu.edu; hillem@ohsu.edu; simpsone@ohsu.edu

© Springer International Publishing AG 2018
P.S. Yamauchi (ed.), *Biologic and Systemic Agents in Dermatology*, https://doi.org/10.1007/978-3-319-66884-0_31

309

molecular pathways, a variety of experimental biologics are targeting these pathways with the hope of less toxicity and greater efficacy.

Identifying Extracellular Targets in AD

Complex immunobiological dysfunction including both innate and adaptive immune responses drives the cutaneous inflammatory response in AD. Alterations in T-cell number and function have been the focus of study, although altered function of various immune cell subtypes have been observed in AD such as mast cells, eosinophils, innate lymphoid cells, and dendritic cells [15]. Enhanced PDE4 activity has been observed in AD monocytes and represents an attractive explanation for the wide variety of immune cell hyper-reactivity [16].

For many years, textbooks often described a biphasic immune pathobiology in AD where acute skin lesions of AD were thought to be initiated by Th2 cytokines (IL-4,5,13) and chronic lesions were thought to be Th1 dominant (IFN-gamma) [17]. This Th1/Th2 paradigm was reinforced by the findings of an atopy patch test study [18, 19]. Atopy patch testing involves assessing skin reactions to topically applied proteins- a testing procedure not endorsed by current AD guidelines because of a lack of evidence of clinical relevance in AD [20]. Recent whole transcriptome analyses paint a more complex picture of AD inflammation that identifies a central role for type 2 cytokines in both acute and chronic AD with increased expression of Th1 and Th22 cytokines with more chronic disease [21]. Recently, the Asian AD phenotype appears to have important elevations in Th17 cytokine pathways [22]. Thus, the immune pathways in AD, like the AD phenotype, are complex and heterogeneous and provide many opportunities for therapeutic intervention. What follows is a narrative review highlighting both early and more recent studies of biologic therapy in AD organized by immunological target. Our search strategy included searching the English literature using PUBMED for the use of biologics in AD. We primarily reviewed trials and reports that were the highest-level evidence available.

T-Cell Inhibition

Efalizumab is a monoclonal antibody targeting CD11a. There are multiple case reports and case series suggesting efalizumab's effectiveness in AD [23–27]. In some case series and case reports, patients experienced an approximately 50% improvement in EASI and IGA scores as well as improvement in quality of life (QoL). Efalizumab was taken off the market in 2009 due to its side effects that include bacterial sepsis, viral meningitis, invasive fungal disease, and progressive multifocal leukoencephalopathy. Although it is currently off the market, these studies provided proof-of-concept that targeting T-cell functions could be of clinical benefit to patients with AD.

Anti-IgE Therapy

Omalizumab is a humanized IgG1κ monoclonal antibody that selectively binds with high affinity to free IgE, preventing allergen-specific IgE from attaching to of the high-affinity IgE-binding site (FcεRI). Additionally, it reduces the expression of the IgE receptor on mast cells and basophils [28–31]. The Food and Drug Administration (FDA) approved omalizumab in 2003 to treat patients 12 years and older with moderate-to-severe persistent asthma and with chronic idiopathic urticaria (CIU) who are not adequately controlled with conventional therapy [30–34]. The role of IgE in the pathogenesis of AD is not clear, but most experts view elevated IgE levels in AD as an epi-phenomenon possibly reflecting transcutaneous sensitization through a defective barrier or a marker of Th2 dysfunction [35]. Nevertheless, because IgE is present in 80% of patients with AD, and generally associated with a personal or family history of atopy, anti-IgE therapy has been tested in AD in several studies.

Initial case reports and case series reported promising results with an average response close to 50% as well as improvement in some QoL measures [36–39]. Randomized controlled trials (RCTs), however, failed to confirm these effects. Iyengar SR and colleagues reported an RCT that evaluated eight children between 4 and 22 years old with severe, refractory AD. Patients received omalizumab (150–375 mg SC) every 2–4 weeks for 24 weeks or placebo. At 24 weeks, SCORAD reductions of approximately 20–50% and 45–80% were observed in the omalizumab and placebo groups, respectively. [40] The second RCT was reported by Heil M and colleagues that evaluated 20 patients that were treated with placebo vs 0.016 mg/kg/IgE (IU/mL) omalizumab SC every 4 weeks. Changes in IGA and EASI scores from baseline were not different between groups. [41] Most recently, a randomized controlled trial of ligelizumab, a high-affinity anti-IgE antibody failed to show significant improvement in a phase II RCT [42]. Overall, despite the presence of elevated IgE in many cases of AD, IgE-targeted therapy is unlikely to provide benefit for AD.

Anti-CD20: Rituximab

Rituximab is a chimeric monoclonal IgG1 anti-CD20 antibody that induces cell-mediated/antibody-dependent cytotoxicity, apoptosis, and complement-mediated cytotoxicity of B-cells. It has shown promise in the treatment of several autoimmune skin diseases such as pemphigus, bullous pemphigoid, and epidermolysis bullosa aquisita.

In contrast to autoimmune diseases, the role of B-cells, however, is not clear in AD pathogenesis; however, activated B-cells are clearly present [43].

CD20 is expressed by pre-B-cells and mature B-cells, but not plasma cells. Rituximab likely exerts various immunologic effects primarily through B-lymphocyte depletion and secondarily through the loss of the antigen-presenting and immunomodulatory functions of B-cells [44].

Simon and colleagues were the first group to report on the use of rituximab in patients with AD—a case series of six patients receiving two doses of IV rituximab 1000 mg 2 weeks apart. All patients had significant improvement of their disease within 4–8 weeks of treatment, with an initial EASI score mean of 29 and a reduction to mean EASI score of 10 (data approximated from tables). They also noted that all patients reduced the amount of TCS applications (average frequency of application before treatment: 6 times per week, to 3 times per week at week 8). Effects of the drug appeared to be long-lasting with reductions in disease severity continuing up to 22 weeks after the last injection [45]. Ponte and colleagues reported a case of a pregnant patient that had a good response with a single dose of rituximab during her first trimester of pregnancy with a baseline BSA 80% that improved to 5% BSA after the first infusion with no additional flares [46].

In contrast to these positive case reports, McDonald and colleagues reported a case series of three adult patients that received rituximab and none of the patients experienced clinical improvement of their disease [47]. Sediva and colleagues [48] reported two patients that received rituximab and found that SCORAD improved slightly initially; however, this partial improvement only lasted until the 10th week, at which point both patients experienced worsening of their disease. Thus responses to the B-cell depletion therapy rituximab are conflicting and larger controlled studies will be needed to better understand the safety and efficacy of rituximab in this patient population. Given the safety of novel emerging therapies, the feasibility and need of such a trial becomes questionable.

Interferon-Gamma

Interferon-gamma (IFN-gamma), thought to suppress Th2 activity represents the first engineered biologic studied for the treatment of AD. IFN-gamma has shown somewhat mixed results in the treatment of severe AD. Several studies (including two randomized trials) demonstrated improvement with IFN-gamma therapy. Hanifin and colleagues reported that 45% of the treatment group and 21% of the patients in the placebo group achieved at least 50% improvement in physicians'

overall response evaluations ($p = 0.016$). They also measured the response assessed by patients and found a significant improvement in the IFN-gamma group versus the placebo group (53 vs 21% $p = 0.002$) [49]. Another paper published by Schneider and colleagues showed similar results with a baseline mean total body surface area involvement of 61.6% that decreased to 18.5% at 24 months ($p < 0.001$) [50]. Response rates were low in an open-label study [51]. Potential side effects with interferon-gamma include granulocytopenia, fever/chills, myalgias, headache, and pain at the injection site. Most side effects in AD trials were mild headaches, myalgias, or chills that were effectively prevented by pretreatment with acetaminophen and by dosing at bedtime. Unpublished data, however, suggests that IFN-gamma may have only a limited role in the treatment of severe AD. In 1997, a press release available online describes the results of a phase 3 trial of IFN-gamma for AD that included 555 patients. The press release stated that analysis of the study did not show an acceptable therapeutic response with respect to the primary clinical endpoint [52]. It is possible that a subset of patients with AD, such as those with recurring eczema herpeticum or genetic deficiencies in IFN signaling, may benefit from this therapy. The authors experience confirms that some patients do appear to benefit from IFN-g therapy when other treatments have failed.

Type 2 Cytokine Inhibition

Anti-IL-4 and -IL-13 (Dupilumab)

Dupilumab is a fully human, monoclonal antibody targeting the alpha subunit of the IL-4 receptor that blocks downstream signaling of both IL-4 and IL-13. IL-4Rα is a shared subunit of the IL-4 and IL-13 receptor. Early phase I and II studies in adults with AD found dupilumab provides dose-dependent improvement in the signs and symptoms of AD [53–55].

More in-depth studies of lesional and non-lesional skin during Dupilumab therapy found that modulating IL-4/IL-13 signaling through IL-4Rα antagonism in patients with AD has statistically significant and dose-dependent improvement in the AD transcriptome after 4 weeks of treatment with dupilumab compared with placebo. The authors also demonstrated that dupilumab was able to suppress mRNA expression in lesional skin of genes related to activation of T-cells, DCs, eosinophils, inflammatory pathways, and type 2 cytokines. Furthermore, by using microarrays and qRT-PCR they demonstrated that genes responsible for epidermal hyperplasia (S100A and K16 genes) were also downregulated by dupilumab. The authors speculated that blocking IL-4/IL-13 may not only improve inflammation in AD but also may restore skin barrier function as a result of significant increases in claudin and lipid product levels and a trend of dose-dependent increases in expression of LOR and FLG that were not found in the placebo group. These results show promising new insights into the role of type 2 cytokines in AD and suggest that inhibition of IL4/IL13 has the potential to reverse multiple molecular defects in patients with AD.

Most recently Simpson and colleagues confirmed the findings of early stage studies in two-identically designed phase III randomized controlled studies named SOLO 1 and SOLO 2. (Table 31.1) [56] The population under study were adult patients with long-standing (>3 years) moderate-to-severe AD (IGA 3 or 4) who had failed topical treatment or for whom topical treatment was contraindicated. Over 1350 patients were enrolled. Concomitant topical corticosteroids (TCS) were not allowed during this 16-week study. The authors found statistically significant differences compared to placebo in all efficacy endpoints. The primary endpoint was the proportion of patients with Investigators Global Assessment (IGA) score of 0 or 1 (clear or almost clear). The proportion of patients achieving clear or almost clear skin by IGA ranged between 36 and 37% in the 300 mg SQ weekly group and 36–38% in the 300 mg qoweek, all doses showing significant improvement over placebo groups. EASI score reductions of 70–75% were seen in dupilumab-treated groups. Patient-reported symptoms of AD (including effect on sleep, anxiety, depression, quality of life) were significantly decreased in dupilumab cohorts compared with placebo with all effect sizes providing clinically meaningful effects taking into account the known minimal clinically important difference. The rates of rescue treatment were lower in all dupilumab groups compared with placebo. More recently, data from a 1-year controlled trial with TCS named CHRONOS were presented showing sustained improvement with a favorable safety profile with longer-term use [57].

The adverse events of note that were increased over placebo rates reported in the SOLO trials were injection-site reactions and conjunctivitis. Approximately 14% of patients experienced conjunctivitis in the CHRONOS 1 year study at the every other week dosing. Topical ophthalmic anti-inflammatory medications are at times necessary to control eye symptoms in the authors' experience. Some cases may be long-lasting and some may spontaneously resolve. Further studies regarding the etiology of the conjunctivitis and natural course are needed.

The Food and Drug Administration granted Breakthrough Therapy designation to dupilumab for the treatment of adults with moderate-to-severe AD who are not adequately controlled with topical prescription therapies or for whom these treatments are not appropriate. A biologics license application (BLA) for the drug was submitted on 26 September 2016, and dupilumab was FDA approved in April [58].

Other inhibitors of IL-4 and IL4Rα are currently being studied in patients with asthma such as pascolizumab, pitrakinra, and altrakincept. There are no ongoing clinical trials to evaluate their use in AD. Overall dupilumab represents a long-awaited major breakthrough for patients with moderate-to-severe disease and points to the importance of type 2 signaling in AD pathophysiology.

Anti-IL-13 (Lebrikizumab/Tralokinumab)

IL-13 is overproduced in the skin of AD patients and has been shown to play an important role in the pathogenesis of the disease. IL-13 reduces epidermal integrity through a decrease in gene expression of loricrin and involucrin [59]. Further, polymorphisms in the gene encoding IL-13 have been associated with AD [60–62].

According to data that was presented at the 2016 European Academy of Dermatology and Venereology (EADV) congress [42], the authors released the results of a RCT that assessed the efficacy and safety of lebrikizumab in patients with AD. Four dosing regimens were evaluated, a single dose of 125 mg + TCS, a single dose of 250 mg of lebrikizumab + TCS BID, 125 mg of lebrikizumab every 4 weeks + TCS BID and placebo. The primary endpoint was to assess the percent of patients achieving EASI-50 at week 12. EASI-50 was achieved by 82.4% of patients in the q4 week dosing group compared to 62.3% of the patients on placebo, $p = 0.03$. Adverse event rates were generally similar between treatment groups and most were mild or moderate in severity. The investigators concluded that that blocking IL-13 with lebrikizumab in moderate-to-severe AD provides significant improvements in a number of severity outcomes. Dosing every 4 weeks appeared to provide benefit over the single dose groups and markedly improved the percentage of patients achieving the primary and secondary endpoints. It is important to note that these improvements were seen on top of intensive TCS application explaining the very high placebo response rates.

Tralokinumab is a human monoclonal antibody also targeting IL-13. A poster presentation at the American Academy

Table 31.1 Dupilumab efficacy endpoints at 16 weeks.

	IGA 0/1 SOLO 1	$P**$	EASI 75	$P**$	IGA 0/1 SOLO 2	$P**$	EASI 75	$P**$
300 mg QW	37%	$p < 0.001$	52%	$p < 0.001$	36%	$p < 0.001$	48%	$p < 0.001$
300 mg QOW	38%	$p < 0.001$	51%	$p < 0.001$	36%	$p < 0.001$	44%	$p < 0.001$
Placebo	10%		15%		8%		12%	

^EASI 75 at week 16
**P value compared to placebo

of Dermatology in 2017 showed some improvement at higher dose, but large improvements in the placebo groups, similar to the lebrikizumab trials, likely blunted the statistical significance.

In sum, blockade of IL-13 alone appears to have an effect but interpreting the results of trials of lebrikizumab and tralokinumab are obscured by the heavy background use of TCS. It is unknown whether the effect size of blocking IL-13 alone will be similar to IL-4/IL-13 dual blockade until further studies are performed.

Anti-IL-5 (Mepolizumab)

IL-5 is another cytokine produced by Th2 cells and Langerhans cells and is important for eosinophil differentiation, growth, activation, mobilization, survival and induces eosinophil release into the peripheral circulation [63]. Eosinophils have been thought to be important mediators of the inflammatory process in AD, thus blocking this cytokine was hypothesized to be effective in the treatment of patients with AD. Oldhoff and colleagues performed a randomized double-blind, placebo-controlled, parallel group study based at six centers in Europe evaluating mepolizumab, a monoclonal antibody targeting IL-5, in adults with AD [64]. The authors evaluated the efficacy of two single doses of 750 mg mepolizumab intravenously, given 1 week apart, versus placebo in patients with moderate-to-severe AD. The primary endpoint was the percentage of patients who achieved marked improvement of their PGA score on Day 14. Secondary endpoints included SCORAD, pruritus scoring, number of blood eosinophils and serum thymus and activation-regulated chemokine (TARC) values. The authors found a statistically significant reduction in blood eosinophils compared with placebo ($p < 0.05$) although no correlation with the clinical findings was shown. There was no statistical significance for the primary or the other secondary endpoints between the treatment group and the placebo. The authors concluded that this dose was not effective in treating patients with moderate-to-severe AD, although dosing and endpoint measurement (2 weeks after initial dose) may not have been optimal for observing an effect.

Anti-IL-31 (Nemolizumab)

IL-31 is a cytokine produced by Th2 cells that is believed to be a major pruritogenic inflammatory cytokine [65]. It also amplifies proinflammatory cytokine secretion, disrupts epidermal barrier function by affecting epidermal terminal differentiation and lipid constituents [66], and recently has found to activate signal transduction cascades, such as the Janus kinase-STAT (JAK-STAT) pathway. Hence it was hypothesized that blocking IL-31 or its receptor would be effective in the treatment of patients with AD.

Nemolizumab is a humanized anti-human-IL-31-receptor-A (IL-31RA) monoclonal antibody and was studied in a phase II controlled trial [67]. This study evaluated the efficacy and safety of nemolizumab in 264 patients with moderate-to-severe AD. The primary endpoint was the improvement in the percent change in pruritus VAS from baseline at week 12 compared with placebo. Concomitant TCS were not allowed. Secondary efficacy outcomes at week 12 included improvement from baseline in the EASI, SCORAD, IGA, body surface area, pruritus verbal rating scale, and sleep disturbance VAS. At 12 weeks, there was a significant, dose-dependent reduction in the mean percentage from baseline in the pruritus VAS compared with placebo. In the two highest dosing groups, participants experienced 59–63% improvements in sleep disturbance on the VAS. The signs of the disease also reduced, although the reductions in the signs of the disease were not as robust as the reductions in pruritus with a mean EASI reduction of 40.9–42.3% in the 2 highest dosing groups. Overall nemolizumab was well-tolerated; important adverse effects were AD exacerbations, even in treatment groups, and peripheral edema of unknown cause. Targeting IL-31R appears to provide significant itch relief in patients with AD in a dose-dependent manner. Further studies are warranted to better clarify the effects on skin inflammatory lesions and to further understand the side effect profile.

Targeting Th17/IL12/IL-23 Pathway

Ustekinumab blocks both IL-12 and IL-23 by targeting the common p40 subunit shared by these cytokines, thereby inhibiting Th1 and Th17, respectively. Ustekinumab is currently approved for the treatment of psoriasis and psoriatic arthritis and has been studied in AD. Studies have shown higher expression of both IL-17 and IL-22 in the lesional skin of AD compared to non-lesional and normal controls [68]. A few case series and case reports demonstrated positive results when using ustekinumab for AD, including improvement in VAS, EASI, and SCORAD measures [69–71]. However, one report documents flaring of AD with ustekinumab [72]. Another case series that described 2 patients did not find it effective for the treatment of AD [73].

A recent phase II, double-blind, placebo-controlled study evaluated 33 patients with moderate-to-severe AD that were randomly assigned to either ustekinumab or placebo, with subsequent crossover at 16 weeks, and last dose occurring at 32 weeks. The authors concluded that there was no statistical significance between groups suggesting ustekinumab may not be beneficial for patients with AD [74]. Given the trend toward improvement in the study however, further studies may be warranted in subtypes of patients where

IL-17 may play a more important role, such as in Japanese populations.[22].

Anti-IL-6R

Tocilizumab is an IL-6 receptor antagonist, FDA approved in 2008 for the treatment of rheumatoid arthritis. Recent reports of off-label usage included other systemic inflammatory disorders, such as psoriasis, psoriatic arthritis, Behçet's disease, systemic lupus erythematous, systemic sclerosis, relapsing polychondritis, vasculitis, and AD [75]. IL-6 is produced by eosinophils, mast cells, T- and B-cells, monocytes, and fibroblasts. It has been found to have induced T-cell activation and induction of immunoglobulin secretion. A case series by Navarini and colleagues reported three AD patients who were resistant to phototherapy, topical steroids, calcineurin inhibitors, and oral cyclosporine (two patients) and had more than 50% improvement measured by EASI score within 3 months of treatment with tocilizumab (8 mg/kg SQ monthly) [76]. However, two of them developed colonization with *Staphylococcus aureus* and one developed bursitis of the left heel with a hemolytic *streptococcus Group G*. The authors concluded that even though anti-IL6 may play a role in the treatment of AD, further studies are needed to evaluate the safety of this drug and the risk of infection in patients with AD.

Anti-Tumor Necrosis Factor Alpha (TNF-α) Agents

Anti-TNF biologics are well-established safe and effective therapies for moderate-to-severe psoriasis. The role of TNF-α is well-established in psoriasis, but its role in AD is unclear. In the pathogenesis of AD, tumor necrosis factor-α (TNF-α) is thought to be released by infiltrating mast cells and T-helper lymphocytes as well as epidermal keratinocytes. TNF-α is involved in the upregulation of proinflammatory cytokines, such as interleukins (ILs)-1, -6, -8, and helps facilitate the migration and adhesion of inflammatory cells in the epidermis. Patients with AD have significantly elevated serum and tissue concentrations of TNF-α and, thus, may be responsive to treatment with TNF-α-inhibitors [77].

Some case series and case reports did not find anti-TNF approaches effective [78, 79], although one case series did show improvement of pruritus scores and QoL [78]. There have been several reports of eczema occurring as an adverse event during treatment of psoriasis and other Th1-mediated diseases such as inflammatory arthritis and inflammatory bowel disease. Nakamura and colleagues reported a litera-

ture search that reviewed 15 total publications describing eczema during anti-TNFα therapy. The studies and case reports described new onset or exacerbation of preexisting AD, "psoriasiform eczema," and "eczematiform lesions" in varying proportions ranging from 5.4 to 20.6% of patients on a biologic agent. Overall, TNF antagonism does not appear effective for AD and may promote eczematous lesions [80].

Conclusions

The future of targeted biologic therapy is bright for AD. Blockade of the type 2 cytokine pathways appears to provide the most benefit thus far, but other novel pathways are being revealed and targeted in this complex disease. In reality, biologic therapy for AD is still in its infancy, much like the treatment for psoriasis was over a decade ago. The intricacies of study design, endpoints, and the confounding role of concomitant TCS are still being worked out and need to be standardized.

Case Report
34-year-old male with a lifelong history of very severe and recalcitrant atopic dermatitis, recurrent methicillin-resistant *S. aureus* skin infections who experienced severe symptoms of itch (rated 10/10), difficulty sleeping (sleep disturbance scale 10/10), and widespread and intense skin lesions (Eczema Area and Severity Index (EASI) of 66 and total body surface area of over 90% (Fig. 31.1). His disease had a severe impact of his quality of life (DLQI 23/25).

Past Medical History
– Asthma

Previous Therapies
He did not respond consistently to conventional therapy such as topical corticosteroids, phototherapy, methotrexate, and cyclosporine and thus he had to be treated with frequent cycles of systemic prednisone, oral antibiotics, and was using daily topical steroids with minimal improvement.

Management
He underwent a clinical trial with dupilumab and thus qualified for the long-term extension and received dupilumab 300 mg every week for 2 years. After 6 months of therapy his skin was almost clear per his Investigator Global Assessment. After 6 months, his body surface area of involvement ranged from 3 to 5% (Fig. 31.2), his EASI score ranged from 3 to 7, and his quality of life improved significantly (DLQI 3/25).

Fig. 31.1 Initial evaluation before starting trial with dupilumab

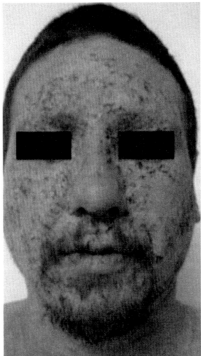
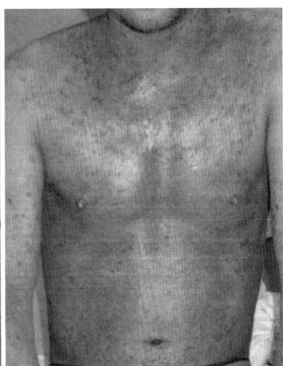

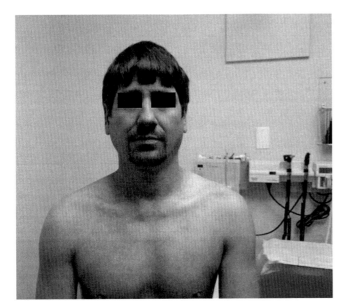

Fig. 31.2 Six months after starting open label extension with dupilumab

References

1. Flohr C, Mann J. New insights into the epidemiology of childhood atopic dermatitis. Allergy. 2014;69(1):3–16.
2. Silverberg JI, Hanifin JM. Adult eczema prevalence and associations with asthma and other health and demographic factors: a US population-based study. J Allergy Clin Immunol. 2013;132(5):1132–8.
3. Drucker AM, Wang AR, Qureshi AA. Research gaps in quality of life and economic burden of atopic dermatitis: the National Eczema Association burden of disease audit. JAMA Dermatol. 2016;152(8):873–4.
4. Leung DY. New insights into atopic dermatitis: role of skin barrier and immune dysregulation. Allergol Int. 2013;62(2):151–61.
5. Williams HC. Is the prevalence of atopic dermatitis increasing? Clin Exp Dermatol. 1992;17(6):385–91.
6. Werfel T, et al. Cellular and molecular immunologic mechanisms in patients with atopic dermatitis. J Allergy Clin Immunol. 2016;138(2):336–49.
7. Simpson EL, et al. Emollient enhancement of the skin barrier from birth offers effective atopic dermatitis prevention. J Allergy Clin Immunol. 2014;134(4):818–23.
8. Horimukai K, et al. Application of moisturizer to neonates prevents development of atopic dermatitis. J Allergy Clin Immunol. 2014;134(4):824–30.e6.
9. Mason JM, et al. Improved emollient use reduces atopic eczema symptoms and is cost neutral in infants: before-and-after evaluation of a multifaceted educational support programme. BMC Dermatol. 2013;13:7.
10. Sidbury R, et al. Guidelines of care for the management of atopic dermatitis: section 3. Management and treatment with phototherapy and systemic agents. J Am Acad Dermatol. 2014;71(2):327–49.
11. Schmitt J, et al. Prednisolone vs. ciclosporin for severe adult eczema. An investigator-initiated double-blind placebo-controlled multicentre trial. Br J Dermatol. 2010;162(3):661–8.
12. Guttman-Yassky E, Nograles KE, Krueger JG. Contrasting pathogenesis of atopic dermatitis and psoriasis—Part II: Immune cell subsets and therapeutic concepts. J Allergy Clin Immunol. 2011;127(6):1420–32.
13. Novak N, Simon D. Atopic dermatitis—from new pathophysiologic insights to individualized therapy. Allergy. 2011;66(7):830–9.
14. Akdis CA, et al. Diagnosis and treatment of atopic dermatitis in children and adults: European academy of Allergology and clinical immunology/American Academy of allergy, asthma and immunology/PRACTALL consensus report. Allergy. 2006;61(8):969–87.

15. Rho NK, et al. Immunophenotyping of inflammatory cells in lesional skin of the extrinsic and intrinsic types of atopic dermatitis. Br J Dermatol. 2004;151(1):119–25.

16. Hanifin JM, et al. Relationship between increased cyclic AMP-phosphodiesterase activity and abnormal adenylyl cyclase regulation in leukocytes from patients with atopic dermatitis. J Invest Dermatol. 1992;98(6 Suppl):100s–5s.

17. Hamid Q, Boguniewicz M, Leung DY. Differential in situ cytokine gene expression in acute versus chronic atopic dermatitis. J Clin Invest. 1994;94(2):870–6.

18. Dhingra N, et al. Molecular profiling of contact dermatitis skin identifies allergen-dependent differences in immune response. J Allergy Clin Immunol. 2014;134(2):362–72.

19. Grewe M, et al. A role for Th1 and Th2 cells in the immunopathogenesis of atopic dermatitis. Immunol Today. 1998;19(8):359–61.

20. Visitsunthorn N, et al. Atopy patch test in children with atopic dermatitis. Ann Allergy Asthma Immunol. 2016;117(6):668–73.

21. Gittler JK, et al. Progressive activation of T(H)2/T(H)22 cytokines and selective epidermal proteins characterizes acute and chronic atopic dermatitis. J Allergy Clin Immunol. 2012;130(6):1344–54.

22. Noda S, et al. The Asian atopic dermatitis phenotype combines features of atopic dermatitis and psoriasis with increased TH17 polarization. J Allergy Clin Immunol. 2015;136(5):1254–64.

23. Weinberg JM, Siegfried EC. Successful treatment of severe atopic dermatitis in a child and an adult with the T-cell modulator efalizumab. Arch Dermatol. 2006;142(5):555–8.

24. Takiguchi R, et al. Efalizumab for severe atopic dermatitis: a pilot study in adults. J Am Acad Dermatol. 2007;56(2):222–7.

25. Ibler K, et al. Efalizumab for severe refractory atopic eczema: retrospective study on 11 cases. J Eur Acad Dermatol Venereol. 2010;24(7):837–9.

26. Hassan AS, et al. Clinical and immunopathologic findings during treatment of recalcitrant atopic eczema with efalizumab. J Am Acad Dermatol. 2007;56(2):217–21.

27. Farshidi A, Sadeghi P. Successful treatment of severe refractory atopic dermatitis with efalizumab. J Drugs Dermatol. 2006;5(10):994–8.

28. Kaplan, A.P., A.M. Gimenez-Arnau, and S.S. Saini, Mechanisms of action that contribute to efficacy of omalizumab in chronic spontaneous urticaria.. Allergy, 2016.

29. Beck LA, et al. Omalizumab-induced reductions in mast cell Fce psilon RI expression and function. J Allergy Clin Immunol. 2004;114(3):527–30.

30. MacGlashan DW Jr, et al. Down-regulation of fc(epsilon)RI expression on human basophils during in vivo treatment of atopic patients with anti-IgE antibody. J Immunol. 1997;158(3):1438–45.

31. Presta LG, et al. Humanization of an antibody directed against IgE. J Immunol. 1993;151(5):2623–32.

32. FDA. Omalizumab. Available from: https://www.fda.gov/Drugs/DrugSafety/ucm414911.htm.

33. FDA. Omalizumab (marketed as Xolair) Information. 2003; Available from: https://www.fda.gov/Drugs/DrugSafety/Postmarket DrugSafetyInformationforPatientsandProviders/ucm103291.htm.

34. Siegfried EC. Long-term follow-up of a child treated with efalizumab for atopic dermatitis. Arch Dermatol. 2007;143(8):1077–8.

35. Cipriani F, et al. Autoimmunity in atopic dermatitis: biomarker or simply epiphenomenon? J Dermatol. 2014;41(7):569–76.

36. Fernandez-Anton Martinez MC, et al. Omalizumab for the treatment of atopic dermatitis. Actas Dermosifiliogr. 2012;103(7):624–8.

37. Ramirez del Pozo ME, et al. Omalizumab (an anti-IgE antibody) in the treatment of severe atopic eczema. J Investig Allergol Clin Immunol. 2011;21(5):416–7.

38. Lane JE, et al. Treatment of recalcitrant atopic dermatitis with omalizumab. J Am Acad Dermatol. 2006;54(1):68–72.

39. Velling P, et al. Improvement of quality of life in patients with concomitant allergic asthma and atopic dermatitis: one year follow-up of omalizumab therapy. Eur J Med Res. 2011;16(9):407–10.

40. Iyengar SR, et al. Immunologic effects of omalizumab in children with severe refractory atopic dermatitis: a randomized, placebo-controlled clinical trial. Int Arch Allergy Immunol. 2013;162(1):89–93.

41. Heil PM, et al. Omalizumab therapy in atopic dermatitis: depletion of IgE does not improve the clinical course - a randomized, placebo-controlled and double blind pilot study. J Dtsch Dermatol Ges. 2010;8(12):990–8.

42. Guttman-Yassky, E., Emerging treatments for atopic dermatitis: Phase 2 Data in 25th European Academy of Dermatology and Venereology, 2016: Viena, Austria .

43. Czarnowicki T, et al. Alterations in B-cell subsets in pediatric patients with early atopic dermatitis. J Allergy Clin Immunol. 2016;

44. Silverman GJ, Weisman S. Rituximab therapy and autoimmune disorders: prospects for anti-B cell therapy. Arthritis Rheum. 2003;48(6):1484–92.

45. Simon D, et al. Anti-CD20 (rituximab) treatment improves atopic eczema. J Allergy Clin Immunol. 2008;121(1):122–8.

46. Ponte P, Lopes MJ. Apparent safe use of single dose rituximab for recalcitrant atopic dermatitis in the first trimester of a twin pregnancy. J Am Acad Dermatol. 2010;63(2):355–6.

47. McDonald BS, Jones J, Rustin M. Rituximab as a treatment for severe atopic eczema: failure to improve in three consecutive patients. Clin Exp Dermatol. 2016;41(1):45–7.

48. Sediva A, et al. Anti-CD20 (rituximab) treatment for atopic eczema. J Allergy Clin Immunol. 2008;121(6):1515–6. author reply 1516-7

49. Hanifin JM, et al. Recombinant interferon gamma therapy for atopic dermatitis. J Am Acad Dermatol. 1993;28(2 Pt 1):189–97.

50. Schneider LC, et al. Long-term therapy with recombinant interferon-gamma (rIFN-gamma) for atopic dermatitis. Ann Allergy Asthma Immunol. 1998;80(3):263–8.

51. Noh GW, Lee KY. Blood eosinophils and serum IgE as predictors for prognosis of interferon-gamma therapy in atopic dermatitis. Allergy. 1998;53(12):1202–7.

52. Connetics, Phase III results of gamma interferon for AD. The Free Library; 1997.

53. Beck LA, et al. Dupilumab treatment in adults with moderate-to-severe atopic dermatitis. N Engl J Med. 2014; 371(2):130–9.

54. Simpson EL, et al. Dupilumab therapy provides clinically meaningful improvement in patient-reported outcomes (PROs): a phase IIb, randomized, placebo-controlled, clinical trial in adult patients with moderate to severe atopic dermatitis (AD). J Am Acad Dermatol. 2016;75(3):506–15.

55. Thaci D, et al. Efficacy and safety of dupilumab in adults with moderate-to-severe atopic dermatitis inadequately controlled by topical treatments: a randomised, placebo-controlled, dose-ranging phase 2b trial. Lancet. 2016;387(10013):40–52.

56. Simpson EL, et al. Two phase 3 trials of Dupilumab versus placebo in atopic dermatitis. N Engl J Med. 2016;375(24):2335–48.

57. Blauvelt, A., Abstract #5267. In: Long-Term management of moderate-to-severe atopic dermatitis (AD) with Dupilumab up to 1 Year with concomitant topical corticosteroids (TCS): a randomized, placebo-controlled Phase 3 Trial (CHRONOS). 2017: annual meeting of the American Academy of Dermatology (AAD) in Orlando, FL, March 3-7; 2017.

58. FDA. Dupilumab biologics liscence application; 2016. Available from: http://www.prnewswire.com/news-releases/regeneron-and-sanofi-announce-dupilumab-biologics-license-application-accepted-for-priority-review-by-us-fda-300333529.html).

59. Kim BE, et al. Loricrin and involucrin expression is down-regulated by Th2 cytokines through STAT-6. Clin Immunol. 2008;126(3):332–7.

60. He JQ, et al. Genetic variants of the IL13 and IL4 genes and atopic diseases in at-risk children. Genes Immun. 2003;4(5):385–9.

61. Kim ST, et al. Topical delivery of interleukin-13 antisense oligonucleotides with cationic elastic liposome for the treatment of atopic dermatitis. J Gene Med. 2009;11(1):26–37.

62. Ultsch M, et al. Structural basis of signaling blockade by anti-IL-13 antibody Lebrikizumab. J Mol Biol. 2013;425(8):1330–9.

63. Sanderson CJ. Interleukin-5, eosinophils, and disease. Blood. 1992;79(12):3101–9.

64. Oldhoff JM, et al. Anti-IL-5 recombinant humanized monoclonal antibody (mepolizumab) for the treatment of atopic dermatitis. Allergy. 2005;60(5):693–6.

65. Sonkoly E, et al. IL-31: a new link between T cells and pruritus in atopic skin inflammation. J Allergy Clin Immunol. 2006;117(2):411–7.

66. Cornelissen C, et al. IL-31 regulates differentiation and filaggrin expression in human organotypic skin models. J Allergy Clin Immunol. 2012;129(2):426–33. 433.e1-8

67. Ruzicka T, et al. Anti-interleukin-31 receptor a antibody for atopic dermatitis. N Engl J Med. 2017;376(9):826–35.

68. Esaki H, et al. Early-onset pediatric atopic dermatitis is TH2 but also TH17 polarized in skin. J Allergy Clin Immunol. 2016;138(6): 1639–51.

69. Fernandez-Anton Martinez MC, et al. Ustekinumab in the treatment of severe atopic dermatitis: a preliminary report of our experience with 4 patients. Actas Dermosifiliogr. 2014;105(3):312–3.

70. Puya R, et al. Treatment of severe refractory adult atopic dermatitis with ustekinumab. Int J Dermatol. 2012;51(1):115–6.

71. Shroff A, Guttman-Yassky E. Successful use of ustekinumab therapy in refractory severe atopic dermatitis. JAAD Case Rep. 2015;1(1):25–6.

72. Lis-Swiety A, et al. Atopic dermatitis exacerbated with ustekinumab in a psoriatic patient with childhood history of atopy. Allergol Int. 2015;64(4):382–3.

73. Samorano LP, et al. Inadequate response to ustekinumab in atopic dermatitis - a report of two patients. J Eur Acad Dermatol Venereol. 2016;30(3):522–3.

74. Khattri S, et al. Efficacy and safety of ustekinumab treatment in adults with moderate-to-severe atopic dermatitis. Exp Dermatol. 2017;26(1):28–35.

75. Koryurek OM, Kalkan G. A new alternative therapy in dermatology: tocilizumab. Cutan Ocul Toxicol. 2016;35(2):145–52.

76. Navarini AA, French LE, Hofbauer GF. Interrupting IL-6-receptor signaling improves atopic dermatitis but associates with bacterial superinfection. J Allergy Clin Immunol. 2011;128(5):1128–30.

77. Danso MO, et al. TNF-alpha and Th2 cytokines induce atopic dermatitis-like features on epidermal differentiation proteins and stratum corneum lipids in human skin equivalents. J Invest Dermatol. 2014;134(7):1941–50.

78. Jacobi A, et al. Infliximab in the treatment of moderate to severe atopic dermatitis. J Am Acad Dermatol. 2005;52(3 Pt 1):522–6.

79. Buka RL, et al. Etanercept is minimally effective in 2 children with atopic dermatitis. J Am Acad Dermatol. 2005;53(2):358–9.

80. Nakamura M, et al. Eczema as an adverse effect of anti-TNFalpha therapy in psoriasis and other Th1-mediated diseases: a review. J Dermatolog Treat. 2016:1–5.

Oral Agents for Atopic Dermatitis: Current and in Development

Julia Mayba and Melinda Gooderham

Abbreviations

AD	Atopic dermatitis
AZA	Azathioprine
CRTH2	Chemoattractant receptor-homologous molecule expressed on T-helper type 2 cells
CsA	Cyclosporine
DGLA	Dihomo-gamma-linolenic acid
EASI	Eczema Area and Severity Index
EC-MPS	Enteric-coated mycophenolate sodium
FDA	U.S. Food and Drug Administration
H4R	Histamine H4 receptor
HTN	Hypertension
IGA	Investigator's Global Assessment
IL	Interleukin
JAK	Janus kinase
MMF	Mycophenolate mofetil
MPS	Mycophenolate sodium
MTX	Methotrexate
NK-1R	Neurokinin 1 receptor
OGCs	Oral glucocorticoids
PDE4	Phosphodiesterase-4
PGD1	Prostaglandin D1
PGD2	Prostaglandin D2
SASSAD	Six area six sign atopic dermatitis
SCORAD	Scoring for atopic dermatitis
TPMT	Thiopurine methyltransferase
VAS	Visual analog scale

J. Mayba, BSc
University of Manitoba, Winnipeg, MB, Canada

SKiN Centre for Dermatology, 775 Monaghan Rd., Peterborough, ON, Canada, K9J 5K2

M. Gooderham, MD, MSc, FRCPC (✉)
SKiN Centre for Dermatology,
775 Monaghan Rd., Peterborough, ON, Canada, K9J 5K2

Probity Medical Research, Waterloo, ON, Canada

Queen's University, Kingston, ON, Canada
e-mail: mgooderham@centrefordermatology.com

Introduction

Atopic dermatitis (AD) is a chronic, pruritic inflammatory skin disease due to a defective skin barrier and aberrant immune responses that results in a reduced quality of life for those affected. Patients with moderate-to-severe AD may require treatment beyond topical therapy [1]. It has been shown that in certain populations, over 10% of patients with AD require more intensive therapy than topical treatment alone [2]. There are many oral immunosuppressive agents currently used off-label for the treatment of AD, since only cyclosporine is approved for use in AD in Europe and Japan [3, 4]. In addition to cyclosporine, azathioprine, methotrexate, mycophenolate mofetil, and systemic corticosteroids are also used for the treatment of AD [1, 5]. A systematic review on systemic therapy for AD reviewed 34 RCTs on a total of 1653 patients [1]. Based on the best available evidence, cyclosporine was recommended first line, azathioprine second line, and methotrexate third line. Although these agents have demonstrated efficacy in the treatment of moderate-to-severe AD in both the adult and pediatric population, they have a narrow margin of safety and their use is limited by toxicity. There still exists a need for therapies with a favorable risk-to-benefit ratio. Targeted biologic therapies have shown promise in the treatment of AD and will be reviewed in a separate chapter. As new targets are identified while we learn more about the pathophysiology of AD, new oral agents are also under investigation for the treatment of AD with both promising and disappointing results.

Cyclosporine

Mechanism of Action

Cyclosporine (CsA) is a calcineurin inhibitor that functions by inhibiting T-lymphocyte-driven immune responses and production of interleukin (IL)-2, which ultimately blunts immunoreactivity [5, 6].

© Springer International Publishing AG 2018
P.S. Yamauchi (ed.), *Biologic and Systemic Agents in Dermatology*, https://doi.org/10.1007/978-3-319-66884-0_32

Clinical Efficacy

CsA is the best-studied systemic agent for the treatment of AD with multiple placebo-controlled randomized controlled trials published [1, 6]. It has been recommended to be the first-line systemic agent used for short-term therapy [1]. Numerous clinical trials have shown CsA to be highly effective in treating AD with an average 50% reduction in disease severity after 6–8 weeks of treatment, as well as a marked improvement in patient quality of life [7–19]. CsA demonstrates dose-related treatment improvements in AD severity. Specifically, two weeks into treatment, patients receiving low-dose therapy (≤3 mg/kg) showed a mean decrease in disease severity of 22%, whereas patients on higher dose therapy (≤4 mg/kg) showed a 40% reduction in disease severity [7]. Cyclosporine is unique for its rapid onset of action compared to other systemic AD treatments [5]. It has been shown to be equally effective in children as in adults, with children possibly exhibiting better tolerability of CsA [7]. Unfortunately, AD relapse rates are quite high after stopping CsA, with 50% of patients relapsing after 2 weeks and 80% by 2 months [20].

Dosage

With respect to dosing, CsA is administered twice daily [21] and is often started at a dose of 3 mg/kg/day and titrated upward as necessary for control [1]. Although higher dosing of CsA, such as 5 mg/kg/day, has been shown to be more effective in treating AD, most CsA side effects are dose related, and therefore dosing is often reduced to the lowest effective dose [1]. In general, the consensus regarding safe pediatric and adult dosing of CsA is 3–6 mg/kg/day, such that the lowest effective dose required to achieve the desired clinical result is given [22]. A 6-month, open-label, randomized trial in patients with moderate-to-severe AD treated with CsA showed a benefit of concomitant topical therapy over CsA monotherapy [23]. Data on long-term use (over 12 months) of CsA is not available, so it is recommended patients taper and eventually discontinue the drug once their disease is in remission [22].

Adverse Events and Drug Monitoring

Adverse events generally related to increased systemic CsA exposure, either through high dosage [6] or long-term treatment [24], include infection, nephrotoxicity, hypertension, gingival hyperplasia, tremor, hypertrichosis, headache, and increased risk of cancer and lymphoma [6, 22]. Reversible side effects that may be resolved by decreasing CsA dosage include increased blood pressure, decreased renal function, gastrointestinal symptoms, infections, headache, and paresthesia [20].

Consequently, therapy with CsA requires baseline blood pressure reading and laboratory testing, including hepatic and renal function, as well as regular monitoring of these parameters [22]. CsA also may exhibit drug interactions with other systemic medications, so consulting up-to-date product information and drug reference resources is imperative for patients prescribed CsA or when adding other medications in conjunction with CsA [22].

Treatment Duration

With respect to treatment duration, CsA is useful for short course treatment or courses of 12 weeks with intermission periods [7]. Long-term safety of CsA cannot be concluded from clinical trials [1] and it is recommended that CsA use is limited to 1 or 2 years [25]. In the pediatric population, CsA has been shown to be well tolerated over a one year period [12].

Overall Recommendation

Overall, CsA is recommended as first-line systemic therapy for AD for short-term use [1]. With the exception of Europe and Japan, where CsA is approved for use in AD, it is used off-label in other jurisdictions [3, 4].

Azathioprine

Mechanism of Action

Azathioprine (AZA) is a purine analog that inhibits DNA proliferation [22]. AZA is converted into 6-mercaptopurine, which produces metabolites that incorporate into DNA [26]. Consequently, this preferentially affects cells with high proliferation rates, such as B- and T-cells in inflammatory states. Initially developed in the 1960s to prevent organ transplant rejection, it has also been used to treat other immunologic conditions such as pemphigus vulgaris, rheumatoid arthritis, and inflammatory bowel disease [24]. AZA can be used off-label to treat other inflammatory and cutaneous disorders, including AD [22].

Clinical Efficacy

A review of 8 studies of AD treatment in adults with AZA found clinical improvement in the majority of patients in 7 of the 8 trials [27–34]. A subsequent publication of a placebo-controlled clinical trial in 37 adult patients also showed that AZA is effective and useful for the treatment of severe AD [35]. In patients treated with AZA, their six area six sign atopic dermatitis (SASSAD) sign score decreased by 26% during their treatment course, compared to a 3% decrease in patients treated with placebo. Furthermore, pruritus, sleep disturbance, and disruption of work/daytime activity improved significantly on active treatment with AZA, but not on placebo. With respect to adverse effects, 14 patients treated with AZA experienced gastrointestinal disturbances, with four patients withdrawing from the study due to these side effects. Overall, however, in patients who tolerated AZA, it offered a reasonably safe and effective therapy in the treatment of severe AD [35].

Another clinical trial in adult patients with AD showed a 37% improvement in mean disease activity at week 12 in patients treated with AZA, compared to a 20% improvement with placebo. Also, patients treated with AZA exhibited significant improvements in patient-reported itch, area of involvement, global assessment, and quality of life [36].

AZA takes several weeks to reach a steady state in the bloodstream and therefore is relatively slow to take effect compared to CsA. Once patients are established on AZA treatment, it is generally well tolerated and can be continued for a longer treatment course than CsA [5].

Adverse Events and Dosage

Common side effects of AZA treatment include nausea, vomiting, and other gastrointestinal symptoms (bloating, anorexia, cramping). Other reported side effects include headache, hypersensitivity reactions, and elevated liver enzymes [22, 37]. A study that examined the outcomes of nearly 200 children treated with AZA revealed no fatal adverse events and various mild side effects, such as cutaneous viral infections, nausea, lethargy, indigestion, and mildly elevated hepatic transaminases [38].

The most common serious adverse events with AZA treatment are dose-dependent myelotoxicity and hepatotoxicity. Myelotoxicity has been shown to correlate with the activity of thiopurine methyltransferase (TPMT), an enzyme required for the metabolism of azathioprine. Homozygous deficiency of TPMT, found in 0.33% of the population, can often result in profound myelosuppression with AZA treatment. Roughly 10% of the population is heterozygous at the TPMT locus and demonstrates intermediate TPMT activity. These patients can also be at risk for myelosuppression when treated with AZA [27]. One clinical trial dosed heterozygous TPMT patients with 1.0 mg/kg per day for AD treatment, while patients with normal TPMT activity received 2.5 mg/kg per day. Patients with heterozygous TPMT activity responded to azathioprine in similar proportion to other participants, without developing bone-marrow toxicity. Overall, it was found that TPMT-based dosing appeared to reduce predicted toxicity while maintaining drug efficacy [36]. Consequently, it is recommended that

AZA dosing is determined based on patient TPMT activity in order to prevent myelosuppression [1]. In adults, this can range from 1 to 3 mg/kg/day and in pediatrics it may range from 1 to 4 mg/kg/day [22]. Graduated dosing to maximize clinical benefit and minimize adverse events is ideal [36].

Long-term immunosuppressive therapy with AZA in transplant patients has shown increased incidence of squamous cell carcinoma and non-Hodgkin's lymphoma [26], however, short and medium course treatment with AZA has not demonstrated this increased risk of carcinogenicity [27].

Drug Monitoring and Treatment Duration

It has also been recommended that patients treated with AZA have their full blood count monitored weekly for the first 8 weeks of treatment. Liver enzymes should be monitored at 2, 4, and 8 weeks of treatment, followed by every 2 months thereafter [35]. There is no concrete recommendation regarding maximum treatment duration; however, it is recommended that once the patient is clear or almost clear and this is maintained, AZA should be tapered or discontinued, maintaining remission with emollients and topical agents [22].

Overall Recommendation

Currently, AZA is recommended as a second-line treatment option for short-term induction treatment and long-term treatment up to 24 weeks. The indirect comparison suggests that AZA is less efficacious than CsA for the treatment of AD [1].

Methotrexate

Mechanism of Action

Methotrexate (MTX) is widely known and approved by the U.S. Food and Drug Administration (FDA) for the treatment of various dermatologic conditions, including advanced mycosis fungoides and psoriasis [22]. However, treatment of AD with MTX is currently off-label [6]. MTX is a dihydrofolate reductase inhibitor used for the treatment of many oncologic and autoimmune disorders, as it suppresses DNA and RNA synthesis and T-cell function [6].

Clinical Efficacy

The true clinical efficacy of MTX in the treatment of refractory AD is unknown, due to a lack of consistency between clinical trials concerning methods, dosing, and duration of therapy [22]. Consequently, what is known about the treatment of moderate-to-severe AD with MTX can only be extrapolated from some clinical trials. In a retrospective review of 31 children and adolescents with a variable treatment duration (2–38 months), 75% of patients found low-dose MTX to be an effective or very effective treatment for AD, while 25% found MTX to be ineffective. Overall, it was found that low-dose MTX appeared to be effective for AD treatment in children and adolescents and exhibited a good safety/tolerability profile in this population [39]. With respect to the adult population, a small prospective open-label clinical trial of MTX for the treatment of moderate-to-severe AD in twelve adults showed that MTX was an effective and well-tolerated treatment during a 24-week treatment period. On average, patient disease activity improved 52% from baseline, along with significant improvement in quality of life, body surface area involved and loss of sleep and itch scores. Importantly, 8 out of 9 patients experienced persistent improvement 12 weeks after stopping MTX. In addition, it appeared that response to MTX compared favorably with other second-line therapies [40].

Another study of 20 adult patients with refractory AD demonstrated clinical improvement in disease severity in 75% of patients after 3 months of treatment with MTX. In addition, the first signs of improvement occurred between weeks 4 and 8 after treatment initiation [41]. Further comparative study to determine the actual clinical efficacy of MTX for the treatment of AD is required.

In the treatment of severe pediatric AD, there was no statistically significant difference in the reduction of severity scoring for atopic dermatitis (SCORAD) scores between patients treated with CsA and those treated with MTX [42]. Interestingly, CsA showed a more rapid response than MTX, while MTX had a longer lasting treatment effect. Nonetheless, overall it was found that both MTX and CsA in low doses are clinically effective, relatively safe and well tolerated for severe AD in children [42]. A separate trial compared the efficacy of MTX to that of AZA in the treatment of severe AD in adults. At week 12 of the study, it was demonstrated that both the patients in the MTX treatment group and those in the AZA group experienced statistically significant reductions in their mean SCORAD scores, 42% and 39%, respectively. Furthermore, no statistically significant differences were found in the number and severity of adverse events in the two groups, nor did any serious adverse events occur [43]. It appears that MTX may be of similar efficacy as AZA in the treatment of severe AD; however, this necessitates further investigation.

Dosage

MTX is usually given as a single weekly dose and can be administered as a subcutaneous injection or in oral tablet form [22]. Dosing of MTX for AD has been extrapolated from what is known about MTX for the treatment of psoriasis and is between 7.5 mg and 25 mg weekly for adults [25]. As is the case with other systemic therapies, dosing should be tailored to each patient's unique situation, such that adequate disease control is achieved and maintained while minimizing the occurrence of dose-related adverse events [22]. In patients unresponsive to MTX, studies have shown that there is no improved clinical efficacy observed after 12–16 weeks of treatment with further dose escalation. The average time maximum effect of MTX on AD treatment is ten weeks [22].

Adverse Events

Possible adverse events caused by treatment with MTX include nausea, elevated liver enzymes, and more rarely, pancytopenia, hepatotoxicity, and pulmonary toxicity. These side effects can be mitigated with proper dosage titration [6, 26]. In psoriasis patients, the cumulative dose of MTX received is recorded to monitor for hepatic toxicity. This has not yet been proven necessary in AD treatment with MTX [6, 22]. It is recommended that all patients taking MTX for the treatment of AD be supplemented with folic acid, to reduce the likelihood of hematologic and gastrointestinal toxicities. The consensus among experts suggests 1 mg/day of folic acid, but depending on the patient's individual needs this may increase up to 5 mg/day. On the day of MTX ingestion, patients should not take their folic acid supplementation [22].

Current Recommendations

Current recommendations suggest MTX as a third-line systemic treatment option for short-term induction treatment and long-term treatment up to 24 weeks [1]. This recommendation is primarily based on a clinical trial that found MTX to be of similar efficacy as AZA for the treatment of severe AD [43].

Mycophenolate Mofetil

Mechanism of Action

Mycophenolate mofetil (MMF) is a selective reversible inhibitor of inosine monophosphate dehydrogenase, an enzyme required for the de novo synthesis of purines. Lymphocytes lack the salvage pathway found in other inflammatory cells and consequently are solely dependent on the de novo synthesis pathway. Thus, inosine monophosphate dehydrogenase inhibition by MMF results in selective suppression of lymphocytes, namely B- and T-cells [6, 26]. Recently, another form of MMF has emerged called mycophenolate sodium (MPS), which is available in an enteric-coated form (EC-MPS). The latter formulation has been designed to minimize the gastrointestinal side effects caused by mycophenolic acid [5].

Clinical Efficacy

In adults with AD, studies have shown that MMF can be effective in treating moderate-to-severe AD resistant to conventional therapy. In particular, a retrospective chart review of 20 patients found that 17 patients improved with MMF therapy within 4 weeks of treatment initiation. Furthermore, 10 patients experienced disease remission and were able to taper and subsequently discontinue treatment. Generally, MMF was well tolerated by the patients, as the most common side effects included mild headache, gastrointestinal complaints, and fatigue. Four patients developed herpes zoster, one developed herpes simplex, and two developed cutaneous infections with *Staphylococcus aureus*. It was determined that MMF had a better safety profile than cyclosporine and oral systemic steroids for long-term treatment [44].

In the pediatric population, a retrospective analysis of 14 patients with severe, recalcitrant AD was conducted. It found that 13 out of the 14 patients exhibited clinical improvement of their AD with MMF treatment, with only one patient who failed to respond. Initial responses to therapy occurred within 8 weeks of treatment (with a mean time of 4 weeks), and maximal effects at 8–12 weeks of treatment (with a mean of 9 weeks). All patients tolerated MMF therapy well, with no complaints of infection, nor any development of leukopenia, anemia, thrombocytopenia, or elevated aminotransferases [45].

Nonetheless, further prospective controlled studies are required in both the pediatric and adult population to assess the true benefit of MMF treatment for recalcitrant AD.

The efficacy of MMF compared to other more established AD treatments is limited to a few clinical trials and retrospective studies. Specifically, a clinical trial in adults with AD comparing EC-MPS to CsA found that EC-MPS was equally as effective as CsA as maintenance therapy in patients with AD. It was also found that clinical improvement with EC-MPS was delayed in comparison with CsA. However, clinical remission after stopping EC-MPS lasted longer compared with CsA [46]. When comparing the clinical efficacy of MMF and AZA, a retrospective case series found that 61% of pediatric patients treated with AZA experienced significant clinical improvement in their AD, compared to 66% of pediatric patients treated with MMF [47].

Dosage

In young children, recommended dosing of MMF is 40–50 mg/kg/day and in adolescents, 30–40 mg/kg/day [6]. In adults, MMF is administered twice daily, and dosing may range from 0.5 to 3.0 g/day [44]. Currently, there is insufficient data for recommendations on optimal dosing of MMF for AD treatment in adults [22].

Adverse Events

With respect to adverse effects related to MMF treatment, common side effects reported in the pediatric population include nausea, vomiting, and abdominal cramping. As of yet, there are no established long-term side effects in children treated with MMF [22]. In adults, MMF is also well tolerated, with nausea, vomiting, and abdominal cramping also being the most common side effects of treatment. Gastrointestinal symptoms, headache, and fatigue are not correlated with dosage increase and tend not to affect patient compliance significantly. In rare instances, hematologic and genitourinary symptoms have been reported with MMF treatment. Based on findings in transplant patients, MMF has a theoretical risk of increasing susceptibility to infections, bacterial and viral; however, how this translates to AD patients is unknown at this time [22].

Current Recommendations

Currently, recommendations for AD treatment with EC-MPS are as follows; due to a lack of controlled trials, only a very weak recommendation is possible for EC-MPS as a maintenance treatment for severe AD after induction of remission by CsA for long-term use up to 30 weeks [1]. MMF/EC-MPS is also used off-label for the treatment of AD.

Systemic Corticosteroids

Mechanism of Action

Oral glucocorticoids (OGCs) affect the transcription of numerous mediators involved in the pathogenesis of AD, which include chemokines, cytokines, and adhesion molecules. The binding of regulatory elements of various genes via their receptors results in the inhibition of cell proliferation, vasoconstriction, and resolution of inflammation [48]. However, these immunomodulatory effects also contribute to many unique toxicities associated with OGC use.

Clinical Efficacy

Although OGCs are quickly effective as short-term therapy for the interruption of acute flare-ups in patients with severe atopic dermatitis, they are associated with a high risk of relapse upon discontinuation [22, 49]. In adults with severe

AD, a clinical trial comparing the treatment efficacy of prednisolone versus CsA found that stable remission was achieved in only 1 of 21 patients receiving prednisolone, compared to 6 of 17 patients treated with CsA [50]. A high rate of relapse was observed in this study, where 10 out of 21 patients treated with prednisolone and 5 out of 17 treated with CsA experienced significant exacerbations of eczema after termination of active treatment, and therefore the study was terminated early by an independent safety board [50].

Two small clinical trials have studied the use of systemic corticosteroids in children with moderate-to-severe and severe AD. Children with moderate-to-severe AD were given 4 weeks of treatment with combined oral plus nasal beclomethasone diproprionate which led to significant improvement of their AD compared to placebo; however, this was based on non-validated outcome measures. No adverse events were observed in the treatment group, except for slight reductions in the 24-h urinary cortisol excretion compared to the placebo group [51]. Another trial compared systemic flunisolide to placebo and found that after 2 weeks of flunisolide treatment, total clinical severity scores indicated a significant improvement in symptoms compared to the placebo group. This study was also based on non-validated outcome measures. Furthermore, after the completion of flunisolide treatment, no worsening of symptoms or AD relapse occurred, and no adverse events were observed [52].

Dosage

An initial prednisone dosage of 0.75–1 mg/kg per day should be tapered in 7–10 days, to minimize the risk of severe AD relapse [48]. However, dosages may vary depending on the type of corticosteroid, patient comorbidities, and AD severity [49]. Nonetheless, regardless of the taper schedule, an AD flare may still be expected. Commonly used OGC formulations include prednisone and prednisolone. Triamcinolone acetonide is administered as an intramuscular injection and is also used as a systemic corticosteroid [22].

Adverse Events and Drug Monitoring

OGCs have numerous side effects associated with their administration that more typically arise with long-term use, which includes diabetes, hypertension, gastric ulcers, osteoporosis, glaucoma, and Cushing's syndrome [49]. Patients requiring long-term treatment are more susceptible to opportunistic infections [22]. Unique to the pediatric population is the possibility of decreased linear growth while being treated

with OGCs [53]. Long-term treatment with OGCs may require blood pressure monitoring, ophthalmologic examination, hypothalamic-pituitary-adrenal axis suppression testing, bone density evaluation in adults, and growth velocity measurement in children [22]. Laboratory monitoring of blood counts and blood sugar levels should also be considered [49].

Treatment Duration

Although treatment of AD with OGCs is not recommended, when used, treatment may last from 3 days to 3 weeks depending on the severity of the flare-up episode. Long-term treatment with OGCs is not recommended because of numerous well-described side effects including risk of relapse [49].

Overall Recommendation

OGCs have a mostly unfavorable risk-to-benefit ratio for the treatment of adult AD. Specifically, long-term treatment of adult AD with OGCs is not recommended, while short-term treatment (preferably up to 1 week duration) can be considered as salvage therapy for an acute flare in extraordinary and severe cases [49]. With respect to the pediatric population, small studies have demonstrated the potential benefit of short-term OGC treatment of moderate and severe AD. However, overall OGCs are not recommended for the pediatric population unless used to treat comorbid conditions, such as asthma exacerbations, or as part of a short-term transition protocol to a steroid-sparing systemic immunomodulatory agent [22].

Alitretinoin

Currently, alitretinoin is recognized as an effective and safe treatment modality for chronic hand dermatitis in both controlled clinical trials and the real-world setting [54–56]. Not only is hand dermatitis more common in patients with AD [57], there is some speculation that alitretinoin may also be of benefit in extra-palmar AD [5]. In a small clinical trial of 6 patients, alitretinoin led to a substantial clinical improvement of both palmar and extra-palmar lesions and was well tolerated [58]. Further study to confirm the clinical efficacy of extra-palmar AD treatment with alitretinoin is required. This agent may be of benefit to AD patients who suffer from the burden of hand dermatitis and can be used with concomitant topical therapy and phototherapy.

New Agents in Development: Promising and Not

Phosphodiesterase-4 (PDE4) Inhibitors

PDE4 regulates the inflammatory response by degrading cyclic adenosine

3′,5′-monophosphate (cAMP), an intracellular second messenger. Inhibition of PDE4 increases the level of cAMP, which results in decreased production of inflammatory mediators and an increase in anti-inflammatory mediators [59]. It has been shown that PDE4 inhibition is an effective means of reducing inflammation associated with atopic dermatitis [60]. PDE4 inhibitors are under investigation for the treatment of AD with both promising and disappointing results reported from phase 2 clinical development thus far [61, 62]. The recent approval of a topical boron-based PDE4 inhibitor, crisaborole (Eucrisa, Pfizer), for mild-to-moderate AD also highlights the benefit of blocking PDE4 in the treatment of AD. A small open label pilot study of 16 adults with moderate-to-severe AD showed the oral PDE4 inhibitor, apremilast, at 20–30 mg BID provided an improvement in the clinical signs of AD as measured by Eczema Area and Severity Index (EASI) score, as well as improvement in pruritus and quality of life [61]. A second proof of concept trial on 10 patients with either AD or allergic contact dermatitis over 12 weeks showed only minimal benefit; however, the lower dose of 20 mg BID was provided [62]. A randomized placebo-controlled phase 2 trial investigating the use of apremilast, 30 mg or 40 mg PO BID, in moderate-to-severe atopic dermatitis is now complete with disappointing results posted (NCT02087943, ClinicalTrials.gov) [63]. The primary endpoint of percent reduction in EASI score was significant for apremilast 40 mg PO BID vs. placebo (p = 0.03) but was not significant at the 30 mg PO BID dose. The secondary endpoints, the percentage of patients reaching Investigator's Global Assessment (IGA) score 0/1 and EASI 50, were not met with either the 30 mg or 40 mg BID dosing groups (NCT02087943, ClinicalTrials.gov) [63].

Janus Kinase (JAK) Inhibitors

The JAK-STAT pathway is essential for the inflammatory signaling pathways of AD [64]. It has been shown that application of topical JAK inhibitors improves the signs and symptoms of atopic dermatitis [65, 66]. Furthermore, a small case series of six patients with recalcitrant AD treated with oral tofacitinib 5 mg OD – BID had a 66% reduction in SCORAD after 8–29 weeks of therapy [67]. Systemic JAK inhibition is now formally being investigated in the management of moderate-to-severe AD. A Phase 2b randomized trial is investigating the JAK 1 inhibitor, PF 04965842, given once daily in four doses (10, 30, 100, 200 mg) compared to placebo over 12 weeks in subjects with moderate-to-severe AD. This study is designed to assess the efficacy of PF 04965842 as measured by the IGA and EASI scores, as well as to monitor safety (NCT02780167, ClinicalTrials.gov) [68].

Other Novel Agents

Fevipiprant (QAW039), an oral antagonist of the receptor for prostaglandin D2 (PGD2), also called the chemoattractant receptor-homologous molecule expressed on T-helper type 2 cells (CRTh2), is being investigated in the management of allergic diseases including asthma and AD [69]. The CRTh2 receptor is a G-protein coupled receptor whose ligand, PGD2, induces inflammatory cytokine release from the Th2 cell. Phase 3 trials are currently ongoing in severe asthma. Phase 2 trials in AD reported discouraging results with no difference noted between fevipiprant 450 mg PO OD and placebo in the change from baseline in EASI score after 12 weeks (NCT01785602, ClinicalTrials.gov) [70].

As pruritus is a significant symptom associated with the burden of atopic dermatitis, targeting the neuronal pathways responsible for pruritus in AD has been approached via both topical and oral routes. The topical application of CT327, which targets tropomyosin receptor kinase A, in a proof of concept trial showed significant benefit [71]. Another target is the neurokinin 1 receptor (NK-1R) and its ligand, substance P. The NK-1R antagonist, tradipitant (VLY-686, LY686017), is being investigated in a randomized placebo-controlled trial in the control of pruritus as measured by the visual analog scale (VAS) as the primary endpoint (NCT02651714, ClinicalTrials.gov) [72].

A phase 2a randomized placebo-controlled clinical trial investigating the oral histamine selective H4 receptor (H4R) antagonist, ZPL-3893787 (ZPL-389), for the treatment of moderate-to-severe AD in adults (N = 98) has been completed. Following 8 weeks of therapy, a 50% reduction in the EASI score was noted compared to 27% (p = 0.01) for ZPL-389 at 30 mg PO OD vs. placebo, respectively [73]. A previous trial for another H4R antagonist, JNJ-39758979, was terminated early due to cases of neutropenia, although it showed numerical improvement in AD scores [74]. Neutropenia was not noted in the phase 2a trial with ZPL-389 [73].

Another approach being trialed is treatment with dihomo-γ-linolenic acid (DGLA, DS107) which was shown to be beneficial as oral therapy in AD in a Phase 2 trial ((NCT02864498) press release) [75], through the regulation of prostaglandin D1 (PGD1) [76]. DGLA is also currently being investigated in mild-to-moderate AD in a trial with a topical formulation, DS107E cream (NCT02925793, ClinicalTrials.gov) [77].

Conclusions

It is clear that there exists some evidence for the effective treatment of recalcitrant or severe AD with CsA in both pediatric and adult populations [7]. CsA is generally well tolerated, and its rapid onset of action makes it an attractive first-line treatment option for patients with recalcitrant AD [5]. CsA has a well-established side effect profile [22], which allows for vigilant monitoring for dose adjustments in AD patients treated with CsA [6]. Nonetheless, there remains a lack of long-term effectiveness and safety data regarding patients requiring long-term treatment with CsA. Further data collection from long-term registries would be beneficial [7]. Currently, CsA is recommended for first-line short-term therapy [1].

Other systemic agents, such as AZA, MTX, and MMF, have also shown clinical efficacy with acceptable safety profiles; however, the margin is narrow [1]. There is literature supporting the use of these agents to treat refractory AD; however, their use remains off-label [22]. Recommended second-line therapy is with AZA, and third-line with methotrexate based on the best available evidence [1]. Though effective, treatment of AD with OGCs is not recommended due to their unfavorable risk-to-benefit ratio [49]. A comprehensive summary of traditional oral systemic therapies for AD treatment is included in Table 32.1. Not all patients will respond to these immunosuppressive agents, so new therapies are needed to provide patients with higher treatment efficacy and fewer safety concerns [78]. Some promising agents, including the PDE-4 inhibitor, apremilast, and the PGD2 receptor antagonist, fevipiprant, showed discouraging results as key primary and secondary endpoints were not met in phase 2 trials. It is unclear at this point whether further studies are planned. Other novel agents, including those targeting the neuronal pathways of pruritus, are also undergoing investigation. An overview of new and upcoming oral systemic therapies for AD is included in Table 32.2. Most promising at this point are the biologic agents targeting cytokines and this will be covered in a separate chapter. Further study of these agents, their long-term efficacy in treating AD, their role in AD maintenance, and their long-term safety is necessary for concrete treatment recommendations.

Table 32.1 Summary of recommendations for adult and pediatric atopic dermatitis treatment with systemic therapy

Treatment	Population	Dosing	Duration of treatment	Side effects	Overall recommendation
Cyclosporine	Adult and pediatric	Twice daily dosing [21]: 3–6 mg/kg/day, such that the lowest effective dose is given [22]	Maximum: 1–2 years [25] Minimum: has shown clinical improvement as early as 2 weeks into treatment [7]	Nausea, headache, paresthesia, renal impairment, HTN, sequelae of chronic immunosuppression	First-line short-term treatment for moderate-to-severe AD because of moderate- and high-quality studies based on the GRADE approach and the efficacy and safety shown for short-term use, including large patient numbers [1]
Azathioprine	Adult and pediatric	Ideally based on TPMT activity level [1]. Can range from 1–3 mg/kg/day [22], with graduated dosing [36].	Maximum: there is no official recommendation. However, when disease clearance is achieved, AZA should be tapered and discontinued if possible [22] Minimum: clinical improvement can take a minimum 12 weeks of treatment, or more [36]	Common: nausea, vomiting, gastrointestinal symptoms (bloating, anorexia, cramping) [22] Less common: headache, hypersensitivity, reactions and elevated liver enzymes [22]	Second-line treatment for moderate-to-severe AD because of a moderate-quality study based on the GRADE approach and the efficacy and safety shown for short- and long-term use (24 weeks), including large patient numbers [1]
Methotrexate	Adult	Single weekly dose: 7.5–25 mg/week [22] Folic acid supplementation: 1 mg/day [22]	Minimum: clinical improvement has been shown as early as 4 weeks after treatment initiation [41]	Nausea, elevated liver enzymes, pancytopenia, pulmonary toxicity	Third-line treatment for adults because of a moderate quality study based on the GRADE approach and the efficacy and safety shown for short- and long-term use (24 weeks), including large patient numbers [1]
	Pediatric	Single weekly dose: 0.2–0.7 mg/kg/week [6] Folic acid supplementation: 1 mg/day [6]			

Table 32.1 (continued)

Treatment	Population	Dosing	Duration of treatment	Side effects	Overall recommendation
Mycophenolate mofetil	Adult	No official recommendations [22]. *Anecdotally* Twice daily dosing: 0.5–3.0 g/day [44]	Maximum: no official recommendation [22] Minimum: clinical improvement has been noted within 4 weeks of treatment [44]	Common: mild headache, gastrointestinal disturbances, fatigue [44] Rare: hematologic and genitourinary symptoms [22]	*For EC-MPS specifically* Very weak recommendation is possible for EC-MPS as a maintenance treatment for severe AD after induction of remission by CsA for long-term use up to 30 weeks [1]
	Pediatric	*Young children* Twice daily dosing [45]: 40–50 mg/kg/day [6] Adolescents Twice daily dosing [45]: 30–40 mg/kg/day [6]			
Oral corticosteroids	Adult and pediatric	0.75–1 mg/kg per day (prednisone, prednisolone)	Minimum: 3 days Maximum: 3 weeks	Diabetes, hypertension, gastric ulcers, osteoporosis, glaucoma, opportunistic infections and Cushing syndrome Pediatric: decreased growth velocity	Not recommended. May be used in short-term (up to 1 week, maximum 3 weeks) for acute flares in exceptional and severe cases of AD

Table 32.2 Oral agents in development for atopic dermatitis.

New agent	Mechanism of action	Phase of development	Current trials
Apremilast	PDE4 inhibitor	Phase 2, completed	NCT02087943
Fevipiprant (QAW 039)	CRTH2 antagonist	Phase 2, completed	NCT01785602
PF 04965842	JAK 1 inhibitor	Phase 2	NCT02780167
DGLA	Regulation of PGD1	Phase 2	NCT02864498
Tradipitant (VLY-686, LY686017)	NK-1R antagonists	Phase 2	NCT02004041 NCT02651714
ZPL-389 (ZPL-3803787)	H4R antagonist	Phase 2	NCT02424253

CRTH2 chemoattractant receptor-homologous molecule expressed on T-helper type 2 cells, *DGLA* dihomo-gamma-linolenic acid, *H4R* histamine H4 receptor, *JAK* Janus kinase, *PDE4* phosphodiesterase-4, *PGD1* prostaglandin D1, *NK-1R* neurokinin 1 receptor

Case Report

A 42-year-old white male presents with a lifelong history of "eczema," which has flared over the past few years. He was previously managed with topical agents but these have not been working for him lately. He complains of severe itching, which interrupts his sleep. Given the night shift at work, he finds it difficult to sleep during the day with ongoing itch and has been having difficulty coping. He notes he has been "short" and "moody" with his family and attributes this to lack of sleep. There is a family history of atopic dermatitis in his daughter as well.

Past Medical History

- Hypertension
- Anxiety
- Asthma

Social History

- Drinks socially
- Married, 2 children
- Floor manager at a distribution plant, working shift work, mainly night shifts

Previous Therapies

- Topical steroids

Physical Exam

- Erythematous excoriated lichenified plaques on the wrists, antecubital and popliteal fossae; facial erythema and scaling with Dennie-Morgan folds noted

Management

Due to the severity of his atopic dermatitis flare and his difficulty coping, systemic therapy with cyclosporine was initiated at 150 mg PO BID. He is also managed with topical tacrolimus 0.1% ointment BID for the face/body and betamethasone valerate 0.1% ointment for the body flares prn. He has good control of his skin with improved sleep while taking cyclosporine but because of his hypertension, his dose is reduced to 100 mg PO BID when possible. To manage flares in symptoms he intermittently increases back to 150 mg PO BID with close monitoring.

References

1. Roekevisch E, Spuls PI, Kuester D, Limpens J, Schmitt J. Efficacy and safety of systemic treatments for moderate-to-severe atopic dermatitis: a systematic review. J Allergy Clin Immunol. 2014;133(2):429–38. https://doi.org/10.1016/j.jaci.2013.07.049.
2. Schmitt J, Schmitt NM, Kirch W, Meurer M. Outpatient care and medical treatment of children and adults with atopic

eczema. J Ger Soc Dermatol. 2009;7(4):345–52. https://doi.org/10.1111/j.1610-0387.2008.06967.x.

3. Bieber T, Straeter B. Off-label prescriptions for atopic dermatitis in Europe. Allergy Eur J Allergy Clin Immunol. 2015;70(1):6–11. https://doi.org/10.1111/all.12498.

4. Saeki H, Nakahara T, Tanaka A, et al. Clinical practice guidelines for the Management of Atopic Dermatitis 2016. J Dermatol. 2016;126(February):1–29. https://doi.org/10.1111/1346-8138.13392.

5. Cookson H, Smith C. Systemic treatment of adult atopic dermatitis. Clin Med (Northfield Il). 2012;12(2):172–6. https://doi.org/10.7861/clinmedicine.12-2-172.

6. Notaro ER, Sidbury R. Systemic agents for severe atopic dermatitis in children. Pediatr Drugs. 2015;17(6):449–57. https://doi.org/10.1007/s40272-015-0150-4.

7. Schmitt J, Schmitt N, Meurer M. Cyclosporin in the treatment of patients with atopic eczema—a systematic review and meta-analysis. J Eur Acad Dermatol Venereol. 2007;21(5):606–19. https://doi.org/10.1111/j.1468-3083.2006.02023.x.

8. Sowden J, Berth-Jones J, Ross J, et al. Double-blind, controlled, crossover study of cyclosporin in adults with severe refractory atopic dermatitis. Lancet. 1991;338(8760):137–40.

9. Munro C, Levell N, Shuster S, Friedmann P. Maintenance treatment with cyclosporin in atopic eczema. Br J Dermatol. 1994;130(3):376–80. http://www.ncbi.nlm.nih.gov/entrez/query.fcgi?cmd=Retrieve&db=PubMed&dopt=Citation&list_uids=9580834

10. Van Joost T, Heule F, Korstanje M, Van Den Broek MJTB, Stenveld HJ, Van Vloten WA. Cyclosporin in atopic dermatitis: a multicentre placebo-controlled study. Br J Dermatol. 1994;130(5):634–40. https://doi.org/10.1111/j.1365-2133.1994.tb13111.x.

11. Zonneveld IM, De Rie MA, Beljaards RC, et al. The long-term safety and efficacy of cyclosporin in severe refractory atopic dermatitis: a comparison of two dosage regimens. Br J Dermatol. 1996;135(Suppl):15–20. https://doi.org/10.1111/j.1365-2133.1996.tb00704.x.

12. Harper JI, Ahmed I, Barclay G, et al. Cyclosporin for severe childhood atopic dermatitis: short course versus contiuous therapy. Br J Dermatol. 2000;142(1):52–8.

13. Czech W, Bräutigam M, Weidinger G, Schöpf E. A body-weight-independent dosing regimen of cyclosporine microemulsion is effective in severe atopic dermatitis and improves the quality of life. J Am Acad Dermatol. 2000;42(4):653–9. https://doi.org/10.1016/S0190-9622(00)90180-4.

14. Pacor ML, Di Lorenzo G, Martinelli N, Mansueto P, Rini GB, Corrocher R. Comparing tacrolimus ointment and oral cyclosporine in adult patients affected by atopic dermatitis: a randomized study. Clin Exp Allergy. 2004;34(4):639–45. https://doi.org/10.1111/j.1365-2222.2004.1907.x.

15. Granlund H, Erkko P, Sinisalo M, Reitamo S. Cyclosporin in atopic dermatitis: time to relapse and effect of intermittent therapy. Br J Dermatol. 1995;132(1):106–12. https://doi.org/10.1111/j.1365-2133.1995.tb08633.x.

16. Berth-Jones J, Finlay AY, Zaki I, et al. Cyclosporine in severe childhood atopic dermatitis: a multicenter study. J Am Acad Dermatol. 1996;34(6):1016–21. https://doi.org/10.1016/S0190-9622(96)90281-9.

17. Atakan N, Erdem C. The efficacy, tolerability and safety of a new oral formulation of Sandimmun®-Sandimmun Neoral® in severe refractory atopic dermatitis. J Eur Acad Dermatol Venereol. 1998;11(3):240–6. https://doi.org/10.1016/S0926-9959(98)00085.

18. Bunikowski R, Staab D, Kussebi F, et al. Low-dose cyclosporin a microemulsion in children with severe atopic dermatitis: clinical and immunological effects. Pediatr Allergy Immunol. 2001;12(4):216–23. http://www.ncbi.nlm.nih.gov/pubmed/11555319

19. Berth-Jones J, Graham-Brown R. A, marks R, et al. long-term efficacy and safety of cyclosporin in severe adult atopic dermatitis. Br J Dermatol. 1997;136(1):76–81. http://www.ncbi.nlm.nih.gov/pubmed/9039299

20. Schmitt J, Schäkel K, Schmitt N, Meurer M. Systemic treatment of severe atopic eczema: a systematic review. Acta Derm Venereol. 2007;87(2):100–11. https://doi.org/10.2340/00015555-0207.

21. Silverberg J. Long-term use of ciclosporin in a real-world setting. Br J Dermatol. 2015:1483–4. https://doi.org/10.1111/bjd.13809.

22. Sidbury R, Davis DM, Cohen DE, et al. Guidelines of care for the management of atopic dermatitis: section 3. Management and treatment with phototherapy and systemic agents. J Am Acad Dermatol. 2014;71(2):327–49. https://doi.org/10.1016/j.jaad.2014.03.030.

23. Kim JE, Shin JM, Ko JY, Ro YS. Importance of concomitant topical therapy in moderate-to-severe atopic dermatitis treated with cyclosporine. Dermatol Ther. 2016;29(2):120–5. https://doi.org/10.1111/dth.12333.

24. Denby KS, Beck LA. Update on systemic therapies for atopic dermatitis. 2012:421–426. doi:https://doi.org/10.1097/ACI.0b013e3283551da5.

25. Menter A, Korman NJ, Elmets CA, et al. Guidelines of care for the management of psoriasis and psoriatic arthritis. Section 4. Guidelines of care for the management and treatment of psoriasis with traditional systemic agents. J Am Acad Dermatol. 2009;61(3):451–85. https://doi.org/10.1016/j.jaad.2009.03.027.

26. Gelbard CM, Hebert AA. New and emerging trends in the treatment of atopic dermatitis. Patient Prefer Adherence. 2008;2:387–92.

27. Meggitt SJ, Reynolds NJ. Azathioprine for atopic dermatitis. Clin Exp Dermatol. 2001;26(5):369–75. https://doi.org/10.1046/j.1365-2230.2001.00837.x.

28. Gunnar S, Johansson O, Juhlin L. Immunoglobulin E in "healed" atopic dermatitis and after treatment with corticosteroids and azathioprine. Br J Dermatol. 1970;82(1):10–3. https://doi.org/10.1111/j.1365-2133.1970.tb02185.x.

29. Younger I, Harris D, Colver G. Azathioprine in dermatology. J Am Acad Dermatol. 1991;25(2):281–6. https://doi.org/10.1016/0190-9622(91)70196-9.

30. Lear JT, English JS, Jones P, Smith AG. Retrospective review of the use of azathioprine in severe atopic dermatitis. J Am Acad Dermatol. 1996;35(4):642–3.

31. Buckley DA, Baldwin P, Rogers S. The use of azathioprine in severe adult atopic eczema. J Eur Acad Dermatol Venereol. 1998;11(2):137–40. https://doi.org/10.1016/S0926-9959(98)00074-9.

32. Scerri L. Azathioprine in dermatological practice: an overview with special emphasis on its use in non-bullous inflammatory dermatoses. Adv Exp Med Biol. 1999;455:343–8.

33. Murphy L, Atherton D. Azathioprine in severe childhood eczema: value of TPMT as a predictor of outcome and safety in treatment. Br J Dermatol. 2001;144:927. https://doi.org/10.1111/bjd.14580.

34. August P. Azathioprine in the treatment of eczema and actinic reticuloid. Br J Dermatol. 1982;107(Supplement 22):23.

35. Berth-Jones J, Takwale A, Tan E, et al. Azathioprine in severe adult atopic dermatitis: a double-blind, placebo-controlled, crossover trial. Br J Dermatol. 2002;147(2):324–30. https://doi.org/10.1046/j.1365-2133.2002.04989.x.

36. Meggitt SJ, Gray JC, Reynolds NJ. Azathioprine dosed by thiopurine methyltransferase activity for moderate-to-severe atopic eczema: a double-blind, randomised controlled trial. Lancet. 2006;367(9513):839–46. https://doi.org/10.1016/S0140-6736(06)68340-2.

37. Aleissa M, Nicol P, Godeau M, et al. Azathioprine hypersensitivity syndrome: two cases of febrile neutrophilic dermatosis induced by azathioprine. Case Rep Dermatol. 2017:6–11. https://doi.org/10.1159/000454876.

38. Fuggle NR, Bragoli W, Mahto A, Glover M, Martinez AE, Kinsler VA. The adverse effect profile of oral azathioprine in pediatric atopic dermatitis, and recommendations for monitoring. J Am Acad Dermatol. 2015;72(1):108–14. https://doi.org/10.1016/j.jaad.2014.08.048.

39. Deo M, Yung A, Hill S, Rademaker M. Pharmacology and thera-peutics methotrexate for treatment of atopic dermatitis in children and adolescents. Int J Dermatol. 2014;53:1037–41.

40. Weatherhead SC, Wahie S, Reynolds NJ, Meggitt SJ. An open-label, dose-ranging study of methotrexate for moderate-to-severe adult atopic eczema. Br J Dermatol. 2007;156(2):346–51. https://doi.org/10.1111/j.1365-2133.2006.07686.x.

41. Goujon C, Bérard F, Dahel K, et al. Methotrexate for the treat-ment of adult atopic dermatitis. Eur J Dermatol. 2006;16(2):155–8. http://www.ncbi.nlm.nih.gov/pubmed/16581567

42. El-Khalawany MA, Hassan H, Shaaban D, Ghonaim N, Eassa B. Methotrexate versus cyclosporine in the treatment of severe atopic dermatitis in children: a multicenter experience from Egypt. Eur J Pediatr. 2013;172(3):351–6. https://doi.org/10.1007/s00431-012-1893-3.

43. Schram ME, Roekevisch E, Leeflang MMG, Bos JD, Schmitt J, Spuls PI. A randomized trial of methotrexate versus azathioprine for severe atopic eczema. J Allergy Clin Immunol. 2011;128(2):353–9. https://doi.org/10.1016/j.jaci.2011.03.024.

44. Murray ML, Cohen JB. Mycophenolate mofetil therapy for moder-ate to severe atopic dermatitis. Clin Exp Dermatol. 2007;32(1):23–7. https://doi.org/10.1111/j.1365-2230.2006.02290.x.

45. Heller M, Shin HT, Orlow SJ, Schaffer JV. Mycophenolate mofetil for severe childhood atopic dermatitis: experience in 14 patients. Br J Dermatol. 2007;157(1):127–32. https://doi.org/10.1111/j.1365-2133.2007.07947.x.

46. Haeck IM, Knol MJ, Berge O, Van Velsen SGA, De Bruin-Weller MS, Bruijnzeel-Koomen CAFM. Enteric-coated mycopheno-late sodium versus cyclosporin A as long-term treatment in adult patients with severe atopic dermatitis: a randomized controlled trial. J Am Dermatol. 2011;64(6):1074–84. https://doi.org/10.1016/j.jaad.2010.04.027.

47. Waxweiler WT, Agans R, Morrell DS. Systemic treatment of pediatric atopic dermatitis with azathioprine and Mycophenolate Mofetil. Pediatr Dermatol. 2011;28(6):689–94. https://doi.org/10.1111/j.1525-1470.2011.01488.x.

48. Simon D, Bieber T. Systemic therapy for atopic dermatitis. Allergy. 2014;69:46–55. https://doi.org/10.1111/all.12339.

49. Megna M, Napolitano M, Patruno C, et al. Systemic treatment of adult atopic dermatitis: a review. Dermatol Ther (Heidelb). 2016. https://doi.org/10.1007/s13555-016-0170-1.

50. Schmitt J, Schäkel K, Fölster-Holst R, et al. Prednisolone vs. ciclo-sporin for severe adult eczema. An investigator-initiated double-blind placebo-controlled multicentre trial. Br J Dermatol. 2010;162(3):661–8. https://doi.org/10.1111/j.1365-2133.2009.09561.x.

51. Heddle R, Soothill J, Bulpitt C, Atherton D. Combined oral and nasal beclomethasone diproprionate in children with atopic eczema: a randomised controlled trial. Br Med J. 1984;289(6446):651–4. https://doi.org/10.1136/bmj.289.6446.651.

52. La Rosa M, Musarra I, Ranno C, et al. A randomized, double-blind, placebo-controlled, crossover trial of systemic flunisolide in the treatment of children with severe atopic dermatitis. Curr Ther Res. 1995;56(7):720–6. https://doi.org/10.1016/0011-393X(95)85143-7.

53. Daley-Yates PT, Richards DH. Relationship between systemic cor-ticosteroid exposureand growth velocity: development and valida-tion of a pharmacokinetic/pharmacodynamic model. Clin Ther. 2004;26(11):1905–19. https://doi.org/10.1016/j.clinthera.2004.11.017.

54. Schmitt-Hoffmann AH, Roos B, Sauer J, et al. Pharmacokinetics, efficacy and safety of alitretinoin in moderate or severe chronic hand eczema. Clin Exp Dermatol. 2011;36(Suppl. 2):29–34. https://doi.org/10.1111/j.1365-2230.2011.04035.x.

55. Dirschka T, Reich K, Bissonnette R, Maares J, Brown T, Diepgen TL. An open-label study assessing the safety and efficacy of ali-tretinoin in patients with severe chronic hand eczema unrespon-sive to topical corticosteroids. Clin Exp Dermatol. 2011;36(2):149–54. https://doi.org/10.1111/j.1365-2230.2010.03955.x.

56. Ham K, Maini P, Gooderham MJ. Real-world experience with Alitretinoin in a community dermatology practice setting in patients with chronic hand dermatitis. J Cutan Med Surg. 2014;18(5):332–6. https://doi.org/10.2310/7750.2014.13195.

57. Agner T. Hand eczema. In: Johansen JD, Frosch PJ, Lepoittevin J-P, editors. Contact dermatitis. Berlin, Heidelberg: Springer; 2011. p. 395–406. https://doi.org/10.1007/978-3-642-03827-3_20.

58. Grahovac M, Molin S, Prinz JC, Ruzicka T, Wollenberg A. Treatment of atopic eczema with oral alitretinoin. Br J Dermatol. 2010;162(1):217–8. https://doi.org/10.1111/j.1365-2133.2009.09522.x.

59. Gooderham M, Papp K. Selective phosphodiesterase inhibitors for psoriasis: focus on Apremilast. BioDrugs. 2015;29(5):327–39. https://doi.org/10.1007/s40259-015-0144-3.

60. Hanifin JM, Chan SC, Cheng JB, et al. Type 4 phosphodiesterase inhibitors have clinical and in vitro anti-inflammatory effects in atopic dermatitis. J Invest Dermatol. 1996;107(1):51–6. https://doi.org/10.1111/1523-1747.ep12297888.

61. Samrao A, Berry TM, Goreshi R, Simpson EL. A pilot study of an oral phosphodiesterase inhibitor (apremilast) for atopic der-matitis in adults. Arch Dermatol. 2012;148(8):890–7. https://doi.org/10.1001/archdermatol.2012.812.

62. Volf EM, Au S-C, Dumont N, Scheinman P, Gottlieb AB. A phase 2, open-label, investigator-initiated study to evaluate the safety and efficacy of apremilast in subjects with recalcitrant allergic contact or atopic dermatitis. J Drugs Dermatol. 2012;11(3):341–6.

63. Celgene Corporation. A Phase 2, Multicenter, Randomized, Double-blind, Placebo-controlled, Parallel-group, Efficacy and Safety Study of Apremilast (CC-10004) in Subjects With Moderate to Severe Atopic Dermatitis. In: ClinicalTrials.gov [Internet]. Bethesda (MD): National Library of Medicine (US). 2000- [cited 2017 Feb 2]. Available from: http://clinicaltrials.gov/show/NCT02087943 NLM Identifier: NCT02087943.

64. Bao L, Zhang H, Chan LS. The involvement of the JAK-STAT sig-naling pathway in chronic inflammatory skin disease atopic dermati-tis. Jak-Stat. 2013;2(3):e24137. https://doi.org/10.4161/jkst.24137.

65. Fukuyama T, Ehling S, Cook E, Bäumer W. Topically administered Janus-kinase inhibitors Tofacitinib and Oclacitinib display impres-sive antipruritic and anti-inflammatory responses in a model of allergic dermatitis. J Pharmacol Exp Ther. 2015;354(3):394–405. https://doi.org/10.1124/jpet.115.223784.

66. Bissonnette R, Papp K, Poulin Y, et al. Topical tofacitinib for atopic dermatitis: a phase 2a randomised trial. Br J Dermatol. 2016. https://doi.org/10.1111/bjd.14871.

67. Levy LL, Urban J, King BA. Treatment of recalcitrant atopic der-matitis with the oral Janus kinase inhibitor tofacitinib citrate. J Am Acad Dermatol. 2015;73(3):395–9. https://doi.org/10.1016/j.jaad.2015.06.045.

68. Pfizer. A Phase 2b Randomized, Double-Blind, Placebo-controlled, Parallel, Multicenter, Dose-ranging, Study To Evaluate The Efficacy And Safety Profile Of Pf-04965842 In Subjects With Moderate To Severe Atopic Dermatitis. In: ClinicalTrials.gov [Internet]. Bethesda (MD): National Library of Medicine (US). 2000- [cited 2017 Feb 2]. Available from: https://clinicaltrials.gov/ct2/show/NCT02780167 NLM Identifier: NCT02780167.

69. Sykes D, Bradley M, Riddy D, Willard E, Reilly J, Miah A, Bauer C, Watson S, Sandhog D, Dubois GCS. Fevipiprant (QAW039), a slowly dissociating CRTh2 Antagonistwith the potential for improved clinical efficacy. Mol Pharmacol. 2016;1(89):593–605. https://doi.org/10.1124/mol.115.101832.

70. Novartis Pharmaceuticals. A Randomized, Double-blind, Placebo-controlled, Parallel Group Study Evaluating Efficacy and Safety of QAW039 in the Treatment of Patients With Moderate to Severe Atopic Dermatitis. In: ClinicalTrials.gov [Internet]. Bethesda (MD): National Library of Medicine (US). 2000- [cited 2017 Feb 2]. Available from: https://clinicaltrials.gov/ct2/show/NCT01785602 NLM Identifier: NCT01785602.

71. Creabilis S. Creabilis announces positive phase IIa results for TrkA kinase inhibitor CT327 in atopic dermatitis; 2010.

72. Vanda Pharmaceuticals. A Multicenter, Randomized, Double-blind, Placebo-controlled Study to Assess the Safety and Efficacy of Tradipitant in Treatment-resistant Pruritus Associated With Atopic Dermatitis. In: CLinicalTrials.gov [Internet]. Bethesda (MD): National Library of Medicine (US). 2000- [cited 2017 Feb 2]. Available from: https://clinicaltrials.gov/ct2/show/NCT02651714 NLM Identifier: NCT02651714.

73. Werfel T, Lynch V, Asher A, et al. A phase 2a proof of concept clinical trial to evaluate ZPL-3893787 (ZPL-389), a potent, oral histamine H4 receptor antagonist for the treatment of moderate to severe atopic dermatitis (AD) in adults. Allergy Eur J Allergy Clin Immunol. 2016;71(102):95–117.

74. Murata Y, Song M, Kikuchi H, et al. Phase 2a, randomized, double-blind, placebo-controlled, multicenter, parallel-group study of a H4 R-antagonist (JNJ-39758979) in Japanese adults with moderate atopic dermatitis. J Dermatol. 2015;42(2):129–39. https://doi.org/10.1111/1346-8138.12726.

75. DS Biopharma. A Randomised, Double-blind, Placebo-controlled, Phase 2b Study to Assess the Efficacy and Safety of Orally Administered DS107 in Patients With Moderate to Severe Atopic Dermatitis. In: Clinical Trials.gov [Internet]. Bethesda (MD): National Library of Medicine (US). 2000- [cited 2017 Feb 2]. Available from: https://clinicaltrials.gov/ct2/show/NCT02864498 NLM Identifier: NCT02865598.

76. Amagai Y, Oida K, Matsuda A, et al. Dihomo-γ-linolenic acid prevents the development of atopic dermatitis through prostaglandin D1 production in NC/Tnd mice. J Dermatol Sci. 2015;79(1):30–7. https://doi.org/10.1016/j.jdermsci.2015.03.010.

77. DS Biopharma. A Randomised, Double-blind, Vehicle-Controlled, Phase IIb Study to Assess the Efficacy and Safety of Topically Applied DS107 Cream to Adults With Mild to Moderate Atopic Dermatitis. In: ClinicalTrials.gov [Internet]. Bethesda (MD): National Library of Medicine (US). 2000- [cited 2017 Feb 2]. Available from: https://clinicaltrials.gov/ct2/show/NCT02925793 NLM Identifier: NCT02925793.

78. Gooderham M, Lynde CW, Papp K, et al. Review of systemic treatment options for adult atopic dermatitis. J Cutan Med Surg. 2017;21(1):31–9. https://doi.org/10.1177/1203475416670364.

Cutaneous T-Cell Lymphoma

33

Catherine G. Chung, Brian Poligone, and Peter W. Heald

Introduction

Mycosis fungoides and Sézary syndrome (MF/SS) represent the most common types of cutaneous T-cell lymphomas (CTCL). The typically indolent nature of MF/SS makes the disease a chronic illness and one of the consistent clinical observations is that of immunologic failure with the leading cause of death due to infections and secondary malignancies. Indeed in one series, the most common cause of mortality was second malignancy [1]. Second malignancies, including other lymphomas, are more common in MF/SS patients [1, 2]. In addition, viral and bacterial infections appear to be more severe in MF/SS patients and represent another common cause of mortality [3]. Defective adaptive immunity was even noted in Sézary's initial report of his syndrome with the affected patients dying from infection [4]. While our understanding of all of the immune defects observed in MF/SS remains incomplete, the immune dysregulation and immunodeficiency associated with the disease are clinically significant.

Compromise of adaptive immunity is particularly problematic in MF/SS patients since the T-cell compartment is responsible for the antitumor response. The disease appears to have the ability to disarm the immune response responsible for controlling CTCL. The importance of an intact immunity in MF/SS patients has been emphasized by the progression of disease brought on by adaptive immunity suppression, when cyclosporine is administered to MF/SS patients [5]. Moreover

the shifting observed between T helper and T cytotoxic milieus during cancer progression further highlights the effect of MF/SS on the adaptive immunity [6].

The immune dysregulation associated with MF/SS type CTCL is an evolving story that has been largely dependent on the technologies available to visualize the anomalies. The first insight into the magnitude of immunocompromise came from clone-specific antibody testing of peripheral blood lymphocytes. These antibodies could enumerate malignant T-cells in the peripheral blood of select patients. This then allowed the numbers of nonmalignant T-cells to be determined by subtraction of the malignant T-cell number from the total T-cell pool. Using this methodology, in six patients with advanced MF/SS, it was observed that the nonmalignant T-cell population was decreased in some patients to the same level as that seen with advanced HIV patients [7]. Even though antibodies that recognize all CTCL clones do not exist, the normal T-cell population can also be estimated by measurement of the CD8+ population. Increases in the CD4/CD8 ratio and decreases in the numbers of CD8+ T-cells are readily assessed by flow cytometry as measures of the immunocompetence of the patient. Assessing lymphocyte subsets by flow cytometry is a rapid and reproducible staging technique that lends insight into the immune status of the patient.

Another technique that furthered our understanding of MF/SS was the RNAse protection assay. This assay measures the messenger RNA for different T-cell receptors in peripheral blood lymphocytes. In normal controls, the presence of messenger RNA for the diverse T-cell receptor components are represented by multiple bands for the different subunits of the T-cell receptor (Fig. 33.1). In contrast, the loss of T-cell diversity in patients with advanced MF/SS is demonstrated with the loss of the multiple bands with a single band representing the malignant clone (monoclonal banding). The disappearance of this RNA represents a loss of nonmalignant T-cells and the rise of a singular malignant clone. More recently this loss of diversity was shown with high throughput sequencing (HTS) of polymerase chain reaction products. This most sensitive and specific method for detecting and

C.G. Chung, MD (✉)
The Ohio State Wexner Medical Center,
410 W 10th Ave, Columbus, OH 43210, USA
e-mail: catherinechung@gmail.com

B. Poligone, MD, PhD
Rochester Skin Lymphoma Medical Group,
6800 Pittsford Palmyra Rd, Fairport, NY 14450, USA

P.W. Heald, MD
Yale University School of Medicine,
212 Sawyer Hill Road, New Milford, CT 06776, USA

© Springer International Publishing AG 2018
P.S. Yamauchi (ed.), *Biologic and Systemic Agents in Dermatology*, https://doi.org/10.1007/978-3-319-66884-0_33

Fig. 33.1 : Example of the RNase protection assay for assessing clonality. The level of expression of the variable region of the T-cell receptor beta gene (TCRBV) from peripheral mononuclear cells was assayed using three RNase multi-probe sets. The first two lanes show healthy volunteers. The numbers (e.g. 2.1, 5.1, etc.) shown in other lanes identify over-represented TCRBV due to CD4+ clonal expansion in patients with Sézary Syndrome. Cβ identifies the loading control for the gel electrophoresis, which is the expression of the constant region of the T cell receptor beta gene (TCRBC)

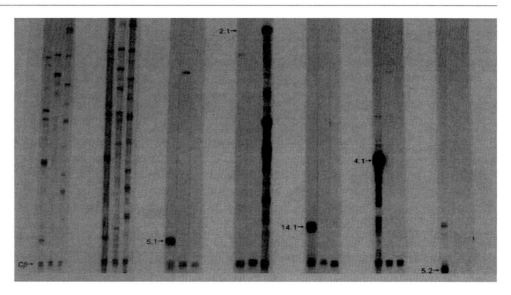

Table 33.1 Summary of biologic therapies in the treatment of MF/SS

Therapy	Drug class	Mechanism of action in MF/SS
Bexarotene	Retinoid/rexinoid	• Terminal differentiation of malignant cells • Arrest of cell cycle • Activation of apoptotic pathway
Vorinostat, Romidepsin, Panobinostat	Histone deacetylase (HDAC) inhibitors	• Modification of gene transcription → cell death, inhibition of cell growth
Denileukin Diftitox, E7777	CD25-Diphtheria fusion immunotoxin	• Apoptosis of activated T_{reg} cells
Alemtuzumab	Anti-CD52 monoclonal antibody	• Antibody-dependent cell-mediated cytotoxicity
Brentuximab	Anti-CD30 monoclonal antibody	• Antibody-dependent cell-mediated cytotoxicity
Mogamulizumab	Anti-CCR4 monoclonal antibody	• Antibody-dependent cell-mediated cytotoxicity • Depletion of T_{reg} cells
Ipilimumab, Nivolumab, Pembrolizumab	Checkpoint inhibitor therapy	• Promotion of cytotoxic antitumor response • Inhibition of immune tolerance
Interferons		• Activation of innate immunity
Imiquimod, Resiquimod, CPG ODN	Toll-like receptor agonists	• Activation of innate and adaptive immunity
Photopheresis		• Dendritic cell (DC) activation • Apoptosis of malignant T-cells
Allogeneic stem cell transplant		• Graft-versus-lymphoma

monitoring unique T-cell receptor clonal rearrangements demonstrates not only the dominance of the malignant clone but the loss of diversity of the other nonmalignant T-cells. The loss of adaptive immunity becomes an accelerating factor in the progression of the disease and a risk factor for mortality from malignancy and infection.

Therefore, a patient's immunocompetence is an important consideration in the treatment of MF/SS. The choice of therapeutics, which may affect the immune system and may cause or correct the marked immune dysregulation that characterizes MF/SS type CTCL is more important than ever considering the wide array of biologic therapies available in MF/SS (see Table 33.1). In this chapter we will highlight current and emerging therapies that can promote a patient's immunocompetence or can target the malignant T-cells without destroying healthy T-cells.

Bexarotene

Background

The retinoids are a group of natural and synthetic compounds structurally and functionally derived from vitamin A (retinol) [8]. Retinoids bind to two groups of nuclear receptors, the retinoic acid receptors (RARs) and retinoic X receptors (RXRs), subsequently affecting gene transcription that results in terminal differentiation of malignant cells [8–11]. Bexarotene is a third-generation synthetic retinoid with selective binding to the RXRs, and therefore is often referred to as a rexinoid. Bexarotene was approved by the Food and Drug Administration (FDA) for treatment of CTCL in 1999. Discussion of other retinoids utilized in dermatologic therapy is covered elsewhere in this book (*see Retinoids*).

Mechanisms of Action

In addition to inducing terminal differentiation of malignant cells, bexarotene may exert its antitumoral effects through other mechanisms. Activation of the RXR receptor is associated with activation of the tumor suppressor p53, promoting arrest of the cell cycle. Bexarotene also exerts influence on the apoptotic pathway, including regulation of Bcl-2 and bax proteins and activation of the pathway through actions on caspase-3 [12, 13]. Other downstream antitumor effects may also include inhibition of tumor cell migration and invasion through inhibition of growth factors [14].

Use and Efficacy in CTCL

Approval of bexarotene for its use in CTCL was based on two phase II–III trials [15, 16]. Clinical responses in these trials were dose dependent. Bexarotene is administered as oral 75 mg capsules. Initial starting dose is often 3–4 capsules daily, with titration upwards as tolerance allows. The use of bexarotene in combination with interferons, phototherapy, extracorporeal photopheresis (ECP), and other agents used in the treatment of CTCL has been investigated in small studies with varying results [17–20]; nonetheless, it is frequently employed in combination with other systemic or skin-directed therapies due to potential synergism given its unique mechanism of action [8]. Adverse side effects (ASEs) of bexarotene include central hypothyroidism, hypertriglyceridemia and dyslipidemia, hepatotoxicity, headache, photosensitivity, and leukopenia [8, 21].

Histone Deacetylase Inhibitors: Vorinostat, Romidepsin, and Panobinostat

Background

Nucleosomes are units consisting of chromatin wrapped around histone octamers; modification of the nucleosome is controlled in large part by the actions of histone acetyltransferases and deacetylases [22]. In general, histone deacetylation results in compaction of chromatin around histones, with subsequent decrease in gene expression [23]. The histone deacetyl transferase (HDAC) inhibitors are a class of drugs that prevent histone deacetylation, thus allowing chromatin to maintain and open configuration with activation of gene transcription, including those involved in apoptosis and inhibition of cell growth [24, 25]. There are several classes of histone deacetylases, including zinc-dependent enzymes (class I, II, and IV) and class III enzymes, which are zinc independent and not currently targeted by any of the available HDAC inhibitors [25–28].

Mechanisms of Action

As mentioned above, the HDAC inhibitors function through modification of gene transcription and resultant cell death as well as inhibition of cell growth. The vast mechanisms by which this occurs are still being elucidated, and are summarized in detail by Bose et al. [22] and include inhibition of DNA repair, increased expression of pro-apoptotic proteins and decreased expression of anti-apoptotic proteins, elevation in DNA damage and generation of reactive oxygen species, cell-cycle checkpoint disruption, diminished chaperone protein function, and induction of autophagy among others. More specifically, HDAC inhibitors inhibit cell-cycle progression through upregulation of p21, p27, and p16 proteins, which lead to G1 arrest [29, 30]. HDAC inhibitors may also prevent cell-cycle progression through S phase through inhibition of the DNA synthesis enzymes cytidine triphosphate synthase and thymidylate synthetase [31]. With regard to apoptosis, HDAC inhibitors upregulate expression of pro-apoptotic proteins such as BH3 while downregulating anti-apoptotic proteins, including Bcl-2, Bcl-XL, and Mcl-1 [30]. In addition to its regulatory actions on the cell cycle and programmed cell death, HDAC inhibitors may exert some of its efficacy in CTCL through immunoregulatory mechanisms. For example, the STAT family of transcription factors (STAT-3, -4, -5, -6) are believed to play a principal role in T-cell pathogenicity, with change in STAT expressions contributing to phenotype switching of aberrant T-cells from a type 1 T-helper (T_{H1}) phenotype to a type 2 T-helper (T_{H2}) phenotype in disease progression. HDAC inhibitors may influence STAT expression in a beneficial manner in patients with CTCL [29, 32, 33].

Use and Efficacy in CTCL

Vorinostat, an oral suberoylanilide hydroxamic acid derivative class I/II HDAC inhibitor [25, 34, 35] was the first HDAC inhibitor approved by the FDA in 2006 for the treatment of CTCL. Its approval was based on the response observed in two phase II single-arm clinical trials of patients with refractory MF/SS of various stages in which the overall response rates (ORR) were 24% and 29%, respectively [29, 35, 36]. **Romidepsin**, a class I HDAC inhibitor with a unique bicyclic structure is administered intravenously typically at a dose of 14 mg/m^2 on days 1, 8, and 15 of a 28-day cycle. It was approved in 2009 for CTCL in patients who have failed at least one prior systemic therapy. Romidepsin also received FDA approval for treatment of refractory or relapsed peripheral T-cell lymphoma (PTCL) in 2011. In addition to its efficacy in CTCL, Kim et al. observed that a significant number of patients treated with romidepsin experienced a clinically meaningful reduction in pruritus severity, including in some individuals who did not achieve any objective clinical response of their skin disease [37]. **Panobinostat** is a broad spectrum hydroxamic acid HDAC inhibitor with activity against all class I, II, and IV HDAC enzymes [29, 38, 39] that is administered orally in 3 weekly doses of 20 mg. Panobinostat is FDA approved for the treatment of multiple myeloma; it is however undergoing evaluation in the setting of CTCL. A 2013 phase II trial of 79 MF/SS patients demonstrated ORR 17%, with 15% of bexarotene-exposed patients demonstrating a clinical response and 20% of bexarotene-naïve patients showing improvement [38]. The HDAC inhibitors demonstrate similar adverse side effect profiles, including fatigue, thrombocytopenia, nausea, vomiting, and diarrhea. Vorinostat may also be associated with dysgeusia [29].

Immunotoxins: Denileukin Diftitox and E7777

Denileukin diftitox is a fusion protein that was approved by the FDA, under the name Ontak, for the treatment of refractory CTCL in 1999. Ontak was placed in a clinical hold by the FDA in 2011 due to impurities identified from the production in E. coli. An improved purity Ontak was devised and phase 3 testing of the new product, entitled E7777, are ongoing as of mid-2017. Therefore denileukin diftitox will likely return to the market.

Denileukin diftitox is a 58 kD recombinant fusion protein of the CD25 subunit of the interleukin-2 (IL-2) protein and the diphtheria toxin. The high affinity IL-2 receptor is mainly expressed on activated T-cells, and binding of IL-2 leads to internalization. When the IL-2 receptor is bound by denileukin, internalization leads to introduction of the diphtheria toxin intracellularly. The toxin causes inhibition of protein synthesis and cell death via apoptosis.

The pivotal phase III study for Ontak established that response rates were dose dependent with an overall response rate of 38% for advanced staged patient with MF/SS at 18 mcg/kg/day and 10% at 9 mcg/kg/day [40]. The median time to first response was 6 weeks, although some first responses did not occur until later cycles, some at cycle 8. Another phase III study, which only examined patients with Stage I–III (no SS), was also placebo controlled. This study identified the relative risk, which is not available for most CTCL therapies. 18 mcg/kg/d of Ontak results in a 73% reduction in relative risk of disease progression or death compared to placebo, while 9 mcg/kg/day reduced risk by 58% [41]. A caveat is that no Stage IV patients were included in this trial. Similar to efficacy, the most common adverse events, which were fever, nausea, and rigors, were also dose dependent. More serious adverse events, including capillary leak syndrome, infusion reactions, and loss of visual acuity occurred in 11%, 8%, and 4%, respectively. Introduction of pretreatment with acetaminophen and diphenhydramine has likely decreased the incidence of fevers, rigors, and infusion reactions. Liver function test abnormalities and bone marrow suppression were also noted, although these typically do not interfere with therapy. It remains to be seen if the E7777 fusion protein, which has the same amino acid sequence of Ontak only a better purity and therefore better bioavailability, will have similar efficacy and safety profile. An early phase I study has shown the maximum tolerated dose was 9 mcg/kg/day with an overall response rate in 1 of 3 patients with CTCL [42].

Monoclonal Antibodies: Alemtuzumab, Brentuximab, Mogamulizumab, and Checkpoint Inhibitors

Background

A variety of monoclonal antibodies have been engineered to target a broad range of cellular targets in hematologic and solid tumors, with promising results. Currently, most approved monoclonal antibodies exert antitumor effects through complement-dependent or antibody-dependent cell-mediated cytotoxicity [43]. The monoclonal antibodies utilized in CTCL are discussed below.

Anti-CD52: Alemtuzumab

Alemtuzumab is a humanized IgG1 anti-CD52 monoclonal antibody that is FDA-approved for the treatment of B-cell chronic lymphocytic leukemia (CLL) as well as relapsing multiple sclerosis (MS). Its use in CTCL is currently off-label. CD52 is a glycoprotein expressed by both B and T lymphocytes as well as monocytes and macrophages [43]. Alemtuzumab causes cell lysis via antibody-dependent cell-mediated cytotoxicity (ADCC); since this leads to depletion of both B and T lymphocytes, alemtuzumab is associated with profound immunosuppression [43]. In a 2003 phase II study for the treatment of MF/SS with alemtuzumab, the investigators observed better responses in erythrodermic SS patients compared to those with plaque or tumor MF [44]. Clark and colleagues elucidated the mechanisms behind this phenomenon, namely that alemtuzumab acts on circulating central memory T-cells (T_{CM}) but not skin-homing effector memory T-cells (T_{EM}), supporting that SS and MF are diseases of different T-cell subsets, and therefore separate entities altogether [45, 46]. While alemtuzumab is typically administered three times weekly, intravenously for CLL and MS, alternate routes and dosing schedules have been investigated in its use in CTCL to combat immunosuppressive side effects and infectious complications. Multiple studies have demonstrated efficacy of 10 mg subcutaneous administration three times per week in MF/SS, without significant increased risk in infectious complications [45, 47, 48]. In general, side effects of alemtuzumab include lymphopenia, infections, acute coronary syndrome, ischemic colitis, deep venous thrombosis, serum sickness-like reaction, and infusion site reactions [25].

Anti-CD30: Brentuximab

CD30 is a transmembrane cell surface leukocyte activation protein belonging to the tumor necrosis factor receptor superfamily. It is expressed on activated B and T lymphocytes as well as various malignant hematopoietic cells in Hodgkin lymphoma, systemic and primary cutaneous anaplastic large cell lymphoma (ALCL), lymphomatoid papulosis (LyP), and MF with large cell transformation (LCT) [43, 49]. Brentuximab vedotin is a chimeric anti-CD30 monoclonal antibody conjugated to mono-methyl auristatin E (vedotin), which increases brentuximab's antitumoral activity [43]. In two recent phase II trials of brentuximab vedotin in MF/SS [50] and CD30-positive lymphoproliferative disorder or MF/SS [51], brentuximab demonstrated efficacy of ORR 70 and 73%, respectively. Of note, not all patients who responded in the trial in MF/SS were characterized by CD30-positive disease, although those with less than 5% CD30 expression had a lower likelihood of response than those with greater than 5% CD30 expression. The investigators observed that there were abundant CD163-positive tumor-associated macrophages in responders, suggesting that brentuximab may target these cells in addition to CD30-expressing T lymphocytes [50, 52]. Adverse side effects of brentuximab include cytopenia, hyperkalemia, fatigue, nausea and vomiting, upper respiratory infection, diarrhea, fever, skin eruption, and cough. Additionally, progressive and possibly irreversible neuropathy may occur [43, 52]. One death due to progressive multifocal leukoencephalopathy has been reported [53].

Future Directions: Mogamulizumab, Checkpoint Inhibitor Therapy

Mogamulizumab is a humanized IgG1 monoclonal antibody that targets CC chemokine receptor 4 (CCR4). It is approved for the treatment of CCR4-positive adult T-cell leukemia (ATLL), peripheral T-cell lymphoma (PTCL) and CTCL in Japan. CCR4 is expressed by malignant CD4+ cells in CTCL and thus presents an attractive therapeutic target through ADCC [54]. CCR4 is also expressed by Treg cells; therefore, in addition to ADCC, mogamulizumab may improve host antitumor responses through depletion of Treg cells [55]. Results of a phase III study of mogamulizumab for the treatment of refractory CTCL in the US are currently awaited.

Malignant cells express immune checkpoint molecules on their surfaces that allow them to mimic healthy cells and evade antitumor host immune responses. Checkpoint inhibitor therapy leads to downregulation of checkpoint proteins with resultant enhanced antitumor responses; recently, checkpoint inhibitor therapy has gained wide attention in the treatment of metastatic melanoma. Ipilimumab, a fully humanized monoclonal antibody to cytotoxic T-lymphocyte antigen 4 (CTLA-4), was the first checkpoint inhibitor FDA-approved for treatment of metastatic melanoma. CTLA-4 is expressed by T lymphocytes; activation of CTLA-4 by antigen-presenting cells inhibits the cytotoxic antitumor response and promotes immune tolerance. CTLA-4 has been shown to be overexpressed by malignant T-cells in CTCL, making it an attractive therapeutic target in MF/SS [56]. Sekulic and colleagues [57] recently identified an SS patient with a novel *CTLA-CD28* gene fusion within malignant cells who responded to treatment with ipilimumab, suggesting additional therapeutic roles of anti-CTLA therapy in MF/SS. Additional checkpoint inhibitor targets include the programmed death-1 (PD-1) pathway (nivolumab, pembrolizumab). A phase II clinical trial evaluating the efficacy of pembrolizumab in MF/SS was recently reported in the United States [52].

Interferons

Background

The interferons, so-named for their ability to interfere with viral replication [58, 59], are naturally occurring polypeptides produced by human cells as part of the innate immune response [60]. Interferon alfa (IFNα) is produced by leukocytes and lymphoblastoid cells in response to viruses, B-cell mitogens, foreign cells, and tumor cells [58, 61], while interferon gamma (IFNγ) is produced by T lymphocytes and natural killer (NK) cells in response to the T-cell mitogen, interleukin-2, and other antigens. Interferon beta is produced by fibroblasts in response to viruses and foreign DNA [62].

Use and Efficacy in CTCL

Interferon alfa (IFNα) is available in the United States as recombinant IFN alfa-2b (Intron) and in pegylated forms IFN alfa-2a and IFN alfa-2b. The pegylated forms are more resistant to breakdown by proteolytic enzymes, and therefore have longer elimination half-lives compared to non-pegylated forms [58]. Malignant T-cells in MF/SS typically exhibit a T_{H2} phenotype [63–66], which results in increased production in T_{H2} cytokines IL-4, IL-5, and IL-10. These may suppress the T_{H1}-mediated immune response [63–67]. Observations that patients with MF/SS have decreased production of the T_{H1} cytokines IFNα, IFNγ, and IL-12 offer further support for this pathomechanism [63, 68, 69]. The administration of IFNα suppresses the T_{H2} imbalance observed in MF/SS through its activation of CD8 T lymphocytes and NK cells [58, 70–72]. While dosing and regimens of IFNα in MF/SS is widely varied in the literature, standard dosing is typically 1.5–6 million units daily, three times weekly [73, 74]. It has also been used successfully intralesionally, possibly with diminished systemic absorption [58]. IFNα has been evaluated in combination with PUVA, oral retinoids, ECP, and total skin electron beam therapy (TSEBT) with varying results [20, 58, 75, 76]; nonetheless, it continues to be used as a mainstay in the treatment of MF/SS, both as monotherapy (see Fig. 33.2) and in combination with other systemic and/or skin-directed treatments [74].

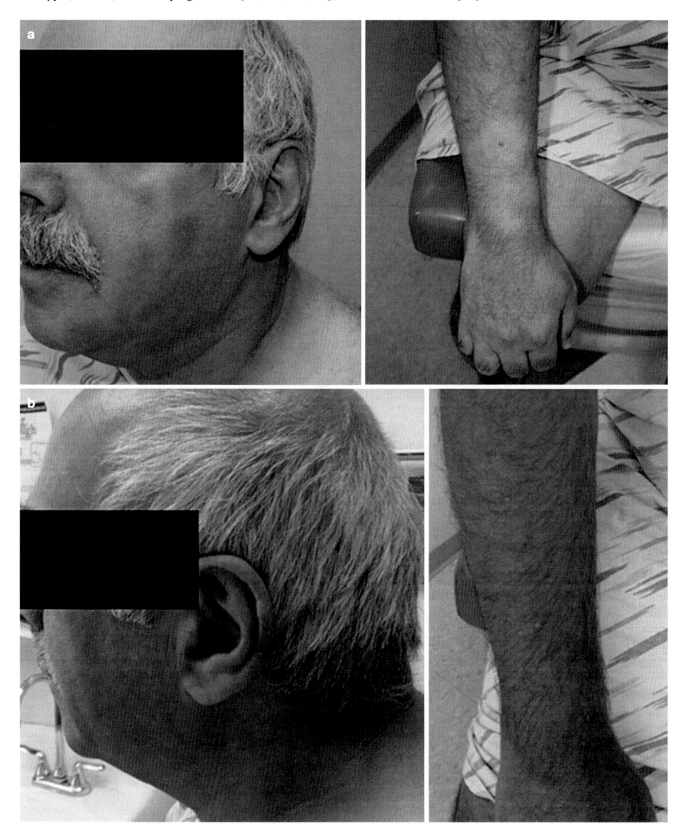

Fig. 33.2 (a) Plaque-stage folliculotropic mycosis fungoides with infiltrated plaques on the face and alopecic plaque of the forearm. (b) Same patient six months after subcutaneous IFNα therapy

Interferon gamma (IFNγ) is available in the United States as recombinant IFN gamma-1b (Actimmune). It is FDA-approved for the treatment of chronic granulomatous disease and osteoporosis [58, 59]. Similar to IFNα, IFNγ functions in the host immune response, improving CD8- and NK-mediated cytotoxicity, reducing T$_{H2}$ immune activity and enhancing the T$_{H1}$ response [58, 77]. Additional actions of IFNγ include stimulation of antigen-presenting cells and inhibition of tumor cell proliferation; some authors have argued that this particular function of IFNγ may lend it to greater synergism with PUVA, ECP, and TSEBT (therapies that induce apoptosis) over IFNα [58].

The most common side effects of the interferons include flu-like symptoms (fever, malaise, myalgias, arthralgias, and headache), which often diminishes after a few weeks of therapy; gradually increasing the dose is recommended to ameliorate these effects. Chronic side effects most commonly include fatigue, and decreased appetite with subsequent weight loss [59]. These adverse effects are also dose-related and tend to improve over time. Cytopenia, depressed mood, thyroid dysfunction, dygeusia, diarrhea, hepatotoxicity, and cardiotoxicity are additional reported side effects that should be monitored. Severe peripheral neuropathy as well as exacerbation of autoimmune disease may also occur. IFNγ appears to have a slightly more favorable side effect profile compared to IFNα, with less risk of mood changes, autoimmune exacerbation, and peripheral neuropathy [58].

Toll-Like Receptor Agonists

Toll-like receptor (TLR) agonists such as imiquimod and resiquimod have the potential of overcoming some of the immune dysregulation in patients with CTCL (Fig. 33.1). Unmethylated oligodeoxynucleotide CPG is a potent TLR-9 agonist that can stimulate dendritic cells (DC) and T-cells. CPG oligodeoxynucleotide (CPG ODN) is a synthetic, nuclease-resistant, TLR9-activating oligodeoxynucleotide that mimics unmethylated CPG. With activating effects on both innate and adaptive immunity, there is the potential to facilitate the host antitumor response against CTCL. By triggering TLR9, there is maturation and enhancement of DC to present antigens and to increase the number of antigen-presenting cells. In response to CPG ODN the DC upregulate costimulatory molecules CD80 and CD86, which enhance the capacity of these cells to present antigens [78]. In the pilot study of weekly CPG ODN injections, the most common adverse events were flu-like symptoms (fatigue, rigors, myalgia, and pyrexia), and injection-site reactions (pain, erythema, edema, and induration). In that initial study of 28 patients with refractory MF type CTCL, there were three complete

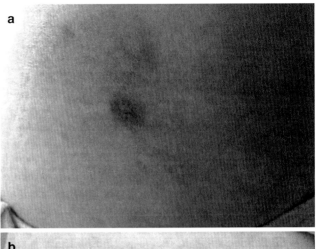

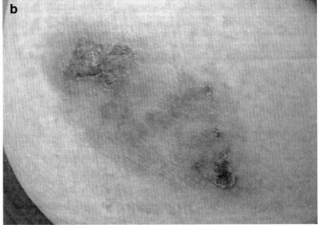

Fig. 33.3 Treatment of patch stage mycosis fungoides on the hip with imiquimod. (**a**) before therapy; (**b**) inflammation with erosion, crusting, and erythema during therapy, indicating activation of the host immune response

responses and six partial responses [79]. As has been observed with other immunotherapies, febrile and flu-like responses were often seen in responders. The most commonly reported treatment-related hematologic toxicities were lymphopenia, leukopenia, neutropenia, anemia, and thrombocytopenia. Given the ability of TLR-9 stimulation to facilitate antigen presentation and the generation of adaptive immune cells to fight the CTCL cells, this modality would theoretically synergize with radiotherapy. There has been one preliminary study of using adjunctive radiation that should provide abundant antigens from dying cells to be presented via dendritic cells activated by CPG ODN. Indeed in that small series the authors noted the disappearance of lesions not impacted directly by radiotherapy [80].

Currently CPG ODN is not being developed for clinical use by Pfizer so it remains an academic interest, even though it does have potential to completely clear the disease in select patients and has the potential to synergize with other immune modulating therapies for CTCL (Fig. 33.3).

Photopheresis

Photopheresis is a three-step procedure. First a leukapheresis is performed to collect approximately 10^{10} peripheral blood mononuclear cells. These cells are dosed with 8-methoxypsoralen and exposed to 1–2 J of ultraviolet A light extracorporeally. The final step is a gradual reinfusion of the treated material. In the end, there is no true "pheresis" (removal from the patient) since everything is reinfused. A treatment session lasts approximately 3 h and is performed twice every 4 weeks, typically on consecutive days and sometimes at 2-week intervals. The major toxicity associated with photopheresis is from the addition of saline a patient receives during the leukapheresis. There have not been signs of immunosuppression such as zoster infection, opportunistic infections, or opportunistic malignancies.

Psoralen in the presence of UVA light has phototoxic effects on cells in the leukapheresis sample. Perhaps the most important observation that supports this modality as an immunotherapy is that only a small portion of the circulating malignant lymphocyte population is treated yet widespread systemic improvement may ensue. In addition to inducing malignant T-cell apoptosis, photopheresis also induces monocytes to differentiate into DCs capable of phagocytosing and processing the apoptotic tumor cell antigens.

A shift in the profile of cytokine production and the balance of T-helper type 1 and type 2 responses after photopheresis may also facilitate a more effective antitumor response [63, 64]. While evaluating the immune regulatory events induced by photopheresis, several studies have observed an increase in T regulatory (Tregs) cells and their function [81, 82]. Since the erythrodermic form of CTCL is known to be associated with a reduction of Tregs [83], it appears that these cells can be upregulated to suppress the malignant lymphocytes of CTCL. In one series, the increase in Tregs paralleled both the clinical response and the diminution of the circulating malignant cells [84].

Photopheresis has been found to be reliably palliative for all forms of erythrodermic CTCL including Sézary syndrome. Response rates in erythrodermic patients range from 31 to 86% [85]. Photopheresis, however, is also effective in early stage mycosis fungoides [86]. While monotherapy trials were needed to document efficacy initially, the current usage of photopheresis is almost always as a component of a multimodality regimen [87]. As with the toll receptor agonists, dendritic cell activating therapies like photopheresis should synergize with radiotherapy and there have been preliminary studies suggesting this [88]. The immune activating effects of interferon should also theoretically synergize with photopheresis and this is often incorporated with the non-immunosuppressing oral bexarotene for a multimodality regimen that has been described as moderately successful in a small series [89]. The future development of photopheresis will involve utilization of immune modulators to improve responses and to extend therapeutic responses into patients with plaque and tumor phases of the disease.

Hematopoietic Stem Cell Transplantation

A discussion on systemic and biologic therapies in MF/SS would not be complete without mention of stem cell transplantation (SCT), the "ultimate" biologic therapy, via an immune-mediated graft-versus-lymphoma effect on the patient. While autologous SCT confers the advantage of diminished transplant-associated risk of death [90, 91], it is associated with higher rates of disease relapse. Unfortunately, responses to autologous SCT in patients with MF/SS are generally discouraging, with progression-free survival (PFS) typically <6 months [92–95]. Although limited, there is some data that supports allogeneic SCT in select patients with MF/SS [90]. A recent prospective study of 47 MF/SS patients demonstrated overall survival (OS) and PFS at 4 years of 51 and 26%, respectively [92]. Patients with SS without large cell transformation responded significantly better, with 4-year PFS of 73%. Of note, many patients who experienced relapse following allogeneic SCT responded to immunomodulatory therapy, including photopheresis, topical therapy, localized radiation, donor lymphocyte infusion, and/or chemotherapy.

Summary

The broad spectrum of immune dysregulation in MF/SS has provided a broad target for biologic therapies that have been developed for topical, oral, subcutaneous, intramuscular, and intravenous administration. Often the improvement in the immune response is dramatic with increased inflammation, redness, and discomfort of lesions as has been reported with all of the TLR agonists, interferon, photopheresis, and denileukin diftitox. Those agents that modulate the malignant phenotype tend to work more slowly with gradual improvement and signs and symptoms over months. The improved outcomes being observed have two possible origins. In many patients the improvement in their skin and immune system can only help with preventing some of the infectious complications that are often their demise. The other improvement is in interrupting the natural progression of the disease. Currently, durable remissions are the best evidence for therapy having had this type of significant impact.

The future of these modalities and understanding their combinations will be defined by their ability to achieve that goal.

Case Report

A 62-year-old Caucasian male diagnosed with patch-plaque mycosis fungoides (see Fig. 33.2) 2 years prior has been undergoing treatment with psoralen-UVA (PUVA) therapy three times weekly for 4 months. He has had improvement of patches, but recalcitrant plaques on the buttocks, abdomen, back, and lower extremities. He complains of an 8 out of 10 pruritus on a visual analog scale (VAS). His review of systems is otherwise negative.

Past Medical History

- Hyperlipidemia
- Hypertension

Social History

- Nonsmoker
- Drinks socially, 5–8 beers per week
- Married
- High school principal

Previous Therapies

- High-potency topical steroids
- PUVA

Physical Exam

- Red-brown plaques with overlying fine scale on the buttocks, abdomen, back and lower extremities, involving 15% of the body surface area
- No cervical, axillary, or inguinal lymphadenopathy
- No hepatosplenomegaly
- Stage T2b N0 M0 B0 = Stage IB

Management

Because of recalcitrant plaques, IFNα was added to his regimen. His initial dosing was 1.5 million units (mU) three days per week, and titrated to 3 mU three days per week. He was unable to tolerate higher doses due to flu-like symptoms and fatigue. Baseline and periodic laboratory monitoring included complete blood count, liver function tests, and thyroid function tests. A baseline electrocardiogram was unremarkable. Oral bexarotene was considered, but chosen for next-line therapy given his history of hyperlipidemia. Given his report of severe pruritus, HDAC inhibitor therapy is also a future consideration for this patient should he fail to respond combination therapy with PUVA and IFNα. Additional options could be identified in the National Comprehensive Cancer Network guidelines for mycosis fungoides in Category A Systemic Therapies (SYST-CAT A) (Fig. 33.4).

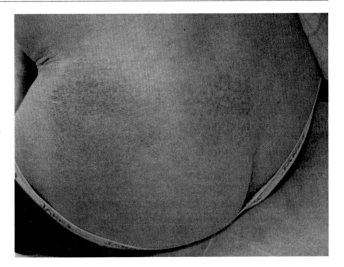

Fig. 33.4 Typical patch-plaque mycosis fungoides on the lower back and buttocks

References

1. Lindahl LM, Fenger-Gron M, Iversen L. Subsequent cancers, mortality, and causes of death in patients with mycosis fungoides and parapsoriasis: a Danish nationwide, population-based cohort study. J Am Acad Dermatol. 2014;71(3):529–35.
2. Kantor AF, Curtis RE, Vonderheid EC, van Scott EJ, Fraumeni JF, Jr. Risk of second malignancy after cutaneous T-cell lymphoma. Cancer 1989;63(8):1612–1615.
3. Posner LE, Fossieck BE, Jr., Eddy JL, Bunn PA, Jr, Septicemic complications of the cutaneous T-cell lymphomas. Am J Med 1981;71(2):210–216.
4. Sezary ABY. Erythrodermie avec presence de cellules monstreuses dans le derme et le sang circulant. Bull Soc Fr Dermatol Syph. 1938;45:254–60.
5. Zackheim HS, Koo J, LeBoit PE, McCalmont TH, Bowman PH, Kashani-Sabet M, et al. Psoriasiform mycosis fungoides with fatal outcome after treatment with cyclosporine. J Am Acad Dermatol. 2002;47(1):155–7.
6. Kim EJ, Hess S, Richardson SK, Newton S, Showe LC, Benoit BM, et al. Immunopathogenesis and therapy of cutaneous T cell lymphoma. J Clin Invest. 2005;115(4):798–812.
7. Heald P, Yan SL, Edelson R. Profound deficiency in normal circulating T cells in erythrodermic cutaneous T-cell lymphoma. Arch Dermatol. 1994;130(2):198–203.
8. Huen AO, Kim EJ. The role of systemic retinoids in the treatment of cutaneous T-cell lymphoma. Dermatol Clin. 2015;33(4):715–29.
9. Kempf W, Kettelhack N, Duvic M, Burg G. Topical and systemic retinoid therapy for cutaneous T-cell lymphoma. Hematol Oncol Clin North Am. 2003;17(6):1405–19.
10. Sokolowska-Wojdylo M, Lugowska-Umer H, Maciejewska-Radomska A. Oral retinoids and rexinoids in cutaneous T-cell lymphomas. Postep Dermatol Alergol. 2013;30(1):19–29.
11. Heller EH, Shiffman NJ. Synthetic retinoids in dermatology. Can Med Assoc J. 1985;132(10):1129–36.
12. Zhang C, Hazarika P, Ni X, Weidner DA, Duvic M. Induction of apoptosis by bexarotene in cutaneous T-cell lymphoma cells: relevance to mechanism of therapeutic action. Clin Cancer Res. 2002;8(5):1234–40.

13. Burg G, Dummer R. Historical perspective on the use of retinoids in cutaneous T-cell lymphoma (CTCL). Clin Lymphoma. 2000;1(Suppl 1):S41–4.

14. Yen WC, Prudente RY, Corpuz MR, Negro-Vilar A, Lamph WW. A selective retinoid X receptor agonist bexarotene (LGD1069, targretin) inhibits angiogenesis and metastasis in solid tumours. Br J Cancer. 2006;94(5):654–60.

15. Duvic M, Martin AG, Kim Y, Olsen E, Wood GS, Crowley CA, et al. Phase 2 and 3 clinical trial of oral bexarotene (Targretin capsules) for the treatment of refractory or persistent early-stage cutaneous T-cell lymphoma. Arch Dermatol. 2001;137(5):581–93.

16. Duvic M, Hymes K, Heald P, Breneman D, Martin AG, Myskowski P, et al. Bexarotene is effective and safe for treatment of refractory advanced-stage cutaneous T-cell lymphoma: multinational phase II-III trial results. J Clin Oncol. 2001;19(9):2456–71.

17. McGinnis KS, Ubriani R, Newton S, Junkins-Hopkins JM, Vittorio CC, Kim EJ, et al. The addition of interferon gamma to oral bexarotene therapy with photopheresis for Sezary syndrome. Arch Dermatol. 2005;141(9):1176–8.

18. Aviles A, Neri N, Fernandez-Diez J, Silva L, Nambo MJ. Interferon and low doses of methotrexate versus interferon and retinoids in the treatment of refractory/relapsed cutaneous T-cell lymphoma. Hematology. 2015;20(9):538–42.

19. Straus DJ, Duvic M, Kuzel T, Horwitz S, Demierre MF, Myskowski P, et al. Results of a phase II trial of oral bexarotene (Targretin) combined with interferon alfa-2b (intron-A) for patients with cutaneous T-cell lymphoma. Cancer. 2007;109(9):1799–803.

20. McGinnis KS, Junkins-Hopkins JM, Crawford G, Shapiro M, Rook AH, Vittorio CC. Low-dose oral bexarotene in combination with low-dose interferon alfa in the treatment of cutaneous T-cell lymphoma: clinical synergism and possible immunologic mechanisms. J Am Acad Dermatol. 2004;50(3):375–9.

21. Graeppi-Dulac J, Vlaeminck-Guillem V, Perier-Muzet M, Dalle S, Orgiazzi J. Endocrine side-effects of anti-cancer drugs: the impact of retinoids on the thyroid axis. Eur J Endocrinol. 2014;170(6):R253–62.

22. Bose P, Dai Y, Grant S. Histone deacetylase inhibitor (HDACI) mechanisms of action: emerging insights. Pharmacol Ther. 2014;143(3):323–36.

23. Rosato RR, Grant S. Histone deacetylase inhibitors: insights into mechanisms of lethality. Expert Opin Ther Targets. 2005;9(4):809–24.

24. Poligone B, Lin J, Chung C. Romidepsin: evidence for its potential use to manage previously treated cutaneous T cell lymphoma. Core Evid. 2011;6:1–12.

25. Chung CG, Poligone B. Cutaneous T cell lymphoma: an update on pathogenesis and systemic therapy. Curr Hematol Malig Rep. 2015;10(4):468–76.

26. Konstantinopoulos PA, Vandoros GP, Papavassiliou AG. FK228 (Depsipeptide): a HDAC inhibitor with pleiotropic antitumor activities. Cancer Chemother Pharmacol. 2006;58(5):711–5.

27. Glaser KB. HDAC inhibitors: clinical update and mechanism-based potential. Biochem Pharmacol. 2007;74(5):659–71.

28. Prince HM, Bishton MJ, Harrison SJ. Clinical studies of histone deacetylase inhibitors. Clin Cancer Res. 2009;15(12):3958–69.

29. Duvic M. Histone deacetylase inhibitors for cutaneous T-cell lymphoma. Dermatol Clin. 2015;33(4):757–64.

30. Jain S, Zain J, O'Connor O. Novel therapeutic agents for cutaneous T-cell lymphoma. J Hematol Oncol. 2012;5:24.

31. Luchenko VL, Litman T, Chakraborty AR, Heffner A, Devor C, Wilkerson J, et al. Histone deacetylase inhibitor-mediated cell death is distinct from its global effect on chromatin. Mol Oncol. 2014;8(8):1379–92.

32. Litvinov IV, Cordeiro B, Fredholm S, Odum N, Zargham H, Huang Y, et al. Analysis of STAT4 expression in cutaneous T-cell lymphoma (CTCL) patients and patient-derived cell lines. Cell Cycle. 2014;13(18):2975–82.

33. Netchiporouk E, Litvinov IV, Moreau L, Gilbert M, Sasseville D, Duvic M. Deregulation in STAT signaling is important for cutaneous T-cell lymphoma (CTCL) pathogenesis and cancer progression. Cell Cycle. 2014;13(21):3331–5.

34. Mann BS, Johnson JR, He K, Sridhara R, Abraham S, Booth BP, et al. Vorinostat for treatment of cutaneous manifestations of advanced primary cutaneous T-cell lymphoma. Clin Cancer Res. 2007;13(8):2318–22.

35. Olsen EA, Kim YH, Kuzel TM, Pacheco TR, Foss FM, Parker S, et al. Phase IIb multicenter trial of vorinostat in patients with persistent, progressive, or treatment refractory cutaneous T-cell lymphoma. J Clin Oncol. 2007;25(21):3109–15.

36. Duvic M, Talpur R, Ni X, Zhang C, Hazarika P, Kelly C, et al. Phase 2 trial of oral vorinostat (suberoylanilide hydroxamic acid, SAHA) for refractory cutaneous T-cell lymphoma (CTCL). Blood. 2007;109(1):31–9.

37. Kim YH, Demierre MF, Kim EJ, Lerner A, Rook AH, Duvic M, et al. Clinically meaningful reduction in pruritus in patients with cutaneous T-cell lymphoma treated with romidepsin. Leuk Lymphoma. 2013;54(2):284–9.

38. Duvic M, Dummer R, Becker JC, Poulalhon N, Ortiz Romero P, Grazia Bernengo M, et al. Panobinostat activity in both bexarotene-exposed and -naive patients with refractory cutaneous T-cell lymphoma: results of a phase II trial. Eur J Cancer. 2013;49(2):386–94.

39. Atadja P. Development of the pan-DAC inhibitor panobinostat (LBH589): successes and challenges. Cancer Lett. 2009;280(2):233–41.

40. Olsen E, Duvic M, Frankel A, Kim Y, Martin A, Vonderheid E, et al. Pivotal phase III trial of two dose levels of denileukin diftitox for the treatment of cutaneous T-cell lymphoma. J Clin Oncol. 2001;19(2):376–88.

41. Prince HM, Duvic M, Martin A, Sterry W, Assaf C, Sun Y, et al. Phase III placebo-controlled trial of denileukin diftitox for patients with cutaneous T-cell lymphoma. J Clin Oncol. 2010;28(11):1870–7.

42. Maruyama DTK, Ando K, Ohmachi K, Ogura M, Uchida T, Nakanishi T, Namiki M. Phase I study of E7777, a diphtheria toxin fragment-Interleukin-2 fusion protein, in Japanese patients with relapsed or refractory peripheral and cutaneous T-cell lymphoma. Blood. 2015;126(23):2724.

43. Geskin LJ. Monoclonal Antibodies. Dermatol Clin. 2015;33(4):777–86.

44. Lundin J, Hagberg H, Repp R, Cavallin-Stahl E, Freden S, Juliusson G, et al. Phase 2 study of alemtuzumab (anti-CD52 monoclonal antibody) in patients with advanced mycosis fungoides/Sezary syndrome. Blood. 2003;101(11):4267–72.

45. Clark RA, Watanabe R, Teague JE, Schlapbach C, Tawa MC, Adams N, et al. Skin effector memory T cells do not recirculate and provide immune protection in alemtuzumab-treated CTCL patients. Sci Transl Med. 2012;4(117):117ra7.

46. Campbell JJ, Clark RA, Watanabe R, Kupper TS. Sezary syndrome and mycosis fungoides arise from distinct T-cell subsets: a biologic rationale for their distinct clinical behaviors. Blood. 2010;116(5):767–71.

47. Bernengo MG, Quaglino P, Comessatti A, Ortoncelli M, Novelli M, Lisa F, et al. Low-dose intermittent alemtuzumab in the treatment of Sezary syndrome: clinical and immunologic findings in 14 patients. Haematologica. 2007;92(6):784–94.

48. Watanabe R, Teague JE, Fisher DC, Kupper TS, Clark RA. Alemtuzumab therapy for leukemic cutaneous T-cell lymphoma: diffuse erythema as a positive predictor of complete remission. JAMA Dermatol. 2014;150(7):776–9.

49. Edinger JT, Clark BZ, Pucevich BE, Geskin LJ, Swerdlow SH. CD30 Expression and proliferative fraction in nontransformed mycosis fungoides. Am J Surg Pathol. 2009;33(12):1860–8.

50. Kim YH, Tavallaee M, Sundram U, Salva KA, Wood GS, Li S, et al. Phase II Investigator-Initiated Study of Brentuximab Vedotin in mycosis Fungoides and Sezary syndrome with variable CD30 expression level: a multi-institution collaborative project. J Clin Oncol. 2015;33(32):3750–8.

51. Duvic M, Tetzlaff MT, Gangar P, Clos AL, Sui D, Talpur R. Results of a Phase II trial of Brentuximab Vedotin for CD30+ cutaneous T-cell lymphoma and Lymphomatoid Papulosis. J Clin Oncol. 2015;33(32):3759–65.

52. Khodadoust M, Rook A, Porcu P, et al. Pembrolizumab for treatment of relapsed/refractory mycosis fungoides and Sezary syndrome: clinical efficacy in a CITN multicenter phase 2 study [abstract]. Blood. 2016;125. Abstract 181

53. Carson KR, Newsome SD, Kim EJ, Wagner-Johnston ND, von Geldern G, Moskowitz CH, et al. Progressive multifocal leukoencephalopathy associated with brentuximab vedotin therapy: a report of 5 cases from the Southern Network on Adverse Reactions (SONAR) project. Cancer. 2014;120(16):2464–71.

54. Duvic M, Evans M, Wang C. Mogamulizumab for the treatment of cutaneous T-cell lymphoma: recent advances and clinical potential. Ther Adv Hematol. 2016;7(3):171–4.

55. Ni X, Jorgensen JL, Goswami M, Challagundla P, Decker WK, Kim YH, et al. Reduction of regulatory T cells by Mogamulizumab, a defucosylated anti-CC chemokine receptor 4 antibody, in patients with aggressive/refractory mycosis fungoides and Sezary syndrome. Clin Cancer Res. 2015;21(2):274–85.

56. Wong HK, Wilson AJ, Gibson HM, Hafner MS, Hedgcock CJ, Berger CL, et al. Increased expression of CTLA-4 in malignant T-cells from patients with mycosis fungoides—cutaneous T cell lymphoma. J Invest Dermatol. 2006;126(1):212–9.

57. Sekulic A, Liang WS, Tembe W, Izatt T, Kruglyak S, Kiefer JA, et al. Personalized treatment of Sezary syndrome by targeting a novel CTLA4:CD28 fusion. Mol Genet Genomic Med. 2015;3(2):130–6.

58. Spaccarelli N, Rook AH. The use of Interferons in the treatment of cutaneous T-cell lymphoma. Dermatol Clin. 2015;33(4):731–45.

59. Olsen EA. Interferon in the treatment of cutaneous T-cell lymphoma. Dermatol Ther. 2003;16(4):311–21.

60. Strander H. Interferon treatment of human neoplasia. Adv Cancer Res. 1986;46:1–265.

61. Roth MS, Foon KA. Alpha interferon in the treatment of hematologic malignancies. Am J Med. 1986;81(5):871–82.

62. Ross C, Tingsgaard P, Jorgensen H, Vejlsgaard GL. Interferon treatment of cutaneous T-cell lymphoma. Eur J Haematol. 1993;51(2):63–72.

63. Vowels BR, Cassin M, Vonderheid EC, Rook AH. Aberrant cytokine production by Sezary syndrome patients: cytokine secretion pattern resembles murine Th2 cells. J Invest Dermatol. 1992;99(1):90–4.

64. Vowels BR, Lessin SR, Cassin M, Jaworsky C, Benoit B, Wolfe JT, et al. Th2 Cytokine mRNA expression in skin in cutaneous T-cell lymphoma. J Invest Dermatol. 1994;103(5):669–73.

65. Asadullah K, Haeussler A, Sterry W, Docke WD, Volk HD. Interferon gamma and tumor necrosis factor alpha mRNA expression in mycosis fungoides progression. Blood. 1996;88(2):757–8.

66. Asadullah K, Docke WD, Haeussler A, Sterry W, Volk HD. Progression of mycosis fungoides is associated with increasing cutaneous expression of interleukin-10 mRNA. J Invest Dermatol. 1996;107(6):833–7.

67. Guenova E, Watanabe R, Teague JE, Desimone JA, Jiang Y, Dowlatshahi M, et al. Th2 Cytokines from malignant cells suppress TH1 responses and enforce a global TH2 bias in leukemic cutaneous T-cell lymphoma. Clin Cancer Res. 2013;19(14):3755–63.

68. French LE, Huard B, Wysocka M, Shane R, Contassot E, Arrighi JF, et al. Impaired CD40L signaling is a cause of defective IL-12 and TNF-alpha production in Sezary syndrome: circumvention by hexameric soluble CD40L. Blood. 2005;105(1):219–25.

69. Wysocka M, Zaki MH, French LE, Chehimi J, Shapiro M, Everetts SE, et al. Sezary syndrome patients demonstrate a defect in dendritic cell populations: effects of CD40 ligand and treatment with GM-CSF on dendritic cell numbers and the production of cytokines. Blood. 2002;100(9):3287–94.

70. Yoo EK, Cassin M, Lessin SR, Rook AH. Complete molecular remission during biologic response modifier therapy for Sezary syndrome is associated with enhanced helper T type 1 cytokine production and natural killer cell activity. J Am Acad Dermatol. 2001;45(2):208–16.

71. Suchin KR, Cassin M, Gottleib SL, Sood S, Cucchiara AJ, Vonderheid EC, et al. Increased interleukin 5 production in eosinophilic Sezary syndrome: regulation by interferon alfa and interleukin 12. J Am Acad Dermatol. 2001;44(1):28–32.

72. Rook AH, Heald P. The immunopathogenesis of cutaneous T-cell lymphoma. Hematol Oncol Clin North Am. 1995;9(5):997–1010.

73. Olsen EA, Rosen ST, Vollmer RT, Variakojis D, Roenigk HH Jr, Diab N, et al. Interferon alfa-2a in the treatment of cutaneous T cell lymphoma. J Am Acad Dermatol. 1989;20(3):395–407.

74. Whittaker S, Hoppe R, Prince HM. How I treat mycosis fungoides and Sezary syndrome. Blood. 2016;127(25):3142–53.

75. Chiarion-Sileni V, Bononi A, Fornasa CV, Soraru M, Alaibac M, Ferrazzi E, et al. Phase II trial of interferon-alpha-2a plus psoralen with ultraviolet light a in patients with cutaneous T-cell lymphoma. Cancer. 2002;95(3):569–75.

76. Wagner AE, Wada D, Bowen G, Gaffney DK. Mycosis fungoides: the addition of concurrent and adjuvant interferon to total skin electron beam therapy. Br J Dermatol. 2013;169(3):715–8.

77. Olsen EA, Rook AH, Zic J, Kim Y, Porcu P, Querfeld C, et al. Sezary syndrome: immunopathogenesis, literature review of therapeutic options, and recommendations for therapy by the United States cutaneous lymphoma consortium (USCLC). J Am Acad Dermatol. 2011;64(2):352–404.

78. Speiser DE, Lienard D, Rufer N, Rubio-Godoy V, Rimoldi D, Lejeune F, et al. Rapid and strong human CD8+ T cell responses to vaccination with peptide, IFA, and CpG oligodeoxynucleotide 7909. J Clin Invest. 2005;115(3):739–46.

79. Kim YH, Girardi M, Duvic M, Kuzel T, Link BK, Pinter-Brown L, et al. Phase I trial of a toll-like receptor 9 agonist, PF-3512676 (CPG 7909), in patients with treatment-refractory, cutaneous T-cell lymphoma. J Am Acad Dermatol. 2010;63(6):975–83.

80. Kim YH, Gratzinger D, Harrison C, Brody JD, Czerwinski DK, Ai WZ, et al. In situ vaccination against mycosis fungoides by intratumoral injection of a TLR9 agonist combined with radiation: a phase 1/2 study. Blood. 2012;119(2):355–63.

81. Rao V, Saunes M, Jorstad S, Moen T. Cutaneous T cell lymphoma and graft-versus-host disease: a comparison of in vivo effects of extracorporeal photochemotherapy on Foxp3+ regulatory T cells. Clin Immunol. 2009;133(3):303–13.

82. Schmitt S, Johnson TS, Karakhanova S, Naher H, Mahnke K, Enk AH. Extracorporeal photophoresis augments function of CD4+CD25+FoxP3+ regulatory T cells by triggering adenosine production. Transplantation. 2009;88(3):411–6.

83. Klemke CD, Fritzsching B, Franz B, Kleinmann EV, Oberle N, Poenitz N, et al. Paucity of FOXP3+ cells in skin and peripheral blood distinguishes Sezary syndrome from other cutaneous T-cell lymphomas. Leukemia. 2006;20(6):1123–9.

84. Shiue LH, Couturier J, Lewis DE, Wei C, Ni X, Duvic M. The effect of extracorporeal photopheresis alone or in combination therapy on circulating CD4(+) Foxp3(+) CD25(−) T cells in patients with leukemic cutaneous T-cell lymphoma. Photodermatol Photoimmunol Photomed. 2015;31(4):184–94.

85. Quaglino P, Knobler R, Fierro MT, Savoia P, Marra E, Fava P, et al. Extracorporeal photopheresis for the treatment of erythrodermic cutaneous T-cell lymphoma: a single center clinical experience with long-term follow-up data and a brief overview of the literature. Int J Dermatol. 2013;52(11):1308–18.

86. Talpur R, Demierre MF, Geskin L, Baron E, Pugliese S, Eubank K, et al. Multicenter photopheresis intervention trial in early-stage mycosis fungoides. Clin Lymphoma Myeloma Leuk. 2011;11(2):219–27.

87. Atzmony L, Amitay-Laish I, Gurion R, Shahal-Zimra Y, Hodak E. Erythrodermic mycosis fungoides and Sezary syndrome treated with extracorporeal photopheresis as part of a multimodality regimen: a single-centre experience. J Eur Acad Dermatol Venereol. 2015;29(12):2382–9.

88. Wilson LD, Licata AL, Braverman IM, Edelson RL, Heald PW, Feldman AM, et al. Systemic chemotherapy and extracorporeal photochemotherapy for T3 and T4 cutaneous T-cell lymphoma patients who have achieved a complete response to total skin electron beam therapy. Int J Radiat Oncol Biol Phys. 1995;32(4):987–95.

89. Richardson SK, McGinnis KS, Shapiro M, Lehrer MS, Kim EJ, Vittorio CC, et al. Extracorporeal photopheresis and multimodality immunomodulatory therapy in the treatment of cutaneous T-cell lymphoma. J Cutan Med Surg. 2003;7(4 Suppl):8–12.

90. Virmani P, Zain J, Rosen ST, Myskowski PL, Querfeld C. Hematopoietic stem cell transplant for mycosis Fungoides and Sezary syndrome. Dermatol Clin. 2015;33(4):807–18. Epub 2015/10/05

91. DeFor TE, Majhail NS, Weisdorf DJ, Brunstein CG, McAvoy S, Arora M, et al. A modified comorbidity index for hematopoietic cell transplantation. Bone Marrow Transplant. 2010;45(5):933–8. Epub 2009/10/06

92. Hosing C, Bassett R, Dabaja B, Talpur R, Alousi A, Ciurea S, et al. Allogeneic stem-cell transplantation in patients with cutaneous lymphoma: updated results from a single institution. Ann Oncol. 2015;26(12):2490–5. Epub 2015/09/30

93. Russell-Jones R, Child F, Olavarria E, Whittaker S, Spittle M, Apperley J. Autologous peripheral blood stem cell transplantation in tumor-stage mycosis fungoides: predictors of disease-free survival. Ann N Y Acad Sci. 2001;941:147–54. Epub 2001/10/12

94. Olavarria E, Child F, Woolford A, Whittaker SJ, Davis JG, McDonald C, et al. T-cell depletion and autologous stem cell transplantation in the management of tumour stage mycosis fungoides with peripheral blood involvement. Br J Haematol. 2001;114(3):624–31. Epub 2001/09/13

95. Bigler RD, Crilley P, Micaily B, Brady LW, Topolsky D, Bulova S, et al. Autologous bone marrow transplantation for advanced stage mycosis fungoides. Bone Marrow Transplant. 1991;7(2):133–7. Epub 1991/02/01

Anti-CD20 Agents and Potential Novel Biologics in Pemphigus Vulgaris and Other Autoimmune Blistering Diseases

Amy Huang, Raman K. Madan, Lauren Bonomo, and Jacob Levitt

Abbreviations

ADCC	Antibody-dependent cellular cytotoxicity
APRIL	A proliferation-inducing ligand
BAFF	B-cell activating factor of the tumor necrosis factor family
BAFF-R	BAFF receptor
BCMA	B-cell maturation antigen
BP	Bullous pemphigoid
CDC	Complement-dependent cytotoxicity
EBA	Epidermolysis bullosa acquisita
HACA	Human anti-chimeric antibodies
IV	Intravenous
IVIG	High-dose intravenous immunoglobulin
mAb	Monoclonal antibody
MMP	Mucous membrane pemphigoid
PAIA	Protein A immunoadsorption
PV	Pemphigus vulgaris
RA	Rheumatoid arthritis
SLE	Systemic lupus erythematosus
SLO	Secondary lymphoid organ
TACI	Transmembrane activator and calcium modulator ligand interactor
TNF	Tumor necrosis factor
T_{Reg}	Regulatory T cells

A. Huang, MD • R.K. Madan, MD
Department of Dermatology, State University of New York Downstate Medical Center, Brooklyn, NY, USA

L. Bonomo, BA • J. Levitt, MD (✉)
Department of Dermatology,
Icahn School of Medicine at Mount Sinai,
5 East 98th Street, Fifth Floor, Box 1048,
New York, NY 10029, USA
e-mail: jacoblevittmd@gmail.com

Anti-CD20 Therapy in Pemphigus Vulgaris

Autoimmune blistering diseases are an immunopathologically and clinically heterogenous group of disorders characterized by autoantibodies to intercellular adhesion proteins within the epidermis and dermo-epidermal junction. In the pemphigus group, antibodies are made to desmosome components, while in sub-epidermal blistering diseases like bullous pemphigoid (BP), antibodies are made to hemidesmosome components [1, 2]. The first-line approach to pemphigus vulgaris (PV) varies, but often includes some combination of systemic corticosteroid, mycophenolate mofetil, rituximab, or intravenous immuno-globulin (IVIG). Second-line agents include azathioprine, methotrexate, cyclophosphamide, plasmapheresis, and more recently, protein A immunoadsorption (PAIA) [1].

B cell-specific biologics have been increasingly used in the past decade to treat autoimmune diseases. There are many populations of B cells in the human body, and the site and properties of the B cells differ according to their stage of development. B cells originate from hematopoietic stem cells in the bone marrow and develop into immature B cells, each stage marked by changes in cell surface markers and immunoglobulin heavy and light chains. The immature B cells migrate to the secondary lymphoid organs (SLOs), such as the spleen and lymph nodes, to complete its development. Major populations in the SLOs are the transitional B cells, follicular B cells, and the marginal zone B cells, while peripheral blood is home to the activated B cells, such as memory B cells and antibody-secreting B cells, which are categorized into short-lived, proliferating plasmablasts and long-lived, non-proliferating plasma cells. The most important cell surface marker in this discussion, CD20, is found in Pre-B cells up to memory B cells, and is targeted by current anti-B cell biologics. Another important marker, CD19, is found in earlier in Pro-B cells up to memory B cells, but is not a current target of biologics.

Rituximab (Rituxan®/Mabthera®) is a potent B cell-depleting, chimeric monoclonal antibody (mAb) to CD20, a transmembrane glycoprotein expressed on the surface of

P.S. Yamauchi (ed.), *Biologic and Systemic Agents in Dermatology*, https://doi.org/10.1007/978-3-319-66884-0_34

most B lymphocytes, from late pro-B cell to memory B cell, and is lost upon plasma cell differentiation [3]. Rituximab only affects CD20-bearing B cells, which include pro-B, pre-B cells, and immature B cells in the bone marrow, B cells in the SLOs, and memory B cells in the peripheral blood. However, as only a small fraction of differentiated plasma cells express CD20, the effect of rituximab on immune function is minimal [4]. For instance, immunity to diseases, such as influenza, after vaccine administration has been shown to be preserved in rituximab-treated rheumatoid arthritis patients and comparable to controls [5].

Rituximab was first approved in 1997 for the treatment of relapsed or refractory low-grade follicular B-cell lymphoma, but has since expanded to become a major treatment modality of B cell neoplasms and refractory rheumatoid arthritis. In addition, it is increasingly used off-label in the treatment of a variety of autoimmune diseases, including PV.

PV is characterized by autoantibodies to desmoglein 1 and desmoglein 3, causing intraepidermal acantholysis. Mucocutaneous lesions and extensive flaccid blisters of PV lead to severe pain and infections and can be difficult to treat. Rituximab therapy has been well studied in PV and has demonstrated efficacy in five independent, nonrandomized studies, where, in the majority of patients, rituximab was administered as adjuvant with immunosuppressive therapies [6–10]. A 2015 analysis showed a remission rate of 90–95% of patients in less than 6 weeks and complete resolution within 3–4 months [11]. Although relapse requiring retreatment was common, rituximab has shown success in inducing remission when conventional immunosuppressive therapies have failed.

Rituximab Mechanism of Action and Resistance

Upon binding of rituximab to B cells, the B cells are destroyed by a combination of mechanisms, including antibody-dependent cellular cytotoxicity (ADCC), complement-dependent cytotoxicity (CDC), and direct apoptosis. In ADCC, natural killer cell CD16, or FcγRIII, recognizes and binds the Fc region on rituximab, triggering the release of lytic enzymes that kill the attached B cell. In CDC, C1q, a complement protein, attaches to the Fc region of rituximab, triggering activation of the classical complement pathway. As CD20 is highly expressed in B cells and does not become internalized or shed from the cell membrane, rituximab exerts a long-lasting depleting effect after infusion, frequently lasting more than 6 months [3]. Rituximab interrupts the generation of plasmablasts from memory B cells and interfere with the survival of long-lived, CD20+ plasma cells in SLOs [12, 13].

Rituximab also has an effect on autoreactive T cells, as demonstrated by one study that showed a significant decrease in autoreactive T cell function in a PV patient treated with rituximab [9]. This effect is likely due to a disruption of T-cell-B-cell costimulatory signals through a significant reduction of CD40 and CD80 expression on B cells and other costimulatory ligands on CD4+ T cells, as well as induction of regulatory T cells (T_{Reg}) [14]. Pathogenic B cell lineages are profoundly depleted from circulation for 6–12 months [2, 15], enabling a shift to a normal, polyclonal B cell repertoire starting at the early pro-B cell and leading to repopulation occurring 5–13 months post-infusion [16]. The repopulated cells will contain novel light and heavy chains that will ideally eliminate the remaining autoreactive B cells. However, rituximab does not target CD20-, antibody-secreting plasma cells. Relapse and resistance after treatment with rituximab may be due to presence of long-lived plasma cells, which can persist for many years.

Variable response to rituximab has been attributed to several host factors, including (1) incomplete B cell depletion in bone marrow, spleen, and lymph nodes, (2) long-lived plasma cells that continue to generate autoantibodies, (3) autoreactive CD4+ Th cells, (4) generation of antibodies to rituximab, or human anti-chimeric antibodies (HACA), that interfere with rituximab binding [17], (5) changes in rituximab pharmacokinetics due to dose and schedule, and (6) FcγRIIIα polymorphisms and lipid raft signaling alterations that lead to rituximab-mediated ADCC resistance [18]. HACA have been associated with poor clinical outcome and infusion adverse events in PV patients treated with rituximab [17]. Relapse can be confirmed clinically or through measurement of anti-desmoglein 3 antibody titers in patients.

Rituximab Therapeutic Regimens in Pemphigus

Although no definitive treatment protocol of rituximab exists for pemphigus vulgaris, rituximab has most often been administered as four weekly infusions of 375 mg/m² on days 1, 8, 15, and 22, which is the recommended dose and schedule for non-Hodgkin's lymphoma [16]. However, a lower dose is approved for use in rheumatoid arthritis (two 1000 mg IV infusions separated by 2 weeks) and has successfully been used in patients with pemphigus [19–21]. An even lower dose has been shown to be effective and safe, in one recent prospective open case series, at a single course of two 500 mg infusions of rituximab at an interval of 2 weeks [22]. Currently, there are no dose-optimization or cost-effectiveness studies of rituximab therapy in pemphigus. Rituximab may be combined with other adjuvant therapies, such as immunoadsorption, high-dose IVIG (2 g/kg per course), or immunosuppressive therapies.

According to manufacturer's instructions, administration of rituximab requires diluting 375 mg/m² rituximab in 500 mL of 0.9% sodium chloride (final concentration: 1 4 mg/mL) and infused intravenously (IV) over 4–5 h [23, 24]. This is administered on days 1, 8, 15, and 22. For the first infusion, rituximab is administered at 50 mg/h and escalated by 50 mg/h at 30-min intervals to a maximum of 400 mg/h (an infusion rate of 500 mL/h). To prevent adverse infusion reactions, it is advisable to provide prophylactic treatment with an antipyretic, antihistamine, and 100 mg IV methylprednisolone about 30 min prior to each infusion. In subsequent infusions, infusions are initiated at 100 mg/h, with a 30-min escalation of 100 mg/h to a maximum infusion rate of 400 mg/h.

Other immunomodulators, such as IVIG, are also used to supplement rituximab therapy. The use of IVIG for pemphigus has been previously described, although for some time, there has been no consensus on how to optimize immunomodulation: should IVIG be administered to keep levels high for an extended period of time, or should IVIG be administered intermittently in high-dose spikes [25]? A 2003 consensus statement on the use of IVIG in blistering disease recommended a dose of 2 g/kg/cycle, given monthly until clinical control, with a subsequent increase in the time between cycles to 6, 8, 10, 12, and 14 weeks [26]. However, these guidelines did not address differences in commercial preparation, management of partial responders, and differences in concomitant therapies. Currently, clinicians are using various strategies in IVIG supplementation.

Autoimmune blistering diseases are rare in the pediatric population, but can be potentially fatal conditions. Although treatment regimens of rituximab for autoimmune blistering diseases have been well characterized in adult patients, treatment regimens for pediatric patients have, thus far, consisted of anecdotal evidence and case reports. Most case reports of pediatric PV treated with rituximab described refractory cases managed with at least one concomitant drug and the administration of rituximab using the lymphoma protocol (375 mg/m² weekly for 4 weeks) [27–30]. One recent study examined the efficacy and safety of rituximab as monotherapy in pediatric PV [30]. In most cases, a positive, robust response was observed, following addition of rituximab.

Rituximab in Other Autoimmune Blistering Diseases

Rituximab has been used off-label in a variety of autoimmune blistering diseases. Multiple case reports and retrospective studies have documented clinical efficacy of rituximab therapy in bullous pemphigoid, epidermolysis bullosa acquisita, mucous membrane pemphigoid, paraneoplastic pemphigus,

pemphigus foliaceous, and pemphigus erythematosus. However, due to the rarity of these conditions, data is limited to case reports and small prospective or retrospective studies. Significant variations in clinical response rates and durations may be due to variable rituximab administration regimens and doses and different adjunctive immunosuppressive agents applied in these studies.

Bullous Pemphigoid

Bullous pemphigoid is characterized by autoantibodies to BPAG1 and BPAG2, components of hemidesmosomes in the dermo-epidermal junction, and the development of tense blisters in the skin. A recent retrospective case-control study evaluated rituximab (four weekly infusions of 500 mg) as a first-line therapy in combination with corticosteroids for severe bullous pemphigoid (BP) [31]. Complete remission was achieved in more than 90% of patients, with no established or new lesions for at least 2 months. Relapse rate was low and reported to be mild and easily controlled. Other retrospective studies have also demonstrated significant reduction in disease activity and low to negative autoantibody titers in recalcitrant BP [32, 33]. Two case reports have demonstrated successful treatment of severe, intractable BP in infants [34, 35].

Epidermolysis Bullosa Acquisita

Epidermolysis bullosa acquisita (EBA) is a rare chronic, severe subepidermal blistering disease of the skin and mucous membranes, most commonly characterized by autoantibodies to type VII collagen and tense blisters at sites of trauma. Many case reports have documented good clinical response of rituximab in recalcitrant EBA, in combination with immunosuppressant or immunoadsorption [36–43]. In most cases, patients exhibited a dramatic decrease in lesions within a few weeks, and complete to near-complete resolution of the disease at 10–12 month follow-ups.

Mucous Membrane Pemphigoid

Mucous membrane pemphigoid (MMP), or cicatricial pemphigoid, is a rare, chronic subepithelial blistering disease characterized by blistering lesions affecting the mucous membranes. As with previous autoimmune blistering skin diseases, MMP presents a major therapeutic challenge, due to possible life-threatening ocular, laryngeal, pharyngeal, or esophageal complications, and severe post-inflammatory scarring [44]. In the largest prospective study of rituximab in refractory MMP, rituximab appeared to have rapid and dramatic efficacy at an 88% complete response rate [45]. Other case reports and retrospective studies have shown similar clinical response, but one study noted that rituximab did not appear to induce long-term remission in all patients with MMP, though it was useful in stabilizing the disease and preventing progression [46–48]. However, relapse continues to be a problem in rituximab therapy across all autoimmune blistering diseases.

Rituximab Adverse Effects in Autoimmune Blistering Disease

Rituximab is generally well tolerated and serious side effects are rare. However, adverse effects, including infection and infusion reaction can be life-threatening. In a recent comprehensive review of PV treated with rituximab, infection and septicemia were observed in 4.8% and 2.1% of patients treated with the lymphoma protocol and rheumatoid arthritis protocol, respectively [11]. In a meta-analysis of 153 PV patients treated with rituximab, 7% developed serious infections, with two reported deaths (1.3%) [49]. Fatal bacterial sepsis, fatal *Pneumocystis jirovecii* pneumonia, pulmonary embolism, persistent hypogammaglobulinemia, bacterial arthritis, *Varicella zoster* infection, and *Listeria monocytogenes* sepsis were observed in autoimmune blistering disease patients treated with rituximab [2, 50]. The rate of serious adverse events reported in rituximab-treated autoimmune blistering disease patients was higher (22%) than that of patients with rheumatoid arthritis (RA) (12%), systemic lupus erythematosus (SLE) (17%), and dermatomyositis (0%).

As with any biologic therapy, risk of tuberculosis reactivation is of concern, especially since many patients on biologic therapy are concurrently on other immunosuppressive agents. A 2014 meta-analysis noted that there have been no reports of tuberculosis in rituximab-treated patients, although most of the reports of tuberculosis reactivation were linked to TNF inhibitor therapy [51]. Only one report described knee tuberculosis in a rituximab-treated patient [52]. There is currently not enough evidence to support tuberculosis screening in rituximab monotherapy. In addition, hepatitis C reactivation is also a concern with rituximab therapy. Though most literature on hepatitis C reactivation are from oncology studies [53] using the R-CHOP protocol (rituximab, cyclophosphamide, vincristine, doxorubicin, and glucocorticoids), which itself is hepatotoxic, a few cases of hepatitis C reactivation has been described in rheumatology literature [54]. However, rituximab has been safely used in three patients with pemphigus and coexisting hepatitis B and C [55]. Thus, risk of infection remains a serious consideration when treating an autoimmune blistering disease patient with rituximab.

Future studies are needed to compare conventional immunosuppressive therapies to various rituximab protocols in the treatment of autoimmune blistering diseases.

Infusion-related reactions, including anaphylaxis, hypotension, dyspnea, fever, chills, nausea, dizziness, and urticaria, can also occur, but can be prevented with slow infusions and administration of antihistamines, corticosteroids, and antipyretics prior to rituximab infusion. Onset of symptoms is usually within 2 h of first infusion, but immediate reactions must be controlled with medications and stopping the infusion [23]. Arrhythmia, including atrial fibrillation, has been associated with rituximab use as well (personal observation in two cases).

Other Therapeutics Targets

Autoimmunity requires a complex interplay of genes, cytokines, and effector cells, all of which are potential targets in the treatment of autoimmune bullous diseases. Two B cell mediators, B-cell activating factor of the tumor necrosis factor family (BAFF) and a proliferation-inducing ligand (APRIL), are promising targets in the treatment of autoimmune blistering diseases. BAFF is a protein mainly produced by antigen-presenting cells that acts as an essential B cell maturation and survival factor and co-stimulator of immunoglobulin production. It binds to three receptors, transmembrane activator and calcium modulator ligand interactor (TACI), B cell maturation antigen (BCMA), and BAFF receptor (BAFF-R) [56]. APRIL binds only to TACI and BCMA. BAFF and APRIL have been shown to be elevated in patients with SLE, RA, Sjögren's syndrome, and bullous pemphigoid. In patients with bullous pemphigoid, elevated serum BAFF/APRIL levels have been demonstrated to decrease quickly in response to treatment [56, 57]. In PV, treatment with immunosuppressants does not affect serum levels of BAFF/APRIL; conversely, rituximab therapy induces a strong elevation of BAFF, but not of APRIL, likely due to dramatic B cell depletion [58].

Selective inhibitors of BAFF and APRIL are currently under investigation for autoimmune diseases, including belimumab, a fully human anti-BAFF antibody that binds soluble BAFF, and atacicept, a recombinant fusion protein that blocks both BAFF and APRIL. Anti-BAFF and APRIL biologics have demonstrated mixed responses from current clinical trials. Tabalumab, another anti-BAFF antibody, has been discontinued for failing to show statistical improvement in SLE and RA [59]. Belimumab, however, was successful in two large Phase III trials in SLE [60]. Further studies are required to elucidate anti-BAFF dosing and administration regimens. A combination of rituximab and BAFF antagonists may be helpful in preventing relapse and ensuring long-term clinical remission.

TNF-α, an inflammatory cytokine, is another therapeutic target that has been studied in the treatment of pemphigus. Although not as extensively studied as rituximab, TNF-α inhibitors, such as infliximab, etanercept, and adalimumab, have indicated clinical efficacy in pemphigus patients in several case reports. Infliximab, a chimeric mAb with high binding specificity to TNF-α, has shown good clinical response in two case reports [61, 62]. Etanercept was successful in two reports of cicatricial pemphigoid and pemphigus foliaceus [63, 64], though a limited, double-blinded, randomized, placebo-controlled trial for PV showed mixed results [65]. Non-biologic, nonselective TNFα inhibitors, sulfasalazine and pentoxifylline, have recently been studied as adjuvants with immunosuppressants in a prospective, controlled, double-blinded study for PV, and were shown to be well tolerated and clinically effective [66].

Other anti-CD20 biologics, such as veltuzumab, ofatumumab, ocrelizumab, and obinutuzumab, are possible treatments for autoimmune blistering diseases. Anti-CD20 antibodies are diverse and possess different pharmacologic properties, and possibly, different clinical responses. Type I anti-CD20 mAbs (rituximab, ofatumumab, veltuzumab, ocrelizumab) have a more potent CDC response and increased B cell binding than Type II mAbs (obinutuzumab/GA101), while Type II mAbs exhibit stronger induction of apoptosis [67, 68]. One randomized, placebo-controlled clinical trial is currently active in evaluating the efficacy and safety of subcutaneous ofatumumab in the treatment of PV (NCT01920477).

Subcutaneous injection is a suitable alternative to infusion in the administration of biologics, preventing infusion reactions and potentially decreasing the cost of administration. Subcutaneous veltuzumab has been shown to be effective in one PV patient, with complete remission after two administrations [69]. A subcutaneous formulation of rituximab is also currently available in Europe for the treatment of chronic lymphocytic leukemia.

Case Report: Bullous Disorder Treated with a Biologic Agent

A 50-year-old African-American male presented with an eruption of blisters over his chest that had worsened dramatically over the previous week. He was initially diagnosed with pemphigus foliaceus 4 years prior to presentation and was receiving monthly IV immunoglobulin infusions. The lesions were causing the patient moderate itch and significant emotional stress. Family history was notable for hypertension and hyperlipidemia but negative for dermatologic or autoimmune disease.

Past Medical History:

- Pemphigus vulgaris
- Vitamin D deficiency

Social History:

- Social alcohol use (1 day per month)
- Former smoker (5 pack-years)
- Married
- Warehouse manager

Previous Therapies and Most Recent Dose:

- Prednisone 5 mg daily
- Mycophenolate mofetil 1 g by mouth twice daily
- IV immunoglobulin 2 g/kg monthly

Physical Exam:

- Erosions and flaccid bullae of the chest accompanied by hyperpigmented patches of the scalp, face, trunk, and extremities

Management

Because of the severity of the patient's lesions and history of failure on oral steroids, IV immunoglobulin, and mycophenolate mofetil, the biologic agent rituximab was chosen for the next line of therapy. Labs drawn prior to treatment included a complete blood count, complete metabolic panel, CD19, desmoglein 1 and 3 antibodies, hepatitis B and C serologies, and interferon-gamma release assay for TB. Results were significant for desmoglein 1 antibody level of 136 (normal range < 20). All other labs were within normal limits. The patient received an IV infusion of rituximab 1 mg at week 0 and week 2. At a follow-up visit 2 months after the second infusion, the patient was clear of bullae and no longer complained of itch.

References

1. Kolesnik M, et al. Treatment of severe autoimmune blistering skin diseases with combination of protein a immunoadsorption and rituximab: a protocol without initial high dose or pulse steroid medication. J Eur Acad Dermatol Venereol. 2014;28(6):771–80.
2. Schmidt E, et al. Rituximab in treatment-resistant autoimmune blistering skin disorders. Clin Rev Allergy Immunol. 2008;34(1):56–64.
3. Zambruno G, Borradori L. Rituximab immunotherapy in pemphigus: therapeutic effects beyond B-cell depletion. J Invest Dermatol. 2008;128(12):2745–7.
4. Cooper N, Arnold DM. The effect of rituximab on humoral and cell mediated immunity and infection in the treatment of autoimmune diseases. Br J Haematol. 2010;149(1):3–13.
5. Arad U, et al. The cellular immune response to influenza vaccination is preserved in rheumatoid arthritis patients treated with rituximab. Vaccine. 2011;29(8):1643–8.
6. Ahmed AR, et al. Treatment of pemphigus vulgaris with rituximab and intravenous immune globulin. N Engl J Med. 2006;355(17):1772–9.
7. Joly P, et al. A single cycle of rituximab for the treatment of severe pemphigus. N Engl J Med. 2007;357(6):545–52.
8. Cianchini G, et al. Treatment of severe pemphigus with rituximab: report of 12 cases and a review of the literature. Arch Dermatol. 2007;143(8):1033–8.

9. Eming R, et al. Rituximab exerts a dual effect in pemphigus vulgaris. J Invest Dermatol. 2008;128(12):2850–8.
10. Lunardon L, et al. Adjuvant rituximab therapy of pemphigus: a single-center experience with 31 patients. Arch Dermatol. 2012;148(9):1031–6. [PMC3658473]
11. Ahmed AR, Shetty S. A comprehensive analysis of treatment outcomes in patients with pemphigus vulgaris treated with rituximab. Autoimmun Rev. 2015;14(4):323–31.
12. Hoyer BF, et al. Long-lived plasma cells and their contribution to autoimmunity. Ann N Y Acad Sci. 2005;1050:124–33.
13. Withers DR, et al. T cell-dependent survival of CD20+ and CD20- plasma cells in human secondary lymphoid tissue. Blood. 2007;109(11):4856–64. [PMC1885535]
14. Nagel A, et al. B-cell-directed therapy for inflammatory skin diseases. J Invest Dermatol. 2009;129(2):289–301.
15. Mouquet H, et al. B-cell depletion immunotherapy in pemphigus: effects on cellular and humoral immune responses. J Invest Dermatol. 2008;128(12):2859–69.
16. Lunardon L, Payne AS. Rituximab for autoimmune blistering diseases: recent studies, new insights. G Ital Dermatol Venereol. 2012;147(3):269–76. [PMC3621036]
17. Schmidt E, et al. Immunogenicity of rituximab in patients with severe pemphigus. Clin Immunol. 2009;132(3):334–41.
18. Rezvani AR, Maloney DG. Rituximab resistance. Best Pract Res Clin Haematol. 2011;24(2):203–16. [PMC3113665]
19. Kasperkiewicz M, et al. Rituximab for treatment-refractory pemphigus and pemphigoid: a case series of 17 patients. J Am Acad Dermatol. 2011;65(3):552–8.
20. Jensen AO, et al. Treatment of treatment-resistant autoimmune blistering skin disorders with rituximab. Br J Dermatol. 2009;160(6):1359–61.
21. Kanwar AJ, et al. Efficacy and safety of rituximab treatment in Indian pemphigus patients. J Eur Acad Dermatol Venereol. 2013;27(1):e17–23.
22. Horvath B, et al. Low-dose rituximab is effective in pemphigus. Br J Dermatol. 2012;166(2):405–12.
23. Hertl M, et al. Recommendations for the use of rituximab (anti-CD20 antibody) in the treatment of autoimmune bullous skin diseases. J Dtsch Dermatol Ges. 2008;6(5):366–73.
24. Biogen Idec Inc. and Genentech USA I. Rituxan 2016. Available from: http://www.rituxan.com/hem/hcp/non-hodgkins/rituxan-infusion.
25. Sinha AA, et al. Pemphigus vulgaris: approach to treatment. Eur J Dermatol. 2015;25(2):103–13.
26. Ahmed AR, Dahl MV. Consensus statement on the use of intravenous immunoglobulin therapy in the treatment of autoimmune mucocutaneous blistering diseases. Arch Dermatol. 2003;139(8):1051–9.
27. Hoffman MB, et al. Rituximab use in pediatric dermatology. J Drugs Dermatol. 2016;15(7):821–9.
28. Fuertes I, et al. Rituximab in childhood pemphigus vulgaris: a long-term follow-up case and review of the literature. Dermatology. 2010;221(1):13–6.
29. Kanwar AJ, et al. Childhood pemphigus vulgaris successfully treated with rituximab. Indian J Dermatol Venereol Leprol. 2012;78(5):632–4.
30. Vinay K, et al. Successful use of rituximab in the treatment of childhood and juvenile pemphigus. J Am Acad Dermatol. 2014;71(4):669–75.
31. Cho YT, et al. First-line combination therapy with rituximab and corticosteroids provides a high complete remission rate in moderate-to-severe bullous pemphigoid. Br J Dermatol. 2015;173(1):302–4.
32. Ahmed AR, et al. Treatment of recalcitrant bullous pemphigoid (BP) with a novel protocol: a retrospective study with a 6-year follow-up. J Am Acad Dermatol. 2016;74(4):700–8. e3
33. Hall RP 3rd, et al. Association of serum B-cell activating factor level and proportion of memory and transitional B cells with clinical response after rituximab treatment of bullous pemphigoid patients. J Invest Dermatol. 2013;133(12):2786–8.
34. Schulze J, et al. Severe bullous pemphigoid in an infant--successful treatment with rituximab. Pediatr Dermatol. 2008;25(4):462–5.
35. Fuertes I, et al. Refractory childhood pemphigoid successfully treated with rituximab. Pediatr Dermatol. 2013;30(5):e96–7.
36. Sadler E, et al. Treatment-resistant classical epidermolysis bullosa acquisita responding to rituximab. Br J Dermatol. 2007;157(2):417–9.
37. Schmidt E, et al. Successful adjuvant treatment of recalcitrant epidermolysis bullosa acquisita with anti-CD20 antibody rituximab. Arch Dermatol. 2006;142(2):147–50.
38. Wallet-Faber N, et al. Epidermolysis bullosa acquisita following bullous pemphigoid, successfully treated with the anti-CD20 monoclonal antibody rituximab. Dermatology. 2007;215(3):252–5.
39. Saha M, et al. Refractory epidermolysis bullosa acquisita: successful treatment with rituximab. Clin Exp Dermatol. 2009;34(8):e979–80.
40. Li Y, et al. Sustained clinical response to rituximab in a case of life-threatening overlap subepidermal autoimmune blistering disease. J Am Acad Dermatol. 2011;64(4):773–8.
41. Niedermeier A, et al. Clinical response of severe mechanobullous epidermolysis bullosa acquisita to combined treatment with immunoadsorption and rituximab (anti-CD20 monoclonal antibodies). Arch Dermatol. 2007;143(2):192–8.
42. Crichlow SM, et al. A successful therapeutic trial of rituximab in the treatment of a patient with recalcitrant, high-titre epidermolysis bullosa acquisita. Br J Dermatol. 2007;156(1):194–6.
43. McKinley SK, et al. A case of recalcitrant epidermolysis bullosa acquisita responsive to rituximab therapy. Pediatr Dermatol. 2014;31(2):241–4.
44. Hertl M, et al. Rituximab for severe mucous membrane pemphigoid: safe enough to be drug of first choice? Arch Dermatol. 2011;147(7):855–6.
45. Le Roux-Villet C, et al. Rituximab for patients with refractory mucous membrane pemphigoid. Arch Dermatol. 2011;147(7):843–9.
46. Wollina U, et al. Rituximab therapy of recalcitrant bullous dermatoses. J Dermatol Case Rep. 2008;2(1):4–7. [PMC3157775]
47. Heelan K, et al. Treatment of mucous membrane pemphigoid with rituximab. J Am Acad Dermatol. 2013;69(2):310–1.
48. Maley A, et al. Rituximab combined with conventional therapy versus conventional therapy alone for the treatment of mucous membrane pemphigoid (MMP). J Am Acad Dermatol. 2016;74(5):835–40.
49. Feldman RJ, Ahmed AR. Relevance of rituximab therapy in pemphigus vulgaris: analysis of current data and the immunologic basis for its observed responses. Expert Rev Clin Immunol. 2011;7(4):529–41.
50. Zakka LR, et al. Rituximab in the treatment of pemphigus vulgaris. Dermatol Ther (Heidelb). 2012;2(1):17. [PMC3510419]
51. Souto A, et al. Risk of tuberculosis in patients with chronic immune-mediated inflammatory diseases treated with biologics and tofacitinib: a systematic review and meta-analysis of randomized controlled trials and long-term extension studies. Rheumatology (Oxford). 2014;53(10):1872–85.

52. Ottaviani S, et al. Knee tuberculosis under rituximab therapy for rheumatoid arthritis. Jt Bone Spine. 2013;80(4):435–6.

53. Sagnelli E, et al. Rituximab-based treatment, HCV replication, and hepatic flares. Clin Dev Immunol. 2012;945950:2012. [PMC3420110]

54. Lin KM, et al. Rituximab-induced hepatitis C virus reactivation in rheumatoid arthritis. J Microbiol Immunol Infect. 2013;46(1):65–7.

55. Kanwar AJ, et al. Use of rituximab in pemphigus patients with chronic viral hepatitis: report of three cases. Indian J Dermatol Venereol Leprol. 2014;80(5):422–6.

56. Watanabe R, et al. Increased serum levels of a proliferation-inducing ligand in patients with bullous pemphigoid. J Dermatol Sci. 2007;46(1):53–60.

57. Asashima N, et al. Serum levels of BAFF are increased in bullous pemphigoid but not in pemphigus vulgaris. Br J Dermatol. 2006;155(2):330–6.

58. Nagel A, et al. Rituximab mediates a strong elevation of B-cell-activating factor associated with increased pathogen-specific IgG but not autoantibodies in pemphigus vulgaris. J Invest Dermatol. 2009;129(9):2202–10.

59. Genovese MC, et al. Tabalumab, an anti-BAFF monoclonal antibody, in patients with active rheumatoid arthritis with an inadequate response to TNF inhibitors. Ann Rheum Dis. 2013;72(9):1461–8.

60. Targeting DA. BAFF in autoimmunity. Curr Opin Immunol. 2010;22(6):732–9. [PMC2997938]

61. Jacobi A, et al. Rapid control of therapy-refractory pemphigus vulgaris by treatment with the tumour necrosis factor-alpha inhibitor infliximab. Br J Dermatol. 2005;153(2):448–9.

62. Pardo J, et al. Infliximab in the management of severe pemphigus vulgaris. Br J Dermatol. 2005;153(1):222–3.

63. Sacher C, et al. Treatment of recalcitrant cicatricial pemphigoid with the tumor necrosis factor alpha antagonist etanercept. J Am Acad Dermatol. 2002;46(1):113–5.

64. Gubinelli E, et al. Pemphigus foliaceus treated with etanercept. J Am Acad Dermatol. 2006;55(6):1107–8.

65. Fiorentino DF, et al. A pilot study of etanercept treatment for pemphigus vulgaris. Arch Dermatol. 2011;147(1):117–8.

66. el-Darouti M, et al. The use of sulfasalazine and pentoxifylline (low-cost antitumour necrosis factor drugs) as adjuvant therapy for the treatment of pemphigus vulgaris: a comparative study. Br J Dermatol. 2009;161(2):313–9.

67. Klein C, et al. Epitope interactions of monoclonal antibodies targeting CD20 and their relationship to functional properties. MAbs. 2013;5(1):22–33. [PMC3564883]

68. Niederfellner G, et al. Epitope characterization and crystal structure of GA101 provide insights into the molecular basis for type I/II distinction of CD20 antibodies. Blood. 2011;118(2):358–67.

69. Ellebrecht CT, et al. Subcutaneous veltuzumab, a humanized anti-CD20 antibody, in the treatment of refractory pemphigus vulgaris. JAMA Dermatol. 2014;150(12):1331–5.

Oral Systemic Agents for Immunobullous Disorders

35

Timothy Patton and Neil J. Korman

Introduction

The immunobullous diseases are a group of cutaneous auto-immune conditions in which antibodies produced by the immune system are directed against proteins present in the skin and/or mucous membranes. The immunobullous diseases are divided into the intraepidermal group of diseases (variants of pemphigus), in which the antibodies are directed against proteins present in the epidermis (or mucosal epithelium), and the subepidermal group of diseases (which includes variants of pemphigoid, as well as other conditions), in which antibodies are directed against proteins present at the dermal-epidermal (or mucosal-submucosal) junction. Options for systemic therapy include systemic corticosteroids, anti-inflammatory agents, and immunosuppressive medications, either as monotherapy or in combination with one another. In the first section of the chapter, each of the medications used in the treatment of immunobullous diseases will be reviewed in terms of their mechanism of action, potential side effects, and recommendations for long-term monitoring. The second section of the chapter will discuss each of the immunobullous diseases separately and review the evidence available for each of the oral agents used in disease management.

In the last decade, rituximab has emerged as an extremely effective therapy in many autoimmune blistering diseases and should be considered as either first- or second-line therapy for any patient with severe autoimmune bullous disease. The focus of this chapter is on oral agents used in autoimmune blistering diseases, and therefore rituximab will not be discussed in detail.

T. Patton, DO (✉)
Department of Dermatology, University of Pittsburgh, Pittsburgh, PA, USA
e-mail: pattontj@UPMC.EDU

N.J. Korman, MD, PhD
Case Western Reserve University, Cleveland, OH 44106, USA
e-mail: Neil.Korman@UHhospitals.org

The Medications

Systemic Corticosteroids

Systemic corticosteroids (CS) act as transcription factors which upregulate and downregulate a number of different proteins that are involved in diverse functions in the body. CS bind to glucocorticoid receptors in the cell, and the glucocorticoid/glucocorticoid receptor complex binds to glucocorticoid response elements present on DNA, affecting the transcription of downstream proteins [1]. The effects of CS are the result of upregulation or downregulation of varying proteins involved in autoimmunity and inflammation. In addition to their effects as direct transcription factors, systemic CS have additional anti-inflammatory and immunosuppressive effects by acting on other transcription factors such as NF-kB and AP-1 [2, 3]. CS remain the first-line therapy for many immunobullous diseases due to their consistent efficacy in both establishing control of disease progression and reduction of disease activity.

Different formulations of systemic corticosteroids exist, each with differing glucocorticoid and mineralocorticoid activity (Table 35.1). The most commonly studied systemic CS in the treatment of immunobullous diseases are prednisone/prednisolone, usually administered as an oral daily dose. Dexamethasone, a more potent and longer-acting CS, has been studied in the management of immunobullous diseases as well, particularly in pulse steroid regimens [4].

The extensive potential side effects of corticosteroids preclude their long-term use at moderate to high doses, and working closely with the patient's primary care providers to manage CS toxicities is essential in the care of these patients. The potential side effects and monitoring recommendations for corticosteroids are reviewed in Table 35.2 [5–7].

© Springer International Publishing AG 2018
P.S. Yamauchi (ed.), *Biologic and Systemic Agents in Dermatology*, https://doi.org/10.1007/978-3-319-66884-0_35

Table 35.1 Systemic corticosteroid comparisons

Corticosteroid	Biologic half-life (h)	Equivalent dose (mg)	Relevant glucocorticoid potency	Relevant mineralocorticoid potency
Hydrocortisone	8–12	20	1	1
Prednisone/prednisolone	20–30	5	4	0.8
Methylprednisolone	20–30	4	5	0.5
Dexamethasone	35–50	0.75	25	0

Table 35.2 Systemic corticosteroid side effects and management recommendations

Glucocorticoid side effect	Recommendations for management
Glucocorticoid-induced osteoporosis	Baseline DEXA
	Minimize risk factors (smoking, excessive EtOH)
	Calcium and vitamin D supplementation
	Bisphosphonates in appropriate settings
Peptic ulcer disease (PUD)	Proton pump inhibitors
	• Initiate in patients taking NSAIDS
	• Consider in patients with other risk factors (previous PUD, smokers, excessive EtOH)
Hyperglycemia	Baseline and routine glucose monitoring
	PCP or endocrinology referral where appropriate
Adrenal insufficiency	For patients on >20 mg/day for >3 weeks
	• Gradual taper of steroids
	• Consider AM cortisol prior to discontinuing steroids to assess for adrenal function
Pneumocystis pneumonia	Consider prophylaxis in select patients
	• Patients on >20 mg and another risk factor (interstitial lung disease, additional immunosuppression, hematologic malignancy)
Tuberculosis (TB) reactivation	Baseline TB testing (interferon gamma release assays such as QuantiFERON Gold or tuberculin skin testing)
	Treatment with isoniazid if latent disease is detected
Hepatitis B and C reactivation	Baseline testing and appropriate referral if positive

Anti-inflammatory Treatments

Tetracycline Group Antibiotics

The tetracycline group of antibiotics includes tetracycline, doxycycline, and minocycline, and all of these medications have been reported to be effective therapy for the management of the immunobullous diseases, most likely due to the anti-inflammatory activity that these antibiotics possess through their inhibition of chemotaxis and certain proteases [8].

The tetracyclines can be attractive options in the management of immunobullous diseases due to their lack of any immunosuppressive effects. Side effects of these medications include less serious reactions such as gastrointestinal upset, photosensitivity, cutaneous hyperpigmentation, and vertigo [9]. More serious side effects such as drug reaction with eosinophilia and systemic symptoms (DRESS) can occur rarely in patients taking minocycline [10, 11]. No specific monitoring is required for patients taking the tetracycline group of medications.

Nicotinamide

Nicotinamide or niacinamide is the amide ester of niacin, also known as vitamin B3. Nicotinamide is believed to possess anti-inflammatory activity through a number of different physiologic pathways [12]. Nicotinamide has been studied in some of the immunobullous diseases, typically in combination with the tetracycline group of antibiotics. Similar to the tetracycline group of antibiotics, nicotinamide is non-immunosuppressive and specific monitoring is not required in patients taking this agent.

Dapsone

Dapsone was originally found to be efficacious in treating leprosy because it is a sulfonamide antibiotic, but it also has anti-inflammatory effects as well. The exact mechanism by which dapsone exerts its anti-inflammatory activity is not completely understood, but in certain experimental conditions, it has been shown to have activity against reactive oxygen species, leukocyte adhesion, neutrophil chemotaxis, and inflammatory proteins [13, 14]. Dapsone is a very effective medication in the IgA-mediated immunobullous diseases, particularly dermatitis herpetiformis (DH) [15] and linear IgA bullous disease (LABD) [16].

Dapsone has some potential serious side effects. Agranulocytosis is a rare side effect of dapsone and can happen early in the course of therapy [17, 18]. Red blood cell hemolysis occurs in almost all patients to varying degrees secondary to the effect that some dapsone metabolites have on erythrocytes [19]. Patients with a glucose-6-phosphate dehydrogenase (G-6-PD) deficiency are more prone to this side effect [20]. Because of the potential adverse effects that dapsone can have on the peripheral blood, it is recommended to screen all patients for G-6-PD deficiency prior to the initiation of dapsone and to closely monitor blood counts while patients are taking dapsone. Methemoglobinemia also occurs to varying degrees in many patients [21]. Typically, the degree of methemoglobinemia is not sufficient to cause symptoms, although if patients taking dapsone develop symptoms of methemoglobinemia including chest pain or shortness of breath, this level should be checked and treated appropriately if significantly elevated [22]. Dapsone can also cause serious side effects such as DRESS and Stevens-Johnson syndrome/toxic epidermal necrolysis (SJS/TEN) [23, 24].

Methotrexate

Methotrexate was initially used for its antimetabolite activity due to its inhibitory effect on the enzyme dihydrofolate reductase. At lower doses, methotrexate was noted to have mostly anti-inflammatory activity and has been shown to be effective in a number of inflammatory and autoimmune conditions [25]. While the exact anti-inflammatory mechanism of methotrexate is unknown, many studies suggest that increased adenosine levels induced by methotrexate are the main pathway by which it exerts its anti-inflammatory effects [26, 27].

Methotrexate is typically administered as a once-weekly dose ranging from 5 mg up to 25 mg. Common side effects include nausea and gastrointestinal upset. Side effects related to folate antagonism such as marrow suppression or mucositis may be alleviated by the concurrent administration of folate on days that the patient does not take the methotrexate [28]. Long-term potential serious side effects include liver fibrosis. Patients who are overweight or who have a history of high alcohol intake or diabetes are at higher risk for liver

fibrosis and should be counseled accordingly [29]. Baseline blood counts, liver enzymes, and kidney function should be checked prior to the initiation of therapy and should be followed regularly during therapy. The gold standard for the measurement of hepatic fibrosis is a liver biopsy and should be considered in patients who have reached a cumulative methotrexate dose of 1.5–4.0 g of methotrexate, depending on their individual risk factors [30]. Less invasive tests exist which may accurately determine the degree of hepatic fibrosis [31, 32], but a consensus regarding these has not been established in terms of monitoring for methotrexate hepatotoxicity.

Colchicine

Colchicine is FDA approved for the treatment of acute gout and familial Mediterranean fever. It seems to exert its anti-inflammatory effects via its action on cellular microtubules, which appear to play a role in multiple inflammatory pathways of the immune response [33].

Colchicine is typically taken twice a day, and the most common reasons for discontinuation are gastrointestinal side effects such as diarrhea, abdominal pain, or nausea.

Immunosuppressive Therapy

Patients who do not respond to less aggressive anti-inflammatory medications or who have severe disease may require immunosuppressive agents in order to control their disease. Patients taking immunosuppressive therapy may be at higher risk of infections and should have appropriate screening for infectious diseases such as hepatitis B and C, as well as tuberculosis testing prior to initiating therapy with this group of medications. Ideally, patients should receive up-to-date vaccinations prior to initiation of immunosuppressive therapy and should avoid receiving any live vaccines while taking these medications. Should patients develop serious infections while taking these medications, it is reasonable to hold therapy until the infection is completely resolved.

In addition to the increased risk of infection, there is also a potential increased risk of malignancy in patients being treated with immunosuppressive agents. Much of the data on malignancy and immunosuppression is in solid organ transplant recipients [34], but nonetheless an increased risk of developing malignancy has been demonstrated in patients taking immunosuppressive agents for immunobullous diseases as well [35]. The degree of immunosuppression in immunobullous diseases is much lower than what is seen in patients with solid organ transplants, and as such the overall risk of malignancy in patients with immunobullous disease is likely to be low, similar to what is seen in other autoimmune conditions where single-agent immunosuppression is common [36–38]. Individual risk factors for the development of malignancy need to be carefully considered and weighed against the risks of inadequately controlled immunobullous disease.

Azathioprine

Azathioprine is a purine analog that can be used as a steroid-sparing agent in many of the immunobullous diseases [39]. Azathioprine is nonenzymatically converted to 6-mercaptopurine (6-MP), which is further broken down into active and inactive metabolites. The active metabolite thiopurine interferes with cellular DNA, inhibiting purine synthesis. Because lymphocytes lack a salvage pathway for purine synthesis, T cells and B cells are preferentially inhibited by azathioprine, leading to immunosuppression [40]. One of the enzymes which metabolizes 6-MP is thiopurine methyltransferase (TPMT), and patients with a decreased TPMT activity may be at higher risk for azathioprine side effects [41].

Azathioprine is taken as a daily dose ranging from 1 to 3 mg/kg/day. In patients with low TPMT activity, azathioprine should not be prescribed. Lower doses should be used for patients with intermediate TPMT activity, while higher doses can be considered in patients with normal TPMT activity [42]. Less serious side effects include fatigue and nausea, while more serious side effects include cytopenias [43], Sweet's syndrome [44], or hypersensitivity reactions such as DRESS [45]. Patients with lower TPMT levels may be more at risk for the former. In addition to TPMT activity, screening for patients who are being considered for azathioprine therapy should include baseline complete blood count with differential and comprehensive metabolic panel. Complete blood counts should be performed frequently during the first few months of therapy and less frequently once the patient has been on a stable dose.

Mycophenolate Mofetil

Mycophenolate mofetil (MMF) is another inhibitor of purine synthesis through its action on the enzyme inosine monophosphate dehydrogenase type II [46]. Similar to azathioprine, mycophenolate has a preferential immunosuppressive effect on T cells and B cells. Mycophenolate is typically dosed at 40 mg/kg with an upper limit of 4 g daily. Gastrointestinal upset is a relatively common early side effect, while cytopenias occur less commonly. Baseline complete blood count with differential and comprehensive metabolic panel should be obtained prior to therapy, and monthly monitoring is recommended initially, followed by monitoring every 3 months once patients are on a stable dose.

Cyclophosphamide

Cyclophosphamide is an alkaloid chemotherapeutic agent that, when used in lower doses, has potent immunosuppressive effects. The oral daily dose of cyclophosphamide is usually between 1 and 2 mg/kg/day. Cytopenias and bladder toxicity in the form of hemorrhagic cystitis can occur in patients taking cyclophosphamide [47]. Patients should be encouraged to drink generous amounts of water while taking the medication and complete blood count with differential, and urinalysis (including microscopic exam looking for the presence of red blood cells) should be performed weekly during the first 8 weeks of therapy. Cyclophosphamide should be used with caution in younger patients because of the possibility of azoospermia or anovulation [48].

Cyclosporine

Cyclosporine is a calcineurin inhibitor that has been studied in some of the immunobullous diseases. By inhibiting calcineurin, cyclosporine prevents the dephosphorylation of nuclear factor of activated T cells (NFAT), which in turn downregulates the formation of several proinflammatory molecules [49]. Cyclosporine is not generally used in most of the immunobullous diseases, although it appears to have some efficacy in the treatment of epidermolysis bullosa acquisita [50].

Cyclosporine is administered as a daily dose ranging from 3 to 5 mg/kg/day. Potential side effects include hypertrichosis and gingival enlargement. With long-term use, patients on cyclosporine are at increased risk for the development of renal toxicity [51]. Creatinine and blood pressure need to be monitored closely during therapy, and reductions in dose are necessary when creatinine becomes elevated or hypertension develops. The use of cyclosporine should be limited to no more than 1 year due to the risk of nephrotoxicity with long-term use.

The Immunobullous Diseases

Pemphigus Subtype

There are two main subtypes of pemphigus, pemphigus vulgaris and pemphigus foliaceus.

Pemphigus Vulgaris

Pemphigus vulgaris (PV) is an autoimmune bullous disease in which antibodies are directed against proteins present in the epidermis and mucosal epithelium. The target antigens, desmogleins 1 and 3, are components of desmosomes, proteins that are involved in keratinocyte adhesion. In PV, patients usually have antibodies directed against desmoglein 3 alone or both desmogleins 1 and 3 and can present with erosions and flaccid bullae on the skin and/or mucous membranes [52] (Fig. 35.1). In severe disease, widespread erosions can develop, placing the patient at risk for developing sepsis (Fig. 35.2). Prior to the advent of systemic corticosteroids, PV was almost universally fatal; however, with the judicious use of systemic corticosteroids in combination with other medications, both IV and oral, mortality has improved significantly.

The mainstay of therapy for PV is systemic corticosteroids. Doses of 1 mg/kg/day are prescribed initially, followed by a slow taper over several months [53]. In patients that are

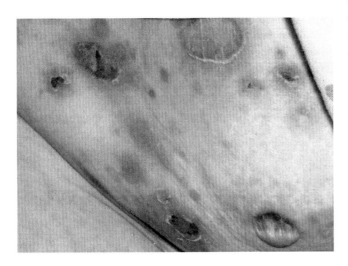

Fig. 35.1 Pemphigus vulgaris. Flaccid bullae, erosions, and hemorrhagic crusts on the lower abdomen

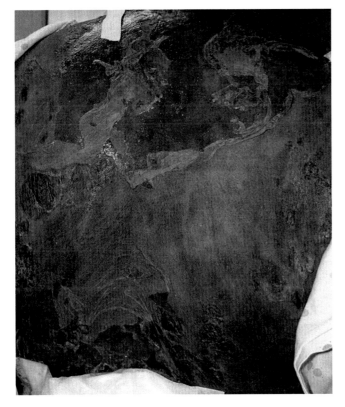

Fig. 35.2 Pemphigus vulgaris. Widespread epidermal sloughing in severe disease

primarily treated with corticosteroids, the taper should be gradual, with reductions of 10–20 mg every 2 weeks early in the course of therapy, followed by reductions of 10 mg every month when disease control is maintained on lower doses of corticosteroids (≤20 mg daily). Corticosteroid tapers may be performed more rapidly in patients receiving adjuvant therapy. While pulse doses of dexamethasone have been studied, their addition to a standard regimen of steroids did not seem to have significant effects on remission [4].

Immunosuppressive agents are frequently added to the corticosteroid regimen in order to decrease or eliminate the dose of corticosteroids used to place patients into a remission. Comparative studies of mycophenolate, azathioprine, and cyclophosphamide have not demonstrated consistent superiority of one agent compared to another in terms of their steroid-sparing ability or adverse effects [54]. Azathioprine at doses of 2–3 mg/kg/day and mycophenolate mofetil at doses of 2–3 g/day are commonly used as first-line adjuvant immunosuppressive therapy. Cyclophosphamide, due to its more immunosuppressive activity, is usually reserved as oral adjuvant therapy for only the most resistant cases. Some physicians advocate the addition of adjuvant immunosuppression at the same time that corticosteroids are initiated for the treatment of pemphigus vulgaris, while others advocate waiting to add adjuvant immunosuppression only if the patient doesn't respond to high-dose corticosteroids or if the dose of corticosteroids to maintain adequate control of disease is too high to be safely administered for a long term [55]. Placebo-controlled studies have demonstrated that the addition of mycophenolate to a standard corticosteroid regimen did not lead to a higher percentage of patients responding to treatment, although faster and longer-lasting responses to initial therapy seemed to be higher in the mycophenolate group [56]. In patients that are unable to tolerate either mycophenolate or azathioprine, or in patients who are not able to taper the corticosteroid dose to an acceptable long-term level, the addition cyclophosphamide as adjuvant therapy can be considered.

While there is some limited evidence for more conservative therapies in the treatment of pemphigus vulgaris, given the potential morbidity and mortality of poorly managed disease, less aggressive therapies are generally not favored as initial therapy. Tetracycline group antibiotics with or without the addition of nicotinamide [57], methotrexate [58, 59], and dapsone [60, 61] have demonstrated limited efficacy as steroid-sparing agents and are generally not favored for the management of pemphigus vulgaris over more proven therapies.

Pemphigus Foliaceous

Classically, patients with pemphigus foliaceous produce antibodies against only one of the desmoglein proteins—desmoglein 1, which leads to the development of superficial erosions on the skin. Mucous membranes are not involved. The lesions of PF tend to be superficial crusted erosions and blisters are typically absent (Fig. 35.3). Because of the superficial nature of the erosions in PF, patients tend to be at less risk for sepsis and are therefore often managed less aggressively when compared to patients with PV.

Treatment for PF, especially more severe cases (Fig. 35.4), is similar to the treatment for PV—systemic corticosteroids in moderate to high doses, followed by a gradual taper over several months, with the addition of steroid-sparing adjuvant therapy as needed. In localized disease, clinicians may try a less aggressive approach such as dapsone [61, 62] or tetracycline antibiotics with nicotinamide [63].

Less Common Pemphigus Subtypes

Paraneoplastic pemphigus (PNP) can be associated with severe mucositis, widespread cutaneous erosions, lung involvement, and a high fatality rate [64]. PNP is most commonly associated with lymphoproliferative malignancies [65], a clinical setting in which immunosuppressant medications such as azathioprine or mycophenolate mofetil would be somewhat contraindicated. The disease can be recalcitrant to systemic corticosteroids, even in high doses. The use of IV rituximab may be associated with improved mortality for what was an almost universally fatal disease [66].

IgA pemphigus is associated with the production of IgA antibodies to epidermal proteins desmocollins 1 and 3. Patients usually do not have oral disease and can present with vesiculopustules (Fig. 35.5). Dapsone is considered to be first-line therapy in these patients [67].

Pemphigus vegetans is a form of pemphigus vulgaris and if widespread (Neumann subtype) is managed similarly to patients with pemphigus vulgaris. A localized form of pemphigus vegetans (the Hallopeau subtype) sometimes can be managed more conservatively.

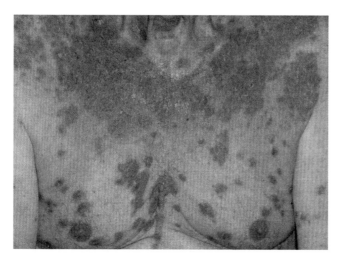

Fig. 35.3 Crusted erosions present on the anterior trunk of a patient with pemphigus foliaceous

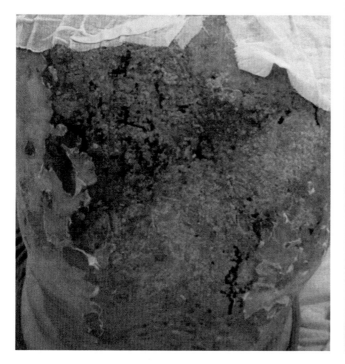

Fig. 35.4 Widespread cutaneous erosions on the posterior trunk in a pemphigus foliaceous patient

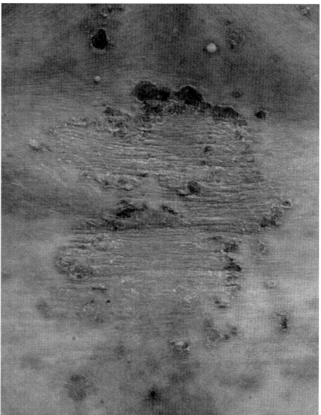

Fig. 35.5 Vesiculopustules, erosions, and hemorrhagic crusting on the posterior trunk of an IgA pemphigus patient

Pemphigoid Group

Bullous Pemphigoid

Bullous pemphigoid (BP) is the most common immunobullous disease. Antibodies are directed against proteins in the hemidesmosome, a transmembrane protein present at the dermoepidermal junction that plays a role in anchoring the epidermis to the basement membrane zone [68, 69]. Following the binding of antibodies BPAg-1 and/or BPAg-2, subsequent inflammation leads to urticarial-like plaques, tense bullae, and erosions (Fig. 35.6).

The first-line therapy for BP depends on the severity of disease. The most consistent responses are seen with systemic corticosteroids, and for severe diseases, they remain the mainstay of therapy. Doses of 0.5–0.75 mg/kg/day—lower than what is typically used for pemphigus patients—can be used initially, followed by a slow taper of 10 mg every 2–4 weeks to control disease [70]. Addition of adjuvant immunosuppressive therapy with either azathioprine or mycophenolate mofetil can be added as needed, although the steroid-sparing effect of these therapies has not been conclusively demonstrated [71]. BP often requires less aggressive therapy to control disease when compared to pemphigus, and for this reason, cyclophosphamide is not commonly used. If a patient fails to tolerate azathioprine or mycophenolate as

steroid-sparing agents, it is reasonable to attempt more conservative therapies prior to initiating cyclophosphamide.

Methotrexate has been demonstrated to be an effective therapy for BP in small case series, particularly elderly patients that may not tolerate more aggressive immunosuppression [72]. The anti-inflammatory activity of methotrexate is enough to control mild to moderate cases of BP and is a good option in some instances. In patients with overlap of BP and psoriasis, methotrexate is a particularly good option because of the activity that it has in treating both diseases [73, 74].

The combination of tetracycline and nicotinamide was found to be as effective as prednisone in one study [75], although for more aggressive disease, tetracycline and nicotinamide may not be effective enough to adequately control blistering. In elderly patients, especially with localized or milder disease, this combination may be a reasonable option to try in place of more aggressive therapies.

Dapsone has been studied in BP, both as a first- and second-line agent. In a small study, dapsone was used as a first-line agent and was effective in controlling disease in 44% of patients [76]. In practice, dapsone is not commonly used in the management of BP, but could be considered in instances where more proven therapies (corticosteroids +/− adjuvant immunosuppressive medications) are contraindicated or have failed to maintain adequate control of disease.

Mucous Membrane Pemphigoid

When compared to the other immunobullous diseases, mucous membrane pemphigoid demonstrates the most heterogeneity in terms of antigenic targets and clinical presentation [77, 78]. Patients with certain variants of mucous membrane pemphigoid can develop scarring of critical mucosal surfaces including the conjunctiva, larynx, and esophagus (Fig. 35.7). Because of the possible sequelae of scarring in these areas (e.g., blindness, complete laryngeal or esophageal closure), more aggressive therapy is warranted. Patients with MMP that have scarring in these areas should be treated with combination therapy, particularly prednisone at doses of 1 mg/kg/day combined with an aggressive immunosuppressive agent, preferably cyclophosphamide 1–2 mg/kg/day [79]. Azathioprine at higher doses (2–3 mg/kg/day) can be used in some instances in place of cyclophosphamide [79].

Milder forms of mucous membrane pemphigoid exist in which patients do not present with scarring, but instead develop vesicles, erosions, and sloughing of the mucous membranes, mostly in the oral mucosa (Fig. 35.8). For these less aggressive forms of MMP, topical therapy may suffice in controlling symptoms [80]. When topical therapy fails to control symptoms, oral systemic therapy can be considered, but less aggressive measures such as the tetracycline group antibiotics [81, 82], dapsone [83], or colchicine [84] may be more reasonable first-line systemic agents in these cases.

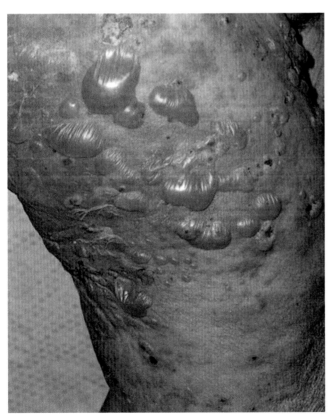

Fig. 35.6 Bullous pemphigoid. Tense vesicles and bullae on an erythematous base

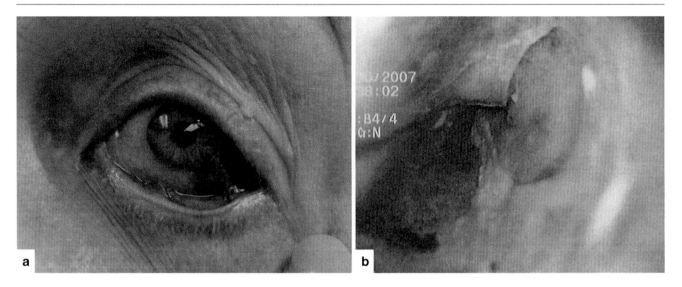

Fig. 35.7 Mucous membrane pemphigoid patients with scarring present in the (**a**) conjunctiva and (**b**) esophagus

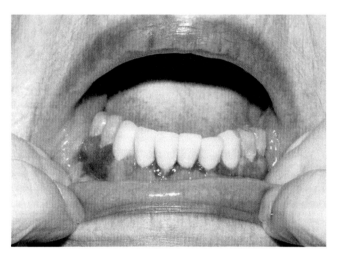

Fig. 35.8 Erosions of the lower gingiva in a patient with mucous membrane pemphigoid

Should patients fail to improve on these less aggressive therapies, other, more aggressive therapies can be initiated, with the understanding that risk of immunosuppressive therapies may outweigh the risk of not treating the disease as aggressively as possible.

Epidermolysis Bullosa Acquisita

Patients with epidermolysis bullosa acquisita (EBA) produce antibodies directed against type VII collagen, a protein present in the sublamina densa [85]. The two main subtypes of EBA are the non-inflammatory and inflamma-

tory subtypes. Patients with the inflammatory subtype of EBA can present in a similar fashion to other immunobullous diseases such as bullous pemphigoid, MMP, or linear IgA disease [86]. In patients with these subtypes of EBA, it is reasonable to treat them as one would treat the clinical disease they most closely resemble. For instance, in patients whose EBA clinically resembles BP (the most common inflammatory subtype of EBA), it is reasonable to treat those patients with moderate doses of systemic corticosteroids in combination with immunosuppressive adjuvant therapy, if needed [87]. Scarring EBA involving critical areas such as the conjunctiva, larynx, and esophagus should be treated aggressively with combination systemic corticosteroids and cyclophosphamide, as one would treat a scarring form of MMP.

The non-inflammatory form of EBA, also known as the mechanobullous form of EBA, is more resistant to conventional therapy [86]. Patients with mechanobullous form of EBA present with bulla and erosions on areas of the skin prone to trauma, such as the elbows, knees, and volar aspects of the palms and soles (Fig. 35.9). Resistance to conventional therapy such as systemic corticosteroids, azathioprine, and mycophenolate mofetil is common in these patients, and rituximab has been used with some success in these patients [88, 89]. Two therapies not commonly used in other immunobullous diseases deserve mention: cyclosporine and colchicine.

Cyclosporine at high doses has been reported as an effective therapy in patients with mechanobullous EBA [90],

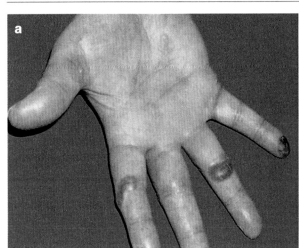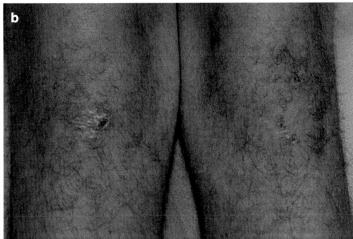

Fig. 35.9 Mechanobullous EBA. (**a**) Multiple bullae present on the palms (**b**) erosions, erythema, and hemorrhagic crusts on the bilateral knees

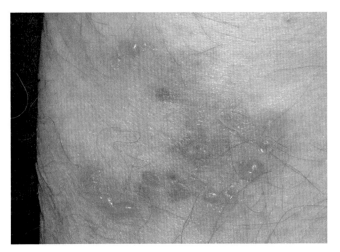

Fig. 35.10 Linear IgA disease with the "string of pearls" distribution of vesicles along the periphery of the lesion

although nephrotoxicity at these doses is expected. Colchicine has also been reported as an effective therapy and should be considered before proceeding to more aggressive options [91].

Linear IgA Disease

Patients with linear IgA disease (LAD) can present with blisters having the distinct clinical finding of smaller vesicles around the periphery of the lesion which coalesce to form a "string of pearls" morphology (Fig. 35.10). Antibodies are of the IgA subtype and commonly directed against a cleaved portion of bullous pemphigoid antigen-1 (BPAg-1) [92]. Linear IgA disease can present in children and is known as

chronic bullous disease of childhood (CBDC). Drug-induced LAD can be induced by exposure to vancomycin, [93].

The first-line therapy for patients with LAD is dapsone [94]. In cases resistant to dapsone, LAD can be managed similar to other immunobullous diseases—moderate doses of systemic corticosteroids in combination with adjuvant immunosuppressive therapy, if needed [95].

Pemphigoid Gestationis

Pemphigoid gestationis shares histologic and immunofluorescent characteristics with BP but occurs in pregnant women. Patients produce antibodies against BPAg-1 and present with urticarial plaques and bullae (Fig. 35.11). Prednisone is the first-line therapy for patients with moderate to severe disease [96]. Doses vary but can range from 0.5 mg to 1 mg/kg/day. The pregnancy classes of the other immunosuppressive agents limit their use in treating gestational pemphigoid while the pregnancy is still active. Once the pregnancy is over, patients can be treated similar to patients with BP.

Bullous Lupus

Bullous lupus is usually seen in patients with uncontrolled systemic lupus [97]. Antibodies are directed against type VII collagen, and patients can present with tense bullae on an erythematous base [98] (Fig. 35.12). Because bullous lupus sometimes occurs in patients that are undergoing a flare of systemic lupus, therapy is often directed against the systemic manifestations of their disease. In addition to these therapies, dapsone has been reported as an extremely effective therapy for skin disease that does not respond to the therapies employed for the systemic disease [97].

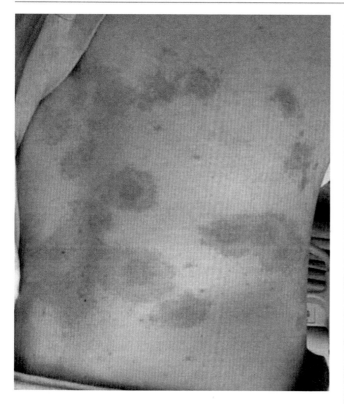

Fig. 35.11 Annular, urticarial-like plaques on the trunk of a patient with gestational pemphigoid

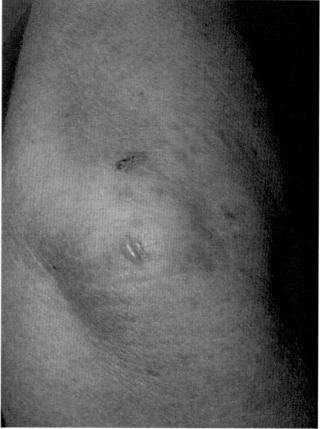

Fig. 35.13 Excoriations, erythematous papules, and vesicles on the elbow of a patient with dermatitis herpetiformis

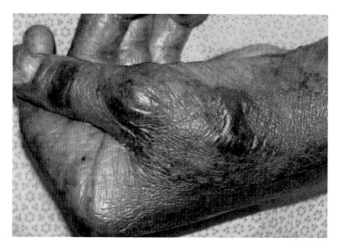

Fig. 35.12 Acral bullae in a patient with systemic lupus erythematosus. A subepidermal blister with predominantly neutrophils was seen on histology

Other Immunobullous Diseases

Dermatitis Herpetiformis

Dermatitis herpetiformis (DH) is the cutaneous manifestation of gluten-sensitive enteropathy (GSE) [99]. Antibodies in DH are directed against both gluten and the enzyme transglutaminase [100]. Circulating IgA antibody-antigen complexes become deposited in the vessels of the dermal papillae, leading to predominant neutrophilic inflammation within the dermal papillae [101]. Patients present with severe pruritus

and small, superficial vesicles on the elbows, knees, lower back, and scalp (Fig. 35.13). Because of the superficial nature of the vesicles and the extreme pruritus, often times only excoriations are visible on exam.

A gluten-free diet can provide long-term resolution of the skin lesions in patients with DH in those patients who are able to successfully follow this restrictive diet [102, 103]. Even with a strict gluten-free diet, it may take several months for patients to see the effect. Dapsone is an extremely effective therapy for DH, and the majority of patients are managed with dapsone.

Case Report

A 66-year-old male was referred to our practice for the management of a 6-month dermatitis. The patient had a history of blisters and pruritus on his hands that progressed to involve the trunk and more proximal extremities. A biopsy was performed prior to referral which demonstrated a subepidermal blister with predominant eosinophilic infiltrate. Direct immunofluorescence was positive for IgG and C3 in a linear pattern along the dermoepidermal junction, indirect immunofluorescence (IIF) studies revealed circulating IgG antibodies binding to the roof of salt-split skin, and ELISA studies were positive for the presence of BP180 and BP230 antibodies. In all three of these studies, a diagnosis of bullous pemphigoid was made. The patient had consistent improvement with higher doses of prednisone (50–60 mg) but would flare when the dose of prednisone was decreased. Doxycycline and nicotinamide was added to his regimen, but the patient would still develop blisters when the prednisone dose was tapered to less than 50 mg.

Past Medical History
- Hypertension

Social History
- Drinks socially (5 beers per week)
- Smokes ½ ppd
- Works as an X-ray repair technician
- Married

Previous Therapies
- Prednisone
- Doxycycline and nicotinamide

Medications
- Furosemide 20 mg daily (has been taking for years prior to the development of the rash)
- Prednisone 40 mg qAM

Physical Exam
- Scattered on the extensor and flexural aspects of bilateral upper and lower extremities, the patient had numerous tense 2–5 cm bullae, erosions, and hemorrhagic crusts. On the trunk there were several 3–5 cm urticarial plaques.

Management
The patient continued to have active disease despite a moderate dose of systemic corticosteroids. A more conservative approach with doxycycline and nicotinamide did not permit a lowering of the systemic corticosteroid dose. A hepatitis panel and QuantiFERON Gold test were negative. Baseline CBC and CMP were within acceptable limits. Mycophenolate mofetil, 500 mg BID, was initiated and titrated up to a dose of 1500 mg bid (based upon patient's weight of 75 kg and a desired dose of approximately 40 mg/kg), and CBC and CMP were monitored on a monthly basis. The patient was placed on calcium and vitamin D supplement, and a baseline DEXA scan was ordered with the results to be reviewed by the patient's primary care physician. Over the next few months, the prednisone was gradually tapered by 10 mg a month to 20 mg daily and then slowly tapered by 5 mg a month until the prednisone was able to be discontinued completely, while the mycophenolate was continued at a dose of 1500 mg BID. Throughout this time, the patient remained completely lesion-free. After 6 months of mycophenolate mofetil 1500 mg BID and no signs of active disease, the mycophenolate was tapered down in 500 mg increments every 3 months until he reached 500 mg daily and he continued to remain lesion-free. At this time, repeat DIF of normal skin, IIF on salt-split skin, and BP ELISA studies were all repeated and were all totally negative. Based upon the findings of both clinical and immunologic remission, the mycophenolate mofetil was discontinued and the patient was considered to be in remission.

References

1. Barnes PJ. Anti-inflammatory actions of glucocorticoids: molecular mechanisms. Clin Sci. 1998;94:557–72.
2. Vacca A, Felli MP, Farina AR, Martinotti S, Maroder M, Screpanti I, et al. Glucocorticoid receptor-mediated suppression of the interleukin 2 gene expression through impairment of the cooperativity between nuclear factor of activated T cells and AP-1 enhancer elements. J Exp Med. 1992;175(3):637–46.
3. Beato M, Chávez S, Truss M. Transcriptional regulation by steroid hormones. Steroids. 1996;61(4):240–51.
4. Mentink LF, Mackenzie MW, Tóth GG, Laseur M, Lambert FPG, Veeger NJGM, et al. Randomized controlled trial of adjuvant oral dexamethasone pulse therapy in pemphigus vulgaris: PEMPULS trial. Arch Dermatol. 2006;142(5):570–6. http://archderm.jama-network.com/article.aspx?doi=10.1001/archderm.142.5.570.
5. Caplan A, Fett N, Rosenbach M, Werth VP, Micheletti RG. Prevention and management of glucocorticoid-induced side effects: a comprehensive review: a review of glucocorticoid pharmacology and bone health. J Am Acad Dermatol. 2017;76(1):1–9. http://dx.doi.org/10.1016/j.jaad.2016.01.062.
6. Caplan A, Fett N, Rosenbach M, Werth VP, Micheletti RG. Prevention and management of glucocorticoid-induced side effects: a comprehensive review: gastrointestinal and endocrinologic side effects. J Am Acad Dermatol. 2017;76(1):11–6. http://dx.doi.org/10.1016/j.jaad.2016.02.1239.
7. Caplan A, Fett N, Rosenbach M, Werth VP, Micheletti RG. Prevention and management of glucocorticoid-induced side effects: a comprehensive review Infectious complications and vaccination recommendations glucocorticoids and immunity key point. J Am Acad Dermatol. 2017;76(2):191–8.
8. Webster G. Anti-inflammatory activity of Tetracyclines. Dermatol Clin. 2007;25(2):133–5.
9. Lebrun-Vignes B, Kreft-Jais C, Castot A, Chosidow O, French Network of Regional Centers of Pharmacovigilance. Comparative analysis of adverse drug reactions to tetracyclines: results of a French national survey and review of the literature. Br J Dermatol. 2012;166(6):1333–41. http://www.ncbi.nlm.nih.gov/pubmed/22283782.
10. Lan J, Lahoti A, Lew DB. A severe case of minocycline-induced DRESS resulting in liver transplantation and autoimmune sequelae. Vol. 116, Annals of Allergy, Asthma & Immunology. 2016.
11. Kanno K, Sakai H, Yamada Y, Iizuka H. Drug-induced hypersensitivity syndrome due to minocycline complicated by severe myocarditis. J Dermatol. 2014;41(2):160–2. http://doi.wiley.com/10.1111/1346-8138.12378.
12. Fivenson DP. The mechanisms of action of nicotinamide and zinc in inflammatory skin disease. Cutis. 2006;77(1 Suppl):5–10. http://www.ncbi.nlm.nih.gov/pubmed/16871773.
13. Wozel G, Blasum C. Dapsone in dermatology and beyond. Arch Dermatol Res. 2014;306(2):103–24. http://www.ncbi.nlm.nih.gov/pubmed/24310318.
14. Zhu YI, Stiller MJ. Dapsone and sulfones in dermatology: overview and update. J Am Acad Dermatol. 2001;45(3):420–34. http://www.ncbi.nlm.nih.gov/pubmed/11511841.
15. Cardones ARG, Hall RP. Management of dermatitis herpetiformis. Immunol Allergy Clin North Am. 2012;32(2):275–81, vi–vii. http://www.ncbi.nlm.nih.gov/pubmed/22560140.

16. Lings K, Bygum A. Linear IgA bullous dermatosis: a retrospective study of 23 patients in Denmark. Acta Dermatol Venereol. 2015;95(4):466–71. http://www.medicaljournals.se/acta/content/?doi=10.2340/00015555-1990.

17. Andersohn F, Konzen C, Garbe E. Systematic review: agranulocytosis induced by nonchemotherapy drugs. Ann Intern Med. 2007;146(9):657. http://annals.org/article.aspx?doi=10.7326/0003-4819-146-9-200705010-00009.

18. Coleman MD. Dapsone-mediated agranulocytosis: risks, possible mechanisms and prevention. Toxicology. 2001;162(1):53–60.

19. Bluhm RE, Adedoyin A, McCarver DG, Branch RA. Development of dapsone toxicity in patients with inflammatory dermatoses: activity of acetylation and hydroxylation of dapsone as risk factors. Clin Pharmacol Ther. 1999;65(6):598–605.

20. Degowin RL, Eppes RB, Powell RD, Carson PE. The haemolytic effects of diaphenylsulfone (DDS) in normal subjects and in those with glucose-6-phosphate-dehydrogenase deficiency. Bull World Health Organ. 1966;35(2):165–79. http://www.ncbi.nlm.nih.gov/pubmed/5297001.

21. Barclay JA, Ziemba SE, Ibrahim RB. Dapsone-induced methemoglobinemia: a primer for clinicians. Ann Pharmacother. 2011;45(9):1103–15.

22. Toker I, Yesilaras M, Tur FC, Toktas R. Methemoglobinemia caused by dapsone overdose: which treatment is best? Turkish J Emerg Med. 2015;15(4):182–4. http://www.ncbi.nlm.nih.gov/pubmed/27239625.

23. Wang N, Parimi L, Liu H, Zhang F. A review on dapsone hypersensitivity syndrome among Chinese patients with an emphasis on preventing adverse drug reactions with genetic testing. Am J Trop Med Hyg. 2017;96(5):1014–8. http://www.ncbi.nlm.nih.gov/pubmed/28167593.

24. Agrawal S, Agarwalla A. Dapsone hypersensitivity syndrome: a clinico-epidemiological review. J Dermatol. 2005;32(11):883–9. http://www.ncbi.nlm.nih.gov/pubmed/16361748.

25. Ward JR. Historical perspective on the use of methotrexate for the treatment of rheumatoid arthritis. J Rheumatol Suppl. 1985;12(Suppl 12):3–6. http://www.ncbi.nlm.nih.gov/pubmed/3913774.

26. Cronstein BN, Naime D, Ostad E. The antiinflammatory mechanism of methotrexate. Increased adenosine release at inflamed sites diminishes leukocyte accumulation in an in vivo model of inflammation. J Clin Invest. 1993;92(6):2675–82. http://www.ncbi.nlm.nih.gov/pubmed/8254024.

27. Haskó G, Cronstein BN. Adenosine: an endogenous regulator of innate immunity. Trends Immunol. 2004;25(1):33–9.

28. Al-Dabagh A, Davis SA, Kinney MA, Huang K, Feldman SR. The effect of folate supplementation on methotrexate efficacy and toxicity in psoriasis patients and folic acid use by dermatologists in the USA. Am J Clin Dermatol. 2013;14(3):155–61. http://link.springer.com/10.1007/s40257-013-0017-9.

29. Roenigk HH, Auerbach R, Maibach H, Weinstein G, Lebwohl M. Methotrexate in psoriasis: consensus conference. J Am Acad Dermatol. 1998;38(3):478–85.

30. Osuga T, Ikura Y, Kadota C, Hirano S, Iwai Y, Hayakumo T. Significance of liver biopsy for the evaluation of methotrexate-induced liver damage in patients with rheumatoid arthritis. Int J Clin Exp Pathol. 2015;8(2):1961–6. http://www.ncbi.nlm.nih.gov/pubmed/25973089.

31. Lynch M, Higgins E, McCormick PA, Kirby B, Nolan N, Rogers S, et al. The use of transient elastography and FibroTest for monitoring hepatotoxicity in patients receiving methotrexate for psoriasis. JAMA Dermatol. 2014;150(8):836. http://www.ncbi.nlm.nih.gov/pubmed/24964792.

32. Martyn-Simmons CL, Rosenberg WMC, Cross R, Wong T, Smith CH, JNWN B. Validity of noninvasive markers of methotrexate-induced hepatotoxicity: a retrospective cohort study. Br J Dermatol. 2014;171(2):267–73. http://www.ncbi.nlm.nih.gov/pubmed/24942271.

33. Ben-Chetrit E, Bergmann S, Sood R. Mechanism of the anti-inflammatory effect of colchicine in rheumatic diseases: a possible new outlook through microarray analysis. Rheumatology. 2005;45(3):274–82. https://academic.oup.com/rheumatology/article-lookup/doi/10.1093/rheumatology/kei140.

34. Chapman JR, Webster AC, Wong G. Cancer in the transplant recipient. Cold Spring Harb Perspect Med. 2013;3(7). http://www.ncbi.nlm.nih.gov/pubmed/23818517.

35. Mabrouk D, Gorcan HM, Keskin DB, Christen WG, Ahmed AR. Association between cancer and immunosuppressive therapy-analysis of selected studies in pemphigus and pemphigoid. Ann Pharmacother 2010;44(11):1770-1776. http://journals.sagepub.com/doi/pdf/10.1345/aph.1P309.

36. Farrell RJ, Ang Y, Kileen P, O'Briain DS, Kelleher D, PWN K, et al. Increased incidence of non-Hodgkin's lymphoma in inflammatory bowel disease patients on immunosuppressive therapy but overall risk is low. Gut. 2000;47:514–9. http://gut.bmj.com/content/gutjnl/47/4/514.full.pdf.

37. Asten P, Barrett J, Symmons D. Risk of developing certain malignancies is related to duration of immunosuppressive drug exposure in patients with rheumatic diseases. J Rheumatol. 1999;26(8):1705–14. http://www.ncbi.nlm.nih.gov/pubmed/10451066.

38. Bernatsky S, Joseph L, Boivin J-F, Gordon C, Urowitz M, Gladman D, et al. The relationship between cancer and medication exposures in systemic lupus erythematosus: a case-cohort study. Ann Rheum Dis. 2008;67(1):74–9. http://www.ncbi.nlm.nih.gov/pubmed/17545189.

39. Patel AA, Swerlick RA, McCall CO. Azathioprine in dermatology: the past, the present, and the future. J Am Acad Dermatol. 2006;55(3):369–89.

40. Maltzman JS, Koretzky GA. Azathioprine: old drug, new actions. J Clin Invest. 2003;111(8):1122–4. http://www.ncbi.nlm.nih.gov/pubmed/12697731

41. Lennard L, Van Loon JA, Weinshilboum RM. Pharmacogenetics of acute azathioprine toxicity: Relationship to thiopurine methyltransferase genetic polymorphism. Clin Pharmacol Ther. 1989;46(2):149–54. http://doi.wiley.com/10.1038/clpt.1989.119.

42. Snow JL, Gibson LE. The role of genetic variation in thiopurine methyltransferase activity and the efficacy and/or side effects of azathioprine therapy in dermatologic patients. Arch Dermatol. 1995;131(2):193. http://archderm.jamanetwork.com/article.aspx?doi=10.1001/archderm.1995.01690140077013.

43. Konstantopoulou M, Belgi A, Griffiths KD, Seale JRC, Macfarlane AW. Azathioprine-induced pancytopenia in a patient with pompholyx and deficiency of erythrocyte thiopurine methyltransferase. BMJ. 2005;330(7487):350.

44. McNally A, Ibbetson J, Sidhu S. Azathioprine-induced Sweet's syndrome: a case series and review of the literature. Australas J Dermatol. 2017;58(1):53–7. http://doi.wiley.com/10.1111/ajd.12383.

45. Sinico RA, Sabadini E, Borlandelli S, Cosci P, Di Toma L, Imbasciati E. Azathioprine hypersensitivity: report of two cases and review of the literature. J Nephrol. 2017;16(2):272–6. http://www.ncbi.nlm.nih.gov/pubmed/12768076.

46. Allison AC, Eugui EM. Mycophenolate mofetil and its mechanisms of action. Immunopharmacology. 2000;47(2):85–118.

47. Monach PA, Arnold LM, Merkel PA. Incidence and prevention of bladder toxicity from cyclophosphamide in the treatment of rheumatic diseases: a data-driven review. Arthritis Rheum. 2010;62(1):9–21. http://doi.wiley.com/10.1002/art.25061.

48. Gajjar R, Miller SD, Meyers KE, Ginsberg JP. Fertility preservation in patients receiving cyclophosphamide therapy for renal dis-

ease. Pediatr Nephrol. 2015;30(7):1099–106. http://link.springer.com/10.1007/s00467-014-2897-1.

49. Ho S, Clipstone N, Timmermann L, Northrop J, Graef I, Fiorentino D, et al. The mechanism of action of cyclosporin A and FK506. Clin Immunol Immunopathol. 1996;80(3 Pt 2):S40–5. http://www.ncbi.nlm.nih.gov/pubmed/8811062.

50. Khatri ML, Benghazeil M, Shafi M. Epidermolysis bullosa acquisita responsive to cyclosporin therapy. J Eur Acad Dermatol Venereol. 2001;15(2):182–4. http://www.ncbi.nlm.nih.gov/pubmed/11495534.

51. Naesens M, Kuypers DRJ, Sarwal M. Calcineurin inhibitor nephrotoxicity. Clin J Am Soc Nephrol. 2009;4(2):481–508. http://www.ncbi.nlm.nih.gov/pubmed/19218475.

52. Payne AS, Ishii K, Kacir S, Lin C, Li H, Hanakawa Y, et al. Genetic and functional characterization of human pemphigus vulgaris monoclonal autoantibodies isolated by phage display. J Clin Invest. 2005;115(4):888–99. http://www.pubmedcentral.nih.gov/articlerender.fcgi?artid=1070425&tool=pmcentrez&rendertype=abstract.

53. Mimouni D, Anhalt GJ. Pemphigus. Dermatol Ther. 2002;15(4):362–8. http://doi.wiley.com/10.1046/j.1529-8019.2002.01545.x.

54. Martin LK, Agero AL, Werth V, Villanueva E, Segall J, Murrell DF. Interventions for pemphigus vulgaris and pemphigus foliaceus. In: Murrell DF, editor. Cochrane database of systematic reviews. Chichester: Wiley; 2009. p. CD006263. http://www.ncbi.nlm.nih.gov/pubmed/19160272.

55. Mimouni D, Nousari CH, Cummins DL, Kouba DJ, David M, Anhalt GJ, et al. Differences and similarities among expert opinions on the diagnosis and treatment of pemphigus vulgaris. J Am Acad Dermatol. 2003;49(6):1059–62.

56. Beissert S, Mimouni D, Kanwar AJ, Solomons N, Kalia V, Anhalt GJ. Treating pemphigus vulgaris with prednisone and mycophenolate mofetil: a multicenter, randomized, placebo-controlled trial. J Invest Dermatol. 2010;130(8):2041–8. http://www.ncbi.nlm.nih.gov/pubmed/20410913.

57. McCarty M, Fivenson D. Two decades of using the combination of tetracycline derivatives and niacinamide as steroid-sparing agents in the management of pemphigus: Defining a niche for these low toxicity agents. J Am Acad Dermatol. 2014;71(3):475–9. http://www.ncbi.nlm.nih.gov/pubmed/24906610.

58. Tran KD, Wolverton JE, Soter NA. Methotrexate in the treatment of pemphigus vulgaris: experience in 23 patients. Br J Dermatol. 2013;169(4):916–21. http://www.ncbi.nlm.nih.gov/pubmed/23772610.

59. Baum S, Greenberger S, Samuelov L, Solomon M, Lyakhovitsky A, Trau H, et al. Methotrexate is an effective and safe adjuvant therapy for pemphigus vulgaris. Eur J Dermatol. 2017;22(1):83–7. http://www.ncbi.nlm.nih.gov/pubmed/22266247.

60. Heaphy MR, Albrecht J, Werth VP. Dapsone as a glucocorticoid-sparing agent in maintenance-phase pemphigus vulgaris. Arch Dermatol. 2005;141(6):699–702. http://www.ncbi.nlm.nih.gov/pubmed/15967915.

61. Gürcan HM, Ahmed AR. Efficacy of dapsone in the treatment of pemphigus and pemphigoid. Am J Clin Dermatol. 2009;10(6):383–96. http://link.springer.com/10.2165/11310740-000000000-00000.

62. Cianchini G, Lembo L, Colonna L, Puddu P. Pemphigus foliaceus induced by radiotherapy and responsive to dapsone. J Dermatol Treat. 2006;17(4):244–6. http://www.ncbi.nlm.nih.gov/pubmed/16971322.

63. Chen S, Lu X, Zhou G. Mild pemphigus foliaceus responding to combination therapy with niacinamide and tetracycline. Int J Dermatol. 2003;42(12):981–2. http://www.ncbi.nlm.nih.gov/pubmed/14636199.

64. Anhalt GJ, Kim S, Stanley JR, Korman NJ, Jabs DA, Kory M, et al. Paraneoplastic pemphigus. N Engl J Med. 1990;323(25):1729–35. http://www.ncbi.nlm.nih.gov/pubmed/2247105.

65. Kaplan I, Hodak E, Ackerman L, Mimouni D, Anhalt GJ, Calderon S. Neoplasms associated with paraneoplastic pemphigus: a review with emphasis on non-hematologic malignancy and oral mucosal manifestations. Oral Oncol. 2004;40(6):553–62. http://www.ncbi.nlm.nih.gov/pubmed/15063382.

66. Barnadas M, Roe E, Brunet S, Garcia P, Bergua P, Pimentel L, et al. Therapy of paraneoplastic pemphigus with Rituximab: a case report and review of literature. J Eur Acad Dermatol Venereol. 2006;20(1):69–74. https://doi.org/10.1111/j.1468-3083.2005.01345.x.

67. Carulina Moreno AL, Santi CG, Gabbi TV, Aoki V, Hashimoto T, Maruta CW. IgA pemphigus: case series with emphasis on therapeutic response. J Am Dermatol. 2014;70:200–1.

68. Mueller S, Vera BK, Stanley JR. A 230-kD basic protein is the major bullous pemphigoid antigen. J Invest Dermatol. 1989;92:33–8.

69. Diaz LA, Ratrie H, Saunders WS, Futamura S, Squiquera HL, Anhalt GJ, et al. Isolation of a human epidermal cDNA corresponding to the 180-kD autoantigen recognized by bullous pemphigoid and herpes gestationis sera. Immunolocalization of this protein to the hemidesmosome. J Clin Invest. 1990;86(4):1088–94. http://www.ncbi.nlm.nih.gov/pubmed/1698819.

70. Mutasim DF. Therapy of autoimmune bullous diseases. Ther Clin Risk Manag. 2007;3(1):29–40. http://www.ncbi.nlm.nih.gov/pubmed/18360613.

71. Kirtschig G, Middleton P, Bennett C, Murrell DF, Wojnarowska F, Khumalo NP. Interventions for bullous pemphigoid. In: Kirtschig G, editor. Cochrane database of systematic reviews. Chichester: Wiley; 2010. p. CD002292. http://www.ncbi.nlm.nih.gov/pubmed/20927731.

72. Gürcan HM, Razzaque Ahmed A. Analysis of current data on the use of methotrexate in the treatment of pemphigus and pemphigoid. Br J Dermatol. 2009;161(4):723–31. http://www.ncbi.nlm.nih.gov/pubmed/19548961.

73. Gunay U, Gunduz K, Türel Ermertcan A, Kandiloğlu AR. Coexistence of psoriasis and bullous pemphigoid: remission with low-dose methotrexate. Cutan Ocul Toxicol. 2013;32(2):168–9. http://www.ncbi.nlm.nih.gov/pubmed/22429144.

74. Si X, Ge L, Xin H, Cao W, Sun X, Li W. Erythrodermic psoriasis with bullous pemphigoid: combination treatment with methotrexate and compound glycyrrhizin. Diagn Pathol. 2014;9(1):102. http://www.ncbi.nlm.nih.gov/pubmed/24885087.

75. Fivenson DP, Breneman DL, Rosen GB, Hersh CS, Cardone S, Mutasim D. Nicotinamide and tetracycline therapy of bullous pemphigoid. Arch Dermatol. 1994;130(6):753. http://archderm.jamanetwork.com/article.aspx?doi=10.1001/archderm.1994.01690060083010.

76. Venning VA, Millard PR, Wojnarowska F. Dapsone as first line therapy for bullous pemphigoid. Br J Dermatol. 1989;120(1):83–92. http://www.ncbi.nlm.nih.gov/pubmed/2700666.

77. Scully C, Carrozzo M, Gandolfo S, Puiatti P, Monteil R. Update on mucous membrane pemphigoid: a heterogeneous immune-mediated subepithelial blistering entity. Oral Surg Oral Med Oral Pathol Oral Radiol Endod. 1999;88:56–68.

78. Xu H-H, Werth VP, Parisi E, Sollecito TP. Mucous membrane pemphigoid. Dent Clin North Am. 2013;57(4):611–30. http://www.ncbi.nlm.nih.gov/pubmed/24034069.

79. Chan LS, Ahmed AR, Anhalt GJ, Bernauer W, Cooper KD, Elder MJ, et al. The first international consensus on mucous membrane pemphigoid: definition, diagnostic criteria, pathogenic factors, medical treatment, and prognostic indicators. Arch Dermatol. 2002;138(3):370–9. http://www.ncbi.nlm.nih.gov/pubmed/11902988.

80. Aufdemorte TB, De Villez RL, Parel SM. Modified topical steroid therapy for the treatment of oral mucous membrane pemphigoid.

Oral Surg Oral Med Oral Pathol. 1985;59(3):256–60. http://www.ncbi.nlm.nih.gov/pubmed/3885134.

81. Dragan L, Eng AM, Lam S, Persson T. Tetracycline and niacinamide: treatment alternatives in ocular cicatricial pemphigoid. Cutis. 1999;63(3):181–3. http://www.ncbi.nlm.nih.gov/pubmed/10190074.

82. Reiche L, Wojnarowska F, Mallon E. Combination therapy with nicotinamide and tetracyclines for cicatricial pemphigoid: further support for its efficacy. Clin Exp Dermatol. 1998;23(6):254–7. http://www.ncbi.nlm.nih.gov/pubmed/10233619.

83. Ciarrocca KN, Greenberg MS. A retrospective study of the management of oral mucous membrane pemphigoid with dapsone. Oral Surg Oral Med Oral Pathol Oral Radiol Endod. 1999;88(2):159–63. http://www.ncbi.nlm.nih.gov/pubmed/10468458.

84. Chaidemenos G, Sidiropoulos T, Katsioula P, Koussidou-Eremondi T. Colchicine in the management of mucous membrane pemphigoid. Dermatol Ther. 2011;24(4):443–5. http://www.ncbi.nlm.nih.gov/pubmed/21910802.

85. Woodley DT, Briggaman RA, O'Keefe EJ, Inman AO, Queen LL, Gammon WR. Identification of the skin basement-membrane autoantigen in epidermolysis bullosa acquisita. N Engl J Med. 1984;310(16):1007–13. http://www.nejm.org/doi/abs/10.1056/NEJM198404193101602.

86. Gupta R, Woodley DT, Chen M. Epidermolysis bullosa acquisita. Clin Dermatol. 2012;30:60–9.

87. Iranzo P, Herrero-González JE, Mascaró-Galy JM, Suárez-Fernández R, España A. Epidermolysis bullosa acquisita: a retrospective analysis of 12 patients evaluated in four tertiary hospitals in Spain. Br J Dermatol. 2014;171(5):1022–30. http://doi.wiley.com/10.1111/bjd.13144.

88. Crichlow SM, Mortimer NJ, Harman KE. A successful therapeutic trial of rituximab in the treatment of a patient with recalcitrant, high-titre epidermolysis bullosa acquisita. Br J Dermatol. 2007;156(1):194–6. http://doi.wiley.com/10.1111/j.1365-2133.2006.07596.x.

89. Schmidt E, Benoit S, Bröcker E-B, Zillikens D, Goebeler M. Successful adjuvant treatment of recalcitrant epidermolysis bullosa acquisita with anti-CD20 antibody rituximab. Arch Dermatol. 2006;142(2):147–50. http://www.ncbi.nlm.nih.gov/pubmed/16490841.

90. Crow LL, Finkle JP, Gammon WR, Woodley DT. Clearing of epidermolysis bullosa acquisita with cyclosporine. J Am Acad Dermatol. 1988;19(5 Pt 2):937–42. http://www.ncbi.nlm.nih.gov/pubmed/3057000.

91. Megahed M, Scharffetter-Kochanek K. Epidermolysis bullosa acquisita—successful treatment with colchicine. Arch Dermatol Res. 1994;286(1):35–46. http://www.ncbi.nlm.nih.gov/pubmed/8141610.

92. Zillikens D, Herzele K, Georgi M, Schmidt E, Chimanovitch I, Bröcker E-B, et al. Autoantibodies in a subgroup of patients with linear IgA disease react with the NC16A domain of BP1801. J Invest Dermatol. 1999;113(6):947–53. http://www.ncbi.nlm.nih.gov/pubmed/10594735.

93. Navi D, Michael DJ, Fazel N. Drug-induced linear IgA bullous dermatosis. Dermatol Online J. 2006;12(5):12. http://www.ncbi.nlm.nih.gov/pubmed/16962027.

94. Lings K, Bygum A. Linear IgA bullous dermatosis: a retrospective study of 23 patients in Denmark. Acta Derm Venereol. 2015;95(4):466–71. http://www.ncbi.nlm.nih.gov/pubmed/25350667.

95. Fortuna G, Marinkovich MP. Linear immunoglobulin A bullous dermatosis. Clin Dermatol. 2012;30(1):38–50.

96. Lu PD, Ralston J, Kamino H, Stein JA. Pemphigoid gestationis. Dermatol Online J. 2010;16(11):10. http://www.ncbi.nlm.nih.gov/pubmed/21163161.

97. Hall RP, Lawley TJ, Smith HR, Katz SI. Bullous eruption of systemic lupus erythematosus. Ann Intern Med. 1982;97(2):165. http://annals.org/article.aspx?doi=10.7326/0003-4819-97-2-165.

98. Vassileva S. Bullous systemic lupus erythematosus. Clin Dermatol. 2004;22(2):129–38.

99. Marks J, Shuster S, Watson AJ. Small-bowel changes in dermatitis herpetiformis. Lancet. 1966;2(7476):1280–2.

100. Alaedini A, Green PHR. Narrative review: celiac disease: understanding a complex autoimmune disorder. Ann Intern Med. 2005;142(4):289–98.

101. Zone JJ, Egan CA, Taylor TB, Meyer LJ. Iga autoimmune disorders: development of a passive transfer mouse model. J Investig Dermatol Symp Proc. 2004;9(1):47–51.

102. Fry L, McMinn RM, Cowan JD, Hoffbrand AV. Effect of gluten-free diet on dermatological, intestinal, and haematological manifestations of dermatitis herpetiformis. Lancet. 1968;1(7542):557–61.

103. Reunala T, Kosnai I, Karpati S, Kuitunen P, Torok E, Savilahti E. Dermatitis herpetiformis: jejunal findings and skin response to gluten free diet. Arch Dis Child. 1984;59(6):517–22. http://adc.bmj.com/cgi/doi/10.1136/adc.59.6.517.

Biologic and Systemic Agents in Hidradenitis Suppurativa

Martin M. Okun

Abbreviations

HiSCR   Hidradenitis suppurativa clinical response
HS   Hidradenitis suppurativa
HSS   Hidradenitis suppurativa score
STEEP   Skin-tissue-saving excision with electrosurgical peeling

Introduction

Hidradenitis suppurativa (HS) is a chronic inflammatory disease, typically localizing to the axilla, groin, or inframammary regions, characterized by recurrent nodules or abscesses, carrying the risk of scarring or sinus tract formation [1]. Despite the pain and potentially severe impact on quality of life from HS, and despite the fact that it is not rare, with a recent population-based survey reporting a prevalence of 2.10% in Denmark [2], HS has not attracted the same level of investigational attention as other dermatologic diseases such as acne or psoriasis. Consequently, a limited understanding exists about basic questions concerning HS pathogenesis, epidemiology, natural history, comorbidities, and effectiveness and safety of treatments. The latter limitation frequently obliges clinicians caring for HS patients to choose therapies that lack a robust evidence base; though more than 50 types of HS treatment have been described, there are few randomized controlled studies in HS providing high-quality evidence [3, 4]. This chapter evaluates the evidence for the efficacy and safety of commonly used and promising new systemic therapies for HS. It is intended to be more comprehensive than a meta-analysis of randomized controlled trials in HS [3], because so many commonly used therapies have not been studied in randomized controlled trials. It is not intended to be a compendium of every described HS therapy, because many such therapies have only been described in case reports or very small case series that serve better to generate scientific hypotheses than to influence treatment decisions.

A rational evaluation of the systemic therapies for HS must begin by considering what is known or hypothesized about the pathogenesis of the disease, followed by considering the scientific rationale for the therapeutic options, and then evaluating the quality and quantity of evidence supporting the use of that therapy. The pathogenic trigger of the disease is hypothesized to be occlusion of the infundibulum by follicular keratinocytes, followed by rupture of the hair follicle wall. Leakage of the pilosebaceous unit contents, including commensal bacteria, into the dermis then initiates an intense foreign body-like reaction mediated by resident dermal immune cells secreting pro-inflammatory cytokines and chemokines, which help recruit and activate other arms of the immune system [5]. Blocking the different steps of this disease—via modifying keratinocyte maturation (retinoids) or sebaceous gland activity (retinoids or antiandrogens), via anti-inflammatory effects (antibiotics or immunosuppressants), or via direct alteration of the HS microbiome (antibiotics)—is the rationale for including these medication types in the HS therapeutic armamentarium.

Limitations in the quality of clinical evidence interfere with our ability to reliably assess the efficacy and safety of many therapies. Interpretation of uncontrolled studies is problematic because the few placebo-controlled trials in HS have revealed that approximately 25% of moderate to severe placebo-treated HS patients experience clinically relevant spontaneous improvement in their disease [6], and the placebo response for patients with mild HS is likely higher. This may be due to a true placebo response or due to selection bias: disease activity of many HS patients is volatile, perhaps more than in other dermatologic diseases, and HS patients may be more willing to enroll in clinical trials or start new investigational therapies when their disease activity is peaking.

M.M. Okun, MD, PhD
Fort HealthCare Department of Dermatology,
611 Sherman Avenue East, Fort Atkinson, WI 53538, USA
e-mail: martin.okun@forthc.com

© Springer International Publishing AG 2018
P.S. Yamauchi (ed.), *Biologic and Systemic Agents in Dermatology*, https://doi.org/10.1007/978-3-319-66884-0_36

Table 36.1 Hurley stage classification for HS patients

Stage I	Abscess formation, single or multiple, without sinus tracts or scarring
Stage II	Recurrent abscesses with sinus tract formation or scarring
	Single or multiple, widely separated lesions
Stage III	Diffuse or near-diffuse involvement or multiple interconnected sinus tracts and abscesses across entire anatomic region

Modified from: Hurley H. Axillary hyperhidrosis, apocrine bromhidrosis, hidradenitis suppurativa, and familial benign pemphigus. In: Roenigk RK and Roenigk HH Jr., editors. Dermatologic Surgery: Principles and Practice. New York: Marcel Dekker; 1989. pg. 631–643

As a result, patients' improvement from their "baseline" disease activity, assessed at the time of initiation of an investigational therapy, may represent random fluctuation back toward their typical disease activity. In studies or case series without a placebo group, it is not possible to determine reliably how much improvement is due to therapy and how much is due to spontaneous improvement, but a reasonable heuristic would be to judge a therapy effective if substantially more than 25% of patients with moderate to severe HS experience clinically relevant improvement. In studies using an unvalidated endpoint (i.e., an endpoint lacking evidence of reliability and of clinical relevance), the reported improvement may not be reproducible in clinical practice or may not be meaningful to patients. From studies with few subjects or with limited follow-up, it is not possible to reliably determine the incidence of serious but low probability or long-term adverse events.

The first attempt to categorize HS disease stage within each involved anatomic region was proposed by Hurley [7] (Table 36.1). By convention, a patient's overall Hurley stage corresponds to the Hurley stage of his or her most advanced anatomic region: if a patient has at least one anatomic region with Hurley stage III disease, he or she is a Hurley stage III patient. The Hurley staging system was originally intended to help physicians classify patients as candidates for medical therapy (Hurley stage I), limited surgical intervention (e.g., excision of a sinus tract) (Hurley stage II), or more extensive surgical intervention (e.g., *en bloc* excision of an entire anatomic region) (Hurley stage III). It is not practical to use Hurley staging to classify disease severity, which is determined by a constellation of factors in addition to sinus tract formation or scarring, such as number and severity of inflammatory lesions, pain, and impact of the disease on quality of life. Hurley stage I patients may have severe disease, and Hurley stage III patients with no active inflammation may have mild disease. It is also not practical to use Hurley staging to assess the efficacy of a systemic therapy because it is insufficiently dynamic: the presence and extent of scars and sinus tracts differentiate among the Hurley stages, but once scars or sinus tracts are formed, no systemic medical therapy can reasonably be expected to reverse or downgrade the Hurley stage.

Two HS-specific objective endpoints have been validated and are therefore potentially useful tools for evaluating systemic therapy efficacy: the hidradenitis suppurativa score (HSS) or Sartorius score, which has undergone modifications from its original iteration [8], and the hidradenitis suppurativa clinical response (HiSCR) [6]. The modified Sartorius score is a composite score comprising the number of involved anatomic regions, the numbers and types of lesions for each region, and the extent and severity of involvement within each region. Reproducibility and inter-rater reliability of the modified Sartorius score have been established. The modified Sartorius score suffers from a lack of definition of what constitutes clinically meaningful improvement and contains disparate elements that reflect disease activity (e.g., nodules) and also disease damage (e.g., Hurley stage). As medical therapies can be expected to reduce disease activity but not affect disease damage, change in the modified Sartorius score may not be optimally sensitive to detect clinically relevant improvement. HiSCR response is defined as at least a 50% reduction in total abscess and/or inflammatory nodule count, so long as the abscess count is not increased and the draining fistula count is not increased. Reproducibility and inter-rater reliability of HiSCR have also been established, and achievement of HiSCR response has been demonstrated to be clinically meaningful for patients [9]. US and European regulatory authorities recognize HiSCR as a valid endpoint, as it has been used successfully in phase III clinical trials to achieve regulatory approval of adalimumab for treatment of moderate to severe HS. HiSCR exclusively focuses on disease activity, with no assessment of disease damage included in the measure. In addition to these HS-specific objective endpoints, treatment response can be evaluated using subjective health-related quality of life measures, including validated dermatology-specific measures such as the dermatology life quality index (DLQI) and/or pain VAS scores.

Immunosuppressants

Overexpression of tumor necrosis factor alpha (TNF-α) and interleukin-1 beta (IL-1β) in HS lesional tissue [10] provides the scientific rationale for targeting these pro-inflammatory cytokines. The cellular sources of TNF-α and IL-1β in lesional tissue are uncertain but may include monocytes and macrophages, which are abundantly present in HS lesions and may be activated by pro-inflammatory signals from keratins released followed follicular unit rupture, or from commensal bacteria.

TNF Antagonists

Numerous case reports and series describe the successful use of adalimumab, etanercept, and infliximab for treatment of HS, but an uncontrolled prospective open-label trial of etanercept at a dose of 50 mg weekly demonstrating a clinical response in 3 of 15 patients [11] led to etanercept falling into disfavor relative to other TNF antagonists.

Adalimumab

Adalimumab is a self-injectable monoclonal antibody specific for TNF-α. A phase II dose ranging trial [12] and two confirmatory phase III placebo-controlled trials [6] demonstrated that adalimumab was significantly effective for treatment of HS. The outcomes from these studies resulted in the approval of adalimumab for treatment of moderate to severe HS in the USA, Canada, and the EU, with a dosing regimen of 160 mg at week 0, 80 mg at week 2, and 40 mg weekly starting at week 4. Figure 36.1a, b depicts an affected crural

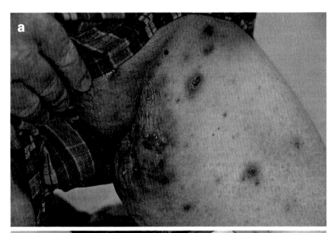

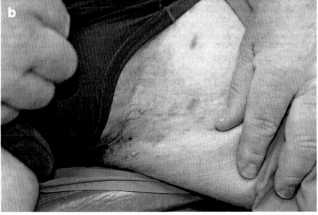

Fig. 36.1 Clinical photographs of the left groin of a patient with severe HS before (**a**) and after (**b**) six months of adalimumab 40 mg weekly dosing therapy. Clinical photographs are courtesy of Dr. Marc Bourcier, Moncton, New Brunswick, Canada

fold before and after 6 months of therapy with adalimumab 40 mg weekly dosing.

The two phase III trials, dubbed PIONEER I and II, randomized 633 patients to adalimumab or placebo. To enter these trials, patients were required to have failed oral antibiotic therapy, have Hurley stage II or III disease in at least one anatomic region, and have at least three abscesses or inflammatory nodules. PIONEER I patients were not allowed concomitant oral medications for treatment of HS; PIONEER II patients who were concomitantly taking a stable dose of minocycline or doxycycline for HS were permitted to continue these oral antibiotics but no other systemic HS therapies. Patients were randomized 1:1 in a double-blind manner either to adalimumab at the above dosing regimen or to placebo, with the validated HiSCR response rate measured at week 12 serving as the primary efficacy endpoint. At week 12, patients who had originally been randomized to adalimumab were rerandomized to continue adalimumab 40 mg weekly, or to receive adalimumab 40 mg every other week dosing, or to receive placebo, with the studies concluding at week 36.

In PIONEER I and II, week 12 HiSCR response rate was 41.8 and 58.9% for adalimumab-treated subjects versus 26.0 and 27.6% for placebo-treated subjects, corresponding to a significant treatment effect [difference in response between adalimumab- and placebo-treated subjects] of 15.8–31.3%. Compared to the treatment effect observed with adalimumab 40 mg every other week dosing in moderate to severe psoriasis patients, the treatment effect of adalimumab 40 mg weekly dosing in moderate to severe HS patients was smaller. The higher treatment effect noted in PIONEER II compared to PIONEER I was partially a consequence of the higher treatment effect in the stratum of patients receiving concomitant oral antibiotics (in PIONEER II, the treatment effect among patients receiving concomitant oral antibiotics for HS was 42.6% vs. 28.6% for patients not on concomitant oral antibiotics) and partially a consequence of milder baseline disease state in PIONEER II. In PIONEER I and II, mean improvements from baseline to week 12 in DLQI scores for adalimumab-treated patients (5.4, 5.1) exceeded the minimal clinically important difference in inflammatory skin diseases for DLQI of 4 [13] and were significantly better versus placebo-treated patients (2.9, 2.3) [$p < 0.001$ in both studies]. While the studies were inadequately powered to test statistical significance of the different dosing regimens from weeks 12 to 36, the numerical trend favored the weekly dosing treatment arm, corroborating the results from the adalimumab phase II dose ranging trial which demonstrated that 40 mg every other week dosing did not result in meaningful improvement above what was observed in placebo patients. The adalimumab safety profile across the phase II and III trials was consistent with what has been observed for adalimumab in clinical trials in other disease states, with no notable increase in the frequency of serious infections among adalimumab-treated versus placebo-treated patients.

Infliximab

Infliximab is a monoclonal antibody specific for TNF-α administered by intravenous infusion. A double-blind phase II trial randomized 15 patients to receive infliximab at a dose of 5 mg per kg at weeks 0, 2, and 6 or 23 patients to placebo [14]. The primary efficacy endpoint was the percentage of patients achieving at least 50% improvement in the hidradenitis suppurativa severity index (HSSI), an unvalidated endpoint, at week 8. There was no significant difference in the primary efficacy endpoint between the infliximab and placebo arms. Post hoc analysis demonstrated that 60% of infliximab-treated patients achieved between 25 and 50% improvement in HSSI compared to 5.6% of placebo patients ($p < 0.001$). Mean change in DLQI for infliximab-treated patients was 10.0, compared with 1.6 for placebo-treated patients ($p = 0.003$). The observed adverse event profile was consistent with what would be expected in a population receiving infliximab infusions for other indications.

Anakinra

Anakinra is an antagonist to the interleukin-1 receptor, capable of binding to and blocking the biological activity of IL-1α and IL-1β. In a placebo-controlled double-blind trial of 20 subjects with Hurley stage II or III disease, subjects were randomized 1:1 in a double-blind manner to anakinra 100 mg administered subcutaneously or to placebo [15]. Anakinra therapy was associated with a significantly higher proportion of patients experiencing reduction from baseline in their disease activity score (determined by the size and degree of inflammation of the two largest lesions in each involved anatomic region) and a significantly higher HiSCR response rate (78% of anakinra-treated patients vs. 30% of placebo-treated patients). Adverse events reported in the anakinra group included diarrhea and vaginal candidiasis.

Ustekinumab

Ustekinumab is a monoclonal antibody approved for treatment of psoriasis that binds the p40 subunit common to il-12 and il-23. Based on evidence that the il-23 pathway is activated in HS, an open-label prospective trial in which 17 HS patients were treated with ustekinumab at the dosing regimen approved for psoriasis [16]. The week 40 HiSCR response was 47% (8 of 17 patients), and 41% of patients experienced a reduction in DLQI of at least 5 points. The

HiSCR response rate was intermediate between reported from adalimumab treatment groups in PIONEER I (41.8%) and PIONEER II (58.9%) trials, but results from these trials cannot be compared directly because of notable differences in baseline demographics, with patients in the ustekinumab trial having substantially lower body mass index than patients in the PIONEER trials.

Antibiotics

Clindamycin and Rifampicin

The scientific rationale for treating HS with clindamycin and rifampin derives from their direct antimicrobial activity against *S. aureus*, coagulase-negative staphylococci, and anaerobic bacteria, which are occasionally cultured from HS lesions [17]. Using these antibiotics in combination reduces the risk of selecting for resistant organisms. Their mechanism of action in HS may not depend strictly upon their antimicrobial properties, as clindamycin modulates oxidative activity of mononuclear cells in a mouse model [18] and rifampin inhibits human neutrophil activity [19].

Three retrospective case series [20–22] and one prospective case series [23], which together report on the experiences of 141 patients, describe the efficacy and safety of combination clindamycin and rifampin in HS. The most commonly employed treatment regimen was a 10-week course of oral rifampin at a dose of 300 mg twice daily and oral clindamycin at a dose of 300 mg twice daily. Efficacy outcomes among the studies were variable, possibly related to differences in patient baseline characteristics or efficacy endpoints across the study populations, but between 56.5% and 85% of patients experienced clinically relevant improvement. Mendonça and Griffiths performed their retrospective analysis of 14 patients, 10 of whom entered "clinical remission" (not defined) after a 10-week treatment course, with remission duration of 1–4 years. All ten patients who experienced remission had disease in the perineal area at baseline, with some of these patients having disease in additional areas. Six patients could not tolerate clindamycin therapy due to the GI side effects of diarrhea: four discontinued the treatment regimen and two were switched to minocycline 100 mg per day. Van der Zee et al. performed their retrospective analysis on 34 patients, 23 of whom received clindamycin 300 mg po bid and rifampicin 300 mg po bid for different treatment durations. A physician's global assessment (PGA) was utilized to evaluate disease severity. Total remission was defined as more than 75% improvement in PGA relative to baseline. Most patients had Hurley stage II or III disease at baseline. Slightly more than half of patients (56.5%) treated with this regimen experienced total remission, and prolonging treatment duration beyond 10 weeks was not associated with a meaningfully higher likelihood of remission. Total remission rates were higher for patients with Hurley stage II disease at baseline (60%) compared to patients with Hurley stage III disease at baseline (29%). Two-thirds of patients with total remission experienced relapse (not defined), with 5.0 months being the mean time to relapse for the relapsers. Approximately one-quarter (26%) of patients discontinued therapy due to side effects. In Gener et al.'s retrospective report on 116 HS patients treated for 10 weeks with clindamycin (300 mg po bid) and rifampin (600 mg po bid), for whom follow-up data on 70 patients were available, statistically significant improvement in Sartorius scores was noted, with median Sartorius score decreasing 50% (from 29 to 14.5). Pain and frequency of purulent drainage decreased significantly, and 66% of patients self-rated the result of treatment as "very good." Unfortunately, week 10 data was missing for 40% of the treated patients. Among the patients with available week 10 data, the discontinuation rate was 11.4%, mostly due to GI symptoms. The 23 HS patients treated prospectively by Bettoli et al. with combination clindamycin-rifampicin experienced a mean reduction in Sartorius score from 132.05 at baseline to 71.50 at week 10, corresponding to a mean decrease of 45.85%. The authors arbitrarily chose 25% improvement in Sartorius score as clinically meaningful; by this criterion, 85% of patients experienced clinically meaningful improvement. Three of 23 patients discontinued treatment, and 3 of 23 patients noted GI side effects. Shortcomings of these studies include absence of a placebo group, variable availability of follow-up data (with incomplete and limited follow-up for patients who experienced remission), and the use of endpoints that were either unvalidated or, in the case of Sartorius score, lacking a validated threshold for clinically meaningful improvement.

Other Antibiotics

Oral tetracycline (500 mg twice daily) was compared with topical clindamycin (1% lotion twice daily) in a double-blind, double-dummy 3-month randomized control trial of 46 Hurley stage I and II patients [24]. Compared to baseline, both treatment arms experienced significant improvement in a variety of efficacy measures. No significant differences were noted between the treatment arms, but the study did not provide power calculations, making it possible that the study lacked power to detect a significant difference. Based on the available data, it is not possible to determine the percentage of subjects who experienced clinically relevant improvement. At baseline, subjects had less than three abscesses and less than five nodules. In both treatment groups, median abscess count and nodule count were approximately halved after 3 months of treatment.

Based on a smaller case series describing successful treatment of HS with dapsone [25], outcomes from 24 HS patients treated with dapsone, at doses ranging from 50 to 200 mg per day for up to 48 months, were reported [26]. With 100% ascertainment at follow-up, "clinically significant improvement" (defined as "drastic relief and major clinical improvement") was observed in six patients (25%). One patient with clinically significant improvement experienced disease recurrence rapidly after treatment discontinuation, but responded again to dapsone when it was reinstituted, suggesting that the improvement observed with dapsone therapy was not coincidental. Two of 24 patients discontinued due to dapsone-related adverse events. The principal strength of this series is the complete ascertainment of treatment outcomes; weaknesses include absence of a placebo control group and lack of a validated endpoint. Interestingly, the reported rate of clinically significant improvement was not notably different from the placebo HiSCR response rate in adalimumab clinical trials (25.0–26.7%), suggesting that at least some of the patients experiencing clinically significant improvement may instead have been undergoing spontaneous, random fluctuation in disease activity.

In a retrospective study, 28 HS patients were treated with a combination of rifampin (10 mg per kg per day), moxifloxacin (400 mg per day), and metronidazole (500 mg tid), sometimes preceded by a 2-week course of intravenous ceftriaxone (1 g per day) and oral metronidazole (500 mg tid) [27]. Metronidazole was administered for 6 weeks, but rifampin and moxifloxacin were continued until disease remitted (i.e., inflammatory lesions were absent at two consecutive visits). Complete remission was achieved by 16 patients (57%), though most Hurley stage III patients failed to remit. Patients achieving complete remission were maintained on trimethoprim-sulfamethoxazole (400 mg/80 mg daily) or doxycycline (100 mg daily). Among the 14 patients who entered remission and had long-term follow-up, 7 experienced relapse. Nausea and diarrhea affected the majority of patients, and four experienced moxifloxacin-associated tendinitis necessitating treatment discontinuation.

In an improved treatment algorithm, 30 patients were treated with intravenous ertapenem (1 g daily) for 6 weeks, followed by the rifampin/moxifloxacin/metronidazole combination described above until disease remitted [28]. Sixteen patients adhered to this treatment regimen; their median Sartorius score decreased from 50.5 at baseline to 12.0 at month 6. Patient remission rates were not provided; remission rates by body region were 100% for Hurley stage I, 96% for Hurley stage II, and 27% for Hurley stage III. Most of the patients required repeat treatment to maintain disease control. During the ertapenem induction, oral and/or vaginal candidiasis was reported for 27% of ertapenem-treated patients, and one patient experienced lymphangitis.

Other Therapies

Zinc

Because zinc salts have been hypothesized to have anti-inflammatory properties and because efficacy with zinc gluconate in treatment of mild to moderate acne has been described, a pilot open-label study of zinc gluconate to treat predominantly Hurley stage I and II patients was conducted [29]. Subjects received 90 mg zinc gluconate per day, which was decreased by 15 mg every 2 months once complete remission (defined as resolution of inflammatory lesions or no new lesions for at least 6 months), or once partial remission (defined as at least 50% reduction in inflammatory lesions or a shorter duration for inflammatory lesions), had been achieved. Eight of 22 patients (36%) achieved complete remission, with the remaining patients achieving partial remission. Treatment was not remittive following dose reduction. One patient discontinued due to nausea and vomiting. Shortcomings of this study include absence of a placebo group, few subjects (one subject with Hurley stage III disease), ambiguity about follow-up duration and endpoint definition, and lack of information about efficacy for different Hurley stages. A subsequent open-label study of 66 patients treated with oral zinc gluconate combined with topical 2% triclosan reported improvements in median Sartorius and DLQI scores [30].

Hormonal Therapy

Clues pointing to a hormonal influence on HS pathogenesis include female preponderance, onset typically after puberty, rarity among postmenopausal women, reports of HS exacerbations associated with menses, and possible association with the hyperandrogenic state of polycystic ovary syndrome [31]. However, no consistent evidence of abnormal serum levels of sex hormones exists, though this does not preclude abnormalities in sex hormone metabolism peripherally, in hair follicles or sebaceous glands.

If hyperandrogenism can trigger HS, then antiandrogens are rational treatment options. Lee and Fischer [32] reported an uncontrolled retrospective analysis of 20 female patients treated with spironolactone 100 mg per day, using an unvalidated PGA scale modified from Kimball et al. [12] that classifies patients into grades of clear, mild, moderate, or severe based on counts of abscesses, draining fistulas, and inflammatory nodules. Response rate was 85% (17 of 20 patients experiencing at least 1 grade improvement relative to baseline); if more stringent response criteria are employed to assess outcomes (i.e., improvement by more than 1 grade relative to baseline), 7 of 12 moderate patients became clear and 1 of 3 severe patients became mild, for a response rate of 53% (8 of 15). Response was typically observed by month 5 or 6. No information was provided about whether any of these patients had clinical or biochemical evidence of hyperandrogenism prior to starting spironolactone. One patient discontinued treatment due to altered mood and dizziness. Shortcomings of this study include its retrospective nature, absence of a placebo control, and concomitant use of potentially beneficial medications (five patients were on concomitant minocycline and seven patients were on concomitant oral contraceptives). The antiandrogen cyproterone acetate (unavailable in the USA) combined with ethinyl estradiol was compared with norgestrel and ethinyl estradiol in a double-blind crossover trial of 24 female HS patients [33]. Both treatment regimens reduced disease activity comparably. Seven of 24 patients experienced disease clearance as assessed by physicians; by patient self-assessment, approximately twice as many patients experienced improvement compared to worsening with one of the regimens. The small number of enrolled patients, the high dropout rate (25%), and the absence of a placebo control limit the study's generalizability. Interestingly, in a case series of 29 patients treated with different types of antiandrogens, evidence of biochemical androgenism was not a factor predictive for responsiveness [31]. Finasteride was tested in seven male and female HS patients who had failed oral antibiotics [34], based on the hypothesis that hair follicle-mediated conversion of testosterone to dihydrotestosterone by type II 5α reductase drives HS pathogenesis. Three patients experienced no new lesions within 2–8 weeks of treatment initiation, and three had fewer or smaller lesions. The small size of this study limits its generalizability.

Metformin

Metformin is typically used for treatment of type II diabetes and polycystic ovary syndrome and reduces plasma glucose levels through a variety of mechanisms including reduced glucose production from hepatocytes, reduced intestinal absorption of glucose, and heightened insulin sensitivity. Its precise mechanism of action is unknown. As type II diabetes and polycystic ovary syndrome are common comorbidities in HS patients, Verdolini et al. [35] conducted an uncontrolled case series of 25 HS patients treated with metformin for 24 weeks. At doses up to 500 mg tid, 18 patients experienced an improvement in the Sartorius score relative to baseline, with 7 of these patients (28%) experiencing at least a 50% improvement in Sartorius score relative to baseline. If it is assumed, based on how the Sartorius score is derived, that a 50% improvement in Sartorius scale is the threshold for clinically meaningful improvement, then the 28% response rate is not markedly higher than the HiSCR placebo response rate of 25–27% reported by

Kimball et al. [6]. Assessment of plasma glucose levels was not performed in these patients, so it is unknown whether those patients with a clinically relevant response had elevated glucose levels prior to starting metformin or a marked reduction in their levels after starting metformin. Minor GI disturbances at the beginning of treatment were the only recorded side effects.

Systemic Retinoids

Systemic retinoids reduce epithelial proliferation, normalize differentiation, and are anti-inflammatory. Isotretinoin was first tested for efficacy in HS by Boer and van Gemert [36], who published retrospective results from 68 patients treated for 4–6 months with isotretinoin (mean daily dose of 0.56 mg per kg). Sixteen patients (23.5%) were "virtually clear" at the end of treatment, all of whom had mild or moderate HS at baseline. The authors concluded that isotretinoin had "limited value" in HS management. This study was followed by a retrospective series of 12 patients with Hurley stage II or III disease treated with acitretin at a mean dose of 0.59 mg per kg for 9–12 months [37]. Nine patients entered total remission, defined as at least 75% improvement in inflammation as measured with a physician's global assessment scale. All but one of the patients experienced clinically meaningful reduction in pain severity. Remission duration lasted between 6 and 45 months. The side effect profile was similar to what is seen for acitretin in psoriasis patients. Marked objective improvement observed in the majority of patients, coupled with substantial improvement in pain, must be tempered by the considerations that this was an uncontrolled retrospective study without a validated objective endpoint, and that acitretin is not practical to use in women of childbearing potential, who comprise the majority of HS patients.

Surgery

Surgical intervention is a complementary approach to managing HS, with potential advantages and disadvantages relative to medical therapy. Because sinus tracts are not expected to resolve with medical therapy, surgery is the only possible means by which these lesions can be definitively eliminated. Successful surgery may, by permanently removing skin prone to abscesses or inflammatory nodules, obviate the need for chronic medical therapy. Disadvantages of surgery are the postoperative morbidity, the risk of complications (e.g., wound infections or dehiscence, bleeding, and scarring limiting the range of motion), and the risk of recurrence (which is less acceptable than recurrence for patients who discontinue medical therapy because medical therapy is generally more tolerable). Surgical outcomes reported in case series or trials cannot be comprehensively evaluated unless the degree of postoperative morbidity; the risk, duration, and severity of surgical complications; and the risk of recurrence are included in the evaluation, and the risk of recurrence may be underestimated if follow-up duration is short.

Excision is the most commonly reported surgical technique employed to manage HS. After excision, surgical wounds may be closed primarily if they are relatively small or may be left to heal via secondary intention, flaps, or grafts if relatively large. Based on case series in which these different closure methods were employed, wounds that underwent primary closure had a higher recurrence risk, presumably because excisions small enough to undergo primary closure were too small to excise all diseased tissue (but to prove this presumption would require a study examining recurrence risk after mandating that methods other than primary closure be used for small wounds, which would be ethically ambiguous). Mandal and Watson [38] noted that among 100 of their patients treated with excision and primary closure, 70% had recurrences requiring additional surgery, but among 43 patients treated with excision and flap or graft, none experienced recurrence [38]. Median follow-up was 4 years; no information about the degree of postoperative pain or duration of postoperative recovery was provided. In a separate series of 31 patients treated with drainage, limited excision, or "radical wide excision" (defined as "all hair-bearing skin (with or without signs of HS) of the affected region with a clear margin of at least 1 cm"), recurrence rates requiring repeat surgery were 100%, 42.8%, and 27%, respectively (with a mean follow-up of 72 months) [39]. Further evidence about the potentially high risk of recurrence in HS wounds undergoing primary closure comes from a 200-patient placebo-controlled trial evaluating the efficacy and safety of placing a collagen matrix containing gentamicin (or placebo) in the wound bed of HS lesions excised and closed with primary intention healing [40]. Three-month recurrence rates were 40% in the gentamicin group and 42% in the control group. van Rappard et al.'s [41] recurrence rate following excision and primary closure was 23% (after a mean follow-up of 10 months). With recurrence rates following local excision and primary closure ranging from 23 to 70%, local cure with this approach is possible but unpredictable.

Larger-scale excisions can result in low recurrence rates, so long as diseased tissue is adequately removed and the surgeon and patient have the capability to manage wounds too large to undergo primary closure, and can manage and tolerate postoperative complications. Rompel and Petres [42] analyzed data from 106 of their HS patients who underwent excision after identification of all communicating branches of sinus tracts via intraoperative injection of methyl violet solution. Excision with this technique typically reached deep subcutaneous tissue or fascia. The different methods used for closure (primary closure, secondary intention, flaps, or grafts) did not influence the risk of complications, which were low (e.g., wound infections were observed in 3.7% of patients). The recurrence rate across the different closure methods was also low at 2.5%, with a median follow-up of 36 months. No information was provided about the extent or duration of postoperative morbidity such as time to wound healing, nor was recurrence defined. Similarly, among another set of 57 HS patients who underwent excision, followed either by primary closure, secondary intention healing, or skin grafting, no local recurrences were noted after a follow-up of 8.4–21.2 months [43]. Postoperative morbidity was not reported. Bohn and Svensson [44] summarized their experiences with 116 HS patients who received excisions extending down to fascia and out to 2 cm beyond the margin of clinically involved skin. Most patients needed split skin grafting. With an 8-year median postoperative follow-up, no patient experienced a relapse in the grafted sites. Anesthesia or paresthesia lasting longer than 3 months was common, and seven patients had limited range of motion of their shoulder persisting up to 5 months. Not all surgical series reporting on excisions replicated such good outcomes: complete clearance was noted in only 59.7% of 57 HS patients who underwent excision in one series [45] and Ritz et al.'s 27% recurrence risk with "radical wide excision" is noted above. Other than closure type (functioning as a proxy for wound size), factors reported to affect recurrence risk include location (axillary and perianal HS less likely to recur compared to inguinal or genital HS) [39] and female gender [46].

Surgical techniques other than scalpel excision have also been described. The STEEP technique ("skin-tissue-saving excision with electrosurgical peeling") is a series of tangential passes designed to progressively remove exclusively diseased tissue with electrosurgery. Blok et al. [46] report a recurrence rate of 29.2% and a wound infection rate of 1.8% after 482 operations and a median follow-up of 43 months [46].

For isolated, chronic lesions in patients with Hurley stage I or II disease, deroofing is a tissue-saving alternative to radical wide excision, as reported by van der Zee et al. [47]. Under local anesthesia, sinus tracts were delineated with a blunt probe, and the skin overlying the sinus tracts was removed with scalpel or electrosurgery. Debris within the sinus tracts was curetted, and the defect was allowed to heal via secondary intention. No recurrence was noted in 83% of the 88 treated lesions, with a median follow-up of 34 months. Mean healing time was 14 days.

The long-pulsed 1064 nm Nd:YAG laser has demonstrated significant efficacy in a prospective trial of patients with multiple involved anatomic regions, who had 4 monthly laser or control treatments randomized to different regions within the same patient [48]. Its mechanism of action in HS is unknown. For regions receiving laser therapy, the entire anatomic region was treated with a single pulse and inflammatory lesions received double pulses. One month after the last laser treatment, percentage improvement in modified Sartorius score among laser-treated regions was 63.6%, compared to 5.3% for control regions ($p < 0.001$). Seventeen of 22 patients (77%) completed all 4 treatments, and treated inflammatory lesions healed within 2–7 days. Recurrence rate after laser therapy completion was not studied.

Ablation of diseased tissue with a CO_2 laser is a relatively bloodless and tissue-sparing alternative to scalpel excision [49]. In this case series, ablation was performed in stages on 24 Hurley stage II patients, with the procedure repeated until all tissue not identified as normal subcutaneous fat was removed. Recurrence rate was 8% (2 of 24 treated sites) over a mean follow-up period of 24 months. Despite generating wound areas of 6–40 cm^2, postoperative pain requiring analgesics lasted no more than 4 days and most patients could resume daily activities within 3 weeks. The same group later improved upon this technique by using a scanner-assisted CO_2 laser, which automatically varies the direction of the laser beam and thereby makes the ablation less operator-dependent than the prior "freehand" method [50]. For more severely affected patients (Hurley stage III), CO_2 laser therapy to excise diseased tissue in cutting mode has been described in a retrospective case series of nine patients with 1-year follow-up [51]. Depending upon defect size, wounds underwent primary closure or secondary intention healing. One patient developed a local recurrence, and one developed postoperative wound dehiscence. A subsequent 61-patient series also reported low incidence of recurrence (with 2 patients experiencing recurrence at the edges of laser-treated areas) and low incidence of complications (3 postoperative cellulitis cases). Wounds averaged approximately 2 months to heal by secondary intention. Compared to scalpel excisions, CO_2 laser therapy is relatively bloodless, making it technically easier to visualize and eradicate subcutaneous sinus tracts. While these reports are promising, small patient numbers and follow-up limit inferences about long-term effectiveness and safety, and few surgeons have the equipment, expertise, or interest to perform CO_2 laser surgery on HS lesions.

Conclusions

Gulliver et al. have proposed an evidence-based approach to HS management (Fig. 36.2) [52]. Recommended first-line therapy for mild disease is twice daily topical clindamycin 1% lotion. For more widespread or severe disease, oral therapy is advised: tetracycline 500 mg twice daily for at least 4 months or, in case of more severe or recalcitrant disease, a 10-week course of clindamycin 300 mg twice daily and rifampin 600 mg once daily. For patients with an inadequate response to oral antibiotics, adalimumab at the HS-approved dose

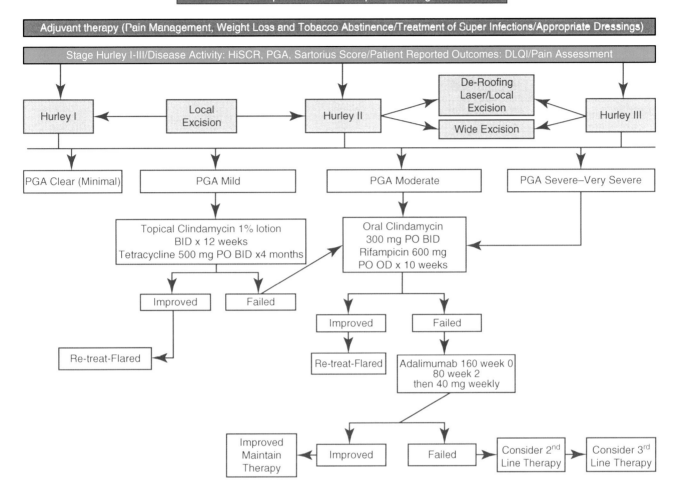

Fig. 36.2 Evidence-based HS treatment algorithm. Published in Gulliver W, Zouboulis CC, Prens E, Jemec GBE, and Tzellos T. Evidence-based approach to the treatment of hidradenitis suppura-tiva/acne inversa, based on the European guidelines for hidradenitis suppurativa. Rev Endocr Metab Disord. 2016;17:343–51

(160 mg at week 0, 80 mg at week 2, 40 mg weekly starting at week 4) is recommended. Surgical interventions personalized to the extent and severity of scarring or sinus tract formation, including options such as radical excision, deroofing, CO_2 laser, and Nd:YAG laser, are recommended to address those disease aspects not expected to respond to medical therapy.

The two therapeutic classes for which evidence is best are oral antibiotics and TNF monoclonal antibodies. The proportion of patients experiencing improvement with antimicrobial therapy are far higher than the proportion of patients with evidence from bacteriologic cultures of the presence of pathogenic bacteria. Because the reports on use of antimicrobial therapy are not placebo-controlled, it is possible that many of those patients who experienced improvement in their HS while receiving antimicrobial therapy may really be experiencing spontaneous waning in their disease severity that is unrelated to their antimi-

crobial therapy. Alternatively, the antimicrobial therapy may be exerting an anti-inflammatory effect or may be altering the proportions of commensal bacteria that are triggering inflammation in HS lesions, bacteria that are not easily cultured with routine bacteriological methods. Placebo-controlled trials of antimicrobial therapy in HS, preferably coupled with assessments of the cutaneous microbiomes before and after antimicrobial therapy, are needed to resolve this question. Antimicrobial therapy use in HS differs from use with true infectious dermatoses such as furunculosis because routine cultures are not warranted and should not be used to guide antimicrobial choice. The antibiotic therapy with the largest available efficacy and safety dataset in HS is combination clindamycin and rifampicin, which is typically administered for no more than 10 weeks because of the risk of inducing *C. difficile* colitis. Therapy with antibiotics in the tetracycline class or zinc gluconate is recommended to maintain disease control after completion of the 10-week clindamycin-rifampicin treatment regimen [20]. TNF monoclonal antibody therapy, particularly adalimumab, has the largest evidence base supporting efficacy and safety for treatment of HS. In the absence of head-to-head trials, it is not possible to use the adalimumab and other biologic trial outcomes to infer comparative efficacy and safety: there are confounding differences in the baseline population, in the primary efficacy measure, and in the endpoint. Among therapies other than oral antibiotics and TNF monoclonal antibodies, retrospective series for zinc gluconate and acitretin report efficacy results that are higher than what would be expected to occur with placebo.

Limited surgical interventions may complement medical therapies to remove isolated, intermittently inflamed sinus tracts, with the surgery expected to be technically easier after inflammation is better controlled. The benefits and risks of larger-scale excision and of Nd:YAG or CO_2 laser surgery are uncertain because of variability in the recurrence risk and insufficient information about their postoperative morbidity.

Given the many limitations in the evidence base for HS treatments, and the real-world constraints dictated by payors about which treatments can be used, clinicians may be obliged to utilize a treatment algorithm without having confidence that all the choices in the algorithm are effective. It is reasonable to engage in empiric trials of unproven medical therapies, so long as the clinician and patient have the discipline to abandon therapies that are not resulting in clinically relevant improvement, or, if response is partial, to supplement with additional therapies expected to act through different mechanisms (e.g., oral antibiotics and TNF monoclonal antibodies). The absence of evidence of toxicity from combining these two classes in the PIONEER II trial further supports this treatment tactic. Two practical means of assessing if clinically relevant improvement is occurring are to collect at baseline and at each follow-up visit abscess plus inflammatory nodule counts and DLQI scores, neither of which are burdensome to collect. Clinically relevant improvement corresponds to at least 50% reduction in abscess plus inflammatory nodule count relative to baseline and/or a decrease from baseline in DLQI scores of at least 4. The severe quality of life impairment resulting from HS, and the risk of disease progression in patients whose inflammatory disease is inadequately controlled, should spur clinicians to change therapies for patients who are languishing on suboptimal therapy.

Case Report

A 45-year-old white female presents with a history of inflammatory lesions in the perianal area and medial thighs that have been present since she was a teenager. Some of the lesions drain fluid. Once to twice per month, she develops severely painful abscesses which persist for approximately a week. The abscesses are more likely to appear during the last week of her menses. Past treatment with doxycycline 100 mg twice daily helped reduce the pain and drainage but failed to resolve the lesions. She denies arthritis, abdominal pain, or diarrhea.

Past medical history: Noncontributory

Social History

- Drinks socially (a few glasses of wine per week)
- Nonsmoker
- Single
- Office worker

Previous therapies: Oral doxycycline

Physical Exam

- Axilla and inframammary folds are clear
- Three draining fistulas on bilateral medial buttock cheeks
- Hypertrophic bridging scars, bilateral medial thighs
- DLQI score of 11

Management

Doxycycline 100 mg po twice daily was continued, and twice daily clindamycin lotion to affected areas was prescribed. Because of the history of flaring during menses, the patient was started on spironolactone 25 mg po bid, which was ultimately increased to a dose of 100 mg po bid. These interventions further reduced her drainage, but because she complained of persistent flares of her abscesses, adalimumab was initiated. The QuantiFERON Gold assay test was negative and she had negative hepatitis B serologies. Adalimumab dosing was 160 mg at week 0, 80 mg at week 2, and then 40 mg weekly starting at week 4. The patient noted pain reduction within the first week of therapy and has remained on topical clindamycin, doxycycline, spironolactone, and adalimumab for several months.

References

1. Kurzen H, Kurokawa I, Jemec GB, Emtestam L, Sellheyer K, Giamarellos-Bourboulis EJ, et al. What causes hidradenitis suppurativa? Exp Dermatol. 2008;17:455–6.
2. Vinding GR, Miller IM, Zarchi K, Ibler KS, Ellervik C, Jemec GBE. The prevalence of inverse recurrent suppuration: a population-based study of possible hidradenitis suppurativa. Br J Dermatol. 2014;170:884–9.
3. Ingram JR, Woo PN, Chua SL, Ormerod AD, Desai N, Kai AC, et al. Interventions for hidradenitis suppurativa: a Cochrane systematic review incorporating GRADE assessment of evidence quality. Br J Dermatol. 2016;174:970–8.
4. Rambhatla PV, Lim HW, Hamzavi I. A systematic review of treatments for hidradenitis suppurativa. Arch Dermatol. 2012;148:439–46.
5. Prens EP, Deckers I. Pathophysiology of hidradenitis suppurativa: an update. J Am Acad Dermatol. 2015;73:S8–11.

6. Kimball AB, Okun MM, Williams DA, Gottlieb AB, Papp KA, Zouboulis CC, et al. Two phase 3 trials of adalimumab for hidradenitis suppurativa. N Engl J Med. 2016;375:422–34.

7. Hurley H. Axillary hyperhidrosis, apocrine bromhidrosis, hidradenitis suppurativa, and familial benign pemphigus. In: Roenigk RK, Roenigk Jr HH, editors. Dermatologic surgery: principles and practice. New York: Marcel Dekker; 1989. p. 623–45.

8. Sartorius K, Emtestam L, Jemec GBE, Lapins J. Objective scoring of hidradenitis suppurativa reflecting the role of tobacco smoking and obesity. Br J Dermatol. 2009;161:831–9.

9. Kimball AB, Jemec GB, Yang M, Kageleiry A, Signorovitch JE, Okun MM, et al. Assessing the validity, responsiveness and meaningfulness of the hidradenitis suppurativa clinical response (HiSCR) as the clinical endpoint for hidradenitis suppurativa treatment. Br J Dermatol. 2014;171:1434–42.

10. van der Zee HH, de Ruiter L, van den Broecke DG, Dik WA, Laman JD, Prens EP. Elevated levels of tumor necrosis factor (TNF)-α, interleukin (IL)-1β, and IL-10 in hidradenitis suppurativa skin: a rationale for targeting TNF-α and IL-1β. Br J Dermatol. 2011;164:1292–8.

11. Lee RA, Dommasch E, Treat J, Sciacca-Kirby J, Chachkin S, Williams J, et al. A prospective clinical trial of open-label etanercept for the treatment of hidradenitis suppurativa. J Am Acad Dermatol. 2009;60:565–73.

12. Kimball AB, Kerdel F, Adams D, Mrowietz U, Gelfand JM, Gniadecki R, et al. Adalimumab for the treatment of moderate to severe hidradenitis suppurativa: a parallel randomized trial. Ann Intern Med. 2012;157:846–55.

13. Basra MK, Salek MS, Camilleri L, Sturkey R, Finlay AY. Determining the minimal clinically important difference and responsiveness of the dermatology life quality index (DLQI): further data. Dermatology. 2015;230:27–33.

14. Grant A, Gonzalez T, Montgomery MO, Cardenas V, Kerdel FA. Infliximab monotherapy for patients with moderate to severe hidradenitis suppurativa: a randomized, double-blind, placebo-controlled cross-over trial. J Am Acad Dermatol. 2010;62:205–17.

15. Tzanetakou V, Kanni T, Giatrakou S, Katoulis A, Papadavid E, Netea MG, et al. Safety and efficacy of anakinra in severe hidradenitis suppurativa. JAMA Dermatol. 2016;152:52–9.

16. Blok JL, Li K, Brodmerkel C, Horvátovich P, Jonkman MF, Horváth B. Ustekinumab in hidradenitis suppurativa: clinical results and a search for potential biomarkers in serum. Br J Dermatol. 2016;174:839–46.

17. Nikolakis G, Join-Lambert O, Karagiannidis I, Guet-Revillet H, Zouboulis CC, Nassif A. Bacteriology of hidradenitis suppurativa/acne inversa: a review. J Am Acad Dermatol. 2015;73:S12–8.

18. Wijaya A, Wulansari R, Amo H, Makimura S. Effect of clindamycin therapy on phagocytic and oxidative activity profiles of spleen mononuclear cells in *Babesia rodhaini*-infected mice. J Vet Med Sci. 2001;63:563–6.

19. Yerramasetti R, Gollapudi S, Gupta S. Rifampicin inhibits CD95-mediated apoptosis of Jurkat T cells via glucocorticoid receptors by modifying the expression of molecules regulating apoptosis. J Clin Immunol. 2002;22:37–47.

20. Gener G, Canoui-Poitrine F, Revuz JE, Faye O, Poli F, Gabison G, et al. Combination therapy with clindamycin and rifampicin for hidradenitis suppurativa: a series of 116 consecutive patients. Dermatology. 2009;219:148–54.

21. Mendonça CO, Griffiths CEM. Clindamycin and rifampin combination therapy for hidradenitis suppurativa. Br J Dermatol. 2006;154:977–8.

22. van der Zee HH, Boer J, Prens EP, Jemec GBE. The effect of combined treatment with oral clindamycin and oral rifampicin in patients with hidradenitis suppurativa. Dermatology. 2009;219:143–7.

23. Bettoli V, Zauli S, Borghi A, Toni G, Minghetti S, Ricci M, et al. Oral clindamycin and rifampicin in the treatment of hidradenitis suppurativa-acne inversa: a prospective study on 23 patients. J Eur Acad Dermatol Venereol. 2014;28:125–6.

24. Jemec GBE, Wendelboe P. Topical clindamycin versus systemic tetracycline in the treatment of hidradenitis suppurativa. J Am Acad Dermatol. 1998;39:971–4.

25. Kaur MR, Lewis HM. Hidradenitis suppurativa treated with dapsone: a case series of five patients. J Dermatolog Treat. 2006;17:211–3.

26. Yazdanyar S, Boer J, Ingvarsson G, Szepietowski JC, Jemec GBE. Dapsone therapy for hidradenitis suppurativa: a series of 24 patients. Dermatology. 2011;222:342–6.

27. Join-Lambert O, Coignard H, Jais JP, Guet-Revillet H, Poirée S, Fraitag S, et al. Efficacy of rifampin-moxifloxacin-metronidazole combination therapy in hidradenitis suppurativa. Dermatology. 2011;222:49–58.

28. Join-Lambert O, Coignard-Biehler H, Jais JP, Delage M, Guet-Revillet H, Poirée S, et al. Efficacy of ertapenem in severe hidradenitis suppurativa: a pilot study in a cohort of 30 consecutive patients. J Antimicrob Chemother. 2016;71:513–20.

29. Brocard A, Knol AC, Khammari A, Dréno B. Hidradenitis suppurativa and zinc: a new therapeutic approach. Dermatology. 2007;214:325–7.

30. Hessam S, Sand M, Meier NM, Gambichler T, Scholl L, Bechara FG. Combination of oral zinc gluconate and topical triclosan: an anti-inflammatory treatment modality for initial hidradenitis suppurativa. J Dermatol Sci. 2016;84:197–202.

31. Kraft JN, Searles GE. Hidradenitis suppurativa in 64 female patients: retrospective study comparing oral antibiotics and antiandrogen therapy. J Cutan Med Surg. 2007;11:125–31.

32. Lee A, Fischer G. A case series of 20 women with hidradenitis suppurativa treated with spironolactone. Australas J Dermatol. 2015;56:192–6.

33. Mortimer PS, Dawber RPR, Gales MA, Moore RA. A double-blind controlled cross-over trial of cyproterone acetate in females with hidradenitis suppurativa. Br J Dermatol. 1986;115:263–8.

34. Joseph MA, Jayaseelan E, Ganapathi B, Stephen J. Hidradenitis suppurativa treated with finasteride. J Dermatolog Treat. 2005;16:75–8.

35. Verdolini R, Clayton N, Smith A, Alwash N, Mannello B. Metformin for the treatment of hidradenitis suppurativa: a little help along the way. J Eur Acad Dermatol Venereol. 2013;27:1101–8.

36. Boer J, van Gemert MJP. Long-term results of isotretinoin in the treatment of 68 patients with hidradenitis suppurativa. J Am Acad Dermatol. 1999;40:73–6.

37. Boer J, Nazary M. Long-term results of acitretin therapy for hidradenitis suppurativa. Is acne inversa also a misnomer? Br J Dermatol. 2011;164:170–5.

38. Mandal A, Watson J. Experience with different treatment modules in hidradenitis suppurativa: a study of 106 cases. Surgeon. 2005;3:23–6.

39. Ritz JP, Runkel N, Haler J, Buhr HJ. Extent of surgery and recurrence rate of hidradenitis suppurativa. Int J Colorect Dis. 1998;13:164–8.

40. Buimer MG, Ankersmit MFP, Wobbes T, Klinkenbijl JHG. Surgical treatment of hidradenitis suppurativa with gentamicin sulfate: a prospective randomized study. Dermatol Surg. 2008; 34:224–7.

41. van Rappard DC, Mooij JE, Mekkes JR. Mild to moderate hidradenitis suppurativa treated with local excision and primary closure. J Eur Acad Dermatol Venereol. 2012;26:898–902.

42. Rompel R, Petres J. Long-term results of wide surgical excision in 106 patients with hidradenitis suppurativa. Dermatol Surg. 2000;26:638–43.

43. Kagan RJ, Yakuboff KP, Warner P, Warden GD. Surgical treatment of hidradenitis suppurativa: a 10-year experience. Surgery. 2005;138:734–41.

44. Bohn J, Svensson H. Surgical treatment of hidradenitis suppurativa. Scand J Plast Reconstr Surg Hand Surg. 2001;35:305–9.

45. Bienik A, Matusiak L, Okulewicz-Gojlik D, Szepietowski JC. Surgical treatment of hidradenitis suppurativa: experiences and recommendations. Dermatol Surg. 2010;36:1998–2004.

46. Blok JL, Boersma M, Terra JB, Spoo JR, Leeman FWJ, van den Heuvel ER, et al. Surgery under general anaesthesia in severe hidradenitis suppurativa: a study of 363 primary operations in 113 patients. J Eur Acad Dermatol Venereol. 2015;29:1590–7.

47. van der Zee HH, Prens EP, Boer J. Deroofing: a tissue-saving surgical technique for the treatment of mild to moderate hidradenitis suppurativa lesions. J Am Acad Dermatol. 2010;63:475–80.

48. Tierney E, Mahmoud BH, Hexsel C, Ozog D, Hamzavi I. Randomized control trial for the treatment of hidradenitis suppurativa with a neodymium-doped yttrium aluminum garnet laser. Dermatol Surg. 2009;35:1188–98.

49. Lapins J, Marcusson JA, Emtestam L. Surgical treatment of chronic hidradenitis suppurativa: CO_2 laser stripping-secondary intention technique. Br J Dermatol. 1994;131:551–6.

50. Lapins J, Sartorius K, Emtestam L. Scanner-assisted carbon dioxide laser surgery: a retrospective follow-up study of patients with hidradenitis suppurativa. J Am Acad Dermatol. 2002;47:280–5.

51. Madan V, Hindle E, Hussain W, August PJ. Outcomes of treatment of nine cases of recalcitrant severe hidradenitis suppurativa with carbon dioxide laser. Br J Dermatol. 2008;159:1309–14.

52. Gulliver W, Zouboulis CC, Prens E, Jemec GBE, Tzellos T. Evidence-based approach to the treatment of hidradenitis suppurativa/acne inversa, based on the European guidelines for hidradenitis suppurativa. Rev Endocr Metab Disord. 2016;17:343–51.

Systemic and Biologic Agents for Lupus Erythematosus

Daniel J. Wallace

Introduction

Lupus erythematosus is an autoimmune, pleomorphic disorder that afflicts over 500,000 individuals in the United States. Approximately half meet established criteria for a systemic disorder or SLE (systemic lupus erythematosus). Most of the remainder have variations of cutaneous lupus [1]. Table 37.1 lists the types of lupus. This chapter will restrict itself to systemic and biologic agents used in the management of LE. Clinical descriptions of subsets of LE are outside of the scope of this review.

Table 37.1 Lupus erythematosus

1. Lupus affecting the skin (prevalence in the United States about 300,000)
(a) Chronic cutaneous lupus erythematosus (CCLE)
• Classic discoid lupus erythematosus (DLE)—localized and generalized
• Hypertrophic/verrucous DLE
• Lupus panniculitis/profundus (dermal rather than epidermal)
• Mucous membrane involvement (oral cavity, nasal, genital, conjunctival)
• Tumid/papulomucinous lupus
• Chilblain lupus
• Lichenoid DLE (LE-lichen planus overlap)
(b) Subacute cutaneous lupus erythematosus (SCLE)
• Annular SCLE
• Papulosquamous/psoriasiform
• Vesiculobullous annular SCLE
• Toxic dermal necrolysis-like SCLE
(c) Acute cutaneous lupus erythematosus (ACLE)—nearly all have SLE
• Localized (malar rash)
• Generalized (morbilliform)
• Bullous LE
• Toxic epidermal necrolysis-like ACLE
(d) Lupus nonspecific skin disease
• Photosensitivity
• Alopecia
• Vasculitis—urticarial, purpuric, subcutaneous nodules, small vessel
• Vasculopathy
− Ischemic/vasomotor—Raynaud's, erythromelalgia, telangiectasias, dysautonomic
− Thromboembolic—related to antiphospholipid antibodies, cryoglobulins, calciphylaxis, or cholesterol crystals
• Miscellaneous—calcinosis, nail changes
2. Systemic lupus erythematosus <SLE> (US prevalence, approximately 250,000)
(a) Non-organ threatening
• Skin (see above)
• Musculoskeletal
• Constitutional (e.g., fatigue, fevers, weight loss)
• Serositis (pleural, pericardial, peritoneal)
(b) Organ threatening
• Cardiopulmonary
• Renal
• Central nervous system
• Hepatic/mesenteric vasculitis involvement
• Hematologic (e.g., hemolytic anemia, thrombocytopenia)
• Ophthalmic (e.g., retinal vasculitis)
3. Drug-induced lupus (15,000 new cases a year; 90% due to five drugs)
(a) Cases that disappear after withdrawal of offending agent (e.g., anti-TNFs, antiarrhythmics)
(b) Cases that can be long lasting (e.g., minocycline, DRESS syndrome)

(continued)

D.J. Wallace, MD, FACP, MACR
Cedars-Sinai Medical Center,
David Geffen School of Medicine Center at UCLA,
Attune Health 8750 Wilshire Blvd, Suite 350,
Beverly Hills, CA 90211, USA
e-mail: drdanielwallace@attunehealth.com

Table 37.1 (continued)

4.	Neonatal lupus (transient if no congenital heart block, <1000 cases a year, patients do not fulfill criteria for SLE)
5.	Overlap syndromes
(a)	Mixed connective tissue disease—must have antibodies to ribonucleoprotein (RNP); approximately 10,000 cases in the United States
(b)	Patients fulfilling criteria for lupus and scleroderma, rheumatoid arthritis, inflammatory myositis without anti RNP—prevalence not known
(c)	Lupus with Sjogren's syndrome (20% of SLE cases)

General Concepts of Managing Lupus Without Prescribing Anti-inflammatory Medication

A newly diagnosed lupus patient should have an educational session with their rheumatologist/primary caregiver that explains the complicated process [2]. It includes a review of physical and lifestyle measures, sun avoidance, distribution of written materials, and/or how to obtain access to responsible online information. The importance of adherence and compliance to treatment regimens should be emphasized. The discussion includes a review of the causes of fatigue (e.g., inflammatory, metabolic, medication, psychological) and how to deal with it, the role of exercise, and conditioning. Patients should be caused regarding tobacco avoidance, using alcohol in moderation, cold avoidance, and protective measures to manage Raynaud's. The role of a well-balanced diet is important, but there is no "anti-inflammatory" diet per se. Fifty percent with SLE use complementary and alternative medicine approaches. Only those that affect the sympathetic nervous system (e.g., stress reduction, meditation) have been shown to have any ameliorative effect [3].

Several preventive strategies have been shown to improve outcome in controlled studies. This includes sunscreens, being properly vaccinated, and regular health maintenance including screening for hypertension, diabetes, hyperlipidemia, and osteoporosis.

Topical Management for Cutaneous Lupus

The best-documented preventive interventions include sun avoidance and sun protection measures. Commercially available sunscreens consist of ultraviolet light-absorbing chemical agents in cream, oil, lotion, alcohol, gel, or foam vehicles that can block UVA, UVB, or both. An agent with a sun protection factor (SPF) of 15 blocks 93% of UVB rays, and a sunscreen with a UVB of 50 blocks only 5% more. Sun exposure is greatest midday and at higher altitudes. Up to 80% of UV rays penetrate cloud cover and can be reflected from water, concrete, sand, snow, tile, and reflective glass in buildings. Clothing provides more sun protection if it is loose fitting, lightweight in dark clothing, and accompanied by sunglasses and broad-brimmed hats [4].

Topical corticosteroids can be fluorinated or non-fluorinated and are sold in differing potencies in a variety of vehicles as ointments, gels, creams, adhesives, and lotions. Fifty years of experience have guided practitioners to the following regimen: (a) non-fluorinated (over the counter) creams are weak but safe for long-term use, especially for facial lesions, (b) fluorinated steroids are quite effective but should be used with caution for longer than 2 weeks on a facial lesion (possibly leading to cutaneous atrophy or telangiectasias), and (c) ointments are 80% absorbed and creams 20% and other vehicles fall in between. Creams are better tolerated but are drying; ointments are moisturizing. (d) Intralesional injections or occlusive dressings ameliorate focal areas of inflammation [5]. There has been surprisingly little evidence-based investigation in this area. For example, the Cochrane Database review for discoid lupus in 2009 could only find two trials for inclusion [6]. The development of the CLASI (Cutaneous Lupus Disease Area and Severity Index) in 2005 should change this outlook over the next few years [7]. Available topical steroid preparations in the United States are summarized below. The Food and Drug Administration (FDA) has seven levels of potency; agents can be in more than one level based on their concentration and vehicle. See Table 37.2.

Table 37.2 Examples of topical agents used for managing cutaneous lupus

1.	Calcinuerin inhibitors: pimecrolimus cream, tacrolimus ointment
2.	Corticosteroids (available as creams, ointments, gels, foams, lotions, sprays)
(a)	Class I (superhigh potency) betamethasone dipropionate, clobetasol propionate, halobetasol propionate
(b)	Class II (high potency): amcinonide, betamethasone dipropionate, desoximetasone, diflorasone diacetate, fluocinonide, halcinonide, mometasone furoate, triamcinolone acetonide
(c)	Class III (medium-high potency): amcinonide, betamethasone dipropionate, betamethasone valerate, desoximetasone, diflorasone diacetate, fluocinonide emollient, fluticasone propionate, triamcinolone acetonide, triamcinolone acetonide
(d)	Class IV (medium potency): betamethasone valerate, fluocinolone acetonide, hydrocortisone valerate, mometasone furoate, triamcinolone acetonide
(e)	Class V (medium-low potency): betamethasone dipropionate, betamethasone valerate, desonide, fluocinolone, flurandrenolide, fluticasone
(f)	Class VI (medium-low potency): hydrocortisone butyrate, hydrocortisone valerate, prednicarbate, triamcinolone acetonide
(g)	Class VII (low potency): alclometasone dipropionate, betamethasone valerate, clocortolone, desonide, fluocinolone, triamcinolone acetonide, hydrocortisone

Several calcineurin inhibitors have been studied for cutaneous lupus: tacrolimus ointment and pimecrolimus cream. Working by inhibiting T cells, these agents are widely available for eczema and are utilized for resistant lesions when steroids are not advisable.

Management of Systemic Lupus

Nonsteroidal Anti-inflammatory Agents (NSAIDs)

NSAIDs are used by 70–80% of all lupus patients, on at least an intermittent basis. Many do not realize that these over-the-counter agents (e.g., naproxen, ibuprofen) warrant additional scrutiny. None of these drugs are Food and Drug Administration approved for lupus, and there are only a handful of evidence-based studies that document their effectiveness. NSAIDs are not disease modifying and can be a bridge therapy until other agents are on board [8]. Patients with nephritis and other forms of organ involvement should be very careful with NSAIDs and limit their use to topical applications for joint discomfort (diclofenac gel is only 6% systemically absorbed) or short-term use for specific circumstances (less than a week for acute gout). There does not appear to be any adverse issues to taking an occasional ibuprofen for a headache and menstrual cramp, for example, if considered on a case-by-case basis.

A landmark National Institutes of Health study documented that ibuprofen and aspirin help fever associated with SLE, and lupus patients report amelioration of headache, fever, adenopathy, serositis, and musculoskeletal complaints [9]. Patients with non-organ-threatening disease who take NSAIDs on a regular basis should be monitored at least three to four times a year with blood pressure monitoring, a complete blood count, and chemistry panel. Aseptic meningitis has rarely been reported in lupus patients taking ibuprofen.

Antimalarials for Lupus

Antimalarials are a cornerstone in the management of lupus. Approximately 80% of all patients with systemic or cutaneous lupus have been prescribed one of these agents in the course of their disease. Over 95% of prescriptions are for hydroxychloroquine (HC), and the remainder for chloroquine and quinacrine. The latter is only available from compounding pharmacists.

Pharmacology
Chloroquine and HC are weakly basic 4-aminoquinoloine compounds, the latter differing by an –OH group attached to a side chain. Quinacrine is an acridine compound that differs from chloroquine by the presence of an extra benzene ring. Chloroquine is two to three times more potent than HC and more retinotoxic. Approximately 50% of HC contains the S-enantiomer, which has greater bioavailability, is eliminated more quickly, and is less toxic to the eyes. HC is nearly entirely absorbed by the gastrointestinal tract, 50% in 2–10 h and 50% bound by serum proteins. Some is conjugated with glucuronide and excreted in the bile, but 30–60% is biotransformed in the liver. HC is broken down to desethylchloroquine, desethyl hydroxychloroquine, and bidesthylchloroquine in two stages: a rapid one with a half-life of 3 days and a slower one with a half-life of 40 days. 45% is renally excreted, 3% by the skin, and 20% fecally. 21–47% of the drug is excreted without being metabolized. It takes 6 months to reach a 96% steady state. Much of HC is deposited into tissues and can be detected for up to 5 years after drug cessation. The dose of HC should be modestly reduced in patients with kidney failure, but patients on dialysis are more susceptible to ocular toxicity. Overdosage is not always ameliorated by dialysis as the drug is extensively sequestered into tissues. HC can interact with digoxin and salicylates and may have a quinidine-like effect. Blood concentrations of HC roughly correlate with response to therapy but are primarily most useful in assessing adherence and compliance [10, 11].

Mechanisms of Action
The effectiveness of antimalarials in lupus stems from a remarkable set of seemingly unrelated pathways, and the two most important are elaborated upon below [12].

Interference with lysosomal function: HC and chloroquine are weak bases with affinity for lysosomes. In order to function, intracellular toll-like receptors require an acidic pH. Antimalarials can prevent the functional transformation of intracellular toll-like receptors, which inhibit their activation. They can also accumulate in lysosomal structures, which decrease surface receptor areas available for cell signaling (especially with IL-6 with monocyte/macrophage-T cell activation) and hence have an anti-inflammatory effect.

Toll-like receptor (TLR)-associated mechanisms: Ineffective clearance of apoptotic cellular material provokes an inflammatory response. TLRs 3, 7, 8, and 9 can sense nucleic acids in intracellular compartments. Plasmacytic dendritic cells have a unique ability to couple the signaling pathways of TLR-7 and TLR-9 which leads to the production of large quantities of type I interferons and substantially increases transcription of type I interferon genes. HC can block the activation of TLRs, and thus this agent plays a major role in the innate immune process.

Table 37.3 summarizes these and other mechanisms of action relevant to antimalarials.

Table 37.3 Actions of antimalarials relevant to lupus

1.	Shown in well-designed studies to be clinically important
	(a) Effect of raising cellular pH on cell signaling and inflammatory pathways
	(b) Blocking activation of TLRs
	(c) Inhibition of ultraviolet light absorption
	(d) Ability to lower lipid levels via its lysosomotropic actions
	(e) Antithrombotic effects
	(f) Decreases serum glucose
	(g) Quinidine-like cardiac actions
	(h) Antimicrobial effects
2.	Theoretic mechanisms in at least pharmacologic doses
	(a) Anti-angiogenic effects (blocks vascular endothelial growth factor)
	(b) Matrix metalloproteinases and tissue inhibitors of metalloproteinases modulation
	(c) Inhibition of phospholipase A2, phospholipase C, and BLyS (B lymphocyte stimulation factor)
	(d) Decreases production of estrogen
	(e) Blockade of graft versus host reactions
	(f) Antiproliferative actions
	(g) Dissolution of circulating immune complexes
	(h) Antioxidant actions; blocks superoxide release
	(i) Induces apoptosis

Clinical Effects in Lupus

In seven controlled studies enrolling over 3000 patients, HC has been shown to demonstrate sustained beneficial effects on overall survival in a time-dependent manner, disease-free survival, and damage accrual [12, 13]. This includes a protective effect against renal damage and major infections. Further, antimalarials may delay the onset of SLE and reduces the number of and severity of clinical flares. The early use of HC maximizes the above benefits. All three antimalarials have lipid-lowering properties that are especially apparent in patients taking corticosteroids and can be beneficial on glycemic status (which increases with duration of use). Tobacco smoking reduces the efficacy of antimalarial doses, and HC appears safe with pregnancy and lactation.

In the cutaneous lupus literature, HC is the initial agent of choice, and more than 50% of patients respond to HC alone. If HC monotherapy fails, the addition of quinacrine can be beneficial. Infrequently, a combination of chloroquine and quinacrine improves the CLASI score and is steroid sparing. More than 70% of lupus patients with non-organ-threatening disease have a favorable response to HC. Usually, patients are started on 5 mg/kg/day dosing for a 12–16-week trial. Sometimes, flares or refractory cases respond to 7 mg/kg dosing for no more than 3 months' use [14]. See Fig. 37.1.

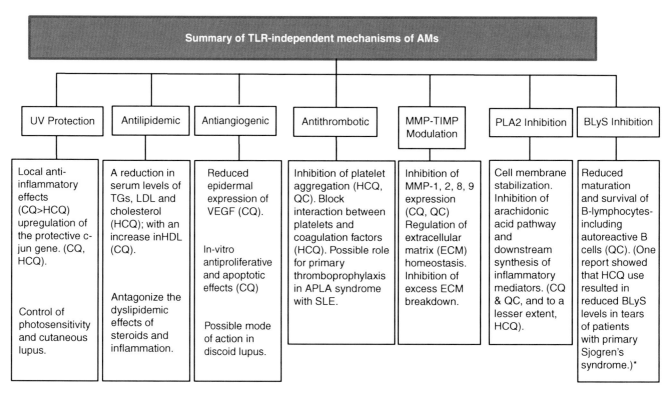

Fig. 37.1

Adverse Reactions

From 1 to 10% of lupus patients prescribed hydroxychloroquine experience skin (dryness, pigment, pruritus, urticarial, rashes, or hair loss) or gastrointestinal (anorexia, distention, cramping, nausea, vomiting, diarrhea, weight loss) complications. Non-retinal eye changes can be related to corneal edema or visual changes. Rare but important side effects include mental status alterations, cardiomyopathy, and cytopenias. Toxicity tends to be dose and duration and related to hepatic and renal function. Improved drug tolerance is associated with splitting or lowering the dose [15].

Corneal edema with light sensitivity is a common but easily reversible finding that normalizes within days of drug withdrawal and may occur on rechallenge. New and improved imaging techniques, especially the SD OCT (spectral domain optical coherence tomography), have changed the way antimalarials should be monitored for retinal eye toxicity. At recommended doses (using no more than 5 mg/kg/day), the risk of toxicity up to 5 years is less than 1%, under 2% at 10 years, but up to 20% after 20 years. Most damage to the retinal is parafoveal but infrequently can be extramacular. After 10 years, the alterations are often irreversible [16]. In 2016, the American Academy of Ophthalmology published monitoring guidelines. In the absence of significant renal impairment, screening should involve the SD OCT, multifocal electroretinogram, and fundus autofluorescence during the first year of therapy, at 5 years and annually thereafter. Chloroquine is more toxic than hydroxychloroquine and quinacrine rarely if ever affects the eyes [17].

Corticosteroids

Corticosteroid therapy is the cornerstone for managing SLE, with up to 80% of patients having taken the drug during the course of their disease. Although available as dexamethasone (sometimes used for central nervous system disease), prednisolone (especially in children), and hydrocortisone (for adrenal insufficiency, refractory fevers or for rapid onset in emergency settings), prednisone accounts for over 90% of steroid prescriptions. For lupus patients with organ-threatening disease (heart, lung, kidney, liver, central nervous system, bone marrow), the usual dose is 0.5–1 mg/kg/day for 4–12 weeks at induction, followed by tapering by up to 10% a week once a response is achieved. In some cases, a steroid sparing agent, either an immune suppressive or a targeted therapy is added to the regimen in the first 1–2 months [18]. Interestingly, there had only been a handful of studies in the last 40 years documenting the efficacy of corticosteroids until targeted therapy trials used steroid sparing as a secondary outcome measure [19, 20].

Half with SLE have manifestations including fatigue, fever, arthritis, serositis, rash, oral ulcers, and adenopathy. These individuals who do not have organ involvement respond to prednisone therapy in doses ranging from 5 to 20 mg daily in the majority of cases. Each person with lupus has a different set of individual circumstances that warrant specialized consideration of what the optimal dose should be. Evidence has shown that the long-term complications of corticosteroids in lupus (e.g., cataracts, glaucoma, bone demineralization, bloating, weight gain, mood changes) occur infrequently if prednisone dosing is kept below adrenal replacement levels (6 mg of prednisone daily or less). Inability to do this is an indication for introduction of an immune suppressive or targeted therapy. Patients who tolerate steroids poorly due to concomitant diabetes, metabolic syndrome, and propensity for developing avascular necrosis should be more aggressively managed to minimize their use [21].

Mild lupus flares can be managed with steroid injections (e.g., triamcinolone or methylprednisolone 40–120 mg IM) or with intraarticular use. Serious systemic flares may be ameliorated by pharmacologic dosing, or "pulse medrol," where patients are infused with 1G of methylprednisolone for at least one and up to 5 days [22, 23].

Corticosteroids work within hours to days and are very effective in the short term, but long-term studies suggest that over time they accelerate renal scarring in nephritis patients, promote accelerated atherogenesis, and raise the lupus damage index [24]. Table 37.4 summarizes the actions and use of glucocorticoids in SLE.

Table 37.4 Glucocorticoids for systemic lupus erythematosus

1.	Important anti-inflammatory and immune suppressive effects on cell types
	(a) Neutrophils: Inhibits adhesion to endothelial cells and migration to tissues, mobilization from bone marrow and neutrophilia, inhibits apoptosis and leukoagglutination
	(b) Eosinophils: Apoptosis and eosinopenia
	(c) Basophils and mast cells: Inhibits mast cell degranulation and cytokine production
	(d) Monocytes and macrophages: Decreases activation, cytokine, and destructive enzyme secretion. Blocks type I interferon signaling, phagocytosis of apoptotic neutrophils, acts as antioxidant, monocytopenia, migration of anti-inflammatory macrophages to sites of inflammation

(continued)

Table 37.4 (continued)

(e)	Dendritic cells and plasmacytic dendritic cells: Apoptosis, blocks migration to lymph nodes, inhibition of plasmacytic cell differentiation, induction of tolerance	
(f)	Lymphocytes: Lymphopenia especially at CD4 T cells, T-cell apoptosis, blockade of T-cell receptor signaling, less T-cell migration to tissues, suppression of Th1 and to a lesser extent Th2 cells and Th17 and IL-17, increase in T-reg cell development	
2.	Usual regimens of systemic glucocorticoid therapy	
(a)	Pulse glucocorticoid regimen: >250 mg methylprednisolone for 1–5 days parenterally for life- or organ-threatening indications (e.g., myelopathy, vasculitis, alveolar hemorrhage)	
(b)	Very-high-dose glucocorticoid: 100–249 mg methylprednisolone or prednisone daily IV or oral for life- or organ-threatening disease (e.g., hemolytic anemia, optic neuritis, severe nephritis)	
(c)	High-dose glucocorticoid: 30–100 mg daily methylprednisolone or prednisone for < 6–8 weeks (e.g., acute lupus pneumonitis, thrombocytopenia)	
(d)	Moderate-dose glucocorticoids: 7.5–30 mg of prednisone equivalent orally used for example for myositis, pleuritis, thrombocytopenia	
(e)	Low-dose glucocorticoids: <7.5 mg prednisone daily orally for maintenance therapy, arthritis, mild constitutional symptoms especially if underresponsive to analgesics, nonsteroidals, and antimalarials	
(f)	Alternate-day glucocorticoids: Used during tapering or complications of lupus when patient has no symptoms (e.g., nephritis) to preserve hypothalamic pituitary axis	
(g)	Lupus flare bursts: Oral methylprednisolone dosepak or injection of triamcinolone/methylprednisolone/betamethasone for mild flares	
3.	Examples of side effects of glucocorticoids in different systems	
(a)	Fluid/electrolyte: Sodium retention, edema, increased potassium excretion	
(b)	Gastrointestinal: Nausea/vomiting, weight gain, distension, pancreatitis, ulceration, gastritis	
(c)	Endocrine: Adrenal insufficiency, altered menses, glucose intolerance, hyperlipidemia, metabolic syndrome	
(d)	Cardiovascular: Hypertension, accelerated atherogenesis	
(e)	Hematologic: Hypercoagulability, leukocytosis	
(f)	Ocular: Posterior subcapsular cataracts, glaucoma	
(g)	Musculoskeletal: Muscle pain/weakness, osteoporosis/fractures, avascular necrosis	
(h)	Neuropsychiatric: Psychosis, mood disturbances, seizures, insomnia	
(i)	Dermatologic: Acne, impaired wound healing, hirsutism, ecchymoses, and skin fragility	
(j)	Other: Increase susceptibility to infection	

Immune-Suppressive Therapies Used in Lupus Patients

Although methotrexate has been available since 1948, and azathioprine and cyclophosphamide since the 1960s, no immune suppressives are approved for use in SLE. However, they are highly effective and steroid sparing in many lupus clinical settings. Interestingly, over any given year in the United States, only 5–10% of all lupus patients are taking an immune-suppressive therapy, as opposed to 30–50% being on nonsteroidal anti-inflammatory agents, corticosteroids, or antimalarials [25].

Cyclophosphamide

Cyclophosphamide (Cytoxan) contributes alkyl groups to DNA, forming covalent linkages. Metabolized to 4-hydroxycyclophosphamide and aldophosphamide by liver cytochrome P450 enzyme, this alkylating agent is a powerful agent that depletes T and B cells, alters macrophage production as well as gene transcription, and suppresses antibody production [26]. A predecessor prodrug drug, nitrogen mustard, became available in 1947 and was initially used to manage cutaneous lupus. Cyclophosphamide became available in 1965. The drug is almost always used intravenously but was widely administered orally until about 1990 until this method of administration was found to be less safe. There are still parts of the world, especially Asia, where it used orally as the parenteral forms are either not available or prohibitively expensive. Twenty percent of cyclophosphamide is excreted by the kidney, and 80% is processed in the liver. It has a half-life of 6 h, and favorable responses are noted within several weeks.

Cyclophosphamide is used in the clinic in low dosages (Eurolupus regimen or 500 mg every 2 weeks for 6 cycles), high dosages (National Institutes of Health regimen of 750 mg/M2 for 6 months with an option of every 2–3 months for 2–3 years), or ablative regimens (e.g., 50 mg/kg/day for 4 days for stem cell induction) [27–29]. It can be employed as monotherapy or in combination with corticosteroids and other agents. The most common uses in SLE are nephritis, alveolitis, generalized systemic vasculitis, central nervous system vasculitis, and hematologic complications such as hemolytic anemia, thrombocytopenia, and thrombotic thrombocytopenic purpura [30]. The nadir of blood counts is between day 7 and 14, and there increased infection risk during this time.

The most common side effects are nausea, vomiting, hair thinning, and reversible alopecia. Less commonly seen are mucosal ulcerations, gynecologic dysplasias, hepatotoxicity, and significant bone marrow suppression. Patients receiving cyclophosphamide must be well hydrated, and the oral form is associated with an increased risk for hemorrhagic cystitis and ultimately bladder cancer if this precaution is not undertaken [31]. Antiemetics such as ondansetron often are helpful, and 2-mercaptoethane intravenous administration is used if hematuria is present to protect the bladder. There is evidence that the administration of leuprolide acetate (3.75 mg subcutaneously q 4 weeks) decreases the risk of premature ovarian failure (estimated to occur in at least 80% in females over the age of 30 receiving the drug) [32].

Azathioprine

Azathioprine (Imuran) is a purine synthesis inhibitor converted to the active metabolites 6-mercaptopurine and 6-thionosinic acid. It reduces numbers of circulating B and T lymphocytes, immunoglobulin synthesis, and CD28-mediated costimulation. Azathioprine is transformed to 6-mercaptopurine by glutathione, and this agent is commonly used for inflammatory bowel disease. It is 20–30% protein bound, is 98% renally excreted, and has a biological half-life of 3–5 h [33].

Azathioprine is mostly prescribed as a steroid-sparing agent. Its primary use is for inflammatory arthritis, nephritis, severe cutaneous disease, pneumonitis, hepatitis, autoimmune hemolytic anemia, and thrombocytopenia [34]. A poor agent for induction therapy, it is frequently prescribed in combination with corticosteroids and other immune suppressives. Therapy is usually initiated at 50 mg daily orally for the first week and built up to 150 mg daily or about 3 mg/kg/day over several weeks, and favorable responses are apparent in 8–12 weeks. About 10% of patients are unable to tolerate the drug due to deficiency of the enzyme thiopurine methyltransferase (TPMT) that can be pretested for where they experience nausea, bone marrow toxicity, rash, or fever [35]. Generally, azathioprine is very well tolerated, but 10–20% report nausea. Cytopenias and transaminase elevations are common but do not cause symptoms and require monitoring. Azathioprine is associated with an increased prevalence of cervical dysplasias and, after 10–20 years of use, lymphoma [36]. The agent has an excellent safety record for patients who wish to conceive. Patients usually have laboratory testing performed monthly for the first 3 months and every 2–3 months thereafter. Concomitant use of allopurinol is a contraindication to the use of azathioprine.

Very few studies have evaluated the use of azathioprine as monotherapy for lupus. However, it has been shown to decrease inflammation in general and has been approved for rheumatoid arthritis, and numerous studies have documented its efficacy in combination with other agents for nephritis [37, 38].

Methotrexate

Methotrexate has been available since 1948 and is used for a wide variety of diseases, ranging from cancer to psoriasis to autoimmune inflammatory disorders such as vasculitis, inflammatory bowel disease, and rheumatoid arthritis. In the latter category, the drug works by inhibiting dihydrofolate reductase, and primarily inhibition of enzymes thought to be involved with purine metabolism, leading to the accumulation of adenosine, inhibition of T-cell activation, and selective downregulation of B cells [39]. In rheumatic diseases, methotrexate is administered orally, subcutaneously, or intramuscularly once a week. It is 35–50% protein bound, metabolized hepatically and intracellularly, and 80–100% excreted in the urine. Dosing should be reduced by 50–75% if renal impairment is present [40].

Methotrexate is administered in doses of 7.5–25 mg weekly, and favorable responses can be seen in 4–12 weeks. Two controlled lupus trials have demonstrated that it is steroid sparing, reduces disease activity, and slows the damage index [41, 42]. It is primarily effective for inflammatory arthritis and cutaneous, serosal, and constitutional symptoms. It is not recommended for interstitial lung disease, hepatitis, cytopenias, or nephritis. In large published controlled trials with belimumab, tabalumab, epratuzumab, rituximab, and abatacept enrolling over 5000 patients, approximately 10–15% of the patients were also taking methotrexate [43–47]. In these trials, 30–50% of patients receiving standard of care (e.g., prednisone, antimalarials, nonsteroidals) with or without a study drug had improvement in clinical indices [48].

Methotrexate is contraindicated in pregnancy, and patients should not drink alcohol or severely restrict its use due to hepatotoxicity. Common adverse effects include nausea, oral ulcerations, hair loss, fatigue, fever, and headache.

Very few studies have evaluated methotrexate as monotherapy for SLE, but several clinical trials enrolling several thousand patients have allowed this agent to be a concomitant medication in doses ranging from 10 to 25 mg weekly.

Mycophenolic Acid

Mycophenolate mofetil (MMF, Cell Cept) is a prodrug of mycophenolic acid that inhibits inosine-5′-monophosphate dehydrogenase. By preferentially depleting guanosine nucleotides in T and B lymphocytes, it inhibits their proliferation, thereby suppressing cell-mediated immune responses and antibody formation. Over 90% protein bound, MMF is hepatically metabolized, and 93% excreted in the urine. Its biologic half-life is approximately 18 h [49]. Taken orally, its anti-inflammatory actions become apparent in 2–4 weeks. Mycophenolate sodium (Myfortic) minimizes gastrointestinal side effects of mycophenolic acid. Dosing in lupus ranges from 500 mg a day (renal transplant rejection protection) to 3000 mg a day (severe nephritis).

MMF has been used since 1990, but lupus studies were not published until the early 2000s. It appears to be very effective for nephritis, modestly helpful for interstitial lung disease, vasculitis, and chronic cutaneous lupus [50, 51]. Some evidence suggests that it is ameliorative in lupus pemphigoid and lichen planus. MMF did not fare well in rheumatoid arthritis trials and is probably weakly effective in lupus arthritis [52, 53]. In clinical trials, it is well tolerated with other lupus agents and may be synergistic with belimumab.

Between 10 and 30% have gastrointestinal complaints (nausea, vomiting diarrhea), and half of these patients are unable to take it as a result. MMF is contraindicated in pregnancy. Bone marrow suppression is monitored by obtaining monthly labs for the first 3 months and every 3 months thereafter [54].

Less Commonly Used Systemic Agents: Used by Less Than 1% of SLE Patients in a Given Year

Calcineurin inhibitors include *cyclosporine A*, *tacrolimus*, and *rapamycin*. These preparations inhibit the transcription of interleukin 2 and other cytokines in T cells. They decrease T-cell proliferation and reduce antigen preparation and T-cell autoantibody production. All three preparations are given daily, orally, work within days, and have multiple drug interactions that should be reviewed prior to initiating therapy. All are used in post-organ transplant rejection regimens, which included lupus patients. Cyclosporine is used in doses of 50–200 mg a day for lupus nephritis, refractory rashes (especially psoriasiform or eczematous), or bone marrow hypoplasias [55, 56]. Tacrolimus is available as a topical preparation for cutaneous lupus and is used with other agents for nephritis, especially in Asia [57, 58]. Rapamycin is an antirenal allograft rejection drug and is being evaluated in ongoing clinical trials for generalized lupus [59]. All these agents raise blood pressure, have neurologic complications such as paresthesias, increase uric acid levels which can induce gout, and induce generalized gastrointestinal upset. Infectious complications are rare.

Leflunomide (Arava) is approved in the United States for rheumatoid arthritis. It is 80% bioavailable, 99% protein bound, metabolized in the GI mucosa and liver, and is equally excreted in the feces and urine. A pyrimidine synthesis inhibitor that works by inhibiting dihydroorotate dehydrogenase, this potent agent is as effective as methotrexate in head-to-head rheumatoid arthritis trials [60]. Effective in 30 days, it is contraindicated in pregnancy and can stay in the system for up to 6 months after its discontinuation. Leflunomide is approved in China for lupus nephritis and, in small-scale lupus arthritis trials in the United States, appears to have some efficacy [61, 62]. At least 20% of users experience diarrhea or loose stools.

Antileprosy drugs such as *dapsone*, *thalidomide*, and *lenalidomide* are infrequently used for refractory cutaneous lupus complications including cutaneous lupus, bullous lupus, cutaneous vasculitis, and urticarial [63, 64]. *Dehydroepiandrosterone (DHEA)* is available over the counter or via a compounding pharmacist and has modest effects on fatigue and disease activity but can have undesirable androgenic effects [65].

The removal of plasma using a centrifugation cell separator or a membrane device and its replacement with albumin or protein is known as *plasmapheresis*. It is used for lupus patients with life- or organ-threatening complications of the disease such as cryoglobulinemia, hyperviscosity syndrome, alveolar hemorrhage, neuromyelitis optica, and alveolar hemorrhage [66].

Table 37.5 Immune-suppressive and other nonbiologic regimens for SLE

Agent	Comment
Cyclophosphamide	Most powerful agent available, cytotoxic, used for life- or organ-threatening involvement
Azathioprine	Well-tolerated agent popular for maintenance therapy and in steroid-sparing regimens
Methotrexate, leflunomide	Mostly used for lupus arthritis
Mycophenolic acid	Highly effective for nephritis and used for interstitial lung disease and selected cutaneous manifestations
Calcineurin inhibitors	Mostly used in nephritis, anti-transplant rejection regimens
Antileprosy drugs	Used primarily for forms of cutaneous lupus
Apheresis	Cryoglobulinemia, hyperviscosity, TTP, alveolar hemorrhage
Dehydroepiandrosterone	Fatigue and aching in patients with mild disease
Intravenous immune globulin, ITP, polyneuritis, hypogammaglobulinemia	

Intravenous immune globulin (IVIg) binds to receptors on antigen-presenting cells and increases expression of an inhibitory Fc receptor that shortens the life of autoreactive antibodies. In SLE, it has been used for severe hypogammaglobulinemia, idiopathic thrombocytopenic purpura, and acute inflammatory polyneuropathies [67, 68].

Immune-suppressive regimens for SLE are summarized in Table 37.5.

Targeted Therapies for Lupus

Targeted or biologic therapies for SLE consist of those approved by the Food and Drug Administration for the disease and those that are available for other disorders but have not received approval for lupus.

Belimumab

Belimumab was approved in March 2011 for autoantibody-positive SLE on the basis of two pivotal trials that demonstrated that it met the previously set conditions of the SRI (Systemic Lupus Responder Index). This included a four-point reduction in the SLEDAI (Systemic Lupus Erythematosus Disease Activity Index) score, no new organ domain involvement as measured by the BILAG (British Isles Lupus Assessment Group), and no more than a 10% change in the physicians' global assessment that was statistically significant when compared to a group of patients also receiving standard of care but not belimumab [45, 69, 70]. Retrospectively, nearly all the patients had musculoskeletal or cutaneous disease. Central nervous system and anything more than mild disease was an exclusion from participation. It is a human monoclonal antibody to soluble (but not membrane bound) B-lymphocyte stimulator given intravenously over 1–2 h and is very well tolerated.

Since its approval, approximately 30,000 patients have received the drug as of 2016. No significant safety signals have been noted, and a pregnancy registry to date has recorded no problems. Seven-year follow-ups continue to demonstrate effectiveness of this drug. Belimumab is given at week 0, 2, and 4 followed by monthly dosing, and clinical improvement is usually noted by the 5th dose [71]. Its clinical use is most common or in patients with active disease despite the use of nonsteroidals, antimalarials, low-dose prednisone, and immune suppressives in patients who have difficulty tolerating any combination of these agents [72]. The agent's effectiveness for other organ systems or in children is currently under study, and a subcutaneous version is expected to be available in 2017 or 2018.

Targeted Therapies Approved for Other Rheumatic Diseases But Not Lupus

Abatacept, rituximab, and anti-IL-6 and anti-TNF (tumor necrosis factor) agents have been studied and are occasionally used in refractory cases of SLE. Abatacept (Orencia) is approved for rheumatoid arthritis and works by blocking co-stimulation of the CTLA4-Ig pathway of T cells. It did not meet its primary endpoint in nephritis and non-nephritis trials, but several secondary endpoints and improvement signals were apparent in post hoc analyses suggesting it may be beneficial in certain subsets of patients (e.g., arthritis, nephritis) [45, 73, 74]. Further studies are ongoing. Rituximab is an anti-CD 20 chimeric monoclonal antibody that failed to meet its primary endpoints in both nephritis and non-nephritis trials. This agent is widely used for rheumatoid arthritis, but both lupus studies mandated that the placebo and rituximab arms of the protocol include the administration of highly effective therapies: corticosteroids and immune suppressives. Both groups improved, and this underpowered study and its open-label follow-up were discontinued prematurely. There is evidence from cohort studies and case series that selected patients with lupus nephritis (given with cyclophosphamide and MMF for example), lupus arthritis, hemolytic anemia, and thrombocytopenia respond to this agent. Agents blocking interleukin-6 may have some promise [47, 75–77]. Tocilizumab had a positive phase I trial at the

National Institutes of Health, but efforts by two pharmaceutical companies with different preparations did not meet their primary endpoints. However, one dosing regimen of PF-04236921 did significantly improve several secondary outcome measures [78, 79]. Antibodies to TNF such as infliximab and etanercept used for rheumatoid arthritis have been studied in SLE with generally disappointing results and can increase formation of anti-dsDNA and antiphospholipid antibodies [80].

Targeted Therapies Under Study

As of January 2017, approximately 30 biologic agents are under study for SLE. Some of the most promising include those that target T cells (e.g., anti CD-40L), toleragens, B cells (two agents similar to belimumab), blockers of complement activation, anticytokines (anti-IL-6, IL-17, anti-IL-23), agents targeting the innate immune system (e.g., those that block interferon or toll receptor activation), or the human kinome (e.g., BTK and JAK inhibitors) [81].

Management of Additional Organ Domains

Constitutional Manifestations

Fatigue, fever, weight loss, and malaise resulting from active inflammation if infection is ruled out respond to nonsteroidal anti-inflammatory agents, antimalarials, and 0.5 mg/kg of prednisone equivalent for at least several weeks.

Cutaneovascular Disease

The management of cutaneous lupus was reviewed earlier. Raynaud's, chilblains, and cutaneous vasculitis are treated with vasodilators (e.g., calcium channel blockers, 5-phosphodiesterase blockers, prostaglandins) in addition to managing the underlying disease [82].

Musculoskeletal Lupus

Nonsteroidals, antimalarial drugs, and corticosteroids all improve synovitis and inflammatory arthritis seen in SLE. The choice of therapy depends on the areas of involvement, duration, and severity of symptoms and amount and degree of disease activity outside of the musculoskeletal system. When indicated, methotrexate or leflunomide is helpful. Low-dose corticosteroids and belimumab are also effective [83].

Nervous System Lupus

Central nervous system vasculitis responds to high-dose corticosteroids (often given in pharmacologic doses, or pulse steroids at 1000 mg of methylprednisolone daily for 3 days). The addition of cyclophosphamide, rituximab, or apheresis is often beneficial [84].

Patients with antiphospholipid antibodies may have cerebrovascular accidents and should be anticoagulated. Individuals who have never had a thromboembolic event but are considered at risk are often placed on platelet antagonists, such as low-dose aspirin (81 mg daily) [85].

Peripheral or cranial neuritis, including mononeuritis multiplex, responds to 0.5 mg of prednisone daily for several weeks, followed by tapering [86].

Cognitive dysfunction, or "lupus fog," is a vasculopathy, and if a lumbar puncture rules out vasculitis (i.e., normal cell count, protein, oligoclonal bands, IgG synthesis rate, myelin basic protein), it is treated with biofeedback, cognitive behavioral therapy, mindfulness, anxiety reduction measures, and management of the underlying disease [87].

Lupus Nephritis

Assuming most patients with SLE and renal disease undergo a biopsy, Class I (normal histology, minor electron microscopy changes) is not treated. Mesangial nephritis (Class II) responds to 20 mg of prednisone equivalent daily for 3 months. Patients with proliferative nephritis (Classes III and IV) have a significant risk of evolving renal failure over a 10-year period of observation. A variety of protocols including high-dose corticosteroid for at least 2–3 months alongside immune suppression with cyclophosphamide, azathioprine, mycophenolate, tacrolimus, or rituximab alone or in combination are used tailored to the patient's specific needs [88, 89]. Membranous nephritis represents 15% of renal disease and has a more indolent course [90]. The above regimens are used but less aggressively. Additionally, hypertension and other comorbidities should be managed with medications that are vasodilators and antiatherogenic. Interstitial changes may be more important than glomerular changes, and new metrics to define and stage this finding are in development [91].

Cardiopulmonary Disease

Serositis responds to nonsteroidals and corticosteroids. Immune suppressives are rarely needed. Serious complications including lupus pneumonitis and pulmonary hemorrhage are managed with corticosteroids, cyclophosphamide, or mycophenolate and rarely apheresis. Interstitial lung disease frequently overlaps with Sjogren's syndrome and may be ameliorated by mycophenolate or rituximab in addition to corticosteroids. Pulmonary embolism (treated with anticoagulation) and pulmonary hypertension (treated with endothelial cell activation antagonists, sildenafil, or other vasodilators) are found in about 5% with SLE [92, 93]. Lupus patients have up to a 50-fold increase in myocardial infarctions and show evidence for accelerated atherogenesis. Patients should be screened for hypertension, hyperlipidemia, and hyperglycemia and, when indicated, baseline electrocardiograms, 2D echo, and carotid duplex scanning should be obtained [94, 95].

Cytopenias in SLE

If low blood counts due to medications are ruled out, cytopenias are common in lupus. Anemia is managed according to its cause (e.g., low vitamin B12, folic acid, iron deficiency, heavy periods, inflammation leading to bone marrow suppression). Hemolytic anemias require aggressive management with high-dose corticosteroids and respond well to rituximab [96]. Leukopenias are usually due to active disease and medication. Qualitative platelet disorders are common but do not require treatment. Autoimmune thrombocytopenia responds to corticosteroids and immune suppression, rituximab, intravenous immune globulin, or splenectomy as needed [97]. Thrombotic thrombocytopenic purpura is a very serious complication of SLE (up to 50% mortality) that is managed with combinations of corticosteroids, apheresis, and rituximab [98].

Summary

SLE is a complex, multisystem inflammatory process. Its management warrants staging the patient for organ domain activity and coordinating considerations of a diverse array of medications and managing comorbidities. Although little has changed over the last 50 years, many new therapeutic approaches are being studied in ongoing clinical trials.

Case Report for Biologic and Systemic Therapies in Dermatology

A 46-year-old African American female presented with diffuse joint aches and malar rash 3 years ago. Laboratory testing showed a positive antinuclear antibody (1:160, homogeneous), sedimentation rate of 30, and CRP three times normal, and C3 complement was 10 points below the normal range. A diagnosis of systemic lupus erythematosus was made. She was started on hydroxychloroquine 400 mg a day. Although her joints ached less, her rash spread to sun-exposed areas, and she became increasingly fatigued.

Prednisone 10 mg a day was started, but her blood sugars rose into diabetic ranges, and metformin was started. Methotrexate was initiated but she vomited every time she took it.

Past Medical History

Hypertension

Obesity

Cholecystectomy

Social History

Pack-a-day smoker

Single mother of two young children

Works as an administrative assistant

Physical Examination

Malar rash, discoid lesions in "V" area of the chest and in forearms

Mild synovitis at both MCP and MTP joints of the hands and feet

Weighs 220 pounds with bp of 150/95

Management

Hydroxychloroquine was maintained, and her prednisone was reduced to 5 mg a day. Because of ongoing but non-organ-threatening disease, belimumab was begun after a loading period of 10 mg/kg at week 0, 2, and 4. Monthly doses were administered thereafter. By month 6, her joint pain, swelling, fatigue, and rashes had disappeared. She was tapered off steroids and maintained on antimalarial therapy. Her blood pressure normalized off prednisone, and blood sugars remained normal with metformin.

References

1. Tsokos G. Systemic lupus erythematosus. N Engl J Med. 2011;365:2110–21.
2. Wallace DJ. The lupus book: a guide for lupus patients and their families. New York: Oxford University Press; 2013.
3. Ishimori M, Weisman MH, Setoodeh M, Wallace DJ. Management of SLE: principles of therapy, local measures, and nonsteroidals. In: Wallace DJ, Hahn BH, editors. Dubois lupus erythematosus and related syndromes. 8th ed. Philadelphia: Elsevier; 2013. p. 582–90.
4. Ting WW, Sontheimer RD. Local therapy for cutaneous and systemic lupus erythematosus: practical and theoretical considerations. Lupus. 2001;10:171–84.
5. Barikbin B, Givrad S, Yousefi M, Eskandari F. Pimecrolimus cream 1% versus betamethasone 17-valerate 0.1% cream in the treatment of facial discoid lupus erythematosus: a double-blind, randomized, pilot study. Clin Exp Dermatol. 2009;34:776–80.
6. Jessop S, Whitelaw DA, Delamere FM. Drugs for discoid lupus erythematosus. Cochrane Database Syst Rev. 2009;4:CD002954. https://doi.org/10.1002/14651858.CD002954.pub2.
7. Krathen MS, Dunham J, Gaines E, Junkins-Hopkins J, Kim E, Kolasinski SL, Kovarik C, Kwan-Morley J, Okawa J, Propert K, Rogers N, Rose M, Thomas P, Troxel AB, Van Voorhees A, Feldt JV, Weber AL, Werth VP. The cutaneous lupus erythematosus disease activity and severity index: expansion for rheumatology and dermatology. Arthritis Rheum. 2008;59(3):338–44. https://doi.org/10.1002/art.2331.
8. Horizon AA, Wallace DJ. Risk:benefit ratio of nonsteroidal anti-inflammatory drugs in systemic lupus erythematosus. Expert Opin Drug Saf. 2004;3(4):273.
9. Karsh J, Kimberly RP, Stahl NI, Plotz PH, Decker JL. Comparative effects of aspirin and ibuprofen in the management of systemic lupus erythematosus. Arthritis Rheum. 1980;23:1401–4.
10. Wallace DJ. Antimalarial agents and lupus. Rheum Dis Clin North Am. 1994;20:243–63.
11. Aruba-Zubieta J, Esdaile JM. Antimalarial medications. In: Wallace DJ, Hahn BH, editors. Dubois lupus erythematosus and related syndromes. 8th ed. Philadelphia: Elsevier; 2013. p. 601–8.
12. Wallace DJ, Goodsoorkar VS, Weisman MH, Venuturupalli SR. New insights of mechanisms of therapeutic effects of antimalarials agents in SLE. Nature Rev Rheumatol. 2012;8:522–33.
13. Bykerk V, the Canadian Hydroxychloroquine Study Group. A randomized study of the effect of withdrawing hydroxychloroquine sulfate in SLE. N Engl J Med. 1991;324:150–4.
14. Alarson GS, McGwin C, Bertoli AM, Fessler BJ, Calvo-Alen J, et al. Effect of hydroxychloroquine on the survival of patients with SLE: data from LUMINA; a multiethnic US cohort. Ann Rheum Dis. 2007;66:1168–72.
15. Ruiz-Irastorza G, Ramos-Casals M, Brito-Zeron P, Khamashta M. Clinical efficacy and side effects of antimalarials in systemic lupus erythematosus: a systemic review. Annals Rheum Dis. 2010;69:20–8.
16. Sivaraj RR, Durrani OM, Denniston AK, Murray PI, Gordon C. Ocular manifestations of systemic lupus erythematosus. Rheumatology (Oxford). 2007;46(12):1757–62.
17. Marmor MF, Kellner U, Lai TY, Melles RB, Mieler WF. Recommendations on screening for chloroquine and hydroxychloroquine retinopathy (2016 revision): American Academy of Ophthalmology. Ophthalmology. 2016;123(6):1386–94. https://doi.org/10.1016/j.ophtha.2016.01.058.
18. Kirou KA, Boumpas DT. Systemic glucocorticoid therapy in SLE. In: Wallace DJ, Hahn BH, editors. Dubois' lupus erythematosus and related syndromes. 8th ed. Philadelphia: Elsevier; 2012. p. 591–600.
19. Albert DA, Hadler NM, Ropes MW. Does corticosteroid therapy affect the survival of patients with SLE? Arthritis Rheum. 1979;22:945–53.
20. Tseng CE, Buyon JP, Kim M, Belmont HM, Mackay MM. The role of moderate dose corticosteroids in preventing severe flares in patients with moderately-active but clinically stable systemic lupus erythematosus. Arthritis Rheum. 2006;54:3623–32.
21. Thamer M, Hernan MA, Cotter P, Petri MA. Prednisone, lupus activity and permanent damage. J Rheumatol. 2009;36:560–5.
22. Danowski A, Magder L, Petri M. Flares in lupus: outcome assessment trial (FLOAT), a comparison between oral methylprednisolone and intramuscular triamcinolone. J Rheumatol. 2006;33(1):57–60.
23. Ilei GG, Austin Ham Crane M, Collins L, Gourley MF, et al. Combination therapy with pulse cyclophosphamide plus pulse methylprednisolone improves long-term renal outcome without adding toxicity to patients with lupus nephritis. Ann Intern Med. 2001;135:248–57.
24. Grootschalten C, Bajema IM, Florquin S, Steenberger EJ, Peutz-Kootsara CJ, et al. Treatment with cyclophosphamide delays the progression of chronic lesions more effectively than does treatment with azathioprine and methylprednisolone in patients with proliferative lupus nephritis. Arthritis Rheum. 2007;67:924–37.
25. Kan H, Nagar S, Patel J, Wallace DJ, Molta C, Chang DJ. Longitudinal treatment patterns and associated outcomes in patients with newly diagnosed systemic lupus erythematosus. Clin Ther. 2016;38(3):610–24.

26. Frangou EA, Bertsias G, Boumpas DT. Cytotoxic-immunosuppressive drug treatment. In: Tsokos GS, editor. Systemic lupus erythematosus: basic, applied and clinical aspects. San Diego: Academic Press; 2016. p. 533–41.

27. Houssiau FA, Vasconelos C, D'Cruz D, Sebastiani GD, de Ramon GE, et al. Early response to immunosuppressive therapy predicts good renal outcome in lupus nephritis: lessons from long-term follow-up of patients in Euro-Lupus Nephritis Trial. Arthritis Rheum. 2004;50:3934–040.

28. Illei GG, Takada K, Parkin D, Austin HA, Crane M, Yarboro CH, Vaughan EM, Kuroiwa T, Danning CL, Pando J, Steinberg AD, Gourley MF, Klippel JH, Balow JE, Boumpas DT. Renal flares are common in patients with severe proliferative lupus nephritis treated with pulse immunosuppressive therapy: long-term followup of a cohort of 145 patients participating in randomized controlled studies. Arthritis Rheum. 2002;46(4):995–1002.

29. Brodsky RA, Petri M, Smith BD, et al. Immunoablative cyclophosphamide without stem cell rescue for refractory, severe, autoimmune disease. Ann Intern Med. 1998;129:1031–5.

30. Takada K, Illei GG, Boumpas DT. Cyclophosphamide for the treatment of systemic lupus erythematosus. Lupus. 2001;10:154–61.

31. Talar-Williams C, Hijazi YM, Walther MM, Lineham WM, Hallahan CW, et al. Cyclophosphamide induced cystitis and bladder cancer in patients with Wegener's granulomatosis. Ann Intern Med. 1996;124:477–84.

32. Dooley MA, Nair MR. Therapy insight: preserving fertility in cyclophosphamide treated patients with rheumatic disease. Nat Clin Prac Rheumatol. 2008;4:250–7.

33. Abu-Shakra M, Schoenfeld Y. Azathioprine therapy for patients with systemic lupus erythematosus. Lupus. 2001;10:152–3.

34. Griffiths B, Emery P, Ryan V, Isenberg D, Akil M, et al. The BILAG multi-centre, randomized, controlled trial comparing ciclosporin vs azathioprine in patients with severe SLE. Rheumatology. 2010;49:723–32.

35. Leopold G, Shutz E, Haas JP, Oellerich M. Azathioprine-induced severe pancytopenia due to a homozygous two-point mutation of the thiopurine methyltransferase gene in a patient with juvenile HLA-B27 spondyloarthritis. Arthritis Rheum. 1997;40:1896–8.

36. Nero P, Rahman A, Isenberg DA. Does long term treatment with azathioprine predispose to malignancy and death in patients with systemic lupus erythematosus? Ann Rheum Dis. 2004;63(3):325–6.

37. Askanase AD, Wallace DJ, Weisman MH, Tseng CE, Bernstein L, Belmont HM, Seidman E, Ishimori M, Izmirly PM, Buyon JP. Use of pharmacogenetics, enzymatic phenotyping and metabolite monitoring to guide treatment with azathioprine in patients with systemic lupus erythematosus. J Rheumatol. 2009;36(1):89–95.

38. Houssiau FA, d'Cruz D, Sangle S, Remy P, Vasconcelos C, et al. Azathioprine versus mycophenolate mofetil for long term immunosuppression in lupus nephritis: results from the MAINTAIN nephritis trial. J Am Soc Nephrol. 2009;20:1103–12.

39. Wong JM, Esdaile JM. Methotrexate in systemic lupus erythematosus. Lupus. 2005;14(2):101–5.

40. Walker UA. Immunomodulation of rheumatologic disorders with non-biologic disease modifying antirheumatic drugs. Semin Hematol. 2016;53(Suppl 1):S58–60.

41. Fortin PR, Abrahamowicz M, Ferland D, Lacaille D, Smith CD, Zummer M, Canadian Network for Improved Outcomes in Systemic Lupus. Steroid-sparing effects of methotrexate in systemic lupus erythematosus: a double-blind, randomized, placebo-controlled trial. Arthritis Rheum. 2008;59(12):1796–804.

42. Carneiro JR, Sato EI. Double blind, randomized, placebo controlled clinical trial of methotrexate in systemic lupus erythematosus. J Rheumatol. 1999;26(6):1275–9.

43. Clowse ME, Wallace DJ, Furie RA, Petri MA, Pike MC, Leszczyński P, Neuwelt CM, Hobbs K, Keiserman M, Duca L, Kalunian KC, Galateanu C, Bongardt S, Stach C, Beaudot C,

Kilgallen B, Gordon C, EMBODY Investigator Group. Efficacy and safety of epratuzumab in moderately to severely active systemic lupus erythematosus: results from the phase 3, randomized, double-blind, placebo-controlled trials, EMBODY 1 and EMBODY 1. Arthritis Rheumatol. 2017;69(2):362–75. https://doi.org/10.1002/art.39856.

44. Isenberg DA, Petri M, Kalunian K, Tanaka Y, Urowitz MB, Hoffman RW, Morgan-Cox M, Iikuni N, Silk M, Wallace DJ. Efficacy and safety of subcutaneous tabalumab in patients with systemic lupus erythematosus: results from ILLUMINATE-1, a 52 week, phase III, multicenter, randomized, double-blind, placebo controlled study. Ann Rheum Dis. 2016;75(2):323–31.

45. Wallace DJ, Stohl W, Furie RA, Lisse JR, McKay JD, Merrill JT, Petri MA, Ginzler EM, Chatham WW, McCune WJ, Fernandez V, Chevrier MR, Zhong ZJ, Freimuth WW. A phase II, randomized, double-blind, placebo-controlled, dose-ranging study of belimumab in patients with active systemic lupus erythematosus. Arthritis Rheum. 2009;61(9):1168–78.

46. ACCESS Trial Group. Treatment of lupus nephritis with abatacept: the abatacept and cyclophosphamide combination efficacy and safety study. Arthritis Rheumatol. 2014;66(11):3096–104.

47. Merrill JT, Neuwelt CM, Wallace DJ, Shanahan JC, Latinis KM, Oates JC, Utset TO, Gordon C, Isenberg DA, Hsieh HJ, Zhang D, Brunetta PG. Efficacy and safety of rituximab in moderate-to-severely active systemic lupus erythematosus: the randomized, double-blind, phase II/III systemic lupus evaluation of rituximab tial. Arthritis Rheum. 2010;62(1):222–33.

48. Contis A, Vanquaethem H, Truchetet ME, Couzi L, Rigothier C, Richez C, Lazaro E, Duffau P. Analysis of the effectiveness and safety of rituximab in patients with refractory lupus nephritis: a chart review. Clin Rheumatol. 2016;35(2):517–22.

49. Wallace DJ. Management of non-renal and non-central nervous system lupus. In: Hochberg MC, et al., editors. Rheumatology. 6th ed. Philadelphia, PA: Elsevier; 2014. p. 1099–106.

50. Liu Z, Zhang H, Liu Z. Multitarget therapy for induction treatment of lupus nephritis: a randomized trial. Ann Intern Med. 2015;162:18–26.

51. Appel GB, Contreras G, Dooley MA, Ginzler EM, Isenberg D. Mycophenolate mofetil versus cyclophosphamide for induction treatment of lupus nephritis, Aspreva Lupus Management Study Group. J Am Soc Nephrol. 2009;20:1103–12.

52. Mak A, Cheak AA, Tan JY, Su HC, Ho RC, Lau CS. Mycophenolate mofetil is as efficacious as, but safer than, cyclophosphamide in the treatment of proliferative lupus nephritis: a meta-analysis and meta-regression. Rheumatology. 2009;48:944–052.

53. Ginzler EM, Wofsy D, Isenberg D, Gordon C, Lisk L, Dooley MA. Nonrenal disease activity following mycophenolate mofetil or intravenous cyclophosphamide as induction treatment for lupus nephritis. Findings in a multicenter randomized, prospective, open-label, parallel-group clinical trial. Arthritis Rheum. 2010;62:211–21.

54. Mok CC. Therapeutic monitoring of the immune-modulating drugs in systemic lupus erythematosus. Expert Rev Clin Immunol. 2016;22:1–7.

55. Moroni G, Doria A, Mosca M, Alberghi OK, Ferraccili OD, et al. A randomized pilot trial comparing cyclosporine and azathioprine as maintenance therapy in diffuse proliferative lupus nephritis over four years. Clin J Am Soc Nephrol. 2006;1:925–32.

56. Singh NP, Prakash A, Garg D, Makhija A, Pathania A, Prakash N, Kubba S, Aggrawal DK. Aplastic anemia complicating systemic lupus erythematosus: successful management with cyclosporine. Rheumatol Int. 2004;24(1):40–2.

57. Wang X, Zhang L, Luo J, Wu Z, Mei Y, Wang Y, Li X, Wang W, Zhou H. Tacrolimus 0.03% ointment in labial discoid lupus erythematosus: a randomized, controlled, clinical trial. J Clin Pharmacol. 2015;55(11):1221–8.

58. Mok CC, Ying KY, Yim CW, Siu YP, Tong KH, To CH, Ng WL. Tacrolimus versus mycophenolate mofetil for induction therapy of lupus nephritis: a randomized controlled trial and long term follow-up. Ann Rheum Dis. 2016;70:30–6.

59. Lai ZW, Hanczko R, Bonilla E, Caza TN, Clair B, Bartos A, Miklossy G, Jimah J, Doherty E, Tily H, Francis L, Garcia R, Dawood M, Yu J, Ramos I, Coman I, Faraone SV, Phillips PE, Perl A. N-acetylcysteine reduces disease activity by blocking mammalian target of rapamycin in T cells from systemic lupus erythematosus patients: a randomized, double-blind, placebo-controlled trial. Arthritis Rheum. 2012;64(9):2937–46.

60. Cao H, Rao Y, Liu L, Lin J, Yang H, Zhang X, Chen Z. The efficacy and safety of leflunomide for the treatment of lupus nephritis in Chinese patients: systematic review and meta-analysis. PLoS One. 2015;10(12):e0144548.

61. Remer CF, Weisman MH, Wallace DJ. Benefits of leflunomide in systemic lupus erythematosus: a pilot observational study. Lupus. 2001;10(7):480–3.

62. Tam LS, Li EK, Wong CK, Lam CW, Szeto CC. Double-blind, randomized, placebo-controlled pilot study of leflunomide in systemic lupus erythematosus. Lupus. 2004;13(8):601–4.

63. Lindskov R, Reymann F. Dapsone in the treatment of cutaneous lupus erythematosus. Dermatologica. 1986;172(4):214–7.

64. Knop J, Bonsmann G, Happle R, Ludolph A, Matz DR, Mifsud EJ, Macher E. Thalidomide in the treatment of sixty cases of chronic discoid lupus erythematosus. Br J Dermatol. 1983;108(4):461–6.

65. Petri MA, Lahita RG, Van Vollenhoven RF, Merrill JT, Schiff M, Ginzler EM, Strand V, Kunz A, Gorelick KJ, Schwartz KE, GL601 Study Group. Effects of prasterone on corticosteroid requirements of women with systemic lupus erythematosus: a double-blind, randomized, placebo-controlled trial. Arthritis Rheum. 2002;46(7):1820–9.

66. Wallace DJ. Apheresis for lupus erythematosus—state of the art. Lupus. 2001;10:193–6.

67. Bayry J, Negi VS, Kaveri SV. Intravenous immunoglobulin therapy in rheumatic diseases. Nat Rev Rheumatol. 2011;7:349–59.

68. Sakthiswary R, D'Cruz D. Intravenous immunoglobulin in the therapeutic armamentarium of systemic lupus erythematosus: a systemic review and meta-analysis. Medicine (Baltimore). 2014;93(16):e86. https://doi.org/10.1097/MD.0000000000000086.

69. Furie R, Petri M, Zamani O, Cervera R, Wallace DJ, Tegzová D, Sanchez-Guerrero J, Schwarting A, Merrill JT, Chatham WW, Stohl W, Ginzler EM, Hough DR, Zhong ZJ, Freimuth W, van Vollenhoven RF, BLISS-76 Study Group. A phase III, randomized, placebo-controlled study of belimumab, a monoclonal antibody that inhibits B lymphocyte stimulator, in patients with systemic lupus erythematosus. Arthritis Rheum. 2011;63(12):3918–30.

70. Navarra SV, Guzman RM, Gallacher AE, Hall S, Levy RA, et al. Efficacy and safety of belimumab in patients with active systemic lupus erythematosus: a randomized, placebo-controlled, phase 3 trial. Lancet. 2011;377(9767):721–31. https://doi.org/10.1016/S0140-6736(10)61354-2.

71. Hui-Yuen JS, Reddy A, Taylor J, Li X, Eichenfield AH, Bermudez LM, Starr AJ, Imundo LF, Buyon J, Furie RA, Kamen DL, Manzi S, Petri M, Ramsey-Goldman R, van Vollenhoven RF, Wallace DJ, Askanase A. Safety and efficacy of belimumab to treat systemic lupus erythematosus in academic clinical practices. J Rheumatol. 2015;42(12):2288–95.

72. Hahn BH. Belimumab for systemic lupus erythematosus. N Engl J Med. 2013;368(16):1528–35.

73. Furie R, Nicholls K, Cheng TT, Houssiau F, Burgos-Vargas R, Chen SL, Hillson JL, Meadows-Shropshire S, Kinaszczuk M, Merrill JT. The efficacy and safety of abatacept in lupus nephritis: a twelve-month, randomized, double-blind study. Arthritis Rheumatol. 2014;66(2):379–89.

74. Merrill JT, Burgos-Vargas R, Westhovens R, Chalmers A, D'Cruz D, Wallace DJ, Bae SC, Sigal L, Becker JC, Kelly S, Raghupathi K, Li T, Peng Y, Kinaszczuk M, Nash P. The safety and efficacy of abatacept in patients with non-life threatening manifestations of systemic lupus erythematosus: results of a twelve-month, multicenter, exploratory, phase IIb, randomized, double-blind, placebo-controlled trial. Arthritis Rheum. 2010;62(10):3077–87.

75. Mok CC. Current role of rituximab in systemic lupus erythematosus. Int J Rheum Dis. 2015;18(2):154–63.

76. Condon MB, Ashby D, Pepper RJ, Cook HT, Levy JB, Griffith M, Cairns TD, Lightstone L. Prospective observational single-centre cohort study to evaluate the effectiveness of treating lupus nephritis with rituximab and mycophenolate mofetil but no oral steroids. Ann Rheum Dis. 2013;72(8):1280–6.

77. Rovin BH, Furie R, Latinis K, Looney RJ, Fervenza FC, Sanchez-Guerrero J, Maciuca R, Zhang D, Garg JP, Brunetta P, Appel G, LUNAR Investigator Group. Efficacy and safety of rituximab in patients with active proliferative lupus nephritis: the lupus nephritis assessment with rituximab study. Arthritis Rheum. 2012;64(4):1215–26.

78. Illei GG, Shirota Y, Yarboro CH, Daruwalla J, Tackey E, Takada K, Fleisher T, Balow JE, Lipsky PE. Tocilizumab in systemic lupus erythematosus: data on safety, preliminary efficacy, and impact on circulating plasma cells from an open-label phase I dosage-escalation study. Arthritis Rheum. 2010;62(2):542–52.

79. Wallace DJ, Strand V, Merrill JT, Popa S, Spindler AJ, Eimon A, Petri M, Smolen JS, Wajdula J, Christensen J, Li C, Diehl A, Vincent MS, Beebe J, Healey P, Sridharan S. Efficacy and safety of an interleukin-6 monoclonal antibody for the treatment of systemic lupus erythematosus: a phase II dose-ranging randomized controlled trial. Ann Rheum Dis. 2017;76(3):534–42. https://doi.org/10.1136/annrheumdis-2016-209668.

80. Aringer M, Houssiau F, Gordon C, Graninger WB, Voll RE, Rath E, Steiner G, Smolen JS. Adverse events and efficacy of TNF-alpha blockade with infliximab in patients with systemic lupus erythematosus: long term follow-up of 13 patients. Rheumatology (Oxford). 2009;48(11):1451–4.

81. Wallace DJ, editor. Special issue: biologic therapies. Lupus. 2016;25(10).

82. Herrick AL. Recent advances in the pathogenesis and management of Raynaud's phenomenon and digital ulcers. Curr Opin Rheumatol. 2016;28(6):577–85.

83. Navarra SV, Torralba TP. The musculoskeletal system and bone metabolism. In: Wallace DJ, Hahn BH, editors. Dubois lupus erythematosus. 8th ed. Philadelphia, PA: Elsevier; 2013. p. 333–40.

84. Boumpas DT, Yamada H, Patronas NJ, et al. Pulse cyclophosphamide for severe neuropsychiatric lupus. Q J Med. 1991;81:975–84.

85. Pons-Estel GJ, Andreoli L, Scanzi F, Cervera R, Tincani A. The antiphospholipid syndrome in patients with systemic lupus erythematosus. J Autoimmun. 2017;76:10–20. https://doi.org/10.1016/j.jaut.2016.10.004.

86. Florica B, Aghdassi E, Su J, Gladman DD, Urowitz MB, Fortin PR. Peripheral neuropathy in patients with systemic lupus erythematosus. Semin Arthritis Rheum. 2011;41(2):203–11.

87. Gao Y, Lau EY, Wan JH, Lau CS, Mok MY. Systemic lupus erythematosus patients with past neuropsychiatric involvement are associated with worse cognitive impairment: a longitudinal study. Lupus. 2016;25(6):637.

88. Venuturupalli S. Rethinking biologics in lupus nephritis. Lupus. 2016;25(10):1102–10.

89. Anders HJ, Rovin B. A pathophysiology-based approach to the diagnosis and treatment of lupus nephritis. Kidney Int. 2016;90(3):493–501.

90. Radhakrishnan J, Moutzouris DA, Ginzler EM, et al. Mycophenolate mofetil and intravenous cyclophosphamide are similar as induction therapy for class V lupus nephritis. Kidney Int. 2010;77:152–60.

91. Clark MR, Trotter K, Chang A. The pathogenesis and therapeutic implications of tubulointerstitial inflammation in human lupus nephritis. Semin Nephrol. 2015;35(5):455–64.

92. Mc Mahon M, Hahn BH, Skaggs BI. Systemic lupus erythematosus and cardiovascular disease: prediction and potential for therapeutic intervention. Expert Rev Clin Immunol. 2011;7:227–41.

93. Robles-Perez A, Molina-Molina M. Treatment considerations of lung involvement in rheumatologic disease. Respiration. 2015;90(4):265–74.

94. Urowitz MB, Gladman D, Ibañez D, Bae SC, Sanchez-Guerrero J, Gordon C, Clarke A, Bernatsky S, Fortin PR, Hanly JG, Wallace DJ, Isenberg D, Rahman A, Alarcón GS, Merrill JT, Ginzler E, Khamashta M, Nived O, Sturfelt G, Bruce IN, Steinsson K, Manzi S, Ramsey-Goldman R, Dooley MA, Zoma A, Kalunian K, Ramos M, Van Vollenhoven RF, Aranow C, Stoll T, Petri M, Maddison P, Systemic Lupus International Collaborating Clinics. Atherosclerotic vascular events in a multinational cohort of systemic lupus erythematosus. Arthritis Care Res (Hoboken). 2010;62(6):881–7.

95. Manzi S, Meilahn EN, Rairie JE, Conte CG, Medsger TA Jr, Jansen-McWilliams L, D'Agostino RB, Kuller LH. Age-specific incidence rates of myocardial infarction and angina in women with systemic lupus erythematosus: comparison with the Framingham study. Am J Epidemiol. 1997;145(5):408–15.

96. González-Naranjo LA, Betancur OM, Alarcón GS, Ugarte-Gil MF, Jaramillo-Arroyave D, Wojdyla D, Pons-Estel GJ, Rondón-Herrera F, Vásquez-Duque GM, Quintana-López G, Da Silva NA, Tavares Brenol JC, Reyes-Llerena G, Pascual-Ramos V, Amigo MC, Massardo L, Alfaro-Lozano J, Segami MI, Esteva-Spinetti MH, Iglesias-Gamarra A, Pons-Estel BA. Features associated with hematologic abnormalities and their impact in patients with systemic lupus erythematosus: data from a multiethnic Latin American cohort. Semin Arthritis Rheum. 2016;45(6): 675–83.

97. Levine AB, Erkan D. Clinical assessment and management of cytopenias in lupus patients. Curr Rheumatol Rep. 2011;13(4):291–9.

98. Abu-Hishmeh M, Sattar A, Zarlasht F, Ramadan M, Abdel-Rahman A, Hinson S, Hwang C. Systemic lupus erythematosus presenting as refractory thrombotic thrombocytopenic purpura: a diagnostic and management challenge. A case report and concise review of the literature. Am J Case Rep. 2016;17:782–7.

Anti-IgE Therapy

Andrea D. Maderal and Brian Berman

Introduction

Omalizumab is an anti-immunoglobulin E (anti-IgE) therapy indicated for moderate to severe persistent asthma and chronic spontaneous or idiopathic urticaria. It is the only anti-IgE therapy currently available. Though only licensed for chronic spontaneous or idiopathic urticaria, it has several additional uses in dermatology. And with an overall good safety profile, it can represent a safe treatment option for often corticosteroid-dependent diseases.

Mechanism of Action and Pharmacology

Immunoglobulin E (IgE) is an antibody class implicated in the allergic response that signals by binding to two different receptors: the high-affinity receptor (FcεRI) and the low-affinity receptor (FcεRII). In normal allergic response, upon exposure to an environmental allergen, the allergen is taken up by antigen-presenting cells to the lymph nodes and presented to lymphocytes, where then a B-lymphocyte is activated and, in the presence of appropriate cytokines, undergoes differentiation to produce allergen-directed IgE by plasma cells. IgE then binds to its receptors and, upon cross-linking of antigen and IgE to the receptors, activates mast cells leading to release of inflammatory mediators, such as histamine [1]. The FcεRI can also be activated by self-reactive IgE

A.D. Maderal, MD
Department of Dermatology and Cutaneous Surgery,
University of Miami Miller School of Medicine,
Miami, FL, USA

B. Berman, MD, PhD (✉)
Department of Dermatology and Cutaneous Surgery,
University of Miami Miller School of Medicine,
Miami, FL, USA

Center for Clinical and Cosmetic Research,
Aventura, FL, USA
e-mail: bbmdphd@gmail.com

autoantibodies that either bind to self-antigens or cross-react with environmental substances [2]. These have been demonstrated in conditions such as chronic spontaneous urticaria (CSU), atopic dermatitis, and bullous pemphigoid.

Omalizumab is a recombinant, 95% humanized monoclonal antibody that selectively binds to the receptor-binding site of circulating human IgE [3]. It originates from a murine monoclonal antibody, which was then humanized, and overall contains 5% nonhuman amino acid residues [4]. Omalizumab binds to circulating IgE with a greater affinity than IgE does to the FcεRI, thereby reducing circulating IgE levels and inhibiting binding of IgE to FcεRI on basophils and mast cells [4]. This leads to inhibition of mast cell response to allergenic stimuli [5]. Omalizumab has also been demonstrated to decrease the expression of FcεRI on the surface of mast cells, reducing the effect of IgE autoantibodies [6, 7]. It is thought that in CSU patients, the downregulation of FcεRI expression is sufficient to prevent cross-linking of anti-FcεRI IgG antibodies and thereby prevent mast cell activation [8].

Omalizumab has a rapid onset of action, with reduction of free IgE within hours of the first dose [9]. Peak serum concentrations are often reached after 7–8 days of administration, with an estimated serum elimination half-life of 24 days [10]. It is excreted through hepatic degradation and may be secreted through bile. In clinical studies evaluated for approval of asthma, <0.1% patients treated with omalizumab developed autoantibodies (Genentech). No autoantibodies to omalizumab have been demonstrated in trials for CSU [11–13].

Dosages

Omalizumab is licensed for the treatment of CSU at a dose of 150 and 300 mg subcutaneously every 4 weeks in the United States and 300 mg subcutaneously every 4 weeks in the European Union [10, 14]. Unlike for patients with asthma, dosing is not based on body weight or serum IgE levels.

© Springer International Publishing AG 2018
P.S. Yamauchi (ed.), *Biologic and Systemic Agents in Dermatology*, https://doi.org/10.1007/978-3-319-66884-0_38

Doses greater than 150 mg should be divided into more than one injection site to minimize injection site reaction [10]. The medication is supplied either as a prefilled syringe or as a lyophilized formulation for reconstitution. When provided as a lyophilized sterile powder, it should be reconstituted with 1.4 mL of sterile water using clean technique, mixed for 5–10 s every 5 min for 15–20 min or longer if needed for the solution to dissolve. After reconstitution, the solution should be used within 8 h if kept refrigerated, and within 4 h if stored at room temperature, and should be protected from sunlight. To administer the medication, 1.2 mL (150 mg of omalizumab) should be aspirated into a 3 mL syringe and administered slowly via subcutaneous injection with a 25-gauge needle.

The maximum tolerated dose has not yet been determined, though single doses of up to 4000 mg have been administered without toxicity, and the highest cumulative dose received was 44,000 mg over 20 weeks, without toxicity [10].

Due to reports of anaphylaxis in clinical trials for asthmatic patients, administration of the medication should be performed by a healthcare professional where treatment for anaphylaxis is available. It is recommended that patient should be observed following administration for 2 h following the first three doses and for 30 min for all subsequent doses.

As none of the three pivotal trials for omalizumab in the treatment of CSU have demonstrated a risk of anaphylaxis [15–17], some authors have advocated for home administration in the appropriate setting. Denman et al. described a home administration protocol where the patients received first and second doses in the healthcare setting, and if there were no complications, subsequent doses were performed at home [18]. The patients were all provided epinephrine autoinjectors. Of 123 patients treated using this protocol, there were no cases of anaphylaxis or other serious adverse effects, and patients reported a preference for at home treatment.

Indications in Dermatology

Chronic Spontaneous Urticaria

Chronic spontaneous urticaria (CSU), or chronic idiopathic urticaria, is defined as hives and swelling lasting greater than or equal to 6 weeks without an identifiable cause [19]. It is a debilitating disease with a significant impact on quality of life, with similar impact to triple-vessel coronary artery disease [20]. Though the exact pathophysiology of CSU is unknown, the final result of urticaria and angioedema is caused by activation of mast cells [21]. Approximately 40% of CSU patients have IgG autoantibodies that target and activate FcεRI, IgE, or both, and these patients tend to have a longer disease duration and poorer response to antihistamines [22].

Omalizumab became licensed for CSU in 2014 and is indicated for chronic idiopathic (or spontaneous) urticaria in adults and adolescents 12 years of age and older who remain symptomatic despite H1 antihistamine treatment. It is not currently indicated for other allergic conditions or other forms of urticaria.

Currently, omalizumab is recommended as a third-line treatment in the European Union and fourth-line treatment in the United States in the management of CSU [23]. Per the European Academy of Allergy and Clinical Immunology, it is recommended that patients first receive a trial of second-generation H1 antihistamines; if symptoms persist at 2 weeks, the medication should be increased to 4× the licensed dose. If symptoms persist after 1–4 additional weeks, then third-line options should be considered in addition to antihistamines, which include omalizumab, cyclosporine, or montelukast [23].

Omalizumab has been extensively studied and shown benefit in the management of CSU in patients refractory to antihistamines. Three pivotal double-blind, placebo-controlled, phase III randomized trials demonstrated benefit in urticaria activity score (UAS7) and itch severity score (ISS), as well as a favorable safety profile, with similar incidence and severity of adverse events as placebo [15–17]. Pooled data from a systematic review demonstrated a reduction in UAS7 of 11.58 points in patients treated with omalizumab as compared with placebo [24]. Complete symptom control was seen in 38.1% of patients in treatment group (vs. 5.6% placebo, $p < 0.001$), and partial response was seen in 55.1% of treatment (vs. 13.7% placebo, $p < 0.001$). There was also an improvement in quality of life and in angioedema-free days, when compared with placebo.

Greatest clinical efficacy was noted for the 300 mg dose group, which met all secondary endpoints, as compared to 75 mg and 150 mg doses, though with a slightly greater frequency of adverse events [15, 16]. The 300 mg dose has consistently demonstrated the most efficacy in reducing weekly ISS and wheal scores, as well as the highest rate of complete responders (36%) in a meta-analysis [25]. In a phase II study, the 75 mg dose did not show any difference from placebo [26].

There is no correlation between urticaria type, presence of associated diseases, serum level of IgE, total body weight, or age with response to omalizumab [27]. There is no difference in response to omalizumab between autoimmune positive and autoimmune negative patients [28]. A phase II randomized, double-blinded, placebo-controlled trial of 49 subjects with CSU and IgE autoantibodies against thyroid peroxidase refractory to antihistamine therapy demonstrated a mean reduction in weekly UAS, as well as complete protection from wheal development was seen in 70.4% of patients [29].

The timing of response to therapy after omalizumab treatment was analyzed from phase III trials [30]. The median time to response was between 8 and 10 weeks in the 300 mg dose group. It was noted that while some patients responded early to therapy (within 4 weeks), others did not achieve response until 24 weeks, and patients could be divided into "fast responders" and "slow responders." "Fast responders" had complete response and well-controlled urticaria after 4–6 weeks of treatment initiation. "Slow responders" responded more gradually by week 12–16 and even up to week 24. Therefore, it is recommended not to discontinue therapy until after 24 weeks of failure, as patients may still respond [30].

In real-world practice, response to omalizumab has been shown to be similar to, if not better than the results from randomized controlled trials [31]. Patients who are "fast responders" often respond within 1 month, with 57% responding within 1 week and 86% within 4 weeks in one study [32]. As well, some patients in real-world practice require higher doses, and some advocate for patients without response at 6 months to have dose increases to 450 mg or 600 mg subcutaneously every 4 weeks [31]. For patients with disease activity just prior to their upcoming injection, the dosing interval can be decreased, and doses of 300 mg every 2 weeks in clinical experience has demonstrated better efficacy than every 4 weeks [33]. Fixed dosing schedules are likely superior to "as needed" administration, which failed to be an effective management strategy in one case series [34].

Long-term usage of omalizumab has not yet been studied. In randomized controlled trials for CSU, data is provided for up to 6 months, though use >1 year has been shown to be safe in two small retrospective studies and individual case studies [35–37] and up to 4 years in individual case reports [35, 36].

There are no guidelines presently for when to discontinue or reduce therapy in patients who are well controlled. It may be possible to decrease the dose, as dose reductions from 300 to 150 mg have been shown to maintain disease remission, [38] or dosing intervals can be lengthened. Treatment discontinuation, on the other hand, has demonstrated a high rate of relapse in previously well-controlled patients and should not be performed abruptly [39]. Retreatment in this setting though is efficacious, and patient often has a rapid and complete response shortly after restarting therapy.

Off-Label Uses in Dermatology

Physical Urticaria

Physical urticarias are a group of inducible urticarias where wheals and/or angioedema can be triggered by different physical stimuli, including sunlight, heat, and cold. Though omalizumab has not been studied in randomized controlled trials for inducible forms of urticaria, it has demonstrated some efficacy in reports for different types of physical urticaria.

Solar urticaria is a rare form of physical urticaria where wheals are triggered within 5–10 min of sun exposure. It is thought to represent a type I hypersensitivity reaction to an unknown photoallergen, and diagnosis can be made with elicitation of wheals on phototesting [7]. Though initiation therapy should begin with sun avoidance and antihistamines, some patients are resistant to these and other adjunctive therapies, including phototherapy, plasmapheresis, and cyclosporine. Several cases have demonstrated efficacy of omalizumab in patients with solar urticaria refractory to antihistamines, including cases triggered by visible light, where complete photoprotection is difficult [3, 7]. A phase II study of ten patients with solar urticaria treated with omalizumab 300 mg subcutaneously every 4 weeks for a total of three injections demonstrated 40% improvement in baseline solar urticaria severity, and 20% of patients reached the primary endpoint of absence of urticaria triggered by a UV dose greater than 10× the baseline minimal urticaria dose [40].

Cold contact urticaria is a form of physical urticaria where urticarial lesions and/or angioedemas occur with exposure to cold objects, liquids, or gases [41]. The urticaria develops typically after rewarming and can even result in life-threatening anaphylaxis. It is seen most commonly in young adults. Treatment for cold contact urticaria is the same as CSU, with antihistamines as first-line therapy [23]. In one case series of five adolescents with cold contact urticaria refractory to antihistamine therapy, treatment with omalizumab 300 mg demonstrated significant improvement in quality of life of all patients [42].

Heat urticaria is a physical urticaria that is triggered by a hot stimulus. Three cases of heat urticaria have been successfully treated with omalizumab, though one required higher than normal doses for complete remission [43, 44].

Delayed pressure urticaria is a form of physical urticaria that is often unresponsive to high doses of antihistamines. Other treatment options, including dapsone, are often ineffective or limited by long-term toxicity [45]. Several cases of delayed pressure urticaria have demonstrated response to omalizumab [45–47].

Other forms of physical urticaria that have responded to omalizumab include cholinergic urticaria and dermographism [48, 49]. Additional studies are needed to better evaluate the role of omalizumab in patients with physical forms of urticaria.

Urticarial Vasculitis

Urticarial vasculitis presents with urticarial lesions that often last longer than 24 h, is associated with burning more so than pruritus, and can leave behind dyspigmentation after the individual lesions resolve. Urticarial vasculitis tends to be unresponsive to traditional antihistamine therapy and often requires treatment with more high-risk medications with unfavorable long-term side effect profiles (e.g., systemic steroids, dapsone). Omalizumab has been reported in several case reports and series to be effective in the management of normocomplementemic urticarial vasculitis [34, 50–52] and may represent a promising treatment option in the future.

Angioedema

Angioedema is the correlate of urticaria in deeper tissues and demonstrates edema within the subcutaneous, mucosal, and submucosal tissue. It can occur anywhere on the body, often affecting the face, and can lead to respiratory insufficiency in severe cases [53]. In patients with CSU with angioedema, omalizumab has demonstrated efficacy in controlling angioedema at the 300 mg dose only [16]. Omalizumab decreases number of angioedema attacks and reduces the size of swelling with attacks [54]. Omalizumab demonstrated clinical efficacy in one patient with angioedema not in the setting of CSU [55]. More rigorous studies are needed to clarify the role of omalizumab for angioedema in non-CSU patients.

Atopic Dermatitis

The benefit of omalizumab in atopic dermatitis is controversial. Overall, two randomized controlled trials and 13 case series have been conducted, which have yielded conflicting results. Both randomized controlled trials demonstrated reductions in Th2 cytokines and IgE but no significant clinical improvement as compared with control [56, 57]. The failure of omalizumab in atopic dermatitis may be due to the less prominent role that IgE has in the pathogenesis of disease, as various mutations in epidermal proteins have been found to underlie atopic dermatitis. In one study of omalizumab in atopic dermatitis, only patients that lacked a filaggrin mutation benefited from omalizumab, whereas none of the patients with a filaggrin mutation responded to therapy [58].

In a systematic review of the data from trials and case series, where 60.5% of patients had severe atopic dermatitis and 67% had asthma, overall, 43% of patients achieved excellent clinical response, while 27.2% showed satisfying results and 30.1% showed irrelevant clinical changes or even worsening [59]. Dosing in these studies was based on the original asthma dosages, which varied depending on body weight and serum IgE levels, but originally only accounted for IgE up to 700 IU/mL. Asthma dosing guidelines have since been expanded to include higher doses for patients with IgE levels >700 IU/mL. In this meta-analysis, patients with lower serum IgE levels (<700 IU/mL) at baseline were associated with more favorable clinical responses, and the authors hypothesized that as many patients enrolled in the study had significantly elevated IgE levels (75% had IgE levels exceeding 700 IU/mL), the doses provided were likely insufficient to account for these values [59]. Interestingly, one investigator-initiated pilot study using combination of immunoadsorption (immunoglobulin apheresis) followed by omalizumab administration for patients with atopic dermatitis showed significant reductions in SCORAD (Scoring Atopic Dermatitis) index in all patients, supporting the notion that possibly higher doses of omalizumab are needed for patients with atopic dermatitis and elevated IgE [60].

Omalizumab has demonstrated efficacy in case reports of genodermatoses with an atopic diathesis, including a case of Netherton syndrome, where treatment with omalizumab resulted in improvement in pruritus, erythema, and desquamation [61] and two cases of Hyper-IgE syndrome, where the dermatitides improved with omalizumab [62, 63].

Whether or not there is a role for omalizumab in the treatment of atopic dermatitis is still unclear, and further trials with additional dosing regimens are needed to fully elucidate.

Bullous Pemphigoid

Bullous pemphigoid (BP) is an autoimmune blistering disease characterized by autoantibodies directed against two hemidesmosomal proteins: bullous pemphigoid antigen 2 (BP180 or type XVII collagen) and bullous pemphigoid antigen 1 (BP230) [64]. IgG antibodies directed against these proteins are important for pathogenesis of disease, diagnosis, and management, as levels can be monitored as markers of disease activity. Therapy presently for widespread bullous pemphigoid includes nonspecific immunosuppressant therapies targeted to decrease antibody production, such as systemic corticosteroids, methotrexate, azathioprine, mycophenolate mofetil, and rituximab. These therapies carry significant risk of infection, malignancy, and many other side effects with long-term use.

The role of IgE antibodies in BP has been explored, as BP lesions often occur as urticarial plaques which can then progress to develop tense blisters, and even an urticarial-only form of BP can exist. It has been demonstrated that patients with BP often have elevated total IgE levels in the sera [65–67]. As well, IgE antibodies targeting BP180 have also been identified [68–70]. The frequency of positivity in patients with BP is variable, ranging from 41 to 90% of patients [67, 71–73]. In a recent study, only 40.2% of patients with BP had anti-BP180 IgE antibodies, but these antibodies did correlate with disease activity [64].

Omalizumab has demonstrated in several case reports to be efficacious in the treatment of bullous pemphigoid and to additionally produce a steroid-sparing effect [74–78]. In the future, testing for presence of IgE antibodies could aid in selection of therapy, as it may indicate patients more likely to respond to omalizumab [64]. Further trials are needed to evaluate the full potential of omalizumab in the treatment of BP.

Mastocytosis

Mastocytosis is a rare mast cell activation disorder that can be limited to the skin or involve systemic organs. The main risk of cutaneous disease includes mast cell activation, resulting in anaphylaxis. Omalizumab has been reported in several cases of both cutaneous and systemic mastocytosis to be beneficial in lessening the severity of skin symptoms, decreasing episodes of anaphylaxis, and reducing GI symptoms in patients with systemic disease [79–88].

Latex Allergy

Latex allergy is a common type I hypersensitivity reaction, seen in particular in healthcare workers frequently exposed to latex products (e.g., gloves or other medical supplies). A double-blind, randomized, placebo-controlled study of the effect of omalizumab on 18 healthcare workers with clinical symptoms and positive skin testing for occupational latex allergy demonstrated efficacy as compared to placebo in clinically relevant ocular and skin antiallergic activity [89].

Other Reports

Additional case reports have demonstrated benefit of omalizumab in type I hypersensitivity drug reactions [90] and toxic epidermal necrolysis (TEN) in combination with systemic steroids [91].

Future Directions

Hypereosinophilic syndromes are a heterogeneous group of disorders characterized by marked eosinophilia in the peripheral blood, tissues, or both, without a secondary cause [92]. Omalizumab has demonstrated in asthmatic patients to reduce peripheral eosinophil counts [92] and may represent a treatment option in the future for patients that are refractory to conventional therapies.

Systemic lupus erythematosus (SLE) has demonstrated elevated IgE levels, which have been shown to correlate with more severe disease [2]. It is thought that some of the IgE antibodies are self-reactive and thus contribute to the disease pathogenesis [93]. As well, IgE antibodies directed against double-stranded DNA (dsDNA) are the most significant antibodies associated with disease activity [94]. In vitro, IgE blockade in serum of patients with + dsDNA IgE was demonstrated to reduce interferon-α (IFN-α) secretion, a cytokine critically important in the pathogenesis of SLE [95]. Clinical trials are currently ongoing to determine the benefit of omalizumab in patients with SLE. (https://clinicaltrials.gov/ct2/show/NCT01716312?term=omalizumab+lupus&rank=1)

Adverse Events

Adverse events from phase III trials were overall mild. In studies for CSU, the most common adverse reactions involving ≥2% omalizumab-treated patients and more frequently occurring than in placebo included nausea, nasopharyngitis, sinusitis, upper respiratory infection, viral upper respiratory infection, arthralgia, headache, and cough [10]. Additional reactions that were reported during the longer 24-week treatment periods included toothache, fungal infection, urinary tract infection, myalgia, pain in extremity, musculoskeletal pain, peripheral edema, pyrexia, migraine, sinus headache, anxiety, oropharyngeal pain, asthma, urticaria, and alopecia (Genentech). Urticaria has been reported in patients with asthma and in one patient required early treatment discontinuation [12]. The hair loss reported in one case series was noted to be transient and only last 4 months [96]. Serum sickness-like reaction has been reported in post-approval use. Monitoring for parasitic infection in patients treated in endemic areas is recommended, though no significant increase in risk has been demonstrated [10]. There is insufficient data to determine the length of monitoring required. Serum total IgE levels increase following administration of omalizumab, secondary to the formation of omalizumab/IgE complexes. Several reports of onset of eosinophilic granulomatosis with polyangiitis occurring during treatment with omalizumab for asthma have been reported [97–101].

Injection site reactions are overall not uncommon, occurring in 2.7% of omalizumab-treated patients at the 300 mg dose, as compared to 0.8% of placebo [10]. Injection site reactions typically included swelling, erythema, pain, bruising, itching, bleeding, and urticaria. In the trials, it did not result in any study discontinuation or treatment interruption.

A black box warning exists for omalizumab for risk of anaphylaxis. This is as a result of an incidence of 0.1–0.2% of patients in clinical trials for asthma [102, 103]. However, no cases of anaphylaxis occurred in the phase III trials of omalizumab for CSU [15–17]. Anaphylaxis has been reported in two patients with CSU in real-world experience, though one patient had recurrent anaphylaxis prior to omalizumab, and the second patient had symptoms that were not consistent with anaphylaxis [104]. In asthma trials, in cases where anaphylaxis occurred, most (70%) occurred within 1 h of omalizumab dosing, with a median time of 30 min [105]. 39.3% of patients experienced anaphylaxis within the first 3 doses of omalizumab, though 32% occurred after more than 20 doses. No deaths or disabilities occurred as a result of the events, though several patients did require hospitalization. All patients should be counseled on signs and symptoms of anaphylaxis and how to seek immediate care if the symptoms occur [10].

Original pooled data from phase I–III studies demonstrated an increase in malignancy in omalizumab-treated patients (0.5%) as compared to controls (0.2%). Upon further review and with more extensive patient population, 11,459 patients in all randomized, double-blinded, placebo-controlled trials were pooled and found similar incidence rates of malignancy in omalizumab-treated patients (4.14 per 1000 patient-years) and controls (4.45 per 1000 patient-years) [106]. Additionally, there was no histologic overrepresentation in either group. There does not appear to be any increased risk of malignancy with omalizumab therapy.

Contraindications

Omalizumab is contraindicated in patients with severe hypersensitivity reaction to omalizumab or any of its ingredients [10].

Pregnancy and Lactation

Omalizumab is pregnancy category B. Monoclonal antibodies, including omalizumab, are able to transport across the placenta as pregnancy progresses. In animal studies of cynomolgus monkeys treated with subcutaneous doses up to 10× the maximum recommended human doses, no fetal harm was demonstrated [107]. There are no randomized controlled trials on the use of omalizumab during pregnancy. A case series of four female subjects with refractory CSU treated with omalizumab demonstrated efficacy in all patients and resulted in full-term deliveries with no negative pregnancy or fetal outcomes [108]. An omalizumab pregnancy registry (EXPECT), a post-marketing commitment to the United States Food and Drug Administration, has been monitoring the incidence of congenital anomalies in pregnant women, and their infants, who were treated with omalizumab [109]. In EXPECT, the prevalence and rates of major congenital anomalies, fetal deaths, small for gestation age births, and preterm births are similar to the general population.

There is no information regarding the presence of omalizumab in human milk or effects that treatment with omalizumab may have on milk production or a breastfed infant [10]. Omalizumab has been demonstrated in breastmilk at levels 0.15% of maternal serum concentration.

Drug Interactions

No formal drug interaction studies have been performed and there are no known drug interactions. In CSU patients, the use of omalizumab in combination with corticosteroids has not been evaluated [10].

Case Report

The patient is a 43-year-old woman with a 3-year history of recurrent bouts of idiopathic urticaria. She failed cetirizine, an H1 antihistamine, in approved doses, as well as four times the FDA-approved doses, and failed the addition of montelukast, the leukotriene antagonist. She was started on omalizumab at 300 mg subcutaneously once monthly with resulting complete reduction in itch and hives. At 12 weeks, her treatment was discontinued, but she developed recurrence in her hives within 2 months. She was restarted on omalizumab at 300 mg monthly, with resolution of her symptoms.

References

1. Godse K, Mehta A, Patil S, et al. Omalizumab-A review. Indian J Dermatol. 2015;60:381–4.
2. Sanjuan MA, Sagar D, Kolbeck R. Role of IgE in autoimmunity. J Allergy Clin Immunol. 2016;137:1651–61.
3. Bruning JH, Ziemer M, Pemler S, et al. Successful treatment of solar urticarial with omalizumab. J Dtsch Dermatol Ges. 2016;14:936–7.
4. Belliveau PP. Omalizumab: a monoclonal anti-IgE antibody. MedGenMed. 2005;7:27.
5. Chang TW, Chen C, Lin CJ, et al. The potential pharmacologic mechanisms of omalizumab in patients with chronic spontaneous urticaria. J Allergy Clin Immunol. 2015;135:337–42.
6. Lin H, Boesel KM, Griffith DT, et al. Omalizumab rapidly decreases nasal allergic response and FcepsilonRI on basophils. J Allergy Clin Immunol. 2004;113:297–302.

7. Moncourier M, Assikar S, Matei I, et al. Visible light-induced solar urticaria is improved by omalizumab. Photodermatol Photoimmunol Photomed. 2016;32:314–6.

8. Kaplan AP, Joseph K, Maykut RJ, et al. Treatment of chronic autoimmune urticaria with omalizumab. J Allergy Clin Immunol. 2008;122:569–73.

9. Djukanovic R, Wilson SJ, Kraft M, et al. Effects of treatment with anti-immunoglobulin E antibody omalizumab on airway inflammation in allergic asthma. Am J Respir Crit Care Med. 2004;170:583–93.

10. Genentech Inc. Xolair: FDA Prescribing Information. 2016. http://www.gene.com/download/pdf/xolair_prescribing.pdf. Accessed 23 Jan 2017.

11. Soler M, Matz J, Townley R, et al. The anti-IgE antibody omalizumab reduces exacerbations and steroid requirement in allergic asthmatics. Eur Respir J. 2001;18:254–61.

12. Berger W, Gupta N, McAlary M, et al. Evaluation of long-term safety of the anti-IgE antibody, omalizumab, in children with allergic asthma. Ann Allergy Asthma Immunol. 2003;91:182–8.

13. Lanier BQ, Corren J, Lumry W, et al. Omalizumab is effective in the long-term control of severe allergic asthma. Ann Allergy Asthma Immunol. 2003;91:154–9.

14. European Medicines Agency. Omalizumab (Xolair) summary of product characteristics. 2014. http://www.ema.europa.eu/ema/index.jsp?curl=pages/medicines/human/medicines/000606/human_med_001162.jsp&mid=WC0b01ac058001d124. Accessed 23 Jan 2017.

15. Saini SS, Bindslev-Jensen C, Maurer M, et al. Efficacy and safety of omalizumab in patients with chronic idiopathic/spontaneous urticaria who remain symptomatic on H1 antihistamines: a randomized, placebo-controlled study. J Invest Dermatol. 2015;135:67–75.

16. Maurer M, Rosen K, Hsieh HJ, et al. Omalizumab for the treatment of chronic idiopathic or spontaneous urticaria. N Engl J Med. 2013;368:924–35.

17. Kaplan A, Ledford D, Ashby M, et al. Omalizumab in patients with symptomatic chronic idiopathic/spontaneous urticaria despite standard combination therapy. J Allergy Clin Immunol. 2013;132:101–9.

18. Denman S, Ford K, Toolan J, et al. Home self-administration of omalizumab for chronic spontaneous urticaria. Br J Dermatol. 2016;175:1405–7.

19. O'Donnell BF, Lawlor F, Simpson J, et al. The impact of chronic urticaria on the quality of life. Br J Dermatol. 1997;136:197–201.

20. Poon E, Seed PT, Greaves MW, et al. The extent and nature of disability in different urticarial conditions. Br J Dermatol. 1999;140:667–71.

21. Ferrer M, Nunez-Cordoba JM, Luquin E, et al. Serum total tryptase levels are increased in patients with active chronic urticaria. Clin Exp Allergy. 2010;40:1760–6.

22. Konstantinou GN, Asero R, Maurer M, et al. EAACI/GA(2)LEN task force consensus report: the autologous serum skin test in urticaria. Allergy. 2009;64:1256–68.

23. Zuberbier AW, Asero R, et al. The EAACI/GA(2) LEN/EDF/WAO guideline for the definition, classification, diagnosis and management of urticaria: the 2013 revision and update. Allergy. 2014;69:868–87.

24. Urgert MC, van den Elzen MT, Knulst AC, et al. Omalizumab in patients with chronic spontaneous urticaria: a systematic review and GRADE assessment. Br J Dermatol. 2015;172:404–15.

25. Zhao ZT, Ji CM, Yu WJ, et al. Omalizumab for the treatment of chronic spontaneous urticaria: a meta-analysis of randomized clinical trials. J Allergy Clin Immunol. 2016;137:1742–50.

26. Saini S, Rosen KE, Hsieh HJ, et al. A randomized, placebo-controlled, dose-ranging study of single-dose omalizumab in patients with H1-antihistamine-refractory chronic idiopathic urticaria. J Allergy Clin Immunol. 2011;128:567–73.

27. Uysal P, Eller E, Mortz GC, et al. An algorithm for treating chronic urticaria with omalizumab: dose interval should be individualized. J Allergy Clin Immunol. 2014;133:914–5.

28. Viswanathan RK, Moss MH, Mathur SK. Retrospective analysis of the efficacy of omalizumab in chronic refractory urticaria. Allergy Asthma Proc. 2013;34:446–52.

29. Maurer M, Altrichter S, Bieber T, et al. Efficacy and safety of omalizumab in patients with chronic urticaria who exhibit IgE against thyroperoxidase. J Allergy Clin Immunol. 2011;128:202–9.

30. Kaplan A, Ferrer M, Bernstein JA, et al. Timing and duration of omalizumab response in patients with chronic idiopathic/spontaneous urticaria. J Allergy Clin Immunol. 2016;137:474–81.

31. Gimenez-Arnau AM, Toubi E, Marsland AM, et al. Clinical management of urticaria using omalizumab: the first licensed biological therapy available for chronic spontaneous urticaria. J Eur Acad Dermatol Venereol. 2016;30:25–32.

32. Maurer M, Weller K, Bindslev-Jensen C, et al. Unmet clinical needs in chronic spontaneous urticaria. A GA2LEN task force report. Allergy. 2011;66:317–30.

33. Clark JJ, Secrest AM, Hull CM, et al. The effect of omalizumab dosing and frequency in chronic idiopathic urticaria: retrospective chart review. J Am Acad Dermatol. 2016;74:1274–6.

34. Kai AC, Flohr C, Grattan CE. Improvement in quality of life impairment followed by relapse with 6-monthly periodic administration of omalizumab for severe treatment-refractory chronic urticaria and urticarial vasculitis. Clin Exp Dermatol. 2014;39:651–2.

35. Fiorino I, Loconte F, Rucco AS, et al. Long-term treatment of refractory severe chronic urticaria by omalizumab: analysis of two cases. Postepy Dermatol Alergol. 2014;31:332–4.

36. Silva PM, Costa AC, Mendes A, et al. Long-term efficacy of omalizumab in seven patients with treatment-resistant chronic spontaneous urticaria. Allergol Immunopathol (Madr). 2015;43:168–73.

37. Har D, Patel S, Khan DA. Outcomes of using omalizumab for more than 1 year in refractory chronic urticaria. Ann Allergy Asthma Immunol. 2015;115:126–9.

38. Romano C, Sellitto A, De Fanis U, et al. Maintenance of remission with low-dose omalizumab in long-lasting, refractory chronic urticaria. Ann Allergy Asthma Immunol. 2010;104:95–7.

39. Metz M, Ohanyan T, Church MK, et al. Retreatment with omalizumab results in rapid remission in chronic spontaneous and inducible urticaria. JAMA Dermatol. 2014;150:288–90.

40. Aubin F, Avenel-Audran M, Jeanmougin M, et al. Omalizumab in patients with severe and refractory solar urticaria: a phase II multicentric study. J Am Acad Dermatol. 2016;74:574–5.

41. Katsarou-Katsari A, Makris M, Lagogianni E, et al. Clinical features and natural history of acquired cold urticaria in a tertiary referral hospital: a 10-year prospective study. J Eur Acad Dermatol Venereol. 2008;22:1405–11.

42. Kitsioulis NA, Xepapadaki P, Kostoudi S, et al. Omalizumab in pediatric cold contact urticaria: warm blanket for a cold bath? Pediatr Allergy Immunol. 2016;27:752–5.

43. Carballada F, Nunez R, Martin-Lazaro J, et al. Omalizumab treatment in 2 cases of refractory heat urticaria. J Investig Allergol Clin Immunol. 2013;23:519–21.

44. Bullerkotte U, Wieczorek D, Kapp A, et al. Effective treatment of refractory severe heat urticaria with omalizumab. Allergy. 2010;65:931–2.

45. Muller S, Rafei-Shamsabadi D, Technau-Hafsi K, et al. Bullous delayed pressure urticaria responding to omalizumab. Acta Derm Venereol. 2016;96:416–7.

46. Metz M, Altrichter S, Ardelean E, et al. Anti-immunoglobulin E treatment of patients with recalcitrant physical urticaria. Int Arch Allergy Immunol. 2011;154:177–80.

47. Groffik A, Mitzel-Kaoukhov H, Magerl M, et al. Omalizumab—an effective and safe treatment of therapy-resistant chronic spontaneous urticaria. Allergy. 2011;66:303–5.

48. Metz M, Bergmann P, Zuberbier T, et al. Successful treatment of cholinergic urticaria with anti-immunoglobulin E therapy. Allergy. 2008;63:247–9.

49. Krause K, Ardelean E, Kessler B, et al. Antihistamine-resistant urticaria factitia successfully treated with anti-immunoglobulin E therapy. Allergy. 2010;65:1494–5.

50. Diez LS, Tamayo LM, Cardona R. Omalizumab: therapeutic option in chronic spontaneous urticaria difficult to control with associated vasculitis, report of three cases. Biomedica. 2013;33:503–12.

51. Sussman G, Hebert J, Barron C, et al. Real-life experiences with omalizumab for the treatment of chronic urticaria. Ann Allergy Asthma Immunol. 2014;112:170–4.

52. Ghazanfar MN, Thomsen SF. Omalizumab for urticarial vasculitis: case report and review of the literature. Case Rep Dermatol Med. 2015;2015:576893.

53. Greaves M. Chronic urticaria. J Allergy Clin Immunol. 2000;105:664–72.

54. Staubach P, Metz M, Chapman-Rothe N, et al. Effect of omalizumab on angioedema in H1-antihistamine-resistant chronic spontaneous urticaria patients: results from X-ACT, a randomized controlled trial. Allergy. 2016;71:1135–44.

55. Kutlu A, Karabacak E, Aydin E, et al. Efficacy of omalizumab in a patient with angioedema clinically resembling a hereditary angioedema. Ann Dermatol. 2016;28:381–2.

56. Heil PM, Maurer D, Klein B, et al. Omalizumab therapy in atopic dermatitis: depletion of IgE does not improve the clinical course— a randomized, placebo-controlled and double blind pilot study. J Dtsch Dermatol Ges. 2010;8:990–8.

57. Iyengar SR, Hoyte EG, Loza A, et al. Immunologic effects of omalizumab in children with severe refractory atopic dermatitis: a randomized, placebo-controlled clinical trial. Int Arch Allergy Immunol. 2013;162:89–93.

58. Hotze M, Baurecht H, Rodriguez E, et al. Increased efficacy of omalizumab in atopic dermatitis patients with wild-type filaggrin status and higher serum levels of phosphatidylcholines. Allergy. 2014;69:132–5.

59. Wang HH, Li YC, Huang YC. Efficacy of omalizumab in patients with atopic dermatitis: a systematic review and meta-analysis. J Allergy Clin Immunol. 2014;138:1719–22.

60. Zink A, Gensbaur A, Zirbs M, et al. Targeting IgE in severe atopic dermatitis with a combination of immunoadsorption and omalizumab. Acta Derm Venereol. 2016;96:72–6.

61. Yalcin AD. A case of netherton syndrome: successful treatment with omalizumab and pulse prednisolone and its effects on cytokines and immunoglobulin levels. Immunopharmacol Immunotoxicol. 2016;38:162–6.

62. Chularojanamontri L, Wimoolchart S, Tuchinda P, et al. Role of omalizumab in a patient with hyper-IgE syndrome and review dermatologic manifestations. Asian Pac J Allergy Immunol. 2009;27:233–6.

63. Bard S, Paravisini A, Aviles-Izquierdo JA, et al. Eczematous dermatitis in the setting of hyper-IgE syndrome successfully treated with omalizumab. Arch Dermatol. 2008;144:1662–3.

64. van Beek N, Luttmann N, Huebner F, et al. Correlation of serum levels of IgE autoantibodies against BP180 with bullous pemphigoid disease activity. JAMA Dermatol. 2017;153:30–8.

65. Kippes W, Schmidt E, Roth A, et al. Immunopathologic changes in 115 patients with bullous pemphigoid. Hautarzt. 1999;50:866–72.

66. Arbesman CE, Wypych JI, Reisman RE, et al. IgE levels in sera of patients with pemphigus or bullous pemphigoid. Arch Dermatol. 1974;110:378–81.

67. Dimson OG, Guidice GJ, Fu CL, et al. Identification of a potential effector function for IgE autoantibodies in the organ-specific autoimmune disease bullous pemphigoid. J Invest Dermatol. 2003;120:784–8.

68. Dopp R, Schmidt E, Chimanovitch I, et al. IgG4 and IgE are the major immunoglobulins targeting the NC16A domain of BP180 in bullous pemphigoid: serum levels of these immunoglobulins reflect disease activity. J Am Acad Dermatol. 2000;42:577–83.

69. Christophoridis S, Budinger L, Borradori L, et al. IgG, IgA and IgE autoantibodies against the ectodomain of BP180 in patients with bullous and cicatricial pemphigoid and linear IgA bullous dermatosis. Br J Dermatol. 2000;143:349–55.

70. Ishiura N, Fujimoto M, Watanabe R, et al. Serum levels of IgE anti-BP180 and anti-BP230 autoantibodies in patients with bullous pemphigoid. J Dermatol Sci. 2008;49:153–61.

71. Yayli S, Pelivani N, Beltraminelli H, et al. Detection of linear IgE deposits in bullous pemphigoid and mucous membrane pemphigoid: a useful clue for diagnosis. Br J Dermatol. 2011;165:1133–7.

72. Messingham KA, Noe MH, Chapman MA, et al. A novel ELISA reveals high frequencies of BP180-specific IgE production in bullous pemphigoid. J Immunol Methods. 2009;346:18–25.

73. Messingham KA, Holahan HM, Fairley JA. Unraveling the significance of IgE autoantibodies in organ-specific autoimmunity: lessons learned from bullous pemphigoid. Immunol Res. 2014;59:273–8.

74. Balakirski G, Alkhateeb A, Merk HF, et al. Successful treatment of bullous pemphigoid with omalizumab as corticosteroid-sparing agent: report of two cases and review of literature. J Eur Acad Dermatol Venereol. 2016;30:1778–82.

75. Yalcin AD, Genc GE, Celik B, et al. Anti-IgE monoclonal antibody (omalizumab) is effective in treating bullous pemphigoid and its effects on soluble CD200. Clin Lab. 2014;60:523–4.

76. London VA, Kim GH, Fairley JA, et al. Successful treatment of bullous pemphigoid with omalizumab. Arch Dermatol. 2012;148:1241–3.

77. Dufour C, Souillet AL, Chaneliere C, et al. Successful management of severe infant bullous pemphigoid with omalizumab. Br J Dermatol. 2012;166:1140–2.

78. Yu KK, Crew AB, Messingham KA, et al. Omalizumab therapy for bullous pemphigoid. J Am Acad Dermatol. 2014;71:468–74.

79. Lieberoth S, Thomsen SF. Cutaneous and gastrointestinal symptoms in two patients with systemic mastocytosis successfully treated with omalizumab. Case Rep Med. 2015;2015:903541.

80. Carter MC, Robyn JA, Bressler PB, et al. Omalizumab for the treatment of unprovoked anaphylaxis in patients with systemic mastocytosis. J Allergy Clin Immuno. 2007;119:1550–1.

81. Pitt TJ, Cisneros N, Kalicinsky C, et al. Successful treatment of idiopathic anaphylaxis in an adolescent. J Allergy Clin Immunol. 2010;126:415–6.

82. Kontou-Fili K, Filis CI, Voulgari C, et al. Omalizumab monotherapy for bee sting and unprovoked "anaphylaxis" in a patient with systemic mastocytosis and undetectable specific IgE. Ann Allergy Asthma Immunol. 2010;104:537–9.

83. Douglass JA, Carroll K, Voskamp A, et al. Omalizumab is effective in treating systemic mastocytosis in a nonatopic patient. Allergy. 2010;65:926–7.

84. Paraskevopoulos G, Sifnaios E, Christodoulopoulos K, et al. Successful treatment of mastocytic anaphylactic episodes with reduction of skin mast cells after anti-IgE therapy. Eur Ann Allergy Clin Immunol. 2013;45:52–5.

85. Kibsgaard L, Skjold T, Deleuran M, et al. Omalizumab induced remission of idiopathic anaphylaxis in a patient suffering from indolent systemic mastocytosis. Acta Derm Venereol. 2014;94:363–4.

86. Siebenhaar F, Kuhn W, Zuberbier T, et al. Successful treatment of cutaneous mastocytosis and Meniere disease with anti-IgE therapy. J Allergy Clin Immunol. 2007;120:213–5.

87. Matito A, Blazquez-Goni C, Morgado JM, et al. Short-term omalizumab treatment in an adolescent with cutaneous mastocytosis. Ann Allergy Asthma Immunol. 2013;111:425–6.

88. Sokol KC, Ghazi A, Kelly BC, et al. Omalizumab as a desensitizing agent and treatment in mastocytosis: a review of the literature and case report. J Allergy Clin Immunol Pract. 2014;2:266–70.

89. Leynadier F, Doudou O, Gaouar H, et al. Effect of omalizumab in health care workers with occupational latex allergy. J Allergy Clin Immunol. 2004;113:360–1.

90. Matheu V, Franco A, Perez E, et al. Omalizumab for drug allergy. J Allergy Clin Immunol. 2007;120:1471–2.

91. Uzun R, Yalcin AD, Celik B, et al. Levofloxacin induced toxic epidermal necrolysis: successful therapy with omalizumab (anti-IgE) and pulse prednisolone. Am J Case Rep. 2016;17:666–71.

92. Wechsler ME, Fulkerson PC, Bochner BS, et al. Novel targeted therapies for eosinophilic disorders. J Allergy Clin Immunol. 2012;130:563–71.

93. Zhu H, Luo H, Yan M, et al. Autoantigen microarray for high-throughput autoantibody profiling in systemic lupus erythematosus. Genomics Proteomics Bioinformatics. 2015;13:210–8.

94. Dema B, Pellefigues C, Hasni S, et al. Autoreactive IgE is prevalent in systemic lupus erythematosus and is associated with increased disease activity and nephritis. PLoS One. 2014;9:e90424.

95. Henault J, Riggs JM, Karnell JL, et al. Self-reactive IgE exacerbates interferon responses associated with autoimmunity. Nat Immunol. 2016;17:196–203.

96. Konstantinou GN, Chioti AG, Daniilidis M. Self-reported hair loss in patients with chronic spontaneous urticaria treated with omalizumab: an under-reported, transient side effect? Eur Ann Allergy Clin Immunol. 2016;48:205–7.

97. Bekcibasi M, Barutcu S, Celen MK, et al. Churg-Strauss syndrome occurring during omalizumab treatment. Eur J Rheumatol. 2015;2:129–30.

98. Winchester DE, Jacob A, Murphy T. Omalizumab for asthma. N Engl J Med. 2006;355(12):1281–2.

99. Giavina-Bianchi P, Giavina-Bianchi M, Agondi R, et al. Administration of anti-IgE to a Churg-Strauss syndrome patient. Int Arch Allergy Immunol. 2007;144:155–8.

100. Bargagli E, Rottoli P. Omalizumab treatment associated with Churg-Strauss vasculitis. Int Arch Allergy Immunol. 2008;145:268.

101. Weschler ME, Wong DA, Miller MK, et al. Churg-strauss syndrome in patients treated with omalizumab. Chest. 2009;136:507–18.

102. Corren J, Casale TB, Lanier B, et al. Safety and tolerability of omalizumab. Clin Exp Allergy. 2009;39:788–97.

103. Limb SL, Starke PR, Lee CE, et al. Delayed onset and protracted progression of anaphylaxis after omalizumab administration in patients with asthma. J Allergy Clin Immunol. 2007;120: 1378–81.

104. Savic S, Marsland A, McKay D, et al. Retrospective case note review of chronic spontaneous urticaria outcomes and adverse effects in patients treated with omalizumab or ciclosporin in UK secondary care. Allergy Asthma Clin Immunol. 2015;11:21.

105. Lieberman PL, Umetsu DT, Carrigan GJ, et al. Anaphylactic reactions associated with omalizumab administration: analysis of a case-control study. J Allergy Clin Immunol. 2016;138:913–5.

106. Busse W, Buhl R, Fernandez Vidaurre C, et al. Omalizumab and the risk of malignancy: results from a pooled analysis. J Allergy Clin Immunol. 2012;129:983–9.

107. Schatz M, Zeiger RS. Asthma and allergy in pregnancy. Clin Perinatol. 1997;24:407–32.

108. Cuervo-Pardo L, Barcena-Blanch M, Radojicic C. Omalizumab use during pregnancy for CIU: a tertiary care experience. Eur Ann Allergy Clin Immunol. 2016;48:145–6.

109. Namazy J, Cabana MD, Scheuerle AE, et al. The Xolair pregnancy registry (EXPECT): the safety of omalizumab use during pregnancy. J Allergy Clin Immunol. 2015;135:407–12.

Kyle T. Amber, Jessica Shiu, Katherine Ferris,
and Sergei A. Grando

Introduction

Intravenous immunoglobulin (IVIg) represents polyclonal natural antibodies pooled from sera of healthy donors. It has been successfully used to treat a variety of autoimmune and inflammatory disorders. Historically, IVIg was used to treat immune deficiencies and was first described in 1952 by Bruton who infused a child with congenital agammaglobulinemia suffering from recurrent infections [1]. Following expansion of its use in primary antibody deficiencies, the use of IVIg in autoimmune disease was described in 1981 [2], and has since been approved by the United States Food and Drug Administration (FDA) for several autoimmune disorders, including immune thrombocytopenic purpura, Grave's disease and multifocal motor neuropathy, and also used off-label in a variety of immune-mediated dermatologic diseases, which is the focus of this chapter.

IVIg is a collection of pooled antibodies, mainly of the immunoglobulin G (IgG) isotype, targeting microbial antigens, as well as anti-idiotypic antibodies and autoantibodies [3]. IgG is the most abundant immunoglobulin and has several subclasses in humans: IgG1, IgG2, IgG3, and IgG4. Other isotypes include immunoglobulin M (IgM), immunoglobulin A (IgA), immunoglobulin D (IgD), and immunoglobulin E (IgE), which are present in very small amounts in IVIg preparations. Structurally, antibodies are large Y-shaped molecules that contain two identical heavy chains and two identical light chains linked by disulfide bonds. Both heavy and light chains are composed of variable domains and constant domains—the variable domains (designated V_H and V_L, respectively) confer specificity of antigen binding while the constant domains (C_H and C_L, respectively) make up the parts of the antibody molecule that allow it to bind and interact with effector cells via cell-surface to the Fragment crystallizable (Fc) receptor. Proteolytic cleavage of IgG yields two dichotomous fragments: Fragment antigen binding (Fab) and Fc. Fab contains the antigen binding portion of antibodies while Fc contains C regions that differentiate various isotypes and allow antibodies to interact with effector cells. For example, Fc receptors on macrophages and neutrophils bind IgG Fc portions to allow phagocytosis of pathogens; mast cells and eosinophils bind the Fc portion of IgE to release inflammatory mediators in allergic responses.

The amount of IgG varies among individual batches and different brands of IVIg products. The number of donors used to prepare a single IVIg batch can vary from a minimum of 1000 donors up to 100,00 [4]. Not surprisingly, there is high variability between individual batches of IVIg and differing brands. The IVIg products are distributed as 50 mg/mL (5%) or 100 mg/mL (10%) [5]. As mentioned earlier, the proportion of IgG subclasses varies between each preparation. Small amounts of albumin, IgA, IgE, IgM, sugars, and salts can be found, with varying concentration [6].

To avoid transmission of infectious agents and minimize immune-related complications, following isolation of donor's sera, the specimens are put through a complex fractionation, chromatography and viral inactivation procedure which has been reviewed in detail by Barahona et al. [5]. IVIg preparations are routinely screened for hepatitis B, hepatitis C and HIV [7], and a maximum safe titer of ABO blood group antibodies is set to reduce the risk of hemolytic complication [8].

K.T. Amber, BA • J. Shiu, MD, PhD • K. Ferris, MD
Departments of Dermatology, University of California,
Irvine, CA 92697, USA
e-mail: kamber@uci.edu

S.A. Grando, MD, PhD, DSc (✉)
Departments of Dermatology, University of California,
Irvine, CA 92697, USA

Biological Chemistry, University of California,
Irvine, CA 92697, USA

Institute for Immunology, University of California Irvine,
118 Med Surg 1, Irvine, CA 92697, USA
e-mail: sgrando@uci.edu

© Springer International Publishing AG 2018
P.S. Yamauchi (ed.), *Biologic and Systemic Agents in Dermatology*, https://doi.org/10.1007/978-3-319-66884-0_39

Following infusion, IVIg requires 3–5 days to equilibrate between the intra- and extravascular components. The total amount of serum IgG thus rapidly declines in the first week, followed by a slower decrease thereafter. This initial rapid decline of IgG is due to the shift of IgG from the vascular system to lymph and extracellular compartments, while the subsequent slower decline is secondary to catabolism [9]. IVIg has a half-life of approximately 3 weeks in humans, though immunodeficient patients can have a half-life of up to 6 weeks [10, 11]. The long half-life of human IgG is notable when compared to other isotypes such as IgM and IgA ($T_{1/2}$ = ~5 days) and is attributed to the presence of the neonatal Fc receptor (FcRn) that binds IgG intracellularly, within an endosome, and then recycle it back to circulation thus protecting it from lysosomal degradation [9, 12].

IVIg exhibits multiple effects on the immune system, which has been harnessed to treat different diseases. Our current understanding of IVIg is dependent on the underlying disease process, and the model used to study these diseases. Significant variation in responses have been noted using different animal models, even within a single disease model such as immune thrombocytopenic purpura (ITP) [13]. This chapter will focus on immune mechanisms of therapeutic actions of IVIg in different dermatologic diseases.

Mechanism of Therapeutic Action of IVIg

It is important to note that IgG antibodies play diverse roles in the immune system. Autoreactive IgG antibodies that target self-tissue antigens can cause an autoimmune disease. Conversely, pooled IgG in IVIg has anti-inflammatory properties exploited in clinical medicine to treat patients. A wide variety of mechanisms have been proposed to explain the anti-inflammatory activities of IVIg, which can be mediated by different structural components of IgG molecule [14]. The antigen binding Fab component can bind and neutralize pathogenic autoantibodies, whereas the Fc portion can interact with Fc receptors on various cell types regulating distinct cell functions. These mechanisms will be detailed below, and are summarized in Fig. 39.1.

Blockade of Fc Receptor

A variety of immune cells express Fc receptors that interact with the Fc component of IgG molecules in IVIg. Phagocytic cells such as macrophages and dendritic cells express Fc receptors that are responsible for opsonization of IgG. IVIg can saturate these Fc receptors, decreasing the overall immune response to antibody-coated cells. However, the blockade of Fc receptors is not required for IVIg function[15]

as the Fab component of IgG also has immunomodulatory effects (see below). The efficacy of pure Fc in ITP, however, does suggest a role of Fcγ receptor blockade in the mechanism of ITP [16].

Natural Antibodies and Anti-idiotypic Antibodies

IVIg contains numerous autoantibodies that account for a large proportion of antibodies present in IVIg preparations. These autoantibodies are termed "natural antibodies," as they are not a result of foreign antigen stimulation [17]. These natural antibodies tend to be polyreactive and have a lower affinity than pathogenic autoantibodies [18–21]. Due to their polyreactivity, these natural autoantibodies appear to have a role in natural host defense due to their reactivity with microbes and microbial toxins in addition to their role in immune homeostasis [22].

Antibodies to Sialic acid-binding Ig-like lectin (SIGLEC)8 have also been identified in IVIg [23]. SIGLEC8 can be activated by anti-SIGLEC8 antibody, resulting in both caspase dependent and independent cell death. SIGLEC8 has been shown to mediate apoptosis of eosinophils [24]. Adsorption of anti-SIGLEC8 antibody leads to a loss of caspase independent neutrophil death [25]. Interestingly, when used in the treatment of eosinophilic granulomatosis with polyangiitis (formerly Churg-Strauss disease), IVIg significantly reduces the number of circulating eosinophils as well as required systemic steroid doses [26]. Accordingly, variation in anti-SIGLEC8 antibodies results in differences in clinical outcomes [27]. Residual eosinophilia following treatment with IVIg has been used as a marker of IVIg resistance in Kawasaki's disease [28].

Anti-idiotypic antibodies are those that are directed against antigenic determinates within or in proximity to another antibody's binding site [29]. These anti-idiotypic antibodies can interfere with antibody-antigen binding and can also precipitate autoantibodies in a column [30–33], thereby decreasing the autoantibody response in multiple ways. Anti-idiotypic antibodies may additionally bind to autoreactive B-cells. Neutralizing or inhibitory anti-idiotypic against antibodies targeting ANCA, DNA, and ribosomal P protein have been demonstrated in patients with vasculitis [34–36]. In fact, there is a significantly higher presence of anti-idiotypic antibodies in patients with ANCA-associated vasculitis in remission compared to active cases [37], suggesting clinical significance of anti-idiotypic antibodies. When IgG from pemphigus foliaceus patients are injected in mice to cause disease, anti-idiotype antibodies to desmoglein 1 abrogate the blistering effect of pathogenic IgG [38]. Antibodies in IVIg targeting Fcγ may

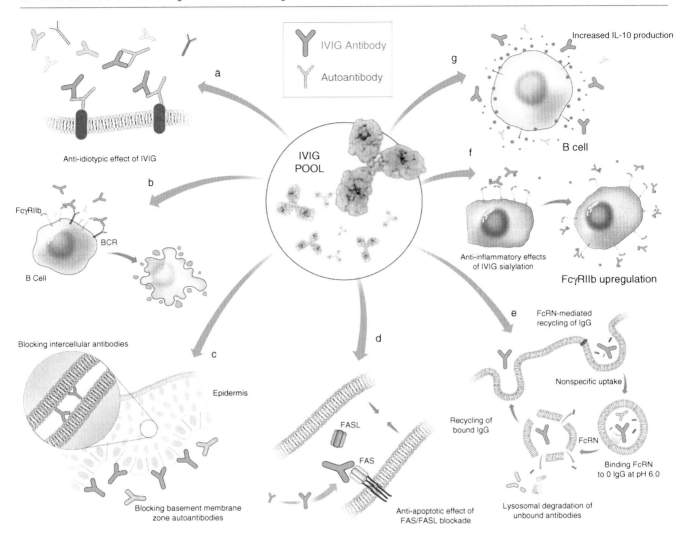

Fig. 39.1 Summary of different therapeutic mechanisms of IVIG in dermatologic diseases with a focus on autoimmune blistering disease. (**a**) IVIG has anti-idiotypic activity and reduces the pathogenicity of autoantibodies. (**b**) Binding of the Fc portion of IVIG to FcγRIIB with simultaneous binding of IVIG Fab portion to BCR leads to anergy by abolishing the BCR-induced stimulation of antibody production. (**c**) Self antigens in bullous pemphigoid and pemphigus vulgaris are protected by blocking IVIG antibodies from autoantibodies. (**d**) IVIG binds Fas and prevents the interaction with FasL, leading to blockade of keratinocyte apoptosis. (**e**) Binding of IVIG to FcRN in endosomes leads to recycling of IVIG molecules with degradation of pathogenic autoantibodies. (**f**) Sialylation of the Fc portion of IVIG molecules leads to interaction with SIGN-R1 and upregulation of the inhibitory receptor FcγRIIB and attenuation of inflammation and tissue damage. (**g**) IVIG increases production of the immunosuppressive cytokine, IL-10, in B-cells

additionally block these receptors from interacting with pathogenic autoantibodies[39]. Functional autoantibodies against FcγRII and FcγRIII capable of blocking immunoglobulin rosette formation have been identified within IVIg [39].

Complement Inhibition

IVIg also affects different arms of the complement system. IVIg has been shown to activate the classical complement pathway, resulting in a significant consumption of C4

following infusion [40]. This is a surprising finding as IVIg clinically exerts an anti-inflammatory effect. In the same study, the authors also showed that IVIg decreased $C3b_2$ containing complexes, resulting in overall complement attenuation. Overall, complement inhibition was short-lived and $C3b_2$ levels returned to the baseline after 2–4 weeks [41].

$C3b_2$ complexes maintain complement amplification to a far greater degree than the short-lived C3b. IVIg reduces the half-life of $C3b_2$-IgG complexes from 3–4 to 1–2 min [42]. In a study of patients with dermatomyositis, the concentration of $C3b_2$ complexes dropped significantly with the use of IVIg. This reduction was dose dependent [40]. There are significant variations in C3b attenuation between IVIg formulations, likely due to variations in anti-C3 antibodies contained within IVIg

IVIg also blocks deposition of early complement activation products C4b and C3b on cellular targets in various diseases, interrupting the classical complement cascade [43]. This may account for the decrease in complement deposition seen in mice with experimental epidermolysis bullosa acquisita treated with IVIg [44].

IVIg can additionally interfere with the deposition of the complement membrane attack complex on capillaries by preventing the incorporation of activated C3 into C5 convertase [45]. This has therapeutic implications in the treatment of dermatomyositis, where the deposition of complement terminal attack components in intramuscular capillaries is pathogenic. When used in murine models of dermatomyositis, IVIg resulted in a dose-dependent inhibition of C1q, C3 and C4 binding. This occurred in an Fc dependent manner[46]. The Fab portion of IgG additionally has different complement inhibiting properties, as it can scavenge the anaphylotoxins C3a and C5a [47].

Apoptosis: Fas-FasL Interaction, Caspases and Bcl-2

IVIg contains antibodies that block Fas-mediated keratinocyte death in vitro [48, 49]. This is of clinical importance in the treatment of toxic epidermal necrolysis. IVIg can induce apoptosis in lymphocytes via antibodies against Fas [50]. As purified anti-Fas antibodies had a 120-fold higher anti-apoptotic potential than unpurified IVIg, ant-Fas antibodies appear to have a significant effect on lymphocyte and monocyte apoptosis [50]. IVIg can contain both agonistic and antagonist ligands for Fas [51]. Agonistic antibodies induce apoptosis in neutrophils, lymphocytes, and monocytes in a caspase dependent manner [50–52]. While high doses of IVIg increase neutrophil apoptosis, perhaps through activation of Fas, the low doses of IVIg can prevent anti-Fas mediated neutrophil apoptosis, perhaps by blocking this pathway due to an antagonist action [50, 53].

In addition to the mode of pharmacologic action of IVIg, the cell type in question as well as its sensitivity to Fas appears to have a role [54]. In keratinocytes, IVIg can prevent Fas-FasL mediated keratinocyte apoptosis in toxic epidermal necrolysis (TEN) [48]. Keratinocytes treated with IVIg demonstrate upregulation of caspase inhibitors which has implications in decreasing pemphigus IgG induced acantholysis [55]. IVIg results in a decrease in the expression of caspases, thus marking a decrease in apoptosis [56–58].

Finally, IVIg's effect on Bcl-2 expression, an anti-apoptotic protein, has varied depending on the cell type studied [59–61]. While endothelial cells demonstrate an IVIg mediated decrease in Bcl-2 expression, monocytes and neural cells in ischemic conditions experience upregulation of Bcl-2.

FcγRIIβ

IVIg has a significant anti-inflammatory effect via FcγRIIβ, an inhibitory Fc receptor expressed on myeloid as well as B-cells [62]. In fact, B-cells contain only the inhibitory FcR, FcγRIIβ, in contrast to macrophages which contain all pro-inflammatory Fcγ receptors [63]. FcγRIIβ increases the B-cell receptor activation threshold and suppresses B-cell mediated antigen presentation to T-cells [64, 65]. FcγRIIβ knockout mice demonstrate increased antibody levels to T-cell dependent antigens [66]. Moreover, FcγRIIβ inhibits FcγR-dependent internalization of antigens, leading to a decrease in dendritic cell-mediated T-cell priming [67]. FcγRIIβ also leads to a reduction of FcγR-mediated phagocytosis and inflammatory cytokine release (TNF-a, IL-6, IL-1) by macrophages [68, 69]. FcγRIIβ additionally inhibits IL-4 production and IgE-receptor mediated histamine release [70, 71]. In FcγRIIβ knockout mice, IVIg is not effective in ameliorating autoimmunity, underlining the importance of this inhibitory receptor in the IVIg's therapeutic effects [72, 73].

IVIg can indirectly increase FcγRIIβ through a direct effect on colony-stimulating factor 1 (CSF1) dependent macrophages [74, 75]. Knockout studies of FcγRIIβ have yielded convincing evidence towards its role in systemic lupus erythematosus (SLE). FcγRIIβ contributes to the development of different lupus-like end organ damage in differing autoimmune models [68, 76]. Restoration of FcγRIIβ in fact resulted in return of tolerance and the prevention of autoimmunity [77]. It has been noted that levels of FcγRIIβ are significantly decreased on B-cells from patients with SLE [78]. Autoantibodies targeting FcγRIIβ have been implicated in systemic sclerosis as well [79]. In chronic inflammatory demyelinating polyneuropathy (CIDP), FcγRIIβ is also significantly decreased at baseline and is then upregulated in patients who are successfully treated with IVIg [62].

In a murine model of ITP, FcγRIIβ was proven to be responsible for IVIg's ability to prevent hemolysis [72]. FcγRIIβ in this model was involved in the late phase of therapeutic action of IVIg, but was not required for immediate therapeutic effect [80, 81]. This is congruent with the finding that FcγRIIβ is dispensable in the inhibition of Fcγ-R mediated phagocytosis seen with IVIg [82]. Even without FcγRIIβ, IVIg can still inhibit antigen-specific T-cell responses [83].

FcRn Saturation

IVIg additionally causes saturation of FcRn, leading to an increase in the rate of catabolism of circulating IgG. Thus pathogenic IgG in circulation can be cleared more quickly. FcRn protects IgG by placing it into recycling endosomes, serving as a refuge from lysosomal degradation [84].

FcRn appears to have an important role in autoimmune bullous disease as FcRn deficient mice were resistant to experimental bullous pemphigoid, pemphigus vulgaris, or pemphigus foliaceus, though the ex vivo suprabasilar blistering models were based on a monopathogenic model which has come into question [85, 86]. FcRn is required for the internalization of pemphigus vulgaris associated anti-mitochondrial IgG which can complex with anti-desmoglein antibodies leading to acantholysis and apoptosis [87]. Deficiency of FcRn or saturation can inhibit experimental arthritis [88]. In contrast, FcRn was, however, not required for therapeutic response to IVIg in a murine model of ITP [89]. Together, these findings indicate that the role of FcRn in mediating the therapeutic effects of IVIg depends on the disease and particular pathogenic mechanisms.

IgG Sialylation

Sialylation refers to the attachment of sialic acid to either the Fc or Fab component of IgG. The presence of sialic acids on IgG has been associated with anti-inflammatory properties and a return to immunologic tolerance [90–93]. Sialylation of IVIg results in a far more potent and anti-inflammatory product [75, 91, 92, 94]. Low baseline levels of sialylation are likewise associated with numerous autoimmune diseases including SLE [95–97].

Sialylation of the Fc portion of IgG promotes anti-inflammatory responses by decreasing the affinity of Fc binding to type I Fc receptors, while enhancing binding to type II Fc receptors[98, 99]. This occurs through interaction with SIGNR1 (specific intercellular adhesion molecule 3-grabbing nonintegrin-related 1). SIGNR1 is a specific C-type lectin adhesion molecule located on splenic marginal zone macrophages that preferentially bind to sialylated IgG [75]. The interaction of sialylated IgG Fc and SIGN-R1 leads to an upregulation of FcγRIIβ through an increase in basophil produced IL-4 [100]. In fact, only FcγRIIβ and terminal sialylation were required for prevention of autoimmunity in several in vivo models [101]. Thus, sialylation of the Fc portion results in an FcγRIIβ dependent protective effect [91, 92]. Other studies have found the interaction between sialylated IgG and SIGN-R1 to be dispensable in IVIg's anti-inflammatory function [102, 103]. Of note, the human orthologue of SIGN-RA, dendritic cell-specific ICAM3-grabbing nonintegrin (DC-SIGN), has a different cellular distribution compared to SIGN-R1 [104] and IVIg may have different effects in various species [105, 106]. Finally, sialylation of the Fc component of IgG can also impair complement-dependent cytotoxicity in a FcγRIIβ independent manner [107].

Sialylation can occur not just on the Fc fragment, but also on Fab [108]. De-glycosylation of IVIg results in a loss of anti-inflammatory activity, while increasing sialylation results in an increase in anti-inflammatory activity [91]. A tetra-Fc-Sialylated was used in an animal model of epidermolysis bullosa acquisita, demonstrating 10-fold enhanced efficacy [94]. Sialylated Fc was not necessary for the down-regulation of DC-SIGN, suggesting that alternative sialylation may play a stronger role [102, 103].

Further studies have also investigated the effects of sialylation on T-cell function. Sialylation appears to be dispensable in inhibiting T-cell activation or inducing Treg [109, 110]. Sialylation is not required for the alteration in Th17 and Treg differentiation [111].

Cell Adhesion

IVIg decreases the adhesion of T-cells to the extracellular matrix [112]. It can reduce serum ICAM-1 as well as ELAM-1 levels in patients with atopic dermatitis [113]. IVIg can also block integrin binding through antibodies targeting the Arg-Gly-Asp motif, which mediates adhesions between extracellular matrix proteins and integrin beta1, beta3m, and beta5 [114].

Modulation of the Glucocorticoid Receptor

Research has demonstrated a steroid sparing effect of IVIg through enhancing glucocorticoid receptor-binding affinity, synergistically leading to decreased lymphocyte interaction [115, 116]. The exact underlying mechanism, however, remains unclear.

Effects on Dendritic Cells

Dendritic cells are a heterogeneous group of antigen-presenting cells that are essential in shaping the adaptive immune response. Dendritic cells prime different arms of the adaptive immune response and can also induce regulatory T-cells resulting peripheral T-cell tolerance. IVIg leads to the development antibody-antigen complexes resulting in activation of FcγR on dendritic cells [80, 117]. This is independent of FCγRIIB, which appears to only have an effect in the late phase of therapeutic action of IVIg [80, 81]. IVIg inhibits dendritic cell maturation and differentiation, decreasing their ability to secrete IL-12, while increasing IL-10 production [118, 119]. This occurs due to interaction of both the Fc and Fab fragments with dendritic cells.

CD11c+ dendritic cells appear to be the primary dendritic cell targeted by IVIg [80]. Interestingly, in immunosuppressed transplant patients, CD11c+ cells are significantly decreased, while the number of Langerhans cells remains unchanged [120]. However, a CD1a+/CD11c+ subset of dendritic cells acts as a direct precursor to Langerhans cells, thus having potential added value in IVIg's role in the treatment cutaneous disease [121]

Crow et al. demonstrated that despite knocking out the common cytokine receptor gamma chain and other receptors for cytokines IL-1R, IL-4, IL-10, IL-12b, TNFα, IFN-y, or MIP-1a, IVIg-treated dendritic cells can still inhibit ITP [122]. Thus, cytokine modulation in isolation does not appear to have a direct role in dendritic cells inhibition by IVIg. In fact, Aubin et al. demonstrated that dendritic cell inhibition was independent of any changes in cytokine profiles [123]. Given these findings, it has been proposed that IVIg creates an IFN-γ refractory state without causing an apparent drop in IFN-γ [124].

IVIg causes a downregulation as well as decrease in function of MHC Class II molecules on dendritic cells [83, 125], while enhancing CD1d, a dendritic cell molecule involved in presentation of bacterial and endogenous lipid antigen complexes to T-cells and natural killer cells [126]. Decreased antigen-presenting abilities can account for IVIg's function in an FcγRIIβ independent fashion[83].

Cytokine Modulation

IVIg modifies the production of numerous pro- and anti-inflammatory cytokines. This can be through the presence of anti-cytokine antibodies, or through regulation of immune cells. IVIg contains numerous anti-cytokine antibodies at various concentrations based on the donor pool, including IL-1α, TNF-α, IL-8, and IFN-γ [127–131].

Changes in cytokine production vary based on the cellular assay used and are thus challenging to translate to clinical disease. For example, mitogen-stimulated PBMCs demonstrated no significant changes in IL-2, IL-10, TNF-a, or IFN y [132, 133], while a study using protein kinase C activator and ionomycin stimulated PBMCs demonstrated a significant decrease in IL-1, IL-2,IL-6, IFN-γ, and TNF-α [134]. Many studies have, however, demonstrated significant reductions in the level of TNF-α in a Fc dependent manner [127, 128]

Levels of IL-10 are convincingly enhanced following treatment with IVIg [135]. Clinically, levels of IL-10 have become elevated following treatment with IVIg in numerous diseases [136, 137]. Increases in IL-1Ra have additionally been confirmed in human studies [138, 139].

Effects on IgE

IVIg inhibits IgE production in a dose dependent manner by decreasing B-cell proliferation in an IL-4 and anti-CD40 state [140]. The Fab portion of IgG is a more potent inhibitor of IgE production than the Fc component [141]. In a disease such as bullous pemphigoid where tissue targeting IgE antibodies are detected [142, 143], this may act as an additional mechanism in achieving therapeutic response.

Effects on B-Cells

IVIg can overall reduce the number of B-cells, while modulating expression of CD19, CD20, and CD40. This reduction in B-cells is primarily due to apoptosis [144]. IVIg also contains antibodies targeting CD5, a T-cell marker which is also a marker for autoantibody secreting B-cells [145].

IVIg contains antibodies against BAFF and APRIL, which normally exert an anti-apoptotic effect on B-cells [146]. Elevations in BAFF and/or APRIL have been noted in myriad dermatologic conditions including atopic dermatitis, graft-versus-host disease, cutaneous and systemic lupus, sarcoidosis, dermatomyositis, Behcet's, psoriasis, systemic and localized scleroderma, and bullous pemphigoid [147–157]. Unlike these diseases, pemphigus vulgaris does not demonstrate elevated levels of BAFF or APRIL. Yet following successful treatment with rituximab, an elevation of BAFF is noted [158, 159].

IVIg's role in pemphigus may be rather due to increasing IL-10 producing B-cells. Increased levels of IL-10 producing B-cells were found in pemphigus patients achieving remission following IVIg, but not in those with active disease [160]. Thus, this may be an additional mechanism of an anti-inflammatory effect on B-cells.

Effects on T-Cells

IVIg has inhibitory effects on T-cell proliferation in several models, including mitogen, anti-CD3 antibody and tetanus toxoid induced T-cells [161, 162]. IVIg contains antibodies that interact with human CD4, inhibiting CD4+ T-cell function [163]. IVIg likewise contains low levels of antibodies that react with both the variable and constant region of the T-cell receptor B chain [164].

IVIg can lead to T-cell apoptosis, though to a smaller degree than B-cell apoptosis [144]. IVIg also inhibits the proliferation of antigen-specific T-cells without the induction of apoptosis [165]. This has been demonstrated to occur through arrest of the cell cycle at the G0 and G1 phase of the cell cycle, partially through an upregulation of p21/WAF-1 and Bcl-2 [61, 166]. IVIg additionally decreases antigen-specific CD8 activation [167]. Long-term treatment efficacy has been associated with a reduction in autoreactive T-cell responses [168].

Effects on Th17 Cells

Th17 is noted to be increased in numerous dermatologic diseases including alopecia areata, pemphigus, pemphigoid, and SLE [169–172]. Th17 is known to be directly involved in the pathogenesis of alopecia areata [169, 173]. Interestingly, epidermal filaggrin deficiency is associated with an increased Th17 response [174].

Treatment with IVIg results in a reduction in Th17. This is mediated by the Fab portion of IgG[175]. Th17 levels are inversely related to levels of Treg [176]. This has also been noted in pemphigus, occurring due to a dysfunctional CCR4-CCL2 interaction[170, 177]. While anti-IL-17 antibodies can be found in IVIg, these are not responsible for the inhibition of IL-17 secretion; rather a decrease in Th17 mediates this finding [178]. IL-17 has been shown to increase IgE production by B-cells which may also account for IVIg's IgE inhibiting properties [179].

Effects on Treg Cells

Regulatory T-cells (Tregs) are characterized by the presence of the transcription factor forkhead box P3 (FOXP3) [180]. Its expression marks a more regulatory phenotype [181]. Depleting Tregs in vivo can lead to a lupus-like phenotype [182] and decreases in Tregs lead to loss of self-tolerance [183]. The frequency of Treg is significantly decreased during the acute phase of Kawasaki disease and improved following IVIg [184]. Likewise, in eosinophilic granulomatosis with polyangiitis, IVIg restores Treg populations [185]. Low levels of Tregs have been identified in numerous dermatologic diseases including pemphigus vulgaris, chronic idiopathic urticaria, bullous pemphigoid, alopecia areata, cutaneous lupus, dermatitis herpetiformis, generalized vitiligo, systemic sclerosis, and polymorphous light eruption [169, 181, 186–194].

IVIg results in an increase in Tregs with improved regulatory function of these cells which can prevent T-cell and B-cell responses[195–197]. Treg expansion occurs through induction of cyclooxygenase-2 dependent prostaglandin E2 in human dendritic cells which only require the Fab component of IgG [175, 198]. IVIg can additionally enhance phosphorylation of ZAP70, increasing the suppressive function of Tregs [199]. In SLE, treatment with IVIg results in a significant increase in Treg [194, 200]. Likewise, in Kawasaki's disease, transcription levels of FOXp3 are enhanced following treatment with IVIg [196, 201]. These IVIg-induced subsets of Tregs demonstrate higher levels of CTLA-4 and secrete IL-10. These Tregs respond only to Fc and not Fab fragments [202].

Tregitopes are epitopes on both the Fc and Fab region that can bind to multiple HLA class 2 molecules, causing activation of FoxP3 [203]. These are also seen in IVIg which may further drive towards an increase in Treg [204].

Effects on Natural Killer Cells and Toll-Like Receptors (TLRs)

Dendritic cells are known to interact with natural killer (NK) cells [205]. NK cells decrease significantly following treatment with IVIg [206]. Inhibition of NK cells has been proposed to occur through CD200, a tolerance signaling molecule on other immune cells that acts on NK cells [207]. This suppression varies based on the formulation of IVIg used [208].

NK cells can interact with TLR3 and TLR9[205] which are both expressed on normal human keratinocytes [209]. Patients with SLE demonstrate a significantly higher level of TLR9, particularly in steroid resistant cases [210]. IVIg can attenuate TLR9 activation in patients with SLE [211]. TLR9 additionally has a role in chronic idiopathic urticaria, where plasmacytoid dendritic cells have an impaired response to TLR9 [212]. In psoriasis, keratinocytes have been shown to express TLR9 which is increased with elevated expression of the cathelicidin antimicrobial peptide LL-37, resulting in increased production of type-I IFN [213]. TLR7 and TLR9 induced IFN-α production can be inhibited by the Fc component of IgG and is mediated by PGE2 production [214].

Dermatologic Diseases Treatable with IgG

The dosage of IVIg can be split into two groups, high-dose IVIg which is 2–3 g/kg/cycle and low dose which is less than 2 g/kg/cycle. The main dermatologic diseases in which the therapeutic effects IVIg has been well established are discussed below.

Stevens Johnson Syndrome (SJS)/Toxic Epidermal Necrolysis (TEN)

IVIg is a commonly used therapy with 1/3 of surveyed physicians using it for the treatment of SJS and 2/3 of surveyed physicians using it for TEN [215]. Measurements of its efficacy have been limited by the retrospective nature of these studies and limited sample sizes. A meta-analysis of patients with TEN trended towards superiority of high-dose IVIg to low-dose IVIg (mortality of 18.9% vs. 50%%) [216]. In pediatric patients, there was a significantly decreased mortality in TEN patients treated with IVIg (0% compared to 21.6%) [216]. An updated meta-analysis demonstrated a significant correlation with IVIg dose and improved survival

[217]. Nevertheless, the use of IVIg in SJS/TEN remains controversial due to limited prospective data. Recent data suggesting superiority of cyclosporine also necessitates future prospective comparative studies [218]. Perhaps, these two treatment modalities can be combined.

IVIg appears to treat TEN through inhibition of the death receptor Fas [48]. Following treatment with IVIg, Fas and Fas-L expression becomes undetectable [219]. IVIg also results in deposition of IgG in both involved and uninvolved skin compared to untreated patients, suggesting a direct protective effect [220].

Autoimmune Blistering Disorders

Pemphigus Vulgaris and Pemphigus Foliaceus

IVIg is an efficacious treatment in pemphigus with significant steroid-sparing potential [221–228]. It can be used as an adjuvant to corticosteroids or as a monotherapy when corticosteroids and conventional immunosuppressives are contraindicated [229, 230]. IVIg is also a safe and efficacious treatment in pregnant women with pemphigus vulgaris as well as in juvenile patients [231, 232]. IVIg is typically given as a monthly dose of 2 g/kg divided into 5 infusions. Following disease quiescence, the frequency of therapy can be titrated down.

IVIg can lead to a rapid decline in circulating serum intercellular autoantibodies without disturbing normal IgG levels [221–227]. Normal degradation and removal from the body of all kinds of IgG antibodies after IVIg infusion results in a selective decrease of relative titer of pathogenic antibodies, because the level of normal antibodies is maintained by those present in the IVIg preparation. This appears to be due to saturation of FcRn [85]. This decrease can be enhanced with the addition of a cytotoxic drug, which can prevent a rebound in pathogenic antibodies following return of serum IgG levels to baseline [221, 222]. Affinity-purified anti-desmoglein antiidiotypic antibodies found in IVIg further inhibit the binding of anti-desmoglein 1 and 3 antibodies to recombinant desmoglein 1 and 3, respectively [233]. Several changes in inflammatory cytokine profiles have been noted in patients with pemphigus treated with IVIg. IVIg can additionally downregulate production of IL-1a and IL-1b while enhancing production of IL-Ra in pemphigus vulgaris patients [138]. While both IVIg and conventional immunosuppressive therapies result in an overall decrease in pro-inflammatory cytokines, only IVIg results in a greater decrease in circulating TNF-α [234].

The use of IVIg as a monotherapy following disease quiescence can lead to sustained long-term clinical remissions with eventual discontinuation of all therapies. This has been particularly well demonstrated in patients treated with both rituximab and IVIg [235–237]. The use of IVIg in combination with rituximab has led to long-lasting disease-free periods, with follow-up time exceeding 10 years [235–237]. These regimens include repeat IVIg infusions following cessation of rituximab after approximately 6 months with continuation of IVIg to approximately 3 years [235, 237]. These combined rituximab and IVIg regimens appear to lead to a more sustained clinical response than single cycles of rituximab [238, 239]. IVIg can also be combined with plasmapheresis or immunoadsorption to prevent rebound increases in pathogenic autoantibodies [228, 240].

Mucous Membrane Pemphigoid

Like in other immunobullous diseases, IVIg can be combined with the use of rituximab in patients with mucous membrane pemphigoid. Foster et al. demonstrated significant reduction in the development of blindness in patients with ocular cicatricial pemphigoid compared to the use of other immunosuppressives [241]. In oral pemphigoid, IVIg resulted in a prolonged and sustained clinical remission compared to patients with traditional immunosuppressives [242, 243]. Patients treated with IVIg had a statistically significant shorter treatment duration, fewer relapses, fewer adverse events, higher remission rate, better quality of life, and no development of extra-oral disease compared to controls who received traditional immunosuppression [243]. While a decrease in antibody titers is similarly noted in oral pemphigoid patients on traditional immunosuppressives and IVIg after 4 months of therapy, patients on IVIg have a significantly faster rate of decline in α6-integrin antibodies [242]. In ocular pemphigoid, similar decreases in α6-integrin antibody titer were noted with patients receiving IVIg as a monotherapy [244].

Likewise in a study of 15 patients with recalcitrant multisite mucous membrane pemphigoid, all patients were able to discontinue previous immunosuppressives and achieved prolonged and sustained remission [245].

Bullous Pemphigoid and Pemphigoid Gestationis

A randomized controlled trial of high-dose IVIg demonstrated significant improvement in disease activity scores in patients with steroid resistant bullous pemphigoid [246]. In A study of 15 bullous pemphigoid patients who had significant side effects from previous immunosuppressive therapies, it was demonstrated that all 15 patients achieved sustained clinical remission with a steroid sparing effect [247]. Other reviews of cases and small case series have shown that approximately 80% of patients improve with IVIg. Delay of treatment, the use of low-dose IVIg, or failure to give multiple infusions is associated with a lower response rate to IVIg [248, 249]. The use of concomitant immunosuppressive agents is recommended, as it prevents rebound of autoantibodies [250].

IVIg at a dose of 2 g/kg/month has been used successfully as a monotherapy in the treatment of pemphigoid gestationis in a patient unable to tolerate corticosteroids due to gestational diabetes [251]. Thus, IVIg can be safely used in recalcitrant cases of pemphigoid gestationis [252].

Epidermolysis Bullosa Acquisita (EBA)

While numerous cases have been reported demonstrating IVIg's efficacy in EBA, the largest retrospective study in EBA followed 10 patients. All patients were recalcitrant to conventional immunosuppression. Following 5–9 months of IVIg, all were able to discontinue all other immunosuppressives including glucocorticoids, and were subsequently maintained on IVIg monotherapy. No patients experienced recurrence of disease during a mean follow-up period of 54 months [253]. A small retrospective study following EBA patients who received IVIg combined with rituximab also demonstrated positive outcomes [254].

Data from mouse studies in experimental EBA showed superior clinical response from IVIg compared to methylprednisolone, associated with autoantibody reduction, a switch to non-complement fixing autoantibody isotypes as well as overall less complement deposition on immunofluorescence [44].

Dermatomyositis

IVIg is an effective treatment in dermatomyositis, lowering cumulative corticosteroid consumption and resulting in symptomatic improvement [255]. In particular, IVIg results in significantly improved muscular remission rates, as well as fewer muscular relapses compared to traditional immunosuppressives [256]. Response to therapy in muscle disease has been associated with downregulation of TGF-$\beta 1$ [257]. A systematic review of 153 patients with amyopathic dermatomyositis noted that IVIg was the most likely treatment to lead to improvement or remission compared to other therapies [258]. Strikingly, improvement with IVIg was noted following the first treatment cycle and a majority of patients were able to discontinue concomitant immunosuppression [259, 260]. An insufficient number of infusions may lead to short-lived remission, thus decreasing overall efficacy [261]. Soluble IL-2R is associated with response to IVIg in patients with extensive cutaneous disease, while concomitant autoantibodies or malignancy were associated with a failure in response[262].

IVIg is also effective in juvenile dermatomyositis, though unequal control groups limited further analysis of the degree of improved efficacy compared to traditional immunosuppression [263, 264]. Children appear to have more variability in regard to tolerating different formulations of IVIg, primarily due to IgA content [265]. Thus, low IgA formulations should be particularly sought after in this patient population.

IVIg can also be used for the treatment of dermatomyositis-associated dystrophic calcinosis, however, given the paucity of cases and mixed results, further data are needed [266–271].

Recent German guidelines recommend the use of IVIg in dermatomyositis cases refractory to corticosteroids plus steroid sparing immunosuppressives before rituximab [272]. The use of pulse IVIg was not associated with any difference in mean therapeutic strength or cumulative corticosteroid dose over a 36-month period compared to methotrexate, mycophenolate mofetil, or azathioprine [273]. IVIg is also recommended in severe esophageal involvement in dermatomyositis [274].

Atopic Dermatitis

Current evidence is insufficient to support the role of IVIg in atopic dermatitis as there are many conflicting clinical studies [275–277]. Particularly, IVIg's effect appears short lived, improving after 3 months of therapy but declining by 6 months [278]. A small study comparing cyclosporine to IVIg noted cyclosporine to be superior as assessed by the Scoring Atopic Dermatitis (SCORAD) measure [279]. Additionally a double-blind randomized controlled trial demonstrated disappointing results with 15% improvement at 30 months and 22% improvement at 60 days using SCORAD [280].

While treatment with IVIg was associated with a decrease in the inflammatory markers ICAM-1, ELAM-1 and eosinophil cationic protein, IVIg did not result in alterations of the elevated Th1/Th2 ratio seen in atopic patients [113].

Cutaneous Lupus Erythematosus

IVIg has been well established in the treatment of SLE [281]. It can, however, also be used in cutaneous disease [282]. In a proof of concept study, patients with cutaneous lupus were treated with 3 monthly cycles of 2 g/kg/month of IVIg as a monotherapy over 4 days and monitored for 6 months off therapy. Patients achieved improvement in their Cutaneous Lupus Erythematosus Disease Area and Severity Index (CLASI-A), with only 3 of 16 patients experiencing mild short-lived relapses [283]. A study of low-dose IVIg also demonstrated efficacy, however, to an apparent lesser degree than high-dose IVIg [284]. IVIg's efficacy has been described in a case of lupus panniculitis[285].

Urticaria

High-dose IVIg in chronic idiopathic urticaria, which is an autoimmune disease associated with autoantibodies to receptor of the Fc region of IgE (FcεRIα) [286], leads to benefit in a majority of patients with 3/10 patients experiencing complete remission following a single cycle, 2 with temporary remissions, and symptom improvement in the remaining patients [287]. A different study of 6 patients noted 4/6 patients achieved complete remission after 2–4 cycles [288]. An additional study demonstrated 19/26 patients with complete remission, with 20 patients remaining disease free at 12-month follow-up after receiving low-dose IVIg (0.15 kg/kg monthly) for at least 6 months of treatment [289].

IVIg's efficacy in solar urticaria is limited. In a retrospective study of 9 patients, only 2 showed remission on phototesting. Half of patients additionally experienced headache [290]. In an alternative study of 7 patients, 5 patients experience complete remission; however, these patients still required antihistamines [291].

A single study has evaluated IVIg's utility in pressure urticaria, with high-dose IVIg given to 8 patients with pressure urticaria. Three of eight patients achieved remission with 2 others showing improvement [292].

Scleroderma

IVIg is effective in numerous facets of scleroderma, though studies remain limited in sample size [293]. IVIg is fairly efficacious in recalcitrant diffuse cutaneous systemic sclerosis [294, 295], though its efficacy remains similar to that of mycophenolate mofetil [296]. IVIg appears to function in part by causing recovery of Th1 cytokines in both sera and skin of patients with scleroderma [297]. IVIg has been shown to improve gastrointestinal dysfunction [298]. Gastrointestinal dysfunction in scleroderma has been associated with autoantibodies targeting the muscarinic-3 receptor. IVIg may reverse this cholinergic dysfunction through anti-idiotypic neutralization of these autoantibodies [299].

Kawasaki's Disease

IVIg is recommended at a dose of 2 g/kg as a single cycle within 10 days of disease onset [300]. Lower doses were associated with a greater risk of coronary artery abnormalities as well as longer duration of fever. IVIg resistance is, however, a significant problem in the treatment of Kawasaki's disease. Numerous risk scores have been created to predict IVIg resistance [301–304]. These are, however, predominantly clinical factors which do not provide an understanding of the underlying mechanism conferring resistance. The immunology of Kawasaki's disease and its interaction with IVIg is complex, described in detail by Burns et al. [305]. In IVIg resistant patients, TNF-α inhibitors are recommended [306].

Vascular Disorders

Livedoid Vasculopathy

Few small retrospective studies demonstrate IVIg's efficacy in livedoid vasculopathy. After even one cycle of high-dose IVIg, significant drops in erythema, ulceration, and pain were noted [307–309]. Low-dose IVIG additionally demonstrated immediate benefits [310]. Relapse following treatment with IVIG is common, however, occurring after a median remission of 10–27 months, but these were readily treated with a repeat cycle [308, 309].

Anti-Neutrophil Cytoplasmic Autoantibody (ANCA)-Associated Vasculitides

ANCA-associated vasculitis consists of three diseases: granulomatosis with polyangiitis (formerly Wegner's disease), eosinophilic granulomatosis with polyangiitis (formerly Churg-Strauss disease), and microscopic polyangiitis. IVIg is a valuable adjuvant to corticosteroids or non-steroidal immunosuppressives, with most experiencing a clinical response to IVIG [311–313]. However, the results are often short-lived [314]. In a study of 22 patients with either granulomatosis with polyangiitis or microscopic polyangiitis, 14 experienced complete remission, with 8 maintaining remission at the 2 year point [311]. At the 6 month point, half of patients with any of the ANCA-associated vasculitides experience complete remission [315]. In light of the limited randomized controlled trials, current evidence does not demonstrate IVIg's superiority to corticosteroids plus immunosuppressives in the treatment of granulomatosis with polyangiitis, thus IVIg is typically reserved for recalcitrant cases [316]. Improvement in granulomatosis with polyangiitis appears best in cutaneous or otolaryngological involvement [317].

In patients with eosinophilic granulomatosis with polyangiitis with residual neuropathy, IVIg leads to significant improvement in muscle strength [318]. IVIg is particularly helpful in those patients with myocardial or neurologic manifestations, where corticosteroids and cyclophosphamide are often ineffective [319]. More sustained remission can be attained with combined plasmapheresis and high-dose IVIg administered monthly for the first 6 months, and every other month for an additional 6 months [320].

Behçet's Disease

Few cases of refractory Behçet's disease have described success with intravenous immunoglobulin [321–323]. In a case series of four patients who failed traditional treatment modalities, all with oral apthosis, genital ulceration and other cutaneous manifestations, experienced immediate and sustained responses following treatment with IVIG [321]. A case series of 6 eyes likewise demonstrated IVIg's efficacy [322].

Cutaneous Polyarteritis Nodosa

IVIg has been used effectively in few cases of refractory cutaneous polyarteritis nodosa, improving both ulceration and neuropathy [324–328]. Its use has been most described in pediatric cutaneous polyarteritis nodosa [329]. In a series of three patients with cutaneous polyarteritis with extensive and recalcitrant toe ulceration, all patients experienced on the second cycle of high-dose IVIg, with clearance by the third cycle [330].

Degos' Disease (Malignant Atrophic Papulosis)

Very few cases have reported on IVIg's use in Degos' disease. The results have, however, been inconsistent [331–334].

Leukocytoclastic Vasculitis/Urticarial Vasculitis

IVIg can be efficacious in the treatment of leukocytoclastic vasculitis and urticarial vasculitis in both SLE related and idiopathic cases [335–341]. Clinical improvement has been noted to occur after just one dose of high-dose IVIg [342].

Adverse Effects of IVIg

Minor adverse reactions are common in IVIg, with a majority occurring within the first 6 h of therapy [343]. They are usually related to infusion rate and include headache, flushing, chills, fever, nausea, vomiting, dizziness, sweating, hypertension, feelings of tightness in the chest, back pain, and muscle aches. A retrospective study of 9892 infusions in 174 patients with either pemphigus or pemphigoid evaluated adverse events, noting an incidence of adverse events occurring in 8.9% of infusions and in 70% of patients. However, these side effects were minor, such as fatigue, nausea, vomiting, and chills. Only one major adverse event was noted in one patient: acute renal failure. No patients required hospitalization for medication-related adverse events [344]. Well-documented adverse reactions as well as their respective prevention or management are discussed below.

Headache

Headaches are a common adverse reaction to IVIg and should not be confused for aseptic meningitis. These headaches can be persistent from hours to days and can be delayed in onset up to 12 h following infusion. Strategies to minimize headaches include hydration, decrease in infusion rate, or use of an alternative IVIg product. Sumatriptan, dihydroergotamine, analgesics, or propranolol can be used as premedication to prevent headaches in patients who experience headaches with treatment [345]. With these

therapies, the overwhelming majority of patients do not experience further headaches. Headaches that fail to respond to therapy and that come with associated neck stiffness, photophobia, fever, and myalgia raise concern for aseptic meningitis. There is a higher risk of developing aseptic meningitis in patients with a prior history of migraine headache [346]. It has been suggested that anti-neutrophil antibodies contained within the IVIg may lead to neutrophil activation within the CNS, leading to aseptic meningitis [347]. ANCAs have been identified in IVIg, causing neutrophil degranulation in an Fc independent manner, which can account for some of the side effect profile [347]. Corticosteroids or TNF-α inhibitors can be used in the case that continuation with IVIg is essential [348].

Renal Failure

Renal failure is typically seen in patients with preexisting renal disease who receive sucrose containing IVIg [349]. It results from osmotic injury. As sucrose is not metabolized in the kidneys, it deposits in the proximal tubule leading to edema and osmotic nephrosis [350]. Post-IVIg renal failure begins with an increase in BUN or creatinine, later followed by oliguria, peaking 5–7 days after transfusion [348]. Limiting daily doses to 0.5 g/kg as well as the use of slower infusion rates can help prevent renal toxicity [348]. Diuretics and renin-angiotensin system inhibitors should not be used [351].

Thromboembolism

There is a higher risk of arterial thromboembolism compared to venous thrombosis, with up to 80% of thromboembolic events occurring in the arterial system [348]. This has been attributed to hyperviscosity as well as retained coagulation factors, more common if history of cardiac disease, stroke, myocardial infarction, thrombosis, old age, hypercoagulation, limited mobility. In higher risk patients [348, 352], limiting daily doses to 0.4–0.5 g/day, hydration, slow infusion rates limited to a maximum of 100 mg/kg/hr, as well as premedication with aspirin or heparin can help prevent the development of thromboembolism [343, 348].

Hemolysis

Mild hemolysis can occur as a result of anti-A, anti-B, anti-D, or anti-K antibodies contained within IVIg[348]. Generally, hemolysis is mild. In the case of severe hemolysis, corticosteroids may be of benefit[351].

Cutaneous Manifestations

Adverse cutaneous reactions occur in approximately 6% of patients receiving IVIg. These, however, typically resolve within 1–4 h [351]. These reactions are most commonly urticarial, though eczematous eruptions and pompholyx have also been described [351, 353]. Most of these patients experienced the eruption following their first treatment. IVIg treatment for neurologic conditions accounted for the majority of patients with eczematous eruptions, without underlying atopy being described [353]. Patients can be treated with diphenhydramine and corticosteroids. Patients with recurrent urticaria following treatment can be pre-medicated with diphenhydramine and/or a low dose of corticosteroid [351]. Eczematous eruptions or pompholyx can be managed with topical corticosteroids [353].

Interestingly, antibodies against SSA have been detected in IVIg and were thought to be the cause of a discoid lupus eruption in a patient with common variable immunodeficiency treated with IVIg that contained anti-SSA [354]. This relationship, however, remains unclear.

Anaphylaxis

Anaphylactic reactions to IVIg are rare and generally a result of IgA deficiency. Pre-screening patients for IgA can help to prevent anaphylactic reactions. In a patient with anaphylaxis, the infusion should be stopped; a corticosteroid and antihistamine should be given [348].

Cost Issues with IVIg Therapy

IVIg's high cost is an area of obvious concern. However, given its decreased risk of opportunistic infections, complications and hospitalizations, studies point towards it being an overall cost-saving therapy compared to conventional immunosuppression. A cost analysis using patients with mucous membrane pemphigoid, ocular cicatricial pemphigoid, bullous pemphigoid, and pemphigus vulgaris has demonstrated it to be significantly less expensive than conventional immunosuppressive therapy when taking into account indirect costs such as hospitalizations [355]. Of note, this study was performed in the United States. In mucous membrane pemphigoid, the use of IVIg compared to traditional immunosuppressives resulted in cost savings, as patients had fewer hospitalizations and adverse events [356]. Still in the treatment of immunobullous disorders, IVIg is a major driver of cost [357].

A cost analysis in Thailand for patients with dermatomyositis likewise demonstrated significant cost savings when IVIg was used as an adjuvant compared to other immunosuppressives used in addition to corticosteroids [358].

Case Report of IVIg Monotherapy in Pemphigus Vulgaris Patient
History of Presenting Illness

A 46-year-old man presented to the dermatology clinic with numerous oral mucosal erosions which had persisted for the past 8–10 months. The patient had been seen by an oral surgeon at an outside facility, who performed a biopsy from the right buccal mucosa. Histopathology demonstrated suprabasilar vesiculation and acantholysis, favored to be pemphigus vulgaris (no immunofluorescence studies or serologies were performed at that time). The patient reported a history of oral lesions that would heal on their own, followed by development of new lesions, although he had not received any treatment for his presumed pemphigus. He denied pain, difficulty swallowing, and weight loss at the time of presentation, nor did he endorse ever having skin involvement.

Past Medical History
- None

Medications
- Multivitamins

Social History
- No tobacco
- Occasional alcohol consumption

Previous Therapies
- None

Physical Exam
- Oral cavity: right and left buccal mucosa with three irregularly shaped erosions, 3–6 mm in diameter and minor background hyperemia.
- Skin: no lesions with negative Nikolsky sign

Workup:
This patient presented with a history, exam, and outside biopsy highly suggestive of pemphigus vulgaris. This diagnosis was confirmed in our clinic by ELISA and indirect immunofluorescence (IIF), which showed elevated IgG against desmoglein 3 (99 units, with normal defined as <9) and the presence of cell-surface IgG on monkey esophagus substrate (1:1280), respectively. IgG to desmoglein 1 was negative (1 unit, with normal defined as <9), as was ELISA

for pemphigoid antibodies (IgG BPAg180 = 3 units; IgG BPAg230 = 1 unit, both with normal defined as <9). IgG and IgA antibodies to the basement membrane zone were also negative on IIF. Taken together, these serologic results confirmed the initial diagnosis of pemphigus vulgaris.

Management:

This patient was initially started on a regimen consisting of mycophenolate mofetil 1 g PO BID, tetracycline 500 mg PO TID, and niacinamide 500 mg PO TID. Clobetasol 0.05% gel was applied to mucosal erosions daily. After discussing with the patient pros and cons of systemic corticosteroid and rituximab therapies, the decision was made to try IVIg first. After initiation of IVIg therapy at 2 g/kg/month, the patient's oral lesions healed within weeks. During the ensuing 6 months, however, the patient developed periodic breakthrough erosions, typically one every 2–3 months, which healed within a few weeks. The patient experienced no side effects or adverse reactions from IVIg, and tolerated infusions very well.

After 9 months of uninterrupted IVIg therapy, the patient entered complete and stable remission. After 6 months of a lesion-free period, IVIg was tapered to every other month for 6 months, followed by cessation of all therapy. The patient has been in stable remission for 5 years. The successful outcome of IVIg therapy of pemphigus vulgaris in this patient illustrates feasibility of achieving a prolonged, stable remission off therapy using IVIg in combination with oral cytotoxic immunosuppressive agents, such as mycophenolate mofetil, in addition to mitochondrion-protecting agents, such as a tetracycline antibiotic and niacinamide. This protocol eliminates the need for potentially hazardous systemic therapies with prednisone and/or rituximab.

Conclusion

IVIg is a safe and effective drug to rapidly induce and maintain a prolonged clinical remission in a large variety of dermatological conditions unresponsive to conventional therapy, producing a distinct corticosteroid-sparing effect. Its early use is of significant benefit in patients who may experience life-threatening complications from corticosteroids and immunosuppression. IVIg works better if given together with a cytotoxic drug to prevent a rebound effect. The safety of IVIg therapy is affected by its administration rate, frequency IgA content, concentration—fluid overload if dilute and osmotic overload if concentrated, and sugar content. The known mechanisms of therapeutic action of IVIg include selective elimination of pathogenic antibodies due to blocking (saturation) of FcRn that protects IgG molecules from lysosomal degradation, anti-inflammatory action of sialylated IgG species that upregulate expression of the inhibitory FcγRIIB receptor on immune cells, inactivation of pathogenic antibodies by the anti-idiotypic antibodies, activation of anergic/apoptotic program in B-cells, increase of B-cells producing the immunosuppressive cytokine IL-10 as well as anti-apoptotic and anti-oncotic effects on keratinocytes.

Acknowledgments The authors would like to thank Mark Mazaitis for assistance with Fig. 39.1.

References

1. Bruton OC. Agammaglobulinemia. Pediatrics. 1952;9:722–8.
2. Imbach P, Barandun S, Baumgartner C, Hirt A, Hofer F, Wagner HP. High-dose intravenous gammaglobulin therapy of refractory, in particular idiopathic thrombocytopenia in childhood. Helv Paediatr Acta. 1981;36:81–6.
3. Durandy A, Kaveri SV, Kuijpers TW, Basta M, Miescher S, Ravetch JV, et al. Intravenous immunoglobulins--understanding properties and mechanisms. Clin Exp Immunol. 2009;158(Suppl 1):2–13.
4. Radosevich M, Burnouf T. Intravenous immunoglobulin G: trends in production methods, quality control and quality assurance. Vox Sang. 2010;98:12–28.
5. Barahona Afonso AF, Joao CM. The production processes and biological effects of intravenous immunoglobulin. Biomolecules. 2016;6
6. Prins C, Gelfand EW, French LE. Intravenous immunoglobulin: properties, mode of action and practical use in dermatology. Acta Derm Venereol. 2007;87:206–18.
7. Ballow M. Intravenous immunoglobulins: clinical experience and viral safety. J Am Pharm Assoc (Wash). 2002;42:449–58. quiz 58-9
8. Thorpe SJ. Specifications for anti-A and anti-B in intravenous immunoglobulin: history and rationale. Transfusion. 2015;55(Suppl 2):S80–5.
9. Ghetie V, Hubbard JG, Kim JK, Tsen MF, Lee Y, Ward ES. Abnormally short serum half-lives of IgG in beta 2-microglobulin-deficient mice. Eur J Immunol. 1996;26:690–6.
10. Morell A, Terry WD, Waldmann TA. Metabolic properties of IgG subclasses in man. J Clin Invest. 1970;49:673–80.
11. Wasserman RL, Church JA, Peter HH, Sleasman JW, Melamed I, Stein MR, et al. Pharmacokinetics of a new 10% intravenous immunoglobulin in patients receiving replacement therapy for primary immunodeficiency. Eur J Pharm Sci. 2009;37:272–8.
12. Junghans RP, Anderson CL. The protection receptor for IgG catabolism is the beta2-microglobulin-containing neonatal intestinal transport receptor. Proc Natl Acad Sci U S A. 1996;93:5512–6.
13. Leontyev D, Neschadim A, Branch DR. Cytokine profiles in mouse models of experimental immune thrombocytopenia reveal a lack of inflammation and differences in response to intravenous immunoglobulin depending on the mouse strain. Transfusion. 2014;54:2871–9.
14. Dezsi L, Horvath Z, Vecsei L. Intravenous immunoglobulin: pharmacological properties and use in polyneuropathies. Expert Opin Drug Metab Toxicol. 2016:1–16.
15. Pierangeli SS, Espinola R, Liu X, Harris EN, Salmon JE. Identification of an Fc gamma receptor-independent mecha-

nism by which intravenous immunoglobulin ameliorates antiphospholipid antibody-induced thrombogenic phenotype. Arthritis Rheum. 2001;44:876–83.

16. Debre M, Bonnet MC, Fridman WH, Carosella E, Philippe N, Reinert P, et al. Infusion of Fc gamma fragments for treatment of children with acute immune thrombocytopenic purpura. Lancet. 1993;342:945–9.

17. Kaveri SV. Intravenous immunoglobulin: exploiting the potential of natural antibodies. Autoimmun Rev. 2012;11:792–4.

18. Coutinho A, Kazatchkine MD, Avrameas S. Natural autoantibodies. Curr Opin Immunol. 1995;7:812–8.

19. Watanabe M, Uchida K, Nakagaki K, Trapnell BC, Nakata K. High avidity cytokine autoantibodies in health and disease: pathogenesis and mechanisms. Cytokine Growth Factor Rev. 2010;21:263–73.

20. Casali P, Prabhakar BS, Notkins AL. Characterization of multireactive autoantibodies and identification of Leu-1+ B lymphocytes as cells making antibodies binding multiple self and exogenous molecules. Int Rev Immunol. 1988;3:17–45.

21. Hurez V, Dietrich G, Kaveri SV, Kazatchkine MD. Polyreactivity is a property of natural and disease-associated human autoantibodies. Scand J Immunol. 1993;38:190–6.

22. Lacroix-Desmazes S, Kaveri SV, Mouthon L, Ayouba A, Malanchere E, Coutinho A, et al. Self-reactive antibodies (natural autoantibodies) in healthy individuals. J Immunol Methods. 1998;216:117–37.

23. von Gunten S, Simon HU. Natural anti-Siglec autoantibodies mediate potential immunoregulatory mechanisms: implications for the clinical use of intravenous immunoglobulins (IVIg). Autoimmun Rev. 2008;7(6):453.

24. von Gunten S, Vogel M, Schaub A, Stadler BM, Miescher S, Crocker PR, et al. Intravenous immunoglobulin preparations contain anti-Siglec-8 autoantibodies. J Allergy Clin Immunol. 2007;119:1005–11.

25. von Gunten S, Schaub A, Vogel M, Stadler BM, Miescher S, Simon HU. Immunologic and functional evidence for anti-Siglec-9 autoantibodies in intravenous immunoglobulin preparations. Blood. 2006;108:4255–9.

26. Hamilos DL, Christensen J. Treatment of Churg-Strauss syndrome with high-dose intravenous immunoglobulin. J Allergy Clin Immunol. 1991;88:823–4.

27. Khan S, Dore PC, Sewell WA. Both patient characteristics and IVIG product-specific mechanisms may affect eosinophils in immunoglobulin-treated Kawasaki disease. Pediatr Allergy Immunol. 2008;19:186–7.

28. Kuo HC, Yang KD, Liang CD, Bong CN, HR Y, Wang L, et al. The relationship of eosinophilia to intravenous immunoglobulin treatment failure in Kawasaki disease. Pediatr Allergy Immunol. 2007;18:354–9.

29. Pan Y, Yuhasz SC, Amzel LM. Anti-idiotypic antibodies: biological function and structural studies. FASEB J. 1995;9:43–9.

30. Rossi F, Dietrich G, Kazatchkine MD. Anti-idiotypes against autoantibodies in normal immunoglobulins: evidence for network regulation of human autoimmune responses. Immunol Rev. 1989;110:135–49.

31. Rossi F, Kazatchkine MD. Antiidiotypes against autoantibodies in pooled normal human polyspecific Ig. J Immunol. 1989;143:4104–9.

32. Ronda N, Haury M, Nobrega A, Coutinho A, Kazatchkine MD. Selectivity of recognition of variable (V) regions of autoantibodies by intravenous immunoglobulin (IVIg). Clin Immunol Immunopathol. 1994;70:124–8.

33. Ronda N, Haury M, Nobrega A, Kaveri SV, Coutinho A, Kazatchkine MD. Analysis of natural and disease-associated

34. Zhang W, Reichlin M. Production and characterization of a human monoclonal anti-idiotype to anti-ribosomal P antibodies. Clin Immunol. 2005;114:130–6.

35. Zhang W, Winkler T, Kalden JR, Reichlin M. Isolation of human anti-idiotypes broadly cross reactive with anti-dsDNA antibodies from patients with Systemic lupus erythematosus. Scand J Immunol. 2001;53:192–7.

36. Pall AA, Varagunam M, Adu D, Smith N, Richards NT, Taylor CM, et al. Anti-idiotypic activity against anti-myeloperoxidase antibodies in pooled human immunoglobulin. Clin Exp Immunol. 1994;95:257–62.

37. Pradhan VD, Ghosh K. Anti-idiotype antibodies in immune regulation of anca associated vasculitis. Indian J Dermatol. 2009;54:258–62.

38. Alvarado-Flores E, Avalos-Diaz E, Diaz LA, Herrera-Esparza R. Anti-idiotype antibodies neutralize in vivo the blistering effect of Pemphigus foliaceus IgG. Scand J Immunol. 2001;53:254–8.

39. Bouhlal H, Martinvalet D, Teillaud JL, Fridman C, Kazatchkine MD, Bayry J, et al. Natural autoantibodies to Fcgamma receptors in intravenous immunoglobulins. J Clin Immunol. 2014;34(Suppl. 1):S4–11.

40. Lutz HU, Stammler P, Bianchi V, Trueb RM, Hunziker T, Burger R, et al. Intravenously applied IgG stimulates complement attenuation in a complement-dependent autoimmune disease at the amplifying C3 convertase level. Blood. 2004;103:465–72.

41. Machimoto T, Guerra G, Burke G, Fricker FJ, Colona J, Ruiz P, et al. Effect of IVIG administration on complement activation and HLA antibody levels. Transpl Int. 2010;23:1015–22.

42. Lutz HU, Stammler P, Jelezarova E, Nater M, Spath PJ. High doses of immunoglobulin G attenuate immune aggregate-mediated complement activation by enhancing physiologic cleavage of C3b in C3bn-IgG complexes. Blood. 1996;88:184–93.

43. Basta M, Fries LF, Frank MM. High doses of intravenous Ig inhibit in vitro uptake of C4 fragments onto sensitized erythrocytes. Blood. 1991;77:376–80.

44. Hirose M, Tiburzy B, Ishii N, Pipi E, Wende S, Rentz E, et al. Effects of intravenous immunoglobulins on mice with experimental epidermolysis bullosa acquisita. J Invest Dermatol. 2015;135:768–75.

45. Basta M, Langlois PF, Marques M, Frank MM, Fries LF. High-dose intravenous immunoglobulin modifies complement-mediated in vivo clearance. Blood. 1989;74:326–33.

46. Wada J, Shintani N, Kikutani K, Nakae T, Yamauchi T, Takechi K. Intravenous immunoglobulin prevents experimental autoimmune myositis in SJL mice by reducing anti-myosin antibody and by blocking complement deposition. Clin Exp Immunol. 2001;124:282–9.

47. Basta M, Van Goor F, Luccioli S, Billings EM, Vortmeyer AO, Baranyi L, et al. F(ab)'2-mediated neutralization of C3a and C5a anaphylatoxins: a novel effector function of immunoglobulins. Nat Med. 2003;9:431–8.

48. Viard I, Wehrli P, Bullani R, Schneider P, Holler N, Salomon D, et al. Inhibition of toxic epidermal necrolysis by blockade of CD95 with human intravenous immunoglobulin. Science. 1998;282:490–3.

49. Trautmann A, Akdis M, Schmid-Grendelmeier P, Disch R, Brocker EB, Blaser K, et al. Targeting keratinocyte apoptosis in the treatment of atopic dermatitis and allergic contact dermatitis. J Allergy Clin Immunol. 2001;108:839–46.

50. Prasad NK, Papoff G, Zeuner A, Bonnin E, Kazatchkine MD, Ruberti G, et al. Therapeutic preparations of normal polyspecific

IgG (IVIg) induce apoptosis in human lymphocytes and monocytes: a novel mechanism of action of IVIg involving the Fas apoptotic pathway. J Immunol. 1998;161:3781–90.

51. Altznauer F, von Gunten S, Spath P, Simon HU. Concurrent presence of agonistic and antagonistic anti-CD95 autoantibodies in intravenous Ig preparations. J Allergy Clin Immunol. 2003;112:1185–90.

52. Sooryanarayana PN, Bonnin E, Pashov A, Ben Jilani K, Ameisen JC, et al. Phosphorylation of Bcl-2 and mitochondrial changes are associated with apoptosis of lymphoblastoid cells induced by normal immunoglobulin G. Biochem Biophys Res Commun. 1999;264:896–901.

53. Aoyama-Ishikawa M, Seishu A, Kawakami S, Maeshige N, Miyoshi M, Ueda T, et al. Intravenous immunoglobulin-induced neutrophil apoptosis in the lung during murine endotoxemia. Surg Infect (Larchmt). 2014;15:36–42.

54. von Gunten S, Simon HU. Cell death modulation by intravenous immunoglobulin. J Clin Immunol. 2010;30(Suppl 1):S24–30.

55. Arredondo J, Chernyavsky AI, Karaouni A, Grando SA. Novel mechanisms of target cell death and survival and of therapeutic action of IVIg in Pemphigus. Am J Pathol. 2005;167:1531–44.

56. Winkler J, Kroiss S, Rand ML, Azzouzi I, Annie Bang KW, Speer O, et al. Platelet apoptosis in paediatric immune thrombocytopenia is ameliorated by intravenous immunoglobulin. Br J Haematol. 2012;156:508–15.

57. Inci A, Sahinturk Unal D, Osman Ozes N, Erin N, Akcakus M, Oygur N. The efficacy of intravenous immunoglobulin on lipopolysaccharide-induced fetal brain inflammation in preterm rats. Am J Obstet Gynecol. 2013;209:347. e1-8

58. Kalay S, Oztekin O, Tezel G, Aldemir H, Sahin E, Koksoy S, et al. Role of immunoglobulin in neuronal apoptosis in a neonatal rat model of hypoxic ischemic brain injury. Exp Ther Med. 2014;7:734–8.

59. Nakatani K, Takeshita S, Tsujimoto H, Sekine I. Intravenous immunoglobulin (IVIG) preparations induce apoptosis in TNF-alpha-stimulated endothelial cells via a mitochondria-dependent pathway. Clin Exp Immunol. 2002;127:445–54.

60. Widiapradja A, Vegh V, Lok KZ, Manzanero S, Thundyil J, Gelderblom M, et al. Intravenous immunoglobulin protects neurons against amyloid beta-peptide toxicity and ischemic stroke by attenuating multiple cell death pathways. J Neurochem. 2012;122:321–32.

61. Ekberg C, Nordstrom E, Skansen-Saphir U, Mansouri M, Raqib R, Sundqvist VA, et al. Human polyspecific immunoglobulin for therapeutic use induces p21/WAF-1 and Bcl-2, which may be responsible for G1 arrest and long-term survival. Hum Immunol. 2001;62:215–27.

62. Tackenberg B, Jelcic I, Baerenwaldt A, Oertel WH, Sommer N, Nimmerjahn F, et al. Impaired inhibitory Fcgamma receptor IIB expression on B cells in chronic inflammatory demyelinating polyneuropathy. Proc Natl Acad Sci U S A. 2009;106:4788–92.

63. Pincetic A, Bournazos S, DiLillo DJ, Maamary J, Wang TT, Dahan R, et al. Type I and type II Fc receptors regulate innate and adaptive immunity. Nat Immunol. 2014;15:707–16.

64. Smith KG, Clatworthy MR. FcgammaRIIB in autoimmunity and infection: evolutionary and therapeutic implications. Nat Rev Immunol. 2010;10:328–43.

65. Nikolova KA, Tchorbanov AI, Djoumerska-Alexieva IK, Nikolova M, Vassilev TL. Intravenous immunoglobulin up-regulates the expression of the inhibitory FcgammaIIB receptor on B cells. Immunol Cell Biol. 2009;87:529–33.

66. Takai T, Ono M, Hikida M, Ohmori H, Ravetch JV. Augmented humoral and anaphylactic responses in Fc gamma RII-deficient mice. Nature. 1996;379:346–9.

67. Kalergis AM, Ravetch JV. Inducing tumor immunity through the selective engagement of activating Fcgamma receptors on dendritic cells. J Exp Med. 2002;195:1653–9.

68. Clynes R, Maizes JS, Guinamard R, Ono M, Takai T, Ravetch JV. Modulation of immune complex-induced inflammation in vivo by the coordinate expression of activation and inhibitory Fc receptors. J Exp Med. 1999;189:179–85.

69. Clatworthy MR, Smith KG. FcgammaRIIb balances efficient pathogen clearance and the cytokine-mediated consequences of sepsis. J Exp Med. 2004;199:717–23.

70. Daeron M, Malbec O, Latour S, Arock M, Fridman WH. Regulation of high-affinity IgE receptor-mediated mast cell activation by murine low-affinity IgG receptors. J Clin Invest. 1995; 95:577–85.

71. Fong DC, Malbec O, Arock M, Cambier JC, Fridman WH, Daeron M. Selective in vivo recruitment of the phosphatidylinositol phosphatase SHIP by phosphorylated Fc gammaRIIB during negative regulation of IgE-dependent mouse mast cell activation. Immunol Lett. 1996;54:83–91.

72. Samuelsson A, Towers TL, Ravetch JV. Anti-inflammatory activity of IVIG mediated through the inhibitory Fc receptor. Science. 2001;291:484–6.

73. Kaneko Y, Nimmerjahn F, Madaio MP, Ravetch JV. Pathology and protection in nephrotoxic nephritis is determined by selective engagement of specific Fc receptors. J Exp Med. 2006;203: 789–97.

74. Bruhns P, Samuelsson A, Pollard JW, Ravetch JV. Colony-stimulating factor-1-dependent macrophages are responsible for IVIG protection in antibody-induced autoimmune disease. Immunity. 2003;18:573–81.

75. Anthony RM, Wermeling F, Karlsson MC, Ravetch JV. Identification of a receptor required for the anti-inflammatory activity of IVIG. Proc Natl Acad Sci U S A. 2008;105:19571–8.

76. Nakamura A, Yuasa T, Ujike A, Ono M, Nukiwa T, Ravetch JV, et al. Fcgamma receptor IIB-deficient mice develop Goodpasture's syndrome upon immunization with type IV collagen: a novel murine model for autoimmune glomerular basement membrane disease. J Exp Med. 2000;191:899–906.

77. McGaha TL, Sorrentino B, Ravetch JV. Restoration of tolerance in lupus by targeted inhibitory receptor expression. Science. 2005;307:590–3.

78. Mackay M, Stanevsky A, Wang T, Aranow C, Li M, Koenig S, et al. Selective dysregulation of the FcgammaIIB receptor on memory B cells in SLE. J Exp Med. 2006;203:2157–64.

79. Kadono T, Tomita M, Tamaki Z, Sato S, Asano Y. Serum levels of anti-Fcgamma receptor IIB/C antibodies are increased in patients with systemic sclerosis. J Dermatol. 2014;41:1009–12.

80. Siragam V, Crow AR, Brinc D, Song S, Freedman J, Lazarus AH. Intravenous immunoglobulin ameliorates ITP via activating Fc gamma receptors on dendritic cells. Nat Med. 2006;12:688–92.

81. Bazin R, Lemieux R, Tremblay T. Reversal of immune thrombocytopenia in mice by cross-linking human immunoglobulin G with a high-affinity monoclonal antibody. Br J Haematol. 2006;135:97–100.

82. Nagelkerke SQ, Dekkers G, Kustiawan I, van de Bovenkamp FS, Geissler J, Plomp R, et al. Inhibition of FcgammaR-mediated phagocytosis by IVIg is independent of IgG-Fc sialylation and FcgammaRIIb in human macrophages. Blood. 2014;124:3709–18.

83. Aubin E, Lemieux R, Bazin R. Indirect inhibition of in vivo and in vitro T-cell responses by intravenous immunoglobulins due to impaired antigen presentation. Blood. 2010;115:1727–34.

84. Akilesh S, Christianson GJ, Roopenian DC, Shaw AS. Neonatal FcR expression in bone marrow-derived cells functions to protect serum IgG from catabolism. J Immunol. 2007;179:4580–8.

85. Li N, Zhao M, Hilario-Vargas J, Prisayanh P, Warren S, Diaz LA, et al. Complete FcRn dependence for intravenous Ig therapy in autoimmune skin blistering diseases. J Clin Invest. 2005;115:3440–50.

86. Grando SA, Pittelkow MR. Pseudo pemphigus phenotypes in mice with inactivated desmoglein 3: further insight to the complexity of pemphigus pathophysiology. Am J Pathol. 2015;185:3125–7.

87. Chen Y, Chernyavsky A, Webber RJ, Grando SA, Wang PH. Critical Role of the Neonatal Fc Receptor (FcRn) in the pathogenic action of antimitochondrial autoantibodies synergizing with anti-desmoglein autoantibodies in pemphigus vulgaris. J Biol Chem. 2015;290:23826–37.

88. Akilesh S, Petkova S, Sproule TJ, Shaffer DJ, Christianson GJ, Roopenian D. The MHC class I-like Fc receptor promotes humorally mediated autoimmune disease. J Clin Invest. 2004;113:1328–33.

89. Crow AR, Suppa SJ, Chen X, Mott PJ, Lazarus AH. The neonatal Fc receptor (FcRn) is not required for IVIg or anti-CD44 monoclonal antibody-mediated amelioration of murine immune thrombocytopenia. Blood. 2011;118:6403–6.

90. Dalziel M, Crispin M, Scanlan CN, Zitzmann N, Dwek RA. Emerging principles for the therapeutic exploitation of glycosylation. Science. 2014;343:1235681.

91. Kaneko Y, Nimmerjahn F, Ravetch JV. Anti-inflammatory activity of immunoglobulin G resulting from Fc sialylation. Science. 2006;313:670–3.

92. Anthony RM, Nimmerjahn F, Ashline DJ, Reinhold VN, Paulson JC, Ravetch JV. Recapitulation of IVIG anti-inflammatory activity with a recombinant IgG Fc. Science. 2008;320:373–6.

93. Oefner CM, Winkler A, Hess C, Lorenz AK, Holecska V, Huxdorf M, et al. Tolerance induction with T cell-dependent protein antigens induces regulatory sialylated IgGs. J Allergy Clin Immunol. 2012;129:1647–55. e13

94. Washburn N, Schwab I, Ortiz D, Bhatnagar N, Lansing JC, Medeiros A, et al. Controlled tetra-Fc sialylation of IVIg results in a drug candidate with consistent enhanced anti-inflammatory activity. Proc Natl Acad Sci U S A. 2015;112:E1297–306.

95. Chen XX, Chen YQ, Ye S. Measuring decreased serum IgG sialylation: a novel clinical biomarker of lupus. Lupus. 2015;24:948–54.

96. Parekh RB, Roitt IM, Isenberg DA, Dwek RA, Ansell BM, Rademacher TW. Galactosylation of IgG associated oligosaccharides: reduction in patients with adult and juvenile onset rheumatoid arthritis and relation to disease activity. Lancet. 1988;1:966–9.

97. Fokkink WJ, Selman MH, Dortland JR, Durmus B, Kuitwaard K, Huizinga R, et al. IgG Fc N-glycosylation in Guillain-Barre syndrome treated with immunoglobulins. J Proteome Res. 2014;13:1722–30.

98. Fiebiger BM, Maamary J, Pincetic A, Ravetch JV. Protection in antibody- and T cell-mediated autoimmune diseases by antiinflammatory IgG Fcs requires type II FcRs. Proc Natl Acad Sci U S A. 2015;112:E2385–94.

99. Sondermann P, Pincetic A, Maamary J, Lammens K, Ravetch JV. General mechanism for modulating immunoglobulin effector function. Proc Natl Acad Sci U S A. 2013;110:9868–72.

100. Anthony RM, Kobayashi T, Wermeling F, Ravetch JV. Intravenous gammaglobulin suppresses inflammation through a novel T(H)2 pathway. Nature. 2011;475:110–3.

101. Schwab I, Mihai S, Seeling M, Kasperkiewicz M, Ludwig RJ, Nimmerjahn F. Broad requirement for terminal sialic acid residues and FcgammaRIIB for the preventive and therapeutic activity of intravenous immunoglobulins in vivo. Eur J Immunol. 2014;44:1444–53.

102. Bayry J, Bansal K, Kazatchkine MD, Kaveri SV. DC-SIGN and alpha2,6-sialylated IgG Fc interaction is dispensable for the anti-inflammatory activity of IVIg on human dendritic cells. Proc Natl Acad Sci U S A. 2009;106:E24. author reply E5

103. Yu X, Vasiljevic S, Mitchell DA, Crispin M, Scanlan CN. Dissecting the molecular mechanism of IVIg therapy: the interaction between serum IgG and DC-SIGN is independent of antibody glycoform or Fc domain. J Mol Biol. 2013;425(8): 1253.

104. Caminschi I, Corbett AJ, Zahra C, Lahoud M, Lucas KM, Sofi M, et al. Functional comparison of mouse CIRE/mouse DC-SIGN and human DC-SIGN. Int Immunol. 2006;18:741–53.

105. Gelfand EW. Intravenous immune globulin in autoimmune and inflammatory diseases. N Engl J Med. 2012;367:2015–25.

106. Schwab I, Lux A, Nimmerjahn F. Pathways responsible for human autoantibody and therapeutic intravenous IgG activity in humanized mice. Cell Rep. 2015;13:610–20.

107. Quast I, Keller CW, Maurer MA, Giddens JP, Tackenberg B, Wang LX, et al. Sialylation of IgG Fc domain impairs complement-dependent cytotoxicity. J Clin Invest. 2015;125:4160–70.

108. Kasermann F, Boerema DJ, Ruegsegger M, Hofmann A, Wymann S, Zuercher AW, et al. Analysis and functional consequences of increased Fab-sialylation of intravenous immunoglobulin (IVIG) after lectin fractionation. PLoS One. 2012;7:e37243.

109. Issekutz AC, Rowter D, Miescher S, Kasermann F. Intravenous IgG (IVIG) and subcutaneous IgG (SCIG) preparations have comparable inhibitory effect on T cell activation, which is not dependent on IgG sialylation, monocytes or B cells. Clin Immunol. 2015;160:123–32.

110. Ramakrishna C, Cantin EM. Fc-sialylated IgGs in intravenous immunoglobulins are not responsible for induction of regulatory T cells. J Allergy Clin Immunol. 2014;134:1469.

111. Othy S, Topcu S, Saha C, Kothapalli P, Lacroix-Desmazes S, Kasermann F, et al. Sialylation may be dispensable for reciprocal modulation of helper T cells by intravenous immunoglobulin. Eur J Immunol. 2014;44:2059–63.

112. Jerzak M, Rechberger T, Gorski A. Intravenous immunoglobulin therapy influences T cell adhesion to extracellular matrix in women with a history of recurrent spontaneous abortions. Am J Reprod Immunol. 2000;44:336–41.

113. Huang JL, Lee WY, Chen LC, Kuo ML, Hsieh KH. Changes of serum levels of interleukin-2, intercellular adhesion molecule-1, endothelial leukocyte adhesion molecule-1 and Th1 and Th2 cell in severe atopic dermatitis after intravenous immunoglobulin therapy. Ann Allergy Asthma Immunol. 2000;84:345–52.

114. Vassilev TL, Kazatchkine MD, Duong Van Huyen JP, Mekrache M, Bonnin E, Mani JC, et al. Inhibition of cell adhesion by antibodies to Arg-Gly-Asp (RGD) in normal immunoglobulin for therapeutic use (intravenous immunoglobulin, IVIg). Blood. 1999;93:3624–31.

115. Spahn JD, Leung DY, Chan MT, Szefler SJ, Gelfand EW. Mechanisms of glucocorticoid reduction in asthmatic subjects treated with intravenous immunoglobulin. J Allergy Clin Immunol. 1999;103:421–6.

116. Pashov A, Delignat S, Bayry J, Kaveri SV. Enhancement of the affinity of glucocorticoid receptors as a mechanism underlying the steroid-sparing effect of intravenous immunoglobulin. J Rheumatol. 2011;38:2275.

117. Siragam V, Brinc D, Crow AR, Song S, Freedman J, Lazarus AH. Can antibodies with specificity for soluble antigens mimic the therapeutic effects of intravenous IgG in the treatment of autoimmune disease? J Clin Invest. 2005;115:155–60.

118. Bayry J, Lacroix-Desmazes S, Carbonneil C, Misra N, Donkova V, Pashov A, et al. Inhibition of maturation and function of dendritic cells by intravenous immunoglobulin. Blood. 2003;101:758–65.

119. Bayry J, Lacroix-Desmazes S, Delignat S, Mouthon L, Weill B, Kazatchkine MD, et al. Intravenous immunoglobulin abrogates dendritic cell differentiation induced by interferon-alpha present in serum from patients with systemic lupus erythematosus. Arthritis Rheum. 2003;48:3497–502.

120. Sandvik LF, Skarstein K, Sviland L, Svarstad E, Nilsen AE, Leivestad T, et al. CD11c(+) dendritic cells rather than Langerhans cells are reduced in normal skin of immunosuppressed renal transplant recipients. Acta Derm Venereol. 2014;94:173–8.

121. Ito T, Inaba M, Inaba K, Toki J, Sogo S, Iguchi T, et al. A CD1a+/CD11c+ subset of human blood dendritic cells is a direct precursor of Langerhans cells. J Immunol. 1999;163:1409–19.

122. Crow AR, Song S, Semple JW, Freedman J, Lazarus AH. A role for IL-1 receptor antagonist or other cytokines in the acute therapeutic effects of IVIg? Blood. 2007;109:155–8.

123. Aubin E, Lemieux R, Bazin R. Absence of cytokine modulation following therapeutic infusion of intravenous immunoglobulin or anti-red blood cell antibodies in a mouse model of immune thrombocytopenic purpura. Br J Haematol. 2007;136:837–43.

124. Park-Min KH, Serbina NV, Yang W, Ma X, Krystal G, Neel BG, et al. FcgammaRIII-dependent inhibition of interferon-gamma responses mediates suppressive effects of intravenous immune globulin. Immunity. 2007;26:67–78.

125. Trepanier P, Aubin E, Bazin R. IVIg-mediated inhibition of antigen presentation: predominant role of naturally occurring cationic IgG. Clin Immunol. 2012;142:383–9.

126. Smed-Sorensen A, Moll M, Cheng TY, Lore K, Norlin AC, Perbeck L, et al. IgG regulates the CD1 expression profile and lipid antigen-presenting function in human dendritic cells via FcgammaRIIa. Blood. 2008;111:5037–46.

127. Abe Y, Miyake M, Sagawa T, Kimura S. Enzyme-linked immunosorbent assay (ELISA) for human tumor necrosis factor (hTNF). Clin Chim Acta. 1988;176:213–7.

128. Abe Y, Horiuchi A, Miyake M, Kimura S. Anti-cytokine nature of natural human immunoglobulin: one possible mechanism of the clinical effect of intravenous immunoglobulin therapy. Immunol Rev. 1994;139:5–19.

129. Reitamo S, Remitz A, Varga J, Ceska M, Effenberger F, Jimenez S, et al. Demonstration of interleukin 8 and autoantibodies to interleukin 8 in the serum of patients with systemic sclerosis and related disorders. Arch Dermatol. 1993;129:189–93.

130. Toungouz M, Denys CH, De Groote D, Dupont E. In vitro inhibition of tumour necrosis factor-alpha and interleukin-6 production by intravenous immunoglobulins. Br J Haematol. 1995;89:698–703.

131. Denys C, Toungouz M, Dupont E. Increased in vitro immunosuppressive action of anti-CMV and anti-HBs intravenous immunoglobulins due to higher amounts of interferon-gamma specific neutralizing antibodies. Vox Sang. 1997;72:247–50.

132. Andersson UG, Bjork L, Skansen-Saphir U, Andersson JP. Downregulation of cytokine production and interleukin-2 receptor expression by pooled human IgG. Immunology. 1993;79:211–6.

133. Andersson U, Bjork L, Skansen-Saphir U, Andersson J. Pooled human IgG modulates cytokine production in lymphocytes and monocytes. Immunol Rev. 1994;139:21–42.

134. Andersson J, Skansen-Saphir U, Sparrelid E, Andersson U. Intravenous immune globulin affects cytokine production in T lymphocytes and monocytes/macrophages. Clin Exp Immunol. 1996;104(Suppl 1):10–20.

135. Ghio M, Contini P, Setti M, Ubezio G, Mazzei C, Tripodi G. sHLA-I Contamination, a novel mechanism to explain ex vivo/in vitro modulation of IL-10 synthesis and release in CD8(+) T lymphocytes and in neutrophils following intravenous immunoglobulin infusion. J Clin Immunol. 2010;30:384–92.

136. Cooper N, Heddle NM, Haas M, Reid ME, Lesser ML, Fleit HB, et al. Intravenous (IV) anti-D and IV immunoglobulin achieve acute platelet increases by different mechanisms: modulation of cytokine and platelet responses to IV anti-D by FcgammaRIIa and FcgammaRIIIa polymorphisms. Br J Haematol. 2004;124:511–8.

137. Mouzaki A, Theodoropoulou M, Gianakopoulos I, Vlaha V, Kyrtsonis MC, Maniatis A. Expression patterns of Th1 and Th2 cytokine genes in childhood idiopathic thrombocytopenic purpura (ITP) at presentation and their modulation by intravenous immunoglobulin G (IVIg) treatment: their role in prognosis. Blood. 2002;100:1774–9.

138. Bhol KC, Desai A, Kumari S, Colon JE, Ahmed AR. Pemphigus vulgaris: the role of IL-1 and IL-1 receptor antagonist in pathogenesis and effects of intravenous immunoglobulin on their production. Clin Immunol. 2001;100:172–80.

139. Schwaighofer H, Oberhuber G, Hebart H, Einsele H, Herold M, Nachbaur D, et al. Endogenous interleukin 1 receptor antagonist during human bone marrow transplantation: increased levels during graft-versus-host disease, during infectious complications, and after immunoglobulin therapy. Transplantation. 1997;63:52–6.

140. Sigman K, Ghibu F, Sommerville W, Toledano BJ, Bastein Y, Cameron L, et al. Intravenous immunoglobulin inhibits IgE production in human B lymphocytes. J Allergy Clin Immunol. 1998;102:421–7.

141. Zhuang Q, Mazer B. Inhibition of IgE production in vitro by intact and fragmented intravenous immunoglobulin. J Allergy Clin Immunol. 2001;108:229–34.

142. Hashimoto T, Ohzono A, Teye K, Numata S, Hiroyasu S, Tsuruta D, et al. Detection of IgE autoantibodies to BP180 and BP230 and their relationship to clinical features in bullous pemphigoid. Br J Dermatol. 2016

143. van Beek N, Luttmann N, Huebner F, Recke A, Karl I, Schulze FS, et al. Correlation of Serum Levels of IgE Autoantibodies Against BP180 With Bullous Pemphigoid Disease Activity. JAMA Dermatol. 2017;153:30–8.

144. Toyoda M, Pao A, Petrosian A, Jordan SC. Pooled human gammaglobulin modulates surface molecule expression and induces apoptosis in human B cells. Am J Transplant. 2003;3:156–66.

145. Vassilev T, Gelin C, Kaveri SV, Zilber MT, Boumsell L, Kazatchkine MD. Antibodies to the CD5 molecule in normal human immunoglobulins for therapeutic use (intravenous immunoglobulins, IVIg). Clin Exp Immunol. 1993;92:369–72.

146. Le Pottier L, Sapir T, Bendaoud B, Youinou P, Shoenfeld Y, Pers JO. Intravenous immunoglobulin and cytokines: focus on tumor necrosis factor family members BAFF and APRIL. Ann N Y Acad Sci. 2007;1110:426–32.

147. Mohamed Ezzat MH, Mohammed AA, Ismail RI, Shaheen KY. High serum APRIL levels strongly correlate with disease severity in pediatric atopic eczema. Int J Dermatol. 2016;

148. Chasset F, De Masson A, Le Buanec H, Xhaard A, Sicre de Fontbrune F, Robin M, et al. APRIL levels are associated with disease activity in human chronic graft versus host disease. Haematologica. 2016;

149. Chong BF, Tseng LC, Kim A, Miller RT, Yancey KB, Hosler GA. Differential expression of BAFF and its receptors in discoid lupus erythematosus patients. J Dermatol Sci. 2014;73:216–24.

150. Ueda-Hayakawa I, Tanimura H, Osawa M, Iwasaka H, Ohe S, Yamazaki F, et al. Elevated serum BAFF levels in patients with sarcoidosis: association with disease activity. Rheumatology (Oxford). 2013;52:1658–66.

151. Baek A, Park HJ, Na SJ, Shim DS, Moon JS, Yang Y, et al. The expression of BAFF in the muscles of patients with dermatomyositis. J Neuroimmunol. 2012;249:96–100.

152. Shaker OG, Tawfic SO, El-Tawdy AM, El-Komy MH, El Menyawi M, Heikal AA. Expression of TNF-alpha, APRIL and BCMA in Behcet's disease. J Immunol Res. 2014;2014:380405.

153. Samoud-El Kissi S, Galai Y, Sghiri R, Kenani N, Ben Alaya-Bouafif N, Boukadida J, et al. BAFF is elevated in serum of patients with psoriasis: association with disease activity. Br J Dermatol. 2008;159:765–8.

154. Matsushita T, Fujimoto M, Hasegawa M, Tanaka C, Kumada S, Ogawa F, et al. Elevated serum APRIL levels in patients with systemic sclerosis: distinct profiles of systemic sclerosis categorized by APRIL and BAFF. J Rheumatol. 2007;34:2056–62.

155. Matsushita T, Fujimoto M, Hasegawa M, Matsushita Y, Komura K, Ogawa F, et al. BAFF antagonist attenuates the development of skin fibrosis in tight-skin mice. J Invest Dermatol. 2007;127:2772–80.

156. Matsushita T, Hasegawa M, Matsushita Y, Echigo T, Wayaku T, Horikawa M, et al. Elevated serum BAFF levels in patients with localized scleroderma in contrast to other organ-specific autoimmune diseases. Exp Dermatol. 2007;16:87–93.

157. Qian H, Kusuhara M, Li X, Tsuruta D, Tsuchisaka A, Ishii N, et al. B-cell activating factor detected on both naive and memory B cells in bullous pemphigoid. Exp Dermatol. 2014;23:596–605.

158. Asashima N, Fujimoto M, Watanabe R, Nakashima H, Yazawa N, Okochi H, et al. Serum levels of BAFF are increased in bullous pemphigoid but not in pemphigus vulgaris. Br J Dermatol. 2006;155:330–6.

159. Nagel A, Podstawa E, Eickmann M, Muller HH, Hertl M, Eming R. Rituximab mediates a strong elevation of B-cell-activating factor associated with increased pathogen-specific IgG but not autoantibodies in pemphigus vulgaris. J Invest Dermatol. 2009;129:2202–10.

160. Kabuto M, Fujimoto N, Tanaka T. Increase of interleukin-10-producing B cells associated with long-term remission after i.v. immunoglobulin treatment for pemphigus. J Dermatol 2016.

161. Kawada K, Terasaki PI. Evidence for immunosuppression by high-dose gammaglobulin. Exp Hematol. 1987;15:133–6.

162. Amran D, Renz H, Lack G, Bradley K, Gelfand EW. Suppression of cytokine-dependent human T-cell proliferation by intravenous immunoglobulin. Clin Immunol Immunopathol. 1994;73:180–6.

163. Hurez V, Kaveri SV, Mouhoub A, Dietrich G, Mani JC, Klatzmann D, et al. Anti-CD4 activity of normal human immunoglobulin G for therapeutic use. (Intravenous immunoglobulin, IVIg). Ther Immunol. 1994;1:269–77.

164. Marchalonis JJ, Kaymaz H, Dedeoglu F, Schluter SF, Yocum DE, Edmundson AB. Human autoantibodies reactive with synthetic autoantigens from T-cell receptor beta chain. Proc Natl Acad Sci U S A. 1992;89:3325–9.

165. Aktas O, Waiczies S, Grieger U, Wendling U, Zschenderlein R, Zipp F. Polyspecific immunoglobulins (IVIg) suppress proliferation of human (auto)antigen-specific T cells without inducing apoptosis. J Neuroimmunol. 2001;114:160–7.

166. van Schaik IN, Vermeulen M, Brand A. In vitro effects of polyvalent immunoglobulin for intravenous use. J Neurol Neurosurg Psychiatry. 1994;57(Suppl):15–7.

167. Trepanier P, Chabot D, Bazin R. Intravenous immunoglobulin modulates the expansion and cytotoxicity of CD8+ T cells. Immunology. 2014;141:233–41.

168. Klehmet J, Meisel C, Meisel A. Efficiency of long-term treatment with intravenous immunoglobulins correlates with reduced autoreactive T cell responses in chronic inflammatory demyelinating polyneuropathy patients. Clin Exp Immunol. 2014;178(Suppl 1):149–50.

169. Han YM, Sheng YY, Xu F, Qi SS, Liu XJ, RM H, et al. Imbalance of T-helper 17 and regulatory T cells in patients with alopecia areata. J Dermatol. 2015;42:981–8.

170. Asothai R, Anand V, Das D, Antil PS, Khandpur S, Sharma VK, et al. Distinctive Treg associated CCR4-CCL22 expression profile with altered frequency of Th17/Treg cell in the immunopathogenesis of Pemphigus Vulgaris. Immunobiology. 2015;220:1129–35.

171. Arakawa M, Dainichi T, Ishii N, Hamada T, Karashima T, Nakama T, et al. Lesional Th17 cells and regulatory T cells in bullous pemphigoid. Exp Dermatol. 2011;20:1022–4.

172. Yang J, Chu Y, Yang X, Gao D, Zhu L, Yang X, et al. Th17 and natural Treg cell population dynamics in systemic lupus erythematosus. Arthritis Rheum. 2009;60:1472–83.

173. Elela MA, Gawdat HI, Hegazy RA, Fawzy MM, Abdel Hay RM, Saadi D, et al. B cell activating factor and T-helper 17 cells: possible synergistic culprits in the pathogenesis of Alopecia Areata. Arch Dermatol Res. 2016;308:115–21.

174. Bonefeld CM, Petersen TH, Bandier J, Agerbeck C, Linneberg A, Ross-Hansen K, et al. Epidermal filaggrin deficiency mediates increased systemic Th17 immune response. Br J Dermatol 2016.

175. Othy S, Hegde P, Topcu S, Sharma M, Maddur MS, Lacroix-Desmazes S, et al. Intravenous gammaglobulin inhibits encephalitogenic potential of pathogenic T cells and interferes with their trafficking to the central nervous system, implicating sphingosine-1 phosphate receptor 1-mammalian target of rapamycin axis. J Immunol. 2013;190:4535–41.

176. Yang J, Yang X, Zou H, Chu Y, Li M. Recovery of the immune balance between Th17 and regulatory T cells as a treatment for systemic lupus erythematosus. Rheumatology (Oxford). 2011;50:1366–72.

177. RC X, Zhu HQ, Li WP, Zhao XQ, Yuan HJ, Zheng J, et al. The imbalance of Th17 and regulatory T cells in pemphigus patients. Eur J Dermatol. 2013;23:795–802.

178. Maddur MS, Sharma M, Hegde P, Lacroix-Desmazes S, Kaveri SV, Bayry J. Inhibitory effect of IVIG on IL-17 production by Th17 cells is independent of anti-IL-17 antibodies in the immunoglobulin preparations. J Clin Immunol. 2013;33(Suppl 1):S62–6.

179. Milovanovic M, Drozdenko G, Weise C, Babina M, Worm M. Interleukin-17A promotes IgE production in human B cells. J Invest Dermatol. 2010;130:2621–8.

180. Piccirillo CA, Shevach EM. Naturally-occurring CD4+CD25+ immunoregulatory T cells: central players in the arena of peripheral tolerance. Semin Immunol. 2004;16:81–8.

181. Antiga E, Quaglino P, Pierini I, Volpi W, Lami G, Bianchi B, et al. Regulatory T cells as well as IL-10 are reduced in the skin of patients with dermatitis herpetiformis. J Dermatol Sci. 2015;77:54–62.

182. Hadaschik EN, Wei X, Leiss H, Heckmann B, Niederreiter B, Steiner G, et al. Regulatory T cell-deficient scurfy mice develop systemic autoimmune features resembling lupus-like disease. Arthritis Res Ther. 2015;17:35.

183. Yu J, Heck S, Patel V, Levan J, Yu Y, Bussel JB, et al. Defective circulating CD25 regulatory T cells in patients with chronic immune thrombocytopenic purpura. Blood. 2008;112:1325–8.

184. Olivito B, Taddio A, Simonini G, Massai C, Ciullini S, Gambineri E, et al. Defective FOXP3 expression in patients with acute Kawasaki disease and restoration by intravenous immunoglobulin therapy. Clin Exp Rheumatol. 2010;28:93–7.

185. Tsurikisawa N, Saito H, Oshikata C, Tsuburai T, Akiyama K. High-dose intravenous immunoglobulin treatment increases

regulatory T cells in patients with eosinophilic granulomatosis with polyangiitis. J Rheumatol. 2012;39:1019–25.

186. Sugiyama H, Matsue H, Nagasaka A, Nakamura Y, Tsukamoto K, Shibagaki N, et al. CD4+CD25high regulatory T cells are markedly decreased in blood of patients with pemphigus vulgaris. Dermatology. 2007;214:210–20.

187. Sun RS, Sui JF, Chen XH, Ran XZ, Yang ZF, Guan WD, et al. Detection of CD4+ CD25+ FOXP3+ regulatory T cells in peripheral blood of patients with chronic autoimmune urticaria. Australas J Dermatol. 2011;52:e15–8.

188. Antiga E, Quaglino P, Volpi W, Pierini I, Del Bianco E, Bianchi B, et al. Regulatory T cells in skin lesions and blood of patients with bullous pemphigoid. J Eur Acad Dermatol Venereol. 2014;28:222–30.

189. Gambichler T, Patzholz J, Schmitz L, Lahner N, Kreuter A. FOXP3+ and CD39+ regulatory T cells in subtypes of cutaneous lupus erythematosus. J Eur Acad Dermatol Venereol. 2015;29:1972–7.

190. Tembhre MK, Parihar AS, Sharma VK, Sharma A, Chattopadhyay P, Gupta S. Alteration in regulatory T cells and programmed cell death 1-expressing regulatory T cells in active generalized vitiligo and their clinical correlation. Br J Dermatol. 2015;172:940–50.

191. Wang YY, Wang Q, Sun XH, Liu RZ, Shu Y, Kanekura T, et al. DNA hypermethylation of the forkhead box protein 3 (FOXP3) promoter in CD4+ T cells of patients with systemic sclerosis. Br J Dermatol. 2014;171:39–47.

192. Lili Y, Yi W, Ji Y, Yue S, Weimin S, Ming L. Global activation of CD8+ cytotoxic T lymphocytes correlates with an impairment in regulatory T cells in patients with generalized vitiligo. PLoS One. 2012;7:e37513.

193. Schweintzger N, Gruber-Wackernagel A, Reginato F, Bambach I, Quehenberger F, Byrne SN, et al. Levels and function of regulatory T cells in patients with polymorphic light eruption: relation to photohardening. Br J Dermatol. 2015;173:519–26.

194. Costa N, Pires AE, Gabriel AM, Goulart LF, Pereira C, Leal B, et al. Broadened T-cell repertoire diversity in ivIg-treated SLE patients is also related to the individual status of regulatory T-cells. J Clin Immunol. 2013;33:349–60.

195. Tjon AS, Tha-In T, Metselaar HJ, van Gent R, van der Laan LJ, Groothuismink ZM, et al. Patients treated with high-dose intravenous immunoglobulin show selective activation of regulatory T cells. Clin Exp Immunol. 2013;173:259–67.

196. Ephrem A, Chamat S, Miquel C, Fisson S, Mouthon L, Caligiuri G, et al. Expansion of CD4+CD25+ regulatory T cells by intravenous immunoglobulin: a critical factor in controlling experimental autoimmune encephalomyelitis. Blood. 2008;111:715–22.

197. Vignali DA, Collison LW, Workman CJ. How regulatory T cells work. Nat Rev Immunol. 2008;8:523–32.

198. Trinath J, Hegde P, Sharma M, Maddur MS, Rabin M, Vallat JM, et al. Intravenous immunoglobulin expands regulatory T cells via induction of cyclooxygenase-2-dependent prostaglandin E2 in human dendritic cells. Blood. 2013;122:1419–27.

199. Tha-In T, Metselaar HJ, Bushell AR, Kwekkeboom J, Wood KJ. Intravenous immunoglobulins promote skin allograft acceptance by triggering functional activation of CD4+Foxp3+ T cells. Transplantation. 2010;89:1446–55.

200. Barreto M, Ferreira RC, Lourenco L, Moraes-Fontes MF, Santos E, Alves M, et al. Low frequency of CD4+CD25+ Treg in SLE patients: a heritable trait associated with CTLA4 and TGFbeta gene variants. BMC Immunol. 2009;10:5.

201. Anthony RM, Ravetch JVA. novel role for the IgG Fc glycan: the anti-inflammatory activity of sialylated IgG Fcs. J Clin Immunol. 2010;30(Suppl 1):S9–14.

202. Franco A, Touma R, Song Y, Shimizu C, Tremoulet AH, Kanegaye JT, et al. Specificity of regulatory T cells that modulate vascular inflammation. Autoimmunity. 2014;47:95–104.

203. De Groot AS, Moise L, McMurry JA, Wambre E, Van Overtvelt L, Moingeon P, et al. Activation of natural regulatory T cells by IgG Fc-derived peptide "Tregitopes". Blood. 2008;112:3303–11.

204. Cousens LP, Najafian N, Mingozzi F, Elyaman W, Mazer B, Moise L, et al. vitro and in vivo studies of IgG-derived Treg epitopes (Tregitopes): a promising new tool for tolerance induction and treatment of autoimmunity. J Clin Immunol. 2013;33(Suppl 1):S43–9.

205. Moretta L, Ferlazzo G, Bottino C, Vitale M, Pende D, Mingari MC, et al. Effector and regulatory events during natural killer-dendritic cell interactions. Immunol Rev. 2006;214:219–28.

206. Bohn AB, Nederby L, Harbo T, Skovbo A, Vorup-Jensen T, Krog J, et al. The effect of IgG levels on the number of natural killer cells and their Fc receptors in chronic inflammatory demyelinating polyradiculoneuropathy. Eur J Neurol. 2011;18:919–24.

207. Clark DA, Chaouat G. Loss of surface CD200 on stored allogeneic leukocytes may impair anti-abortive effect in vivo. Am J Reprod Immunol. 2005;53:13–20.

208. Clark DA, Wong K, Banwatt D, Chen Z, Liu J, Lee L, et al. CD200-dependent and nonCD200-dependent pathways of NK cell suppression by human IVIG. J Assist Reprod Genet. 2008;25:67–72.

209. Lebre MC, van der Aar AM, van Baarsen L, van Capel TM, Schuitemaker JH, Kapsenberg ML, et al. Human keratinocytes express functional Toll-like receptor 3, 4, 5, and 9. J Invest Dermatol. 2007;127:331–41.

210. Ghaly NR, Kotb NA, Nagy HM, Rageh el SM. Toll-like receptor 9 in systemic lupus erythematosus, impact on glucocorticoid treatment. J Dermatol Treat. 2013;24:411–7.

211. Kessel A, Peri R, Haj T, Snir A, Slobodin G, Sabo E, et al. IVIg attenuates TLR-9 activation in B cells from SLE patients. J Clin Immunol. 2011;31:30–8.

212. Futata E, Azor M, Dos Santos J, Maruta C, Sotto M, Guedes F, et al. Impaired IFN-alpha secretion by plasmacytoid dendritic cells induced by TLR9 activation in chronic idiopathic urticaria. Br J Dermatol. 2011;164:1271–9.

213. Morizane S, Yamasaki K, Muhleisen B, Kotol PF, Murakami M, Aoyama Y, et al. Cathelicidin antimicrobial peptide LL-37 in psoriasis enables keratinocyte reactivity against TLR9 ligands. J Invest Dermatol. 2012;132:135–43.

214. Wiedeman AE, Santer DM, Yan W, Miescher S, Kasermann F, Elkon KB. Contrasting mechanisms of interferon-alpha inhibition by intravenous immunoglobulin after induction by immune complexes versus Toll-like receptor agonists. Arthritis Rheum. 2013;65:2713–23.

215. Curtis JA, Christensen LC, Paine AR, Collins Brummer G, Summers EM, Cochran AL, et al. Stevens-Johnson syndrome and toxic epidermal necrolysis treatments: An Internet survey. J Am Acad Dermatol. 2016;74:379–80.

216. Huang YC, Li YC, Chen TJ. The efficacy of intravenous immunoglobulin for the treatment of toxic epidermal necrolysis: a systematic review and meta-analysis. Br J Dermatol. 2012;167:424–32.

217. Barron SJ, Del Vecchio MT, Aronoff SC. Intravenous immunoglobulin in the treatment of Stevens-Johnson syndrome and toxic epidermal necrolysis: a meta-analysis with meta-regression of observational studies. Int J Dermatol. 2015;54:108–15.

218. Kirchhof MG, Miliszewski MA, Sikora S, Papp A, Dutz JP. Retrospective review of Stevens-Johnson syndrome/toxic epidermal necrolysis treatment comparing intravenous immunoglobulin with cyclosporine. J Am Acad Dermatol. 2014;71:941–7.

219. Romanelli P, Schlam E, Green JB, Trent JT, Ricotti C, Elgart GW, et al. Immunohistochemical evaluation of toxic epidermal necrolysis treated with human intravenous immunoglobulin. G Ital Dermatol Venereol. 2008;143:229–33.

220. Paquet P, Kaveri S, Jacob E, Pirson J, Quatresooz P, Pierard GE. Skin immunoglobulin deposition following intravenous

immunoglobulin therapy in toxic epidermal necrolysis. Exp Dermatol. 2006;15:381–6.

221. Lolis M, Toosi S, Czernik A, Bystryn JC. Effect of intravenous immunoglobulin with or without cytotoxic drugs on pemphigus intercellular antibodies. J Am Acad Dermatol. 2011;64:484–9.

222. Aoyama Y, Moriya C, Kamiya K, Nagai M, Rubenstein D, Iwatsuki K, et al. Catabolism of pemphigus foliaceus autoantibodies by high-dose IVIg therapy. Eur J Dermatol. 2011;21:58–61.

223. Green MG, Bystryn JC. Effect of intravenous immunoglobulin therapy on serum levels of IgG1 and IgG4 antidesmoglein 1 and antidesmoglein 3 antibodies in pemphigus vulgaris. Arch Dermatol. 2008;144:1621–4.

224. Czernik A, Beutner EH, Bystryn JC. Intravenous immunoglobulin selectively decreases circulating autoantibodies in pemphigus. J Am Acad Dermatol. 2008;58:796–801.

225. Bystryn JC, Jiao D. IVIg selectively and rapidly decreases circulating pathogenic autoantibodies in pemphigus vulgaris. Autoimmunity. 2006;39(7):601.

226. Sami N, Bhol KC, Ahmed RA. Influence of intravenous immunoglobulin therapy on autoantibody titers to desmoglein 3 and desmoglein 1 in pemphigus vulgaris. Eur J Dermatol. 2003;13:377–81.

227. Sami N, Bhol KC, Ahmed AR. Influence of IVIg therapy on autoantibody titers to desmoglein 1 in patients with pemphigus foliaceus. Clin Immunol. 2002;105:192–8.

228. Aoyama Y, Nagasawa C, Nagai M, Kitajima Y. Severe pemphigus vulgaris: successful combination therapy of plasmapheresis followed by intravenous high-dose immunoglobulin to prevent rebound increase in pathogenic IgG. Eur J Dermatol. 2008;18:557–60.

229. Amagai M, Ikeda S, Shimizu H, Iizuka H, Hanada K, Aiba S, et al. A randomized double-blind trial of intravenous immunoglobulin for pemphigus. J Am Acad Dermatol. 2009;60:595–603.

230. Ahmed AR. Intravenous immunoglobulin therapy in the treatment of patients with pemphigus vulgaris unresponsive to conventional immunosuppressive treatment. J Am Acad Dermatol. 2001;45:679–90.

231. Ahmed AR, Gurcan HM. Use of intravenous immunoglobulin therapy during pregnancy in patients with pemphigus vulgaris. J Eur Acad Dermatol Venereol. 2011;25(9):1073.

232. Asarch A, Razzaque Ahmed A. Treatment of juvenile pemphigus vulgaris with intravenous immunoglobulin therapy. Pediatr Dermatol. 2009;26:197–202.

233. Mimouni D, Blank M, Payne AS, Anhalt GJ, Avivi C, Barshack I, et al. Efficacy of intravenous immunoglobulin (IVIG) affinity-purified anti-desmoglein anti-idiotypic antibodies in the treatment of an experimental model of pemphigus vulgaris. Clin Exp Immunol. 2010;162:543–9.

234. Keskin DB, Stern JN, Fridkis-Hareli M, Razzaque Ahmed A. Cytokine profiles in pemphigus vulgaris patients treated with intravenous immunoglobulins as compared to conventional immunosuppressive therapy. Cytokine. 2008;41:315–21.

235. Ahmed AR, Nguyen T, Kaveri S, Spigelman ZS. First line treatment of pemphigus vulgaris with a novel protocol in patients with contraindications to systemic corticosteroids and immunosuppressive agents: Preliminary retrospective study with a seven year follow-up. Int Immunopharmacol. 2016;34:25–31.

236. Feldman RJ, Christen WG, Ahmed AR. Comparison of immunological parameters in patients with pemphigus vulgaris following rituximab and IVIG therapy. Br J Dermatol. 2012;166:511–7.

237. Ahmed AR, Kaveri S, Spigelman Z. Long-term remissions in recalcitrant pemphigus vulgaris. N Engl J Med. 2015;373:2693–4.

238. Wang HH, Liu CW, Li YC, Huang YC. Efficacy of rituximab for pemphigus: a systematic review and meta-analysis of different regimens. Acta Derm Venereol. 2015;95:928–32.

239. Amber KT, Hertl M. An assessment of treatment history and its association with clinical outcomes and relapse in 155 pemphigus

patients with response to a single cycle of rituximab. J Eur Acad Dermatol Venereol. 2015;29:777–82.

240. Shimanovich I, Nitschke M, Rose C, Grabbe J, Zillikens D. Treatment of severe pemphigus with protein A immunoadsorption, rituximab and intravenous immunoglobulins. Br J Dermatol. 2008;158:382–8.

241. Foster CS, Chang PY, Ahmed AR. Combination of rituximab and intravenous immunoglobulin for recalcitrant ocular cicatricial pemphigoid: a preliminary report. Ophthalmology. 2010;117:861–9.

242. Sami N, Bhol KC, Ahmed AR. Treatment of oral pemphigoid with intravenous immunoglobulin as monotherapy. Long-term follow-up: influence of treatment on antibody titres to human alpha6 integrin. Clin Exp Immunol. 2002;129:533–40.

243. Ahmed AR, Colon JE. Comparison between intravenous immunoglobulin and conventional immunosuppressive therapy regimens in patients with severe oral pemphigoid: effects on disease progression in patients nonresponsive to dapsone therapy. Arch Dermatol. 2001;137:1181–9.

244. Letko E, Bhol K, Foster SC, Ahmed RA. Influence of intravenous immunoglobulin therapy on serum levels of anti-beta 4 antibodies in ocular cicatricial pemphigoid. A correlation with disease activity. A preliminary study. Curr Eye Res. 2000;21:646–54.

245. Sami N, Bhol KC, Razzaque Ahmed A. Intravenous immunoglobulin therapy in patients with multiple mucosal involvement in mucous membrane pemphigoid. Clin Immunol. 2002;102:59–67.

246. Amagai M, Ikeda S, Hashimoto T, Mizuashi M, Fujisawa A, Ihn H, et al. A randomized double-blind trial of intravenous immunoglobulin for bullous pemphigoid. J Dermatol Sci. 2017;85:77–84.

247. Ahmed AR. Intravenous immunoglobulin therapy for patients with bullous pemphigoid unresponsive to conventional immunosuppressive treatment. J Am Acad Dermatol. 2001;45:825–35.

248. Gaitanis G, Alexis I, Pelidou SH, Gazi IF, Kyritsis AP, Elisaf MS, et al. High-dose intravenous immunoglobulin in the treatment of adult patients with bullous pemphigoid. Eur J Dermatol. 2012;22:363–9.

249. Engineer L, Ahmed AR. Role of intravenous immunoglobulin in the treatment of bullous pemphigoid: analysis of current data. J Am Acad Dermatol. 2001;44:83–8.

250. Czernik A, Bystryn JC. Improvement of intravenous immunoglobulin therapy for bullous pemphigoid by adding immunosuppressive agents: marked improvement in depletion of circulating autoantibodies. Arch Dermatol. 2008;144:658–61.

251. Nguyen T, Alraqum E, Razzaque Ahmed A. Positive clinical outcome with IVIg as monotherapy in recurrent pemphigoid gestationis. Int Immunopharmacol. 2015;26:1–3.

252. Intong LR, Murrell DF. Pemphigoid gestationis: current management. Dermatol Clin. 2011;29:621–8.

253. Ahmed AR, Gurcan HM. Treatment of epidermolysis bullosa acquisita with intravenous immunoglobulin in patients nonresponsive to conventional therapy: clinical outcome and post-treatment long-term follow-up. J Eur Acad Dermatol Venereol. 2012;26:1074–83.

254. Oktem A, Akay BN, Boyvat A, Kundakci N, Erdem C, Bostanci S, et al. Long-term results of rituximab-intravenous immunoglobulin combination therapy in patients with epidermolysis bullosa acquisita resistant to conventional therapy. J Dermatolog Treat. 2016:1–5.

255. Wang DX, Shu XM, Tian XL, Chen F, Zu N, Ma L, et al. Intravenous immunoglobulin therapy in adult patients with polymyositis/dermatomyositis: a systematic literature review. Clin Rheumatol. 2012;31:801–6.

256. Kampylafka EI, Kosmidis ML, Panagiotakos DB, Dalakas M, Moutsopoulos HM, Tzioufas AG. The effect of intravenous immunoglobulin (IVIG) treatment on patients with dermatomyositis: a 4-year follow-up study. Clin Exp Rheumatol. 2012;30:397–401.

257. Amemiya K, Semino-Mora C, Granger RP, Dalakas MC. Downregulation of TGF-beta1 mRNA and protein in the muscles of patients with inflammatory myopathies after treatment with high-dose intravenous immunoglobulin. Clin Immunol. 2000;94:99–104.

258. Callander J, Robson Y, Ingram J, Piguet V. Treatment of clinically amyopathic dermatomyositis in adults: a systematic review. Br J Dermatol. 2016;

259. Femia AN, Eastham AB, Lam C, Merola JF, Qureshi AA, Vleugels RA. Intravenous immunoglobulin for refractory cutaneous dermatomyositis: a retrospective analysis from an academic medical center. J Am Acad Dermatol. 2013;69:654–7.

260. Saito E, Koike T, Hashimoto H, Miyasaka N, Ikeda Y, Hara M, et al. Efficacy of high-dose intravenous immunoglobulin therapy in Japanese patients with steroid-resistant polymyositis and dermatomyositis. Mod Rheumatol. 2008;18:34–44.

261. Bounfour T, Bouaziz JD, Bezier M, Cordoliani F, Saussine A, Petit A, et al. Clinical efficacy of intravenous immunoglobulins for the treatment of dermatomyositis skin lesions without muscle disease. J Eur Acad Dermatol Venereol. 2014;28:1150–7.

262. Gottfried I, Seeber A, Anegg B, Rieger A, Stingl G, Volc-Platzer B. High dose intravenous immunoglobulin (IVIG) in dermatomyositis: clinical responses and effect on sIL-2R levels. Eur J Dermatol. 2000;10:29–35.

263. Lam CG, Manlhiot C, Pullenayegum EM, Feldman BM. Efficacy of intravenous Ig therapy in juvenile dermatomyositis. Ann Rheum Dis. 2011;70:2089–94.

264. Al-Mayouf SM, Laxer RM, Schneider R, Silverman ED, Feldman BM. Intravenous immunoglobulin therapy for juvenile dermatomyositis: efficacy and safety. J Rheumatol. 2000;27:2498–503.

265. Manlhiot C, Tyrrell PN, Liang L, Atkinson AR, Lau W, Feldman BM. Safety of intravenous immunoglobulin in the treatment of juvenile dermatomyositis: adverse reactions are associated with immunoglobulin A content. Pediatrics. 2008;121:e626–30.

266. Galimberti F, Li Y, Fernandez AP. Intravenous immunoglobulin for treatment of dermatomyositis-associated dystrophic calcinosis. J Am Acad Dermatol. 2015;73:174–6.

267. Touimy M, Janani S, Rachidi W, Etaouil N, Mkinsi O. Calcinosis universalis complicating juvenile dermatomyositis: improvement after intravenous immunoglobulin therapy. Joint Bone Spine. 2013;80:108–9.

268. Shahani L. Refractory calcinosis in a patient with dermatomyositis: response to intravenous immune globulin. BMJ Case Rep 2012;2012.

269. Penate Y, Guillermo N, Melwani P, Martel R, Hernandez-Machin B, Borrego L. Calcinosis cutis associated with amyopathic dermatomyositis: response to intravenous immunoglobulin. J Am Acad Dermatol. 2009;60:1076–7.

270. Kalajian AH, Perryman JH, Callen JP. Intravenous immunoglobulin therapy for dystrophic calcinosis cutis: unreliable in our hands. Arch Dermatol. 2009;145:334. author reply 5

271. Amano H, Nagai Y, Katada K, Hashimoto C, Ishikawa O. Successful treatment of cutaneous lesions in juvenile dermatomyositis with high-dose intravenous immunoglobulin. Br J Dermatol. 2007;156:1390–2.

272. Sunderkotter C, Nast A, Worm M, Dengler R, Dorner T, Ganter H, et al. Guidelines on dermatomyositis--excerpt from the interdisciplinary S2k guidelines on myositis syndromes by the German Society of Neurology. J Dtsch Dermatol Ges. 2016;14:321–38.

273. Johnson NE, Arnold WD, Hebert D, Gwathmey K, Dimachkie MM, Barohn RJ, et al. Disease course and therapeutic approach in dermatomyositis: a four-center retrospective study of 100 patients. Neuromuscul Disord. 2015;25:625–31.

274. Marie I, Menard JF, Hatron PY, Hachulla E, Mouthon L, Tiev K, et al. Intravenous immunoglobulins for steroid-refractory esophageal involvement related to polymyositis and dermato-

myositis: a series of 73 patients. Arthritis Care Res (Hoboken). 2010;62:1748–55.

275. Roekevisch E, Spuls PI, Kuester D, Limpens J, Schmitt J. Efficacy and safety of systemic treatments for moderate-to-severe atopic dermatitis: a systematic review. J Allergy Clin Immunol. 2014;133:429–38.

276. Turner PJ, Kakakios A, Wong LC, Wong M, Campbell DE. Intravenous immunoglobulin to treat severe atopic dermatitis in children: a case series. Pediatr Dermatol. 2012;29:177–81.

277. Jolles S, Sewell C, Webster D, Ryan A, Heelan B, Waite A, et al. Adjunctive high-dose intravenous immunoglobulin treatment for resistant atopic dermatitis: efficacy and effects on intracellular cytokine levels and CD4 counts. Acta Derm Venereol. 2003;83:433–7.

278. Jee SJ, Kim JH, Baek HS, Lee HB, Oh JW. Long-term efficacy of intravenous immunoglobulin therapy for moderate to severe childhood atopic dermatitis. Allergy Asthma Immunol Res. 2011;3:89–95.

279. Bemanian MH, Movahedi M, Farhoudi A, Gharagozlou M, Seraj MH, Pourpak Z, et al. High doses intravenous immunoglobulin versus oral cyclosporine in the treatment of severe atopic dermatitis. Iran J Allergy Asthma Immunol. 2005;4:139–43.

280. Paul C, Lahfa M, Bachelez H, Chevret S, Dubertret L. A randomized controlled evaluator-blinded trial of intravenous immunoglobulin in adults with severe atopic dermatitis. Br J Dermatol. 2002;147:518–22.

281. Sakthiswary R, D'Cruz D. Intravenous immunoglobulin in the therapeutic armamentarium of systemic lupus erythematosus: a systematic review and meta-analysis. Medicine (Baltimore). 2014;93:e86.

282. Lampropoulos CE, Hughes GR, D'Cruz DC. Intravenous immunoglobulin in the treatment of resistant subacute cutaneous lupus erythematosus: a possible alternative. Clin Rheumatol. 2007;26:981–3.

283. Ky C, Swasdibutra B, Khademi S, Desai S, Laquer V, Grando SA. Efficacy of intravenous immunoglobulin monotherapy in patients with cutaneous lupus erythematosus: results of proof-of-concept study. Dermatol Rep. 2015;7:5804.

284. Goodfield M, Davison K, Bowden K. Intravenous immunoglobulin (IVIg) for therapy-resistant cutaneous lupus erythematosus (LE). J Dermatolog Treat. 2004;15:46–50.

285. Espirito Santo J, Gomes MF, Gomes MJ, Peixoto L, CP S, Acabado A, et al. Intravenous immunoglobulin in lupus panniculitis. Clin Rev Allergy Immunol. 2010;38:307–18.

286. Fagiolo U, Kricek F, Ruf C, Peserico A, Amadori A, Cancian M. Effects of complement inactivation and IgG depletion on skin reactivity to autologous serum in chronic idiopathic urticaria. J Allergy Clin Immunol. 2000;106:567–72.

287. O'Donnell BF, Barr RM, Black AK, Francis DM, Kermani F, Niimi N, et al. Intravenous immunoglobulin in autoimmune chronic urticaria. Br J Dermatol. 1998;138:101–6.

288. Mitzel-Kaoukhov H, Staubach P, Muller-Brenne T. Effect of high-dose intravenous immunoglobulin treatment in therapy-resistant chronic spontaneous urticaria. Ann Allergy Asthma Immunol. 2010;104:253–8.

289. Pereira C, Tavares B, Carrapatoso I, Loureiro G, Faria E, Machado D, et al. Low-dose intravenous gammaglobulin in the treatment of severe autoimmune urticaria. Eur Ann Allergy Clin Immunol. 2007;39:237–42.

290. Aubin F, Porcher R, Jeanmougin M, Leonard F, Bedane C, Moreau A, et al. Severe and refractory solar urticaria treated with intravenous immunoglobulins: a phase II multicenter study. J Am Acad Dermatol. 2014;71:948–53. e1

291. Adamski H, Bedane C, Bonnevalle A, Thomas P, Peyron JL, Rouchouse B, et al. Solar urticaria treated with intravenous immunoglobulins. J Am Acad Dermatol. 2011;65:336–40.

292. Dawn G, Urcelay M, Ah-Weng A, O'Neill SM, Douglas WS. Effect of high-dose intravenous immunoglobulin in delayed pressure urticaria. Br J Dermatol. 2003;149:836–40.

293. Cantarini L, Rigante D, Vitale A, Napodano S, Sakkas LI, Bogdanos DP, et al. Intravenous immunoglobulins (IVIG) in systemic sclerosis: a challenging yet promising future. Immunol Res. 2015;61:326–37.

294. Takehara K, Ihn H, Sato SA. randomized, double-blind, placebo-controlled trial: intravenous immunoglobulin treatment in patients with diffuse cutaneous systemic sclerosis. Clin Exp Rheumatol. 2013;31:151–6.

295. Levy Y, Amital H, Langevitz P, Nacci F, Righi A, Conforti L, et al. Intravenous immunoglobulin modulates cutaneous involvement and reduces skin fibrosis in systemic sclerosis: an open-label study. Arthritis Rheum. 2004;50:1005–7.

296. Poelman CL, Hummers LK, Wigley FM, Anderson C, Boin F, Shah AA. Intravenous immunoglobulin may be an effective therapy for refractory, active diffuse cutaneous systemic sclerosis. J Rheumatol. 2015;42:236–42.

297. Kudo H, Jinnin M, Yamane K, Makino T, Kajihara I, Makino K, et al. Intravenous immunoglobulin treatment recovers the down-regulated levels of Th1 cytokines in the sera and skin of scleroderma patients. J Dermatol Sci. 2013;69:77–80.

298. Raja J, Nihtyanova SI, Murray CD, Denton CP, Ong VH. Sustained benefit from intravenous immunoglobulin therapy for gastrointestinal involvement in systemic sclerosis. Rheumatology (Oxford). 2016;55:115–9.

299. Kumar S, Singh J, Kedika R, Mendoza F, Jimenez SA, Blomain ES, et al. Role of muscarinic-3 receptor antibody in systemic sclerosis: correlation with disease duration and effects of IVIG. Am J Physiol Gastrointest Liver Physiol. 2016;310:G1052–60.

300. Oates-Whitehead RM, Baumer JH, Haines L, Love S, Maconochie IK, Gupta A, et al. Intravenous immunoglobulin for the treatment of Kawasaki disease in children. Cochrane Database Syst Rev. 2003:CD004000.

301. Rigante D, Andreozzi L, Fastiggi M, Bracci B, Natale MF, Esposito S. Critical overview of the risk scoring systems to predict non-responsiveness to intravenous immunoglobulin in Kawasaki syndrome. Int J Mol Sci 2016;17.

302. Baek JY, Song MS. Meta-analysis of factors predicting resistance to intravenous immunoglobulin treatment in patients with Kawasaki disease. Korean J Pediatr. 2016;59:80–90.

303. Kawamura Y, Takeshita M, Kanai T, Yoshida Y, Nonoyama S. The combined usefulness of the neutrophil-to-lymphocyte and platelet-to-lymphocyte ratios in predicting intravenous immunoglobulin resistance with Kawasaki disease. J Pediatr 2016.

304. Davies S, Sutton N, Blackstock S, Gormley S, Hoggart CJ, Levin M, et al. Predicting IVIG resistance in UK Kawasaki disease. Arch Dis Child. 2015;100:366–8.

305. Burns JC, Franco A. The immunomodulatory effects of intravenous immunoglobulin therapy in Kawasaki disease. Expert Rev Clin Immunol. 2015;11:819–25.

306. Xue LJ, Wu R, Du GL, Xu Y, Yuan KY, Feng ZC, et al. Effect and safety of TNF Inhibitors in immunoglobulin-resistant Kawasaki disease: a meta-analysis. Clin Rev Allergy Immunol 2016.

307. Kim EJ, Yoon SY, Park HS, Yoon HS, Cho S. Pulsed intravenous immunoglobulin therapy in refractory ulcerated livedoid vasculopathy: seven cases and a literature review. Dermatol Ther. 2015;28:287–90.

308. Monshi B, Posch C, Vujic I, Sesti A, Sobotka S, Rappersberger K. Efficacy of intravenous immunoglobulins in livedoid vasculopathy: long-term follow-up of 11 patients. J Am Acad Dermatol. 2014;71:738–44.

309. Bounfour T, Bouaziz JD, Bezier M, Petit A, Viguier M, Rybojad M, et al. Intravenous immunoglobulins in difficult-to-treat ulcerated livedoid vasculopathy: five cases and a literature review. Int J Dermatol. 2013;52(9):1135.

310. Kreuter A, Gambichler T, Breuckmann F, Bechara FG, Rotterdam S, Stucker M, et al. Pulsed intravenous immunoglobulin therapy in livedoid vasculitis: an open trial evaluating 9 consecutive patients. J Am Acad Dermatol. 2004;51:574–9.

311. Martinez V, Cohen P, Pagnoux C, Vinzio S, Mahr A, Mouthon L, et al. Intravenous immunoglobulins for relapses of systemic vasculitides associated with antineutrophil cytoplasmic autoantibodies: results of a multicenter, prospective, open-label study of twenty-two patients. Arthritis Rheum. 2008;58:308–17.

312. Levy Y, Sherer Y, George J, Langevitz P, Ahmed A, Bar-Dayan Y, et al. Serologic and clinical response to treatment of systemic vasculitis and associated autoimmune disease with intravenous immunoglobulin. Int Arch Allergy Immunol. 1999;119:231–8.

313. Ito-Ihara T, Ono T, Nogaki F, Suyama K, Tanaka M, Yonemoto S, et al. Clinical efficacy of intravenous immunoglobulin for patients with MPO-ANCA-associated rapidly progressive glomerulonephritis. Nephron Clin Pract. 2006;102:c35–42.

314. Jayne DR, Chapel H, Adu D, Misbah S, O'Donoghue D, Scott D, et al. Intravenous immunoglobulin for ANCA-associated systemic vasculitis with persistent disease activity. QJM. 2000;93:433–9.

315. Crickx E, Machelart I, Lazaro E, Kahn JE, Cohen-Aubart F, Martin T, et al. Intravenous Immunoglobulin as an Immunomodulating agent in antineutrophil cytoplasmic antibody-associated vasculitides: a French Nationwide Study of Ninety-Two Patients. Arthritis Rheumatol. 2016;68:702–12.

316. Fortin PM, Tejani AM, Bassett K, Musini VM. Intravenous immunoglobulin as adjuvant therapy for Wegener's granulomatosis. Cochrane Database Syst Rev. 2013:Cd007057.

317. Richter C, Schnabel A, Csernok E, De Groot K, Reinhold-Keller E, Gross WL. Treatment of anti-neutrophil cytoplasmic antibody (ANCA)-associated systemic vasculitis with high-dose intravenous immunoglobulin. Clin Exp Immunol. 1995;101:2–7.

318. Koike H, Akiyama K, Saito T, Sobue G. Intravenous immunoglobulin for chronic residual peripheral neuropathy in eosinophilic granulomatosis with polyangiitis (Churg-Strauss syndrome): a multicenter, double-blind trial. J Neurol. 2015;262:752–9.

319. Tsurikisawa N, Taniguchi M, Saito H, Himeno H, Ishibashi A, Suzuki S, et al. Treatment of Churg-Strauss syndrome with high-dose intravenous immunoglobulin. Ann Allergy Asthma Immunol. 2004;92:80–7.

320. Danieli MG, Cappelli M, Malcangi G, Logullo F, Salvi A, Danieli G. Long term effectiveness of intravenous immunoglobulin in Churg-Strauss syndrome. Ann Rheum Dis. 2004;63:1649–54.

321. Cantarini L, Stromillo ML, Vitale A, Lopalco G, Emmi G, Silvestri E, et al. Efficacy and safety of intravenous immunoglobulin treatment in refractory Behcet's disease with different organ involvement: a case series. Isr Med Assoc J. 2016;18:238–42.

322. Seider N, Beiran I, Scharf J, Miller B. Intravenous immunoglobulin therapy for resistant ocular Behcet's disease. Br J Ophthalmol. 2001;85:1287–8.

323. Rewald E, Jaksic JC. Behcet's syndrome treated with high-dose intravenous IgG and low-dose aspirin. J R Soc Med. 1990;83:652–3.

324. Breda L, Franchini S, Marzetti V, Chiarelli F. Intravenous immunoglobulins for cutaneous polyarteritis nodosa resistant to conventional treatment. Scand J Rheumatol. 2016;45:169–70.

325. Pego PM, Camara IA, Andrade JP, Costa JM. Intravenous immunoglobulin therapy in vasculitic ulcers: a case of polyarteritis nodosa. Auto Immun Highlights. 2013;4:95–9.

326. Lobo I, Ferreira M, Silva E, Alves R, Selores M. Cutaneous poly-arteritis nodosa treated with intravenous immunoglobulins. J Eur Acad Dermatol Venereol. 2008;22:880–2.

327. Asano Y, Ihn H, Maekawa T, Kadono T, Tamaki K. High-dose intravenous immunoglobulin infusion in polyarteritis nodosa: report on one case and review of the literature. Clin Rheumatol. 2006;25:396–8.

328. Uziel Y, Silverman ED. Intravenous immunoglobulin therapy in a child with cutaneous polyarteritis nodosa. Clin Exp Rheumatol. 1998;16:187–9.

329. Bansal NK, Houghton KM. Cutaneous polyarteritis nodosa in childhood: a case report and review of the literature. Arthritis. 2010;2010:687547.

330. Marie I, Miranda S, Girszyn N, Soubrane JC, Vandhuick T, Levesque H. Intravenous immunoglobulins as treatment of severe cutaneous polyarteritis nodosa. Intern Med J. 2012;42:459–62.

331. Umemura M, Miwa Y, Yanai R, Isojima S, Tokunaga T, Tsukamoto H, et al. A case of Degos disease: demonstration of C5b-9-mediated vascular injury. Mod Rheumatol. 2015;25:480–3.

332. Guo YF, Pan WH, Cheng RH, Yu H, Liao WQ, Yao ZR. Successful treatment of neurological malignant atrophic papulosis in child by corticosteroid combined with intravenous immunoglobulin. CNS Neurosci Ther. 2014;20:88–91.

333. De Breucker S, Vandergheynst F, Decaux G. Inefficacy of intra-venous immunoglobulins and infliximab in Degos' disease. Acta Clin Belg. 2008;63:99–102.

334. Zhu KJ, Zhou Q, Lin AH, ZM L, Cheng H. The use of intravenous immunoglobulin in cutaneous and recurrent perforating intesti-nal Degos disease (malignant atrophic papulosis). Br J Dermatol. 2007;157:206–7.

335. Yamazaki-Nakashimada MA, Duran-McKinster C, Ramirez-Vargas N, Hernandez-Bautista V. Intravenous immunoglobulin therapy for hypocomplementemic urticarial vasculitis associated with systemic lupus erythematosus in a child. Pediatr Dermatol. 2009;26:445–7.

336. Filosto M, Cavallaro T, Pasolini G, Broglio L, Tentorio M, Cotelli M, et al. Idiopathic hypocomplementemic urticarial vasculitis-linked neuropathy. J Neurol Sci. 2009;284:179–81.

337. Shah D, Rowbottom AW, Thomas CL, Cumber P, Chowdhury MM. Hypocomplementaemic urticarial vasculitis associated with non-Hodgkin lymphoma and treatment with intravenous immuno-globulin. Br J Dermatol. 2007;157:392–3.

338. Perez C, Guarch R, Rodrigo M, Gallego M, Ormazabal O. Successful treatment of leucocytoclastic vasculitis and pancy-topenia secondary to systemic lupus erythematosus with intrave-nous immunoglobulin. Br J Dermatol. 2002;147:180–2.

339. Wetter DA, Davis MD, Yiannias JA, Gibson LE, Dahl MV, el-Azhary RA, et al. Effectiveness of intravenous immunoglobulin therapy for skin disease other than toxic epidermal necrolysis: a retrospective review of Mayo Clinic experience. Mayo Clin Proc. 2005;80:41–7.

340. Ong CS, Benson EM. Successful treatment of chronic leucocyto-clastic vasculitis and persistent ulceration with intravenous immu-noglobulin. Br J Dermatol. 2000;143:447–9.

341. Sais G, Vidaller A, Servitje O, Jucgla A, Peyri J. Leukocytoclastic vasculitis and common variable immunodeficiency: success-ful treatment with intravenous immune globulin. J Allergy Clin Immunol. 1996;98:232–3.

342. Staubach-Renz P, von Stebut E, Brauninger W, Maurer M, Steinbrink K. Hypocomplementemic urticarial vasculitis syn-drome. Successful therapy with intravenous immunoglobulins. Hautarzt. 2007;58:693–7.

343. Nydegger UE, Sturzenegger M. Adverse effects of intravenous immunoglobulin therapy. Drug Saf. 1999;21:171–85.

344. Gurcan HM, Ahmed AR. Frequency of adverse events associated with intravenous immunoglobulin therapy in patients with pem-phigus or pemphigoid. Ann Pharmacother. 2007;41(10):1604.

345. Thornby KA, Henneman A, Brown DA. Evidence-based strate-gies to reduce intravenous immunoglobulin-induced headaches. Ann Pharmacother. 2015;49:715–26.

346. Sekul EA, Cupler EJ, Dalakas MC. Aseptic meningitis associated with high-dose intravenous immunoglobulin therapy: frequency and risk factors. Ann Intern Med. 1994;121:259–62.

347. Jarius S, Eichhorn P, Albert MH, Wagenpfeil S, Wick M, Belohradsky BH, et al. Intravenous immunoglobulins contain nat-urally occurring antibodies that mimic antineutrophil cytoplasmic antibodies and activate neutrophils in a TNFalpha-dependent and Fc-receptor-independent way. Blood. 2007;109:4376–82.

348. Stiehm ER. Adverse effects of human immunoglobulin therapy. Transfus Med Rev. 2013;27:171–8.

349. Renal insufficiency and failure associated with immune globulin intravenous therapy--United States, 1985–1998. MMWR Morb Mortal Wkly Rep. 1999;48:518–21.

350. Ahsan N, Palmer BF, Wheeler D, Greenlee RG Jr, Toto RD. Intravenous immunoglobulin-induced osmotic nephrosis. Arch Intern Med. 1994;154:1985–7.

351. Cherin P, Marie I, Michallet M, Pelus E, Dantal J, Crave JC, et al. Management of adverse events in the treatment of patients with immunoglobulin therapy: A review of evidence. Autoimmun Rev. 2016;15:71–81.

352. Mizrahi M. The hypercoagulability of intravenous immunoglobu-lin. Clin Adv Hematol Oncol. 2011;9:49–50.

353. Gerstenblith MR, Antony AK, Junkins-Hopkins JM, Abuav R. Pompholyx and eczematous reactions associated with intravenous immunoglobulin therapy. J Am Acad Dermatol. 2012;66:312–6.

354. van der Molen RG, Hamann D, Jacobs JF, van der Meer A, de Jong J, Kramer C, et al. Anti-SSA antibodies are present in immu-noglobulin preparations. Transfusion. 2015;55:832–7.

355. Daoud YJ, Amin KG. Comparison of cost of immune globulin intravenous therapy to conventional immunosuppressive therapy in treating patients with autoimmune mucocutaneous blistering diseases. Int Immunopharmacol. 2006;6:600–6.

356. Daoud Y, Amin KG, Mohan K, Ahmed AR. Cost of intravenous immunoglobulin therapy versus conventional immunosuppressive therapy in patients with mucous membrane pemphigoid: a pre-liminary study. Ann Pharmacother. 2005;39:2003–8.

357. Heelan K, Hassan S, Bannon G, Knowles S, Walsh S, Shear NH, et al. Cost and resource use of pemphigus and pemphigoid disorders pre- and post-rituximab. J Cutan Med Surg. 2015; 19:274–82.

358. Bamrungsawad N, Chaiyakunapruk N, Upakdee N, Pratoomsoot C, Sruamsiri R, Dilokthornsakul P. Cost-utility analysis of intra-venous immunoglobulin for the treatment of steroid-refractory dermatomyositis in Thailand. Pharmacoeconomics. 2015; 33:521–31.

Systemic Antifungals

Allen S.W. Oak, John W. Baddley, and Boni E. Elewski

Abbreviations

5-FC	5-Fluorocytosine
5-FU	5-Fluorouracil
7-DHC	7-Dehydrocholesterol
AAM	Allylamine
AEs	Adverse effects
AGEP	Acute generalized exanthematous pustulosis
AIDS	Acquired immunodeficiency syndrome
AmB	Amphotericin B
CC	Complete cure
CD	Cyclodextrins
CDC	Centers for Disease Control and Prevention
CHF	Congestive heart failure
CI	Confidence interval
CoA	Coenzyme A
CR	Clinical relapse
CTI	ClinicalTrials.gov Identifier
CYP450	Cytochrome P450
EMA	European Medicines Agency
EP	Evaluable patient
FDA	Food and Drug Administration
FdUMP	5-Fluorodeoxyuridine monophosphate
FUTP	5-Fluorouridine triphosphate
GI	Gastrointestinal
GPI	Glycosylphosphatidylinositol
HIV	Human immunodeficiency virus
HMG-CoA	3-Hydroxy-3-methylglutaryl coenzyme A
HR	Hazard ratio
ITT	Intention-to-treat

KOH	Potassium hydroxide
LFT	Liver function test
LION	Lamisil vs. Itraconazole in Onychomycosis
mAbs	Monoclonal antibodies
MC	Mycologic cure
Meltrex	Melt extrusion technology
MFC	Minimum fungicidal concentration
MIC	Minimum inhibitory concentration
MISC	Miscellaneous
MR	Mycologic relapse
NNT	Number needed to treat
PUVA	Psoralen with UVA
ROS	Reactive oxygen species
RR	Relative risk
SCC	Squamous cell carcinoma
SCLE	Subacute cutaneous lupus erythematosus
SJS	Stevens-Johnson syndrome
TEN	Toxic epidermal necrolysis
UVA	Ultraviolet A (320–400 nm)
UVB	Ultraviolet B (280–320 nm)

A.S.W. Oak, MD • B.E. Elewski, MD (✉)
Department of Dermatology, University of Alabama at
Birmingham, Birmingham, AL 35294, USA
e-mail: beelewski@gmail.com

J.W. Baddley, MD, MSPH
Division of Infectious Diseases, Department of Medicine,
University of Alabama at Birmingham,
Birmingham, AL 35294, USA

Introduction

Fungi were identified as pathogens even prior to bacteria. Thrush, now ascribed to *Candida albicans*, was listed as a fatal disease as early as 1665 [1]. In the US, the first reported human case of blastomycosis in 1894 [2, 3] by Thomas Gilchrist, an American dermatologist, marked the beginning of medical mycology, the study of diseases caused by fungal invasion into human or animal tissue.

Fungal infections, or mycoses, are among the most common groups of diseases worldwide. Cutaneous fungal infections were the fourth most prevalent group of diseases worldwide with an estimated global prevalence of 984,290,432 in 2010 [4]. The estimated prevalence of onychomycosis is 6.9–13.8% in the US, 10.0% in Japan, and 20% in Europe with a worldwide incidence that ranges between 2.7

© Springer International Publishing AG 2018
P.S. Yamauchi (ed.), *Biologic and Systemic Agents in Dermatology*, https://doi.org/10.1007/978-3-319-66884-0_40

and 20% [5–7]. Furthermore, the economic burden of cutaneous fungal infections is considerable. In 2004, the total and indirect cost of cutaneous fungal infections exceeded $1.9 billion in the US [8]. The annual Medicare cost of treating onychomycosis alone is estimated to exceed $43 million [9].

Fungal infections are an important cause of morbidity and mortality in not only severely ill individuals, such as those with an underlying malignancy, but also diabetics and immunocompromised individuals, such as patients with human immunodeficiency virus (HIV) and organ transplant recipients. Infections, such as onychomycosis, that are usually well tolerated in healthy individuals can have dire consequences in these susceptible patient populations. About a third of diabetics and 15–44% of HIV-positive patients have onychomycosis [10–12]. Onychomycosis in diabetics form large dystrophic toenails that accumulate subungual debris, a nidus for fungi and bacteria [12]. Even more concerning is the resulting increase in pressure on underlying toes that may go unnoticed by those with diabetic neuropathy. Onychomycosis is a significant predictor (hazard ratio (HR): 1.58, 95% confidence interval (CI): 1.16–2.16) of diabetic foot ulcer [13], a debilitating condition that may lead to osteomyelitis, gangrene, or even amputation [12].

The prevalence of invasive fungal infection in those with solid tumors, hematologic malignancy, acquired immunodeficiency syndrome (AIDS), solid or hematopoietic cell transplantation, or other diagnoses was 8.2% in a postmortem analysis of 2707 patients between 1993 and 2005 [14]. In the US, an overall 12-month cumulative incidence of invasive fungal infection was 3.1% in solid organ [15], and 3.4% in hematopoietic cell transplant recipients [16]. Although many patients with invasive fungal infection have serious underlying disorders, the mortality directly attributable to invasive fungal infection remains high and the mortality rate directly attributable to candidemia alone ranges between 10% and 49% [17, 18]. The estimated total direct cost, a sum of inpatient and outpatient costs, of treating systemic fungal infections is $2.6 billion with an average per-patient attributable cost of $31,200 [19]. Because of the clinical importance of the problem and the growing need to develop more effective therapy, there has been great interest in understanding the pathogenesis of fungal infections.

There has been substantial progress in antifungal therapy, especially over the last two decades. Previously, polyenes and imidazoles were the only classes that were available, along with other miscellaneous compounds, such as griseofulvin. Currently, there are four main classes of systemic antifungal agents. These are polyenes, allylamines, echinocandins, and azoles. Azoles include imidazoles, triazoles, and tetrazoles that are currently under investigation. Other miscellaneous systemic antifungals include flucytosine, a fluorinated pyrimidine analog, and griseofulvin, a fungal mitotic inhibitor. An up-to-date mechanistic understanding of systemic antifungal drugs pertinent to treating dermatomycoses, relevant pharmacologic properties, and future directions, including drugs under investigation, will be discussed.

Classification of Fungal Infections and Indications for Systemic Antifungals

Three distinct parameters help classify fungal infections clinically. These are (1) the pathogen's degree of virulence, (2) the level of tissue involvement, and (3) the route of acquisition.

1. The degree of virulence of a fungal organism determines its classification as either a true or an opportunistic pathogen. While true pathogenic fungi, such as *Coccidioides immitis*, are capable of causing disease even in healthy individuals, opportunistic fungi are only able to infect predisposed immunocompromised individuals [20].

2. Depending on the degree of tissue involvement, cutaneous fungal infections are categorized as superficial, subcutaneous, or systemic. Superficial mycoses, limited to the integument and its appendages, involve the hair, nails, and the stratum corneum. Subcutaneous mycoses, also called mycoses of implantation, often arise as a result of traumatic inoculation and are limited to the subcutaneous tissue. Systemic, or deep, mycoses involve underlying structures, such as the abdominal viscera, the central nervous stem, the lungs, or bones. In true pathogenic fungi, cutaneous lesions signify hematogenous spread or the involvement of underlying tissue, whereas in opportunistic fungi, cutaneous lesions arise as either primary or secondary lesions in an immunocompromised host [20–22]. The gastrointestinal (GI) tract, respiratory tract, and blood vessels serve as the most common portals of entry for systemic mycoses [21].

3. Fungal infections, depending on the route of acquisition, may also be categorized as endogenous or exogenous. Endogenous infections arise as a result of colonization or activation of a latent infection, but exogenous infections are acquired from the external environment through a cutaneous, percutaneous, or airborne route [21].

Most superficial mycoses respond adequately to topical antifungals in an immunocompetent host, but a systemic treatment is warranted under certain conditions. Such conditions include hair or nail involvement, extensive cutaneous involvement, failure of topical treatments, chronic or recurrent cases, and a significant inflammatory reaction secondary to the superficial mycosis. Immunocompromised patients require systemic treatments for superficial mycoses. Systemic antifungals are needed to treat onychomycosis if any of the following conditions are met: involvement of the nail matrix, involvement of both fingernails and toenails, concurrent treatment with an immunosuppressive agent, and any evidence of immunodeficiency. Only itraconazole and terbinafine are approved by the US Food and Drug Administration (FDA) to treat onychomycosis. Fluconazole may be used, but it is not FDA-approved to treat onychomycosis. Oral ketoconazole is no longer indicated to treat skin and nail fungal infections due to hepatotoxicity and adrenal insufficiency [23–25]. Tinea pedis unresponsive to topical therapy also necessitate systemic therapy, as does tinea manuum. In contrast, subcutaneous and systemic mycoses require systemic treatment as first-line therapy [22].

Basic Fungal Biology

The taxonomic kingdom of fungi, a clade consisting of highly diversified species of eukaryotes, emerged about 1.6 million years ago. Although the kingdom is estimated to contain more than five million species, only 120,000 fungal species have been formally described so far. Fungi lack chlorophyll and thus are obligated to obtain carbon compounds from either a living host (e.g., a human) or a nonliving organic substrate [26]. Pathogenic fungi, which may exist as unicellular yeasts or as filamentous molds, are relatively rare. Even of 300 species that are reportedly pathogenic to immunocompetent humans, only a few species are considered common pathogens [27]. However, many species of fungi can be opportunistic invaders in hosts with primary and secondary immunodeficiencies.

Cell Wall

Fungi possess structurally unique cell walls composed of three main components: glucans, chitins, and glycoproteins (Fig. 40.1). The fungal cell wall is a dynamic structure that grants mechanical strength, protects the organism from environmental stress, and provides adequate plasticity that allows the organism to carry out key events during its life cycle (e.g., cell growth and division). Glucans, composed of glucose residues linked by glucan synthase, are considered the major structural polysaccharides. Approximately 65–90% of glucans found in the fungal cell wall are β-1,3-glucans synthesized by β-1,3-glucan synthase. Chitins, linear polymers of N-acetylglucosamine, provide enormous tensile strength due to extensive hydrogen bonds between chitin chains. Glycoproteins are extensively modified oligosaccharides that are often tethered to the plasma membrane by glycosylphosphatidylinositol (GPI) anchors [28].

Ergosterol

The fungal plasma membrane contains ergosterol (Fig. 40.1), a fungal analog of 7-dehydrocholesterol (7-DHC) in animals. Ergosterol plays an important role in regulating membrane function, such as maintaining membrane fluidity and permeability. In addition, ergosterol interacts with sphingolipids to form lipid rafts that are functional microdomains implicated in endocytosis, membrane trafficking, and signal transduction. Ergosterol is found in various intracellular organelles, such as mitochondria, endoplasmic reticulum, and peroxisomes [29, 30]. Since ergosterol plays a critical role in regulating many functions of fungal cells and humans lack ergosterol, the ergosterol biosynthesis pathway serves as a target of many antifungal agents currently available on the market (Fig. 40.2).

Antifungal Efficacy

Two useful criteria for evaluating antifungal activity of a given agent are its range of activity (broad- vs. narrow-spectrum) and its ability to kill the organism (fungistatic vs. fungicidal).

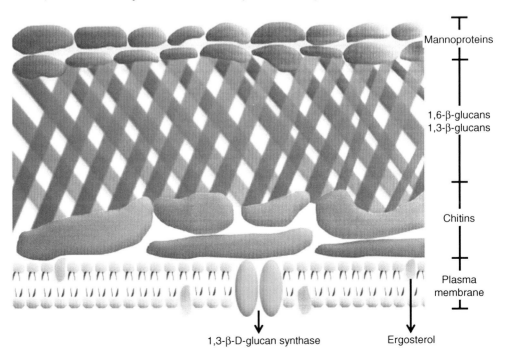

Fig. 40.1 The fungal cell wall

Mannoproteins

1,6-β-glucans
1,3-β-glucans

Chitins

Plasma membrane

1,3-β-D-glucan synthase   Ergosterol

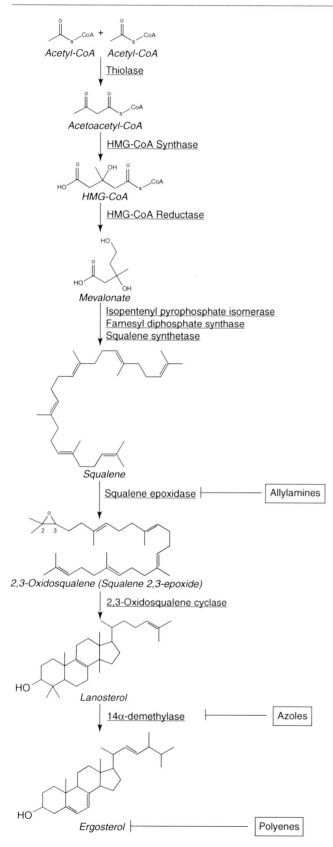

Broad-spectrum antifungals, such as amphotericin B and voriconazole, are able to inhibit a wide variety of organisms, including molds and yeasts. Narrow-spectrum antifungals have a more limited spectrum. For example, griseofulvin is only active against dermatophytes.

Antifungals may also be classified as fungicidal or fungistatic. Fungistatic agents are able to inhibit and arrest fungal growth, whereas fungicidal agents are able to kill the organism. This may be tested in vitro by subjecting a standardized fungal inoculum to a series of drug dilutions. An antifungal agent's minimum inhibitory concentration (MIC) is its lowest concentration that visibly inhibits fungal growth, whereas its minimum fungicidal concentration (MFC) is its lowest concentration that eradicates 99.9% of the original fungal inoculum. The MFC/MIC ratio indicates whether a compound is considered fungicidal (MFC/MIC $\leq$ 4) or fungistatic (MFC/MIC > 4) [31–34]. Time-kill studies have also been used to determine the extent of fungicidal activity, and the pharmacodynamics properties. Time-kill studies may be used to determine potential synergistic/antagonist properties of agents when tested concomitantly [33].

In immunocompetent individuals, treatment with a fungistatic agent, which may be coupled with other therapeutic interventions (e.g., drainage, or removal of foreign body), is often enough to prevent dissemination, and the host immune system eventually eradicates the organism to achieve clinical cure. However, the use of fungicidal agents becomes critical for certain circumstances: (a) the involvement of sites not easily accessible to the immune system (e.g., hair and nails) or sites with essential physiologic function where rapid cure is needed (e.g., central nervous system, or the bone), and (b) treating immunocompromised individuals. Immunocompromised patients are more prone to developing fungal infections and their lack of a functional immune system, especially in neutropenic individuals, necessitate a fungicidal regimen. This is because without a competent immune system, the pathogenic fungi potentially lie dormant until the treatment is discontinued.

The clinical importance of using a fungicidal agent can be illustrated in treating onychomycosis. Three parameters, clinical cure, mycologic cure (MC), and complete cure (CC), are often used when evaluating an antifungal agent's efficacy in treating onychomycosis. A clinical cure is achieved when 100% of the nail plate is visibly clear of infection. MC is achieved when the potassium hydroxide (KOH) smear and fungal culture are both negative. CC requires the attainment of both clinical cure and MC [35]. Comparative trials using either griseofulvin or terbinafine, which are respectively fungistatic or fungicidal, to treat toenail onychomycosis demonstrated that griseofulvin results in a lower rate of CC (2% vs. 42%) with a higher rate of relapse even with a longer course of treatment (48–52 weeks vs. 16–24 weeks) [36, 37]. The rate of relapse for griseofulvin was as high as 70% for toenail onychomycosis [38, 39].

Fig. 40.2 Targets of antifungal agents in the ergosterol biosynthesis pathway. Abbreviations: *CoA* coenzyme A, *HMG-CoA* 3-hydroxy-3-methylglutaryl coenzyme A. Biosynthesis of ergosterol from lanosterol occurs in a series of steps

Antifungal Agents

Fungal organisms were known causes of systemic illnesses in humans since the 1890s, but treatments then were limited to surgical therapy and application of weak acids, such as undecylenic acid and phenolic dyes. The first active and safe antifungal agent, griseofulvin, was successfully isolated from *Penicillium griseofulvum* in 1939 [40] and first used in humans in 1958 [41].

Azoles

Azole antifungals are classified according to the number of nitrogen atoms in their characteristic five-membered heterocyclic rings. An imidazole derivative contains two nitrogens in its azole ring, whereas a triazole derivative contains three (Table 40.1). Azole rings are attached to other aromatic rings via carbon-nitrogen bonds.

Table 40.1 Structure of each systemic antifungal class and its representative member (defining structure highlighted in blue)

Class	Structure	Member
Imidazole[a]		Ketoconazole
Triazole[a]		Itraconazole
Allylamine		Terbinafine
Polyene		Amphotericin B

[a]A member of the azole family

Mechanism: All azole antifungals inhibit a fungal-specific cytochrome P450 (CYP450)-dependent enzyme, 14α-demethylase (CYP51A1), encoded by *ERG11*. Azoles act as metalloenzyme inhibitors that bind the heme cofactor on the active site of CYP51 in a competitive, reversible manner [42]. This inhibition causes a depletion of ergosterol and a buildup of its sterol precursors (Fig. 40.2), such as lanosterol, 24-methylenedihydrolanosterol, and 14-dimethylergosterol, which ultimately compromises the structural integrity of the plasma membrane. However, this CYP450-dependent mode of action is also responsible for many adverse effects (AEs) since the ubiquitous CYP450 superfamily plays crucial roles in hepatic drug metabolism and steroidogenesis.

Imidazole

Imidazoles were the first effective class of drugs that provided an antimicrobial capability beyond the designation of "broad-spectrum" since it exhibited both antifungal and antibacterial capabilities [43].

Ketoconazole

Ketoconazole, an imidazole derivative (Table 40.1), was FDA-approved in 1981. Owing to its superior oral absorption compared to the other imidazoles that were available on the market, ketoconazole remained the only oral antifungal against systemic fungal infections for nearly a decade. However, many significant AEs of ketoconazole, exacerbated by its prolonged treatment course as a fungistatic agent, became apparent as it stayed on the market.

These limitations necessitated the development of other antifungals, including other azoles, and resulted in an effort to significantly reduce ketoconazole use when viable alternatives became available. In 2013, the European Medicines Agency (EMA) withdrew all oral ketoconazole-containing drugs from the EU [44] and the FDA mandated that ketoconazole should not be used as a first-line therapy for any fungal infections, including nail and skin infections [23].

Limitations and AEs:

(a) Hepatotoxicity

Ketoconazole's hepatotoxic properties are thought to be due to metabolic idiosyncrasy. Ketoconazole's primary metabolite, *N*-deacetylketoconazole, is more hepatotoxic than ketoconazole, and capable of undergoing further metabolism by flavin-containing monooxygenase to yield more downstream hepatotoxic metabolites [45]. Ketoconazole use is linked to acute liver injury that occurs with an incidence rate of 134.1 per 100,000 person-months (95% CI: 36.8–488.0) [46]. A cohort study of 69,830 individuals without liver or systemic disease who received at least one prescription for an oral antifungal correlated ketoconazole use with the highest relative risk (RR) of developing acute liver injury (RR: 228.0, 95% CI: 33.9–933.0), more than ten times RRs of itraconazole and terbinafine combined [46]. Furthermore, 20 per 10,000 persons exposed to ketoconazole develop symptomatic hepatitis [47]. Cases of liver cirrhosis [48], fatal hepatitis [49], and liver failure necessitating a liver transplant [50, 51] have all been attributed to ketoconazole use. Finally, multiple deaths have been attributed to ketoconazole-related liver toxicity, including the death of a patient prescribed ketoconazole for onychomycosis, which occurred after the label change in 2013 [24, 49, 51–56].

(b) Inhibitive Effect on Testosterone Synthesis

Ketoconazole inhibits androgen biosynthesis in a dose-dependent manner [57, 58], namely through the inhibition of C17–C20 lyase [59], an enzyme found both in testes and adrenals [60]. For example, although a higher dose (800 mg/day) of oral ketoconazole was highly effective at treating disseminated histoplasmosis than a lower dose (400 mg/day), toxic effects, including a potentially life-threatening adrenal insufficiency, were observed more frequently (79.4% vs. 43.7%) among those receiving a higher dose [61]. This inhibition of testosterone synthesis is also thought to contribute to reported cases of gynecomastia in men taking ketoconazole [62, 63].

(c) Inhibition of CYP3A4

Ketoconazole is not only a potent inhibitor of CYP3A4 [64], which metabolizes more than 50% of all prescribed drugs on the market [65], but also potentially a universal inhibitor of all CYP450 isozymes [66].

(d) Fungistatic

Ketoconazole's limited role in treating immunocompromised individuals, demonstrated by either therapy failure [67, 68] or reduced efficacy [69], represented a critical lack of utility [70]. Since ketoconazole is largely fungistatic, it cannot be utilized effectively in patients with a compromised immune system, including organ transplant patients and patients with AIDS [71]. These patients have an increased risk of developing invasive fungal infections that are potentially life-threatening [72]. Furthermore, using a fungistatic systemic agent, such as ketoconazole, often requires a prolonged treatment course. However, ketoconazole's various AEs made its prolonged use undesirable.

Triazoles

Triazoles were developed to overcome the undesirable traits of imidazoles. Thus, they possess many advantages over imidazoles, including an increased selectivity for fungal

CYP450 enzymes that accounts for their improved toxicity profiles [73]. Itraconazole (Table 40.1) and fluconazole, available since the late 1980s, are now considered first-generation triazoles. The second-generation triazoles, which include voriconazole, posaconazole, and isavocunazole, have an enhanced potency, a broader spectrum, and more favorable pharmacokinetic properties.

Itraconazole

Indications: Three formulations of itraconazole are currently available, each with different indications; oral solution is approved to treat oropharyngeal/esophageal candidiasis in immunocompromised adults [74]. Capsules are approved to treat aspergillosis, blastomycosis, histoplasmosis, and fingernail or toenail onychomycosis [75]. Tablets are approved to treat toenail onychomycosis caused by *Trichophyton rubrum* or *T. mentagrophytes* [76]. Tablets, made using melt extrusion technology (Meltrex), contain a dose equivalent to two capsules, allowing a once-daily dosing regimen [77, 78].

AEs: When used to treat onychomycosis, itraconazole is overall well tolerated and adverse events are reported in only 3% of patients [79, 80]. Common AEs include diarrhea and abdominal pain or discomfort (1.7–4%), rash and pruritus (5%), headache (2.2–10%), and rhinitis (5–9%) [75, 76]. Itraconazole's risk of causing acute liver injury, although much lower than that of ketoconazole, has been reported with an incidence rate of 10.4 per 100,000 person-months (95% CI: 2.9–38.1) with an RR of 17.7 (95% CI: 2.6–72.6) [46]. Two cases of prolonged cholestasis with biliary ductopenia (vanishing bile duct syndrome) have also been reported [47]. Acute generalized exanthematous pustulosis (AGEP) is rarely associated with itraconazole, and the eruption resolves in most cases after treatment cessation and corticosteroid therapy [81–83]. Other significant AEs linked with itraconazole use are as follows.

(a) AEs Due to Cyclodextrin

Cyclodextrins (CDs) are cyclic oligomers of dextrin units with a hydrophobic exterior and a hydrophilic interior [84]. This structure allows CDs to form inclusion complexes with drugs, especially those with poor solubility in water, to enhance their delivery. CD is present in the oral solution formulation of itraconazole, but not present in griseofulvin or fluconazole [85, 86]. CDs of pharmacologic interest are α-, β-, and γ-CDs with 6, 7, and 8 dextrose units in their glucopyranose rings, respectively [87]. Since itraconazole is insoluble in water (solubility <0.0001 g/100 mL) [88], hydroxypropyl-β-CD is used to enhance its solubility to form an oral solution formulation, which comes in cherry and caramel flavors to mask its unpleasant taste [74]. However, CDs appear to account for almost all toxicities reported with this formulation [88]. Nephrotoxicity and GI toxicity have been reported

in animal studies [89]. Vacuolation, as well as swelling, was observed in the bladder cells, pelvic urothelial cells, and renal cortical cells in rats treated with 2-hydroxylpropyl-β-CD in their diet (500–5000 mg/kg body weight per day) [89]. A significant increase in polypoid tumors of the large intestine was observed at higher doses and an increase in exocrine pancreatic tumors was also observed at all dose levels [89]. While daily oral doses of 4–8 g of hydroxypropyl-β-CD for at least 2 weeks are considered safe and well tolerated, higher oral doses of 16–24 g resulted in higher incidence of diarrhea and soft stools [89, 90]. In a study examining the effects of hydroxypropyl-β-CD in 26 pediatric patients with HIV, two patients had to discontinue therapy due to either persistent diarrhea or a maculopapular rash with a decrease in visual acuity [91]. 2-Hydroxypropyl-β-cyclodextrin has been linked to ototoxicity, namely dose-dependent damage to cochlear cells, in animal studies [92–95]. More detailed reviews regarding the toxicological implications of CDs and their derivatives have been published [84, 87, 88, 96].

(b) Cardiotoxicity

Fifty-eight cases of congestive heart failure (CHF) potentially caused by itraconazole were reported between 1992 and 2001 [97]. Of them, 28 were hospitalized and 13 died. This negative inotropic effect appeared to be specific to itraconazole since similar findings were not reported in other members of the azole family. Itraconazole also prolongs the QT interval [98].

(c) Bone Defects

Thinning of the zona compacta, increased fragility of bones, and reduced activity of bone plates have all been reported as itraconazole-induced bone defects at doses as low as 20 mg/kg/day in rats [75]. Dental abnormalities have also been reported with long-term exposure (≥6 months) in rats [75]. Thus, treating children with itraconazole, especially over a prolonged period of time, may be problematic.

Lab Parameters to Monitor: Liver function test (LFT) for those treated longer than 1 month or those with preexisting hepatic dysfunction, renal function, and signs/symptoms of CHF.

Contraindications: Concomitant administration of certain drugs metabolized by CYP3A4 (e.g., lovastatin and ergot alkaloids) is contraindicated since itraconazole and its metabolites are major substrates and inhibitors of CYP3A4 (Table 40.2) [102]. Drugs that prolong the QT interval are also contraindicated during itraconazole use. Evidence of ventricular dysfunction or a history of CHF is a contraindication. Itraconazole use is strongly discouraged in those with active liver disease or those who have experienced liver toxicity with other therapeutic agents.

Table 40.2 Selected pharmacodynamic and pharmacokinetic properties of systemic antifungals

	Pharmacodynamics and pharmacokinetics
Allylamine	
Terbinafine	**Oral bioavailability**: 40% in adults, 36–64% in children **Absorption**: Children and adults: >70%, unaffected by food **Metabolism**: Extensively metabolized in the liver. Inhibitor of CYP2D6 **Half-life elimination**: Children: 27–31 h; adults: ~36 h
Azoles	
Fluconazole	**Oral bioavailability**: >80% [99] **Absorption**: Well absorbed orally. Increases with food **Metabolism**: 80% of dose can be recovered in urine in its unchanged form. 11% can be recovered as glucuronide and N-oxide metabolites, which are products of hepatic metabolism by CYP3A4 [100]. It is a potent inhibitor of CYP2C9, as well as CYP2C19, and is a moderate CYP3A4 inhibitor **Half-life elimination**: Normal renal function: 30 h (range: 20–50 h)
Isavocunazole	**Oral bioavailability**: 98% [101] **Absorption**: Well absorbed orally. Not significantly affected by food **Metabolism**: Substrate of CYP3A4 (moderate inhibitor) and CYP3A5 **Half-life elimination**: 56–104 h
Itraconazole	**Oral bioavailability**: >70% [99] **Absorption**: Requires gastric acidity. Capsule or tablet better absorbed with food, but solution better absorbed without food **Metabolism**: Occurs extensively in the liver. Major substrate and inhibitor of CYP3A4 [102] **Half-life elimination**: 30–40 h
Posaconazole	**Oral bioavailability**: 54% under fasting condition [25] **Absorption**: Well absorbed orally. Increases with food (relative oral bioavailability increased by 400% when given with a high-fat meal) [103]. Affected by gastric pH (higher pH decreases absorption) [104] **Metabolism**: Metabolized by uridine diphosphate glucuronosyltransferase enzyme pathways in the liver. Not metabolized significantly by the CYP isozymes, but is a strong inhibitor of CYP3A4. Substrate of P-glycoprotein efflux [105] **Half-life elimination**: 31 h [106]
Voriconazole	**Oral bioavailability**: 96% in adults, range widely variable in children aged 2–12: 45–80% [107–109] **Absorption**: Well absorbed orally. Decreases with food [110] **Metabolism**: Occurs extensively in the liver, predominantly by CYP2C19, but also by CYP2C9, CYP3A4 **Half-life elimination**: 6 h [111]
Echinocandins	
Anidulafungin	**Metabolism**: Not metabolized. Undergoes slow spontaneous degradation to inactive metabolites **Half-life elimination**: 40–50 h
Caspofungin	**Metabolism**: Undergoes slow hydrolysis and N-acetylation. Some spontaneous hepatic degradation [111] **Half-life elimination**: 40–50 h
Micafungin	**Metabolism**: Metabolized by arylsulfatase and catechol-O-methyltransferase in the liver [111]. A mild inhibitor of CYP3A4 **Half-life elimination**: 11–21 h
Polyene	
AmB	**Metabolism**: Details unknown **Half-life elimination** (triphasic plasma profile): **Conventional AmB** (AmB deoxycholate): 24 h **Liposomal AmB**: 8.6 ± 3.1 h **AmB lipid complex**: 173.4 h
Miscellaneous	
Flucytosine	**Oral bioavailability**: >80% **Absorption**: Well absorbed orally. Food decreases the rate of absorption, although the extent of absorption remains unaffected [112] **Metabolism**: Not metabolized significantly **Half-life elimination**: 3–6 h
Griseofulvin	**Oral bioavailability**: Low and erratic [113, 114] **Absorption**: Poor unless coated with polyethylene glycol or microsized [115]. Increases with food. Almost complete for the ultramicrosize griseofulvin, although it is variable (25–70%) for microsize griseofulvin. Decreases (more prominently in the microsize than the ultramicrosize formulation) with repeated administrations, which may be due to mucosal damage from unabsorbed griseofulvin in the gut [116] **Metabolism**: Undergoes extensive hepatic metabolism (primary metabolite: 6-desmethylgriseofulvin) [117] **Half-life elimination**: 9–24 h

Abbreviations: *AmB* amphotericin B
Information retrieved from the package insert unless otherwise noted

Fluconazole

Indications: Fluconazole is used to treat candidiasis (esophageal, oropharyngeal, peritoneal, urinary tract, vaginal) and systemic *Candida* infections. It may also be used as antifungal prophylaxis in allogeneic bone marrow transplant recipients.

Off-Label Uses:

(a) Onychomycosis

Fluconazole is not FDA-approved to treat onychomycosis. However, fluconazole still was the second most prescribed antifungal agent for onychomycosis between 1995 and 2010 in the US [118]. Fluconazole is approved to treat onychomycosis in Europe. Fluconazole, which has in vivo activity against dermatophytes and *C. albicans*, has been evaluated previously for treating onychomycosis. While *Candida* spp. are frequently isolated in cultures during mycological testing, determining whether they are commensal organisms or true pathogens is difficult. However, *Candida* spp. are significantly associated with some fingernail infections, and they are frequent colonizers of toe webs in diabetics [12]. Terbinafine is not as effective for treating onychomycosis caused by *Candida* spp. since terbinafine's in vitro activity and clinical efficacy data against *Candida* onychomycosis are unpredictable and inconsistent [119, 120]. Both itraconazole and fluconazole are effective against *Candida* onychomycosis, but itraconazole's negative inotropic effect is a significant contraindication in diabetics, a population with an increased prevalence of coronary artery disease [12]. Therefore, fluconazole is the treatment of choice for *Candida* onychomycosis in diabetics, although special attention must be paid to potential drug-drug interactions since fluconazole is metabolized by CYP3A4 (Table 40.2) and appears to interact significantly with certain hypoglycemic agents including a number of sulfonylureas (glyburide, glipizide, and tolbutamide) [12].

In those with subungual dermatophyte onychomycosis of the toenail, a once-weekly regimen of 150, 300, or 450 mg for 12 months resulted in CC and MC rates of 28–36% and 47–62%, respectively [121]. The rate of relapse was 4% after 6 months of follow-up. The regimen was well tolerated with comparable rates of adverse events between the treatment group and the placebo group [121]. However, subsequent onychomycosis trials that compared the rates of cure between fluconazole (150 mg/week for 3 or 4 months, MC: 31.2–51% and CC: 21–31.2%), terbinafine (250 mg/day for 3 months, MC: 75–89% and CC: 62.5–67%), and itraconazole (400 mg/day for 1 week per month for 3 months, MC: 61.2% and CC: 61.1%) showed that intermittent fluconazole is the least effective in achieving cure [122, 123]. Therefore, fluconazole may have a role as a third-line treatment in those unable to tolerate terbinafine or itraconazole.

The efficacy of pulse fluconazole, a weekly regimen that may potentially increase patient compliance, is dependent on its duration of therapy, but not its dose [124]. The rate of clinical cure and MC for toenail dermatophyte onychomycosis increased with a longer duration of pulse fluconazole (>6 months vs. ≤6 months), while varying the dose (150, 300, or 450 mg/week) failed to show any significant changes [124]. This is a considerable advantage since the rate of treatment discontinuation due to adverse reactions is lower for intermittent fluconazole given at 150 mg/week (1.98%, 95% CI: 0.05–3.92%) than that of continuous terbinafine given at 250 mg/day (3.44%, 95% CI: 2.28–4.61%) or continuous itraconazole given at 200 mg/day (4.21%, 95% CI, 2.33–6.09%) [125].

(b) Tinea Capitis

Tinea capitis, which usually presents as scaly patches of alopecia with pruritus in prepubescent children, is a highly communicable dermatophyte infection with a reported prevalence of 3–8% in the US [126] and 1–19.7% in developing countries around the world [127]. The causative organisms are dermatophytes that belong to the genera *Microsporum* and *Trichophyton*. Their relative distribution varies around the globe. *T. tonsurans* is the most common cause in North America and the UK [126], but *M. canis* is the dominant species in the Mediterranean countries [128, 129], such as Italy and Greece, and *T. violaceum* is the most common causative species in places such as Iran [130], Palestine [131], Ethiopia [114] and Libya [132]. However, this distribution is dynamic and is susceptible to selective pressure. Griseofulvin was introduced in North American at a time when *M. canis* and *M. audouinii* were still predominant causes of tinea capitis. Currently, *T. tonsurans* is isolated in more than 95% of cases in the US [133]. Furthermore, *T. tonsurans* is becoming more resistant to griseofulvin, as evidenced by the increase in the recommended dose of griseofulvin and its high rates of failure that range between 24 and 39% in more recent studies [134, 135].

Based on studies that reported fluconazole's high rates of cure, ranging from 89 to 98% [136–138], in treating tinea capitis, clinical trials have been conducted to evaluate its efficacy. A randomized controlled trial of 880 pediatric patients with tinea capitis (isolated dermatophytes on culture: *T. tonsurans*: 86% and *M. canis*: 11%) showed no significant differences in clinical, mycological, or combined outcomes between groups treated with fluconazole (6 mg/kg for 6 weeks) and griseofulvin (11 mg/kg for 6 weeks). Furthermore, the observed rates of MC for children treated with fluconazole were 44–50%, which were less than expected [139]. A clinical study of 113 patients with tinea capitis with positive fungal cultures (*T. violaceum*: 43.4% and *M. canis*: 49.6%) treated with griseofulvin (15 or 25 mg/kg/day) or fluconazole (4 or 6 mg/kg/day) up to 12 weeks or until a negative fungal culture was observed showed no difference between griseofulvin and fluconazole [140]. A study of 75 children with tinea capitis (*T. violaceum*: 68%) showed no difference between intermittent fluconazole for 6 weeks, continuous griseofulvin for 6 weeks, and continuous terbinafine for 2 weeks [141]. Finally, results of a meta-analysis show no significant difference between fluconazole and griseofulvin in achieving a CC when given for 2–4 weeks (41.4% vs. 52.7%, RR: 0.92, 95% CI: 0.81–1.05) or 6 weeks (34.1% vs. 32.1%, RR: 1.06, 95% CI: 0.77–1.46) [142]. No significant difference in achieving CC was observed for fluconazole when given for either 3 weeks or 6 weeks [142].While these findings suggest that fluconazole may not be superior to griseofulvin for treating tinea capitis, they do suggest that it may be a comparable alternative.

AEs: Fluconazole is generally well tolerated and the most common AEs include nausea (3.7%, 2% in children), abdominal pain (1.7%, 3% in children), headache (1.9%), vomiting (1.7%, 5% in children), and diarrhea (1.5%, 2% in children) [85]. Rare cases of AGEP [143, 144], drug eruption [145–148], Stevens-Johnson syndrome (SJS), and toxic epidermal necrolysis (TEN) have been reported [149–151]. Telogen effluvium associated with prolonged use (400 mg/day for 2 months or longer) has been reported [152].

(a) Hepatotoxicity and Cardiotoxicity

A rise in serum aminotransferase is seen in 5–25% of individuals, although most cases are mild to moderate elevations that are transient [47, 153]. The risk of liver injury with fluconazole use is low, but cases of hepatitis and fatal hepatic necrosis have been reported [154–160]. The incidence rate of drug-induced liver injury for fluconazole is 31.6 per 10,000 persons [161]. Fluconazole also prolongs the QT interval [85, 98, 162].

(b) Teratogenic Effects

Fluconazole use during pregnancy has been linked to reports of infants born with craniofacial and skeletal anomalies, as well as congenital heart defects [163–166]. The US Centers for Disease Control and Prevention (CDC) recommended against the use of fluconazole during pregnancy in 2002 and 2006. In 2011, the FDA issued a change in the pregnancy category for fluconazole (other than vaginal candidiasis) from category C to category D based on reports of teratogenicity linked to chronic high doses (400–800 mg/day) [167]. Vaginal candidiasis during pregnancy, estimated to occur in 10% of pregnant women in the US, is attributed to an increase in sex hormones that occur during pregnancy [168–170]. Although fluconazole is effective in treating most cases of vulvovaginal candidiasis, oral fluconazole use should be avoided during pregnancy [171] based on recent epidemiological studies that further substantiate the reported clinical observations of fluconazole's teratogenic effects.

1. A cohort study of 976,300 liveborn infants in Denmark reported a threefold increase in tetralogy of Fallot in those exposed to fluconazole in utero [172].
2. To study the teratogenic effects of a low dose of fluconazole used to treat vulvovaginal candidiasis, the investigators of the National Birth Defects Prevention Study identified 50 mothers reporting fluconazole use during pregnancy. More than 72% of these mothers were prescribed fluconazole to treat vulvovaginal candidiasis. Fluconazole use was linked to a significantly increase in infants born with cleft lip with cleft palate (odds ratio (OR): 5.53, 95% CI: 1.68–18.24) and with d-transposition of the great arteries (OR: 7.56, 95% CI: 1.22–35.45) [173].
3. A nationwide register-based cohort study of 1,405,663 pregnant women in Denmark demonstrated a significant increase in the risk of spontaneous abortion in pregnant women treated with oral fluconazole (HR: 1.48, 95% CI: 1.23–1.77) [168]. A higher risk of spontaneous abortion with oral fluconazole use was observed when compared to that of topical azole use (HR: 1.62, 95% CI: 1.26–2.07) [168]. No increased risk was seen with oral itraconazole use, although there was a much lower number of itraconazole-exposed pregnancies (*n* = 163) than fluconazole-exposed pregnancies (*n* = 3315) [168].

Lab Parameters to Monitor: Periodic LFTs and renal function tests [174].

Contraindications: Concomitant administration of drugs metabolized by CYP3A4 (Table 40.2) that prolong the QT interval (e.g., cisapride and quinidine) is contraindicated. Levels of drugs metabolized by CYP3A4, CYP2C9, and CYP2C19 should be carefully monitored [85]. Fluconazole is contraindicated in those with severe liver disease.

Second-Generation Triazoles (Voriconazole, Posaconazole, and Isavocunazole)

Voriconazole, posaconazole, and isavocunazole are second-generation triazoles with an extended spectrum of activities against non-*albicans Candida* spp., against yeasts, *C. neoformans* and various molds, such as *Fusarium, Aspergillus, Scedosporium* spp. [175].

(a) Voriconazole

Voriconazole is a synthetic derivative of fluconazole. Voriconazole's additional α-methyl group and its fluorinated pyrimidine that replaced one of the triazole rings of fluconazole are responsible for voriconazole's enhanced spectrum

[176]. Compared to fluconazole, voriconazole is a more effective inhibitor of 14α-demethylase and possesses activity against fluconazole-resistant organisms, such as *Candida krusei* and strains of fluconazole-resistant *C. albicans* [177].

Voriconazole use had been linked to phototoxic reactions and, with long-term use, photocarcinogenesis and accelerated photoaging. Voriconazole-associated phototoxicity reportedly occurs in 17.3% of adults and 5–36.5% of children, although the incidence rate is as high as 47% in those treated for 6 months or longer [178]. Voriconazole *N*-oxide, the major hepatic metabolite of voriconazole, and the ultraviolet B (UVB)-photoproduct of voriconazole *N*-oxide are known ultraviolet A (UVA)-sensitizers that induce oxidative DNA damage through reactive oxygen species (ROS) generation [179]. Extensive lentigo formation, reminiscent to a similar phenomenon that occurs with psoralen with UVA (PUVA) therapy, had been observed in those on chronic voriconazole therapy [180–182]. Chronic voriconazole therapy is a risk factor for squamous cell carcinoma (SCC) that increases with longer duration and higher cumulative dose [183–185]. A stepwise progression to SCC that manifested as an acute phototoxicity (year 1), actinic keratosis in sun-exposed skin (year 2–3), and SCC (year 3 or later) had been described [186]. SCCs that arise after chronic voriconazole therapy had observed in a patient as young as nine [180]; aggressive and even metastatic SCCs have been reported [180, 183, 186–189]. Five melanoma in situ lesions that arose from sites of chronic photodamage have been identified in two patients on long-term (≥35 months) voriconazole therapy [182].

(b) Posaconazole

Posaconazole was synthetically derived from itraconazole by replacing its chlorine substituents with fluorine in the phenyl ring and adding a hydroxyl group to the triazolone side chain [190]. Structural differences are responsible for the enhanced potency and spectrum of posaconazole. Posaconazole has more in vitro activity against *Aspergillus* spp. than voriconazole and amphotericin B [191, 192]. Until recently, posaconazole was the only azole with activity against mucormycetes (also called zygomycetes) [193, 194]. Posaconazole use had been evaluated for the treatment of onychomycosis (Table 40.3) [203].

Table 40.3 Reported cure rates, nail pharmacokinetics, route of incorporation into nails of systemic antifungals

	Cure rates		Residual nail concentration after cessation of therapy	Route of incorporation
AAM				
Terbinafine	**Toenails**[a] **CC:** 38%, **MC:** 70% [195] **Fingernails**[a] **CC:** 59%, **MC:** 79%		**250 mg/day for 12 weeks**: >MIC (1–60 µg/g for most dermatophytes) for 6 months after treatment cessation for toenails [196, 197]	• Diffuses from the nail matrix and the nail plate [197]
Azoles				
Fluconazole (off-label)	**Toenails** **CC:** 20–36%, **MC:** 55–62% **Fingernails** **CC:** 78–90%, **MC:** 90–99% [121, 124]		**150 mg/week for 12 months**: > fungicidal concentration for yeasts and dermatophytes in vivo (2000–3000 ng/g) detected 6 months after treatment cessation in toenails [196, 198] $t_{1/2}$ **for healthy nails:** 58 ± 31 days for toenails and 58 ± 30 days for fingernails [196] $t_{1/2}$ **for diseased nails:** 87 ± 22 days for toenails and 50 ± 1 days for fingernails [196]	• Rapidly diffuses from the nail matrix and the nail bed [199] • Detectable in nails within 2 h after a single dose [200]
Itraconazole	C	**Toenails**[a] **CC:** 14%, **MC:** 54% **Fingernails**[a] **CC:** 47%, **MC:** 61%	**100 mg/day for 6 months**: > MIC (100 ng/g nail keratin) of most dermatophytes and *Candida* 2 months after treatment cessation for fingernails and up to 6 months for toenails **200/day for 6 months**: >MIC for 6 months after treatment cessation for fingernails and toenails [201]	• Diffuses from the nail matrix and the nail bed [202]
	T	**Toenails**[a] **CC:** 22%, **MC:** 44%		
Posaconazole (off-label)		**Toenails** [203]	**100, 200 or 400 mg/day for 24 weeks or 400 mg/day for 12 weeks:** Detected in toenails as early as 2 weeks after initiation of therapy and concentrations continued to increase after cessation of therapy. Maximum concentrations (1100–2750 ng/g) were found 18–30 weeks after the cessation of therapy in great toenails. Maximum concentrations (1440–4210 ng/g) were found and 8–16 weeks after the cessation of therapy in other toenails [204]	• Likely diffuses from the nail matrix and the nail bed [204]
	100 mg/day, 24 weeks	**CC:** 23% **MC:** 37%		
	200 mg/day, 24 weeks	**CC:** 54% **MC:** 70%		
	400 mg/day, 24 weeks	**CC:** 46% **MC:** 79%		
	400 mg/day, 12 weeks	**CC:** 20% **MC:** 43%		

(continued)

Table 40.3 (continued)

	Cure rates	Residual nail concentration after cessation of therapy	Route of incorporation
Misc.			
Griseofulvin[b]	**Toenails** **CC**: 2–56%, **MC**: 46–62% **Fingernails** **CC**: 39%, **MC**: 63% [36, 37, 205–207]	**Persists for <2 weeks** [208]	• Taken up by the keratin matrix precursor cells • Higher affinity for diseased tissue [79] • Binds new keratin that become resistant to fungal invasion [196]

Abbreviations: *AAM* allylamine, *C* capsule, *T* tablet, *CC* complete cure, *MC* mycologic cure, *MIC* minimum inhibitory concentration, *MISC* miscellaneous

[a]Rates reported on the package insert

[b]Not commonly used for dermatophyte onychomycosis since itraconazole and terbinafine have better efficacy, tolerability, and safety profiles

(c) Isavuconazole

Isavuconazole, a broad-spectrum triazole, was approved by the FDA in March 2015 to treat invasive aspergillosis and invasive mucormycosis in those older than 18 years of age. Compared to voriconazole, isavuconazole possesses a broader spectrum of activity and fewer CYP450-mediated drug-drug interactions [209]. No evidence of phototoxicity had been demonstrated with isavuconazole use [101, 210].

Allylamine

Mechanism: Allylamines are noncompetitive inhibitors of squalene epoxidase (Fig. 40.2). The resulting deficiency of ergosterol is fungistatic, but the simultaneous intracellular accumulation of squalene, which interferes with both the membrane function and the fungal cell wall synthesis, is fungicidal [211]. Allylamines inhibit CYP450 to a lesser degree than azoles, and do not affect cholesterol biosynthesis in vivo [211].

Terbinafine

Indications: Terbinafine (Table 40.1) tablets are indicated to treat adults with toenail or fingernail onychomycosis caused by dermatophytes [212]. It is minimally effective against yeasts and saprophytes. Terbinafine granules are indicated to treat tinea capitis in patients older than four [25].

(a) Onychomycosis

Terbinafine, the most prescribed antifungal treatment for onychomycosis in the US [118], is the most efficacious systemic antifungal currently FDA-approved to treat onychomycosis (Table 40.3). Terbinafine has a significantly higher rate of CC (Table 40.3), as well as a lower rate of relapse, than griseofulvin for treating toenail onychomycosis. A series of large clinical trials comparing continuous terbinafine and pulse or continuous itraconazole in treating toenail onychomycosis have consistently yielded data favoring terbinafine (Table 40.4).

Pulse regimen: Pulse regimen, while not FDA-approved, is commonly used to treat onychomycosis in clinical practice in the US and other countries [218]. A meta-analysis of nine studies compared the efficacies of pulse regimen and continuous regimen for treating dermatophyte toenail onychomycosis using an intention-to-treat (ITT) analysis and an evaluable patient (EP) analysis. While no significant difference was seen between continuous and pulse regimens for achieving CC, continuous treatment provided a small advantage for achieving MC (pooled RR: 0.87, ITT 95% CI: 0.79–0.96 and EP 95% CI: 0.80–0.96) [219]. On the other hand, the risk of treatment discontinuation due to an adverse event is higher in those on a continuous regimen (pooled risk: 3.44%, 95% CI: 2.28–4.61%) than those on a pulse regimen (pooled risk: 2.09%, 95% CI: 0–4.42%) [125]. Furthermore, pulse therapy may potentially eradicate newly germinating spore structures that arise in between "pulses," providing an opportunity to destroy these structures that are largely responsible for relapse [219].

Onychomycosis in Diabetics and Immunocompromised Individuals: Terbinafine, a fungicidal agent that does not interact with CYP3A4, is a first-line choice for treating onychomycosis in diabetics and immunocompromised individuals. One notable exception is *Candida* onychomycosis, which responds better to fluconazole as discussed above. However, *Candida* onychomycosis is rare since the distribution of causative pathogens is similar to that of a general population in both diabetics (dermatophytes: 88%, *Candida* spp.: 3%, and non-dermatophyte molds: 9%) and HIV-positive patients (dermatophytes: 90–95.5%, *Candida* spp.: 0–3%, and non-dermatophyte molds: 1.5–9%) [12, 220, 221].

CYP3A4 is the predominant hepatic isoenzyme responsible for metabolizing most of the drugs on the market, many that are pertinent to diabetics and HIV-positive individuals (e.g., various HMG-CoA reductase inhibitors, as well as hypoglycemic agents, and all the protease inhibitors)

Table 40.4 Selected clinical trials comparing terbinafine and itraconazole for the treatment of toenail onychomycosis

Study	Design	Summary	Results
De Backer et al. (1998) [213]	Prospective, randomized, multicenter, double-blind, parallel-group	372 adults with dermatophyte onychomycosis, verified by microscopy and culture, were included in an ITT analysis. Subjects were treated for 12 weeks with either **continuous terbinafine** (250 mg/day, n = 186) or **continuous itraconazole** (200 mg/day, n = 186). Outcome assessments were carried out at 4, 8, 12, 24, 36, and 48 weeks	*At week 48* T: CC: 38%, MC: 73% I: CC: 23%, MC: 46%
Bräutigam et al. (1995) [214]	Prospective, randomized, multicenter, double-blind, parallel-group	195 adults with dermatophyte onychomycosis, verified by culture, were included. Subjects were treated for 12 weeks with either **continuous terbinafine** (250 mg/day, n = 86) or **continuous itraconazole** (200 mg/day, n = 84). Outcome assessments were carried out at 2, 4, 8, and 12 weeks, then every 8 weeks until 40 weeks	*At week 40* T: MC: 81% Length of affected nail: 1.3 mm at baseline, 9.4 mm at week 40 I: MC: 63% Length of affected nail: 1.2 mm at baseline, 7.9 mm at week 40
LION Study [215, 216]	Prospective, randomized, double-blind, double-dummy, multicenter, parallel-group	496 adults with dermatophyte onychomycosis, verified by culture and microscopy, were included in an ITT analysis. The treatment groups were as follows: 12 or 16 weeks (T_{12} or T_{16}) of **continuous terbinafine** (250 mg/day, T_{12}: n = 124 and T_{16}: n = 120) or 12 or 16 weeks (I_3 or I_4) of **pulse itraconazole** (400 mg/day for 1 week, every 4 weeks, I_3: n = 126 and I_4: n = 126). Outcome assessments were carried out every 4 weeks during treatment (weeks 0–16), then at weeks 24, 36, 48, and 72	*At week 72* T_{12}: CC: 46%, MC: 76% T_{16}: CC: 55%, MC: 81% I_3: CC: 23%, MC: 38% I_4: CC: 26%, MC: 49%
LION Icelandic Extension Study [217]	5-year prospective follow-up	Of the 496 patients from the LION study group, 144 patients (T: n = 68, I: n = 76) from Iceland were prospectively followed up for 5 years. Starting from the end of the LION study (first intervention), patients with clinical signs of relapse, regardless of the first intervention, were offered additional 12 weeks of terbinafine therapy (second intervention). Outcome assessments were carried out every 6 months for 5 years	*At year 5* **Without second intervention** T: MR: 23%, CR: 21% I: MR: 53%, CR: 48% **With second intervention** **T (first intervention)** CC: 72%, MC: 92% **I (first intervention)** CC: 72%, MC: 85%

Abbreviations: *ITT* intention-to-treat, *T* terbinafine, *I* itraconazole, *CC* complete cure, *MC* mycologic cure, *MR* mycologic relapse, *CR* clinical relapse, *LION*, Lamisil vs. Itraconazole in Onychomycosis

[12, 111]. Furthermore, terbinafine is better suited for treating immunocompromised individuals than itraconazole since (a) itraconazole is largely fungistatic, while terbinafine is fungicidal, against clinical isolates of dermatophytes that cause onychomycosis [222], and (b) itraconazole has negative inotropic effects, a significant contraindication in diabetics and HIV-positive patients since both patient populations are at an increased risk for coronary atherosclerosis [223, 224]. Continuous terbinafine (250 mg/day for 12 weeks) achieved MC of 73% and CC of 48% at the end of the follow-up period (week 48) in 89 diabetic patients (52 non-insulin-dependent and 37 insulin-dependent) with toenail onychomycosis. No severe AEs or hypoglycemic episodes were reported [225]. In a similar study, continuous terbinafine (250 mg/day for 12 weeks) was able to achieve MC in 19 out of 25 (76.0%, week 72) diabetics with dermatophyte onychomycosis of the toenail. No severe AEs or drug-drug interactions were reported [226]. Herranz et al. and Nandwani et al. studied the efficacy of continuous terbinafine (250 mg/day for 12–16 weeks) and reported MC in 7/16 and 3/10 HIV-positive patients with toenail onychomy-

cosis, respectively; in both studies, terbinafine was well tolerated and only one patient withdrew due to a terbinafine-induced event (drug rash) [227, 228].

Tinea Capitis: Griseofulvin, while safe and efficacious, requires a treatment course of at least 6 weeks, a prolonged treatment course that may decrease patient compliance [229]. In 2007, the FDA approved oral granules of terbinafine hydrochloride for the treatment of tinea capitis in children older than four. These miniature granules, which offer the advantage of shorter treatment duration, typically 4 weeks [230], are coated to mask the taste and can be sprinkled over soft food, such as pudding, before consumption. Furthermore, terbinafine is fungicidal, while griseofulvin is fungistatic. Meta-analyses derived from clinical trials [142, 230, 231] reveal the following findings: (a) terbinafine is superior to griseofulvin in achieving CC for tinea capitis caused by *T. tonsurans* (risk ratio (RR): 1.47, 95% CI: 1.22–1.77), but inferior in treating cases caused by *Microsporum* spp. (RR: 0.68, 95% CI: 0.53–0.86), (b) for treating tinea capitis caused by *T. violaceum*, terbinafine and griseofulvin have a similar efficacy (RR: 0.91, 95% CI: 0.68–1.24), and

(c) both terbinafine and griseofulvin are safe with a comparable rate of AEs (RR: 1.11, 95% CI: 0.79–1.57) and a low rate of severe AEs (0.6% for both).

AEs: Terbinafine is generally well tolerated. Approximately 10.5% of patients report AEs, mostly mild and transient events involving the GI system (4.9%) or skin (2.3%) [232–234]. Transient taste disturbance, lasting for an average of 6 weeks, was reported in 0.06% of 10,000 patients in a post-marketing survey of terbinafine [232]. Terbinafine is also well tolerated among HIV-positive patients and diabetics [79].

(a) Liver Injury

Rare cases of liver injury, thought to be idiosyncratic, have been reported, although most cases resolved completely after cessation of therapy. Clinically apparent liver injury is observed in 1:50,000–120,000 individuals that appear after 4–6 weeks of continuous treatment with terbinafine [218]. An asymptomatic elevation in liver enzyme levels is seen in 0.2–0.5% of those taking terbinafine [218]. Only three cases of liver injury have been linked to terbinafine exposure for less than 2 weeks [218].

(b) Cutaneous Reactions

While most cutaneous AEs attributed to terbinafine are mild and transient, more severe reactions, including subacute cutaneous lupus erythematosus (SCLE), erythema multiforme [235, 236], SJS [237], and AGEP [238] have been reported.

Terbinafine-Induced SCLE: More than 31 cases of terbinafine-induced SCLE have been published, representing 26% of all cases of drug-induced SCLE [239, 240]. One proposed mechanism is that terbinafine, lipophilic and keratophilic, deposits in keratinocytes. In susceptible individuals, this changes the configuration of nuclear antigens and results in the formation of antinuclear antibodies [241]. Through an antibody-dependent mechanism, cell-mediated cytotoxicity of SCLE-associated autoantibodies (e.g., anti-Ro autoantibodies) may be enhanced, causing keratinocyte damage [241].

Lab Parameters to Monitor: When administering terbinafine to those with immunodeficiency for more than 6 weeks, complete blood counts should be monitored. The necessity of obtaining LFTs prior to or during terbinafine use had been brought into question since cases of clinically apparent liver injury associated with terbinafine use is very rare, and most cases that occur are reversible with cessation of therapy. Furthermore, obtaining pretreatment tests (e.g., KOH or direct period acid-Schiff) prior to initiating terbinafine may not be cost-effective; the estimated testing costs to prevent one clinically apparent case of liver injury range between $9.62 million and $233.89 million [242].

Contraindications: History of prior liver disease is a relative contraindication. Furthermore, while terbinafine does not interact with CYP3A4, it does competitively inhibit CYP2D6. Thus, potential drug-drug interactions should be carefully monitored if a concomitant use of CYP2D6 substrates is unavoidable (e.g., amitriptyline, metoprolol, codeine, dapoxetine, duloxetine, aripiprazole) [243].

Polyene

Amphotericin B

Amphotericin B is an amphipathic molecule with both hydrophobic and hydrophilic properties due to its polyhydroxyl chain and polyene hydrocarbon chain, respectively (Table 40.1). Amphotericin B's antifungal mechanism is derived from its interaction with plasma membranes containing ergosterol (Fig. 40.1), followed by the intercalation of amphotericin B into the fungal plasma membranes [244]. This intercalation results in the formation of an "amphotericin B channel," which rapidly alters the membrane permeability and causes an efflux of K^+ and Mg^{2+}, an influx of protons, and an inhibition of fungal glycolysis. The result is cell death [245]. Amphotericin B's principal use is to treat systemic mycosis (e.g., disseminated aspergillosis, mucormycosis, cryptococcosis, and candidiasis). It also is used to treat endemic respiratory infections (e.g., histoplasmosis).

Although amphotericin B continues to have the broadest antifungal spectrum out of all the antifungal drugs on the market, its use is hampered by its toxicities, namely acute infusion-related toxicities (i.e., fever, chills, rigors, bronchospasm, nausea, vomiting, headaches, and arthralgia) and nephrotoxicity (i.e., decreased renal clearance and tubular damage). Liposomal amphotericin B and amphotericin B lipid complex are lipid formulations of amphotericin B that were developed in an attempt to increase its tolerability. Lipid-formulated preparations are better suited for parental administration due to their increased solubility. Furthermore, they are (a) protected from enzymatic destruction since they are encapsulated in a lipid bilayer, (b) preferably taken up by members of the mononuclear phagocyte system, which facilitates the targeting of these compounds to sites of infection, and (c) significantly less nephrotoxic compared to conventional amphotericin B (OR: 0.42, 95% CI: 0.33–0.54) [245, 246].

Echinocandins (Caspofungin, Micafungin, and Anidulafungin)

Echinocandins are noncompetitive inhibitors of 1,3-β-D-glucan synthase (Fig. 40.1). 1,3-β-D-Glucan synthase, which are not present in mammalian cells, is responsible for the synthesis of 1,3-β-D-glucan polymers that are essential cross-

Table 40.5 FDA-approved indications for echinocandins [250–252]

	CASPOFUNGIN†	MICAFUNGIN†	ANIDULAFUNGIN
Candidemia and other *Candida* infections	■	░	░
Esophageal candidiasis	▓	▓	▓
Candida prophylaxis in patients undergoing hematopoietic stem cell transplantation		▓	
Invasive *Aspergillus* infections in those refractory or intolerant of other therapies	▓		
Empirical therapy for fungal infections in febrile neutropenic patients	▓		

† *approved for pediatric use*

▓ *approved for indicated use*

■ *abscesses, peritonitis, pleural space infections*

░ *abscesses and peritonitis*

linking structural elements of the fungal cell wall [247]. The inhibition of 1,3-β-D-glucan synthase weakens the fungal cell wall and eventually leads to cell lysis. Three echinocandins, all administered intravenously, are currently available. These include caspofungin, micafungin, and anidulafungin. While subtle differences do exist between these echinocandins, they demonstrate excellent and comparable in vitro activities against invasive isolates of *Aspergillus* spp. ($n = 5346$) and *Candida* spp. ($n = 526$) [248, 249] (Table 40.5).

Griseofulvin

Mechanism: Upon entering a cell in an energy-dependent fashion, griseofulvin binds microtubules, constituents of the mitotic spindle. In doing so, griseofulvin inhibits not only the assembly of microtubules, but also their contraction during mitosis. The end result is the arrest of mitosis at metaphase due to the mitotic spindle's dissociation [253]. As a result, griseofulvin is a fungistatic agent that is only active against growing organisms.

Indications: Griseofulvin is still available in the US, but no longer available in certain European nations (e.g., Greece, Portugal, and Belgium). Griseofulvin is no longer the first-line therapy for dermatophyte onychomycosis since newer agents, itraconazole and terbinafine, have better tolerability and efficacy. Griseofulvin is still widely used to treat tinea capitis and is still the treatment of choice for cases caused by *Microsporum* species. Griseofulvin should be taken after a meal since its absorption increases with food (Table 40.2). It may also be used to treat cutaneous dermatophyte infection not adequately treated by topical therapy. Ultramicrosize and microsize griseofulvin are available.

(a) Tinea Capitis

Variables affecting treatment efficacy have changed drastically since the initial approval of griseofulvin, namely the rise of *T. tonsurans* in North America and its increasing level of resistance to griseofulvin. While terbinafine treatment requires a shorter course, and is superior to griseofulvin in treating tinea capitis caused by *T. tonsurans*, terbinafine is still inferior to griseofulvin for treating cases caused by *Microsporum* species.

Microsporum **spp. Infections**: Griseofulvin's higher efficacy in treating *Microsporum* spp. infections may be attributed to its tendency to be secreted in sweat to the body surface, where it is detectable within 4–8 h after an oral administration [254]. On the other hand, terbinafine is a highly lipophilic drug that is not found in sweat [198]. Since *Microsporum* spp. infections are ectothrix, the drug must reach the hair surface via either sebum or sweat to exert its effect. However, since children have low sebum secretion, the drug has to be delivered by sweat. Sweat acts as a carrier for griseofulvin to the stratum corneum, where it is detectable within 4–8 h when administered orally [254]. Griseofulvin's excretion in sweat, a trait not found in terbinafine, may provide a feasible explanation for its comparative advantage in treating *Microsporum* spp. infections that overcomes its relative lack of fungicidal capabilities [255].

AEs: Griseofulvin (10–20 mg/kg) was well tolerated in pediatric patients (*n* = 509) when used to treat tinea capitis for 6 weeks [231]. No serious adverse events were attributed to griseofulvin. Only mild or moderate AEs (e.g., headache (1.4%), vomiting (1.6%), diarrhea (1%), and upper abdominal pain (1%)) were observed [231]. Nausea and rashes were seen in 8–15% of patients treated with griseofulvin for onychomycosis [79]. Rare AEs include intrahepatic cholestasis and precipitation of acute intermittent porphyria in certain predisposed patients [256]. Griseofulvin had been implicated to trigger SCLE, and exacerbate systemic lupus erythematosus in a small number of cases [257, 258]. A dose-dependent induction of hepatocellular and thyroid tumors had been reported in rodents [259].

(a) **Photosensitivity**: Since more than 37 documented cases of griseofulvin-induced photosensitivity have been reported, prolonged or intense sun exposure is not recommended during griseofulvin use [260, 261]. Griseofulvin's action spectrum for erythema matches its absorption spectrum [261].

(b) **Reproductive Toxicity**: Griseofulvin is a spindle poison that is both embryotoxic and teratogenic. A dose-dependent increase in chromosomal aberrations has been observed in vitro in murine spermatocytes [262]. Cases of conjoined twins, linked to griseofulvin use during the first trimester of pregnancy, have been published [86, 263].

Lab Parameters to Monitor: Periodic liver, renal and hematopoietic function tests, especially with long-term use [86, 237].

Contraindication: Griseofulvin use is contraindicated in pregnant women (Table 40.6) and those with liver failure or porphyria. Men are advised to wait at least 6 months after the conclusion of griseofulvin therapy prior to fathering a child [264].

Table 40.6 Available form(s), antifungal effect and pregnancy category of each systemic antifungal agent

Name	Formulations	Antifungal effect[a] (Fs vs. Fc)	Pregnancy category
Allylamine			
Terbinafine	Oral packet and tablet	**FS** and **FC**	B
Azoles			
Fluconazole	IV, oral suspension and tablet	**FS**	D
Isavuconazole	IV and capsule	**FS. FC** against *Aspergillus* spp.	C
Itraconazole	Oral solution, tablet and capsule	**FS. FC** against *Aspergillus* spp.	C
Ketoconazole	Tablet	**FS**	C
Posaconazole	IV, oral suspension and tablet	**FS. FC** against *Aspergillus* spp.	C
Voriconazole	IV, oral suspension and tablet	**FS. FC** against *Aspergillus* spp.	D
Polyene			
AmB		**FC**	B
Conventional AmB	IV		
Liposomal AmB	IV		
AmB lipid complex	IV		
Echinocandins			
Anidulafungin	IV	**FC** in *Candida* spp. **FS** in *Aspergillus* spp.	B
Caspofungin	IV	**FC** in *Candida* spp. **FS** in *Aspergillus* spp.	C
Micafungin	IV	**FC** in *Candida* spp. **FS** in *Aspergillus* spp.	C
Miscellaneous			
Flucytosine	Capsule	**FS**	C
Griseofulvin		**FS**	X
Microsize	Oral suspension and tablet		
Ultramicrosize	Tablet		

Abbreviations: *FS* fungistatic, *FC* fungicidal, *amB* amphotericin B, *IV* intravenous

[a]General trend, since an antifungal's fungistatic/fungicidal effect is species-dependent

Flucytosine

Flucytosine, also known as 5-fluorocytosine (5-FC), is a synthetic fluorinated pyrimidine currently indicated as an adjunctive treatment (i.e., in combination with amphotericin B) of systemic fungal infections caused by susceptible strains of *Cryptococcus* spp. or *Candida* spp. Fungal cells transport flucytosine using an active transporter, cytosine permease, located on their plasma membrane. Cytosine permease is also responsible for the transport of hypoxanthine, cytosine and adenine. 5-FC undergoes rapid deamination by cytosine deaminase to become 5-fluorouracil (5-FU). 5-FU exhibits two distinct antifungal mechanisms. The first mechanism involves stepwise phosphorylations of 5-FU into its mono (5-fluorouridine monophosphate), di (5-fluorouridine diphosphate), and triphosphate (5-fluorouridine triphosphate) forms. 5-Fluorouridine triphosphate (FUTP) is incorporated into the fungal RNA, which in turn hinders the fungal protein synthesis [265, 266]. The second mechanism involves the uridine monophosphate pyrophosphorylase's conversion of 5-FU into 5-fluorodeoxyuridine monophosphate (FdUMP), a potent inhibitor of thymidylate synthetase that is responsible for thymidine synthesis. Thus, this second mechanism hinders fungal DNA synthesis [265, 266].

Comparative Studies for Specific Indications

Onychomycosis

Onychomycosis in Children: Onychomycosis is uncommon in children with an estimated prevalence of 0.3% [267], but its incidence may be increasing [268]. No FDA-approved treatment for onychomycosis is currently present for the pediatric population. Fluconazole, terbinafine, and itraconazole have been used off-label. Systemic antifungals have similar efficacies in children with high rates of CC for terbinafine (80.4%) and itraconazole (81.3%) [269]. CC for fluconazole is reported to be 66.7%, but with a sample size of only six children [269]. Safety profiles for these antifungals were also similar to those in adults, but a worsening case of ataxia had been reported with itraconazole use [269, 270].

Pharmacoeconomic Analyses: To potentially aid healthcare decision-makers, pharmacoeconomic analyses have been carried out to determine the cost-effectiveness (i.e., cost per designated unit of effectiveness [271]) of various treatment regimens for onychomycosis. A meta-analysis conducted in 2001 concluded that the two most cost-effective regimens were continuous terbinafine and pulse itraconazole with griseofulvin being the least cost-effective regimen. Overall, terbinafine was the most cost-effective agent since its highest success rate, shortest treatment duration, and lowest relapse rate compensated for its highest cost per tablet [272]. A meta-analysis in 2003 that examined the cost-effectiveness of continuous terbinafine, intermittent and continuous itraconazole, and topical ciclopirox reached a similar conclusion that terbinafine was the most cost-effective treatment. Terbinafine had the lowest overall expected cost for both toenail and fingernail infections, as well as the lowest cost per disease-free day ratio [273]. A cost-effectiveness analysis of the Lamisil versus Itraconazole in Onychomycosis (LION) study was carried out to model healthcare costs in Germany, Iceland, the Netherlands, the UK, Italy, and Finland. Barring Finland, continuous terbinafine (250 mg/day for 12 weeks) was more cost-effective, defined as cost per complete patient cure, than intermittent itraconazole (400 mg/day for 1 week every 4 weeks for either 12 weeks or 16 weeks) [274]. Angello and colleagues calculated the cost per mycologically cured infection for continuous terbinafine, itraconazole, and griseofulvin to be $649, $1845, and $2721, respectively [275]. A pulse regimen was more cost-effective than a continuous regimen for both itraconazole and terbinafine in the same study. For patients with dermatophyte onychomycosis with matrix involvement, a combination regimen of an amorolfine nail lacquer and oral terbinafine was able to achieve a higher success rate, defined as negative mycology and clinical cure, with a lower treatment cost per cured patient [276].

Tinea Cruris, Tinea Corporis, and Tinea Pedis

Systemic treatments are used to treat superficial mycoses under certain conditions: infection in an immunocompromised individual, presence of an extensive cutaneous involvement (i.e., involvement of large areas that makes topical treatment impractical), a failed trial of topical treatments, chronic or recurrent cases and presence of a significant inflammatory reaction secondary to the superficial mycosis.

Tinea Cruris and Tinea Corporis: Trials comparing the efficacies of terbinafine, itraconazole, fluconazole against griseofulvin have been conducted with mixed results. A double-blind, parallel group study of 239 patients with tinea corporis and/or tinea cruris treated with griseofulvin (500 mg/day) or fluconazole (150 mg/week) for 4–6 weeks showed no difference in CC or MC at both endpoints (days 25–28 or days 42–44) [277]. A double-blind study of 78 patients with tinea corporis or tinea cruris treated with itraconazole (100 mg/day) or griseofulvin (500 mg/day) for 15 days showed a higher rate of MC for itraconazole (87% vs. 57%) 2 weeks after cessation of treatment [278]. However, a similar study of 40 patients with tinea corporis or tinea cruris treated with itraconazole (100 mg/day) or griseofulvin (500 mg/day) for 15 days showed no difference in CC or MC at the end of treatment and at a follow-up visit after 15 days [279]. A randomized, double-blind comparative study of 64 patients with tinea corporis or tinea cruris treated with terbinafine (250 mg/day) or griseofulvin (500 mg/day) for 2 weeks showed significantly higher rates of both CC and MC for the terbinafine-treated group than those of the griseofulvin-treated group (CC: 83.9% vs. 41.9%, MC: 90.0% vs. 54.8%) at the 4-week follow-up visit with only transient, mild adverse events for both groups [280].

Tinea Pedis: A meta-analysis of 15 trials ($n = 1438$) identified no significant difference between fluconazole and itraconazole, as well as terbinafine and itraconazole. However, terbinafine had a significantly higher rate of cure compared to griseofulvin (pooled RR: 2.26, 95% CI: 1.49–3.44). Both terbinafine and itraconazole were more effective than placebo [281].

Investigational Antifungal Agents

Investigational agents, including potential new members of pre-existing antifungal classes, as well as those with novel mechanisms, are currently under clinical investigation (Table 40.7).

Many preclinical investigational agents are also currently under development. Those with novel mechanisms include (a) E-1210, a selective fungal inhibitor of inositol acylation that is integral to the GPI synthesis pathway [290], (b) sordarins, selective inhibitors of fungal elongation factor 2, a protein necessary to carry out ribosomal translocation during protein synthesis [292] and (c) antifungal antibodies, protective monoclonal antibodies (mAbs) with direct antimicrobial properties that may also enhance the innate immune system through complement activation and opsonization. Antifungal mAbs that may be used as adjuvant agents against species of *Cryptococcus*, *Candida*, *Histoplasma*, *Aspergillus*, *Paracoccidioides*, and *Sporothrix* have been described previously [291–293].

Table 40.7 Selected investigational antifungal agents in clinical trial

	Antifungal activity	Proposed indications
VT-1161 (Viamet) VT-1161 is a tetrazole that was synthesized to (a) lower the interaction with the heme-iron motif of CYP450 enzymes and (b) compensate for the resulting decrease in inhibitor potency by modifying the scaffold, the portion of the inhibitor recognized by the substrate binding site of the target enzyme [282]. VT-1161 exhibited no binding to human CYP51 at concentrations as high as 50 µM [283]	**In vitro**: *C. albicans, T. rubrum, Coccidioides* isolates, *Rhizopus arrhizus* var. *arrhizus* [282–285]	• **Onychomycosis** (Phase 2, CTI: NCT02267356) • **Acute vaginal candidiasis** (Phase 2, CTI: NCT01891331) • **Recurrent vaginal candidiasis** (Phase 2, CTI: NCT02267382) • **Moderate to severe interdigital tinea pedis** (Phase 2, CTI: NCT01891305)
Albaconazole Albaconazole is a new broad-spectrum, second-generation triazole with a long half-life in humans (70.5 h after single oral doses of 240 mg) [286]. Thus, a weekly dosing for systemic treatment is potentially feasible. A phase II, double-blind, placebo-controlled study of 538 adults with distal subungual dermatophyte onychomycosis (affecting at least 1 great toenail, confirmed by culture and microscopy) treated with placebo or albaconazole has been completed [287]. Albaconazole was well tolerated overall. Treatment groups with respective cure rates are as follows	**In vitro**: More than 500 clinical isolates of *Candida* spp. **In vivo**: Filamentous fungi (*Paecilomyces* spp., *Chaetomium* spp., *Fusarium* spp., *Scytalidium* spp. and *Aspergillus* spp.), dermatophytes (*Trichophyton* spp. and *M. canis*), and *C. albicans* [286]	• **Onychomycosis** (Phase 2, CTI: NCT00730405) • **Moccasin-type tinea pedis** (phase 1b, CTI: NCT00509275)
Placebo (36 weeks) **CC**: 0%, **MC**: 6%		
Albaconazole (100 mg/week for 36 weeks) **CC**: 12%, **MC**: 34%		
Albaconazole (200 mg/week for 36 weeks) **CC**: 21%, **MC**: 43%		
Albaconazole (400 mg/week for 36 weeks) **CC**: 33%, **MC**: 71%		
Albaconazole (400 mg/week for 24 weeks, followed by 12 weeks of placebo) **CC**: 26%, **MC**: 54%		
Nikkomycin Z Nikkomycin Z is a novel chitin synthase inhibitor that is more effective against highly chitinous fungi, such as *C. immitis* and *Blastomyces dermatitidis* [288]	**In vitro** and **in vivo**: *C. albicans, C. immitis* and *B. dermatitidis* [288, 289]	• **Coccidioidomycosis** (Phase 1, CTI: NCT00834184)

Abbreviations: *CTI* ClinicalTrials.gov Identifier, *CC* complete cure, *MC* mycologic cure

Case Report

A 5-year-old Caucasian male weighing 22 kg developed an itchy area with associated hair loss on his scalp 3 weeks ago during a month-long trip to Italy. During the trip, the patient and his family visited the patient's aunt who has cats, kittens, and dogs. The rash started while the patient was exposed to these animals. Since then, the area became increasingly scaly and expanded in size. Several more morphologically similar areas appeared near the original site of eruption. The patient and his family returned from their trip 3 days ago. The patient's mother reported that the aunt had "several flat, scaly red spots surrounded by a scaly red border" on her face and neck. The patient had not tried any treatments previously.

Past Medical History

- Mild intermittent asthma (controlled with albuterol inhaler used as needed)

Social History

- Recently returned from a month-long trip from Italy
- Second grade in elementary school
- Immunizations up-to-date

Previous Therapies

- None

Physical Exam

- Several ill-defined, erythematous, dry patches of alopecia (all measuring 2–5 cm in diameter) with overlying scales noted on the scalp. Loose and broken hairs also observed in these areas
- Posterior cervical and auricular lymphadenopathy seen bilaterally
- Yellow-green fluorescence visible with Wood's lamp examination

Management

Empiric treatment for tinea capitis with fluconazole was initiated. Hair samples and scales were collected during the initial visit. Oral fluconazole (reconstituted suspension) was chosen since the patient developed his fluorescent-positive tinea capitis in Italy, where *M. canis* is the dominant species. For 6 weeks, the patient received 6 mg/kg/day of fluconazole (132 mg/day) for tinea capitis. Two percent ketoconazole shampoo was also prescribed for use every other day for the patient and his family members. The patient's family members were counseled to discard combs and brushes used by the patient previously. After 3 weeks, the fungal culture confirmed the diagnosis of *M. canis* tinea capitis, and fluconazole was continued. Complete clearance was observed after treatment, and the areas of alopecia also gradually resolved.

References

1. Gooday BW. Biosynthesis of the fungal wall—mechanisms and implications. The first Fleming lecture. J Gen Microbiol. 1977;99:1–11. https://doi.org/10.1099/00221287-99-1-1.
2. Gilchrist TC. Protozoan dermatitis. J Cutan Gen Dis. 1894;12:496–9.
3. Gilchrist TC, Stokes WR. A case of pseudo-lupus vulgaris caused by a blastomyces. J Exp Med. 1898;3:53–78.
4. Hay RJ, Johns NE, Williams HC, et al. The global burden of skin disease in 2010: an analysis of the prevalence and impact of skin conditions. J Invest Dermatol. 2014;134:1527–34. https://doi.org/10.1038/jid.2013.446.
5. Ghannoum MA, Hajjeh RA, Scher R, et al. A large-scale north American study of fungal isolates from nails: the frequency of onychomycosis, fungal distribution, and antifungal susceptibility patterns. J Am Acad Dermatol. 2000;43:641–8. https://doi.org/10.1067/mjd.2000.107754.
6. Burzykowski T, Molenberghs G, Abeck D, et al. High prevalence of foot diseases in Europe: results of the Achilles project. Mycoses. 2003;46:496–505.
7. Watanabe S, Harada T, Hiruma M, et al. Epidemiological survey of foot diseases in Japan: results of 30,000 foot checks by dermatologists. J Dermatol. 2010;37:397–406. https://doi.org/10.1111/j.1346-8138.2009.00741.x.
8. Bickers DR, Lim HW, Margolis D, et al. The burden of skin diseases: 2004 a joint project of the American Academy of Dermatology Association and the Society for Investigative Dermatology. J Am Acad Dermatol. 2006;55:490–500. https://doi.org/10.1016/j.jaad.2006.05.048.
9. Scher RK. Onychomycosis is more than a cosmetic problem. Br J Dermatol. 1994;130(Suppl 43):15.
10. Millikan LE. Role of oral antifungal agents for the treatment of superficial fungal infections in immunocompromised patients. Cutis. 2001;68:6–14.
11. Surjushe A, Kamath R, Oberai C, et al. A clinical and mycological study of onychomycosis in HIV infection. Indian J Dermatol Venereol Leprol. 2007;73:397–401.
12. Cathcart S, Cantrell W, Elewski B. Onychomycosis and diabetes. J Eur Acad Dermatol Venereol. 2009;23:1119–22. https://doi.org/10.1111/j.1468-3083.2009.03225.x.
13. Boyko EJ, Ahroni JH, Cohen V, et al. Prediction of diabetic foot ulcer occurrence using commonly available clinical information: the seattle diabetic foot study. Diabetes Care. 2006;29:1202–7. https://doi.org/10.2337/dc05-2031.
14. Lehrnbecher T, Frank C, Engels K, et al. Trends in the postmortem epidemiology of invasive fungal infections at a university hospital. J Inf Secur. 2010;61:259–65. https://doi.org/10.1016/j.jinf.2010.06.018.
15. Pappas PG, Alexander BD, Andes DR, et al. Invasive fungal infections among organ transplant recipients: results of the transplant-associated infection surveillance network (TRANSNET). Clin Infect Dis. 2010;50:1101–11. https://doi.org/10.1086/651262.
16. Kontoyiannis DP, Marr KA, Park BJ, et al. Prospective surveillance for invasive fungal infections in hematopoietic stem cell transplant recipients, 2001–2006: overview of the transplant-associated infection surveillance network (TRANSNET) database. Clin Infect Dis. 2010;50:1091–100. https://doi.org/10.1086/651263.
17. Zaoutis TE, Argon J, Chu J, et al. The epidemiology and attributable outcomes of candidemia in adults and children hospitalized in the United States: a propensity analysis. Clin Infect Dis. 2005;41:1232–9. https://doi.org/10.1086/496922.

18. Pfaller MA, Pappas PG, Wingard JR. Invasive fungal pathogens: current epidemiological trends. Clin Infect Dis. 2006;43:S3–S14. https://doi.org/10.1086/504490.

19. Wilson LS, Reyes CM, Stolpman M, et al. The direct cost and incidence of systemic fungal infections. Value Health. 2002;5:26–34. https://doi.org/10.1046/j.1524-4733.2002.51108.x.

20. Elewski BE. Cutaneous fungal infections. 2nd ed. Malden, MA: Blackwell Science; 1998.

21. Baron S. Medical microbiology. 4th ed. Galveston, Tex: University of Texas Medical Branch at Galveston; 1996.

22. Bolognia J, Jorizzo JL, Schaffer JV. Dermatology. Philadelphia/London: Elsevier Saunders; 2012.

23. U.S. Food and Drug Administration. FDA Drug Safety Communication: FDA limits usage of Nizoral (ketoconazole) oral tablets due to potentially fatal liver injury and risk of drug interactions and adrenal gland problems. U.S. Food and Drug Administration; 2013.

24. U.S. Food and Drug Administration. FDA warns that prescribing of Nizoral (ketoconazole) oral tablets for unapproved uses including skin and nail infections continues; linked to patient death. U.S. Food and Drug Administration; 2016.

25. Merck. Noxafil (posaconazole) [package insert]. Kenilworth, NJ; 2015.

26. Garcia-Solache MA, Casadevall A. Global warming will bring new fungal diseases for mammals. MBio. 2010;1:e00061-10. https://doi.org/10.1128/mBio.00061-10.

27. Watkinson S, Boddy L, Money N. The fungi. 3rd ed. Amsterdam: Academic Press; 2016.

28. Bowman SM, Free SJ. The structure and synthesis of the fungal cell wall. BioEssays News Rev Mol Cell Dev Biol. 2006;28:799–808. https://doi.org/10.1002/bies.20441.

29. Jacquier N, Schneiter R. Mechanisms of sterol uptake and transport in yeast. J Steroid Biochem Mol Biol. 2012;129:70–8. https://doi.org/10.1016/j.jsbmb.2010.11.014.

30. Zhang Y-Q, Rao R. Beyond ergosterol: linking pH to antifungal mechanisms. Virulence. 2010;1:551–4.

31. Murray PR, Rosenthal KS, Pfaller MA. Medical microbiology. 8th ed. Philadelphia, PA: Elsevier; 2016.

32. Hazen KC, Wu G. Kill power of oral antifungals against dermatophytes. Pediatr Infect Dis J. 1999;18:200–4.

33. Pfaller MA, Sheehan DJ, Rex JH. Determination of fungicidal activities against yeasts and molds: lessons learned from bactericidal testing and the need for standardization. Clin Microbiol Rev. 2004;17:268–80. https://doi.org/10.1128/CMR.17.2.268-280.2004.

34. Meletiadis J, Antachopoulos C, Stergiopoulou T, et al. Differential fungicidal activities of amphotericin b and voriconazole against aspergillus species determined by microbroth methodology. Antimicrob Agents Chemother. 2007;51:3329–37. https://doi.org/10.1128/AAC.00345-07.

35. Scher RK, Tavakkol A, Sigurgeirsson B, et al. Onychomycosis: diagnosis and definition of cure. J Am Acad Dermatol. 2007;56:939–44. https://doi.org/10.1016/j.jaad.2006.12.019.

36. Faergemann J, Anderson C, Hersle K, et al. Double-blind, parallel-group comparison of terbinafine and griseofulvin in the treatment of toenail onychomycosis. J Am Acad Dermatol. 1995;32:750–3.

37. Hofmann H. Treatment of toenail onychomycosis: a randomized, double-blind study with terbinafine and griseofulvin. Arch Dermatol. 1995;131:919. https://doi.org/10.1001/archderm.1995.01690200057011.

38. Onychomycosis and terbinafine. Lancet. 1990;335:636.

39. Elewski BE. Mechanisms of action of systemic antifungal agents. J Am Acad Dermatol. 1993;28:S28–34. https://doi.org/10.1016/S0190-9622(09)80305-8.

40. Oxford AE, Raistrick H, Simonart P. Studies in the biochemistry of micro-organisms: griseofulvin, C(17)H(17)O(6)cl, a metabolic product of Penicillium griseo-fulvum Dierckx. Biochem J. 1939;33:240–8.

41. Becker L. Griseofulvin. Dermatol Clin. 1984;2:115–20.

42. Podust LM, Poulos TL, Waterman MR. Crystal structure of cytochrome P450 14alpha-sterol demethylase (CYP51) from mycobacterium tuberculosis in complex with azole inhibitors. Proc Natl Acad Sci U S A. 2001;98:3068–73. https://doi.org/10.1073/pnas.061562898.

43. Raab WPE, Kligman AM, Telger TC. The treatment of mycosis with imidazole derivatives. Berlin: Springer; 1980.

44. European Medicines Agency. European Medicines Agency recommends suspension of marketing authorisations for oral ketoconazole. European Medicines Agency; 2013.

45. Rodriguez RJ, Buckholz CJ. Hepatotoxicity of ketoconazole in Sprague-Dawley rats: glutathione depletion, flavin-containing monooxygenases-mediated bioactivation and hepatic covalent binding. Xenobiotica fate foreign. Compd Biol Syst. 2003;33:429–41. https://doi.org/10.1080/0049825031000072243.

46. Rodríguez G, Duque C, et al. A cohort study on the risk of acute liver injury among users of ketoconazole and other antifungal drugs: oral antifungals and acute liver injury. Br J Clin Pharmacol. 2001;48:847–52. https://doi.org/10.1046/j.1365-2125.1999.00095.x.

47. Schiff ER, Maddrey WC, Sorrell MF. Schiff's diseases of the liver: Schiff/Schiff's diseases of the liver. Oxford: Wiley-Blackwell; 2011.

48. Kim T-H, Kim B-H, Kim Y-W, et al. Liver cirrhosis developed after ketoconazole-induced acute hepatic injury. J Gastroenterol Hepatol. 2003;18:1426–9.

49. Duarte PA, Chow CC, Simmons F, Ruskin J. Fatal hepatitis associated with ketoconazole therapy. Arch Intern Med. 1984;144:1069–70.

50. Russo MW, Galanko JA, Shrestha R, et al. Liver transplantation for acute liver failure from drug induced liver injury in the United States. Liver Transpl. 2004;10:1018–23. https://doi.org/10.1002/lt.20204.

51. Knight TE, Shikuma CY, Knight J. Ketoconazole-induced fulminant hepatitis necessitating liver transplantation. J Am Acad Dermatol. 1991;25:398–400. https://doi.org/10.1016/0190-9622(91)70214-M.

52. Boughton K. Ketoconazole and hepatic reactions. South Afr Med J. 1983;63:955.

53. Janssen PA, Symoens JE. Hepatic reactions during ketoconazole treatment. Am J Med. 1983;74:80–5.

54. Bercoff E, Bernuau J, Degott C, et al. Ketoconazole-induced fulminant hepatitis. Gut. 1985;26:636–8.

55. Krivoy N, Bassan L. Ketoconazole-induced acute liver necrosis. Harefuah. 1986;110:346–7.

56. Lake-Bakaar G, Scheuer PJ, Sherlock S. Hepatic reactions associated with ketoconazole in the United Kingdom. Br Med J (Clin Res Ed). 1987;294:419–22.

57. Grosso DS, Boyden TW, Pamenter RW, et al. Ketoconazole inhibition of testicular secretion of testosterone and displacement of steroid hormones from serum transport proteins. Antimicrob Agents Chemother. 1983;23:207–12.

58. Pont A, Williams PL, Azhar S, et al. Ketoconazole blocks testosterone synthesis. Arch Intern Med. 1982;142:2137–40.

59. Santen RJ, Van den Bossche H, Symoens J, et al. Site of action of low dose ketoconazole on androgen biosynthesis in men. J Clin Endocrinol Metab. 1983;57:732–6. https://doi.org/10.1210/jcem-57-4-732.

60. English HF, Santner SJ, Levine HB, Santen RJ. Inhibition of testosterone production with ketoconazole alone and in combination with a gonadotropin releasing hormone analogue in the rat. Cancer Res. 1986;46:38–42.

61. Treatment of blastomycosis and histoplasmosis with ketoconazole. Results of a prospective randomized clinical trial. National Institute of Allergy and Infectious Diseases mycoses study group. Ann Intern Med. 1985;103:861–72.

62. DeFelice R, Johnson DG, Galgiani JN. Gynecomastia with ketoconazole. Antimicrob Agents Chemother. 1981;19:1073–4. https://doi.org/10.1128/AAC.19.6.1073.

63. Pont A, Goldman ES, Sugar AM, et al. Ketoconazole-induced increase in estradiol-testosterone ratio. Probable explanation for gynecomastia. Arch Intern Med. 1985;145:1429–31.

64. Zhang W, Ramamoorthy Y, Kilicarslan T, et al. Inhibition of cytochromes P450 by antifungal imidazole derivatives. Drug Metab Dispos Biol Fate Chem. 2002;30:314–8.

65. Kurreck J, Stein CA. Molecular medicine: an introduction, 1., Auflage. Weinheim: Wiley; 2015.

66. Higashi Y, Omura M, Suzuki K, et al. Ketoconazole as a possible universal inhibitor of cytochrome P-450 dependent enzymes: its mode of inhibition. Endocrinol Jpn. 1987;34:105–15. https://doi.org/10.1507/endocrj1954.34.105.

67. Greene NB, Baughman RP, Kim CK, Roselle GA. Failure of ketoconazole in an immunosuppressed patient with pulmonary blastomycosis. Chest. 1985;88:640–1.

68. Dismukes WE, Stamm AM, Graybill JR, et al. Treatment of systemic mycoses with ketoconazole: emphasis on toxicity and clinical response in 52 patients. National Institute of Allergy and Infectious Diseases collaborative antifungal study. Ann Intern Med. 1983;98:13–20.

69. Balbi C, D'Ajello M, Balbi GC. Treatment with ketoconazole in diabetic patients with vaginal candidiasis. Drugs Exp Clin Res. 1986;12:413–4.

70. Maertens JA. History of the development of azole derivatives. Clin Microbiol Infect. 2004;10(Suppl 1):1–10.

71. Fromtling RA. Overview of medically important antifungal azole derivatives. Clin Microbiol Rev. 1988;1:187–217.

72. Bitar D, Lortholary O, Le Strat Y, et al. Population-based analysis of invasive fungal infections, France, 2001–2010. Emerg Infect Dis. 2014;20:1149–55. https://doi.org/10.3201/eid2007.140087.

73. Matsumoto M, Ishida K, Konagai A, et al. Strong antifungal activity of SS750, a new triazole derivative, is based on its selective binding affinity to cytochrome P450 of fungi. Antimicrob Agents Chemother. 2002;46:308–14. https://doi.org/10.1128/AAC.46.2.308-314.2002.

74. Janssen Pharmaceuticals. SPORANOX (itraconazole) oral solution [package insert]. Beerse, Belgium; 2014.

75. Janssen Pharmaceuticals. SPORANOX (itraconazole) capsules [package insert]. Beerse, Belgium; 2014.

76. Merz Pharma. ONMEL (itraconazole) Tablets [package insert]. Greensboro, North Carolina; 2012.

77. Business Wire. Merz, Inc. Announces the Completion of the Acquisition of ONMEL™ Oral Treatment for Fungal Infections of the Toenail in Patients with a Normal Immune System; 2012.

78. Maddin S, Quiring J, Bulger L. Randomized, placebo-controlled, phase 3 study of itraconazole for the treatment of onychomycosis. J Drugs Dermatol. 2013;12:758–63.

79. Elewski B, Tavakkol A. Safety and tolerability of oral antifungal agents in the treatment of fungal nail disease: a proven reality. Ther Clin Risk Manag. 2005;1:299–306.

80. Scher RK. Onychomycosis: therapeutic update. J Am Acad Dermatol. 1999;40:S21–6.

81. Cançado GGL, Fujiwara RT, Freitas PA, et al. Acute generalized exanthematous pustulosis induced by itraconazole: an immunological approach. Clin Exp Dermatol. 2009;34:e709–11. https://doi.org/10.1111/j.1365-2230.2009.03440.x.

82. Park YM, Kim JW, Kim CW. Acute generalized exanthematous pustulosis induced by itraconazole. J Am Acad Dermatol. 1997;36:794–6. https://doi.org/10.1016/S0190-9622(97)80353-2.

83. Heymann WR, Manders SM. Itraconazole-induced acute generalized exanthemic pustulosis. J Am Acad Dermatol. 1995;33:130–1. https://doi.org/10.1016/0190-9622(95)90038-1.

84. Loftsson T, Duchene D. Cyclodextrins and their pharmaceutical applications. Int J Pharm. 2007;329:1–11. https://doi.org/10.1016/j.ijpharm.2006.10.044.

85. Pfizer DIFLUCAN (Fluconazole) Tablets and oral suspension [package insert]. New York City, NY.

86. Valeant Pharmaceuticals. Gris-PEG [package insert]. Quebec, Canada; 2010.

87. Stella VJ, He Q. Cyclodextrins. Toxicol Pathol. 2008;36:30–42. https://doi.org/10.1177/0192623307310945.

88. Stevens DA. Itraconazole in cyclodextrin solution. Pharmacotherapy. 1999;19:603–11. https://doi.org/10.1592/phco.19.8.603.31529.

89. Gould S, Scott RC. 2-Hydroxypropyl-β-cyclodextrin (HP-β-CD): a toxicology review. Food Chem Toxicol. 2005;43:1451–9. https://doi.org/10.1016/j.fct.2005.03.007.

90. Irie T, Uekama K. Pharmaceutical applications of cyclodextrins. III. Toxicological issues and safety evaluation. J Pharm Sci. 1997;86:147–62. https://doi.org/10.1021/js960213f.

91. Groll AH, Wood L, Roden M, et al. Safety, pharmacokinetics, and pharmacodynamics of cyclodextrin itraconazole in pediatric patients with oropharyngeal candidiasis. Antimicrob Agents Chemother. 2002;46:2554–63. https://doi.org/10.1128/AAC.46.8.2554-2563.2002.

92. Ward S, O'Donnell P, Fernandez S, Vite CH. 2-hydroxypropyl-beta-cyclodextrin raises hearing threshold in normal cats and in cats with Niemann-pick type C disease. Pediatr Res. 2010;68:52–6. https://doi.org/10.1203/PDR.0b013e3181df4623.

93. Crumling MA, Liu L, Thomas PV, et al. Hearing loss and hair cell death in mice given the cholesterol-chelating agent hydroxypropyl-β-cyclodextrin. PLoS One. 2012;7:e53280. https://doi.org/10.1371/journal.pone.0053280.

94. Cronin S, Lin A, Thompson K, et al. Hearing loss and otopathology following systemic and intracerebroventricular delivery of 2-hydroxypropyl-beta-cyclodextrin. J Assoc Res Otolaryngol. 2015;16:599–611. https://doi.org/10.1007/s10162-015-0528-6.

95. Takahashi S, Homma K, Zhou Y, et al. Susceptibility of outer hair cells to cholesterol chelator 2-hydroxypropyl-β-cyclodextrine is prestin-dependent. Sci Rep. 2016;6:21973. https://doi.org/10.1038/srep21973.

96. Kurkov SV, Loftsson T. Cyclodextrins. Int J Pharm. 2013;453:167–80. https://doi.org/10.1016/j.ijpharm.2012.06.055.

97. Ahmad SR, Singer SJ, Leissa BG. Congestive heart failure associated with itraconazole. Lancet. 2001;357:1766–7. https://doi.org/10.1016/S0140-6736(00)04891-1.

98. Yap YG. Drug induced QT prolongation and torsades de pointes. Heart. 2003;89:1363–72. https://doi.org/10.1136/heart.89.11.1363.

99. Scholar EM, Pratt WB. The antimicrobial drugs. 2nd ed. New York: Oxford University Press; 2000.

100. Cousin L. Dosing guidelines for fluconazole in patients with renal failure. Nephrol Dial Transplant. 2003;18:2227–31. https://doi.org/10.1093/ndt/gfg363.

101. Pasqualotto A, Falci DR. Profile of isavuconazole and its potential in the treatment of severe invasive fungal infections. Infect Drug Resist. 2013;163. https://doi.org/10.2147/IDR.S51340.

102. Isoherranen N, Kunze KL, Allen KE, et al. Role of itraconazole metabolites in CYP3A4 inhibition. Drug Metab Dispos Biol Fate Chem. 2004;32:1121–31. https://doi.org/10.1124/dmd.104.000315.

103. Courtney R, Radwanski E, Lim J, Laughlin M. Pharmacokinetics of posaconazole coadministered with antacid in fasting or nonfasting healthy men. Antimicrob Agents Chemother. 2004;48:804–8. https://doi.org/10.1128/AAC.48.3.804-808.2004.

104. Krishna G, Moton A, Ma L, et al. Pharmacokinetics and absorption of posaconazole oral suspension under various gastric conditions in healthy volunteers. Antimicrob Agents Chemother. 2009;53:958–66. https://doi.org/10.1128/AAC.01034-08.

105. Li Y, Theuretzbacher U, Clancy CJ, et al. Pharmacokinetic/pharmaco-dynamic profile of posaconazole. Clin Pharmacokinet. 2010;49:379–96. https://doi.org/10.2165/11319340-000000000-00000.

106. Keating GM. Posaconazole. Drugs. 2005;65:1553–69.

107. Karlsson MO, Lutsar I, Milligan PA. Population pharmacokinetic analysis of voriconazole plasma concentration data from pediatric studies. Antimicrob Agents Chemother. 2009;53:935–44. https://doi.org/10.1128/AAC.00751-08.

108. Neely M, Rushing T, Kovacs A, et al. Voriconazole pharmaco-kinetics and pharmacodynamics in children. Clin Infect Dis. 2010;50:27–36. https://doi.org/10.1086/648679.

109. Friberg LE, Ravva P, Karlsson MO, Liu P. Integrated population pharmacokinetic analysis of voriconazole in children, adolescents, and adults. Antimicrob Agents Chemother. 2012;56:3032–42. https://doi.org/10.1128/AAC.05761-11.

110. Purkins L, Wood N, Kleinermans D, et al. Effect of food on the phar-macokinetics of multiple-dose oral voriconazole: effect of food on voriconazole pharmacokinetics. Br J Clin Pharmacol. 2003;56:17–23. https://doi.org/10.1046/j.1365-2125.2003.01994.x.

111. Goodman LS, Brunton LL, Chabner B, Knollmann BC. Goodman & Gilman's pharmacological basis of therapeutics. 12th ed. New York: McGraw-Hill; 2011.

112. Kirmani N, Woeltje KF, Babcock H, Washington University in St. Louis. The Washington manual infectious diseases subspe-cialty consult. 2nd ed. Philadelphia, PA: Wolters Kluwer Health, Lippincott Williams & Wilkins; 2013.

113. Wong SM, Kellaway IW, Murdan S. Enhancement of the dissolu-tion rate and oral absorption of a poorly water soluble drug by formation of surfactant-containing microparticles. Int J Pharm. 2006;317:61–8. https://doi.org/10.1016/j.ijpharm.2006.03.001.

114. Arida AI, Al-Tabakha MM, Hamoury HAJ. Improving the high variable bioavailability of griseofulvin by SEDDS. Chem Pharm Bull (Tokyo). 2007;55:1713–9.

115. Lin C, Lim J, DiGiore C, et al. Comparative bioavailability of a microsize and ultramicrosize griseofulvin formulation in man. J Int Med Res. 1982;10:274–7.

116. Schäfer-Korting M, Korting HC, Mutschler E. Human plasma and skin blister fluid levels of griseofulvin after its repeated adminis-tration. Eur J Clin Pharmacol. 1985;29:351–4.

117. Lin CC, Magat J, Chang R, et al. Absorption, metabolism and excretion of 14C-griseofulvin in man. J Pharmacol Exp Ther. 1973;187:415–22.

118. Taheri A, Davis SA, Huang KE, Feldman SR. Onychomycosis treatment in the United States. Cutis. 2015;95:E15–21.

119. Rex JH, Walsh TJ, Sobel JD, et al. Practice guidelines for the treatment of candidiasis. Clin Infect Dis. 2000;30:662–78. https://doi.org/10.1086/313749.

120. Elewski BE. Onychomycosis: pathogenesis, diagnosis, and man-agement. Clin Microbiol Rev. 1998;11:415–29.

121. Scher RK, Breneman D, Rich P, et al. Once-weekly fluconazole (150, 300, or 450 mg) in the treatment of distal subungual onycho-mycosis of the toenail. J Am Acad Dermatol. 1998;38:S77–86. https://doi.org/10.1016/S0190-9622(98)70490-6.

122. Havu V, Heikkilä H, Kuokkanen K, et al. A double-blind, ran-domized study to compare the efficacy and safety of terbinafine (Lamisil) with fluconazole (Diflucan) in the treatment of onycho-mycosis. Br J Dermatol. 2000;142:97–102.

123. Arca E, Taştan HB, Akar A, et al. An open, randomized, compara-tive study of oral fluconazole, itraconazole and terbinafine therapy in onychomycosis. J Dermatol Treat. 2002;13:3–9. https://doi.org/10.1080/09546630252775171.

124. Gupta AK, Drummond-Main C, Paquet M. Evidence-based opti-mal fluconazole dosing regimen for onychomycosis treatment. J Dermatol Treat. 2013;24:75–80. https://doi.org/10.3109/0954663 4.2012.703308.

125. Chang C-H, Young-Xu Y, Kurth T, et al. The safety of oral anti-fungal treatments for superficial dermatophytosis and onychomy-cosis: a meta-analysis. Am J Med. 2007;120:791–8. https://doi.org/10.1016/j.amjmed.2007.03.021.

126. Elewski BE. Tinea capitis: a current perspective. J Am Acad Dermatol. 2000;42(1):20–4.

127. World Health Organization. Epidemiology and management of common skin diseases in children in developing countries. World Health Organization; 2005.

128. Ginter-Hanselmayer G, Weger W, Ilkit M, Smolle J. Epidemiology of tinea capitis in Europe: current state and changing patterns. Mycoses. 2007;50(Suppl 2):6–13. https://doi.org/10.1111/j.1439-0507.2007.01424.x.

129. Seebacher C, Bouchara J-P, Mignon B. Updates on the epidemiol-ogy of dermatophyte infections. Mycopathologia. 2008;166:335–52. https://doi.org/10.1007/s11046-008-9100-9.

130. Bassiri Jahromi S, Khaksar AA. Aetiological agents of tinea capitis in Tehran (Iran). Mycoses. 2006;49:65–7. https://doi.org/10.1111/j.1439-0507.2005.01182.x.

131. Ali-Shtayeh MS, Arda HM, Abu-Ghdeib SI. Epidemiological study of tinea capitis in schoolchildren in the Nablus area (West Bank). Mycoses. 1998;41:243–8.

132. Ellabib MS, Agaj M, Khalifa Z, Kavanagh K. Trichophyton violaceum is the dominant cause of tinea capitis in children in Tripoli, Libya: results of a two year survey. Mycopathologia. 2002;153:145–7.

133. Foster KW, Ghannoum MA, Elewski BE. Epidemiologic surveil-lance of cutaneous fungal infection in the United States from 1999 to 2002. J Am Acad Dermatol. 2004;50:748–52. https://doi.org/10.1016/S0190.

134. Bhanusali D, Coley M, Silverberg JI, et al. Treatment outcomes for tinea capitis in a skin of color population. J Drugs Dermatol. 2012;11:852–6.

135. Abdel-Rahman SM, Nahata MC, Powell DA. Response to initial griseofulvin therapy in pediatric patients with tinea capitis. Ann Pharmacother. 1997;31:406–10.

136. Gupta AK, Adam P, Dlova N, et al. Therapeutic options for the treatment of tinea capitis caused by Trichophyton species: griseo-fulvin versus the new oral antifungal agents, terbinafine, itracon-azole, and fluconazole. Pediatr Dermatol. 2001;18:433–8.

137. Solomon BA, Collins R, Sharma R, et al. Fluconazole for the treatment of tinea capitis in children. J Am Acad Dermatol. 1997;37:274–5.

138. Gupta AK, Dlova N, Taborda P, et al. Once weekly fluconazole is effective in children in the treatment of tinea capitis: a prospective, multicentre study. Br J Dermatol. 2000;142:965–8.

139. Foster KW, Friedlander SF, Panzer H, et al. A randomized con-trolled trial assessing the efficacy of fluconazole in the treatment of pediatric tinea capitis. J Am Acad Dermatol. 2005;53:798–809. https://doi.org/10.1016/j.jaad.2005.07.028.

140. Shemer A, Plotnik IB, Davidovici B, et al. Treatment of tinea capitis—riseofulvin versus fluconazole—a comparative study. J Dtsch Dermatol Ges. 2013;11(737–741):737–42. https://doi.org/10.1111/ddg.12095.

141. Grover C, Arora P, Manchanda V. Comparative evaluation of griseofulvin, terbinafine and fluconazole in the treatment of tinea capitis. Int J Dermatol. 2012;51:455–8. https://doi.org/10.1111/j.1365-4632.2011.05341.x.

142. Chen X, Jiang X, Yang M, et al. Systemic antifungal therapy for tinea capitis in children. Cochrane Database Syst Rev. 2016;5:CD004685. https://doi.org/10.1002/14651858.CD004685.pub3.

143. Alsadhan A, Taher M, Krol A. Acute generalized exanthema-tous pustulosis induced by oral fluconazole. J Cutan Med Surg. 2002;6:122–4. https://doi.org/10.1007/s10227-001-0035-8.

144. Di Lernia V, Ricci C. Fluconazole-induced acute generalized exanthematous pustulosis. Indian J Dermatol. 2015;60:212. https://doi.org/10.4103/0019-5154.152572.

145. Beecker J, Colantonio S. Fixed drug eruption due to fluconazole. Can Med Assoc J. 2012;184:675. https://doi.org/10.1503/cmaj.111530.

146. Pai VV, Bhandari P, Kikkeri NN, et al. Fixed drug eruption to fluconazole: a case report and review of literature. Indian J Pharm. 2012;44:643–5. https://doi.org/10.4103/0253-7613.100403.

147. Gaiser CA, Sabatino D. Fluconazole-induced fixed drug eruption. J Clin Aesthetic Dermatol. 2013;6:44–5.

148. Kim CY, Kim JG, Oh CW. Fluconazole induced fixed drug eruption. Ann Dermatol. 2011;23:S1–3. https://doi.org/10.5021/ad.2011.23.S1.S1.

149. Pasmatzi E, Monastirli A, Georgiou S, et al. Short-term and low-dose oral fluconazole treatment can cause Stevens-Johnson syndrome in HIV-negative patients. J Drugs Dermatol. 2011;10:1360.

150. Thiyanaratnam J, Cohen PR, Powell S. Fluconazole-associated Stevens-Johnson syndrome. J Drugs Dermatol. 2010;9:1272–5.

151. Dixit R, Chhabra N, Sharma S, et al. Toxic epidermal necrolysis caused by fluconazole in a patient with human immunodeficiency virus infection. J Pharmacol Pharmacother. 2012;3:276. https://doi.org/10.4103/0976-500X.99445.

152. Pappas PG. Alopecia associated with fluconazole therapy. Ann Intern Med. 1995;123:354. https://doi.org/10.7326/0003-4819-123-5-199509010-00006.

153. Wakelin SH, Maibach HI, Archer CB. Handbook of systemic drug treatment in dermatology. 2nd ed. Boca Raton: CRC Press, Taylor & Francis Group; 2015.

154. Chalasani N, Fontana RJ, Bonkovsky HL, et al. Causes, clinical features, and outcomes from a prospective study of drug-induced liver injury in the United States. Gastroenterology. 2008;135:1924–34. https://doi.org/10.1053/j.gastro.2008.09.011.

155. Ferrajolo C, Capuano A, Verhamme KMC, et al. Drug-induced hepatic injury in children: a case/non-case study of suspected adverse drug reactions in VigiBase. Br J Clin Pharmacol. 2010;70:721–8. https://doi.org/10.1111/j.1365-2125.2010.03754.x.

156. Reuben A, Koch DG, Lee WM, Acute Liver Failure Study Group. Drug-induced acute liver failure: results of a U.S. multicenter, prospective study. Hepatology. 2010;52:2065–76. https://doi.org/10.1002/hep.23937.

157. Jacobson MA, Hanks DK, Ferrell LD. Fatal acute hepatic necrosis due to fluconazole. Am J Med. 1994;96:188–90.

158. Bronstein JA, Gros P, Hernandez E, et al. Fatal acute hepatic necrosis due to dose-dependent fluconazole hepatotoxicity. Clin Infect Dis. 1997;25:1266–7.

159. Fischer MA, Winkelmayer WC, Rubin RH, Avorn J. The hepatotoxicity of antifungal medications in bone marrow transplant recipients. Clin Infect Dis. 2005;41:301–7. https://doi.org/10.1086/431586.

160. Samonis G, Rolston K, Karl C, et al. Prophylaxis of oropharyngeal candidiasis with fluconazole. Rev Infect Dis. 1990;12(Suppl 3):S369–73.

161. Kao W-Y, Su C-W, Huang Y-S, et al. Risk of oral antifungal agent-induced liver injury in Taiwanese. Br J Clin Pharmacol. 2014;77:180–9. https://doi.org/10.1111/bcp.12178.

162. Goldstein EJC, Owens RC, Nolin TD. Antimicrobial-associated QT interval prolongation: pointes of interest. Clin Infect Dis. 2006;43:1603–11. https://doi.org/10.1086/508873.

163. Aleck KA, Bartley DL. Multiple malformation syndrome following fluconazole use in pregnancy: report of an additional patient. Am J Med Genet. 1997;72:253–6.

164. Lopez-Rangel E, Van Allen MI. Prenatal exposure to fluconazole: an identifiable dysmorphic phenotype. Birt Defects Res A Clin Mol Teratol. 2005;73:919–23. https://doi.org/10.1002/bdra.20189.

165. Lee BE, Feinberg M, Abraham JJ, Murthy AR. Congenital malformations in an infant born to a woman treated with fluconazole. Pediatr Infect Dis J. 1992;11:1062–4.

166. Pursley TJ, Blomquist IK, Abraham J, et al. Fluconazole-induced congenital anomalies in three infants. Clin Infect Dis. 1996;22:336–40.

167. FDA. FDA Drug Safety Communication: use of long-term, high-dose Diflucan (fluconazole) during pregnancy may be associated with birth defects in infants. FDA; 2011.

168. Mølgaard-Nielsen D, Svanström H, Melbye M, et al. Association between use of oral fluconazole during pregnancy and risk of spontaneous abortion and stillbirth. JAMA. 2016;315:58. https://doi.org/10.1001/jama.2015.17844.

169. Cotch MF, Hillier SL, Gibbs RS, Eschenbach DA. Epidemiology and outcomes associated with moderate to heavy Candida colonization during pregnancy. Vaginal infections and prematurity study group. Am J Obstet Gynecol. 1998;178:374–80.

170. Sobel JD. Vulvovaginal candidosis. Lancet. 2007;369:1961–71. https://doi.org/10.1016/S0140-6736(07)60917-9.

171. Eckert LO. Acute vulvovaginitis. N Engl J Med. 2006;355:1244–52. https://doi.org/10.1056/NEJMcp053720.

172. Mølgaard-Nielsen D, Pasternak B, Hviid A. Use of oral fluconazole during pregnancy and the risk of birth defects. N Engl J Med. 2013;369:830–9. https://doi.org/10.1056/NEJMoa1301066.

173. Howley MM, Carter TC, Browne ML, et al. Fluconazole use and birth defects in the National Birth Defects Prevention Study. Am J Obstet Gynecol. 2016;214:657.e1–9. https://doi.org/10.1016/j.ajog.2015.11.022.

174. da Silva Barros ME, de Assis SD, Hamdan JS. Evaluation of susceptibility of Trichophyton mentagrophytes and Trichophyton rubrum clinical isolates to antifungal drugs using a modified CLSI microdilution method (M38-a). J Med Microbiol. 2007;56:514–8. https://doi.org/10.1099/jmm.0.46542-0.

175. Chen SCA, Sorrell TC. Antifungal agents. Med J Aust. 2007;187:404–9.

176. Johnson LB, Kauffman CA. Voriconazole: a new triazole antifungal agent. Clin Infect Dis. 2003;36:630–7. https://doi.org/10.1086/367933.

177. Sanati H, Belanger P, Fratti R, Ghannoum M. A new triazole, voriconazole (UK-109,496), blocks sterol biosynthesis in Candida Albicans and Candida Krusei. Antimicrob Agents Chemother. 1997;41:2492–6.

178. Sheu J, Hawryluk EB, Guo D, et al. Voriconazole phototoxicity in children: a retrospective review. J Am Acad Dermatol. 2015;72:314–20. https://doi.org/10.1016/j.jaad.2014.10.023.

179. Ona K, Oh DH. Voriconazole N-oxide and its ultraviolet B photoproduct sensitize keratinocytes to ultraviolet A. Br J Dermatol. 2015;173:751–9. https://doi.org/10.1111/bjd.13862.

180. Cowen EW, Nguyen JC, Miller DD, et al. Chronic phototoxicity and aggressive squamous cell carcinoma of the skin in children and adults during treatment with voriconazole. J Am Acad Dermatol. 2010;62:31–7. https://doi.org/10.1016/j.jaad.2009.09.033.

181. Stern RS. The risk of squamous cell and basal cell cancer associated with psoralen and ultraviolet a therapy: a 30-year prospective study. J Am Acad Dermatol. 2012;66:553–62. https://doi.org/10.1016/j.jaad.2011.04.004.

182. Miller DD, Cowen EW, Nguyen JC, et al. Melanoma associated with long-term voriconazole therapy: a new manifestation of chronic photosensitivity. Arch Dermatol. 2010;146:300–4. https://doi.org/10.1001/archdermatol.2009.362.

183. Vadnerkar A, Nguyen MH, Mitsani D, et al. Voriconazole exposure and geographic location are independent risk factors for squamous cell carcinoma of the skin among lung transplant recipients. J Heart Lung Transplant. 2010;29:1240–4. https://doi.org/10.1016/j.healun.2010.05.022.

184. Feist A, Lee R, Osborne S, et al. Increased incidence of cutaneous squamous cell carcinoma in lung transplant recipients taking

long-term voriconazole. J Heart Lung Transplant. 2012;31:1177–81. https://doi.org/10.1016/j.healun.2012.05.003.

185. Singer JP, Boker A, Metchnikoff C, et al. High cumulative dose exposure to voriconazole is associated with cutaneous squamous cell carcinoma in lung transplant recipients. J Heart Lung Transplant. 2012;31:694–9. https://doi.org/10.1016/j.healun.2012.02.033.

186. Epaulard O, Saint-Raymond C, Villier C, et al. Multiple aggressive squamous cell carcinomas associated with prolonged voriconazole therapy in four immunocompromised patients. Clin Microbiol Infect. 2010;16:1362–4. https://doi.org/10.1111/j.1469-0691.2009.03124.x.

187. McCarthy KL, Playford EG, Looke DFM, Whitby M. Severe photosensitivity causing multifocal squamous cell carcinomas secondary to prolonged voriconazole therapy. Clin Infect Dis. 2007;44:e55–6. https://doi.org/10.1086/511685.

188. Vanacker A, Fabré G, Van Dorpe J, et al. Aggressive cutaneous squamous cell carcinoma associated with prolonged voriconazole therapy in a renal transplant patient. Am J Transplant. 2008;8:877–80. https://doi.org/10.1111/j.1600-6143.2007.02140.x.

189. Ibrahim SF, Singer JP, Arron ST. Catastrophic squamous cell carcinoma in lung transplant patients treated with voriconazole. Dermatol Surg. 2010;36:1752–5. https://doi.org/10.1111/j.1524-4725.2010.01596.x.

190. Schiller D, Fung H. Posaconazole: an extended-spectrum triazole antifungal agent. Clin Ther. 2007;29:1862–86. https://doi.org/10.1016/j.clinthera.2007.09.015.

191. Cuenca-Estrella M, Gomez-Lopez A, Mellado E, et al. Head-to-head comparison of the activities of currently available antifungal agents against 3,378 Spanish clinical isolates of yeasts and filamentous fungi. Antimicrob Agents Chemother. 2006;50:917–21. https://doi.org/10.1128/AAC.50.3.917-921.2006.

192. Sabatelli F, Patel R, Mann PA, et al. In vitro activities of posaconazole, fluconazole, itraconazole, voriconazole, and amphotericin B against a large collection of clinically important molds and yeasts. Antimicrob Agents Chemother. 2006;50:2009–15. https://doi.org/10.1128/AAC.00163-06.

193. Page AV, Liles WC. Posaconazole: a new agent for the prevention and management of severe, refractory or invasive fungal infections. Can J Infect Dis Med Microbiol. 2008;19:297–305.

194. Cornely OA, Arikan-Akdagli S, Dannaoui E, et al. ESCMID and ECMM joint clinical guidelines for the diagnosis and management of mucormycosis 2013. Clin Microbiol Infect. 2014;20(Suppl 3):5–26. https://doi.org/10.1111/1469-0691.12371.

195. Drake LA, Shear NH, Arlette JP, et al. Oral terbinafine in the treatment of toenail onychomycosis: north American multicenter trial. J Am Acad Dermatol. 1997;37:740–5.

196. Debruyne D, Coquerel A. Pharmacokinetics of antifungal agents in onychomycoses. Clin Pharmacokinet. 2001;40:441–72. https://doi.org/10.2165/00003088-200140060-00005.

197. Schatz F, Bräutigam M, Dobrowolski E, et al. Nail incorporation kinetics of terbinafine in onychomycosis patients. Clin Exp Dermatol. 1995;20:377–83.

198. Faergemann J, Zehender H, Jones T, Maibach I. Terbinafine levels in serum, stratum corneum, dermis-epidermis (without stratum corneum), hair, sebum and eccrine sweat. Acta Derm Venereol. 1991;71:322–6.

199. Rich P, Scher RK, Breneman D, et al. Pharmacokinetics of three doses of once-weekly fluconazole (150, 300, and 450 mg) in distal subungual onychomycosis of the toenail. J Am Acad Dermatol. 1998;38:S103–9.

200. Hay R. Pharmacokinetic evaluation of fluconazole in skin and nails. Int J Dermatol. 1992;31:6.

201. Willemsen M, De Doncker P, Willems J, et al. Posttreatment itraconazole levels in the nail. J Am Acad Dermatol. 1992;26:731–5. https://doi.org/10.1016/0190-9622(92)70102-L.

202. Matthieu L, Doncker P, Cauwenbergh G, et al. Itraconazole penetrates the nail via the nail matrix and the nail bed-an investigation in onychomycosis. Clin Exp Dermatol. 1991;16:374–6. https://doi.org/10.1111/j.1365-2230.1991.tb00405.x.

203. Elewski B, Pollak R, Ashton S, et al. A randomized, placebo- and active-controlled, parallel-group, multicentre, investigator-blinded study of four treatment regimens of posaconazole in adults with toenail onychomycosis. Br J Dermatol. 2012;166:389–98. https://doi.org/10.1111/j.1365-2133.2011.10660.x.

204. Krishna G, Ma L, Martinho M, et al. Determination of posaconazole levels in toenails of adults with onychomycosis following oral treatment with four regimens of posaconazole for 12 or 24 weeks. Antimicrob Agents Chemother. 2011;55:4424–6. https://doi.org/10.1128/AAC.01302-10.

205. Baran R, Belaich S, Beylot C, et al. Comparative multicentre double-blind study of terbinafine (250 mg per day) versus griseofulvin (1 g per day) in the treatment of dermatophyte onychomycosis. J Dermatol Treat. 1997;8:93–7. https://doi.org/10.3109/09546639709160278.

206. Korting HC, Schäfer-Korting M, Zienicke H, et al. Treatment of tinea unguium with medium and high doses of ultramicrosize griseofulvin compared with that with itraconazole. Antimicrob Agents Chemother. 1993;37:2064–8.

207. Haneke E, Tausch I, Bräutigam M, et al. Short-duration treatment of fingernail dermatophytosis: a randomized, double-blind study with terbinafine and griseofulvin. LAGOS III study group. J Am Acad Dermatol. 1995;32:72–7.

208. Schlefman BS. Onychomycosis: a compendium of facts and a clinical experience. J Foot Ankle Surg. 1999;38:290–302.

209. Slavin MA, Thursky KA. Isavuconazole: a role for the newest broad-spectrum triazole. Lancet. 2016;387:726–8. https://doi.org/10.1016/S0140-6736(15)01218-0.

210. Astellas. Advisory committee briefing document, isavuconazonium, invasive aspergillosis and invasive mucormycosis. Astellas, Tokyo, Japan; 2015.

211. Ryder NS. Terbinafine: mode of action and properties of the squalene epoxidase inhibition. Br J Dermatol. 1992;126(Suppl 39):2–7.

212. Novartis. LAMISIL (terbinafine hydrochloride) Tablets [package insert]. Basel, Switzerland; 2015.

213. De Backer M, De Vroey C, Lesaffre E, et al. Twelve weeks of continuous oral therapy for toenail onychomycosis caused by dermatophytes: a double-blind comparative trial of terbinafine 250 mg/day versus itraconazole 200 mg/day. J Am Acad Dermatol. 1998;38:S57–63. https://doi.org/10.1016/S0190-9622(98)70486-4.

214. Bräutigam M, Nolting S, Schopf RE, Weidinger G. Randomised double blind comparison of terbinafine and itraconazole for treatment of toenail tinea infection. Seventh Lamisil German Onychomycosis study group. BMJ. 1995;311:919–22.

215. Evans EG, Sigurgeirsson B. Double blind, randomised study of continuous terbinafine compared with intermittent itraconazole in treatment of toenail onychomycosis. The LION study group. BMJ. 1999;318:1031–5.

216. Sigurgeirsson B, Billstein S, Rantanen T, et al. L.I.ON. Study: efficacy and tolerability of continuous terbinafine (Lamisil) compared to intermittent itraconazole in the treatment of toenail onychomycosis. Lamisil vs. Itraconazole in Onychomycosis. Br J Dermatol. 1999;141(Suppl 56):5–14.

217. Sigurgeirsson B, Olafsson JH, Steinsson JB, et al. Long-term effectiveness of treatment with terbinafine vs itraconazole in onychomycosis: a 5-year blinded prospective follow-up study. Arch Dermatol. 2002;138:353–7.

218. Kanzler MH. Reevaluating the need for laboratory testing in the treatment of onychomycosis: safety and cost-effectiveness considerations. JAMA Dermatol. 2016;152:263–4. https://doi.org/10.1001/jamadermatol.2015.4203.

219. Gupta AK, Paquet M, Simpson F, Tavakkol A. Terbinafine in the treatment of dermatophyte toenail onychomycosis: a meta-analysis of efficacy for continuous and intermittent regimens. J Eur Acad Dermatol Venereol. 2013;27:267–72. https://doi.org/10.1111/j.1468-3083.2012.04584.x.

220. Gupta AK, Konnikov N, MacDonald P, et al. Prevalence and epidemiology of toenail onychomycosis in diabetic subjects: a multi-centre survey. Br J Dermatol. 1998;139:665–71.

221. Gupta AK, Taborda P, Taborda V, et al. Epidemiology and prevalence of onychomycosis in HIV-positive individuals. Int J Dermatol. 2000;39:746–53.

222. Hazen KC. Fungicidal versus fungistatic activity of terbinafine and itraconazole: an in vitro comparison. J Am Acad Dermatol. 1998;38:S37–41. https://doi.org/10.1016/S0190-9622(98)70482-7.

223. Goraya TY, Leibson CL, Palumbo PJ, et al. Coronary atherosclerosis in diabetes mellitus. J Am Coll Cardiol. 2002;40:946–53. https://doi.org/10.1016/S0735-1097(02)02065-X.

224. Post WS, Budoff M, Kingsley L, et al. Associations between HIV infection and subclinical coronary atherosclerosis. Ann Intern Med. 2014;160:458. https://doi.org/10.7326/M13-1754.

225. Farkas B, Paul C, Dobozy A, et al. Terbinafine (Lamisil) treatment of toenail onychomycosis in patients with insulin-dependent and non-insulin-dependent diabetes mellitus: a multicentre trial. Br J Dermatol. 2002;146:254–60.

226. Gupta AK, Gover MD, Lynde CW. Pulse itraconazole vs. continuous terbinafine for the treatment of dermatophyte toenail onychomycosis in patients with diabetes mellitus. J Eur Acad Dermatol Venereol. 2006;20:1188–93. https://doi.org/10.1111/j.1468-3083.2006.01698.x.

227. Herranz P, Garcia J, Lucas R, et al. Toenail onychomycosis in patients with acquired immune deficiency syndrome: treatment with terbinafine. Br J Dermatol. 1997;137:577–80. https://doi.org/10.1111/j.1365-2133.1997.tb03789.x.

228. Nandwani R, Parnell A, Youle M, et al. Use of terbinafine in HIV-positive subjects: pilot studies in onychomycosis and oral candidiasis. Br J Dermatol. 1996;134(Suppl 46):22–4; discussion 39.

229. Elewski BE. Treatment of tinea capitis: beyond griseofulvin. J Am Acad Dermatol. 1999;40:S27–30.

230. Tey HL, Tan ASL, Chan YC. Meta-analysis of randomized, controlled trials comparing griseofulvin and terbinafine in the treatment of tinea capitis. J Am Acad Dermatol. 2011;64:663–70. https://doi.org/10.1016/j.jaad.2010.02.048.

231. Elewski BE, Cáceres HW, DeLeon L, et al. Terbinafine hydrochloride oral granules versus oral griseofulvin suspension in children with tinea capitis: results of two randomized, investigator-blinded, multicenter, international, controlled trials*. J Am Acad Dermatol. 2008;59:41–54. https://doi.org/10.1016/j.jaad.2008.02.019.

232. O'Sullivan DP, Needham CA, Bangs A, et al. Postmarketing surveillance of oral terbinafine in the UK: report of a large cohort study. Br J Clin Pharmacol. 1996;42:559–65.

233. Hall M, Monka C, Krupp P, O'Sullivan D. Safety of oral terbinafine: results of a postmarketing surveillance study in 25,884 patients. Arch Dermatol. 1997;133:1213–9.

234. O'Sullivan DP. Terbinafine: tolerability in general medical practice. Br J Dermatol. 1999;141(Suppl 56):21–5.

235. Carstens J, Wendelboe P, Søgaard H, Thestrup-Pedersen K. Toxic epidermal necrolysis and erythema multiforme following therapy with terbinafine. Acta Derm Venereol. 1994;74:391–2.

236. Todd P, Halpern S, Munro DD. Oral terbinafine and erythema multiforme. Clin Exp Dermatol. 1995;20:247–8.

237. Rzany B, Mockenhaupt M, Gehring W, Schöpf E. Stevens-Johnson syndrome after terbinafine therapy. J Am Acad Dermatol. 1994;30:509. https://doi.org/10.1016/S0190-9622(08)81961-5.

238. Beltraminelli HS, Lerch M, Arnold A, et al. Acute generalized exanthematous pustulosis induced by the antifungal terbinafine: case report and review of the literature. Br J Dermatol. 2005;152:780–3. https://doi.org/10.1111/j.1365-2133.2005.06393.x.

239. Kalińska-Bienias A, Kowalewski C, Woźniak K. Terbinafine-induced subacute cutaneous lupus erythematosus in two patients with systemic lupus erythematosus successfully treated with topical corticosteroids. Adv Dermatol Allergol. 2013;4:261–4. https://doi.org/10.5114/pdia.2013.37038.

240. Callen JP, Hughes AP, Kulp-Shorten C. Subacute cutaneous lupus erythematosus induced or exacerbated by terbinafine: a report of 5 cases. Arch Dermatol. 2001;137:1196–8.

241. Bonsmann G, Schiller M, Luger TA, Ständer S. Terbinafine-induced subacute cutaneous lupus erythematosus. J Am Acad Dermatol. 2001;44:925–31. https://doi.org/10.1067/mjd.2001.114565.

242. Mikailov A, Cohen J, Joyce C, Mostaghimi A. Cost-effectiveness of confirmatory testing before treatment of onychomycosis. JAMA Dermatol. 2016;152:276–81. https://doi.org/10.1001/jamadermatol.2015.4190.

243. Vickers AE, Sinclair JR, Zollinger M, et al. Multiple cytochrome P-450s involved in the metabolism of terbinafine suggest a limited potential for drug-drug interactions. Drug Metab Dispos Biol Fate Chem. 1999;27:1029–38.

244. Stewart GG, Russell I, Symposium on Yeasts. Current developments in yeast research. Toronto, New York: Pergamon Press; 1981.

245. Hamill RJ. Amphotericin B formulations: a comparative review of efficacy and toxicity. Drugs. 2013;73:919–34. https://doi.org/10.1007/s40265-013-0069-4.

246. Barrett JP, Vardulaki KA, Conlon C, et al. A systematic review of the antifungal effectiveness and tolerability of amphotericin B formulations. Clin Ther. 2003;25:1295–320.

247. Wiederhold NP, Lewis RE. The echinocandin antifungals: an overview of the pharmacology, spectrum and clinical efficacy. Expert Opin Investig Drugs. 2003;12:1313–33. https://doi.org/10.1517/13543784.12.8.1313.

248. Pfaller MA, Boyken L, Hollis RJ, et al. In vitro susceptibility of invasive isolates of Candida spp. to anidulafungin, caspofungin, and micafungin: six years of global surveillance. J Clin Microbiol. 2008;46:150–6. https://doi.org/10.1128/JCM.01901-07.

249. Pfaller MA, Boyken L, Hollis RJ, et al. In vitro susceptibility of clinical isolates of Aspergillus spp. to Anidulafungin, Caspofungin, and Micafungin: a head-to-head comparison using the CLSI M38-A2 broth microdilution method. J Clin Microbiol. 2009;47:3323–5. https://doi.org/10.1128/JCM.01155-09.

250. Roerig (Pfizer). ERAXIS (anidulafungin) for injection, for IV use only [package insert]. New York, NY; 2013.

251. Merck. CANCIDAS (caspofungin acetate) for injection, for intravenous use [package insert]. Kenilworth, NJ; 2016.

252. Astellas. MYCAMINE (micafungin sodium) for injection, for IV use only [package insert]. Tokyo, Japan; 2013.

253. Ryley JF. Chemotherapy of fungal diseases. Berlin Heidelberg: Springer; 1990.

254. Shah VP, Epstein WL, Riegelman S. Role of sweat in accumulation of orally administered griseofulvin in skin. J Clin Invest. 1974;53:1673–8. https://doi.org/10.1172/JCI107718.

255. Wolverton SE. Comprehensive dermatologic drug therapy. 3rd ed. Edinburgh: Saunders/Elsevier; 2013.

256. Hay RJ. Risk/benefit ratio of modern antifungal therapy: focus on hepatic reactions. J Am Acad Dermatol. 1993;29:S50–4. https://doi.org/10.1016/S0190-9622(08)81838-5.

257. Sontheimer RD, Henderson CL, Grau RH. Drug-induced subacute cutaneous lupus erythematosus: a paradigm for bedside-to-bench patient-oriented translational clinical investigation. Arch Dermatol Res. 2009;301:65–70. https://doi.org/10.1007/s00403-008-0890-x.

258. Madhok R, Zoma A, Capell H. Fatal exacerbation of systemic lupus erythematosus after treatment with griseofulvin. Br Med J (Clin Res Ed). 1985;291:249–50.

259. Rustia M, Shubik P. Thyroid tumours in rats and hepatomas in mice after griseofulvin treatment. Br J Cancer. 1978;38:237–49.

260. Dawe RS, Ibbotson SH. Drug-induced photosensitivity. Dermatol Clin. 2014;32:363–8. https://doi.org/10.1016/j.det.2014.03.014, ix.

261. Kawabe Y, Mizuno N, Miwa N, Sakakibara S. Photosensitivity induced by griseofulvin. Photo-Dermatology. 1988;5:272–4.

262. Fahmy MA, Hassan NH. Cytogenetic effect of griseofulvin in mouse spermatocytes. J Appl Toxicol. 1996;16:177–83. https://doi.org/10.1002/(SICI)1099-1263(199603)16:2<177::AID-JAT330>3.0.CO;2-T.

263. Rosa F, Hernandez C, Carlo W. Griseofulvin teratology, including two thoracopagus conjoined twins. Lancet. 1987;329:171. https://doi.org/10.1016/S0140-6736(87)92015-0.

264. Janssen Pharmaceuticals. Grifulvin V [package insert]. Beerse, Belgium; 2011.

265. Waldorf AR, Polak A. Mechanisms of action of 5-fluorocytosine. Antimicrob Agents Chemother. 1983;23:79–85.

266. Vermes A. Flucytosine: a review of its pharmacology, clinical indications, pharmacokinetics, toxicity and drug interactions. J Antimicrob Chemother. 2000;46:171–9. https://doi.org/10.1093/jac/46.2.171.

267. Gupta AK, Chang P, Del Rosso JQ, et al. Onychomycosis in children: prevalence and management. Pediatr Dermatol. 1998;15:464–71.

268. Lange M, Roszkiewicz J, Szczerkowska-Dobosz A, et al. Onychomycosis is no longer a rare finding in children. Mycoses. 2006;49:55–9. https://doi.org/10.1111/j.1439-0507.2005.01186.x.

269. Gupta AK, Paquet M. Systemic antifungals to treat onychomycosis in children: a systematic review. Pediatr Dermatol. 2013;30:294–302. https://doi.org/10.1111/pde.12048.

270. Heikkilä H, Stubb S. Onychomycosis in children: treatment results of forty-seven patients. Acta Derm Venereol. 2002;82:484–5. https://doi.org/10.1080/000155502762064764.

271. Arenas-Guzman R, Tosti A, Hay R, Haneke E. Pharmacoeconomics—an aid to better decision-making. J Eur Acad Dermatol Venereol. 2005;19:34–9. https://doi.org/10.1111/j.1468-3083.2005.01285.x.

272. Joish VN, Armstrong EP. Which antifungal agent for onychomycosis? A pharmacoeconomic analysis. PharmacoEconomics. 2001;19:983–1002.

273. Casciano J, Amaya K, Doyle J, et al. Economic analysis of oral and topical therapies for onychomycosis of the toenails and fingernails. Manag Care. 2003;12:47–54.

274. Jansen R, Redekop WK, Rutten FF. Cost effectiveness of continuous terbinafine compared with intermittent itraconazole in the treatment of dermatophyte toenail onychomycosis: an analysis of based on results from the L.I.ON. Study. Lamisil versus Itraconazole in Onychomycosis. PharmacoEconomics. 2001;19:401–10.

275. Angello JT, Voytovich RM, Jan SA. A cost/efficacy analysis of oral antifungals indicated for the treatment of onychomycosis: griseofulvin, itraconazole, and terbinafine. Am J Manag Care. 1997;3:443–50.

276. Baran R, Sigurgeirsson B, de Berker D, et al. A multicentre, randomized, controlled study of the efficacy, safety and cost-effectiveness of a combination therapy with amorolfine nail lacquer and oral terbinafine compared with oral terbinafine alone for the treatment of onychomycosis with matrix involvement. Br J Dermatol. 2007;157:149–57. https://doi.org/10.1111/j.1365-2133.2007.07974.x.

277. Faergemann J, Mörk NJ, Haglund A, Odegård T. A multicentre (double-blind) comparative study to assess the safety and efficacy of fluconazole and griseofulvin in the treatment of tinea corporis and tinea cruris. Br J Dermatol. 1997;136:575–7.

278. Bourlond A, Lachapelle JM, Aussems J, et al. Double-blind comparison of itraconazole with griseofulvin in the treatment of tinea corporis and tinea cruris. Int J Dermatol. 1989;28:410–2.

279. Panagiotidou D, Kousidou T, Chaidemenos G, et al. A comparison of itraconazole and griseofulvin in the treatment of tinea corporis and tinea cruris: a double-blind study. J Int Med Res. 1992;20:392–400.

280. Voravutinon V. Oral treatment of tinea corporis and tinea cruris with terbinafine and griseofulvin: a randomized double blind comparative study. J Med Assoc Thail Chotmaihet Thangphaet. 1993;76:388–93.

281. Bell-Syer SE, Khan SM, Torgerson DJ. Oral treatments for fungal infections of the skin of the foot. Cochrane Database Syst Rev. 2012;10:CD003584.

282. Hoekstra WJ, Garvey EP, Moore WR, et al. Design and optimization of highly-selective fungal CYP51 inhibitors. Bioorg Med Chem Lett. 2014;24:3455–8. https://doi.org/10.1016/j.bmcl.2014.05.068.

283. Warrilow AGS, Hull CM, Parker JE, et al. The clinical candidate VT-1161 is a highly potent inhibitor of candida albicans CYP51 but fails to bind the human enzyme. Antimicrob Agents Chemother. 2014;58:7121–7. https://doi.org/10.1128/AAC.03707-14.

284. Gebremariam T, Wiederhold NP, Fothergill AW, et al. VT-1161 protects immunosuppressed mice from Rhizopus arrhizus var. arrhizus infection. Antimicrob Agents Chemother. 2015;59:7815–7. https://doi.org/10.1128/AAC.01437-15.

285. Shubitz LF, Trinh HT, Galgiani JN, et al. Evaluation of VT-1161 for treatment of coccidioidomycosis in murine infection models. Antimicrob Agents Chemother. 2015;59:7249–54. https://doi.org/10.1128/AAC.00593-15.

286. Grayson ML, Kucers A. Kucers' the use of antibiotics: a clinical review of antibacterial, antifungal, antiparasitic and antiviral drugs. 6th ed. London: Hodder Arnold; 2010.

287. Sigurgeirsson B, van Rossem K, Malahias S, Raterink K. A phase II, randomized, double-blind, placebo-controlled, parallel group, dose-ranging study to investigate the efficacy and safety of 4 dose regimens of oral albaconazole in patients with distal subungual onychomycosis. J Am Acad Dermatol. 2013;69:416–25. https://doi.org/10.1016/j.jaad.2013.03.021.

288. Hector RF, Zimmer BL, Pappagianis D. Evaluation of nikkomycins X and Z in murine models of coccidioidomycosis, histoplasmosis, and blastomycosis. Antimicrob Agents Chemother. 1990;34:587–93.

289. Li RK, Rinaldi MG. In vitro antifungal activity of nikkomycin Z in combination with fluconazole or itraconazole. Antimicrob Agents Chemother. 1999;43:1401–5.

290. Watanabe N-A, Miyazaki M, Horii T, et al. E1210, a new broad-spectrum antifungal, suppresses Candida Albicans hyphal growth through inhibition of glycosylphosphatidylinositol biosynthesis. Antimicrob Agents Chemother. 2012;56:960–71. https://doi.org/10.1128/AAC.00731-11.

291. Hodgetts S, Nooney L, Al-Akeel R, et al. Efungumab and caspofungin: pre-clinical data supporting synergy. J Antimicrob Chemother. 2008;61:1132–9. https://doi.org/10.1093/jac/dkn075.

292. Richie DL, Ghannoum MA, Isham N, et al. Nonspecific effect of Mycograb on amphotericin B MIC. Antimicrob Agents Chemother. 2012;56:3963–4. https://doi.org/10.1128/AAC.00435-12.

293. Ostrosky-Zeichner L, Casadevall A, Galgiani JN, et al. An insight into the antifungal pipeline: selected new molecules and beyond. Nat Rev Drug Discov. 2010;9:719–27. https://doi.org/10.1038/nrd3074.

294. Woldeamanuel Y, Leekassa R, Chryssanthou E, et al. Prevalence of tinea capitis in Ethiopian schoolchildren. Mycoses. 2005;48:137–41. https://doi.org/10.1111/j.1439-0507.2004.01081.x.

295. Justice MC. Elongation factor 2 as a novel target for selective inhibition of fungal protein synthesis. J Biol Chem. 1998;273:3148–51. https://doi.org/10.1074/jbc.273.6.3148.

Systemic Antivirals in Dermatology

A. Jarad Peranteau, Ramya Vangipuram, Kevin Sharghi,
and Stephen K. Tyring

Abbreviations

ACV	Acyclovir
AIDS	Acquired immunodeficiency syndrome
CDC	Centers for Disease Control and Prevention
CMV	Cytomegalovirus
EBV	Epstein-Barr virus
eGFR	Estimated glomerular filtration rate
FCV	Famciclovir
FDA	Food and Drug Administration
GCV	Ganciclovir
GI	Gastrointestinal
HSCT	Hematopoietic stem cell transplant
HSV	Herpes simplex virus
HAART	Highly active antiretroviral therapy
HIV	Human immunodeficiency syndrome
HHV	Human herpesvirus family
HPV	Human papillomavirus
IV	Intravenous
PCV	Penciclovir
PEP	Post-exposure prophylaxis
PrEP	Pre-exposure prophylaxis
SOT	Solid organ transplant
TTP	Thrombotic thrombocytopenic purpura
VACV	Valacyclovir
VGCV	Valganciclovir

A. Jarad Peranteau, MD
New York Medical College, New York, NY, USA
e-mail: APeranteau@ccstexas.com

R. Vangipuram, MD
University of Texas Health Science Center at Houston, Houston, TX, USA

K. Sharghi, MD
Virginia Tech Carilion School of Medicine, Roanoke, VA, USA

S.K. Tyring, MD, PhD (✉)
University of Texas Health Science Center at Houston, Houston, TX, USA

Center for Clinical Studies, Houston, TX, USA
e-mail: styring@ccstexas.com

Introduction

Viral infections cause a multitude of diseases with varying clinical presentations and outcomes, which range from benign illnesses to life-threatening conditions. These infections are often difficult to treat and can present with skin-limited disease or with systemic symptoms and cause significant morbidity and mortality. Additionally, viral diseases such as HIV fundamentally alter the immune system and may significantly alter the presentation of dermatological diseases.

This chapter will focus on the systemic antiviral drugs of most relevance to the dermatologist, namely, those used to treat infections caused by the human herpesvirus family (HHV). We will also cover some of the investigational drugs currently being developed along with providing a brief overview of systemic antiviral agents used to treat HIV and chronic viral hepatitis (B and C).

The first line of defense against viral infections should always be good public health and prevention measures. This includes educating patients about the disease and its transmission and encouraging all patients to receive their required vaccinations (including the human papillomavirus (HPV) vaccine). Prevention strategies also include emphasizing proper sewage disposal and the use of clean drinking water (where appropriate), vector control, testing of blood and blood products, non-sharing of needles, hand-washing and the use of disposable gloves, and encouraging condom usage/abstinence. This is especially important in viral infections because once a patient acquires these diseases (i.e., HIV, HHV), there is often no cure and antivirals merely offer symptom/disease control. Another important concept is that antiviral agents are most active during viral replication; therefore, the earlier the treatment is given, the better the results.

Antiviral treatment is also challenging because most therapies work by targeting specific steps in viral replication without interfering with host cellular function. Viruses, however, are intracellular parasites that use host cell metabolism, which often means that antiviral agents have significant host cell toxicity that limits their use. Never has the

© Springer International Publishing AG 2018
P.S. Yamauchi (ed.), *Biologic and Systemic Agents in Dermatology*, https://doi.org/10.1007/978-3-319-66884-0_41

future of antiviral therapy been more promising however, as we are in an age of ever increasing antiviral effectiveness. The pace of development over the past 30 years has accelerated dramatically, largely due to the viral pandemic HIV that, according to 2015 statistics, infects 36.7 million people worldwide. Currently, there are 39 different FDA-approved medications for the treatment of HIV alone. Research into the disease has helped accelerate our basic understanding of both molecular biology and viral pathogenesis and has helped pave the way for newer and greater treatment options in the future for all viral infections.

Drugs for Treatment of Herpesvirus Infections

HHV are double-stranded, linear DNA viruses that cause a wide range of illnesses (Table 41.1). Classically, herpes labialis is caused by herpes simplex virus type 1 (HSV-1), and herpes simplex genitalis is caused by herpes simplex virus type 2 (HSV-2), although it has been shown that both viruses can cause either infection. Human herpesvirus type 3 (HHV-3) or varicella-zoster virus (VZV) primary infection causes varicella or chicken pox, and recurrent infection causes shingles or herpes zoster. The HHV family is also known to cause herpetic whitlow, herpes encephalitis, erythema multiforme, and roseola infantum to name a few. The drugs used to treat HHV infections are discussed below (see Table 41.2 for complete list of drugs and dosages used in the treatment of herpesvirus infections).

Acyclovir

Mechanism of Action

Acyclovir (ACV) (9-[{2-hydroxyethoxy}methyl]-9H-guanine; Zovirax) was the first oral drug to be used for the treatment of herpes simplex virus (HSV) and varicella-zoster virus (VZV) infections and is the most widely used antiviral drug in the world [1]. ACV is a synthetic guanosine analog and works by selectively inhibiting DNA replication in virally infected cells. After initial cellular uptake, acyclovir becomes activated when viral thymidine kinase (TK) phosphorylates it to acyclovir monophosphate. This step does not occur to any significant degree in uninfected cells and is the key component in the drug's selective activity. The remaining two phosphorylation steps occur inside the cell due to host cellular enzymes.

The final product, acyclovir triphosphate, competitively inhibits viral DNA polymerase by acting as an analog to deoxyguanosine triphosphate (dGTP). Incorporation of acyclovir triphosphate into the DNA chain results in chain termination as there is no free 3′ hydroxyl group to which additional nucleosides can bond. This irreversible complex renders DNA polymerase inactive. Acyclovir triphosphate possesses a much higher affinity for viral DNA polymerase (from 30 to 50 times more affinity) which results in its high therapeutic ratio [2].

Resistance

Three basic resistance mechanisms have been identified in ACV-resistant HSV strains which primarily occur only in the immunocompromised. The mechanisms are absent or low

Table 41.1 Herpesviruses causing disease in humans

Subfamily	Genus	Virus	Abbreviation	Associated diseases
Alphaherpesvirinae	Simplexvirus	Human herpesvirus 1/ herpes simplex virus 1	HHV-1/HSV-1	Herpes labialis (cold sores), genital herpes, cutaneous herpes, gingivostomatitis, keratoconjunctivitis, viral meningitis, esophagitis[a], pneumonia[a], hepatitis[a]
		Human herpesvirus 2/ herpes simplex virus 2	HHV-2/HSV-2	Genital herpes, cutaneous herpes, gingivostomatitis, neonatal herpes, viral meningitis, disseminated infection[a], hepatitis[a]
		Varicella-zoster virus		
	Varicellovirus		VZV/HHV-3	Chicken pox, herpes zoster, disseminated herpes zoster[a], varicella pneumonia
Betaherpesvirinae	Cytomegalovirus	Cytomegalovirus	CMV/HHV-4	CMV mononucleosis, hepatitis[a], congenital CMV disease, retinitis[a], pneumonia[a], esophagitis[a], colitis[a]
	Roseolovirus	Human herpesvirus 6	HHV-6	Roseola infantum, otitis media with fever, encephalitis
		Human herpesvirus 7	HHV-7	Roseola infantum, pityriasis rosea[b]
Gammaherpesvirinae	Lymphocryptovirus	Epstein-Barr virus	EBV/HHV-4	Infectious mononucleosis, hepatitis, encephalitis, nasopharyngeal carcinoma, Hodgkin lymphoma, Burkitt lymphoma, lymphoproliferative syndromes[a], oral hairy leukoplakia[a]
	Rhadinovirus	Human herpesvirus 8 (formerly Kaposi sarcoma associated herpesvirus)	HHV-8/KSV	Kaposi sarcoma[a], primary effusion lymphoma[a], Castleman disease

[a]Indicates infection primarily in immunocompromised patients
[b]Exact causal role yet to be determined

Table 41.2 Antiviral therapy for the treatment of herpesvirus infections

Virus	Clinical disease	Drug	Recommended dosage (Immunocompetent)	Comments
Herpes simplex virus	Genital herpes: first episode	Acyclovir (PO)	400 mg tid or 200 mg 5×/day for 7–10 days	
		Famciclovir (PO)	250 mg tid for 7–10 days	
		Valacyclovir (PO)	1 g bid for 7–10 days	
	Genital herpes: recurrent	Acyclovir (PO)	800 mg tid for 2 days or 400 mg tid or 200 mg 5×/day or 800 mg big for 5 days	
		Famciclovir (PO)	125 mg bid for 5 days or 1000 mg repeated once at 12 h for 1 day	
		Valacyclovir (PO)	500 mg bid for 3 days or 1 g/day for 5 days	
	Genital herpes: suppression	Acyclovir (PO)	400 mg bid or 200 mg tid	400 mg bid continued indefinitely or 400 to 800 mb 2–3×/day
		Famciclovir (PO)	250 mg bid	
		Valacyclovir (PO)	500 mg/day or 250 mg bid 1 g/day	Recurrence of <9 episodes/year
				Recurrence of >9 episodes/year
	Encephalitis	Acyclovir (IV)	10–15 mg/kg/8 h in 1-h infusions for 14–21 days	Risk of crystalline nephropathy
	Mucocutaneous disease in immunocompromised hosts	Acyclovir (IV)	5 mg/kg/8 h for 7–14 days	
		Acyclovir (PO)	400 mg 5×/day for 7–14 days	
		Valacyclovir (PO)	500 mg or 1 g bid for 7–10 days	
		Penciclovir (IV)	5 mg/kg/8–12 h 7 days	
		Famciclovir (PO)	500 mg bid for 7–10 days	
	Orolabial herpes: first episode	Acyclovir (PO)	Children: 15 mg/kg 5×/day for 7 days (max. 200 mg/dose)	
			Adults: drugs and doses recommended for first-episode genital herpes have been used	
	Orolabial herpes: recurrent	Valacyclovir (PO)	2 g repeated once at 12 h	
		Famciclovir (PO)	1500 mg once or 750 mg every 12 h for 2 total doses	
		Acyclovir (PO)	400 mg tid/day for 5 days	
	Neonatal HSV	Acyclovir (IV)	10–20 mg/kg/8 h for 14–21 days	
Varicella-zoster virus	Varicella in normal children	Acyclovir (PO)	20 mg/kg (≤800 mg) qid for 5 days	Typically not indicated unless at risk for severe disease
	Varicella in immunocompromised hosts	Acyclovir (IV)	10 mg/kg/8 h or 500 mg/m/8 h for 7–10 days	
	Herpes zoster in immunocompromised hosts	Acyclovir (IV)	10 mg/kg/8 h in 1-h infusion for 7–10 days	
	Herpes zoster in normal hosts	Acyclovir (PO)	800 mg 5×/day for 7–10 days	Poor bioavailability; VACV preferred
		Valacyclovir (PO)	1 g tid for 7 days	Preferred oral therapy for mild or localized disease
		Famciclovir (PO)	500 mg tid for 7 days	
		Brivudin (PO)	120 mg daily for 7 days	
Cytomegalovirus	Cytomegalovirus infection	Ganciclovir (IV)	5 mg/kg/12 h in 1-h infusion for 14–21 days	Can give same dose once daily for CMV prophylaxis in transplant recipients
		Valganciclovir (PO)	900 mg bid	Risk of myelosuppression; can give same dose once daily for CMV prophylaxis in transplant patients
	Retinitis	Valganciclovir (PO)	900 mg bid for 21 days	Induction therapy
			900 mg once daily	Maintenance therapy until immune reconstitution
		Cidofovir (IV)	5 mg/kg once weekly × 2, then every other week	Indicated for GCV-resistant CMV
		Foscarnet (IV)	60 mg/kg/8 h in 1- to 2-h infusion for 14–21 days	Indicated for GCV-resistant CMV

production of viral TK (resulting in an inability to activate ACV), altered TK activity (i.e., phosphorylation of thymidine, but not of acyclovir), and altered viral DNA polymerase. Immunocompetent patients rarely acquire ACV-resistant HSV (0.1–0.7%), but this increases to ~4% to 14% in immunocompromised patients [3–6]. In situations where ACV resistance is suspected, foscarnet is recommended as it similarly inhibits viral DNA polymerase but does not require phosphorylation for its antiviral activity [7].

Pharmacokinetics

ACV has modest oral bioavailability of about 15–30% which decreases with higher doses. The half-life of the drug is between 2.5 and 3.3 h in adults, 4 h in neonates, and 2–3 h in children below 12. The drug is not highly protein bound and as such achieves good penetration into tissues and fluids, including vaginal fluids and the cerebrospinal fluid (CSF), the latter of which contains an ACV concentration approximately 50% of that seen in plasma [8]. Excretion is predominately renal, and dose modifications are required in those with impaired renal function.

Clinical Indications

- Primary, recurrent, or suppressive therapy for HSV-1/2 infections
- HSV encephalitis/disseminated disease
- Primary VZV infection (chicken pox) and VZV recurrence (herpes zoster)
- Treatment of HSV infections in pregnancy and prevention/treatment of neonatal HSV infections
- Prevention/treatment of HSV/VZV infections in immunosuppressed patients (off-label)

Herpesviruses have varying degrees of susceptibility to ACV: HSV-1 is the most susceptible to ACV, followed by HSV-2 and VZV, and to a lesser extent Epstein-Barr virus (EBV). Cytomegalovirus (CMV) is inhibited by high ACV levels; however, these concentrations are often not clinically achievable. As such, ACV is not recommended for the treatment of CMV. It has been used as prophylactic treatment against CMV disease in solid organ and bone marrow transplant recipients but is inferior to other readily available drugs (i.e., ganciclovir and foscarnet).

ACV is FDA-approved for the treatment of primary and recurrent genital HSV infection, mucocutaneous HSV, and primary and recurrent varicella-zoster (chicken pox and herpes zoster, respectively) and prevention of perinatal and treatment of neonatal HSV infections and herpes simplex encephalitis. ACV is also used as suppressive therapy (400 mg twice daily) in patients with frequent recurrences of HSV-1/2 infections and can reduce genital HSV recurrences by 80–90% and reduce asymptomatic viral shedding of HSV-2 by 95% [9]. Treatment of primary, nonprimary, or recurrent genital herpes during pregnancy is essential in minimizing perinatal transmission of

HSV and in reducing the need for cesarean delivery. Therefore, recommendations are that any woman presenting with a genital HSV lesion anytime during pregnancy (no matter whether primary, nonprimary, or recurrent) should initiate ACV therapy (400 mg three times daily) at 36-week gestation and continue through delivery. This regimen has been proven to reduce viral shedding, reduce the number of clinical HSV recurrences at the time of delivery, and reduce the need for cesarean delivery [10].

Oral ACV is frequently used in the off-label treatment of herpes labialis, and doses of either 200 mg 5 times daily for 5 days or 400 mg three times daily typically have only modest benefits. Studies have shown that ACV treatment reduced the time to loss of crusts, but pain or time to complete lesion healing was largely unaffected. However, increasing the dose to 400 mg 5 times daily for 5 days, if started prior to vesicle formation in the prodromal phase, decreased the mean duration of pain by 36% and time to loss of crust by 27% [11]. In patients with more than 2 outbreaks of herpes labialis, suppressive dosing of ACV at 400–1000 mg/day, divided into two doses, reduced the occurrence of new lesions by 50–78% [12]. In 2013, a buccal tablet formulation of ACV was FDA-approved for the treatment of recurrent herpes labialis in immunocompetent adults.

Intravenous (IV) ACV is the first-line treatment for HSV encephalitis and should be started as soon as possible based on clinical suspicion and characteristic imaging findings demonstrating temporal lobe involvement. ACV is also recommended in the treatment of first-episode VZV in adults and children. ACV has been shown to reduce the severity and duration of varicella infections if given within 72 h of the development of skin lesions, although it should ideally be started within 24 h of lesion development for maximal benefit. It is FDA-approved for adults and children over two. Treatment is highly recommended for children who are at an increased risk of complicated disease such as children older than 12 years of age, those with chronic cutaneous or pulmonary disorders, or individuals on steroid or chronic salicylate therapy. For otherwise healthy children presenting with primary varicella infection, the American Academy of Pediatrics (AAP) does not currently recommend ACV treatment [13]. This is based on a systematic review of three randomized, controlled trials that looked at over 988 children and determined that although ACV treatment did accelerate lesion healing and reduction in fever if started within the first 24 h of rash onset, these reductions were not seen if started after 24 h. Additionally, ACV had no effect on secondary complications, did not demonstrate a reduction in the number of days missed from school, and overall failed to show a positive outcome in cost-benefit analysis [14]. Oral antiviral therapy is recommended in all adults with primary VZV infection due to the risk of varicella pneumonia. For acute varicella (chicken pox) and recurrent infection (herpes zoster), dosages of 800 mg five times daily for 7–10 days have proven efficacious. If started within 72 h of herpes zoster symptoms, oral ACV reduces the duration of the rash and zoster-related pain by nearly half and also reduces the mean duration of postherpetic neuralgia (PHN) as well. IV ACV is used in immunocompromised patients, patients presenting with disseminated disease for both HSV and VZV infections, and in pregnant women with any evidence of pneumonia due to the high risk of fetal complications.

Other off-label uses for ACV include treatment of HSV gingivostomatitis, treatment of recurrent erythema multiforme, and prevention of HSV, CMV, or VZV reactivation in hematopoietic stem cell transplant (HSCT) recipients and HIV patients. ACV is also used for prevention of HSV and CMV infections following renal transplantation. It can also be used in the treatment of varicella pneumonia, acute retinal necrosis (associated with HSV, VZV, or HIV), herpes zoster ophthalmicus, eczema herpeticum, oral hairy leukoplakia due to EBV, ocular herpes simplex, and in new-onset Bell's palsy.

Dosing Regimens

Treatment regimens with ACV depend on the indication, age group, and route of administration. For a list of various dosing regimens with ACV, please see Table 41.2.

Dose Modifications

Decreased renal function results in accumulation of ACV and potential toxicity. In all patients with significantly reduced estimated glomerular filtration rate (eGFR), dose modifications are required. For oral dosing, patients with eGFR ≤ 25 mL/min/1.73 m^2 require adjustments, and if administered IV, dosing should be adjusted in any patient with an eGFR ≤ 50 mL/min/1.73 m^2 (see Table 41.3 for renal dose adjustments). Additionally, in obese patients, weight-based dosing should be calculated based on ideal body weight and not actual body weight to avoid an increased risk of toxicity.

Adverse Effects

ACV is remarkably well tolerated in most patients regardless of the formulation. As ACV is primarily eliminated renally, the main toxicities involve renal impairment (5–10% incidence). Elevations in creatinine, acute renal failure, and interstitial nephritis have all been reported with IV therapy and can be minimized by prior IV hydration (with goal urine

output of >75 mL/h) as well as slowly infusing the drug over 1 or 2 h which can help minimize the production of relatively insoluble ACV crystals in the renal tubules. Rare neurological toxicities manifested as lethargy, tremors, agitation, hallucinations, and myoclonus have also been reported primarily in patients with underlying renal failure and in the elderly, and this can be minimized by adjusting ACV doses in those with renal impairment. Gastrointestinal (GI) side effects like nausea/vomiting/diarrhea are common (up to 7% incidence when given parenterally) along with injection site inflammation and phlebitis (9% incidence).

ACV is a pregnancy category B drug meaning it is safe during pregnancy with no documented adverse effects to the fetus. ACV can also safely be used during breastfeeding as long as there are no active lesions around the breast or nipple. Because ACV is not metabolized by hepatic (CYP) enzymes, significant drug interactions are minimal. Notable pharmacological interactions include probenecid, which increases the half-life of ACV resulting in increased bioavailability, and coadministration of zidovudine, which can cause increased somnolence [15]. Extreme care should be taken in patients receiving other drugs known to be nephrotoxic.

Valacyclovir

Mechanism of Action

Valacyclovir (VACV; Valtrex) is an oral prodrug of ACV which provides 3–5 times greater bioavailability (55%) than oral ACV and can achieve plasma concentrations similar to IV ACV in adults [16]. Because VACV is metabolized to ACV, the mechanism of action, efficacy, indications, and safety profile are virtually identical.

Resistance

VACV resistance occurs because of the exact same mechanisms as those previously described for ACV.

Pharmacokinetics

The enhanced bioavailability of VACV is particularly advantageous as it allows patients to dose much less frequently than with ACV which facilitates better treatment compliance and patient satisfaction. Once ingested, VACV undergoes rapid and extensive first-pass hydrolysis to ACV by hepatic and intestinal enzymes, achieving peak serum concentration in 1–3 h. Like ACV, absorption of the drug is not affected by food.

Clinical Indications
- Initial and recurrent therapy for HSV-1/2 infections
- Suppressive therapy and reduction of transmission of genital HSV infections
- Primary (chicken pox) and recurrent (herpes zoster) VZV infections
- Herpes labialis

Table 41.3 Acyclovir dose adjustments in patients with renal failure

Intravenous	
Creatinine clearance (mL/min)	*Dose*
25–50	Normal dose every 12 h
10–25	Normal dose every 24 h
<10	50% of normal dose every 24 h
Oral	
Creatinine clearance (mL/min)	*Dose*
25–50	Normal
10–25	HSV: 200 mg q 8 h; HZ: 800 mg q 8 h
<10	HSV: 200 mg q 12 h; HZ: 800 mg q 12 h

As previously mentioned, the indications for VACV are virtually identical to ACV. The main advantage of VACV over ACV is the convenience of a less frequent dosing regimen (twice daily dosing with VACV compared to either three or five times a day dosing with ACV). However, VACV is considerably more expensive than ACV. Treatment with VACV is most efficacious if started at the onset of symptoms (within 72 h of first diagnosis or 24 h of recurrence). Unlike oral ACV, VACV is FDA-approved for treatment of herpes labialis and can be dosed in a convenient 2 g twice daily for 1-day dosing regimen if started in the prodromal phase. Several randomized, controlled trials demonstrated that 500 mg daily of VACV reduced the recurrence rate of labial herpes among affected study patients from 68 to 40% [17]. Another study also demonstrated that VACV was an effective prophylactic against recurrent labial HSV when started 1 day prior to laser resurfacing and continued for 2 weeks post-procedure [18].

Numerous studies have shown VACV to be of similar efficacy in the treatment of primary and recurrent genital herpes. VACV can also be used for chronic suppressive therapy (500 mg daily) in patients with 9 or fewer genital outbreaks yearly, and the dose can be increased to 1 g daily or 500 mg twice daily in patients experiencing 10 or more episodes yearly. Additionally, daily use of VACV (500 mg daily) has also proven effective in reducing transmission of genital herpes by 53% in heterosexual, HSV-2 discordant couples by reducing asymptomatic viral shedding [19]. In addition to condom use and abstinence during genital HSV outbreaks, daily antiviral therapy should be considered as an additional preventive measure. According to Centers for Disease Control and Prevention (CDC) guidelines, suppressive therapy should also be considered in persons with a history of genital herpes who have multiple sexual partners and by those who are HSV-2 seropositive but have never had a symptomatic outbreak of genital herpes. Suppressive therapy with VACV or ACV may also be helpful in patients who suffer frequent and disabling recurrences of cutaneous herpes infections (i.e., herpetic whitlow, HSV-related erythema multiforme).

VACV shows considerable improvement over ACV in the treatment of herpes zoster. A dosing regimen of 1 g three times daily for 7 days is as effective as ACV in reducing time to crusting, time to 50% lesion healing, and in reducing the appearance of new zoster lesions. However, VACV is more effective in reducing the median duration of pain after lesion healing, with an average time of 40 days of pain compared to 60 days of pain in ACV recipients. Additionally, VACV also reduced the proportion of patients in whom pain persisted for at least 6 months [20]. If on initial presentation, the herpes zoster patient states their pain is ≥4 (on a 10-point scale), the addition of gabapentin (and analgesics) along with VACV therapy has been proven to reduce the incidence and/or severity of PHN and is now the standard of care [21].

VACV prophylaxis (2 g four times daily for 90 days) is used in immunocompromised patients to reduce the risk of CMV transmission following kidney or HSCT transplants and may also reduce the risk of CMV infection in HIV patients. Much like ACV, VACV demonstrates in vitro activity against EBV; however, at present there are no clear indications for its use. Although studies have shown conflicting results, more recent evidence suggests that a combination of antivirals (i.e., VACV, ACV, famciclovir) and corticosteroids is more effective than steroids alone in treating Bell's palsy [22–24].

Dosing Regimens

For a complete list of dosing regimens, please refer to Table 41.2. Normal dosing regimens in adults for HHV infections are typically anywhere from 500 mg to 1 g two to three times daily for 5–10 days although this varies based on the indication. Pediatric dosing below 2 months of age is not recommended due to decreased renal clearance and the potential for renal toxicity. VACV is FDA-approved for chicken pox in immunocompetent patients 2 years of age and older. Currently, VACV is not FDA-approved for any HSV indication in those <12 years of age. However, pharmacokinetic studies in children 3 months through 11 years of age have demonstrated that a twice daily or three times daily dose of 20 mg/kg oral suspension of VACV was safe and effective and produced favorable acyclovir blood levels [25].

In severely immunocompromised patients or in unstable patients presenting with disseminated disease, IV ACV should be used as VACV is only available in oral formulations.

Dose Modifications

As the primary route of elimination of VACV is renal, dose modifications are recommended in patients with a creatinine clearance below 30 mL/min/1.73 m². Dose adjustments are not required in those with hepatic impairment (see Table 41.4 for VACV renal dose adjustments).

Adverse Effects

The adverse effect profile is similar to those with ACV, including a potential for acute renal failure as well as CNS effects. The elderly and patients with chronic renal insufficiency are most susceptible to the CNS effects of VACV which include agitation, hallucinations, confusion, ataxia, myoclonus, seizures, and encephalopathy [26]. These symptoms typically occur within 3 days of starting VACV and resolve within 5 days of drug withdrawal. The most common adverse effects in the majority of clinical trials with VACV were headache, nausea/vomiting, diarrhea, dyspepsia, and fatigue, but only headache, nausea, and dyspepsia were observed more frequently in VACV groups compared to placebo [27].

In one study, high-dose VACV (8 g/day) was associated with an increased risk of a thrombotic microangiopathy-like

Table 41.4 Valacyclovir dosage adjustments in adults with renal insufficiency

Indication	Normal dose (creatinine clearance ≥ 50 mL/min)	Creatinine clearance (mL/min)		
		30–49	10–29	<10
Herpes labialis	Two 2 g doses taken 12 h apart	Two 1 g doses taken 12 h apart	Two 500 mg doses taken 12 h apart	500 mg single dose
Genital herpes: initial episode	1 g every 12 h	No reduction	1 g every 24 h	500 mg every 24 h
Genital herpes: recurrent episode(s)	500 mg every 12 h	No reduction	500 mg every 24 h	500 mg every 24 h
Genital herpes: suppressive therapy				
Immunocompetent patients (≥10 recurrences/year)	1 g every 24 h	No reduction	500 mg every 24 h	500 mg every 24 h
Immunocompetent patients (≤9 recurrences/year)	500 mg every 24 h	No reduction	500 mg every 48 h	500 mg every 48 h
HIV-infected patients	500 mg every 12 h	No reduction	500 mg every 24 h	500 mg every 24 h
Herpes zoster	1 g every 8 h	1 g every 12 h	1 g every 24 h	500 mg every 24 h

syndrome, reported as thrombotic thrombocytopenic purpura or hemolytic-uremic syndrome (TTP/HUS). However, these patients were severely immunocompromised with acquired immunodeficiency syndrome (AIDS) and/or renal transplant recipients receiving numerous concomitant medications, and most had other concomitant illnesses which may have also predisposed to the condition. Because of these circumstances, no causality was able to be determined between VACV dosing in the immunocompromised and TTP/HUS [28]. However, treatment with VACV should be stopped immediately if clinical signs, symptoms, and laboratory abnormalities consistent with TTP/HUS emerge.

VACV, like ACV, is labeled as pregnancy category B risk and is safe during pregnancy, although just like with ACV, breastfeeding mothers should be cautioned to not breastfeed if there are active HSV lesions on breast or around nipples.

Common drugs known to interact with VACV are probenecid and cimetidine which result in increased concentrations of VACV due to reductions in renal clearance of the drug. In patients with normal renal function, dose reductions are typically not indicated but should be made in those patients with renal insufficiency taking the aforementioned drugs to avoid toxicity.

Famciclovir

Mechanism of Action

Famciclovir (FCV; Famvir) is an acyclic guanosine analog that is the prodrug of the more poorly absorbed penciclovir (PCV), (9-[4-hydroxy-3-hydroxymethylbut-1-yl] guanine; Denavir). The mechanism of action is similar to ACV and VACV. After cellular uptake, PCV is converted by first-pass metabolism into a monophosphorylated form by viral thymidine kinase before eventually being converted into penciclovir triphosphate (the active compound) by cellular enzymes. Like ACV, the active triphosphate form preferentially inhibits the DNA polymerase of susceptible viruses with minimal effects on host cellular DNA polymerase thereby minimizing side effects. PCV is active against the same drugs as ACV/VACV, namely, HSV-1/2 and VZV.

Pharmacokinetics

FCV is rapidly absorbed, reaching peak plasma concentrations within 1 h and is unaffected by food. Compared to ACV and VACV, FCV has superior oral bioavailability (77% with FCV compared to 15–30% and 55% with ACV and VACV, respectively) [29]. FCV also reaches higher concentrations in HSV-infected cells than ACV; however, in practical terms, these higher concentrations do not result in increased inhibitory properties. FCV is more stable than ACV, however, and this does confer some advantages in regard to dosing. The added stability of penciclovir triphosphate yields a longer intracellular half-life which allows for less frequent dosing than ACV. The intracellular half-life of penciclovir in HSV-1/2 infected cells is 10–20 h and 7–14 h in VZV infected cells compared with an hour or less with ACV [30]. Excretion of the drug is primarily renal with dose reductions recommended in patients with creatinine clearances under 60 mL/min.

Resistance

The mechanisms of FCV resistance are identical to the ones already described for ACV/VACV. Most ACV-resistant strains of HSV and VZV display cross-resistance to FCV with reduced or absent viral TK being the primary resistance mechanism [29].

Clinical Indications

- Initial and recurrent HSV genital infections
- Suppression of frequently recurring genital HSV infections
- Initial and recurrent HSV labialis (cold sores) infections
- Treatment of recurrent orolabial or genital HSV infections in HIV-positive patients
- Herpes zoster (shingles)
- Varicella infections (chicken pox/herpes zoster) in HIV patients (off-label)

As with all of the antiherpetic antiviral drugs, treatment is most effective if started within 72 h of rash onset. The FDA-approved clinical indications for FCV use are in the treatment of acute herpes zoster, treatment and suppression of recurrent genital herpes in immunocompetent patients, and treatment of recurrent herpes labialis. FCV is also FDA-approved for recurrent orolabial or genital herpes in HIV-infected patients. Frequent off-label uses of FCV include primary episodes of oral and genital herpes, primary varicella, chronic suppressive therapy for HSV infections in HIV-positive adolescents and adults, as well as herpes zoster and varicella infections in HIV-positive patients. Several subsets of HSV infections including herpetic whitlow, eczema herpeticum, and herpes-associated erythema multiforme can also be treated with FCV at doses identical to the ones used for primary and recurrent HSC episodes in adults. Additionally, recent studies have demonstrated promising results with the use of FCV and prednisolone in the treatment of severe idiopathic Bell's palsy [31].

Dosing Regimens

For a list of various FCV dosing regimens, please see Table 41.2. FCV is only available orally, and currently insufficient clinical data exists to recommend pediatric dosing although studies are ongoing. Off-label adolescent dosing is typically similar to adult dosing (i.e., 500 mg 2–3 times daily for 5–10 days). One of the main advantages of FCV is that it allows for single-day treatment of recurrent genital herpes (1000 mg every 12 h) and recurrent herpes labialis (1500 mg single dose) which has been associated with higher patient satisfaction [32].

Accounting to its poor absorption from the GI tract and low bioavailability, PCV (the metabolite of FCV) is available as an FDA-approved topical treatment for herpes labialis. Topical penciclovir 1% applied twice daily during waking hours for 4 days was shown to speed healing and decrease pain duration by about 1 day in recurrent herpes labialis outbreaks.

Dose Modifications

As with ACV/VACV, dose reductions should be made in those with chronic renal insufficiency, and special care should be paid to patients on concomitant medications known to be nephrotoxic. Acute renal failure has occurred in patients taking inappropriately high doses of FCV (see Table 41.5 for dose adjustments in renal insufficiency patients).

Adverse Effects

Adverse events with FCV are rare and are similar to those seen with ACV and VACV. An integrated safety analysis of over 1600 patients receiving FCV for herpes zoster or genital herpes revealed an adverse event profile not significantly different from placebo [33]. The most commonly reported side effects are nausea, diarrhea, and headache. Rare side effects including

Table 41.5 Famciclovir dosage adjustments in adults with renal insufficiency[a]

Indication	Normal dose (creatinine clearance ≥ 50 mL/min)	Creatinine clearance (mL/min)		
		40–59	20–39	<20
Recurrent genital herpes	125 mg every 12 h	Normal dose	125 mg every 24 h	125 mg every 24 h
Suppression of recurrent genital herpes	250 mg every 12 h	No reduction	125 mg every 12 h	125 mg every 24 h
Recurrent orolabial and genital herpes simplex infection in HIV-infected patients	500 mg every 12 h	No reduction	500 mg every 24 h	250 mg every 24 h
Herpes zoster	500 mg every 8 h	500 mg every 12 h	500 mg every 24 h	250 mg every 24 h

[a]Hemodialysis patients should receive same dose as patients with creatinine clearance <20 mL/min but should only be dosed following each dialysis

pruritus, rash, jaundice, and elevation in liver enzymes may be seen in ~2–3% of patients, although frequency varies depending on dose and duration of treatment [33].

FACV is a pregnancy category B drug and based on the available data appears to be well tolerated and safe during pregnancy.

How to Decide Which Antiherpetic Antiviral Is Correct

In general, ACV, VACV, and FCV are roughly equivalent in their efficacy and safety in treating infections caused by HSV-1/2 and VZV. VACV and FCV have proven to be more effective than ACV in reducing the duration of zoster-associated pain, likely due to their higher oral bioavailability. Due to this fact, either drug is preferred over ACV in the treatment of VZV infections. If cost is an issue, ACV is unquestionably the cheapest option with VACV and FCV being considerably more expensive.

All three of the aforementioned antiherpes antivirals appear equally effective in the treatment of recurrent HSV-1/2 infections and in the suppression of future outbreaks. For the treatment of first episode of genital or labial herpes infections, oral ACV and VACV are preferred as the efficacy of FCV for initial HSV-1/2 infections has not been established.

Ultimately, the selection of a specific drug should be based on provider preference, familiarity, cost, and convenience of administration. For primary HSV-1/2 infection, we recommend VACV due to the convenient dose of 1 g twice daily for 7–10 days. As ACV, VACV, and FCV all have similar efficacy in the treatment of symptomatic recurrences, we recommend FCV due to the convenient dosing regimen of 1 g administered orally every 12 h for 2 doses. For suppressive therapy one must consider both the reduction of future outbreaks and the reduction in asymptomatic viral shedding. The reduction in asymptomatic viral shedding is especially important in decreasing transmission rates among discordant, heterosexual couples where the source partner has a history of genital HSV-2 infection. Suppressive therapy should also be considered in patients who have multiple sexual partners and by those who are HSV-2 seropositive without a history of genital herpes, as well as in anyone that experiences frequent or severe recurrences. ACV, FCV, and VACV all appear equally effective in suppressing future outbreaks of HSV; however, FCV appears somewhat less effective for suppression of viral shedding [34]. Based on this, our recommendation for suppressive therapy would be VACV at a dose of 500 mg once daily (or 1000 mg daily if immunosuppressed).

In severely immunocompromised patients, the elderly, or those with widely disseminated disease, internal organ involvement, or those with CNS complications (confusion, inability to swallow, encephalitis), IV acyclovir should be used. In immunocompromised patients (i.e., HIV-positive patients, HSCT recipients) ACV resistance may be a problem. Since cross-resistance to VACV and FCV is common, patients that fail oral and IV ACV therapy should be managed with IV foscarnet or cidofovir.

Other Antivirals for Human Herpesvirus Infections

Cidofovir

Mechanism of Action
Cidofovir (CDV) ([S]-1-[3-hydroxy-2-{phosphomethoxypropyl}] cytosine dihydrate; HPMPC; Vistide) is an acyclic phosphonate nucleotide analog that demonstrates in vitro antiviral activity against a wide variety of DNA viruses including herpesviruses, adenovirus, polyomavirus, papillomavirus, and poxvirus [35]. Unlike other nucleoside analogs, CDV does not require intracellular activation by viral kinases. CDV is phosphorylated to its diphosphate form by host cell enzymes where it then acts as a competitive inhibitor of viral DNA synthesis. Once incorporated into the developing viral DNA strand, the drug slows down viral DNA synthesis by inhibiting viral DNA polymerase and prevents further chain elongation. CDV is much more selective for viral DNA polymerase versus human DNA polymerase. Studies have demonstrated that incorporation of just one CDV molecule into DNA slows down DNA synthesis by 31%, and the addition of two consecutive CDV molecules halts DNA chain elongation and synthesis completely [36].

The mechanism of action of CDV in human papillomavirus (HPV) differs from the previously highlighted mechanism utilized in herpesvirus family infections. Unlike HHV infections which utilize viral kinases, HPV uses host cell DNA polymerase. CDV has been shown to induce cell cycle arrest in S-phase (phase where DNA synthesis occurs) resulting in decreased DNA production. CDV has also been shown to induce DNA fragmentation and apoptosis of HPV-infected cells by activating caspases responsible for programmed cell death [37].

Pharmacokinetics
One of the main advantages of CDV is its long intracellular half-life which allows less frequent dosing than the plasma half-life (2.6 h) would lead one to believe. Although over 80% of the drug is eliminated unchanged in the urine within 24 h of administration, the metabolites (cidofovir monophosphate, diphosphate, and monophosphate-choline) are eliminated more slowly with half-lives of 24, 65, and 87 h, respectively. It is postulated that the accumulation of cidofovir monophosphate-choline acts as an intracellular reservoir, and this property is what allows the drug to be dosed every 1–2 weeks.

CDV is poorly absorbed orally and hence is always given parenterally, usually intravenously, although a topical formulation can be compounded for off-label usage. The drug is excreted renally by tubular secretion. As nephrotoxicity is the main side effect, the drug is contraindicated in those with significant renal disease and CDV should be coadministered with probenecid and IV hydration. Probenecid coadministration reduces renal tubular secretion of the drug which results in higher concentrations. This might reasonably lead one to assume that it could lead to increased toxicity; however, probenecid appears to prevent damage to proximal renal tubular cells by preventing uptake of CDV into these cells.

Resistance
CDV-resistant CMV has been associated with point mutations in the viral DNA polymerase gene. Overall CDV displays low levels of resistance, and prolonged treatment with the drug uncommonly leads to the development of resistance.

Clinical Indications
- CMV retinitis
- Acyclovir-resistant HSV infections (off-label)
- Numerous other off-label indications (discussed below)

The only FDA-approved indication for CDV is in the treatment of CMV retinitis in patients with AIDS although it is also frequently used in ACV-resistant HSV infections. Additionally, because CDV does not rely on viral kinases, it retains activity against ganciclovir- and foscarnet-resistant CMV infections along with the previously mentioned ACV-resistant HSV infections due to TK mutations. Both IV and topical formulations of CDV have proven successful in small series of patients with both genital and labial herpes infections. CDV has also demonstrated efficacy in HIV-positive patients with treatment resistant CMV disease. Other successful off-label treatments based on small case series, case reports, and retrospective analysis include treatment of BK virus-associated hemorrhagic cystitis, JC virus-associated progressive multifocal leukoencephalopathy, adenovirus infections in HSCT patients, papillomavirus infections (i.e., condyloma acuminatum, Bowenoid papulosis, verruca vulgaris, recurrent respiratory papillomatosis), and molluscum contagiosum [38–40]. Due to its activity against poxviruses, CDV has also been studied for its potential use in the therapy and short-term prophylaxis of smallpox in case of a bioterrorism attack. Case reports have also documented the potential efficacy of CDV in the treatment of vaccinia (smallpox) vaccine complications were the vaccine to be reinstituted in the case of a future smallpox outbreak. Additionally, the CDC will provide CDV at no cost to patients with vaccinia vaccine complications unresponsive to VIG (vaccinia immune globulin) as long as their established protocol is used which seeks to investigate if CDV is an effective secondary treatment for smallpox vaccine complications [41]. Given its significant renal metabolism, CDV is contraindicated in those with preexisting renal impairment, as evidenced by serum creatinine >1.5 or >2+ proteinuria.

Dosing Regimens

For adults, CDV may be given at an induction dose of 5 mg/kg once weekly for the first 2 weeks, followed by a 5 mg/kg dose once every 2 weeks (for off-label dosing regimens please see Table 41.2). Adolescent dosing (off-label) is equivalent to adult dosing, and insufficient data exists in pediatric patients to recommend its use in that patient population.

Adverse Effects

Systemic side effects from topical or intralesional CDV administration are rare and are primarily limited to application site reactions. The major toxicity with CDV is renal toxicity which severely limits its use. Renal toxicity developed in 59% of patients receiving 5 mg/kg IV every other week and presented as >1+ proteinuria, serum creatinine elevations ≥ 0.4 mg/dL, and decreased creatinine clearance ≤ 55 mL/min. Maintenance dose reductions from 5 mg/kg to 3 mg/kg were required in 26–29% of patients. Reversible renal damage resulting in a Fanconi-type syndrome has also been associated with CDV use and is characterized by proteinuria, glucosuria, and renal bicarbonate wasting leading to metabolic acidosis.

Due to the high risk of nephrotoxicity, serum creatinine and urine protein should be checked within 48 h prior to each dose of CDV and dose reduction or discontinuation made if evidence of renal dysfunction exists. To minimize nephrotoxicity, patients should receive 1 L of normal saline over 1–2 h immediately preceding CDV dosing, and, if tolerated,

a second liter should be given either during or immediately following IV administration.

Other common adverse effects include nausea (7–69%), asthenia (43%), headache (30%), alopecia (16–27%), unspecified rash (30%), fever (14–50%), diarrhea (26%), anorexia (23%), increased cough (19%), oral candidiasis (18%), and abdominal pain. Neutropenia was noted in about 20% of patients in clinical trials; however, most of these clinical trials were done in severely immunosuppressed patients (i.e., advanced AIDS patients) so causality is difficult to determine and the neutropenia observed in some study patients was not dose related. Additionally, it should be noted that probenecid coadministration is likely the culprit for at least some of the adverse effects as well seen in clinical studies (not to mention many of the patients were on numerous concomitant medications). In one study, 56% of patients had adverse events that were attributable to the probenecid [42].

In animal studies, CDV was found to be carcinogenic in rats and as such should be considered potentially carcinogenic in humans. Animal studies also demonstrated CDV to be spermatogenic and teratogenic and as such is labeled a pregnancy category C drug, suggesting possible teratogenic risk. It is thus recommended that women of childbearing potential use effective contraception during and for 1 month following treatment and that men use barrier contraception during and for 3 months following treatment. CDV therapy should be used in pregnancy only if the potential benefit justifies the potential risk to the fetus and should be avoided in the first trimester if possible. Additionally, due to the potential adverse effects on neonates, breastfeeding while on CDV is contraindicated.

Ganciclovir and Valganciclovir

Mechanism of Action

Ganciclovir (GCV) (9-(1,3-dihydroxy-2-propoxymethyl) guanine; Cytovene) is an acyclic guanine nucleoside analog that is structurally similar to ACV and was the first antiviral agent approved for the treatment of CMV infection. Like ACV, GCV requires triphosphorylation by viral and cellular enzymes before it is activated. However, unlike ACV which uses viral thymidine kinase (TK) for initial phosphorylation, GCV is converted to ganciclovir monophosphate by the CMV UL97 gene product. Cellular kinases then complete the phosphorylation to the di- and triphosphosphorylated ganciclovir, the pharmacologically active form. Levels of ganciclovir triphosphate are 10 to 100 times higher in CMV or HSV-infected cells than uninfected cells [43]. Ganciclovir triphosphate then competes with deoxyguanosine triphosphate for incorporation into DNA. Once GCV incorporates into DNA, it preferentially inhibits viral DNA polymerase more than cellular DNA polymerases. Additionally, GCV disrupts viral DNA synthesis in a second manner by serving as a poor substrate for chain elongation, thus halting further DNA synthesis.

GCV and its oral prodrug valganciclovir (VGCV; Valcyte) are primarily used in the treatment of CMV infections although in vitro it demonstrates activity against HSV-1/2, EBV, VZV, and HHV-6/8.

Pharmacokinetics

The absorption of oral GCV is extremely poor, and early studies demonstrated a bioavailability of only 5–6% following a single oral dose. Thus, the drug is given intravenously, with the oral formulation no longer available in the United States. VGCV, an L-valyl ester of GCV, was developed in response and has received FDA approval as an oral treatment option for CMV infections and prophylaxis in the immunocompromised.

Orally administered VGCV is rapidly hydrolyzed (plasma half-life of 0.47 h) to GCV by hepatic and intestinal wall esterases. Food increases absorption of GCV (from VGCV oral administration) with an absolute bioavailability of approximately 60% when taken with or immediately following a high-fat meal [44]. Systemic exposure of a 900 mg dose of VGCV in adults is similar to that attained by a single dose of 5 mg/kg of IV GCV. The mean plasma half-life of either IV GCV or oral VGCV is approximately 3–4 h, although the intracellular half-life of ganciclovir triphosphate in CMV- or HSV-infected cells is markedly longer (16.5 h).

GCV is eliminated primarily in the urine, with about 90% excreted unchanged by glomerular filtration and active tubular secretion. Due to this property dose adjustments are required in patients with renal insufficiency. Hemodialysis decreases serum concentrations of GCV by 50%, so administration of additional doses after dialysis is necessary. GCV crosses the placenta as well as the blood-brain barrier and produces CSF concentrations that average about 40% of plasma concentrations.

Resistance

Resistance to GCV/VGCV may occur after long-term use and is associated with mutations in either the CMV viral protein kinase gene (UL97) and/or in the viral polymerase gene (UL54). Typically these mutations do not confer resistance to foscarnet which may be used instead [45].

Clinical Indications

- CMV retinitis in immunocompromised patients
- Suppression and prevention of CMV disease in transplant recipients
- CMV esophagitis, colitis, or neurological disease in HIV patients (off-label)
- Congenital CMV infection (off-label)

Intravenous GCV and oral VGCV are both approved for use in the treatment of CMV infections in immunocompromised patients as well as in prevention of CMV disease in transplant patients.

Dosing Regimens

The standard IV GCV induction dose in adolescents and adults is 5 mg/kg/dose every 12 h for 2–3 weeks followed by 5 mg/kg/day dosing every 24 h for maintenance therapy. This regimen is primarily used for the treatment of CMV retinitis. The same maintenance dosing is used in the treatment of CMV end-organ disease; however, induction therapy generally lasts 3–6 weeks. Maintenance therapy may be required indefinitely and is generally only stopped if disease symptoms resolve and CD4+ T-cell counts stabilize at >100 cell/μL for at least 6 months. The equivalent dosing of VGCV is 900 mg twice daily for induction therapy followed by once daily maintenance. Pediatric dosing regimens have not been established as there are not extensive studies in this patient population. Typical doses used in pediatric patients are induction dosing with 7.5–10 mg/kg/day divided into two or three doses and 2.5–5 mg/kg/day for maintenance therapy. However, pediatric dosing is not recommended without prior consultation with a pediatric infectious disease expert.

Dose Modifications/Contraindications

GCV/VGCV is contraindicated in those with a history of hypersensitivity reactions to ACV and VCV or with previous GCV/VGCV hypersensitivities. Both drugs should be used with caution in patients with bone marrow suppression or to those who are receiving other myelosuppressive chemotherapy or radiation therapy. Both drugs are contraindicated in patients with an ANC <500 cells/mm³ or platelet count <25,000 cells/mm³. Dose modifications are required in patients with renal insufficiency, but these will not be detailed as the average dermatologist does not typically prescribe and/or manage these medications.

Adverse Effects

The main toxicity associated with VGCV/GCV is bone marrow suppression resulting in neutropenia, anemia, and thrombocytopenia. The effects on the bone marrow are typically reversible with discontinuation of the drug although it may also require administration of granulocyte colony-stimulating factor. Other common side effects include diarrhea, nausea, abdominal pain, headache, tremor, insomnia, and hypertension, and these have been reported in clinical studies with greater than 10% frequency. Acute renal failure has been reported in patients with predisposing conditions (i.e., chronic renal insufficiency).

Known drug interactions include potentiation of imipenem, mycophenolate, probenecid, reverse transcriptase inhibitors, and tenofovir. It is labeled as pregnancy category C, and patients receiving these medications are recommended to use contraception during and 30–90 days posttreatment. In animal studies, it was also found to be gonadotoxic. Breastfeeding is not recommended, since it is not known if GCV or VGCV are excreted into breast milk.

Foscarnet

Mechanism of Action

Foscarnet is unique from the other previously mentioned antivirals in that it is not a nucleoside analog but rather a pyrophosphate analog that selectively inhibits viral DNA polymerases (both DNA dependent and RNA dependent, the latter of which is usually called reverse transcriptase). Unlike the other antiherpes antivirals, foscarnet does not require initial phosphorylation by viral enzymes but rather binds reversibly near the pyrophosphate-binding site of DNA polymerase (or reverse transcriptase) without requiring further modification. Normally during DNA synthesis when a deoxynucleoside triphosphate is added to the growing DNA chain, a pyrophosphate is cleaved during the process. Because foscarnet blocks this cleavage, further nucleoside addition is prevented which in turn halts DNA chain elongation. Cellular DNA polymerases are not affected as foscarnet must be present in concentrations 100-fold greater than that required to block CMV replication [46]. When intracellular concentrations of foscarnet decrease, foscarnet no longer binds to the DNA polymerase and viral DNA synthesis resumes. This unique mechanism allows it to retain activity against HSV-1/2, VZV, EBV, CMV, and HHV-6/8. It also inhibits the reverse transcriptases present in hepatitis B virus as well as HIV and retains activity against strains of HSV and CMV that are resistant to nucleoside analogs.

Pharmacokinetics

Foscarnet has poor oral bioavailability and is therefore administered by intravenous infusion over 1–2 h. The drug is not significantly metabolized and is excreted unchanged in urine via glomerular filtration and tubular secretion. Elimination has three phases with half-lives of 1 h, 3–6 h, and 88 h or longer [46]. Up to 20% of the cumulative dose may be deposited in bone and cartilage.

Resistance

Resistance mechanisms should be considered in patients with poor clinical response and have been attributed to amino acid substitutions in the viral DNA polymerase. These substitutions have been shown to confer cross-resistance to GCV, ACV, and/or CDV [47].

Clinical Indications

- CMV retinitis in AIDS patients
- Acyclovir-resistant mucocutaneous HSV infections in immunocompromised patients
- Acyclovir-resistant VZV infections in immunocompromised patients (off-label)
- CMV esophagitis or colitis in immunocompromised patients (off-label)
- Ganciclovir-resistant CMV infections (off-label)
- Preemptive or prophylactic treatment of CMV infections in transplant recipients (off-label)

Dosing Regimens

Most common dosing regimen is induction therapy with 60 mg/kg/dose every 8–12 h followed by maintenance therapy of 90–120 mg/kg/day. Patients with renal impairment require dose adjustments, and special care should be taken with coadministration of other nephrotoxic drugs. Renal toxicity appears to be reduced by concomitant IV hydration.

Adverse Effects

Renal toxicity is the major risk with foscarnet, with up to 25% of patients developing dose-limiting renal impairment for which close monitoring of renal function is required [48]. Impairment of renal function typically occurs during the second week of induction therapy and is reversible within 1 week following dose adjustment or discontinuation of therapy. Saline hydration before administration and slow infusion of the drug may reduce the risk of nephrotoxicity. In addition, the drug has been associated with significant electrolyte and metabolic abnormalities including hypocalcemia, hyper/hypophosphatemia, hypomagnesemia, and hypokalemia. Accordingly, electrolytes should be monitored closely during treatment. Other common adverse reactions include nausea/vomiting/diarrhea, anemia, and granulocytopenia (33% and 17% of patients in clinical trials, respectively) [49].

Careful monitoring for renal impairment and seizures (which can be seen in up to 10% of patients) is recommended due to foscarnet's effects on renal function and electrolytes, respectively [49].

Another common side effect of particular importance to the dermatologist is the development of penile and vulvar ulcerations that is thought to be due to the toxic effects of high concentrations of unmetabolized foscarnet in the urine. Ulcerations appear on average 1 week after treatment initiation and tend to resolve approximately 2 weeks after discontinuation of the drug. These effects can be minimized with increased hygiene including washing of area after urination [50].

Foscarnet has been determined as pregnancy category C risk, for which ultrasound monitoring of amniotic fluid volumes is recommended after 20 weeks to detect oligohydramnios. It not known whether foscarnet is excreted in breast milk. Known drug interactions include potentiation of adverse side effects of ACV/VACV, aminoglycosides, amphotericin B, cyclosporine, QTc-prolonging agents, methotrexate, and tacrolimus. Conversely, loop diuretics and pentamidine have been shown to enhance the toxic effect of foscarnet.

Investigational Agents for the Treatment of HHV Infections

There is a major need for the development of new, nontoxic antivirals for HSV infection. Two new agents are approaching licensure that will be very useful in the management of HSCT and SOT patients. The oral lipid conjugate prodrug of cidofovir, CMX001, has improved activity against herpesviruses, poxvirus, and adenovirus compared to parenterally administered cidofovir and a markedly reduced risk of nephrotoxicity [51]. Another novel agent, letermovir (AIC246), is highly orally bioavailable and has a novel mechanism of action, exerting its antiviral effect by interfering with the viral terminase complex. This agent demonstrates substantial promise as a once-daily alternative to more toxic antivirals in patients at high risk for CMV disease, particularly in the transplantation setting. Because it does not inhibit viral DNA polymerase, it retains activity against CMV strains that are otherwise resistant to all other anti-CMV agents. A phase III trial is currently underway to further evaluate its use in preventing CMV infection in HSCT recipients. It is also active against BK virus and poxviruses [52]. Maribavir is an oral agent which shows great promise in the treatment of CMV strains resistant to GCV, CDV, and foscarnet. Maribavir treats CMV infections by inhibition of the UL97 protein kinase and has demonstrated promising results in phase II studies. Although results of phase III studies were disappointing, dosages may have been too low and additional phase III trials are currently underway [53].

Another group of novel agents is currently being investigated for the treatment of HSV-1/2 infections and has shown great promise in providing an alternative to foscarnet (which has many adverse effects and requires IV administration) for HSV strains resistant to nucleoside analogs. These drugs target the viral helicase-primase enzyme complex, which comprises three proteins (helicase, primase, and a scaffold protein shown to promote primer synthesis) crucial for viral DNA replication. In phase II trials, pritelivir (AIC316) and amenamevir (ASP2151) demonstrated low resistance rates and superior efficacy against HSV in animal models with further studies currently ongoing [54, 55].

Other Infections

Drugs for the Treatment of Human Immunodeficiency Virus (HIV)

Treatment for human immunodeficiency virus (HIV) aims to reduce morbidity and mortality, allow people infected with the disease to live longer, healthier lives, and also reduces the risk of further transmission. Although there is no cure for HIV at present, many patients who are compliant with therapy are able to live a full and prosperous life [56].

There are six major categories of antiretroviral classes that are taken in combination with each other to target various points in the pathophysiology of HIV. Highly active antiretroviral therapy, or HAART, is the combination of at least three drugs for the suppression of HIV. Clinical trials haven proven the purpose of HIV treatment is valid: ART reduces the morbidity, mortality, and even behavior-associated transmission of the virus.

It is imperative that HAART is started immediately after the diagnosis of HIV is made, regardless of CD4 count, viral load, or pregnancy status. It is also worthwhile to perform other assessments such as a complete blood count, chemistries, lipids, liver function test, tuberculosis evaluation, and hepatitis testing to assess for any other comorbidities [56].

Replication Cycle

In order to understand the mechanism of action of the different classes of HIV drugs, it is important to understand the replication cycle of the virus. The replication cycle of HIV is as follows [56, 57]:

1. Binding/attachment
   (a) The viruses' envelope glycoprotein binds to the CD4 receptor on CD4+ T cells as well as their co-receptors CC chemokine receptor 5 (CCR5) or CXC chemokine receptor 4 (CXCR4).
2. Fusion
   (a) After binding, the HIV envelope and host cell begin to fuse together, releasing the viral capsid into the host cell.
3. Reverse transcriptase
   (a) Reverse transcriptase, inside the viral capsid, converts the HIV RNA contained in the virus into double-stranded DNA (dsDNA).
4. Integration
   (a) The viral integrase enzyme, also brought from the capsid, integrates the HIV dsDNA into the host DNA.
5. Replication
   (a) The host then begins to transcribe and translate the HIV dsDNA as it is now in the host DNA.
6. Assembly
   (a) The newly synthesized HIV proteins and RNA move toward the surface of the host cell and assemble into immature virions.
7. Budding and maturity
   (a) The new virions begin to bud out of the host cell, and the viral enzyme protease begins to break up the viruses' protein chain.

Prevention

Pre-exposure Prophylaxis (PrEP)

In addition to physical barriers, there are pharmaceutical options to prevent the infection of HIV. PrEP is the use of ART by HIV-negative individuals taken long term to prevent HIV infection. The WHO recommends PrEP for those at higher risk of infection such as those engaging in high-risk sexual behaviors, injection drug use, and sex workers. For HIV-uninfected patients who are at high risk for acquiring HIV and are committed to medication adherence, PrEP using tenofovir disoproxil fumarate-emtricitabine (TDC-FTC) can reduce the risk of HIV transmission by more than 90% [58]. Prior to prescribing, HIV status should be confirmed to be negative, and patients should be educated that this medication is to be taken daily and not as needed. HIV status should be checked regularly while on PrEP. In addition, physical barriers for sexual intercourse should still be emphasized to prevent the transmission of a sexually transmitted infection [59, 60].

Post-exposure Prophylaxis (PEP)

The use of ART by an HIV-negative individual after exposure to either a known or suspected source of HIV is called post-exposure prophylaxis (PEP). Common use of PEP includes after occupational exposure by healthcare workers, unprotected sexual exposure, injection drug use, and post-sexual assault. Table 41.6 lists the WHOs recommendation for PEP regimens. Animal studies have suggested that the efficacy of PEP in preventing infection is time dependent, thus it is impervious that PEP be started as soon as possible after exposure [61].

Entry Inhibitors

There is only one FDA-approved entry inhibitor—maraviroc.

Table 41.6 Post-exposure prophylaxis regimens in HIV-negative patients exposed to HIV virus

Generic name	Dose
Tenofovir (TDF)	300 mg once daily
Lamivudine (3TC)	150 mg twice daily or 300 mg once daily
Emtricitabine (FTC)	200 mg once daily
Lopinavir/ritonavir (LPV/r)	400 mg/100 mg twice daily or 800 mg/200 mg once daily[a]
Atazanavir/ritonavir (ATV/r)	300 mg + 100 mg once daily
Raltegravir (RAL)	400 mg twice daily
Darunavir + ritonavir (DRV/r)	800 mg + 100 mg once daily or 600 mg + 100 mg twice daily
Efavirenz (EFV)	600 mg once daily

[a]Once-daily dosing can be considered as an alternative for adults, but more data are needed for children and adolescents

Pharmacology and Mechanism of Action

Maraviroc works by binding to CCR5 on CD4+ T cells, preventing the interaction of HIV and its ability to enter the host cell.

Adverse Effects

- Allergic reaction
- Abdominal pain
- Hepatotoxicity, including jaundice and dark-colored urine
- Stevens-Johnson syndrome
- Toxic epidermal necrolysis

Fusion Inhibitors

Enfuvirtide is the only FDA-approved fusion inhibitor.

Pharmacology and Mechanism of Action

Enfuvirtide is a synthetic peptide that mimics a portion of glycoprotein 41 (gp41), an HIV envelope glycoprotein that is required for fusion of the viral envelope with the host cell membrane. This drug blocks the formation of a six-helix bundle structure that is critical for fusion. This medication is administered as a subcutaneous injection [62].

Adverse Effects

- Injection site reaction such as induration, erythema, and pain
- Allergic reaction
- Increased risk for bacterial pneumonia

Nucleoside and Nucleotide Reverse Transcriptase Inhibitors (NRTIs)

FDA-approved NRTIs are abacavir, didanosine, emtricitabine, lamivudine, stavudine, tenofovir disoproxil fumarate, and zidovudine.

Pharmacology and Mechanism of Action

NRTIs compete with deoxynucleoside substrates for binding to reverse transcriptase. After diffusing into the cytoplasm, these drugs are phosphorylated by intracellular kinases to their active triphosphate forms. The triphosphate form is incorporated into DNA, resulting in chain termination. NRTIs are well absorbed from the gastrointestinal tract, although there are differences in bioavailability when they are administered with and without food as well as differences in both serum and intracellular half-lives.

Adverse Effects

As a class effect, NRTIs are associated with mitochondrial toxicity, and this presents as hepatic steatosis, peripheral neuropathy, pancreatitis, dyslipidemia, fat maldistribution, and lipoatrophy. All NRTIs have "black box" warnings in their product labeling regarding the possibility of lactic acidosis syndrome, which is potentially fatal. Listed below are specific NRTIs with their adverse events:

- Abacavir: Patients who carry the HLA-B*5701 allele are at a higher risk of experiencing a sometimes fatal hypersensitivity reaction to the drug. Providers should check for this allele and wait for the result prior to prescribing.
- Emtricitabine: Fat redistribution has been seen in patients taking emtricitabine. These changes may include increased amount of fat in the upper back and neck ("buffalo hump"), breast, and around the trunk. Loss of fat from the legs, arms, and face may also happen. Hyperpigmentation primarily of the palms and/or soles, but may include tongue, arms, lip, and nails, has also been seen with this medication. Rash is common and diverse including a hypersensitivity reaction, maculopapular rash, pustular rash, and vesiculobullous rash.
- Didanosine: Rash, pruritus, xerostomia, alopecia, lipodystrophy, Stevens-Johnson syndrome, and vasculitis can occur with didanosine. It can also cause pancreatitis and peripheral neuropathy.
- Lamivudine: Lamivudine is a generally well-tolerated drug but may produce neutropenia as well as alopecia, rash, pruritis, and fat redistribution.
- Stavudine: Fat redistribution has been documented. It is also associated with lipoatrophy and lactic acidosis.
- Tenofovir: Rash including macular, papular, pustular, vesiculobullous, or urticarial, as well as pruritus, and diaphoresis can be seen with tenofovir. It is also associated with headache and nausea. It can elevate didanosine levels and lower those of atazanavir.
- Zidovudine: Lipodystrophy, blue skin/nail pigmentation, Stevens-Johnson syndrome, toxic epidermal necrolysis, urticarial, and morbilliform eruption can be seen. Common side effects of zidovudine include bone marrow suppression and gastrointestinal intolerance.

Of note, the onset of bullous pemphigoid has been reported with the combination of lamivudine + didanosine + nelfinavir [63].

Non-nucleoside Reverse Transcriptase Inhibitors (NNRTIs)

FDA-approved NNRTIs are delavirdine, efavirenz, etravirine, nevirapine, and rilpivirine.

Pharmacology and Mechanism of Action

Although a similar name, NNRTIs are different than NRTIs in that NNRTIs bind near the catalytic site of reverse transcriptase and alter the enzymes' ability to change conformation. This increased enzyme rigidity prevents its normal polymerization function and therefore decreases the viral rate of replication. Nevirapine has greater than 90% bioavailability and a plasma half-life of 24 h. It is metabolized in the liver and induces its own metabolic pathway. As the metabolism of the drug increases, the dose is increased from once a day during the first 2 weeks to twice daily thereafter. Delavirdine has a bioavailability of 85%. It requires an acidic environment for absorption and should not be given with antacids, H2 blockers, or proton pump inhibitors. Its plasma half-life is 6 h, and it is metabolized in the liver. The absorption of efavirenz is increased by food. However, it is generally administered on an empty stomach to minimize side effects. The half-life of efavirenz is 40+ h, and it is metabolized in the liver [62].

Side Effects
A class effect of NNRTIs is hepatitis and central nervous system abnormalities.

- Nevirapine is associated with cutaneous side effects in approximately 20% of patients. Mucosal side effects include whitish plaques, burning, taste disturbance, and xerostomia [63]. Among HIV-infected patients with CD4 counts <250, higher baseline counts are associated with a higher incidence of rash requiring discontinuation of the drug [63]. Treatment should be initiated slowly to minimize the risk of these cutaneous adverse events. This reaction is thought to be due to quinone methide formed in the skin by sulfation of the 12-OH metabolite followed by loss of the sulfate [57]. If the rash is extensive, or if mucous membranes are involved, the drug should be discontinued.
- In addition, nevirapine is generally not recommended for women with CD4+ T-cell counts higher than 250 or for men with CD4+ T-cell counts above 400 because of an increased risk of hepatitis.
- Etravirine is associated with a self-limiting rash in 19% of patients [63].
- Delavirdine is also commonly associated with drug rash.
- Efavirenz is teratogenic.

Integrase Strand Transfer Inhibitors (INSTIs)

FDA-approved INSTIs are dolutegravir, elvitegravir, and raltegravir.

Pharmacology and Mechanism of Action

The HIV integrase enzyme is blocked by INSTIs which then inhibits the integration of the viral dsDNA into the host DNA. This prevents the later formation of HIV provirus and the replication cycle.

Adverse Effects

Adverse events of this class of medication are insomnia, headaches, dizziness, nausea, diarrhea, and fatigue. Raltegravir has been associated with allergic reaction, Stevens-Johnson syndrome, and toxic epidermal necrolysis. Dolutegravir has been associated with rash, constitutional findings, and even organ failure.

Protease Inhibitors (PIs)

FDA-approved protease inhibitors are atazanavir, atazanavir-cobicistat, darunavir, darunavir-cobicistat, fosamprenavir, indinavir, lopinavir/ritonavir boosting, nelfinavir, ritonavir (used as a pharmacokinetic boosting agent), saquinavir, and tipranavir.

Pharmacology and Mechanism of Action

The protease enzyme is the target of protease inhibitors. Blockage of this enzyme prevents the proteolytic cleavage of viral polypeptide precursors. In addition to HIV, this class of drug may be active against other viruses. Bioavailability of PIs vary among the different medications

- Ritonavir has good oral bioavailability but side effects limit the dose in most patients. Ritonavir is used primarily for its CYP effect to inhibit the metabolism of other agents to raise blood levels of the protease inhibitors.
- Saquinavir and lopinavir have poor oral availability and are administered in combination with low-dose ritonavir to improve drug levels.

All PIs are metabolized via the hepatic cytochrome P450 system. The cytochrome P450 system is utilized in many other drug metabolism pathways. Because of this, PIs interfere are known to interfere with numerous other medications.

Adverse Effects

Lipodystrophy is a common side effect of PIs, likely due to the inhibition of ZMPSTE24, an enzyme that removes the farnesylated tail of prelamin A. Buildup of this protein is related to acquired lipodystrophy, conceivably through an interaction with a transcription factor called sterol regulatory element-binding protein-1. Fat distribution may improve with L-acetylcarnitine therapy, and fillers to add volume

have been employed to reduce the social stigma associated with therapy [63]. In addition to lipodystrophy, other side effects include rash, erythema, striae, xerosis, Stevens-Johnson syndrome, nausea, vomiting, diarrhea, hepatitis dyslipidemia, and abnormal glucose metabolism.

Drugs for the Treatment of Hepatitis C

Hepatitis C virus (HCV) infection is a major cause of chronic liver disease and cirrhosis [64]. It is a global health problem with 130–150 million people estimated to be chronically infected worldwide [64]. HCV is predominantly transmitted by exposure to blood or body fluids. The infection progresses to a chronic state in 80% of patients, whereas the virus clears completely after the acute infection in 20% of patients [64, 65]. For these patients, the risk of progression to liver cirrhosis is estimated to be 15–30% within 20 years [65]. HCV is an enveloped, positive-sense RNA virus that belongs to the Flaviviridae family [66]. The lack of a proofreading mechanism during the replication of the HCV RNA genome leads to significant variation [66]. Thus, HCV has been divided into seven genotypes with distinct geographic distribution [67]. Genotype 1 is the most common genotype worldwide and in the United States [67]. Up to 85% of patients with acute HCV infection are unable to clear the infection and become chronically infected if left untreated. These patients are at higher risk of subsequently developing hepatocellular carcinoma [65].

Treatment of patients with chronic HCV infection is determined by genotype, extent of fibrosis or cirrhosis, prior treatment, comorbidities, and potential adverse effects [65]. The goal of therapy is to reduce all-cause mortality and liver-associated complications [68]. Although interferon-based regimens have been the mainstay of treatment for HCV infection, the US Food and Drug Administration recently approved two combination-pill interferon-free treatments (ledipasvir plus sofosbuvir and ombitasvir/paritaprevir/ritonavir plus dasabuvir) for chronic HCV genotype 1. The goal of HCV treatment is the achievement of a sustained virological response (SVR), defined by the absence of HCV RNA on polymerase chain reaction. SVR 24 weeks after cessation of treatment is associated with a 99% chance of being HCV RNA negative during long-term follow-up [69]. SVR 12 weeks after treatment is a new primary end point in many recent drug trials. A small post hoc analysis of patients with HCV genotype 1 found that the SVR at 12 weeks has a 100% positive predictive value for SVR at 24 weeks [70].

PEG-IFNα and Ribavirin Combination Therapy

HCV virus is able to suppress the innate and adaptive immune and pro-inflammatory responses of the host by various mechanisms. Exogenous pegylated interferon alpha

(PEG-IFNα) is used in attempt to counteract that suppression. It inhibits viral replication by antiviral, antiproliferative, and immunomodulatory effects [71]. Ribavirin inhibits viral RNA polymerase, but there is also evidence to suggest that it may have an immunomodulatory effect that mediates increased sensitivity to PEG-IFNα [72]. Patients are treated for 24–48 weeks. Interferon-based therapy is limited by less than optimal response rates and relatively intolerable side effects.

PEG-IFNα is administered subcutaneously and is associated with localized injection site reactions in the majority of treated patients. These include self-limited erythema, tenderness, pruritus, and rashes at the site of injection [73]. Less commonly (<4%), cutaneous necrosis can occur at the injection site, which can be managed with local wound care and usually resolves in 1–2 months [9]. Alternative injection sites can be used for future doses [74]. Alopecia, psoriasis, fixed drug eruptions, eczematous drug reactions, sarcoidosis, lupus, pigmentary changes, and lichenoid eruptions have also been reported [75–77].

Systemic side effects with interferon are also common and often result in discontinuation of the drug. In a majority of patients, flu-like symptoms of fever, chills, tachycardia, malaise, myalgia, and headache may occur within 1–2 h of administration. Other adverse effects include bone marrow suppression, gastrointestinal upset, and hepatotoxicity [75–77]. Interferon-α has caused or exacerbated depression psychosis, cognitive changes, and suicidal and homicidal ideation. Interferon-α should not be used to treat hepatitis B-related cirrhosis or decompensated liver disease because hepatitis flares could lead to further decompensation [75–77]. Interferon is labeled as pregnancy risk factor C; interferon in combination with ribavirin is pregnancy category risk factor X, as it is associated with birth defects.

Direct-Acting Antiviral Agents

First Generation DAAs

The first-generation protease inhibitors include boceprevir (Victrelis) and telaprevir (Incivek), which were both approved by the FDA in 2011. These were later discontinued because of greater efficacy of alternative treatments and higher rates of serious adverse events [77]. They were used for genotype 1 HCV in combination with PEG-IFNα and ribavirin, since they were associated with higher SVR rates. However, compared to PEG-IFNα plus ribavirin alone, these agents were more expensive and were associated with higher incidence of clinically significant adverse events leading to poor adherence and higher rates of premature discontinuation of therapy.

Boceprevir was associated with anemia, neutropenia, and distortion of taste [78, 79]. When compared to PEG-IFNα and ribavirin alone, boceprevir was not associated with a significantly increased incidence of serious skin rash [79]. Conversely, telaprevir was associated with rash, pruritus, anorectal discomfort, diarrhea, and anemia [79]. Around 6–7% of patients receiving telaprevir discontinued therapy due to an eczematous rash. The rash can occur at any time during treatment with telaprevir, but 50% of the cases occurred within the first 4 weeks of initiation of therapy. Moreover, telaprevir has been associated with more serious dermatologic adverse reactions, including drug rash with eosinophilia and systemic symptoms (DRESS) and Stevens-Johnson syndrome (SJS) [79].

Second-Generation DAAs

In 2014, the FDA approved the first combination pill containing ledipasvir and sofosbuvir (Harvoni). It is taken once daily to treat chronic HCV genotype 1 infection. Later in the year, the FDA also approved Viekira Pak, which was a combination of ombitasvir (NS5A inhibitor), paritaprevir (NS3/4A inhibitor), and ritonavir (HIV-1 protease inhibitor) tablets in combination with dasabuvir tablets (NS5B inhibitor) for adults with chronic HCV genotype 1 infection. These drugs work together to inhibit the growth of HCV and may be used with or without RBV.

Treatment with 8 weeks of ledipasvir/sofosbuvir was noninferior to treatment with 12 weeks of ledipasvir/sofosbuvir plus RBV, as reported by a phase 3, randomized, open-label study involving 647 treatment-experienced patients with HCV genotype 1 infection [80]. A multicenter, randomized, double-blind, placebo-controlled trial evaluating 631 patients found an SVR of 96.2%, with a 0.6% discontinuation rate because of adverse events [81]. The most commonly reported adverse events with ledipasvir/sofosbuvir are headache, anemia, fatigue, and nausea [80, 81]. Up to 7% of patients had rash [78]. However, none of the dermatological adverse events required discontinuation of treatment. Rash was not listed as a side effect in patients with HCV/HIV-1 coinfection who were treated with Harvoni [80].

Simeprevir (Olysio) is another second-generation DAA that is effective for genotypes 1, 4, 5, and 6 [80, 81]. It is only indicated in combination with sofosbuvir or PEG-IFNα plus ribavirin. Two randomized controlled trials involving patients with genotypes 1 to 3 reported a superior SVR at 12 weeks with simeprevir combined with pegylated interferon and RBV (80–92%) vs. pegylated interferon and RBV alone (40–50%) [80, 81]. The most common systemic adverse effects include anemia, fatigue, flu-like symptoms, pruritus, headache, and nausea [81].

Cutaneous adverse events associated with simeprevir include rash and photosensitivity. However, the rates of discontinuation of therapy were comparable to those with PEG-IFNα plus ribavirin alone. The skin rash can develop at any time during treatment but most commonly begins within 4 weeks from the initiation of therapy [80, 81].

Case Report

A 24-year-old male third year medical student complains of very painful rash that develop 2 days ago along his right torso. He has never had a rash like this in the past. Prior to the development of the lesion, he began to endorse a burning sensation in the area where the rash developed. Of note, he has been under a great deal of stress as he is preparing to take his country's medical licensing exam.

Past Medical History

* Generalized anxiety disorder, diagnosed at age 22
* Appendicitis status post appendectomy, diagnosed at age 16

Relevant Family Medical History

* Father: herpes zoster, occurred at age 52

Medications

* Escitalopram 5 mg qDay

Social History

* Third year medical student
* Drinks 1–2 oz. of alcohol per week
* Drinks 16 oz. of coffee per day
* Denied tobacco use
* Not sexually active

Physical Exam

* Numerous vesicles superimposed onto a beefy red patch on the right-sided T6 dermatome

Management

A clinical diagnosis of herpes zoster, or shingles, was made. His positive family history of shingles and high level of stress contributes to this diagnosis. His physician swabbed the lesions for varicella-zoster virus/herpes simplex virus DNA PCR. The student was prescribed valacyclovir 1000 mg PO TID × 7 days for treatment of shingles as well as gabapentin 100 mg PO TID PRN for shingles-related pain. Until his lesions crust over, which takes approximately 1–2 weeks, he is considered contagious and should keep his lesions covered, especially around pregnant women, individuals who have not been vaccinated, and the immunosuppressed. His lesions are expected to heal within 1 month and the pain to resolve in around 6–9 months. He was educated that the rest of his blood-related family should consider the herpes zoster vaccination as the disease is associated with a family history.

References

1. Wagstaff AJ, Faulds D, Goak L. Acyclovir, a reappraisal of its antiviral activity, pharmacokinetic properties and therapeutic efficacy. Drugs. 1994;47:153–205.
2. Whitley RJ, Gnann JW Jr. Acyclovir: a decade later. N Engl J Med. 1992;327(11):782.
3. Chatis PA, Crumpacker CS. Resistance of herpesvirus to antiviral drugs. Antimicrob Agents Chemother. 1992;36(8):1589.
4. Levin MJ, Bacon TH, Leary JJ. Resistance of herpes simplex virus infections to nucleoside analogues in HIV-infected patients. Clin Infect Dis. 2004;39(5):S248.
5. Stranska R, Schuurman R, Nienhuis E, et al. Survey of acyclovir-resistant herpes simplex virus in the Netherlands: prevalence and characterization. J Clin Virol. 2005;32:7–18.
6. Gilbert C, Bestman-Smith J, Boivin G. Resistance of herpesviruses to antiviral drugs: clinical impacts and molecular mechanisms. Drug Resist Updat. 2002;5:88–114.
7. Hardy WD. Foscarnet treatment of acyclovir-resistant herpes simplex virus infection in patients with acquired immunodeficiency syndrome: preliminary results of a controlled, randomized, regimen-comparative trial. Am J Med. 1992;92(2A):30S.
8. Laskin OL. Clinical pharmacokinetics of acyclovir. Clin Pharmacokinet. 1983;8(3):187.
9. Wald A, Zeh J, Barnum G, et al. Suppression of subclinical shedding of herpes simplex virus type 2 with acyclovir. Ann Intern Med. 1996;124:8–15.
10. Hollier LM, Wendel GD. Third trimester antiviral prophylaxis for preventing maternal genital herpes simplex virus (HSV) recurrences and neonatal infection. Cochrane Database Syst Rev. 2008;1:CD004946.
11. Spruance SL, Stewart JCB, Rowe NH, et al. Treatment of recurrent herpes simplex labialis with oral acyclovir. J Infect Dis. 1990;161:185–90.
12. Spruance SL. Prophylactic chemotherapy with acyclovir for recurrent herpes simplex labialis. J Med Virol. 1993;1:27–32.
13. Centers for Disease Control and Prevention. Managing people at risk for severe varicella. 2016. https://www.cdc.gov/chickenpox/hcp/persons-risk.html. Accessed 7 Feb 2016.
14. Harris D, Redhead J. Should acyclovir be prescribed for immunocompetent children presenting with chickenpox? Arch Dis Child. 2005;90(6):648–50.
15. Cooper DA, Pehrson PO, Pedersen C, et al. The efficacy and safety of zidovudine alone or as cotherapy with acyclovir for the treatment of patients with AIDS and AIDS-related complex: a double-blind randomized trial. European-Australian Collaborative Group. AIDS. 1993;7:197–207.
16. Hoglund M, Ljungman P, Weller S. Comparable acyclovir exposures produced by oral valaciclovir and intravenous acyclovir in immunocompromised cancer patients. J Antimicrob Chemother. 2001;47(6):855–61.
17. Baker D, Eisen D. Valacyclovir for prevention of recurrent herpes labialis: 2 double-blind placebo-controlled studies. Cutis. 2003;71:239–42.
18. Beeson WH, Rachel JD. Valacyclovir prophylaxis for herpes simplex virus infection or infection recurrence following laser skin resurfacing. Dermatol Surg. 2002;28(4):331–6.
19. Corey L, Wald A, Patel R, et al. Once-daily valacyclovir to reduce the risk of transmission of genital herpes. N Engl J Med. 2004;350:11–20.
20. Beutner KR, Friedman DJ, Forszpaniak C, et al. Valaciclovir compared with acyclovir for improved therapy for herpes zoster in immunocompetent adults. Antimicrob Agents Chemother. 1995;39:1546–53.
21. Lapolla W, Digiorgio C, Haitz K, Magel G, Mendoza N, Grady J, Lu W, Tyring S. Incidence of postherpetic neuralgia after com-

bination treatment with gabapentin and valacyclovir in patients with acute herpes zoster: open-label study. Arch Dermatol. 2011;147(8):901–7.

22. Hato N, Yamada H, Kohno H, Matsumoto S, Honda N, Gyo K, et al. Valacyclovir and prednisolone treatment for Bell's palsy: a multicenter, randomized, placebo-controlled study. Otol Neurotol. 2007;28(3):408–13.

23. Lee HY, Byun JY, Park MS, Yeo SG. Steroid-antiviral treatment improves the recovery rate in patients with severe Bell's palsy. Am J Med. 2013;126(4):336–41.

24. Shahidullah M, Haque A, Islam MR, Rizvi AN, Sultana N, Mia BA. Comparative study between combination of famciclovir and prednisolone with prednisolone alone in acute Bell's palsy. Mymensingh Med J. 2011;20(4):605–13.

25. Kimberlin DW, Jacobs RF, Weller S, et al. Pharmacokinetics and safety of extemporaneously compounded valacyclovir oral suspension in pediatric patients from 1 month through 11 years of age. Clin Infect Dis. 2010;50(2):221 8.

26. Bates D. Valacyclovir neurotoxicity: two case reports and a review of the literature. Can J Hosp Pharm. 2002;55:123–7.

27. Tyring SK, Baker D, Snowden W. Valacyclovir for herpes simplex infection: long-term safety and sustained efficacy after 20 years' experience with acyclovir. J Infect Dis. 2002;186(1):S40–6.

28. Feinberg JE, Hurwitz S, Cooper D, et al. A randomized, double-blind trial of valaciclovir prophylaxis for CMV disease in patients with advanced human immunodeficiency virus infection. AIDS Clinical Trials Group Protocol 204/Glaxo Wellcome 123-014 international CMV Prophylaxis Study Group. J Infect Dis. 1998;177:48–56.

29. Perry CM, Wagstaff AJ. Famciclovir: a review of its pharmacological properties and therapeutic efficacy in herpesvirus infections. Drugs. 1995;50(2):396.

30. Vere Hodge RA. Famciclovir and penciclovir: the mode of action of famciclovir including its conversion to penciclovir. Antivir Chem Chemother. 1993;4:67.

31. Kim HJ, Kim SH, Jung J, et al. Comparison of acyclovir and famciclovir for the treatment of Bell's palsy. Eur Arch Oto-Rhino-Laryngol. 2016;273(10):3083–90.

32. Aoki FY. The continuing evolution of antiviral therapy for recurrent genital herpes: 1-day patient-initiated treatment with famciclovir. Herpes. 2007;14(3):62–5.

33. Saltzman R, Jurewicz R, Boon R. Safety of famciclovir in patients with herpes zoster and genital herpes. Antimicrob Agents Chemother. 1994;38(10):2454.

34. Wald A, Selke S, Warren T, et al. Comparative efficacy of famciclovir and valacyclovir for suppression of recurrent genital herpes and viral shedding. Sex Transm Dis. 2006;33:529–33.

35. De Clercq E. Clinical potential of the acyclic nucleoside phosphonates cidofovir, adefovir, and tenofovir in treatment of DNA virus and retrovirus infections. Clin Microbiol Rev. 2003;16(4):569.

36. Xiong X, Smith JL, Chen MS. Effect of incorporation of Cidofovir into DNA by human cytomegalovirus DNA polymerase on DNA elongation. Antimicrob Agents Chemother. 1997;41(3):594–9.

37. Snoeck R, Andrei G, De Clercq E. Cidofovir in the treatment of HPV-associated lesions. Verh K Acad Geneeskd Belg. 2001;63(2):93–120.

38. Andrei G, Fiten P, Goubau P, et al. Dual infection with polyomavirus BK and acyclovir-resistant herpes simplex virus successfully treated with cidofovir in a bone marrow transplant recipient. Transpl Infect Dis. 2007;9(2):126–31.

39. Coremans G, Snoeck R. Cidofovir: clinical experience and future perspectives on an acyclic nucleoside phosphonate analog of cytosine in the treatment of refractory and premalignant HPV-associated anal lesions. Expert Opin Pharmacother. 2009;10(8):1343–52.

40. Sonvico F, Colombo G, Bortolotti F, et al. Therapeutic paint of cidofovir/sucralfate gel combination topically administered by spraying for treatment of orf virus infections. AAPS J. 2009;11(2):242–9.

41. Cono J, Casey CG, Bell DM. Smallpox vaccination and adverse reactions. Guidance for clinicians. MMWR Recomm Rep. 2003;52:1.

42. Lalezari JP, Stagg RJ, Kuppermann BD, et al. Intravenous cidofovir for peripheral cytomegalovirus retinitis in patients with AIDS. A randomized, controlled trial. Ann Intern Med. 1997;126:257.

43. Sullivan V, Talarico CL, Stanat SC, et al. A protein kinase homologue controls phosphorylation of ganciclovir in human CMV-infected cells [errata in]. Nature. 1992;358:162–4.

44. Brown F, Banken L, Saywell K, et al. Pharmacokinetics of valganciclovir and ganciclovir following multiple oral dosages of valganciclovir in HIV- and CMV-seropositive volunteers. Clin Pharmacokinet. 1999;37:167–76.

45. Jabs DA, Martin BK, Forman MS, et al. Cytomegalovirus resistance to ganciclovir and clinical outcomes of patients with cytomegalovirus retinitis. Am J Ophthalmol. 2003;135:26–34.

46. Wagstaff AJ, Bryson HM. Foscarnet: a reappraisal of its antiviral activity, pharmacokinetic properties and therapeutic use in immunocompromised patients with viral infections. Drugs. 1994;48(2):199.

47. Chou S, Van Wechel LC, Lichy HM, et al. Phenotyping of cytomegalovirus drug resistance mutations by using recombinant viruses incorporating a reporter gene. Antimicrob Agents Chemother. 2005;49:2710.

48. Narimatsu H, Kami M, Kato D, et al. Reduced dose of foscarnet as preemptive therapy for cytomegalovirus infection following reduced-intensity cord blood transplantation. Transpl Infect Dis. 2007;9(1):11–5.

49. Jayaweera DT. Minimising the dosage-limiting toxicities of foscarnet induction therapy. Drug Saf. 1997;16:258–66.

50. Mancini M, Matozzo V, Previtali D, et al. Observational retrospective study on the incidence of haemorrhagic cystitis and genital lesions in allogenic THSC patients treated with foscarnet. Bone Marrow Transpl. 2011;46:S417.

51. Parker S, Touchette E, Oberle C, et al. Efficacy of therapeutic intervention with an oral ether lipid analogue of cidofovir (CMX001) in a lethal mousepox model. Antivir Res. 2008;77:39–49.

52. Sharp M, Corp D. MK_8228 (Leter, movir) versus Placebo in the Prevention of Clinically-Significant Cytomegalovirus (CMV) Infection in Adult, CMV-Seropositive Allogeneic Hematopoietic Stem Cell Transplant Recipients (MK-8228-001). In ClinicalTrials. gov, editors. Bethesda: National Library of Medicine; 2000.

53. Alain S, Revest M, Veyer D, et al. Maribavir use in practice for cytomegalovirus infection in French transplantation centers. Transplant Proc. 2013;45(4):1603–7.

54. Katsumata K, Weinberg A, Chono K, et al. Susceptibility of herpes simplex virus isolated from genital herpes lesions to ASP2151, a novel helicase-primase inhibitor. Antimicrob Agents Chemother. 2012;56:3587–91.

55. Wald A, Corey L, Timmler B, et al. Helicase-primase inhibitor pritelivir for HSV-2 infection. N Engl J Med. 2014;370:201–10.

56. Panel on Antiretroviral Guidelines for Adults and Adolescents. Guidelines for the Use of Antiretroviral Agents in HIV-1-Infected Adults and Adolescents. https://aidsinfo.nih.gov/contentfiles/lvguidelines/adultandadolescentgl.pdf. Accessed 1 Feb 2017.

57. Laskey SB, Siliciano RF. A mechanistic theory to explain the efficacy of antiretroviral therapy. Nat Rev Micro. 2014;12(11):772–80.

58. Anderson PL, Glidden DV, Liu A, et al. Emtricitabine-tenofovir concentrations and pre-exposure prophylaxis efficacy in men who have sex with men. Sci Transl Med. 2012;4(151):151ra125.

59. WHO. Guideline on When to Start Antiretroviral Therapy and on Pre-Exposure Prophylaxis for HIV. Geneva: WHO; 2015. http://www.who.int/hiv/pub/guidelines/earlyrelease-arv/en/.

60. United States Public Health Service, Centers for Disease Control and Prevention (U.S.), National Center for HIV/AIDS, Viral Hepatitis, STD, and TB Prevention (U.S.), et al. Preexposure Prophylaxis for the Prevention of HIV Infection. 2014. A Clinical Practice Guideline. http://stacks.cdc.gov/view/cdc/23109.

61. WHO. News and Events Topics Publications Data and Statistics About Us Guidelines on Post-Exposure Prophylaxis for HIV and the Use of Co-Trimoxazole Prophylaxis for HIV-Related Infections among Adults, Adolescents and Children. Geneva, Switzerland: WHO; 2014. http://www.who.int/hiv/pub/guidelines/arv2013/arvs2013upplement_dec2014/en/.

62. AIDSinfo Drug Database|AIDSinfo. https://aidsinfo.nih.gov/drugs. Accessed 1 Feb 2017.

63. Atzori L, Pinna AL, Pilloni L. Bullous skin eruption in an HIV patient during antiretroviral drugs therapy. Dermatol Ther. 2008;21(2):S30–4.

64. Guidelines for the screening, care and treatment of persons with hepatitis C infection. Geneva: World Health Organization; 2014.

65. Wikins T, Akhtar M, Gititu E, et al. Diagnosis and management of hepatitis C. Am Fam Physician. 2015;91(12):835–42.

66. Bostan N, Mahmood T. An overview about hepatitis C: a devastating virus. Crit Rev Microbiol. 2010;36(2):91–133.

67. Messina JP, Humphreys I, Flaxman A, et al. Global distribution and prevalence of hepatitis C virus genotypes. Hepatology. 2015;61:77–87.

68. American Association for the Study of Liver Diseases; Infectious Diseases Society of America. Recommendations for testing, managing, and treating hepatitis C. http://www.hcvguidelines.org/. Accessed 31 Jan 2017.

69. Kau A, Vermehren J, Sarrazin C. Treatment predictors of a sustained virologic response in hepatitis B and C. J Hepatol. 2008;49(4):634–51.

70. Zeuzem S, Mensa FJ. Concordance between sustained virologic response week 12 (SVR12) and SVR24 in genotype 1 hepatitis C virus patients receiving interferon-free treatment in the SOUND-C2 study. Hepatology. 2013;58(4):1516.

71. Chung RT, et al. Mechanisms of action of interferon and ribavirin in chronic hepatitis C: summary of a workshop. Hepatology. 2008;47:306–20. https://doi.org/10.1002/hep.22070.

72. Negro F. Adverse effects of drugs in the treatment of viral hepatitis. Best Pract Res Clin Gastroenterol. 2010;24:183–92. https://doi.org/10.1016/j.bpg.2009.10.012.

73. Mistry N, Shapero J, Crawford RI. A review of adverse cutaneous drug reactions resulting from the use of interferon and ribavirin. Can J Gastroenterol. 2009;23:677–83.

74. Fried MW. Side effects of therapy of hepatitis C and their management. Hepatology. 2002;36:S237–44. https://doi.org/10.1053/jhep.2002.36810.

75. Cacoub P, et al. Dermatological side effects of hepatitis C and its treatment: patient management in the era of direct-acting antivirals. J Hepatol. 2012;56:455–63. https://doi.org/10.1016/j.jhep.2011.08.006.

76. Belousova V, Abd-Rabou AA, Mousa SA. Recent advances and future directions in the management of hepatitis C infections. Pharmacol Ther. 2015;145:92–102.

77. Jacobson IM, et al. A practical guide for the use of boceprevir and telaprevir for the treatment of hepatitis C. J Viral Hepat. 2012;19(Suppl 2):1–26. https://doi.org/10.1111/j.1365-2893.2012.01590.x.

78. Afdhal N, et al. Ledipasvir and sofosbuvir for previously treated HCV genotype 1 infection. N Engl J Med. 2014;370:1483–93. https://doi.org/10.1056/NEJMoa1316366.

79. Feld JJ, Kowdley KV, Coakley E, et al. Treatment of HCV with ABT-450/ombitasvir and dasabuvir with ribavirin. N Engl J Med. 2014;370(17):1594–603.

80. Naggie S, et al. Ledipasvir and Sofosbuvir for HCV in patients Coinfected with HIV-1. N Engl J Med. 2015;373:705–13. https://doi.org/10.1056/NEJMoa1501315.

81. Lawitz E, Lalezari JP, Hassanein T, et al. Sofosbuvir in combination with peginterferon alfa-2a and ribavirin for non-cirrhotic, treatment-naive patients with genotypes 1, 2, and 3 hepatitis C infection: a randomised, double-blind, phase 2 trial. Lancet Infect Dis. 2013;13(5):401–8.

Anthelmintics in Dermatology

42

Scott Worswick and Sean Dreyer

Scabies

Permethrin and ivermectin are among the most commonly used topical agents for scabies. Permethrin topical 5% cream is the first-line treatment, and should be applied to the entire skin surface from the neck-down. Most practitioners advise patients to apply the entire tube of 30 g at bedtime and leave it in place all night. In the morning patients should wash all bedding and clothing in hot water and then bathe. For all scabies infestations, this process should be repeated 1 week later at the very least; additional weekly applications are frequently necessary for "Norwegian"/crusted scabies [1, 2]. Permethrin is generally well tolerated, occasionally associated with mild skin irritation, and exists as a treatment option for pregnant women [3, 4].

Oral ivermectin (0.2 mg/kg orally once; with a repeat dose 5 days or 2 weeks after the initial dose) is particularly effective for treating crusted scabies, and is the only routinely used oral therapeutic option [1–3]. Oral ivermectin is generally well tolerated, with urticarial rash and pruritus being the most common adverse reactions [1, 3, 5]. However, ivermectin has been shown to have neurotoxic effects in animal studies [6]. Additionally, several cases of altered mental status in patients with *Onchocerca volvulus* and *Loa loa* treated with ivermectin have also been reported, likely due to disruption of the blood–brain barrier [7–9]. There is no consensus on the safety of oral ivermectin during pregnancy, but one study on women inadvertently treated with oral ivermectin during pregnancy showed no effect on developmental status or disease patterns of children of treated mothers [10]. The efficacy of 5% permethrin cream versus single-dose oral ivermectin 200 mcg/kg is comparable, though several trials have demonstrated slight superiority of permethrin over single-dose ivermectin, and similar efficacy between permethrin and two doses of ivermectin [1, 2, 5, 11]. Topical ivermectin is also an effective treatment, with no reported adverse events [3, 12]. A randomized clinical trial of 315 patients reported equal efficacy of 5% permethrin and 1% topical ivermectin, both of which were more effective than oral ivermectin [13].

Other therapeutic agents include topical 1% lindane, benzyl benzoate 10–25% lotion, crotamiton 10% cream, topical 0.5% malathion, sulfur 5–10% ointment, and monosulfram 25%, though all are inferior to treatment with permethrin or ivermectin [11, 14]. Topical 1% lindane is generally considered less effective than permethrin for treatment of scabies, apart from one randomized control trial with 467 patients by Schultz et al., which reported similar efficacy [15–17]. Due to its higher potential for neurotoxicity, lindane is contraindicated for use in epileptics, pregnant women, and infants, and considered a second-line treatment reserved for recalcitrant cases or for patients unable to tolerate other treatment options [3, 4, 15].

Topical benzyl benzoate, available as a 10 or 25% cream or lotion, is a cost-effective option but requires repeated applications over days to weeks [3, 18, 19]. Crotamiton 10% cream requires daily use over several days and has excellent antipruritic effects but is weakly scabicidal [3, 20].

Benzyl benzoate and crotamiton have no serious side effects, other than severe skin irritation with benzyl benzoate [20]. Malathion 0.5% is an effective treatment as an alternative to permethrin or ivermectin, particularly for use in the scalp or hairy areas, but has been less studied compared to more commonly used treatment modalities [21, 22]. Sulfur 5 or 10% ointment is safe and cost effective, but its efficacy is not yet well studied and it must be compounded [20, 23–25]. Monosulfram 25% is available as a lotion and soap, but lacks strong evidence for its efficacy as a treatment for scabies and has the potential to cause disulfiram-like reaction with alcohol consumption [3, 26].

Esdepallethrine is a less-studied option, used in combination with piperonyl butoxide, available as a lotion and a spray

S. Worswick, MD (✉)
Assistant Professor of Dermatology at UCLA,
Los Angeles, CA, USA
e-mail: SWorswick@mednet.ucla.edu

S. Dreyer, BA
MS4 at David Geffen School of Medicine at UCLA, Los Angeles, CA, USA
e-mail: sdreyer@mednet.ucla.edu

© Springer International Publishing AG 2018
P.S. Yamauchi (ed.), *Biologic and Systemic Agents in Dermatology*, https://doi.org/10.1007/978-3-319-66884-0_42

[27]. Several studies have shown inferior efficacy as compared to benzyl benzoate, with many observed treatment failures [28]. Skin stinging and irritation are the most commonly experienced adverse effects [27]. However, the topical spray form of the product may cause bronchospasm, and is contraindicated in asthmatics and children and infants with a history of wheezing bronchitis or bronchiolitis [27, 28].

Leishmaniasis, Cutaneous

Leishmaniasis is caused by *Leishmania* spp. protozoa which is transmitted by infected female sandflies. Cutaneous leishmaniasis is usually characterized by an ulcerating papule following a bite from an infected sandfly, although diffuse cutaneous leishmaniasis presents as nodular lesions that do not ulcerate [29, 30]. Many lesions resolve on their own over months to years, which makes evaluating efficacy of different treatments difficult [29]. There is no one definitive treatment option, and different treatment options may have different levels of efficacy for different species. Choice of treatment depends on number and location of lesions, identification of the infecting organism, and severity of disease [29].

Pentavalent antimonials, including sodium stibogluconate and meglumine antimoniate, are widely considered first-line for systemic treatment, and have had generally favorable outcomes documented in studies [30]. Intravenous sodium stibogluconate 20 mg/kg/day for 20 days demonstrated a 90% cure rate for treatment of American cutaneous leishmaniasis [29]. In addition, pentavalent antimonials are not contraindicated during pregnancy [29, 30]. Adverse effects include arthralgia and myalgia, though older patients are at higher risk of cardiotoxicity and renal failure [30]. Infection with *L. brasiliensis* in particular requires full systemic treatment with either sodium stibogluconate or meglumine antimoniate through either intravenous or intramuscular injection at a dose of 20 mg/kg for 21–28 days [4, 29].

Intravenous amphotericin B (3 mg/kg/day for 7 doses given on days 1–5, 14, and 21) has also been shown to be effective, with a reported cure rate of 84% per a retrospective review by Wortmann et al., though side effects including renal toxicity may limit its use [29–32].

Pentamidine (4 mg/kg/day; maximum dose of 2.0 g) has been shown to have similar efficacy to antimonial drugs, but carries the risk of hypoglycemia and hyperglycemia [30]. Miltefosine (2.5 mg/kg/day for a total of 28 days) has some evidence for its efficacy against several species of *Leishmania*, including *L. v. panamensis*, *L. v. gluyanensis*, and *L. v. braziliensis*, but is contraindicated for use in pregnant women due to teratogenic effects in animal studies [4, 30, 33]. More common side effects include nausea, vomiting, diarrhea, and anorexia [34, 35].

Leishmaniasis, Visceral

Visceral leishmaniasis, also caused by *Leishmania donovani* spp. commonly presents with systemic symptoms and splenomegaly, and may occasionally present with cutaneous manifestations including a primary skin sore, hyperpigmentation, a papular rash, or pruritic necrotic lesions [4, 36, 37]. Preferred treatment is with intravenous liposomal amphotericin B (5–20 mg/kg total, given as 4–10 doses over 10–20 days), which has an efficacy over 97% [38, 39]. Intravenous amphotericin B has an efficacy of over 90%, but carries significant risk of nephrotoxicity, supporting the preferred use of liposomal amphotericin B [39]. Oral miltefosine is an effective but cheaper option, dosed as 1.5–2.5 mg/day for 28 days, with an efficacy between 94 and 97% [39]. However, miltefosine is contraindicated for use in pregnant women due to potential teratogenicity [39]. Miltefosine in combination with amphotericin B (at a maximal dose of 0.5 mg/kg/dose) or paromomycin sulfate (maximal dose of 63 mg/kg/dose) has also been used successfully [40]. Paromomycin sulfate (15 mg/kg/day IM for 21 days) has been found to have 94% efficacy in India, but lower efficacy ranging from 46 to 85% in Africa [39]. Reported adverse effects include ototoxicity, nephrotoxicity, and hepatotoxicity [39]. Pentavalent antimonials including meglumine amnionate and sodium stibogluconate (20 mg/kg/day for 30 days), were long used as preferred treatment, but have fallen out of favor due to significant adverse effect profile, including cardiotoxicity, nephrotoxicity, hepatotoxicity, and pancreatitis, requiring hospitalization and monitoring [39]. Sitamiquine is a newer drug with several studies reporting cure rates ranging from 50 to 100%, given as a dose of 1–3 mg/kg/day orally for approximately 1 month [38]. Headache and abdominal pain are commonly experienced adverse effects, with rare reports of nephrotoxicity at higher doses [38].

Amoebiasis

Cutaneous amoebiasis is a rare condition caused by entry of typically one of three amoebic species, *Entamoeba histolytica*, *Acanthamoeba castellani*, or *Balamuthia mandrillaris*. Cystic forms of the organisms can enter lung or skin tissue but it is the trophozoites (which can also be acquired into open wounds or through sexual contact) that are pathogenic in some immunocompromised patients [41, 42]. Cutaneous amoebiasis can present in many ways but the most common manifestation is an ulceronecrotic nodule. Treatment with antiamoebics is necessary to prevent invasion beyond the skin into the subcutaneous tissues [4, 43].

First-line treatment for *E. histolytica* is with oral metronidazole (750 mg orally every 8 h for 10 days) or IV metronidazole (1500 mg/day in three doses for 10 days, though effective treatment from 3 to 28 days has been reported) for severe or invasive disease [41, 44–46]. Oral metronidazole should be taken with a luminal agent to combat colonization, such as paromomycin (30 mg/kg/day orally in three divided doses for 5–10 days), diloxanide furoate (500 mg orally three times a day for 10 days), diiodohydroxyquin (650 mg orally three times a day for 21 days), or iodoquinol (650 mg orally three times a day for 20 days) [4, 45]. Beyond the more commonly experienced side effects of nausea, vomiting, and diarrhea, patients may experience a disulfiram-like reaction with alcohol consumption, or more rarely peripheral neuropathies or central nervous system toxicity [45].

Alternative treatment options include nitazoxanide (500 mg orally twice daily for age ≥12; 200 mg twice daily for ages 4–11, 100 mg twice daily for ages 1–3; all for 3–10 days), tinidazole (2 g orally daily for 3–5 days), pentamidine (4 mg/kg/day IM until resolution of lesions), emetine hydrochloride (1–1.5 mg/kg daily for up to 90 days if oral, or 5–10 days if IV/SC), and diloxanide (500 mg orally three times per day for 10 days) [47–52].

The treatment of *Balamuthia* is less straightforward, though a review article from Peru suggests first-line therapy with combination miltefosine (2 mg/kg/day), albendazole (800 mg/day), and fluconazole (8 mg/kg/day) [53]. Other suggested therapies for *Balamuthia* have included various combinations of amphotericin B, fluconazole or itraconazole, metronidazole, flucytosine, pentamidine, sulfadiazine, azithromycin or clarithromycin, and albendazole [54, 55]. Eleven cases are detailed in the largest case series to-date, with varying results using combinations of one to all of the aforementioned agents [55]. Documented cases of successful treatment are sparse given the low survival rates with this infection, but the majority of successfully treated cases have occurred as a result of using multidrug therapy.

When dealing with an *Acanthamoeba* infection, most physicians employ two therapies simultaneously: amphotericin B with either itraconazole or voriconazole. However, as is the case with *Balamuthia* infections, many different therapeutic modalities have been attempted, including miconazole, clotrimazole, ketoconazole, fluconazole, itraconazole, pentamidine, sulfadiazine, and 5-flucytosine (Table 42.1).

Table 42.1 Compilation of reported therapies for *Acanthamoeba* infection and outcomes of treatment

Article	Regimen	Number of patients	Outcome
Morrison et al. [56]	Ketoconazole 2% topical cream and topical silver sulfadiazine	1	New lesions developed daily, and it was decided they were too numerous and widespread for surgical debridement.
Galarza et al. [57]	Treatment with itraconazole and amphotericin B (dosages not clarified) has shown partial resolution of skin lesions in several immunocompromised patients	3	Good clinical response and partial remission of lesions, but they succumbed to opportunistic infections (disseminated cryptococcosis and miliary tuberculosis)
Walia et al. [58]	Intravenous amphotericin B lipid complex (ABLC) 7 mg/kg/day and intravenous voriconazole 6 mg/kg twice daily for the first 2 doses, followed by 4 mg/kg twice daily	1	Lead to improvement of symptoms within 1 week (significant reduction in the tenderness and erythema around the lesions and no new lesions erupted on this regimen)
Slater et al. [59]	IV pentamidine isethionate (4 mg/kg/day) for 4 weeks (total dose of 2700 mg). Topical therapy consisted of morning and evening cleansing of all skin lesions with chlorhexidine gluconate, followed by 2% ketoconazole cream	1	Eight months after the start of treatment, all skin lesions were fully healed and there was continued improvement in the patient's stamina and well-being
Aichelburg et al. [60]	Treatment included a combination of parenteral trimethoprim/sulfamethoxazole (later changed to oral sulfadiazine) and parenteral fluconazole. As skin lesions were also gaining size, treatment with miltefosine was initiated topically as a solution, 60 mg/mL, 1 drop applied directly to each skin lesion 2 times a day. After 3 weeks during which dramatic improvement in skin lesions were noted, topical miltefosine was switched to oral miltefosine 100 mg/day (2.5 mg/kg)	1	After 1 year, acanthamoebae could not be detected on PCR, and serologic titers (High IgG and IgM against *Acanthamoeba* spp.) were normal
Helton et al. [61]	40 mg of 5-fluorocytosine per kg for 2 weeks in an AIDS patient with cutaneous and sinus lesions	1	Resolution of all skin lesions within 2 weeks of treatment
Seijo et al. [62]	Sulfadiazine (500 mg four times a day) and pyrimethamine (50 mg once a day), fluconazole (200 mg twice daily), fluconazole (200 mg twice daily) in an AIDS patient	1	Surgical mass removal for granulomatous amebic encephalitis due to *Acanthamoeba castellanii* was performed in addition to medical treatment, with a full recovery other than a left homonymous hemianopsia

Ancylostomiasis, Ascariasis, and Cutaneous Larva Migrans

Ancylostomiasis, also referred to as hookworm infection, is most commonly caused by *Ancyclostoma duodenale* and *Necator americanus*. Cutaneous manifestations caused by larva entry into the skin include severe pruritus and papulovesicular rash [63]. The most common treatments are the benzimidazoles albendazole (400 mg orally daily for 3 days) and mebendazole (100 mg orally twice daily for 3 days) [64, 65]. A meta-analysis examining the efficacy of single-dose oral albendazole, mebendazole, and pyrantel pamoate against hookworm infections determined 72, 15, and 31% efficacy, respectively. All three drugs are generally well tolerated, with abdominal pain, nausea, vomiting, and diarrhea being the most common reported side effects [64]. Albendazole and mebendazole have had teratogenic effects reported in experimental studies [66, 67]; however no significant increase in congenital defects has been established with use of either drug in pregnant patients [68]. Additionally, pruritus can be controlled with oral antihistamines or combination crotamiton and 1% hydrocortisone cream [4].

Both single-dose and triple-dose therapy with albendazole and mebendazole are highly efficacious for treatment of *Ascaris lumbricoides* as well, another parasite known to cause cutaneous larva migrans [65]. More commonly it causes Ascariasis, a helminthic infection in which roundworms cohabitate in the gut and lung of about one billion people worldwide. A meta-analysis of 20 randomized controlled trials examining treatment of ascariasis with single-dose oral albendazole, mebendazole, and pyrantel pamoate, reported 88, 95, and 88% efficacy, respectively [64].

Cutaneous larva migrans is a condition caused by hookworm larvae that migrate through the upper dermis, leaving serpiginous tracks ("creeping eruption" sign) that can cause pain and severe pruritus [41, 69]. Causative organisms include *Ancylostoma brasiliense, Ancylostoma caninum, Ancylostoma ceylonicum, Unicararia stenocephala, Bubostumum phlebotomum*, and occasionally other non-hookworm species including the roundworm, *Ascaris lumbricoides* [4, 41, 69]. Cutaneous larva migrans is a self-limiting condition, but anthelmintic treatment with ivermectin or albendazole is used to definitively treat the underlying helminthic infection and prevent bacterial superinfection from excoriations caused by scratching [41, 69]. Ivermectin is the treatment of choice, given as a single oral dose (200 μg/kg). Occasionally a second dose may be necessary if the first treatment fails. Oral albendazole is a second-line treatment, requiring a longer treatment period (400 mg daily for 5–7 days) and is generally less efficacious as compared to ivermectin [69–71]. Studies evaluating the cure rate of albendazole for cutaneous larva migrans cite a range from 46 to 100% while cure rate for ivermectin has been cited at 77 to 94% [96].

Gnathostomiasis (Larva Migrans Profundus)

Gnathostomiasis, also known as larva migrans profundus, is caused most commonly by *Gnathostoma spinigerum, G. hispidum, and G. binucleatum* nematodes, and may cause both cutaneous and visceral manifestations [72]. Cutaneous gnathostomiasis is commonly characterized by intermittent migratory cutaneous swellings that last for several weeks, most commonly affecting the trunk and upper limbs [72, 73]. Regarding treatment, abscesses or nodules that occur due to superficial larval migration can often be excised [72]. Additionally, albendazole has been shown to be efficacious as treatment at 400 mg orally daily for 21 days, acting both by killing *Gnathostoma* organisms and including outward migration of larvae, facilitating excision [72]. Ivermectin has also been found effective, functioning by paralyzing and killing *Gnathostoma* organisms [72]. A study comparing treatment of albendazole (400 mg orally twice daily for 21 days) versus ivermectin (200 μg/kg daily for 2 days) for gnathostomiasis found similar efficacy between the two drugs (93.8% albendazole, 95.2% ivermectin) [74]. However, one study found higher rates of exacerbation of cutaneous symptoms with ivermectin as compared to albendazole [75].

Toxocariasis (Visceral and Ocular Larva Migrans)

Toxocariasis is an infection from either *Toxocara canis* or *Toxocara cati* roundworms, via ingestion of parasite eggs in dog or cat feces [76, 77]. Children under 5 years of age are most commonly affected [77]. The two main manifestations of toxocariasis are visceral larva migrans and ocular larva migrans [77]. Visceral larva migrans varies in presentation, potentially causing liver necrosis, splenomegaly, central nervous system signs, or abdominal symptoms depending on where larva migrate [76, 77]. Cutaneous features may also be present, most commonly urticaria, prurigo, and papular eruptions [4, 77]. Ocular larva migrans occurs when a single larva migrates into the orbit; loss of vision can occur within weeks.

Some cases of toxocariasis may self-resolve [4]. For symptomatic patients, anthelmintic therapy can be initiated, although evidence in support of its efficacy is lacking [78]. Albendazole (400 mg orally twice daily for 5 days) has traditionally been used as a first-line treatment, found to be superior to mebendazole and thiabendazole [77, 78]. Addition of systemic corticosteroids (oral prednisolone, 1 mg/kg/day for 1 month) has been associated with favorable outcomes, particularly in patients with central nervous system or ocular involvement [4, 78–80]. Either topical or systemic corticosteroids can be used to relieve inflammation-associated symptoms [78]. An alternative therapeutic option is diethylcarbamazine (3–4 mg/kg daily for 21 days), shown to have similar efficacy compared to mebendazole (10–25 mg/kg daily for 10–20 days) in one head-to-head study [81].

Strongyloidiasis (Larva Currens)

Strongyloidiasis is most commonly caused by the nematode *S. stercoralis*, or less commonly by *S. fulleborni* [41]. Infected patients may often be asymptomatic or present with gastrointestinal symptoms, but cutaneous manifestations may occur due to larval migration to the skin, termed "larva currens" [41, 82]. Larva currens typically presents as a linear or serpiginous rash associated with urticaria, which rapidly migrates at a rate significantly faster than larva migrans (up to 10–15 cm/h) [41]. Preferred treatment is with a single dose of oral ivermectin 0.2 mg/kg, although 2 days of treatment may be necessary in some cases to eradicate the infection [41, 82]. Reported cure rates for 2-day treatment with ivermectin range from 70 to 85% [83]. Stercoralis-specific antibodies should be checked for 1–2 years after treatment to evaluate the effectiveness of treatment, since occasionally infections may continue to persist [84]. Alternative treatment options include albendazole or thiabendazole. Commonly used dosing regimens include albendazole 400 mg orally twice a day for 7–14 days and thiabendazole 25 mg/kg orally twice a day for 3–7 days (3000 mg/day maximum) [83, 85, 86]. One comparative trial of single-dose ivermectin (200 µg/kg) versus 3-day treatment with albendazole (400 mg/day for 3 days) found cure rates of 83 and 45%, respectively [87]. Incidence of adverse events between ivermectin and albendazole is comparable [88]. Weak evidence exists suggesting that thiabendazole (50 mg/kg/day divided every 12 h (maximum 3 g/day) for 2 days) may be as effective as ivermectin for treatment of strongyloidiasis, but thiabendazole was associated with higher rates of adverse events [88].

Lymphatic Filariasis

Lymphatic filariasis, also known as dermatolymphangioadenitis, is an infection caused by *Wuchereria bancrofti*, *Brugia malayi*, and *Brugia timori* [89]. Clinical presentations range from asymptomatic to lymphangioadenitis, also known as elephantitis. The most widely used drug for treatment of lymphatic filariasis has long been diethylcarbamazine (given in increasing dosage over a 14 day course), often given with albendazole [89, 90]. Possible adverse effects include fever, rash, arthralgia, visual disturbances, and acute inflammatory reactions due to destruction of microfilariae, which can be managed with anti-inflammatory and antipyretic medications [91].

Oral ivermectin (400 µg/kg) is a second-line treatment, effective in eliminating microfilariae but not adult worms [92]. As a result, recurrence often occurs, necessitating co-treatment with diethylcarbamazine [92]. Doxycycline, dosed at 100–200 mg/day for 6 weeks, is effective against microfilariae, while 200 mg/day doses for 6 weeks showed efficacy against both microfilariae and macrofilariae, without serious side effects [89, 93, 94]. The mechanism of action involves attacking *Wolbachia*, a bacterial symbiont associated with filarial nematodes, resulting in a significant decrease in filarial antigen levels months after treatment [89, 95]. Evidence of the efficacy of albendazole against macrofilariae is mixed, but combined treatment with single-dose albendazole and diethylcarbamazine has been found effective in reducing prevalence of macrofilariae [89].

Treatment with diethylcarbamazine is contraindicated in patients with coexistent onchocerciasis or loiasis, due to the possibility of triggering a severe inflammatory reaction due to rapid killing of high microfilarial loads (the Mazzotti reaction) [89]. In such cases, medical management must be adjusted. Patients with coexistent onchocerciasis may be treated with single-dose ivermectin for treatment of onchocerciasis first, followed by standard treatment for lymphatic filariasis 1 month later [96, 97]. Patients with coexistent loiasis may be treated first for lymphatic filariasis with doxycycline or albendazole, both of which have no effect on *Loa loa*, followed by standard treatment for loiasis after resolution of lymphatic filariasis [89].

Dirofilariasis

Dirofilariasis refers to an infection by zoonotic parasites in the *Dirofilaria* genus (including *D. repens*, *D. immitus*, and *D. tenuis*). Notably, these parasites often have a symbiotic relationship with the bacteria *Wuchereria bancrofti*, one of the known causes of filariasis and hence a source of some confusion given the similar names between these two disorders. Unlike filariasis, in which patients suffer from debilitating lymphedema, there are two main clinical manifestations of dirofilariasis: pulmonary and subcutaneous dirofilariasis [98]. Subcutaneous dirofilariasis, presents as a slowly growing subcutaneous nodule, though it may also present in the ocular conjunctiva [98]. Cutaneous and ocular lesions are treated by surgical removal [98, 99]. Addition of oral diethylcarbamazine (given in increasing doses over a 14 day period), both with and without oral ivermectin has also been reported as an effective treatment [99]. Common side effects of diethylcarbamazine include lymphadenopathy, rash, urticaria, fever, and proteinuria [100].

Schistosomiasis (Bilharziasis)

Schistosomiasis infection may cause several types of cutaneous manifestations. These include a hypersensitivity reaction to a systemic infection that can present as itching, papular dermatitis, petechiae, or urticaria. The reaction can be so severe so as to mimic a serum-sickness-like reaction; in Japan this is called Kotaya fever. When eggs are deposited in the skin (typically in the genital or perianal skin) granulomas can occur, as can vegetating masses, sinus tracts and nodules [4]. In cercarial dermatitis, also known as "swimmer's itch," direct skin penetration by cercariae occurs [41]. Lesions often present as erythematous papules that are pruritic or asymptomatic [41, 101, 102]. Treatment of cercarial dermatitis includes symptomatic relief of pruritus with oral steroids, topical steroid creams, or oral antihistamines [4, 103, 104].

Praziquantel (20 mg/kg orally three times a day for 1 day) remains the most effective drug for definitive treatment of all types of schistosomiasis apart from cercarial dermatitis [105]. Common side effects include nausea and abdominal pain, headache, urticaria, and diaphoresis, while uncommon side effects include a Jarisch-Herxheimer-like reaction, arrhythmia, seizures, and hypersensitivity reaction.

Cysticercosis

Cysticercosis, caused by larval *Taenia solium*, presents with cutaneous manifestations in about half of cases, as subcutaneous nodules primarily on the trunk and extremities containing cysticerci and calcifications [106, 107]. Asymptomatic lesions may be left untreated. There is no consensus for a first-line treatment of cutaneous cysticercosis, but symptomatic nodules may be surgically excised or treated with nonsteroidal anti-inflammatory medications [41]. Albendazole, dosed at 15 mg/kg/day for 30 days has also been shown to resolve or decrease the size of subcutaneous nodules [108]. Presence of skin lesions may indicate further involvement of internal organs, and thus the need for further investigation and treatment [4]. Neurocysticercosis can be treated with albendazole (15 mg/kg/day for 7–14 days) or praziquantel (50–100 mg/kg/day divided every 8 h, for 14 days), with the addition of corticosteroids for severe inflammation and antiepileptics for seizure control [41, 109].

Dracunculiasis

Dracunculiasis, also known as Guinea worm disease, is caused by the Guinea worm *Dracunculus medinsis* [110]. Human infection occurs from consumption of water containing fleas infected with Guinea worm larvae [110]. Patients typically remain asymptomatic for 1 year, at which time the worm migrates towards the skin surface, often forming a cord-like lesion that becomes a papule, nodule, or painful enlarging vesicle blister; it can also present as an urticarial rash. Lesions of all types are most common on the lower limbs [110]. As the guinea worm begins emerging from the skin surface, the worm may be manually extracted by winding a few centimeters of the worm each day onto a stick [110]. This process may take days to weeks, as care must be taken to avoid breaking the worm, which may result in severe allergic cellulitis [4, 110]. Because of the significant pain associated with manual extraction of the worm, oral analgesics may be recommended [110]. One study found that 400 mg orally three times daily of metronidazole improves local inflammation and is a helpful adjunctive therapy as it permits therefore easier removal of the worm during the extraction process [111]. Additionally, ointments containing antibiotics may be helpful in preventing secondary infections [112]. Surgical extraction can also be employed in select cases.

Anthelmintics are generally regarded as unhelpful for eradication of the worm and may even prevent surfacing of the worm and aberrant migration to other areas of the body [110, 113]. Only one placebo-controlled study found that treatment with metronidazole (30–40 mg/kg for 3 days) or thiabendazole (50 or 100 mg/kg for 2 days) resulted in faster elimination of the worm as compared to placebo, but the difference in elimination rates was not statistically significant [114]. It should also be noted that while this study and the aforementioned study showed a trend for improved worm extraction rates in patients on concomitant metronidazole, numerous other studies have been published showing no such benefit.

Loiasis

Loiasis is caused by the filarial parasite *Loa loa*, which is transmitted by *Chrysops* fly bite [115]. While most cases are asymptomatic, some patients manifest with Calabar swellings, which are edematous and often painful and urticarial swellings caused by migration of larvae [115]. As for dracunculiasis, treatment involves surgical removal of large microfilariae, but in contrast this should be done quickly and in conjunction with medical management. Oral diethylcarbamazine 2 mg/kg three times a day for 3 weeks is the preferred treatment, effective against both microfilariae and macrofilariae [89, 115]. Oral albendazole 200 mg twice daily or mebendazole 300 mg daily for 3 weeks can be used as second-line treatments [115]. Oral ivermectin 200 µg/kg for 2 days is a third-line treatment, due to potential for neurologic side effects in patients with high filarial load and lack of effect on macrofilariae [115, 116]. In endemic regions in Africa, diethylcarbamazine is also used prophylactically, at a dose of 300 mg orally weekly [117]. Treatment of patients with loiasis coexistent with lymphatic filariasis or onchocerciasis is discussed below.

Onchocerciasis

Onchocerciasis, also known as "river blindness" and "Robles disease," is caused by infection with the filarial nematode *Onchocerca volvulus*. Skin manifestations vary widely, including but not limited to rashes of different morphologies, lichenification, atrophy, depigmented patches, and subcutaneous nodules [118]. When left untreated about 5% of patients will develop blindness in the end stages of the disease. The mainstay of treatment is with oral ivermectin, given as a single dose of 100–200 μg/kg on an empty stomach and repeated every 3–6 months until the patient is asymptomatic [119, 120]. Doxycycline has also emerged as a useful therapeutic agent by targeting *Wolbachia*, a endobacterial symbiont associated with *Onchocerca volvulus* [121]. Drawbacks of treatment with doxycycline include long course of treatment (daily treatment over 4–6 weeks) and contraindication in pregnant patients and children of the age of 8 or less [121]. Rifampicin has been shown to reduce microfilariae production in animal models, but studies in humans are lacking, and existing studies do not provide a consensus on its efficacy [122–124]. Patients co-infected with loiasis can be treated with albendazole and doxycycline, due to the potential of serious neurological side effects from treatment with ivermectin [115, 125, 126].

Echinococcosis

Echinococcosis is caused by infection from larval *Echinococcus* species cestodes [127]. The most common presentation is enlargement of the liver due to hydatid cyst formation, usually without any changes in the overlying skin [4, 127]. However, several case reports have reported cutaneous findings. Generalized eczema has been reported in one case of a patient with cystic echinococcosis, which resolved with surgical removal of cysts and treatment with albendazole and praziquantel [128]. Abdominal fistulas from larval migration and inflammatory subcutaneous nodules have also been reported in two separate patients, both whom were treated with albendazole, resulting in regression of the lesions [129]. Additionally, urticaria, rash, and angioedema have also been reported following cyst removal [130]. Definitive treatment of echinococcosis consists of surgical removal of cysts and adjuvant chemotherapy with albendazole (400 mg twice daily for 28 days) or mebendazole (40–50 mg/kg per day, administered in three divided doses) [127, 131]. Care must be taken to avoid rupture of the cyst and release of its contents, which may result in allergic reactions, most severely anaphylaxis [127, 130].

Enterobiasis

Enterobiasis, also known as oxyuriasis or pinworm infection, is caused by *Enterobius vermicularis* [67]. This infection primarily affects children and commonly presents with perianal itch [67]. Improvement in hygiene practices may prevent the oral-fecal transmission of the worm [132]. However, pharmacologic therapy is currently the most effective and definitive therapy, regarded as the primary treatment even without changes in hygiene practices [132]. Albendazole, mebendazole, or pyrantel pamoate are the most effective treatments, taken either as a single dose with reported cure rates varying from 60% to over 90%, or preferably as two doses given 2 weeks apart, with cure rates approaching 100% [67, 133, 134].

Alternative treatment options less frequently used include piperazine, ivermectin, and pyrvinium (viprynium) embonate [67]. Single-dose piperazine has been shown to be effective in several studies, with cure rates ranging from 90 to 100% [134–138]. The most common reported side effects include nausea and diarrhea, although urticaria and transient neurological effects have also been reported [132]. Pyrazine is contraindicated in epileptics, can be used with caution in patients with impaired renal function, and should be avoided in pregnant patients [132]. Oral ivermectin is not regularly used, but demonstrated a cure rate of 85% as single-dose treatment in one study, and 100% efficacy when given as two doses taken 10 days apart in another study [139, 140]. Pyrvinium has been shown to be effective as a single dose tablet or suspension with a cure rate of nearly 98%, and also as a double-dose (5.0 mg/kg) taken 2 weeks apart [67, 141–143]. Pyrvinium embonate was well tolerated, but was associated with nausea, vomiting, and diarrhea in several patients [142]. Combination suspension containing piperazine hydrate and pyrvinium pamoate (given as a suspension of 25 mg pyrvinium and 750 mg piperazine per 5 mL teaspoonful, dosed at 0.5 mL/kg, maximum 25 mL/day) was also reported effective in significantly reducing ova count [144].

For close contacts of the infected patient (typically including the patient's family), treatment with a benzimidazole (mebendazole 100 mg tablet, single dose) or pyrantel pamoate (11 mg/kg as a single dose) is also recommended [132]. However, given that it takes 2–3 weeks for eggs to mature into adult worms, these medications are best used 2 weeks after the initial household member is infected [132].

Malaria

Malaria is a parasitic infection caused by members of the protozoan genus *Plasmodium* [145]. Among the many systemic manifestations of the disease, malaria can also present with nonspecific cutaneous manifestations including urticaria, angioedema, erythema, petechiae, and purpura [146]. Cutaneous features often resolve with standard antimalarial treatment, but some may benefit from addition of antihistamines such as cetirizine to hasten resolution of urticaria [146].

Paragonimiasis

Paragonimiasis is a parasitic infection caused by flukes of the *Paragonimus* species (most commonly *P. westermani*), primarily infecting the lung [147]. Patients typically present with acute abdominal and pulmonary symptoms then after 2–3 months develop a cough with sputum production, chest pain, dyspnea, and eosinophilia, though patients over the age of 50 are likelier to be asymptomatic than younger patients [147]. Cutaneous symptoms occur less frequently, but may include pruritic rash and subcutaneous nodules that may progress to cold abscesses, particularly likely with *P. skrjabini* infection [147–149]. The preferred therapeutic agent for pulmonary paragonimiasis is praziquantel, dosed at 75 mg/kg per day in three 8-h doses for 3 days [150]. Three-day treatment has been shown to have a nearly 100% cure rate [83, 149, 151, 152]. However, some patients may require additional treatments with praziquantel or decortication of the lung [149]. Possible side effects of praziquantel include nausea, headache, and dizziness [149, 151]. Triclabendazole (dosed either as 5 mg/kg once daily for 3 days, 10 mg/kg twice on 1 day, or 10 mg/kg in a single dose) has also been shown to be effective, with one study suggesting it is better tolerated than praziquantel (25 mg/kg thrice daily for 3 days) [147, 153]. Unlike praziquantel, triclabendazole also has activity against fascioliasis as well [149, 154]. Patients taking triclabendazole may experience headaches, fevers, nausea, and abdominal pain [154].

Sparganosis

Sparganosis is a parasitic infection caused by tapeworms of the genus *Spirometra*. Larva migration may cause symptoms in various anatomical sites (particularly the eyes and brain), but cutaneous manifestations are the most common presentation [155]. Cutaneous sparganosis typically presents as a slow-growing subcutaneous nodule that may or may not be tender [155, 156]. Complete surgical excision of the lesions is considered curative, and anthelmintic medications have not been proven to be effective [155, 156].

Streptocerciasis

Streptocerciasis is caused by infection with *Mansonella streptocerca*, a parasitic nematode. Most cases are asymptomatic, but cutaneous manifestations may include pruritus, dermatitis, hypopigmented macules, and lymphadenopathy [82]. The absence of subcutaneous nodules is useful for distinguishing streptocerciasis from onchocerciasis, though otherwise the organisms and manifestations are quite similar [82]. Diethylcarbamazine (commonly dosed at 6 mg/kg/day for 12 days) has previously been used as a successful therapeutic option, by killing both microfilariae and adult worms [4, 157]. However, risk of severe systemic reactions in patients co-infected with onchocerciasis has limited its use [157–159]. Now, ivermectin is considered a first-line treatment. Single-dose ivermectin 15 µg/kg has been shown to be effective, with pruritus and dermatitis being common adverse effects [157].

Toxoplasmosis

Toxoplasmosis is caused by consumption of food or water containing *Toxoplasma gondii* cysts [83]. Infected patients may often be asymptomatic, patients may develop lymphadenopathy or a mononucleosis-type syndrome [83]. Congenital infection may lead to chorioretinitis and hydrocephalus, and infection in immunocompromised patients may lead to disseminated disease and encephalitis [160, 161]. Cutaneous manifestations are rare, but reports of a wide variety of clinical presentations of cutaneous toxoplasmosis exists, most commonly diffuse maculopapular rashes on the trunk and extremities and urticaria [4, 162, 163]. Pyrimethamine (100 mg oral loading dose, followed by 25–50 mg/day) with sulfadiazine (2–4 g/day divided 4 times daily) has traditionally been used as first-line treatment for all forms of toxoplasmosis [164]. Pyrimethamine may also be dosed as follows: 200 mg orally once, followed by 50 mg (if <60 kg) or 75 mg (if >60 kg) orally once a day [83].

Combination trimethoprim-sulfamethoxazole (5/25 mg/kg orally or IV every 12 h) is also comparable to pyrimethamine and sulfadiazine for treatment of toxoplasmic encephalitis and chorioretinitis, with the added benefit of being available in intravenous form [83, 164]. Pyrimethamine with clindamycin (600 mg IV every 6 h or 450 mg orally) for toxoplasmic encephalitis and intra-vitreal clindamycin with dexamethasone for ocular toxoplasmosis have both been shown to be comparable to pyrimethamine with sulfadiazine [164]. One randomized double-blind trial found trimethoprim with sulfamethoxazole superior to placebo for treatment of toxoplasmic lymphadenopathy [164]. Treatment with pyrimethamine and/or sulfamethoxazole requires supplementation with folate (10–25 mg orally once per day), as the mechanism of action of these drugs involves interfering with folate metabolism [4, 83]. Case reports of cutaneous toxoplasmosis have documented successful treatment with sulfonamide alone, pyrimethamine with sulfadiazine, and combination pyrimethamine with trimethoprim-sulfamethoxazole [162].

Trichinellosis

Trichinellosis, also called trichinosis, is caused consumption of raw or undercooked meat containing nematodes belonging to the *Trichinella* genus. Most cases present with myalgia, and patients may also dermatologic manifestations including periorbital edema, urticarial exanthem, and nailbed splinter hemorrhages [4, 82]. Most infections resolve on their own without complications, but early treatment is recommended immediately after diagnosis to reduce the incidence of complications, including central nervous system, cardiac, or pulmonary involvement, and prevent maturation of larvae [165]. Treatment is usually with a benzimidazole plus a corticosteroid [165]. Albendazole (400 mg twice daily for 8–14 days) and mebendazole (200–400 mg three times daily for 3 days, followed by 400–500 mg three times daily for 10 days) are effective for treatment of children and adults, but are contraindicated in pregnancy [165]. Albendazole is often preferred as it does not require monitoring of blood levels, unlike treatment with mebendazole which may result in varying plasma levels [165]. Thiabendazole (2 doses per day for 2–4 successive days according to the response of the patient) is an alternative option. It is dosed according to weight. According to the manufacturer's label, dosing of thiabendazole for a 50-pound child would be one tablet (500 mg), or 5 mL (one teaspoon), orally daily. A one-hundred-pound patient would receive a dose of 2 tablets (1 g) or 10 mL (two teaspoons). Any patient who weighs over 150 pounds should receive three pills by mouth (1.5 g), or 15 mL (three teaspoons).

One study comparing thiabendazole (45 ± 7.3 mg/kg daily for 6.1 ± 1.7 days) to albendazole (13 ± 2.6 mg/kg daily for 8 days) found similar efficacy, but albendazole was better tolerated [166]. Thiabendazoles are often used concomitantly with corticosteroids, frequently prednisone, to alleviate allergic reactions and inflammatory responses secondary to larval migration [4, 82].

Trichomoniasis

Trichomoniasis is a common sexually transmitted infection caused by *Trichomonas vaginalis* [83, 167]. The majority of infected patients are asymptomatic. Women may present with dysuria, urethral discharge, and pruritus, while men typically have asymptomatic urethritis, occasionally balani-

tis, epididymitis, prostatitis [167, 168]. Oral single-dose metronidazole has long been used as standard treatment, with a week-long course given as a second-line option [4, 167]. Cure rates of single-dose metronidazole from several studies have ranged from 77.9 to 95%, but recently, other nitroimidazoles have had higher reported success rates [169, 170]. Single-dose tinidazole, ornidazole, and secnidazole have all been shown to have higher cure rates than metronidazole in one comparative study (cure rates of 97.7, 97.7, 80.2% respectively, compared to 77.9% for metronidazole) [170].

However, tinidazole, ornidazole, and secnidazole are typically at least 3–4 times the cost of metronidazole, and thus are used less frequently.

Another study comparing 7-day courses of metronidazole versus tinidazole found similar cure rates, and comparable side effect profiles [170, 171]. As such, use of these newer nitroimidazoles is falling into favor for treatment of trichomoniasis. Additionally, it is important to note that sexual partners should also be treated (single-dose tinidazole 2 g or metronidazole 2 g) to prevent reinfection as well [167].

African Trypansomiasis

Trypanosomiasis manifests as two different forms: African trypanosomiasis caused by *Trypanosoma brucei* subspecies, and American trypanosomiasis caused by *Trypanosoma cruzii*, also known as Chagas disease [83]. Cutaneous manifestations of African trypanosomiasis include a chancre in the first stage, distinctive urticarial, erythematous, or petechial rashes in the second stage, and occasionally pruritus in the third stage [172, 173].

Pentamidine and suramin are effective for treatment of first-stage *T. b. gambiense*, but pentamidine is preferred due to more favorable adverse effect profile as compared to suramin [174]. Pentamidine is typically administered as intramuscular injections dosed at 4 mg/kg daily for 7–10 days [174]. Adverse effects associated with pentamidine include hypotension, hypoglycemia, nephrotoxicity, leukopenia, and rarely hepatitis, pancreatitis, and Stevens-Johnson syndrome [41, 174]. Preferred treatment for first-stage trypanosomiasis caused by *T. b. rhodesiense* is with suramin, which is significantly more effective than pentamidine, with no reports of resistance [41, 174]. Suramin is administered intravenously as 20 mg/kg every 3–7 days over 4 weeks [174]. Potential adverse effects include nausea, anemia, neuropathy, renal failure, and anaphylactic shock, although the risk may be lowered by slow infusion at a rate under 1 g per injection [174]. An alternative option is nifurtimox, which has been shown to be effective against *T. b. gambiense*, but poorly effective against *T. b. rhodesiense* [174]. Nifurtimox for treatment of African trypanosomiasis is commonly dosed at

15 mg/kg/day for 60 days, but one clinical trial found that 30 mg/kg/day for 30 days was more efficacious, but at the expense of significant toxicity (including neurotoxicity and death) [175, 176].

Second-stage disease can be treated with melarsoprol, eflornithine, or nifurtimox. Melarsoprol (most commonly dosed as approximately 2.2 mg/kg per day over a period of 10 days) had previously been the first-line treatment for both subspecies of *T. brucei*, but is being replaced by eflornithine (56 intravenous infusions at 100 mg/kg (150 mg/kg for children) every 6 h a day for a total of 14 days; alternatively, 28 intravenous infusions at 100 mg/kg every 6 h a day for a total of 7 days) and combination eflornithine-nifurtimox (three daily oral doses of nifurtimox for a total of 10 days and 14 infusions of eflornithine for a total of 7 days) for treatment of *T. b. gambiense* due to more favorable safety profiles, as well as increased resistance to melarsoprol [174]. Melarsoprol may be highly toxic as it contains an arsenic group, potentially resulting in post-treatment reactive encephalopathy, characterized by nausea, vomiting, dizziness, and even seizures [174]. Survival rates of post-treatment reactive encephalopathy are near 50%, although potential treatments include corticosteroids, azathioprine, eflornithine, and substance P agonists [174]. Eflornithine is more efficacious than melarsoprol for treatment of *T. b. gambiense*, and more so when given in combination with nifurtimox [174, 177]. Common adverse effects of eflornithine include diarrhea, fever, headaches, dizziness, hypertension, peripheral neuropathy, rash, and myelosuppression, which are usually reversible upon decreasing the dose [41, 174]. Nifurtimox alone is a poorer alternative against *T. b. gambiense* (reported cure rates ranging from 50 to 80%), with significant toxicities [174]. Combination melarsoprol and nifurtimox has been shown to be more effective than melarsoprol monotherapy for second-stage disease, but would benefit from further studies demonstrating its efficacy [178]. Finally, combination eflornithine and melarsoprol may be useful for late-stage disease involving the central nervous system as both drugs can pass the blood–brain barrier, unlike pentamidine and suramin [41].

American Trypanosomiasis

American trypanosomiasis is often asymptomatic during acute infection, but may present with unilateral palpebral edema (Romaña's sign), regional lymphadenopathy, an indurated skin lesion, or a variety of exanthems [4, 41, 179]. Treatment of American trypanosomiasis with benznidazole or nifurtimox has been shown to be effective, though benznidazole is preferred to do a more favorable side effect profile [179]. Benznidazole is dosed at 5 mg/kg orally daily in two divided doses for 60 days, with potential adverse effects including peripheral neuropathy, bone marrow suppression, and skin changes ranging from photosensitive rashes to exfoliative dermatitis [179]. Treatment with nifurtimox lasts between 90 and 120 days, and dosing with nifurtimox varies by age: 8–10 mg/kg orally daily in adults, 10–12.5 mg/kg daily in adolescents, and 15–20 mg/kg daily divided into four doses for children [179].

Drug	Serious side effect(s)	Number of reported cases	Contraindications	Monitoring parameters
Albendazole	Hepatitis/liver injury	8 [220–226]	Pregnancy	CBC and LFTs prior to each 28-day treatment cycle, every 2 weeks during cycle, more frequently if liver disease
	SJS	3 [227, 228]	Hepatic disease	Ophthalmic exam in pts. w/neurocysticercosis. Pregnancy test prior
	Acute renal failure	1 [229]		
	Aplastic anemia/cytopenia	2 [222, 230]		
	Erythema multiforme	5 [227]		
Amphotericin B	Nephrotoxicity/renal failure	–	Severe renal impairment	Baseline and frequent BUN and Cr, CBC, electrolytes, LFTs, PT/PTT
	Seizures	1 [285]		Monitor for signs of hypokalemia
	Arrhythmias	7 [286–291]		
	Hepatotoxicity	40 [292–297]		
	Agranulocytosis (in patients treated with flucytosine concurrently)	1 [298]		
	Hemorrhagic gastroenteritis	–		
	Anaphylaxis	7 [299–304]		
	Cardiac failure/ cardiotoxicity/cardiac arrest	9 [305–309]	Congenital long QT syndrome	BUN/Cr and glucose as baseline, throughout treatment, and periodically after treatment
Benznidazole	Leukopenia	–	Pregnancy	Initial CBC, electrolytes, LFTs
	Thrombocytopenia	–	Hepatic disease	CBC every 2 weeks throughout duration of therapy
	Seizures	–	Renal disease	
Benzyl benzoate	–			–
Crotamiton	–		–	–
Diethylcarbamazine	Orchitis		–	CBC, BMP, UA during first 2 weeks of therapy
	Epididymitis			Ophthalmologic examination in patients with onchocerciasis or Loa loa
	Lymphangitis	2 [249]		
Doxycycline	Vasculitis		Pregnancy	BUN/Cr, CBC, LFTs, UA, chest radiograph for prolonged treatment
	Hepatitis	2 [250, 251]	Age <8	ANA, LFTs if drug-induced lupus
	Transaminitis	6 [252]	Severe hepatic impairment	
	Pseudotumor cerebri	11 [253–256]		
	Jarisch-Herxheimer reaction	2 [257, 258]		
	Esophagitis	24 [259–263]		
	Esophageal ulcer	1 [264]		
	Nephrotoxicity	1 [265]		
	Pancreatitis	7 [266–272]		
	Pericarditis			
	Thrombocytopenia	1 [273]		
	Neutropenia			
	Hemolytic anemia			
	Fungal infection			
Eflornithine	Seizures	9 [405]; 6 patients in study with nifurtimox-eflornithine combination [177]	–	CBC at baseline, twice weekly, and posttreatment
Ivermectin	Hepatitis	2 [180, 181]	Breastfeeding	–
	Leukopenia/anemia		Hepatic disease	
	SJS/TEN		Renal disease	
	Severe neurologic disease (e.g., coma) in patients with onchocerciasis		Children <5 of age or weight <15 kg	
	Seizures		Co-infection with onchocerciasis	

(continued)

Drug	Serious side effect(s)	Number of reported cases	Contraindications	Monitoring parameters
Lindane	Seizures, hypoxemia	1 [182]	Premature neonates	
	Aplastic anemia/ pancytopenia	6 [183–188]	History of uncontrolled seizures	
Malathion	Second-degree burn		Neonates	–
Mebendazole	Seizures	1 [231]	–	CBC prior to each cycle and every 2 weeks if current hepatic disease
	Neutropenia	2 [232, 233]		LFTs prior to each treatment cycle
	Hepatitis	2 [234, 235]		Screen at baseline for retinal lesions if neurocysticercosis infection
	Agranulocytosis	2 [236]		
	Marrow aplasia	1 [237]		
	Angioedema	1 [238]		
Meglumine antimoniate	Arrhythmia	3 [278–280]	–	CBC, LFTs, amylase, lipase, renal function tests prior to treatment and weekly during treatment
	Hepatotoxicity	2 [281]		ECG twice weekly starting 3rd week of treatment
	Pancreatitis	12 [281]		
	Pancytopenia	1 [281]		
	Nephrotoxicity	19 [277, 281–284]		
Melarsoprol	Hepatitis		G6PD	CSF evaluation prior to and during treatment (leukocyte count, protein content, presence of trypanosomes)
	Myocardial damage/heart failure/arrhythmia		During influenza epidemic (risk of RAE)	Continuous CSF evaluation every 6 months for at least 3 years after treatment
	Reactive arsenical encephalopathy (RAE)	118 [399–403] (Haller: 38/588 patients [403]; Kuepfer: 9/78 patients [404])		
	Renal failure			
	Hyperhemolytic reaction in patients with G6PD deficiency			
	Jarisch-Herxheimer-type reaction			
	Hypertension			
	Blood dyscrasias (e.g., agranulocytosis, aplastic anemia)			
	Hemorrhagic encephalopathy			
Metronidazole	Disulfiram-like reaction		1st trimester pregnancy	Baseline Cr and CBC + diff; CBC + diff after treatment
	SJS/TEN (risk higher with concomitant mebendazole use, odds ratio of 9.5 in a study with 46 SJS/TEN patients, 92 controls [195])	5 [190–194]		Closely monitor INR if on warfarin
	Encephalopathy	17 [196–211]		
	Aseptic meningitis	3 [212–214]		
	Cerebellar dysfunction	48 [215]		
	AMS	21 [215]		
	Seizures	9 [215, 216]		
	Leukopenia	17 [217–219]		
Miltefosine	SJS		Pregnancy	Baseline pregnancy test
	Agranulocytosis		Sjogren-Larsson syndrome	BUN/Cr every 4 weeks during and 4 weeks after tx
				Platelet count if used for visceral leishmaniasis
Monosulfram	Disulfiram-like reaction	1 [189]	–	–
Nifurtimox	Peripheral neuropathy	6/53 patients [406]	Pregnancy	

Drug	Serious side effect(s)	Number of reported cases	Contraindications	Monitoring parameters
	Angioedema	1/81 patients [407]	Advanced cardiac progression	
	Acute myocarditis	1/81 patients [407]	Hepatic impairment	
	Anaphylaxis	1/81 patients [407]	Renal impairment	
Ornidazole	Seizure		–	–
	Hepatic impairment	12 [244–246]		
Paromomycin sulfate	Nephrotoxicity	4 [408]	GI obstruction	Bun/Cr and eighth nerve function frequently in patients with suspected renal impairment
	Transaminitis/ hepatotoxicity	41 [408]	Pregnancy	
	Ototoxicity	7 [408]		
	Neurotoxicity	–		
	Neuromuscular blockade	–		
Pentamidine	Hypoglycemia/ hyperglycemia/diabetes	64 [309–314]	Uncorrected electrolyte abnormalities	Ca, CBC, platelets, LFTs, ECG at baseline, periodically during treatment, and after treatment
	Pancreatitis	13 [309, 312, 314–321]		BP during administration, repeat until stable
	Renal failure/nephrotoxicity	58 [310, 322–324]		
	Hypotension	64/82 (78%) IM, 44/66 (67%) IV group [325]	64/82 (78%) IM, 44/66 (67%) IV group	
	Ventricular tachycardia/ torsades dc pointes	4 [326–328]		
	SJS	2 [329, 330]		
	Hepatitis	1 [331]		
	Anaphylaxis	2 [332]		
Permethrin	Seizures		–	–
Piperazine	Hemolytic anemia		Seizure disorders	–
	Seizures		Hepatic impairment	
			Renal impairment	
Praziquantel	Hepatitis		Ocular cysticercosis (hypersensitivity/CSF reaction syndrome), ocular schistosomiasis, seizure hx, CNS lesions	ECG if history of arrhythmia, LFTs, culture urine or feces for ova prior to initiating therapy
	Polyserositis	1 [247]		Monitor for seizures
	Jarisch-Herxheimer reaction			
	Seizures	1 [248]		
	AV block			
	Cardiac arrhythmias			
Pyrantel pamoate	–		Hepatic impairment	Serum AST and ALT
Pyrimethamine	SJS/TEN	2 [333, 334]	Megaloblastic anemia	CBC and platelets twice weekly if high-dose tx for toxoplasmosis
	Anaphylaxis			
	Pancytopenia	4 [335–338]		
	Seizures	2 [339]		
Secnidazole	Transient cytopenias		–	Closely monitor INR if on warfarin
	Seizures			
	QT interval prolongation			
Sodium stibogluconate	Pancreatitis		Severe renal impairment	Lipase and amylase twice weekly
	Venous thrombosis			ECG during injection
	Anaphylaxis			Consider CBC, BMP, LFT in high-risk patients
	ECG changes	[274]		ECG and BMP (for potassium monitoring) at least once per week in pts. >40 of age or with cardiac conditions

(continued)

Drug	Serious side effect(s)	Number of reported cases	Contraindications	Monitoring parameters
	Hepatotoxicity	10 [275–277]		
Sulfadiazine	SJS/TEN	1 [227]	Pregnancy	Frequent CBC, UA
	Anaphylaxis	2 [340, 341]	Children <2 except for tx of congenital toxoplasmosis	Serum drug levels if serious infection
	Hemolytic anemia	3 [342–344]	Nursing mothers	
	Hepatitis	2 [345, 346]		
	Acute renal failure	10 [8, 347–353]		
	C. difficile-associated diarrhea	2 [354, 355]		
	Lupus erythematosus	1 [356]		
	Methemoglobinemia	4 [357, 358]		
	Kernicterus (in neonates)			
Sulfur	Sulfanamide hypersensitivity		–	–
	SJS/TEN			
Suramin	Severe hypotension/shock	3 [395, 396]	Hepatic function impairment	Regular CBC, Cr
	Seizures		Impaired renal function	UA prior to administration of each dose
	Arrhythmias			
	Renal failure	1 [397]		
	Optic atrophy	6 [398]		
Thiabendazole	Seizures	1 [239]	–	
	SJS/TEN	4 [240, 241]		
	Hepatotoxicity/hepatitis	1 [242]		
	Leukopenia			
	Nephrotoxicity			
Tinidazole	Seizures		Pregnancy 1st trimester	Baseline Cr, WBC + diff if retreatment
	Thrombocytopenia	1 [243]	Breastfeeding	Closely monitor INR if on warfarin
	SJS/TEN		Hepatic impairment	
	Angioedema		Blood dyscrasia	
	Bronchospasm		CNS disorder	
	Erythema multiforme			
	Leukopenia/neutropenia			
TMP-SMX	SJS/TEN	3 [359–361]	Megaloblastic anemia/folate deficiency	BUN/Cr, UA baseline and periodically
	Hepatic necrosis/liver failure	5 [362–366]	Pregnancy	Frequent CBCs
	Agranulocytosis	18 [367–369]	Nursing mothers	K if renal impairment or on ACE inhibitor
	Aplastic anemia	1 [370]	Patients age <2 months	
	Pancreatitis	8 [363, 366, 371–376]	Significant hepatic damage	
	Renal failure/nephrotoxicity/AIN	37 [377–380]	Severe renal dysfunction without renal function monitoring	
	Methemoglobinemia	4 [381–384]	History of thrombocytopenia	
	Aseptic meningitis	42 [368, 385]	G6PD deficiency	
	Seizures			
	Lupus erythematosus	2 [386, 387]		
	C. difficile-associated diarrhea	2 [388]		
	Rhabdomyolysis	6 [389–394]		
	Kernicterus (in neonates)			
Triclabendazole	–		–	–

Case Report

A 38-year-old homeless male presents to clinic with intensely pruritic lesions predominantly on his hands, wrists, and elbows bilaterally. He also has some lesions on the groin and axillae, with sparse lesions elsewhere.

Past Medical History

- None

Social History

- 10-year history of homelessness
- Sleeps in shelters, occasionally on the street

Previous Therapies

- Vaseline

Physical Exam

- Numerous excoriations are present, as well as several erythematous crusted burrows
- Some lesions are arranged in a linear distribution along the flexor aspect of the bilateral wrists
- Similar lesions are also present in several of the interdigital web spaces

Management

Scabies was confirmed by positive skin scraping for mites. The patient was treated with 12 mg (200 µg/mg) single-dose oral ivermectin on day 0, with repeat dosing on day 5. Follow-up 2 weeks after treatment showed significant improvement with near resolution of all lesions and decreased surrounding erythema.

References

1. Andrews RM, McCarthy J, Carapetis JR, Currie BJ. Skin disorders, including pyoderma, scabies, and tinea infections. Pediatr Clin N Am. 2009;56(6):1421–40.
2. Strong M, Johnstone P. Interventions for treating scabies. Cochrane Database Syst Rev. 2007;3:CD000320.
3. Hay RJ. Scabies and pyodermas—diagnosis and treatment. Dermatol Ther. 2009;22(6):466–74.
4. Burns T, Breathnach S, Cox N, Griffiths C. Rook's textbook of dermatology. 8th ed. Hoboken, NJ: Wiley-Blackwell; 2010.
5. Panahi Y, Poursaleh Z, Goldust M. The efficacy of topical and oral ivermectin in the treatment of human scabies. Ann Parasitol. 2015;61(1):11–6.
6. Orzechowski KL, Swain MD, Robl MG, et al. Neurotoxic effects of ivermectin administration in genetically engineered mice with targeted insertion of the mutated canine ABCB1 gene. Am J Vet Res. 2012;73(9):1477–84.
7. Burkhart CN, Burkhart CG. Ivermectin: a few caveats are warranted before initiating therapy for scabies. Arch Dermatol. 1999;135(12):1549–50.
8. Allinson J, Topping W, Edwards SG, Miller RF. Sulphadiazine-induced obstructive renal failure complicating treatment of HIV-associated toxoplasmosis. Int J STD AIDS. 2012;23(3):210–2.
9. Edwards G. Ivermectin: does P-glycoprotein play a role in neurotoxicity? Filaria J. 2003;2(Suppl 1):S8.
10. Pacqué M, Muñoz B, Poetschke G, Foose J, Greene BM, Taylor HR. Pregnancy outcome after inadvertent ivermectin treatment during community-based distribution. Lancet. 1990;336(8729):1486–9.
11. Shimose L, Munoz-Price LS. Diagnosis, prevention, and treatment of scabies. Curr Infect Dis Rep. 2013;15(5):426–31.
12. Dourmishev A, Serafimova D, Dourmishev L. Efficacy and tolerance of oral ivermectin in scabies. J Eur Acad Dermatol Venereol. 1998;11(3):247–51.
13. Chhaiya SB, Patel VJ, Dave JN, Mehta DS, Shah HA. Comparative efficacy and safety of topical permethrin, topical ivermectin, and oral ivermectin in patients of uncomplicated scabies. Indian J Dermatol Venereol Leprol. 2012;78(5):605–10.
14. Goldust M, Rezaee E, Raghifar R, Hemayat S. Comparing the efficacy of oral ivermectin vs malathion 0.5% lotion for the treatment of scabies. Skinmed. 2014;12(5):284–7.
15. Schultz MW, Gomez M, Hansen RC, et al. Comparative study of 5% permethrin cream and 1% lindane lotion for the treatment of scabies. Arch Dermatol. 1990;126(2):167–70.
16. Goldust M, Babae Nejad S, Rezaee E, Raghifar R. Comparative trial of permethrin 5% versus lindane 1% for the treatment of scabies. J Dermatolog Treat. 2013;
17. Zargari O, Golchai J, Sobhani A, et al. Comparison of the efficacy of topical 1% lindane vs 5% permethrin in scabies: a randomized, double-blind study. Indian J Dermatol Venereol Leprol. 2006;72(1):33–6.
18. Bachewar NP, Thawani VR, Mali SN, Gharpure KJ, Shingade VP, Dakhale GN. Comparison of safety, efficacy, and cost effectiveness of benzyl benzoate, permethrin, and ivermectin in patients of scabies. Indian J Pharmacol. 2009;41(1):9–14.
19. Heukelbach J, Feldmeier H. Scabies. Lancet. 2006;367(9524):1767–74.
20. Fujimoto K, Kawasaki Y, Morimoto K, Kikuchi I, Kawana S. Treatment for crusted scabies: limitations and side effects of treatment with ivermectin. J Nippon Med Sch. 2014;81(3):157–63.
21. Chosidow O. Scabies and pediculosis. Lancet. 2000;355(9206):819–26.
22. Idriss S, Levitt J. Malathion for head lice and scabies: treatment and safety considerations. J Drugs Dermatol. 2009;8(8):715–20.
23. Alipour H, Goldust M. The efficacy of oral ivermectin vs. sulfur 10% ointment for the treatment of scabies. Ann Parasitol. 2015;61(2):79–84.
24. Kenawi MZ, Morsy TA, Abdalla KF, el Hady HM. Treatment of human scabies by sulfur and permethrin. J Egypt Soc Parasitol. 1993;23(3):691–6.
25. Sharquie KE, Al-Rawi JR, Noaimi AA, Al-Hassany HM. Treatment of scabies using 8% and 10% topical sulfur ointment in different regimens of application. J Drugs Dermatol. 2012;11(3):357–64.
26. Sule HM, Thacher TD. Comparison of ivermectin and benzyl benzoate lotion for scabies in Nigerian patients. Am J Trop Med Hyg. 2007;76(2):392–5.
27. Buffet M, Dupin N. Current treatments for scabies. Fundam Clin Pharmacol. 2003;17(2):217–25.
28. Berthe-Aucejo A, Prot-Labarthe S, Pull L, et al. Treatment of scabies and Ascabiol(®) supply disruption: what about the pediatric population? Arch Pediatr. 2014;21(6):670–5.
29. Hepburn NC. Cutaneous leishmaniasis: an overview. J Postgrad Med. 2003;49(1):50–4.
30. Goto H, Lindoso JA. Current diagnosis and treatment of cutaneous and mucocutaneous leishmaniasis. Expert Rev Anti-Infect Ther. 2010;8(4):419–33.
31. Amato VS, Rabello A, Rotondo-Silva A, et al. Successful treatment of cutaneous leishmaniasis with lipid formulations of

amphotericin B in two immunocompromised patients. Acta Trop. 2004;92(2):127–32.

32. Wortmann G, Zapor M, Ressner R, et al. Lipsosomal amphotericin B for treatment of cutaneous leishmaniasis. Am J Trop Med Hyg. 2010;83(5):1028–33.

33. Dorlo TP, Balasegaram M, Beijnen JH, de Vries PJ. Miltefosine: a review of its pharmacology and therapeutic efficacy in the treatment of leishmaniasis. J Antimicrob Chemother. 2012;67(11):2576–97.

34. Emad M, Hayati F, Fallahzadeh MK, Namazi MR. Superior efficacy of oral fluconazole 400 mg daily versus oral fluconazole 200 mg daily in the treatment of cutaneous leishmania major infection: a randomized clinical trial. J Am Acad Dermatol. 2011;64(3):606–8.

35. Alrajhi AA, Ibrahim EA, De Vol EB, Khairat M, Faris RM, Maguire JH. Fluconazole for the treatment of cutaneous leishmaniasis caused by Leishmania major. N Engl J Med. 2002;346(12):891–5.

36. Khorvash F, Naeini AE, Behjati M, Abdi F. Visceral leishmaniasis in a patient with cutaneous lesions, negative Leishman-Donovan bodies and immunological test: A case report. J Res Med Sci. 2011;16(11):1507–10.

37. Zijlstra EE, Musa AM, Khalil EA, el-Hassan IM, el-Hassan AM. Post-kala-azar dermal leishmaniasis. Lancet Infect Dis. 2003;3(2):87–98.

38. Moore EM, Lockwood DN. Treatment of visceral leishmaniasis. J Glob Infect Dis. 2010;2(2):151–8.

39. Freitas-Junior LH, Chatelain E, Kim HA, Siqueira-Neto JL. Visceral leishmaniasis treatment: what do we have, what do we need and how to deliver it? Int J Parasitol Drugs Drug Resist. 2012;2:11–9.

40. Seifert K, Croft SL. In vitro and in vivo interactions between miltefosine and other antileishmanial drugs. Antimicrob Agents Chemother. 2006;50(1):73–9.

41. Belizario V, Delos Trinos JP, Garcia NB, Reyes M. Cutaneous manifestations of selected parasitic infections in Western Pacific and Southeast Asian Regions. Curr Infect Dis Rep. 2016;18(9):30.

42. Gee SN, Rothschild B, Click J, Sheth V, Saavedra A, Hsu MY. Tender ulceronecrotic nodules in a patient with leukemia. Cutaneous acanthamebiasis. Arch Dermatol. 2011;147(7):857–62.

43. Fernández-Antón Martínez MC, Alfageme Roldán F, Ciudad Blanco C, Suárez Fernández R. Ustekinumab in the treatment of severe atopic dermatitis: a preliminary report of our experience with 4 patients. Actas Dermosifiliogr. 2014;105(3):312–3.

44. Morán P, Rojas L, Cerritos R, et al. Case report: cutaneous amebiasis: the importance of molecular diagnosis of an emerging parasitic disease. Am J Trop Med Hyg. 2013;88(1):186–90.

45. Stanley SL. Amoebiasis. Lancet. 2003;361(9362):1025–34.

46. Kimura M, Nakamura T, Nawa Y. Experience with intravenous metronidazole to treat moderate-to-severe amebiasis in Japan. Am J Trop Med Hyg. 2007;77(2):381–5.

47. Lupi O, Bartlett BL, Haugen RN, et al. Tropical dermatology: tropical diseases caused by protozoa. J Am Acad Dermatol. 2009;60(6):897–925. quiz 926-898

48. Swami B, Lavakusulu D, Devi CS. Tinidazole and metronidazole in the treatment of intestinal amoebiasis. Curr Med Res Opin. 1977;5(2):152–6.

49. Sra KK, Sracic J, Tyring SK. Treatment of protozoan infections. Dermatol Ther. 2004;17(6):513–6.

50. Rossignol JF, Kabil SM, El-Gohary Y, Younis AM. Nitazoxanide in the treatment of amoebiasis. Trans R Soc Trop Med Hyg. 2007;101(10):1025–31.

51. Parshad S, Grover PS, Sharma A, Verma DK. Primary cutaneous amoebiasis: case report with review of the literature. Int J Dermatol. 2002;41(10):676–80.

52. Ortiz JJ, Ayoub A, Gargala G, Chegne NL, Favennec L. Randomized clinical study of nitazoxanide compared to metronidazole in the treatment of symptomatic giardiasis in children from Northern Peru. Aliment Pharmacol Ther. 2001;15(9):1409–15.

53. Cabello-Vílchez AM, Rodríguez-Zaragoza S, Piñero J, Valladares B, Lorenzo-Morales J. Balamuthia mandrillaris in South America: an emerging potential hidden pathogen in Perú. Exp Parasitol. 2014;145(Suppl):S10–9.

54. Bravo FG, Alvarez PJ, Gotuzzo E. Balamuthia mandrillaris infection of the skin and central nervous system: an emerging disease of concern to many specialties in medicine. Curr Opin Infect Dis. 2011;24(2):112–7.

55. Moriarty P, Burke C, McCrossin D, et al. Balamuthia mandrillaris encephalitis: survival of a child with severe meningoencephalitis and review of the literature. J Pediatric Infect Dis Soc. 2014;3(1):e4–9.

56. Morrison AO, Morris R, Shannon A, Lauer SR, Guarner J, Kraft CS. Disseminated acanthamoeba infection presenting with cutaneous lesions in an immunocompromised patient: a case report, review of histomorphologic findings, and potential diagnostic pitfalls. Am J Clin Pathol. 2016;145(2):266–70.

57. Galarza C, Ramos W, Gutierrez EL, et al. Cutaneous acanthamebiasis infection in immunocompetent and immunocompromised patients. Int J Dermatol. 2009;48(12):1324–9.

58. Walia R, Montoya JG, Visvesvara GS, Booton GC, Doyle RL. A case of successful treatment of cutaneous Acanthamoeba infection in a lung transplant recipient. Transpl Infect Dis. 2007;9(1):51–4.

59. Slater CA, Sickel JZ, Visvesvara GS, Pabico RC, Gaspari AA. Brief report: successful treatment of disseminated acanthamoeba infection in an immunocompromised patient. N Engl J Med. 1994;331(2):85–7.

60. Aichelburg AC, Walochnik J, Assadian O, et al. Successful treatment of disseminated Acanthamoeba sp. infection with miltefosine. Emerg Infect Dis. 2008;14(11):1743–6.

61. Helton J, Loveless M, White CR. Cutaneous acanthamoeba infection associated with leukocytoclastic vasculitis in an AIDS patient. Am J Dermatopathol. 1993;15(2):146–9.

62. Seijo Martinez M, Gonzalez-Mediero G, Santiago P, et al. Granulomatous amebic encephalitis in a patient with AIDS: isolation of acanthamoeba sp. Group II from brain tissue and successful treatment with sulfadiazine and fluconazole. J Clin Microbiol. 2000;38(10):3892–5.

63. Chaudhry AZ, Longworth DL. Cutaneous manifestations of intestinal helminthic infections. Dermatol Clin. 1989;7(2):275–90.

64. Keiser J, Utzinger J. Efficacy of current drugs against soil-transmitted helminth infections: systematic review and meta-analysis. JAMA. 2008;299(16):1937–48.

65. Steinmann P, Utzinger J, ZW D, et al. Efficacy of single-dose and triple-dose albendazole and mebendazole against soil-transmitted helminths and Taenia spp.: a randomized controlled trial. PLoS One. 2011;6(9):e25003.

66. de Silva NR, Sirisena JL, Gunasekera DP, Ismail MM, de Silva HJ. Effect of mebendazole therapy during pregnancy on birth outcome. Lancet. 1999;353(9159):1145–9.

67. Cook GC. Enterobius vermicularis infection. Gut. 1994;35(9):1159–62.

68. Bradley M, Horton J. Assessing the risk of benzimidazole therapy during pregnancy. Trans R Soc Trop Med Hyg. 2001;95(1):72–3.

69. Feldmeier H, Schuster A. Mini review: Hookworm-related cutaneous larva migrans. Eur J Clin Microbiol Infect Dis. 2012;31(6):915–8.

70. Caumes E, Carriere J, Datry A, Gaxotte P, Danis M, Gentilini M. A randomized trial of ivermectin versus albendazole for the treatment of cutaneous larva migrans. Am J Trop Med Hyg. 1993;49(5):641–4.

71. Caumes E. Treatment of cutaneous larva migrans and Toxocara infection. Fundam Clin Pharmacol. 2003;17(2):213–6.

72. Herman JS, Chiodini PL. Gnathostomiasis, another emerging imported disease. Clin Microbiol Rev. 2009;22(3):484–92.

73. Rusnak JM, Lucey DR. Clinical gnathostomiasis: case report and review of the English-language literature. Clin Infect Dis. 1993;16(1):33–50.

74. Nontasut P, Bussaratid V, Chullawichit S, Charoensook N, Visetsuk K. Comparison of ivermectin and albendazole treatment for gnathostomiasis. Southeast Asian J Trop Med Public Health. 2000;31(2):374–7.

75. Kraivichian K, Nuchprayoon S, Sitichalernchai P, Chaicumpa W, Yentakam S. Treatment of cutaneous gnathostomiasis with ivermectin. Am J Trop Med Hyg. 2004;71(5):623–8.

76. Lee RM, Moore LB, Bottazzi ME, Hotez PJ. Toxocariasis in North America: a systematic review. PLoS Negl Trop Dis. 2014;8(8):e3116.

77. Despommier D. Toxocariasis: clinical aspects, epidemiology, medical ecology, and molecular aspects. Clin Microbiol Rev. 2003;16(2):265–72.

78. Ahn SJ, Ryoo NK, Woo SJ. Ocular toxocariasis: clinical features, diagnosis, treatment, and prevention. Asia Pac Allergy. 2014;4(3):134–41.

79. Dinning WJ, Gillespie SH, Cooling RJ, Maizels RM. Toxocariasis: a practical approach to management of ocular disease. Eye (Lond). 1988;2(Pt 5):580–2.

80. Magnaval JF, Glickman LT, Dorchies P, Morassin B. Highlights of human toxocariasis. Korean J Parasitol. 2001;39(1):1–11.

81. Magnaval JF. Comparative efficacy of diethylcarbamazine and mebendazole for the treatment of human toxocariasis. Parasitology. 1995;110(Pt 5):529–33.

82. Lupi O, Downing C, Lee M, et al. Mucocutaneous manifestations of helminth infections: Nematodes. J Am Acad Dermatol. 2015;73(6):929–44. quiz 945-926

83. Kappagoda S, Singh U, Blackburn BG. Antiparasitic therapy. Mayo Clin Proc. 2011;86(6):561–83.

84. Satoh M, Kokaze A. Treatment strategies in controlling strongyloidiasis. Expert Opin Pharmacother. 2004;5(11):2293–301.

85. Pungpak S, Bunnag D, Chindanond D, Radmoyos B. Albendazole in the treatment of strongyloidiasis. Southeast Asian J Trop Med Public Health. 1987;18(2):207–10.

86. Schaffel R, Nucci M, Portugal R, et al. Thiabendazole for the treatment of strongyloidiasis in patients with hematologic malignancies. Clin Infect Dis. 2000;31(3):821–2.

87. Marti H, Haji HJ, Savioli L, et al. A comparative trial of a single-dose ivermectin versus three days of albendazole for treatment of Strongyloides stercoralis and other soil-transmitted helminth infections in children. Am J Trop Med Hyg. 1996;55(5):477–81.

88. Henriquez-Camacho C, Gotuzzo E, Echevarria J, et al. Ivermectin versus albendazole or thiabendazole for Strongyloides stercoralis infection. Cochrane Database Syst Rev. 2016;1:CD007745.

89. Katiyar D, Singh LK. Filariasis: Current status, treatment and recent advances in drug development. Curr Med Chem. 2011;18(14):2174–85.

90. Reddy M, Gill SS, Kalkar SR, Wu W, Anderson PJ, Rochon PA. Oral drug therapy for multiple neglected tropical diseases: a systematic review. JAMA. 2007;298(16):1911–24.

91. Haarbrink M, Terhell AJ, Abadi GK, Mitsui Y, Yazdanbakhsh M. Adverse reactions following diethylcarbamazine (DEC) intake in 'endemic normals', microfilaraemics and elephantiasis patients. Trans R Soc Trop Med Hyg. 1999;93(1):91–6.

92. Moulia-Pelat JP, Nguyen LN, Hascoët H, Luquiaud P, Nicolas L. Advantages of an annual single dose of ivermectin 400 micrograms/kg plus diethylcarbamazine for community treatment of bancroftian filariasis. Trans R Soc Trop Med Hyg. 1995;89(6):682–5.

93. Hoerauf A, Volkmann L, Hamelmann C, et al. Endosymbiotic bacteria in worms as targets for a novel chemotherapy in filariasis. Lancet. 2000;355(9211):1242–3.

94. Taylor MJ. Wolbachia bacteria of filarial nematodes in the pathogenesis of disease and as a target for control. Trans R Soc Trop Med Hyg. 2000;94(6):596–8.

95. Sanprasert V, Sujariyakul A, Nuchprayoon SA. single dose of doxycycline in combination with diethylcarbamazine for treatment of bancroftian filariasis. Southeast Asian J Trop Med Public Health. 2010;41(4):800–12.

96. Greene BM, Taylor HR, Cupp EW, et al. Comparison of ivermectin and diethylcarbamazine in the treatment of onchocerciasis. N Engl J Med. 1985;313(3):133–8.

97. Lariviere M, Vingtain P, Aziz M, et al. Double-blind study of ivermectin and diethylcarbamazine in African onchocerciasis patients with ocular involvement. Lancet. 1985;2(8448):174–7.

98. Simón F, Siles-Lucas M, Morchón R, et al. Human and animal dirofilariasis: the emergence of a zoonotic mosaic. Clin Microbiol Rev. 2012;25(3):507–44.

99. Jelinek T, Schulte-Hillen J, Löscher T. Human dirofilariasis. Int J Dermatol. 1996;35(12):872–5.

100. Taylor HR, Greene BM, Langham ME. Controlled clinical trial of oral and topical diethylcarbamazine in treatment of onchocerciasis. Lancet. 1980;1(8175):943–6.

101. Mota LS, Silva SF, Almeida FC, Mesquita LS, Teixeira RD, Soares AM. Ectopic cutaneous schistosomiasis - case report. An Bras Dermatol. 2014;89(4):646–8.

102. Nunes KM, Cardoso AE, Pereira FS, Batista LH, Houly RL. Ectopic cutaneous schistosomiasis—case report. An Bras Dermatol. 2013;88(6):969–72.

103. Hoeffler DF. Cercarial dermatitis. Arch Environ Health. 1974;29(4):225–9.

104. Centers for Disease Control (CDC). Cercarial dermatitis outbreak at a state park—Delaware, 1991. MMWR Morb Mortal Wkly Rep. 1992;41(14):225–8.

105. GY W, Halim MH. Schistosomiasis: progress and problems. World J Gastroenterol. 2000;6(1):12–9.

106. Wolff K, Goldsmith LA, Katz SI, Gilchrest BA, Paller AS, Leffell DJ. Fitzpatrick's dermatology in general medicine, 2 volumes. Transplantation. 2008; 85(654).

107. Wortman PD. Subcutaneous cysticercosis. J Am Acad Dermatol. 1991;25(2 Pt 2):409–14.

108. Schmidt DK, Jordaan HF, Schneider JW, Cilliers J. Cerebral and subcutaneous cysticercosis treated with albendazole. Int J Dermatol. 1995;34(8):574–9.

109. Kraft R. Cysticercosis: an emerging parasitic disease. Am Fam Physician. 2007;76(1):91–6.

110. Greenaway C. Dracunculiasis (guinea worm disease). CMAJ. 2004;170(4):495–500.

111. Pardanani DS, Trivedi VD, Joshi LG, Daulatram J, Nandi JS. Metronidazole ("Flagyl") in dracunculiasis: a double blind study. Ann Trop Med Parasitol. 1977;71(1):45–52.

112. Magnussen P, Yakubu A, Bloch P. The effect of antibiotic- and hydrocortisone-containing ointments in preventing secondary infections in guinea worm disease. Am J Trop Med Hyg. 1994;51(6):797–9.

113. Belcher DW, Wunapa FK, Ward WB. Failure of thiabendazole and metronidazole in the treatment and suppression of guinea worm disease. Am J Trop Med Hyg. 1975;24(3):444–6.

114. Kale OO, Elemile T, Enahoro F. Controlled comparative trial of thiabendazole and metronidazole in the treatment of dracontiasis. Ann Trop Med Parasitol. 1983;77(2):151–7.

115. Padgett JJ, Jacobsen KH. Loiasis: African eye worm. Trans R Soc Trop Med Hyg. 2008;102(10):983–9.

116. Elgart ML. Onchocerciasis and dracunculosis. Dermatol Clin. 1989;7(2):323–30.

117. Nutman TB, Miller KD, Mulligan M, et al. Diethylcarbamazine prophylaxis for human loiasis. Results of a double-blind study. N Engl J Med. 1988;319(12):752–6.

118. Enk CD. Onchocerciasis—river blindness. Clin Dermatol. 2006;24(3):176–80.

119. Aziz MA, Diallo S, Diop IM, Lariviere M, Porta M. Efficacy and tolerance of ivermectin in human onchocerciasis. Lancet. 1982;2(8291):171–3.

120. Gardon J, Boussinesq M, Kamgno J, Gardon-Wendel N, Demanga-Ngangue DBO. Effects of standard and high doses of ivermectin on adult worms of Onchocerca volvulus: a randomised controlled trial. Lancet. 2002;360(9328):203–10.

121. Taylor MJ, Hoerauf A, Townson S, Slatko BE, Ward SA. Anti-Wolbachia drug discovery and development: safe macrofilaricides for onchocerciasis and lymphatic filariasis. Parasitology. 2014;141(1):119–27.

122. Specht S, Mand S, Marfo-Debrekyei Y, et al. Efficacy of 2- and 4-week rifampicin treatment on the Wolbachia of Onchocerca volvulus. Parasitol Res. 2008;103(6):1303–9.

123. Bah GS, Ward EL, Srivastava A, Trees AJ, Tanya VN, Makepeace BL. Efficacy of three-week oxytetracycline or rifampin monotherapy compared with a combination regimen against the filarial nematode Onchocerca ochengi. Antimicrob Agents Chemother. 2014;58(2):801–10.

124. Hoerauf A. Filariasis: new drugs and new opportunities for lymphatic filariasis and onchocerciasis. Curr Opin Infect Dis. 2008;21(6):673–81.

125. Wanji S, Tendongfor N, Nji T, et al. Community-directed delivery of doxycycline for the treatment of onchocerciasis in areas of co-endemicity with loiasis in Cameroon. Parasit Vectors. 2009;2(1):39.

126. Klion AD, Horton J, Nutman TB. Albendazole therapy for loiasis refractory to diethylcarbamazine treatment. Clin Infect Dis. 1999;29(3):680–2.

127. Moro P, Schantz PM. Echinococcosis: a review. Int J Infect Dis. 2009;13(2):125–33.

128. Velasco-Tirado V, Yuste-Chaves M, Belhassen-García M. Cutaneous disease as the first manifestation of cystic echinococcosis. Am J Trop Med Hyg. 2016;95(2):257–9.

129. Bresson-Hadni S, Humbert P, Paintaud G, et al. Skin localization of alveolar echinococcosis of the liver. J Am Acad Dermatol. 1996;34(5 Pt 2):873–7.

130. Ferré-Ybarz L, Galán CG, Palau AT, de la Borbolla JM, Falcó SN. Recurrent angioedema and urticaria in patient with severe osteoporosis. Allergol Immunopathol (Madr). 2011;39(6):379–80.

131. Horton RJ. Albendazole in treatment of human cystic echinococcosis: 12 years of experience. Acta Trop. 1997;64(1–2):79–93.

132. Caldwell JP. Pinworms (enterobius vermicularis). Can Fam Physician. 1982;28:306–9.

133. Lormans JA, Wesel AJ, Vanparus OF. Mebendazole (R 17635) in enterobiasis. A clinical trial in mental retardates. Chemotherapy. 1975;21(3–4):255–60.

134. St Georgiev V. Chemotherapy of enterobiasis (oxyuriasis). Expert Opin Pharmacother. 2001;2(2):267–75.

135. Ragan JT. Single-dose treatment of enterobiasis-use of a new piperazine-senna preparation. Calif Med. 1962;97(6):338–40.

136. Brown HW, Chan KF, Hussey KL. Treatment of enterobiasis and ascariasis with piperazine. J Am Med Assoc. 1956;161(6):515–20.

137. Rachelson M, Ferguson W. Piperazine in the treatment of enterobiasis. AMA Am J Dis Child. 1955;89:346–9.

138. White RH, Standen OD. Piperazine in the treatment of threadworms in children; report on a clinical trial. Br Med J. 1953;2(4839):755–7.

139. Heukelbach J, Wilcke T, Winter B, et al. Efficacy of ivermectin in a patient population concomitantly infected with intestinal helminths and ectoparasites. Arzneimittelforschung. 2004;54(7):416–21.

140. Naquira C, Jimenez G, Guerra JG, et al. Ivermectin for human strongyloidiasis and other intestinal helminths. Am J Trop Med Hyg. 1989;40(3):304–9.

141. Li B, Flaveny CA, Giambelli C, et al. Repurposing the FDA-approved pinworm drug pyrvinium as a novel chemotherapeutic agent for intestinal polyposis. PLoS One. 2014;9(7):e101969.

142. Desai AS. Single-dose treatment of oxyuriasis with pyrvinium embonate. Br Med J. 1962;2(5319):1583–5.

143. Wolfe MS. Oxyuris, trichostrongylus and trichuris. Clin Gastroenterol. 1978;7(1):201–17.

144. Barua AC, Deka P, Das BN. Clinical trial of piperazine hydrate and pyrvinium pamoate in ascariasis and oxyuriasis infestation. Indian J Pediatr. 1979;46(376):182–6.

145. Sinnis P, Zavala F. The skin: where malaria infection and the host immune response begin. Semin Immunopathol. 2012;34(6):787–92.

146. Vaishnani JB. Cutaneous findings in five cases of malaria. Indian J Dermatol Venereol Leprol. 2011;77(1):110.

147. Nagayasu E, Yoshida A, Hombu A, Horii Y, Maruyama H. Paragonimiasis in Japan: a twelve-year retrospective case review (2001-2012). Intern Med. 2015;54(2):179–86.

148. Sogandares-Bernal F, Seed JR. American paragonimiasis. Curr Top Comp Pathobiol. 1973;2:1–56.

149. Procop GW. North American paragonimiasis (Caused by Paragonimus kellicotti) in the context of global paragonimiasis. Clin Microbiol Rev. 2009;22(3):415–46.

150. Saborio P, Lanzas R, Arrieta G, Arguedas A. Paragonimus mexicanus pericarditis: report of two cases and review of the literature. J Trop Med Hyg. 1995;98(5):316–8.

151. Johnson RJ, Jong EC, Dunning SB, Carberry WL, Minshew BH. Paragonimiasis: diagnosis and the use of praziquantel in treatment. Rev Infect Dis. 1985;7(2):200–6.

152. Udonsi JK. Clinical field trials of praziquantel in pulmonary paragonimiasis due to Paragonimus uterobilateralis in endemic populations of the Igwun Basin, Nigeria. Trop Med Parasitol. 1989;40(1):65–8.

153. Calvopiña M, Guderian RH, Paredes W, Chico M, Cooper PJ. Treatment of human pulmonary paragonimiasis with triclabendazole: clinical tolerance and drug efficacy. Trans R Soc Trop Med Hyg. 1998;92(5):566–9.

154. Villegas F, Angles R, Barrientos R, et al. Administration of triclabendazole is safe and effective in controlling fascioliasis in an endemic community of the Bolivian Altiplano. PLoS Negl Trop Dis. 2012;6(8):e1720.

155. Johnson G, Gardner J, Fukai T, Goto K. Cutaneous sparganosis: a rare parasitic infection. J Cutan Pathol. 2015;42(1):1–5.

156. Griffin MP, Tompkins KJ, Ryan MT. Cutaneous sparganosis. Am J Dermatopathol. 1996;18(1):70–2.

157. Fischer P, Bamuhiiga J, Büttner DW. Treatment of human Mansonella streptocerca infection with ivermectin. Tropical Med Int Health. 1997;2(2):191–9.

158. Meyers WM, Moris R, Neafie RC, Connor DH, Bourland J. Streptocerciasis: degeneration of adult Dipetalonema streptocerca in man following diethylcarbamazine therapy. Am J Trop Med Hyg. 1978;27(6):1137–47.

159. Awadzi K, Gilles HM. Diethylcarbamazine in the treatment of patients with onchocerciasis. Br J Clin Pharmacol. 1992;34(4):281–8.

160. Saadatnia G, Golkar M. A review on human toxoplasmosis. Scand J Infect Dis. 2012;44(11):805–14.

161. Beverley JK. Congenital toxoplasma infections. Proc R Soc Med. 1960;53:111–3.

162. Mawhorter SD, Effron D, Blinkhorn R, Spagnuolo PJ. Cutaneous manifestations of toxoplasmosis. Clin Infect Dis. 1992;14(5):1084–8.

163. Leyva WH, Santa Cruz DJ. Cutaneous toxoplasmosis. J Am Acad Dermatol. 1986;14(4):600–5.

164. Rajapakse S, Chrishan Shivanthan M, Samaranayake N, Rodrigo C, Deepika Fernando S. Antibiotics for human toxoplasmosis: a systematic review of randomized trials. Pathog Glob Health. 2013;107(4):162–9.

165. Gottstein B, Pozio E, Nöckler K. Epidemiology, diagnosis, treatment, and control of trichinellosis. Clin Microbiol Rev. 2009;22(1):127–45. Table of Contents

166. Cabié A, Bouchaud O, Houzé S, et al. Albendazole versus thiabendazole as therapy for trichinosis: a retrospective study. Clin Infect Dis. 1996;22(6):1033–5.

167. Kissinger P. Trichomonas vaginalis: a review of epidemiologic, clinical and treatment issues. BMC Infect Dis. 2015;15:307.

168. Lossick JG. Treatment of trichomonas vaginalis infections. Rev Infect Dis. 1982;4:S801–18.

169. Cudmore SL, Garber GE. Prevention or treatment: the benefits of Trichomonas vaginalis vaccine. J Infect Public Health. 2010;3(2):47–53.

170. Thulkar J, Kriplani A, Agarwal N. A comparative study of oral single dose of metronidazole, tinidazole, secnidazole and ornidazole in bacterial vaginosis. Indian J Pharmacol. 2012;44(2):243–5.

171. Schwebke JR, Desmond RA. Tinidazole vs metronidazole for the treatment of bacterial vaginosis. Am J Obstet Gynecol. 2011;204(3):211.e211–6.

172. McGovern TW, Williams W, Fitzpatrick JE, Cetron MS, Hepburn BC, Gentry RH. Cutaneous manifestations of African trypanosomiasis. Arch Dermatol. 1995;131(10):1178–82.

173. Scott JA, Davidson RN, Moody AH, Bryceson AD. Diagnosing multiple parasitic infections: trypanosomiasis, loiasis and schistosomiasis in a single case. Scand J Infect Dis. 1991;23(6):777–80.

174. Babokhov P, Sanyaolu AO, Oyibo WA, Fagbenro-Beyioku AF, Iriemenam NC. A current analysis of chemotherapy strategies for the treatment of human African trypanosomiasis. Pathog Glob Health. 2013;107(5):242–52.

175. Pépin J, Milord F, Meurice F, Ethier L, Loko L, Mpia B. High-dose nifurtimox for arseno-resistant Trypanosoma brucei gambiense sleeping sickness: an open trial in central Zaire. Trans R Soc Trop Med Hyg. 1992;86(3):254–6.

176. Pepin J, Milord F, Mpia B, et al. An open clinical trial of nifurtimox for arseno-resistant Trypanosoma brucei gambiense sleeping sickness in central Zaire. Trans R Soc Trop Med Hyg. 1989;83(4):514–7.

177. Priotto G, Kasparian S, Mutombo W, et al. Nifurtimox-eflornithine combination therapy for second-stage African Trypanosoma brucei gambiense trypanosomiasis: a multicentre, randomised, phase III, non-inferiority trial. Lancet. 2009;374(9683):56–64.

178. Bisser S, N'Siesi FX, Lejon V, et al. Equivalence trial of melarsoprol and nifurtimox monotherapy and combination therapy for the treatment of second-stage Trypanosoma brucei gambiense sleeping sickness. J Infect Dis. 2007;195(3):322–9.

179. Hemmige V, Tanowitz H, Sethi A. Trypanosoma cruzi infection: a review with emphasis on cutaneous manifestations. Int J Dermatol. 2012;51(5):501–8.

180. Sparsa A, Bonnetblanc JM, Peyrot I, Loustaud-Ratti V, Vidal E, Bédane C. Systemic adverse reactions with ivermectin treatment of scabies. Ann Dermatol Venereol. 2006;133(10):784–7.

181. Veit O, Beck B, Steuerwald M, Hatz C. First case of ivermectin-induced severe hepatitis. Trans R Soc Trop Med Hyg. 2006;100(8):795–7.

182. Sudakin DL. Fatality after a single dermal application of lindane lotion. Arch Environ Occup Health. 2007;62(4):201–3.

183. Schimmel M, Abrahamov A, Brama I. A rare complication of aplastic anemia due to Lindane intoxication. Harefuah. 1980;98(8):355–6.

184. Brahams D. Lindane exposure and aplastic anaemia. Lancet. 1994;343(8905):1092.

185. Rauch AE, Kowalsky SF, Lesar TS, Sauerbier GA, Burkart PT, Scharfman WB. Lindane (Kwell)-induced aplastic anemia. Arch Intern Med. 1990;150(11):2393–5.

186. Morgan DP, Roberts RJ, Walter AW, Stockdale EM. Anemia associated with exposure to lindane. Arch Environ Health. 1980;35(5):307–10.

187. Loge JP. Aplastic anemia following exposure to benzene hexachloride (Lindane). JAMA. 1965;193:110–4.

188. Albahary C, Dubrisay J, Guerin H. Obstinate pancytopenia due to lindane (gamma isomer of hexachlorocyclohexane). Arch Mal Prof. 1957;18(6):687–91.

189. Burgess I. Adverse reactions to monosulfiram. Lancet. 1990;336(8719):873.

190. Gursale S, Chargulla S, Khanwelkar C, Thorat V, Gaonkar R, Jadhav S. Metronidazole-Furazolidone induced Stevens-Johnson Syndrome. Indian Medical Gazette. 2010.

191. Piskin G, Mekkes J. Stevens-Johnson syndrome from metronidazole. Contact Dermatitis. 2006;55:192–3.

192. Egan CA, Grant WJ, Morris SE, Saffle JR, Zone JJ. Plasmapheresis as an adjunct treatment in toxic epidermal necrolysis. J Am Acad Dermatol. 1999;40(3):458–61.

193. Magazine R, Chogtu B. Stevens Johnson syndrome and neurotoxic effects of metronidazole. Indian J Pharmacol. 2014;46(5):565.

194. Mazumdar G, Shome K. Stevens-Johnson syndrome following use of metronidazole in a dental patient. Indian J Pharmacol. 2014;46(1):121–2.

195. Chen KT, Twu SJ, Chang HJ, Lin RS. Outbreak of Stevens-Johnson syndrome/toxic epidermal necrolysis associated with mebendazole and metronidazole use among Filipino laborers in Taiwan. Am J Public Health. 2003;93(3):489–92.

196. Hobbs K, Stern-Nezer S, Buckwalter MS, Fischbein N, Finley Caulfield A. Metronidazole-induced encephalopathy: not always a reversible situation. Neurocrit Care. 2015;22(3):429–36.

197. Bahn Y, Kim E, Park C, Park HC. Metronidazole induced encephalopathy in a patient with brain abscess. J Korean Neurosurg Soc. 2010;48(3):301–4.

198. Huang YT, Chen LA, Cheng SJ. Metronidazole-induced encephalopathy: case report and review literature. Acta Neurol Taiwanica. 2012;21(2):74–8.

199. Cheong HC, Jeong TG, Cho YB, et al. Metronidazole-induced encephalopathy in a patient with liver cirrhosis. Korean J Hepatol. 2011;17(2):157–60.

200. Thakkar N, Bhaarat S, Chand R, et al. Metronidazole induced encephalopathy. J Assoc Physicians India. 2016;64(11):72–4.

201. Jang HJ, Sim SY, Lee JY, Bang JH. Atypical metronidazole-induced encephalopathy in anaerobic brain abscess. J Korean Neurosurg Soc. 2012;52(3):273–6.

202. Arik N, Cengiz N, Bilge A. Metronidazole-induced encephalopathy in a uremic patient: a case report. Nephron. 2001;89(1):108–9.

203. Kim H, Kim YW, Kim SR, Park IS, Jo KW. Metronidazole-induced encephalopathy in a patient with infectious colitis: a case report. J Med Case Rep. 2011;5:63.

204. Seok JI, Yi H, Song YM, Lee WY. Metronidazole-induced encephalopathy and inferior olivary hypertrophy: lesion analysis with diffusion-weighted imaging and apparent diffusion coefficient maps. Arch Neurol. 2003;60(12):1796–800.

205. Papathanasiou A, Zouvelou V, Kyriazi S, Rentzos M, Evdokimidis I. Metronidazole-induced reversible encephalopathy in a patient with facioscapulohumeral muscular dystrophy. Clin Neuroradiol. 2013;23(3):217–9.

206. Yagi T, Shihashi G, Oki K, et al. Metronidazole-induced encephalopathy and myoclonus: case report and a review of the literature. Neurol Clin Neurosci. 2015;3:111–3.

207. Onder H, et al. J Neurol Res. 2016;6(4):81–4.

208. Haridas A, Trivedi TH, Moulick ND, Joshi AR. Metronidazole-induced encephalopathy in chronic diarrhoea. J Assoc Physicians India. 2015;63(6):77–9.

209. Godfrey MS, Finn A, Zainah H, Dapaah-Afriyie K. Metronidazole-induced encephalopathy after prolonged metronidazole course for treatment of C. difficile colitis. BMJ Case Rep. 2015;2015:bcr2014206162.

210. Furukawa S, Yamamoto T, Sugiyama A, et al. Metronidazole-induced encephalopathy with contrast enhancing lesions on MRI. J Neurol Sci. 2015;352(1–2):129–31.

211. Kalia V, Vibhuti SK. Case report: MRI of the brain in metronidazole toxicity. Indian J Radiol Imaging. 2010;20(3):195–7.

212. Corson AP, Chretien JH. Metronidazole-associated aseptic meningitis. Clin Infect Dis. 1994;19(5):974.

213. Khan S, Sharrack B, Sewell WA. Metronidazole-induced aseptic meningitis during Helicobacter pylori eradication therapy. Ann Intern Med. 2007;146(5):395–6.

214. Hari A, Srikanth BA, Lakshmi GS. Metronidazole induced cerebellar ataxia. Indian J Pharmacol. 2013;45(3):295–7.

215. Kuriyama A, Jackson JL, Doi A, Kamiya T. Metronidazole-induced central nervous system toxicity: a systematic review. Clin Neuropharmacol. 2011;34(6):241–7.

216. Ogundipe OA. Metronidazole associated seizures: a case report and review of the pharmacovigilance literature. Int J Basic Clin Pharmacol. 2014;3(1):235–8.

217. Smith JA. Neutropenia associated with metronidazole therapy. Can Med Assoc J. 1980;123(3):202.

218. Sanders CV, Hanna BJ, Lewis AC. Metronidazole in the treatment of anaerobic infections. Am Rev Respir Dis. 1979;120(2):337–43.

219. Taylor JA. Metronidazole and transient leukopenia. JAMA. 1965;194(12):1331–2.

220. Choi GY, Yang HW, Cho SH, et al. Acute drug-induced hepatitis caused by albendazole. J Korean Med Sci. 2008;23(5):903–5.

221. Marin Zuluaga JI, Marin Castro AE, Perez Cadavid JC, Restrepo Gutierrez JC. Albendazole-induced granulomatous hepatitis: a case report. J Med Case Rep. 2013;7:201.

222. Ben Fredj N, Chaabane A, Chadly Z, Ben Fadhel N, Boughattas NA, Aouam K. Albendazole-induced associated acute hepatitis and bicytopenia. Scand J Infect Dis. 2014;46(2):149–51.

223. Amoruso C, Fuoti M, Miceli V, et al. Acute hepatitis as a side effect of albendazole: a pediatric case. Pediatr Med Chir. 2009;31(4):176–8.

224. Shah C, Mahapatra A, Shukla A, Bhatia S. Recurrent acute hepatitis caused by albendazole. Trop Gastroenterol. 2013;34(1):38–9.

225. Gözüküçük R, Abci İ, Güçlü M. Albendazole-induced toxic hepatitis: a case report. Turk J Gastroenterol. 2013;24(1):82–4.

226. Ríos D, Restrepo JC. Albendazole-induced liver injury: a case report. Colomb Med (Cali). 2013;44(2):118–20.

227. Sharma R, Mathur MN. Stevens-Johnson syndrome following sulfadiazine, Tri-sulfose and sulfatriad therapy. J Assoc Physicians India. 1965;13(9):727–30.

228. Dewerdt S, Machet L, Jan-Lamy V, Lorette G, Therizol-Ferly M, Vaillant L. Stevens-Johnson syndrome after albendazole. Acta Derm Venereol. 1997;77(5):411.

229. Batzlaff CM, Pupaibool J, Sohail MR. Acute renal failure associated with albendazole therapy in a patient with trichinosis. BMJ Case Rep. 2014;2014:bcr2013200668.

230. Opatrny L, Prichard R, Snell L, Maclean JD. Death related to albendazole-induced pancytopenia: case report and review. Am J Trop Med Hyg. 2005;72(3):291–4.

231. Wilmshurst JM, Robb SA. Can mebendazole cause lateralized occipital seizures? Eur J Paediatr Neurol. 1998;2(6):323–4.

232. Levin MH, Weinstein RA, Axelrod JL, Schantz PM. Severe, reversible neutropenia during high-dose mebendazole therapy for echinococcosis. JAMA. 1983;249(21):2929–31.

233. Kammerer WS, Schantz PM. Long term follow-up of human hydatid disease (Echinococcus granulosus) treated with a high-dose mebendazole regimen. Am J Trop Med Hyg. 1984;33(1):132–7.

234. Junge U, Mohr W. Mebendazole-hepatitis. Z Gastroenterol. 1983;21(12):736–8.

235. Colle I, Naegels S, Hoorens A, Hautekeete M. Granulomatous hepatitis due to mebendazole. J Clin Gastroenterol. 1999;28(1):44–5.

236. Shcherbakov AM, Kozlova TL, Bebris NK. Agranulocytosis–a complication of the chemotherapy of echinococcosis with mebendazole. Med Parazitol (Mosk). 1992;(5-6):9–11.

237. Fernández-Bañares F, González-Huix F, Xiol X, et al. Marrow aplasia during high dose mebendazole treatment. Am J Trop Med Hyg. 1986;35(2):350–1.

238. Ashubu OF, Ademola AD, Asinobi AO. A case report of suspected angioedema in a child after administration of mebendazole, cotrimoxazole and leaf extracts. Ann Ib Postgrad Med. 2016;14(1):41–3.

239. Tchao P, Templeton T. Thiabendazole-associated grand mal seizures in a patient with Down syndrome. J Pediatr. 1983;102(2):317–8.

240. Robinson HM, Samorodin CS. Thiabendazole-induced toxic epidermal necrolysis. Arch Dermatol. 1976;112(12):1757–60.

241. Johnson-Reagan L, Bahna SL. Severe drug rashes in three siblings simultaneously. Allergy. 2003;58(5):445–7.

242. Eland IA, Kerkhof SC, Overbosch D, Wismans PJ, Stricker BH. Cholestatic hepatitis ascribed to the use of thiabendazole. Ned Tijdschr Geneeskd. 1998;142(23):1331–4.

243. Ambroise-Thomas P, Meyer HA. Hepatic amebiasis in the Kilimanjaro region. Serodiagnosis on micro-specimens of dried blood and attempts at treatment with tinidazole (fasigyn). Acta Trop. 1975;32(4):359–64.

244. Tabak F, Ozaras R, Erzin Y, Celik AF, Ozbay G, Senturk H. Ornidazole-induced liver damage: report of three cases and review of the literature. Liver Int. 2003;23(5):351–4.

245. Ersöz G, Vardar R, Akarca US, et al. Ornidazole-induced autoimmune hepatitis. Turk J Gastroenterol. 2011;22(5):494–9.

246. Harputluoglu MM, Demirel U, Karadag N, et al. Severe hepatitis with prolonged cholestasis and bile duct injury due to the long-term use of ornidazole. Acta Gastroenterol Belg. 2007;70(3):293–5.

247. Azher M, el-Kassimi FA, Wright SG, Mofti A. Exudative polyserositis and acute respiratory failure following praziquantel therapy. Chest. 1990;98(1):241–3.

248. Bada JL, Treviño B, Cabezos J. Convulsive seizures after treatment with praziquantel. Br Med J (Clin Res Ed). 1988;296(6622):646.

249. Lima AW, Medeiros Z, Santos ZC, Costa GM, Braga C. Adverse reactions following mass drug administration with diethylcarbamazine in lymphatic filariasis endemic areas in the Northeast of Brazil. Rev Soc Bras Med Trop. 2012;45(6):745–50.

250. Carrascosa MF, Lucena MI, Andrade RJ, et al. Fatal acute hepatitis after sequential treatment with levofloxacin, doxycycline, and naproxen in a patient presenting with acute Mycoplasma pneumoniae infection. Clin Ther. 2009;31(5):1014–9.

251. Selimoglu MA, Ertekin V. Autoimmune hepatitis triggered by Brucella infection or doxycycline or both. Int J Clin Pract. 2003;57(7):639–41.

252. Perlmutter A, Abramovits W, Gupta AK. Oracea (doxycycline monohydrate). Skinmed. 2006;5(5):238–40.

253. Takahashi R, Tsukada T, Hasegawa M. Tetracycline-induced hemolytic anemia. Keio J Med. 1963;12:161–8.

254. Tabibian JH, Gutierrez MA. Doxycycline-induced pseudotumor cerebri. South Med J. 2009;102(3):310–1.

255. Lochhead J, Elston JS. Doxycycline induced intracranial hypertension. BMJ. 2003;326(7390):641–2.

256. Friedman SJ, Winkelmann RK. Familial granuloma annulare. Report of two cases and review of the literature. J Am Acad Dermatol. 1987;16(3 Pt 1):600–5.

257. Kadam P, Gregory NA, Zelger B, Carlson JA. Delayed onset of the Jarisch-Herxheimer reaction in doxycycline-treated disease: a case report and review of its histopathology and implications for pathogenesis. Am J Dermatopathol. 2015;37(6):e68–74.

258. Haney C, Nahata MC. Unique expression of chronic Lyme disease and Jarisch-Herxheimer reaction to doxycycline therapy in a young adult. BMJ Case Rep. 2016;2016:bcr2013009433.

259. Kadayifci A, Gulsen MT, Koruk M, Savas MC. Doxycycline-induced pill esophagitis. Dis Esophagus. 2004;17(2):168–71.

260. Shelat VG, Seah M, Lim KH. Doxycycline induced acute erosive oesophagitis and presenting as acute dysphagia. J Assoc Physicians India. 2011;59:57–9.

261. Kato S, Kobayashi M, Sato H, Saito Y, Komatsu K, Harada Y. Doxycycline-induced hemorrhagic esophagitis: a pediatric case. J Pediatr Gastroenterol Nutr. 1988;7(5):762–5.

262. Amendola MA, Spera TD. Doxycycline-induced esophagitis. JAMA. 1985;253(7):1009–11.

263. Al Mofarreh MA, Al Mofleh IA. Doxycline-induced esophageal ulcerations. Saudi J Gastroenterol. 1998;4(1):20–4.

264. Tahan V, Sayrak H, Bayar N, Erer B, Tahan G, Dane F. Doxycycline-induced ulceration mimicking esophageal cancer. Cases J. 2008;1(1):144.

265. Orr LH, Rudisill E, Brodkin R, Hamilton RW. Exacerbation of renal failure associated with doxycycline. Arch Intern Med. 1978;138(5):793–4.

266. Wachira JK, Jensen CH, Rhone K. Doxycycline-induced pancreatitis: a rare finding. S D Med. 2013;66(6):227–9.

267. Ocal S, Selçuk H, Korkmaz M, Unal H, Yilmaz U. Acute pancreatitis following doxycycline and ornidazole coadministration. JOP. 2010;11(6):614–6.

268. Inayat F, Virk HU, Yoon DJ, Riaz I. Drug-induced pancreatitis: a rare manifestation of doxycycline administration. N Am J Med Sci. 2016;8(2):117–20.

269. Eland IA, van Puijenbroek EP, Sturkenboom MJ, Wilson JH, Stricker BH. Drug-associated acute pancreatitis: twenty-one years of spontaneous reporting in The Netherlands. Am J Gastroenterol. 1999;94(9):2417–22.

270. Moy BT, Kapila N. Probable doxycycline-induced acute pancreatitis. Am J Health Syst Pharm. 2016;73(5):286–91.

271. Achecar Justo L, Rivero Fernández M, Cobo Reinoso J, Ruiz Del Arbol Olmos L. Doxycycline induced-acute pancreatitis. Med Clin (Barc). 2010;134(15):705–6.

272. Pourmorteza M, Virk H, Yoon D, Riaz I, Rai A, Rahman Z. P14: doxycycline: a rare cause of drug induced pancreatitis. J Investig Med. 2016;64(3):822–3.

273. Knox-Macaulay HH, Adil SN, Ahmed EM. Acute thrombotic thrombocytopenic purpura following doxycycline treatment of Chlamydia pneumoniae infection in a patient with dermatomyositis. Clin Lab Haematol. 2004;26(2):147–51.

274. Chulay JD, Spencer HC, Mugambi M. Electrocardiographic changes during treatment of leishmaniasis with pentavalent antimony (sodium stibogluconate). Am J Trop Med Hyg. 1985;34(4):702–9.

275. Hepburn NC, Siddique I, Howie AF, Beckett GJ, Hayes PC. Hepatotoxicity of sodium stibogluconate in leishmaniasis. Lancet. 1993;342(8865):238–9.

276. Hepburn NC, Siddique I, Howie AF, Beckett GJ, Hayes PC. Hepatotoxicity of sodium stibogluconate therapy for American cutaneous leishmaniasis. Trans R Soc Trop Med Hyg. 1994;88(4):453–5.

277. Oliveira AL, Brustoloni YM, Fernandes TD, Dorval ME, Cunha RV, Bóia MN. Severe adverse reactions to meglumine antimoniate in the treatment of visceral leishmaniasis: a report of 13 cases in the southwestern region of Brazil. Trop Dr. 2009;39(3):180–2.

278. Neumayr AL, Walter C, Stoeckle M, Braendle N, Glatz K, Blum JA. Successful treatment of imported mucosal Leishmania infantum leishmaniasis with miltefosine after severe hypokalemia under meglumine antimoniate treatment. J Travel Med. 2012;19(2):124–6.

279. Ortega-Carnicer J, Alcázar R, de la Torre M, Benezet J. Pentavalent antimonial-induced torsade de pointes. J Electrocardiol. 1997;30(2):143–5.

280. Castelló Viguer MT, Echánove Errazti I, Ridocci Soriano F, Esteban Esteban E, Atienza Fernández F, Cuesta Estellés G. Torsades de pointes during treatment of leishmaniasis with meglumine antimoniate. Rev Esp Cardiol. 1999;52(7):533–5.

281. Ezzine Sebai N, Mrabet N, Khaled A, et al. Side effects of meglumine antimoniate in cutaneous leishmaniasis: 15 cases. Tunis Med. 2010;88(1):9–11.

282. Hailu W, Weldegebreal T, Hurissa Z, et al. Safety and effectiveness of meglumine antimoniate in the treatment of Ethiopian visceral leishmaniasis patients with and without HIV co-infection. Trans R Soc Trop Med Hyg. 2010;104(11):706–12.

283. Rodrigues ML, Costa RS, Souza CS, Foss NT, Roselino AM. Nephrotoxicity attributed to meglumine antimoniate (Glucantime) in the treatment of generalized cutaneous leishmaniasis. Rev Inst Med Trop Sao Paulo. 1999;41(1):33–7.

284. Samrao A, Berry TM, Goreshi R, Simpson EL. A pilot study of an oral phosphodiesterase inhibitor (apremilast) for atopic dermatitis in adults. Arch Dermatol. 2012;148(8):890–7.

285. Aruna AS, Al-Samarrai SA, Al-Humaidan AS. Amphotericin B-induced seizures in a patient with AIDS. Ann Pharmacother. 2001;35(9):1037–41.

286. Chongtham DS, Singh MM, Ram T. Amphotericin B induced ventricular arrhythmia and its relation to central venous line. J Postgrad Med. 2001;47(4):282.

287. Thakur CP. Correction of serum electrolyte imbalance prevents cardiac arrhythmia during amphotericin B administration. Natl Med J India. 1995;8(1):13–4.

288. Craven PC, Gremillion DH. Risk factors of ventricular fibrillation during rapid amphotericin B infusion. Antimicrob Agents Chemother. 1985;27(5):868–71.

289. Googe JH, Walterspiel JN. Arrhythmia caused by amphotericin B in a neonate. Pediatr Infect Dis J. 1988;7(1):73.

290. Aguado JM, Hidalgo M, Moya I, Alcazar JM, Jimenez MJ, Noriega AR. Ventricular arrhythmias with conventional and liposomal amphotericin. Lancet. 1993;342(8881):1239.

291. Sanches BF, Nunes P, Almeida H, Rebelo M. Atrioventricular block related to liposomal amphotericin B. BMJ Case Rep. 2014;2014:bcr2013202688.

292. Patel GP, Crank CW, Leikin JB. An evaluation of hepatotoxicity and nephrotoxicity of liposomal amphotericin B (L-AMB). J Med Toxicol. 2011;7(1):12–5.

293. Gill J, Sprenger HR, Ralph ED, Sharpe MD. Hepatotoxicity possibly caused by amphotericin B. Ann Pharmacother. 1999;33(6):683–5.

294. Miller MA. Reversible hepatotoxicity related to amphotericin B. Can Med Assoc J. 1984;131(10):1245–7.

295. Shigemi A, Matsumoto K, Ikawa K, et al. Safety analysis of liposomal amphotericin B in adult patients: anaemia, thrombocytopenia, nephrotoxicity, hepatotoxicity and hypokalaemia. Int J Antimicrob Agents. 2011;38(5):417–20.

296. Ellis M, Shamoon A, Gorka W, Zwaan F, al-Ramadi B. Severe hepatic injury associated with lipid formulations of amphotericin B. Clin Infect Dis. 2001;32(5):E87–9.

297. Mohan UR, Bush A. Amphotericin B-induced hepatorenal failure in cystic fibrosis. Pediatr Pulmonol. 2002;33(6):497–500.

298. Shindo K, Mizuno T, Matsumoto Y, et al. Granulocytopenia and thrombocytopenia associated with combination therapy of amphotericin B and low-dose flucytosine in a patient with cryptococcal meningitis. DICP. 1989;23(9):672–4.

299. Vaidya SJ, Seydel C, Patel SR, Ortin M. Anaphylactic reaction to liposomal amphotericin B. Ann Pharmacother. 2002;36(9):1480–1.

300. Torre I, López-Herce J, Vázquez P. Anaphylactic reaction to liposomal amphotericin B in children. Ann Pharmacother. 1996;30(9):1036–7.

301. Schneider P, Klein RM, Dietze L, Söhngen D, Leschke M, Heyll A. Anaphylactic reaction to liposomal amphotericin (AmBisome). Br J Haematol. 1998;102(4):1108–9.

302. Kauffman CA, Wiseman SW. Anaphylaxis upon switching lipid-containing amphotericin B formulations. Clin Infect Dis. 1998;26(5):1237–8.

303. Laing RB, Milne LJ, Leen CL, Malcolm GP, Steers AJ. Anaphylactic reactions to liposomal amphotericin. Lancet. 1994;344(8923):682.

304. Nath P, Basher A, Harada M, et al. Immediate hypersensitivity reaction following liposomal amphotericin-B (AmBisome) infusion. Trop Dr. 2014;44(4):241–2.

305. Moyssakis I, Vassilakopoulos TP, Sipsas NV, et al. Reversible dilated cardiomyopathy associated with amphotericin B treatment. Int J Antimicrob Agents. 2005;25(5):444–7.

306. Bandeira AC, Filho JM, de Almeida Ramos K. Reversible cardiomyopathy secondary to Amphotericin-B. Med Mycol Case Rep. 2016;13:19–21.

307. Soares JR, Nunes MC, Leite AF, Falqueto EB, Lacerda BE, Ferrari TC. Reversible dilated cardiomyopathy associated with amphotericin B therapy. J Clin Pharm Ther. 2015;40(3):333–5.

308. Chung DK, Koenig MG. Reversible cardiac enlargement during treatment with amphotericin B and hydrocortisone. Report of three cases. Am Rev Respir Dis. 1971;103(6):831–41.

309. Balslev U, Nielsen TL. Adverse effects associated with intravenous pentamidine isethionate as treatment of Pneumocystis carinii pneumonia in AIDS patients. Dan Med Bull. 1992;39(4):366–8.

310. Stahl-Bayliss CM, Kalman CM, Laskin OL. Pentamidine-induced hypoglycemia in patients with the acquired immune deficiency syndrome. Clin Pharmacol Ther. 1986;39(3):271–5.

311. Das VN, Ranjan A, Sinha AN, et al. A randomized clinical trial of low dosage combination of pentamidine and allopurinol in the treatment of antimony unresponsive cases of visceral leishmaniasis. J Assoc Physicians India. 2001;49:609–13.

312. CP L, HP W, Chuang LM, Lin BJ, Chuang CY, Tai TY. Pentamidine-induced hyperglycemia and ketosis in acquired immunodeficiency syndrome. Pancreas. 1995;11(3):315–6.

313. Bouchard P, Sai P, Reach G, Caubarrère I, Ganeval D, Assan R. Diabetes mellitus following pentamidine-induced hypoglycemia in humans. Diabetes. 1982;31(1):40–5.

314. Hauser L, Sheehan P, Simpkins H. Pancreatic pathology in pentamidine-induced diabetes in acquired immunodeficiency syndrome patients. Hum Pathol. 1991;22(9):926–9.

315. Schwartz MS, Cappell MS. Pentamidine-associated pancreatitis. Dig Dis Sci. 1989;34(10):1617–20.

316. Murphey SA, Josephs AS. Acute pancreatitis associated with pentamidine therapy. Arch Intern Med. 1981;141(1):56–8.

317. Sauleda J, Gea JG, Aguar MC, Aran X, Pastó M, Broquetas JM. Probable pentamidine-induced acute pancreatitis. Ann Pharmacother. 1994;28(1):52–3.

318. Klatt EC. Pathology of pentamidine-induced pancreatitis. Arch Pathol Lab Med. 1992;116(2):162–4.

319. Murphy RL, Noskin GA, Ehrenpreis ED. Acute pancreatitis associated with aerosolized pentamidine. Am J Med. 1990;88(5N):53N–6N.

320. Herer B, Chinet T, Labrune S, Collignon MA, Chretien J, Huchon G. Pancreatitis associated with pentamidine by aerosol. BMJ. 1989;298(6673):605.

321. Shen M, Orwoll ES, Conte JE, Prince MJ. Pentamidine-induced pancreatic beta-cell dysfunction. Am J Med. 1989;86(6 Pt 1):726–8.

322. Briceland LL, Bailie GR. Pentamidine-associated nephrotoxicity and hyperkalemia in patients with AIDS. DICP. 1991;25(11):1171–4.

323. Lachaal M, Venuto RC. Nephrotoxicity and hyperkalemia in patients with acquired immunodeficiency syndrome treated with pentamidine. Am J Med. 1989;87(3):260–3.

324. Misíková Z, Kovács L, Foltinová A. Nephrotoxic effect of pentamidine in the treatment of interstitial pneumonia in 2 children with acute lymphoblastic leukemia. Cesk Pediatr. 1979;34(12):715–7.

325. Helmick CG, Green JK. Pentamidine-associated hypotension and route of administration. Ann Intern Med. 1985;103(3):480.

326. Bibler MR, Chou TC, Toltzis RJ, Wade PA. Recurrent ventricular tachycardia due to pentamidine-induced cardiotoxicity. Chest. 1988;94(6):1303–6.

327. Mani S, Kocheril AG, Andriole VT. Case report: pentamidine and polymorphic ventricular tachycardia revisited. Am J Med Sci. 1993;305(4):236–40.

328. Stein KM, Haronian H, Mensah GA, Acosta A, Jacobs J, Kligfield P. Ventricular tachycardia and torsades de pointes complicating pentamidine therapy of Pneumocystis carinii pneumonia in the acquired immunodeficiency syndrome. Am J Cardiol. 1990;66(10):888–9.

329. Wang JJ, Freeman AI, Gaeta JF, Sinks LF. Unusual complications of pentamidine in the treatment of Pneumocystis carinii pneumonia. J Pediatr. 1970;77(2):311–4.

330. Watarai A, Niiyama S, Amoh Y, Katsuoka K. Toxic epidermal necrolysis caused by aerosolized pentamidine. Am J Med. 2009;122(1):e1–2.

331. Picon M, Causse X, Gelas P, Retornaz G, Trépo C, Bouletreau P. Pentamidine-related acute hepatitis during pneumocystosis treatment in acquired immunodeficiency syndrome. Gastroenterol Clin Biol. 1991;15(5):463–4.

332. DeMasi JM, Cox JA, Leonard D, Koh AY, Aquino VM. Intravenous pentamidine is safe and effective as primary pneumocystis pneumonia prophylaxis in children and adolescents undergoing hematopoietic stem cell transplantation. Pediatr Infect Dis J. 2013;32(9):933–6.

333. Caumes E, Bocquet H, Guermonprez G, et al. Adverse cutaneous reactions to pyrimethamine/sulfadiazine and pyrimethamine/clindamycin in patients with AIDS and toxoplasmic encephalitis. Clin Infect Dis. 1995;21(3):656–8.

334. Bamber MG, Elder AT, Gray JA, Minns RA. Fatal Stevens-Johnson syndrome associated with Fansidar and chloroquine. J Infect. 1986;13(1):31–3.

335. Pajor A. Pancytopenia in a patient given pyrimethamine and sulphamethoxidiazine during pregnancy. Arch Gynecol Obstet. 1990;247(4):215–7.

336. Boudes P, Zittoun J, Sobel A. Acute pancytopenia induced by pyrimethamine during treatment of cerebral toxoplasmosis associated with AIDS. Role of dihydrofolate reductase inhibitors. Ann Med Interne (Paris). 1990;141(2):183–6.

337. Mori T, Kato J, Okamoto S. Pancytopenia due to pyrimethamine triggered by transplant-associated microangiopathy after allogeneic bone marrow transplantation. J Infect Chemother. 2011;17(6):866–7.

338. Matthews JI, Molitor JT, Hunt KK. Pyrimethamine-induced leukopenia and thrombocytopenia in a patient with malaria and tropical sprue: case report. Mil Med. 1973;138(5):280–3.

339. Armata J. Letter: pyrimethamine poisoning. Br Med J. 1973;4(5895):783.

340. Zheng X, Fang X, Cai X. Two episodes of anaphylaxis caused by a chlorhexidine sulfadiazine-coated central venous catheter. Chin Med J. 2014;127(12):2395–7.

341. Stephens R, Mythen M, Kallis P, Davies DW, Egner W, Rickards A. Two episodes of life-threatening anaphylaxis in the same patient to a chlorhexidine-sulphadiazine-coated central venous catheter. Br J Anaesth. 2001;87(2):306–8.

342. Boyette DP, London AH. Hemolytic anemia due to sulfadiazine; report of a case. N C Med J. 1949;10(3):132.

343. Ross JF, Paegel BL. Acute hemolytic anemia and hemoglobinuria following sulfadiazine medication. Blood. 1946;1:189–201.

344. Eldad A, Neuman A, Weinberg A, Benmeir P, Rotem M, Wexler MR. Silver sulphadiazine-induced haemolytic anaemia in a glucose-6-phosphate dehydrogenase-deficient burn patient. Burns. 1991;17(5):430–2.

345. Khalili H, Soudbakhsh A, Talasaz AH. Severe hepatotoxicity and probable hepatorenal syndrome associated with sulfadiazine. Am J Health Syst Pharm. 2011;68(10):888–92.

346. Geier B, Nousbaum JP, Cauvin JM, Rosaszkiewick M, Gouérou H. Acute hepatitis probably secondary to the treatment with pyrimethamine-sulfadiazine combination. Gastroenterol Clin Biol. 1992;16(8–9):724–5.

347. Díaz F, Collazos J, Mayo J, Martínez E. Sulfadiazine-induced multiple urolithiasis and acute renal failure in a patient with AIDS and Toxoplasma encephalitis. Ann Pharmacother. 1996;30(1):41–2.

348. Chaby G, Viseux V, Poulain JF, De Cagny B, Denoeux JP, Lok C. Topical silver sulfadiazine-induced acute renal failure. Ann Dermatol Venereol. 2005;132(11 Pt 1):891–3.

349. de la Prada Alvarez FJ, Prados Gallardo AM, Tugores Vázquez A, Uriol Rivera M, Morey Molina A. Acute renal failure due to sulfadiazine crystalluria. An Med Interna. 2007;24(5):235–8.

350. Hein R, Brunkhorst R, Thon WF, Schedel I, Schmidt RE. Symptomatic sulfadiazine crystalluria in AIDS patients: a report of two cases. Clin Nephrol. 1993;39(5):254–6.

351. Simon DI, Brosius FC, Rothstein DM. Sulfadiazine crystalluria revisited. The treatment of Toxoplasma encephalitis in patients with acquired immunodeficiency syndrome. Arch Intern Med. 1990;150(11):2379–84.

352. Oster S, Hutchison F, McCabe R. Resolution of acute renal failure in toxoplasmic encephalitis despite continuance of sulfadiazine. Rev Infect Dis. 1990;12(4):618–20.

353. Guitard J, Kamar N, Mouzin M, et al. Sulfadiazine-related obstructive urinary tract lithiasis: an unusual cause of acute renal failure after kidney transplantation. Clin Nephrol. 2005;63(5):405–7.

354. Jennings LJ, Hanumadass M. Silver sulfadiazine induced clostridium difficile toxic megacolon in a burn patient: case report. Burns. 1998;24(7):676–9.

355. Tan CB, Rajan D, Shah M, et al. Toxic megacolon from fulminant clostridium difficile infection induced by topical silver sulphadiazine. BMJ Case Rep. 2012;2012:bcr2012006460.

356. Arnold HL. Lupus erythematosus disseminatus (response to sulfadiazine?). Arch Dermatol Syphilol. 1946;53:53.

357. Tsai TC, Peng SK, Shih YR, Luk HN. Sulfadiazine-induced methemoglobinemia in a boy with thalassemia. Can J Anaesth. 2005;52(9):1002–3.

358. Kath MA, Shupp JW, Matt SE, et al. Incidence of methemoglobinemia in patients receiving cerium nitrate and silver sulfadiazine for the treatment of burn wounds: a burn center's experience. Wound Repair Regen. 2011;19(2):201–4.

359. Taqi SA, Zaki SA, Nilofer AR, Sami LB. Trimethoprim-sulfamethoxazole-induced Steven Johnson syndrome in an HIV-infected patient. Indian J Pharmacol. 2012;44(4):533–5.

360. Langlois MR, Derk F, Belczyk R, Zgonis T. Trimethoprim-sulfamethoxazole-induced Stevens-Johnson syndrome: a case report. J Am Podiatr Med Assoc. 2010;100(4):299–303.

361. Mistry RD, Schwab SH, Treat JR. Stevens-Johnson syndrome and toxic epidermal necrolysis: consequence of treatment of an emerging pathogen. Pediatr Emerg Care. 2009;25(8):519–22.

362. Muñoz SJ, Martinez-Hernandez A, Maddrey WC. Intrahepatic cholestasis and phospholipidosis associated with the use of trimethoprim-sulfamethoxazole. Hepatology. 1990;12(2):342–7.

363. Abusin S, Johnson S. Sulfamethoxazole/trimethoprim induced liver failure: a case report. Cases J. 2008;1(1):44.

364. Faria LC, Resende CC, Couto CA, Couto OF, Fonseca LP, Ferrari TC. Severe and prolonged cholestasis caused by trimethoprim-sulfamethoxazole: a case report. Clinics (Sao Paulo). 2009;64(1):71–4.

365. Colucci CF, Lo Cicero M. Letter: hepatic necrosis and trimethoprim-sulfamethoxazole. JAMA. 1975;233(9):952–3.

366. Alberti-Flor JJ, Hernandez ME, Ferrer JP, Howell S, Jeffers L. Fulminant liver failure and pancreatitis associated with the use of sulfamethoxazole-trimethoprim. Am J Gastroenterol. 1989;84(12):1577–9.

367. Andrès E, Noel E, Maloisel F. Trimethoprim-sulfamethoxazole-induced life-threatening agranulocytosis. Arch Intern Med. 2003;163(16):1975–6. author reply 1976

368. Jha P, Stromich J, Cohen M, Wainaina JN. A rare complication of trimethoprim-sulfamethoxazole: drug induced aseptic meningitis. Case Rep Infect Dis. 2016;2016:3879406.

369. Keisu M, Wiholm BE, Palmblad J. Trimethoprim-sulphamethoxazole-associated blood dyscrasias. Ten years' experience of the Swedish spontaneous reporting system. J Intern Med. 1990;228(4):353–60.

370. Menger RP, Dossani RH, Thakur JD, Farokhi F, Morrow K, Guthikonda B. Extra-axial hematoma and trimethoprim-sulfamethoxazole induced aplastic anemia: the role of hematological diseases in subdural and epidural hemorrhage. Case Rep Hematol. 2015;2015:374951.

371. Bartels RH, van der Spek JA, Oosten HR. Acute pancreatitis due to sulfamethoxazole-trimethoprim. South Med J. 1992;85(10):1006–7.

372. Park TY, Oh HC, Do JH. A case of recurrent pancreatitis induced by trimethoprim-sulfamethoxazole re-exposure. Gut Liver. 2010;4(2):250–2.

373. Antonow DR. Acute pancreatitis associated with trimethoprim-sulfamethoxazole. Ann Intern Med. 1986;104(3):363–5.

374. Dickey SE, Mabry WA, Hamilton LA. Possible sulfamethoxazole/trimethoprim-induced pancreatitis in a complicated adolescent patient posttraumatic injury. J Pharm Pract. 2015;28(4):419–24.

375. Floris-Moore MA, Amodio-Groton MI, Catalano MT. Adverse reactions to trimethoprim/sulfamethoxazole in AIDS. Ann Pharmacother. 2003;37(12):1810–3.

376. Versleijen MW, Naber AH, Riksen NP, Wanten GJ, Debruyne FM. Recurrent pancreatitis after trimethoprim-sulfamethoxazole rechallenge. Neth J Med. 2005;63(7):275–7.

377. Garvey JP, Brown CM, Chotirmall SH, Dorman AM, Conlon PJ, Walshe JJ. Trimethoprim-sulfamethoxazole induced acute interstitial nephritis in renal allografts; clinical course and outcome. Clin Nephrol. 2009;72(5):331–6.

378. Fraser TN, Avellaneda AA, Graviss EA, Musher DM. Acute kidney injury associated with trimethoprim/sulfamethoxazole. J Antimicrob Chemother. 2012;67(5):1271–7.

379. Smith EJ, Light JA, Filo RS, Yum MN. Interstitial nephritis caused by trimethoprim-sulfamethoxazole in renal transplant recipients. JAMA. 1980;244(4):360–1.

380. Cryst C, Hammar SP. Acute granulomatous interstitial nephritis due to co-trimoxazole. Am J Nephrol. 1988;8(6):483–8.

381. Kawasumi H, Tanaka E, Hoshi D, Kawaguchi Y, Yamanaka H. Methemoglobinemia induced by trimethoprim-sulfamethoxazole in a patient with systemic lupus erythematosus. Intern Med. 2013;52(15):1741–3.

382. Carroll TG, Carroll MG. Methemoglobinemia in a pediatric oncology patient receiving sulfamethoxazole/trimethoprim prophylaxis. Am J Case Rep. 2016;17:499–502.

383. Koirala J. Trimethoprim-sulfamethoxazole—induced methemoglobinemia in an HIV-infected patient. Mayo Clin Proc. 2004;79(6):829–30.

384. Damergis JA, Stoker JM, Abadie JL. Methemoglobinemia after sulfametoxazole and trimethoprim. JAMA. 1983;249(5):590–1.

385. Bruner KE, Coop CA, White KM. Trimethoprim-sulfamethoxazole-induced aseptic meningitis-not just another sulfa allergy. Ann Allergy Asthma Immunol. 2014;113(5):520–6.

386. Naitoh T, Yamamoto M, Kawakami K, et al. Case of systemic lupus erythematosus repeated with various allergic reactions by trimethoprim-sulfamethoxazole. Nihon Rinsho Meneki Gakkai Kaishi. 2009;32(6):492–8.

387. Jose A, Cramer AK, Davar K, Gutierrez G. A case of drug-induced lupus erythematosus secondary to trimethoprim/sulfamethoxazole presenting with pleural effusions and pericardial tamponade. Lupus. 2016;

388. Gordin F, Gibert C, Schmidt ME. Clostridium difficile colitis associated with trimethoprim-sulfamethoxazole given as prophylaxis for Pneumocystis carinii pneumonia. Am J Med. 1994;96(1):94–5.

389. Ainapurapu B, Kanakadandi UB. Trimethoprim-sulfamethoxazole induced rhabdomyolysis. Am J Ther. 2014;21(3):e78–9.

390. Kiel PJ, Dickmeyer N, Schwartz JE. Trimethoprim-sulfamethoxazole-induced rhabdomyolysis in an allogeneic stem cell transplant patient. Transpl Infect Dis. 2010;12(5):451–4.

391. Walker S, Norwood J, Thornton C, Schaberg D. Trimethoprim-sulfamethoxazole associated rhabdomyolysis in a patient with AIDS: case report and review of the literature. Am J Med Sci. 2006;331(6):339–41.

392. Augustyn A, Lisa Alattar M, Naina H. Rhabdomyolysis due to trimethoprim-sulfamethoxazole administration following a hematopoietic stem cell transplant. Case Rep Oncol Med. 2015;2015:619473.

393. Singer SJ, Racoosin JA, Viraraghavan R. Rhabdomyolysis in human immunodeficiency virus—positive patients taking trimethoprim-sulfamethoxazole. Clin Infect Dis. 1998;26(1):233–4.

394. Mancano MA. Trimethoprim-sulfamethoxazole-induced rhabdomyolysis; gabapentin-induced hypoglycemia in diabetic and nondiabetic patients; purple glove syndrome after oral phenytoin administration; acute dystonic reaction after methylphenidate initiation; serotonin syndrome with vilazodone monotherapy; cabozantinib-associated dermatologic adverse reactions. Hosp Pharm. 2015;50(8):662–6.

395. Cottle LE, Peters JR, Hall A, et al. Multiorgan dysfunction caused by travel-associated African trypanosomiasis. Emerg Infect Dis. 2012;18(2):287–9.

396. Awadzi K. Clinical picture and outcome of serious adverse events in the treatment of onchocerciasis. Filaria J. 2003;2(Suppl 1):S6.

397. Smith A, Harbour D, Liebmann J. Acute renal failure in a patient receiving treatment with suramin. Am J Clin Oncol. 1997;20(4):433–4.

398. Thylefors B, Rolland A. The risk of optic atrophy following suramin treatment of ocular onchocerciasis. Bull World Health Organ. 1979;57(3):479–80.

399. Arroz JO. Melarsoprol and reactive encephalopathy in Trypanosoma brucei rhodesiense. Trans R Soc Trop Med Hyg. 1987;81(2):192.

400. Pépin J, Milord F, Khonde AN, et al. Risk factors for encephalopathy and mortality during melarsoprol treatment of Trypanosoma brucei gambiense sleeping sickness. Trans R Soc Trop Med Hyg. 1995;89(1):92–7.

401. Pialoux G, Kernbaum S, Vachon F. Arsenical-induced encephalopathy during the treatment of African trypanosomiasis. Apropos of a case with a favorable outcome. Bull Soc Pathol Exot Filiales. 1988;81(3 Pt 2):555–6.

402. Blum J, Nkunku S, Burri C. Clinical description of encephalopathic syndromes and risk factors for their occurrence and outcome during melarsoprol treatment of human African trypanosomiasis. Tropical Med Int Health. 2001;6(5):390–400.

403. Haller L, Adams H, Merouze F, Dago A. Clinical and pathological aspects of human African trypanosomiasis (T. b. gambiense) with particular reference to reactive arsenical encephalopathy. Am J Trop Med Hyg. 1986;35(1):94–9.

404. Kuepfer I, Schmid C, Allan M, et al. Safety and efficacy of the 10-day melarsoprol schedule for the treatment of second stage Rhodesiense sleeping sickness. PLoS Negl Trop Dis. 2012;6(8):e1695.

405. Milord F, Pépin J, Loko L, Ethier L, Mpia B. Efficacy and toxicity of eflornithine for treatment of Trypanosoma brucei gambiense sleeping sickness. Lancet. 1992;340(8820):652–5.

406. Forsyth CJ, Hernandez S, Olmedo W, et al. Safety profile of nifurtimox for treatment of chagas disease in the United States. Clin Infect Dis. 2016;63(8):1056–62.

407. Jackson Y, Alirol E, Getaz L, Wolff H, Combescure C, Chappuis F. Tolerance and safety of nifurtimox in patients with chronic chagas disease. Clin Infect Dis. 2010;51(10):e69–75.

408. Sundar S, Jha TK, Thakur CP, Sinha PK, Bhattacharya SK. Injectable paromomycin for Visceral leishmaniasis in India. N Engl J Med. 2007;356(25):2571–81.

Systemic Therapies for Scarring and Non-scarring Alopecia

Carolyn Goh

Introduction

Primary scarring (cicatricial) and non-scarring alopecia comprise a diverse group of diseases that range from very common, such as androgenetic alopecia, to very rare, most of the scarring alopecias. The non-scarring alopecias tend to be asymptomatic, without pruritus or pain, while the scarring alopecias are often characterized by intense pruritus and/or pain. Regardless of symptoms, both scarring and non-scarring alopecias can have profound psychological effects on those experiencing the hair loss. One source of particular frustration for patients with alopecia and their physicians is the difficulty in treating these disorders. The presence, type (lymphocytic, neutrophilic, mixed), and location (peri-infundibular vs. peri-bulbar) of inflammation vary in each type of alopecia, dictating the treatment approach. As with other dermatologic conditions, topical or intralesional treatment is preferred due to safety, but may not be sufficient. Topical and intralesional therapy with corticosteroids is a mainstay for treating inflammatory alopecias (e.g., alopecia areata, chronic cutaneous lupus erythematosus, lichen planopilaris). Topical minoxidil is an effective hair growth-promoting therapy for androgenetic alopecia and may be helpful for other types of hair loss, including scarring alopecia in which it may help maintain the existing hair. Low-level laser therapy may be helpful, both targeting the hair growth cycle as well as reducing

inflammation [1]. Platelet-rich plasma therapy has been rising in its popularity, but there is limited evidence to support its use at this time [2, 3].

Systemic therapies, when necessary, can have benefit in treating scarring and non-scarring alopecia, but generally have limited evidence. They are recommended based on our understanding of the pathophysiology of the particular disease being treated and case reports, case series, or expert recommendations. Likewise, no systemic treatments are FDA approved for hair loss except for finasteride for the treatment of androgenetic alopecia in men. See Fig. 43.1 for an algorithm for when to use systemic therapies in hair loss patients.

Scarring Alopecia

Primary scarring alopecia is subdivided based on the type of inflammatory infiltrate that predominates on histopathology: lymphocytic, neutrophilic, or mixed. See Table 43.1 for a list of scarring alopecias. The inflammation typically is peri-infundibular, but can extend more deeply in some variants. Treatment is similar within each subtype, but also overlaps; for example, oral antibiotics can be used for some types of lymphocytic scarring alopecias in addition to those in the neutrophilic group (Table 43.2). Most of the time, systemic therapy should be combined with topical or intralesional corticosteroids or topical calcineurin inhibitors. Adding anti-inflammatory shampoos such as ketoconazole 2% shampoo, zinc pyrithione shampoo, chlorhexidine 4% cleanser, or betadine surgical scrub may be useful adjuncts as well. There are some over the counter shampoos with small amounts of sodium hypochlorite, and these may be useful as well.

Systemic therapy should be considered early in the course, but may be deferred based on patient preference and

C. Goh, MD
David Geffen School of Medicine
at University of California, 200 Medical Plaza Driveway,
Suite 450, Los Angeles, CA 90095, USA
e-mail: cgoh@mednet.ucla.edu

© Springer International Publishing AG 2018
P.S. Yamauchi (ed.), *Biologic and Systemic Agents in Dermatology*, https://doi.org/10.1007/978-3-319-66884-0_43

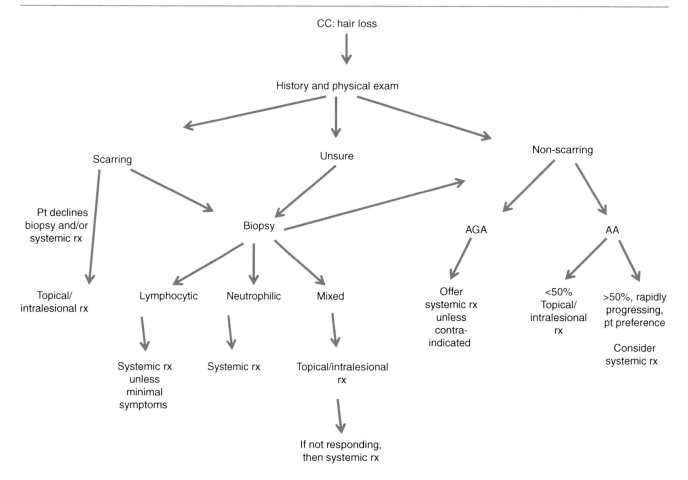

Fig. 43.1 Algorithm for diagnosis and treatment of scarring and non-scarring alopecia

Table 43.1 North American Hair Research Society (NAHRS) working classification of primary cicatricial (scarring) alopecia

Lymphocytic
Chronic cutaneous lupus erythematosus
Lichen planopilaris
Classic lichen planopilaris
Frontal fibrosing alopecia
Graham-Little syndrome
Classic pseudopelade (Brocq)
Central centrifugal cicatricial alopecia
Alopecia mucinosa
Keratosis follicularis spinulosa decalvans
Neutrophilic
Folliculitis decalvans
Dissecting cellulitis/folliculitis
Mixed
Folliculitis (acne) keloidalis
Folliculitis (acne) necrotica
Erosive pustular dermatosis
Nonspecific
Defined as an idiopathic scarring alopecia with inconclusive clinical and histopathologic findings
May include the end stage of a variety of inflammatory cicatricial alopecias

extent of disease symptoms. Lichen planopilaris and frontal fibrosing alopecia are slowly progressive, and many patients may remain stable over years without treatment, with episodes of worsening, then stabilize once more, making it difficult for some patients to accept the potential risks of systemic therapy. If symptoms or hair loss is persistent or progressive, however, systemic therapy should be given stronger consideration.

The goals of treatment for primary scarring alopecia are to reduce or halt progression of hair loss, control any symptoms (burning, pruritus, tenderness), and reduce or eliminate clinical signs of inflammation (erythema, scale) [4]. Of these goals, it is common to control symptoms, but complete elimination of clinical signs of inflammation is rare. Slowing progression of hair loss is difficult to achieve and to confirm, but serial photography can be helpful to determine a treatment's effectiveness.

The effects of treatment may take 6 months or more to appreciate, and disease may resume or flare upon discontinuation of systemic and/or topical therapy. The effectiveness of maintenance therapy with topical and intralesional corticosteroids or topical calcineurin inhibitors has not been established [4].

Table 43.2 Summary of systemic therapies for scarring and non-scarring alopecias

	DLE	LPP	FFA	Graham-Little	Pseudopelade	CCCA	Alopecia mucinosa	KFSD	Folliculitis decalvans	Dissecting cellulitis	Folliculitis keloidalis	Folliculitis necrotica	EPD	AGA	Alopecia areata
Hydroxychloroquine	X	X	X	+/−	+/−	+/−	+/−								−
Prednisone	+	+	−	+/−	+				+	+			X		X
Mycophenolate mofetil	+	+	+		+/−	+/−									−
Cyclosporine	+	X	−	+/−		+/−							+/−		+
Methotrexate	+	+/−	+/−												+
Azathioprine	+		+/−												+
Retinoids	+	+/−	+/−	+/−	+/−		+/−	X	+	+	+	+	+/−		
Dapsone	+						+/−	+	+	+	+	+	+/−		
Other biologics	+	−													+/−
Abatacept	+/−														+/−
Thalidomide	+	+/−													
Tetracyclines		X	X	+/−		X	+/−	+	X	X	X	X	+/−		
Pioglitazone		+	+/−												
TNF-alpha inhibitors	−	+/−							+/−	+					−
5-alpha reductase inhibitors			X											X	
Other antibiotics									X	X	+	+	+/−		
Zinc sulfate									+	+			+/−		
Antiandrogens														X	
Sulfasalazine															+
Simvastatin-ezetimibe															+/−
JAK inhibitors															+

DLE discoid lupus erythematosus, *LPP* lichen planopilaris, *FFA* frontal fibrosing alopecia, *CCCA* central centrifugal cicatricial alopecia, *KFSD* keratosis follicularis spinulosa decalvans, *EPD* erosive pustular dermatosis, *AGA* androgenetic alopecia

X = first-line systemic therapy. + = largely positive results to support use, +/− = mixed results or limited evidence, − = largely negative results

Lymphocytic Scarring Alopecia

Scarring alopecias with lymphocyte predominant inflammation include discoid lupus erythematosus, lichen planopilaris and its variants including frontal fibrosing alopecia, pseudopelade of Brocq (Brocq's alopecia), central centrifugal cicatricial alopecia, alopecia mucinosa, and keratosis follicularis spinulosa decalvans.

Discoid Lupus Erythematosus

Discoid lupus erythematosus (DLE) of the scalp has a female predominance and typically occurs between the ages of 20 and 60 [5]. Lesions are often pruritic and/or tender. Patients often do not have discoid lesions or other types of chronic cutaneous lupus elsewhere on the body, but approximately 14–27% of patients with DLE have extracutaneous signs of disease or will develop systemic lupus erythematosus in the future [6, 7]. Therefore, screening for SLE is important. If treated early in the disease process, the alopecia associated with discoid lupus may be reversible. Early systemic treatment with hydroxychloroquine and possibly of prednisone for patients with one or more American College of Rheumatology (ACR) criteria for SLE, including discoid lupus or alopecia, but less than the four required for diagnosis of SLE, has been associated with delayed onset of SLE [8]. It is unknown if treatment with other systemic agents would have a similar effect or if early treatment prevents development of SLE. Nonetheless, it may be beneficial to implement systemic therapy in DLE earlier in the treatment course than one might consider for a different scarring alopecia.

First-line systemic therapy for DLE of the scalp is hydroxychloroquine (HCQ). HCQ is an antimalarial drug with immunomodulatory properties. There is a wealth of data supporting its use in SLE. In addition to delaying onset of SLE in patients with DLE, HCQ has been shown to reduce or postpone scarring associated with DLE [9]. HCQ is typically started at 200 mg daily for 1 week and then can be increased up to 400 mg daily as tolerated. Common adverse effects include gastrointestinal (GI) intolerance, including nausea, vomiting, and diarrhea, and cutaneous reactions including a blue-gray to black hyperpigmentation and a variety of eruptions including urticarial, morbilliform, eczematous, and lichenoid types [10]. Hemolysis in patients with G6PD deficiency is possible, but not likely in the typical dose range used for DLE. Leukopenia, anemia, pancytopenia, and elevated transaminases are uncommon, but possible. Ophthalmologic toxicity with HCQ tends to be of great concern to patients and physicians. While corneal deposits and neuromuscular eye toxicity are reversible, retinopathy is irreversible, but does not progress if detected early. Recent data suggest the dose should be limited to 5 mg/kg actual weight daily to reduce the risk of retinopathy [11]. Baseline eye examination with automated visual fields and spectral-domain optical coherence tomography is recommended within the first year of use with annual screening recommended after 5 years of exposure unless a patient is at high risk. The major risk factors are dose and duration, underlying maculopathy, renal disease, and tamoxifen use [11].

The new recommendations for dosing mean that many patients may be overdosed at 400 mg daily [12]. However, HCQ doses accumulate, so, for example, for a 55 kg patient, the daily dose should average 275 mg daily. Tablets are supplied in 200 mg, so taking one tablet daily and two tablets alternating every 2–3 days averages 275 mg daily. It is not clear, however, that this dosing would be effective for the uses discussed in this chapter.

If no benefit is seen within 3 months, adding quinacrine 100 mg daily is recommended [4]. This does not increase risk of ocular toxicity. Quinacrine, however, is not commercially available in the USA, but it can be ordered through some compounding pharmacies. Approximately 50% of patients respond to HCQ, but 20% of those may become less responsive over 2 years of continued use [13].

Low-dose prednisone of 10–20 mg daily (≤1 mg/kg/day) tapered over 6–8 weeks can be effective for active disease [4]. Oral retinoids including isotretinoin (40–80 daily) or acitretin (up to 50 mg daily) can be helpful, although adverse effects include telogen effluvium. Acitretin 50 mg daily was shown to be as effective as HCQ in a randomized controlled trial, but had significantly more adverse effects [14]. Dapsone (50–100 mg daily), thalidomide (50–100 mg daily), and methotrexate have shown some efficacy. Azathioprine and cyclosporine are used less commonly, but may be effective in refractory cases. Interestingly, ustekinumab and apremilast have been reported to be effective in a few cases of DLE [15–17].

Lichen Planopilaris

Lichen planopilaris (LPP) typically presents as multifocal patches of scarring alopecia on the scalp with mild to moderate perifollicular erythema and scale, typically on the periphery of the patches. It may be pruritic, tender, or asymptomatic. LPP is most common in Caucasian women in their 50s, but men and women of all ages can be affected [18, 19]. Cutaneous and/or oral lichen planus may be present and, in one series, was seen in as many as 50% of patients, though often after the onset of LPP [4, 18, 20].

Treatment of LPP is challenging, with partial response typical, and spontaneous improvement possible, making it difficult to assess whether our treatments are truly effective [4]. Symptoms of pruritus and pain may be improved with topical and intralesional treatments, but systemic medications may be required for better control [18, 20–22]. Hair loss tends to be progressive, though may be slow at times. Progression or lack thereof can be difficult to assess accurately, even by experts [23]. Nonetheless, data is available regarding the effectiveness of various treatment modalities.

Overall, case series have reported 228 patients treated for LPP with topical and/or systemic medications [24]. It is difficult to compare these studies as the methodology and endpoints differ, but it is possible to generalize the results into groups of "good response, partial response, and no response."

Of the systemic medications, tetracycline antibiotics or HCQ is generally considered first-line. While many practitioners may skip the tetracyclines in favor of HCQ, the safety profile and lack of laboratory monitoring keeps tetracyclines near the top of the list. At least a partial response, defined as improvement of signs and symptoms of disease including stabilization of hair loss, was reported in 54% of patients ($n = 28$) [24]. Tetracycline 500 mg twice daily and doxycycline hyclate 100 mg twice daily have been reported, and doxycycline was found to be similar in efficacy to HCQ [18, 19]. This author has also seen response to treatment with minocycline 100 mg once to twice daily. The mechanism of action is thought to be due to the anti-inflammatory benefits of the tetracycline antibiotics [25, 26]. Due to concerns for antibiotic resistance, it is recommended to limit use to 6 months, if possible [27]. Tapering the dose gradually is recommended to reduce risk for flares.

There are more reports of HCQ use in LPP than tetracyclines ($n = 71$), but the overall percentage of patients with either good or partial response was 53%, comparable to the tetracycline antibiotics [24]. However, Chiang et al. [28] measured response using the Lichen Planopilaris Activity Index (LPPAI), which calculates a score based on symptoms, clinical signs of inflammation, anagen hair pull test, and observed spreading of the condition, and found a significant reduction in the scores in 69% of patients after 6 months of treatment with HCQ and 83% of patients after 12 months ($n = 40$). Dosing is the same as for DLE, ranging from 200 to 400 mg daily.

Cyclosporine at doses of 3–5 mg/kg/day has been reported in 21 patients in the literature with at least a partial response in 83% of patients [24]. Maximum response was reported at 3–5 months, and treatment was discontinued when clinical response was achieved. Recurrence was common after discontinuation of the medication. However, some were able to sustain their response for more than 1 year [29].

Systemic corticosteroids may also be helpful in the short term [20]. Oral prednisone (30–40 mg/day (0.5 mg/kg/day)) tapered slowly over 3–4 months resulted in improvement in 82% of patients ($n = 9/11$) and in 77% of all those reported ($n = 13/17$) [20, 24]. Relapse occurred in most patients within 1 year of discontinuing oral prednisone. As in other conditions, transitioning to a safer long-term treatment, whether systemic or topical, is prudent when using prednisone or cyclosporine.

Pioglitazone is a peroxisome-proliferator gamma agonist (PPAR-gamma) typically used for type 2 diabetes mellitus.

It has been shown that PPAR-gamma is downregulated in patients with LPP [30]. Pioglitazone has been reported to be successful in treating LPP at doses of 15–30 mg daily with the 30 mg dose appearing to be more effective [31–34]. Adverse effects include lower extremity edema, exacerbation of congestive heart failure, and long-term increased risk of bladder cancer. As with other treatments, improvement may not be long-lasting upon discontinuation of the drug.

Mycophenolate mofetil (MMF) use also has been reported in 33 patients with LPP with 48% having at least a partial response [24, 35]. This is similar to HCQ and tetracyclines. Acitretin has also been used at a dose of 25 mg daily with improvement seen in two out of seven patients reported [19, 24]. Griseofulvin has been tried with improvement noted in 5 out of 12 reports (42%) and thalidomide (100–200 mg/day) in 1 out of 5 reports (20%) [20, 24, 36, 37]. Data is limited with methotrexate and other immunosuppressants. Rituximab was effective in one case report [38]. Adalimumab was effective in one patient, but generally TNF-alpha inhibitors have been associated with onset of LPP and other forms of lichen planus, and ustekinumab was ineffective in one case [39–42].

Frontal Fibrosing Alopecia

Frontal fibrosing alopecia (FFA) is considered a variant of LPP and presents with gradual recession of the frontal hairline with or without eyebrow loss (50–95% of cases) [4]. Eyelash and body hair loss may also occur, as well as hair loss along the temporal and/or occipital hairline. LPP on the crown or other areas of the scalp may also occur. Postmenopausal women are most commonly affected, but younger women account for 15% of cases and men may also be affected [4]. Treatment is largely the same as with LPP with the exception of 5-alpha reductase inhibitors, finasteride and dutasteride, in women. It is not known how these work in men with FFA.

Treatments for FFA may have different effectiveness as compared to LPP, possibly related to differences in signs and symptoms of disease and/or pathophysiology [24]. Systemic corticosteroids and cyclosporine do not appear to be beneficial, even in the short term, for FFA [43–46]. The tetracycline antibiotics have been used on occasion with some success [45, 47, 48]. HCQ with or without chloroquine does appear to result in at least partial response or stabilization in the majority of patients and MMF in less than half of patients [28, 43, 49, 50]. There is minimal data published regarding the use of pioglitazone, acitretin, methotrexate, azathioprine, and interferon alfa-2b in FFA; most are negative results or no result as of yet [48, 50].

Finasteride and dutasteride, which inhibit the conversion of testosterone to dihydrotestosterone through 5-alpha reductase, appear to be the most beneficial for FFA with 90% of reported cases resulting in at least partial response [24, 48, 50].

In women with FFA, finasteride is typically used at a dose of 2.5 mg daily and dutasteride can be given with a loading dose of 0.5 mg daily for 1 week, then once weekly as its half-life is 5 weeks. The role of androgens in FFA has not been elucidated, but the effectiveness of these drugs implicates androgens in the pathophysiology of the disease. Hormone replacement therapy, however, has not been effective [43]. It is important to note that there is no clear safety data regarding the use of 5-alpha reductase inhibitors in women and there is no FDA-approved indication in women. Women of childbearing age should be counseled extensively regarding the risk for abnormal development in male fetuses should they become pregnant; pregnancy testing and use of effective contraception are recommended. Review of published data regarding the use of these drugs in women indicates incomplete reporting of adverse effects, but among those reported were decreased libido, breast swelling and tenderness, irregular menstruation, headache, and gastrointestinal discomfort [51, 52]. Dizziness and depression have also been reported.

There is a theoretical concern regarding relative estrogen excess leading to increased risk for breast cancer in men and women taking 5-alpha reductase inhibitors. The inhibition of DHT production can lead to increased testosterone levels, which are converted to estradiol by aromatase. However, one study has suggested that finasteride may actually be protective against some types of breast cancer by inhibiting the production of 5-alpha dihydroprogesterone, which acts as a cancer promoter [53]. Furthermore, although some literature has suggested an increased risk of breast cancer in men taking finasteride or dutasteride, case-control studies in the UK and the USA have shown no increased risk of breast cancer in men who have taken either drug, even with cumulative exposure [54, 55].

Graham-Little Syndrome

Graham-Little syndrome is also considered a variant of LPP in which non-scarring alopecia of the axillae and pubic hair and follicular papules on the trunk and extremities accompany LPP on the scalp [4]. Like LPP and FFA, it is more common in women [56, 57]. There is less data regarding its treatment, but it is typically treated similarly to LPP with some response reported with HCQ in combination with doxycycline, cyclosporine, systemic corticosteroids, and retinoids [58, 59].

Pseudopelade of Brocq

Pseudopelade of Brocq or Brocq's alopecia is a controversial diagnosis, but classified as a lymphocytic primary scarring alopecia. It may represent end-stage lichen planopilaris or other scarring alopecias, but is still treated as a separate entity by some practitioners [4]. It presents with discrete patches of scarring alopecia without follicular hyperkeratosis

or inflammation and is chronic and slowly progressive. Treatment is similar to LPP, but given the rarity of true pseudopelade, the effectiveness of these treatment regimens has not been established. Prednisone 0.5 mg/kg slowly tapered over 2 months may be initiated for actively progressing disease; transitioning to HCQ 200–400 mg daily is considered first-line systemic treatment [60]. Response to HCQ, meaning halting of hair loss, can be seen in the first 3–6 months; if helpful, then the same dose should be continued for 9–12 months, then tapered gradually over the next 6–12 months. Alternative therapies include isotretinoin 1 mg/kg/day for 6–12 months and MMF 1 g twice daily for 3–6 months followed by gradual tapering by 500 mg daily every 2–3 months [60].

Central Centrifugal Cicatricial Alopecia

Central centrifugal cicatricial alopecia (CCCA) is a common form of primary cicatricial alopecia with a prevalence of 3–6% in women of African descent [61–63]. While harsh hair care practices have been associated with CCCA, this association has been found to be inconsistent; thus, the etiology is unknown [61, 64, 65]. Systemic therapy is typically not necessary to control symptoms, which can include pruritus or tenderness, but when needed, tetracycline antibiotics typically are helpful. Improvement may be seen within 2–6 months, after which the dose can be tapered. HCQ, MMF, and cyclosporine have been used as well [4, 66].

Alopecia Mucinosa

Alopecia mucinosa can be considered as follicular mucinosis with associated alopecia. It is typically non-scarring and reversible, presenting as follicular papules and/or indurated plaques most often on the head and neck, but can rarely result in scarring. It is characterized histologically by mucin deposition in the follicular epithelium and may be associated with mycosis fungoides. No specific therapy has been identified as consistently effective for primary alopecia mucinosa. Topical, intralesional and systemic corticosteroids, dapsone, antimalarials, isotretinoin, indomethacin, minocycline, and interferon can be tried [4, 67, 68].

Keratosis Follicularis Spinulosa Decalvans

Keratosis follicularis spinulosa decalvans is a rare genetic form of scarring alopecia on the spectrum of keratosis pilaris atrophicans. It typically begins in childhood with keratosis pilaris on the face, trunk, and extremities followed by cicatricial alopecia on the scalp, eyebrows, and eyelashes. Systemic treatment has been reported with etretinate, isotretinoin, oral antibiotics, and dapsone [4].

In summary, lymphocytic primary scarring alopecias generally can be treated with tetracycline antibiotics, HCQ, or immunosuppressant medications including systemic corticosteroids, cyclosporine, and MMF. Retinoids may have some benefit. Novel treatments for some conditions include pioglitazone for LPP and its variants and 5-alpha reductase inhibitors for FFA. Treatment response can be seen typically between 6 and 12 months, and gradual taper may result in sustained remission after discontinuation of oral therapy.

Neutrophilic Scarring Alopecia

Neutrophil predominant inflammatory primary scarring alopecia includes folliculitis decalvans and dissecting cellulitis of the scalp (perifolliculitis capitis abscedens et suffodiens). Treatment for both conditions start with oral antibiotics, but isotretinoin and TNF-alpha inhibitors have been used with success.

Folliculitis Decalvans

Folliculitis decalvans occurs primarily in young and middle-aged adults with a slight predominance in men [69]. It tends to involve the vertex and occipital areas of the scalp with erythematous papules and pustules that can become quite pruritic and/or tender. Most of the time, *Staphylococcus aureus* can be isolated from these pustules. For that reason, oral antibiotics are considered first-line treatment. Tetracycline, doxycycline, minocycline, erythromycin, clarithromycin, ciprofloxacin, trimethoprim-sulfamethoxazole, dicloxacillin, cephalexin, and clindamycin alone or in combination with rifampin can be used generally with good success, but relapse is commonly seen after discontinuation [70]. Gradual tapering of the antibiotics over the course of many months may help prolong remission [71]. See Table 43.3 for a list of common regimens and recommended dosing.

Any of the antibiotics could be considered first-line, though clindamycin 300 mg twice daily in combination with rifampin 300 mg twice daily for 10 weeks is a classic regimen [72, 73]. Tetracycline 500 mg twice daily, doxycycline 100 mg twice daily, and minocycline 100 mg twice daily are

commonly used as well and have led to sustained remission in some patients, but the course may be required to extend several years, which is less than the ideal given the risk for antibacterial resistance [71]. Rifampin is a highly effective antistaphylococcal agent, but can rapidly induce resistance, so its use is recommended in combination with other antibiotics [74, 75]. A notable side effect of rifampin is turning bodily fluids, including urine, sweat, sputum, and tears, orange or red, which can limit its use in those who wear soft contact lenses, although most soft contacts are now disposable [76]. In addition, rifampin interacts with many drugs as it is a potent cytochrome p450 inducer [74]. Clarithromycin 250 mg twice daily for 3 weeks to 3 months is another potential regimen that may be helpful [70]. As discussed above, transitioning to another treatment after 3–6 months to reduce resistance is recommended in general with antibiotics in inflammatory skin disease.

Dapsone is a sulfone antibiotic that has both antimicrobial activity as well as anti-inflammatory action directed at neutrophil metabolism. It is used in many dermatologic conditions that are neutrophil or eosinophil mediated [77]. Dapsone can be started at a dose of 25–50 mg daily and increased to 100 mg daily if insufficient response is seen at lower doses [4, 69–71]. G6PD levels should be evaluated at baseline, along with complete blood count (CBC) with differential, liver function tests, and creatinine. Screening for hepatitis B or C can also be done as history of hepatitis is associated with higher risk of adverse effects [77]. Hemolytic anemia, methemoglobinemia, and agranulocytosis are expected side effects but vary in intensity. Cyanosis is a sign of mild methemoglobinemia, while more severe methemoglobinemia is characterized by dyspnea and vascular collapse and possibly death. Treatment is with methylene blue, 1–2 mg/kg given by slow injection intravenously [77]. Reticulocyte counts can be followed q2 weeks along with CBC with differential and are increased (2–12%) throughout treatment [69]. Peripheral neuropathy primarily affecting motor neurons is a rare but serious adverse effect and should

Table 43.3 Antibiotic regimens for scarring alopecias

Medication[a]	Dose	Duration[b]
Clindamycin/rifampin	300 mg/300 mg twice daily	10 weeks then taper
Tetracycline	500 mg twice daily	2–4 months, then taper over 6–24 months
Doxycycline	100 mg twice daily	
Minocycline	100 mg twice daily	
Clarithromycin	250 mg twice daily	3 weeks to 3 months
Dapsone	25 mg daily up to 100 mg daily	6–12 months, then taper
Trimethoprim/sulfamethoxazole	1 DS tab twice daily	3–6 months
Cephalexin	500 mg twice daily	1–5 months, then taper
Ciprofloxacin	250–500 mg twice daily	4 weeks at high dose, then 3 weeks low dose

[a]Consider using any of the above with rifampin to reduce risk of antibiotic resistance
[b]Antibiotic use should be limited to 6 months, but in some cases, patients may require a longer course

prompt discontinuation of the medication [77]. Dapsone hypersensitivity syndrome occurs in more than 1% of those taking dapsone [78]. Rash, fever, facial edema, lymphadenopathy, liver function test abnormalities, eosinophilia, and leukocytosis are often seen, and it may occur as long as 5 months after starting dapsone [78]. Dapsone should be discontinued and systemic steroids should be initiated.

Isotretinoin may also be effective for folliculitis decalvans. In one series, it was highly successful with 9/10 patients achieving full remission with 6/10 sustaining that remission off of the medication for up to 2 years. The dose was 0.2–0.5 mg/kg/day (20–40 mg) for 5–7 months followed by slow tapering of the drug to a low dose of 10 mg 2–3 times a week for several months before discontinuation. Some patients were also on dapsone [70]. Other reports are not as promising, and some patients may experience worsening of their symptoms due to the drying effect of isotretinoin [4, 69, 71].

Oral prednisone may be used in conjunction with isotretinoin or oral antibiotics for highly active, rapidly progressing cases [4, 69]. Dosing should be similar to that in severe nodular acne, starting either before or at the same time as isotretinoin or oral antibiotics at a dose of 0.5–1 mg/kg (40–60 mg) tapering over the course of 4 weeks. Oral fusidic acid along with zinc sulfate 400 mg per day for 6 months, followed by 200 mg per day, has also been shown to be effective with more than 1-year follow-up [79]. Zinc is important for normal immune function of the skin, especially innate immunity, and has been found to be helpful for a variety of inflammatory skin conditions [80]. In the USA, zinc sulfate is available in 220 mg tablets, which is equivalent to 50 mg elemental zinc. Fusidic acid is an antistaphylococcal antibiotic that is available in oral and topical forms in many countries, but not in the USA [81]. One case report showed no response to the TNF-alpha inhibitor adalimumab after 3 months, but another showed improvement with adalimumab in two treatment-refractory patients within 2–3 months. The dose used was 40 mg subcutaneous (SC) every 2 weeks after a loading dose of 80 mg SC at day 0 and 40 mg SC at week 1 [40, 82]. Long-term data are unavailable.

Dissecting Cellulitis

Dissecting cellulitis of the scalp (DCS) is a rare chronic inflammatory disease of the scalp leading to scarring alopecia, predominantly in young African American men. It is exquisitely tender, presenting with suppurative nodules and draining sinus tracts, and is considered part of the follicular occlusion triad along with acne conglobata and hidradenitis suppurativa, though patients most often have DCS alone [4]. Lesions are typically sterile, though secondary bacterial infections can occur [83]. Seronegative arthritis is rarely seen in association [84, 85]. Tinea capitis must be ruled out with culture studies, especially if the patient is not in the typical demographic [86].

Treatment of DCS is markedly similar to folliculitis decalvans, but is often refractory to treatment and has a high relapse rate. Oral antibiotics including tetracyclines, ciprofloxacin, trimethoprim/sulfamethoxazole, clindamycin, rifampin, cephalexin, dapsone, and others are often used first-line and may result in moderate improvement or reduction of pain, but relapse occurs with discontinuation of treatment [83, 87]. Ciprofloxacin has been reportedly successful in achieving improvement in several cases at a dose of 250 mg twice daily or 500 mg twice daily for 4 weeks, then 250 mg twice daily for 3 weeks [88, 89]. This result is likely due to immunomodulatory effects of fluoroquinolones, which can induce interleukin (IL)-2 synthesis and inhibit IL-1 and TNF-alpha. Influence on intracellular cyclic adenosine monophosphate and phosphodiesterases and nuclear factor kappa B may be the mechanism for immunomodulation [88]. However, a potential severe adverse effect of fluoroquinolones is tendon rupture (0.14–0.4%), which suggests that it should be prescribed with caution. Tendon rupture is more likely in older patients with comorbid conditions and with concomitant corticosteroid use [90].

Isotretinoin tends to have good results with DCS at doses of 0.5–1 mg/kg/day [87, 91]. One regimen is to continue for at least 4 months after remission is achieved in order to reduce the risk of recurrence [4]. Adding dapsone (50–100 mg daily) or rifampin (300 mg twice daily) has been reported to improve outcomes if monotherapy with isotretinoin is insufficient [92, 93]. In one patient who failed acitretin 20 mg daily, alitretinoin was effective. The dose was 10 mg daily for 2 months, followed by 20 mg daily, and improvement noted after 5 months of therapy. Eventually, treatment was reduced to 10 mg daily [94].

TNF-alpha inhibitors, specifically adalimumab and infliximab, have been used with some success [82, 83, 95, 96]. Adalimumab was administered at the standard plaque psoriasis dosing: 80 mg subcutaneous initially followed by 40 mg subcutaneous at 1 week and every 2 weeks thereafter. Although some patients had sustained remission following discontinuation, others relapsed, suggesting that chronic therapy may be necessary in some cases. Combination therapy with oral antibiotics may be useful in conjunction with TNF-alpha inhibitors.

Use of oral prednisolone has been reported as well, with temporary benefit [88]. Zinc sulfate 220 mg (50 mg elemental zinc) three times daily as monotherapy has been recommended [91]. Dose of 135 mg three times daily followed by 260 mg daily was successful in one case, but relapse occurred upon withdrawal, then 135 mg once or twice daily was resumed and maintained for a year with remission [97]. Another regimen reported was 90 mg elemental zinc three times daily with improvement after 6 weeks of therapy [98]. The absorption of zinc as well as fluoroquinolones and tetracyclines is reduced when taken together. Signs of zinc toxicity include nausea, vomiting, loss of appetite, abdominal cramps, diarrhea, and headaches. Copper levels can be reduced as zinc affects its absorption [99]. Zinc therapy has been ineffective in some cases of DCS [88].

In summary, neutrophilic primary scarring alopecias can be treated with oral antibiotics, isotretinoin or other oral retinoids, or TNF-alpha inhibitors. Zinc therapy may be effective as monotherapy or adjuvant therapy. Combination therapy with multiple systemic medications in addition to topical treatments may be more effective.

Mixed Inflammatory Scarring Alopecia

Folliculitis (acne) keloidalis, folliculitis (acne) necrotica, and erosive pustular dermatosis comprise those scarring alopecias that have mixed inflammation on histopathology. Treatment of these is similar to that of neutrophil predominant primary scarring alopecias.

Folliculitis (Acne) Keloidalis

Folliculitis keloidalis, or acne keloidalis, is also primarily seen in young men of African descent and is characterized by inflamed papules or pustules that develop into keloidal papules and plaques with resultant scarring alopecia. Most commonly, it is on the occipital scalp at the nape of the neck. Typically, topical, intralesional therapy, or surgical therapy suffice, but oral antibiotics (typically tetracyclines or erythromycin) or isotretinoin may be effective if needed [100, 101]. Similar to the neutrophilic scarring alopecias, dosing can be tapered gradually to reduce risk for recurrence [4, 101].

Folliculitis (Acne) Necrotica

Folliculitis necrotica, or acne necrotica, is a rare condition composed of two types: varioliformis and miliaris. Folliculitis necrotica varioliformis results in scarring alopecia and usually involves the anterior hairline and seborrheic areas of the face and trunk. Reddish-brown papulopustules appear and develop central necrosis, eventually leaving atrophic scars. Treatment consists of oral antibiotics or isotretinoin [4].

Erosive Pustular Dermatosis

Erosive pustular dermatosis is an underrecognized primary scarring alopecia that tends to affect elderly patients, particularly those who have had trauma to the scalp via surgery, radiation therapy, or actinic keratosis treatment with cryotherapy, topical imiquimod, photodynamic therapy, or 5-fluorouracil [102–104]. Erosions, crusting, and pustular lesions are characteristic, and patients may be diagnosed as having chronic non-healing wounds. Pruritus may be present [102, 103]. It may also present on other parts of the body [105, 106]. Topical therapy with high potency corticosteroids, calcineurin inhibitors, or dapsone is usually effective, but systemic therapy may be required in some cases [4, 102–104]. Oral prednisone tapered slowly over 3–4 weeks or more can be effective. The use of doxycycline (100 mg twice daily), isotretinoin (0.75 mg/kg/day × 4 months), acitretin (50 mg daily tapered to 25 mg daily over 3 months), oral dapsone (50 mg three times a day, tapered to 50 mg twice daily over 3–4 months), cyclosporine (3 mg/kg/day × 3 weeks), and oral zinc sulfate (60 mg three times daily) has been reported, but with mixed results [4, 102, 106–111].

Non-scarring Alopecia

Non-scarring alopecias are significantly more common than scarring alopecias, and many types have been described [112]. Androgenetic alopecia and alopecia areata are common causes of non-scarring alopecia, and various systemic treatments are available. While the hair follicle is not destroyed, other types of non-scarring alopecia are not medically treatable, such as temporal triangular alopecia and congenital atrichia with papular lesions [113, 114]. Acute telogen effluvium typically does not require treatment either.

Treatment of trichotillomania may require oral medications, but psychiatric management is advised. One case report notes successful treatment of trichotillomania with N-acetylcysteine 1200 mg daily in two patients for 4–6 months with sustained remission for at least 8 months off of medication [115].

Type II vitamin D-dependent rickets is autosomal recessive and sometimes presents with a non-scarring alopecia in the first 6 months of life. Some patients do not regrow hair when treated with the standard 1-alpha-hydroxycholecalciferol and calcium, but this was successful in one case [116, 117].

Chemotherapy-induced anagen effluvium is typically reversible after completion of chemotherapy, but some patients have permanent chemotherapy-induced alopecia. Topical minoxidil may be helpful in this situation, but one case report showed successful treatment with low-dose oral minoxidil 1 mg daily with improvement seen as early as 6 weeks. No adverse effects were reported, specifically there were no changes in blood pressure or hypertrichosis in non-scalp areas [118]. Theoretically, oral minoxidil, a potent antihypertensive agent, may be helpful in other types of hair loss, but there are no published efficacy or safety data in this regard, except one negative study in alopecia areata (5 mg twice daily) that required a strict 2 g sodium diet to reduce the risk of hypernatremia and fluid retention [119]. Cardiac risks preclude its common use in hypertension, but safety of low-dose (1 mg daily) oral minoxidil is unknown.

Androgenetic Alopecia

Androgenetic alopecia (AGA) likely affects at least 80% of Caucasian men and 40–50% of Caucasian women in their lifetime [120, 121]. Although known to be genetic, AGA is a polygenic condition with unclear mode of inheritance—either maternal or paternal relatives may be affected [122]. Male AGA is understood to be clearly androgen dependent, but in females the role of androgens is less clear, hence the use of the term female pattern hair loss (FPHL) instead of AGA [123]. As in scarring alopecia, the primary goal of treatment is to halt progression of hair loss/thinning with a small chance of regrowth. Topical minoxidil 2–5% is a mainstay of treatment, and all patients should be encouraged to use it, if possible, in addition to systemic therapies, should they choose to pursue them. Given possible adverse effects, many patients opt not to treat AGA.

In men, finasteride 1 mg once daily is FDA approved for the treatment of AGA. Finasteride is a type 2 5-alpha reductase inhibitor that decreases the conversion of testosterone to dihydrotestosterone (DHT), a more potent androgen. DHT is responsible for the miniaturization of hair follicles in male AGA. In a systematic review of the literature, long-term use of finasteride in men resulted in improvement in 30% of patients over 2–5 years and found no difference between the 1 mg and 5 mg dose [124]. There was no discussion of stabilization of disease, but some studies have reported halting of the hair loss as shown by hair counts in as many as 70–86% of men as compared to 42% of men on placebo [125–127]. Improvement of AGA can be seen within 6 months and continues at least 5 years. Return to pretreatment status occurs within 1 year of discontinuation [128]. One retrospective study reported that finasteride was effective in boys aged 14–19 with 1 out of 6 patients with decreased sexual function that resolved despite staying on the medication [129]. Safety data is lacking in adolescents, though, so finasteride use in boys younger than 18 is not recommended. While finasteride is generally well tolerated with no reported hepatotoxicity or nephrotoxicity, the main concern for adverse effects is typically regarding sexual function [128]. Decreased libido, erectile dysfunction, and decreased ejaculated volume are reported in approximately 3.8% of patients vs. 2.1% for placebo [124]. The rate is lower in men ages 18–41 (1.8% vs. 1.1%) than in men over 41 (8.7% vs. 5.1%) [125, 130]. Gynecomastia with or without pain can be seen [131]. There can be reduction in sperm motility, and there are reports of infertility associated with long-term finasteride use. This appears to be reversible when the drug is discontinued [132–134]. The half-life of finasteride is 4.7–7.1 h, but it can accumulate with multiple doses [135]. The concentration of finasteride in semen is low, and men taking finasteride do not pose any risk to a pregnant woman or her fetus [136]. Therefore, if a patient is trying to conceive with a female partner, discontinuation may be advised if they are having difficulty. Once pregnant, the patient can resume finasteride.

Permanent sexual side effects are a concern, but have only been reported in post-marketing surveillance (<1%) [137]. Depression and suicidal ideation have also been reported, especially in those with permanent sexual side effects. Androgen levels may be lower in these patients [138]. Post-finasteride syndrome is a term that describes these prolonged adverse effects. It is important to note that most patients with sexual side effects experience them mildly and can continue the drug, while others experience resolution of their symptoms upon discontinuation of the drug [124].

Patients should be advised that their prostate-specific antigen (PSA) levels are reduced by about 50%, which could mask prostate cancer early on. Baseline PSA levels may be considered prior to starting finasteride in men over age 50. Patients taking finasteride are 25% less likely to develop prostate cancer, but if prostate cancer develops, it may be higher-grade disease, likely due to detection bias—as finasteride reduces the size of the prostate, a blind biopsy from the prostate is more likely to show cancer cells [139, 140]. Long-term consequences of finasteride 5 mg daily in the Prostate Cancer Prevention Trial (7 years of medication, with median of 16 years of follow-up, $n = 13,935$) showed a 10% increased risk of depression in the treatment group as compared to the placebo group and a 6% decreased risk of procedures for benign prostatic hyperplasia-related events. No long-term cardiac, endocrine, or sexual adverse effects were seen [141].

In women, the evidence is far weaker to support the use of finasteride. In several case reports and uncontrolled studies, finasteride 2.5–5 mg daily has been effective in pre- and postmenopausal women, but randomized controlled trials of finasteride 1 mg daily in postmenopausal women showed no benefit over placebo [142–146]. Women of childbearing age should utilize effective contraception as it can cause feminization of a male fetus [147]. Furthermore, men taking finasteride should be advised against blood donation given the risk of a pregnant woman receiving the blood products.

Dutasteride is a dual 5-alpha reductase inhibitor (both types 1 and 2) that reduces serum DHT levels by more than 90% as compared to 70% for finasteride [148]. The dose approved in the USA for benign prostatic hyperplasia is 0.5 mg daily. It is approved for use at the same dose for male AGA in a few countries, including Korea and Mexico, but not the USA [149]. A few trials have shown that dutasteride is superior to finasteride in increasing hair counts, though the dosing required to achieve superiority may be as high as 2.5 mg daily [150, 151]. At the very least, dutasteride 0.5 mg daily is as effective as finasteride 1 mg daily. Concomitant therapy may be more effective, and dutasteride may be effective even if finasteride has failed [152, 153]. Adverse effects have been similar to those of finasteride at similar rates [150, 151]. However, the half-life, at 5 weeks, is significantly longer than that of finasteride, which implies that adverse effects may persist for longer as well [132]. In women, a few case reports suggest that dutasteride 0.5 mg daily can be effective [154, 155].

For FPHL, androgen receptor antagonists may be used. Spironolactone, cyproterone acetate (not available in the USA), and flutamide may be used, but overall evidence is limited regarding their effectiveness.

Spironolactone is a synthetic steroidal derivative of aldosterone that works as an aldosterone antagonist. Therefore, it is potassium sparing and has a diuretic effect. It is a competitive inhibitor of the androgen receptor, weakly reduces synthesis of testosterone, and decreases 5-alpha reductase activity [156–159]. Spironolactone 50–200 mg daily may be effective in halting progression of FPHL (26–44%) and improving hair density (44–70%) [160, 161]. Side effects include diuresis, potential hyperkalemia, irregular menstrual periods, breast swelling and tenderness, headache or light-headedness, and fatigue. Combining spironolactone treatment with an oral contraceptive can alleviate the symptoms of irregular menstrual bleeding and ensure pregnancy is avoided given the risk of feminization of a male fetus. The risk of hyperkalemia has been shown to be minimal, even when spironolactone is administered with other aldosterone antagonists (such as drospirenone-containing oral contraceptives) [162]. The rate of hyperkalemia in healthy young females (ages 18–41) taking spironolactone for acne was revealed to be equivalent to that of the general population; therefore, routine monitoring is of low utility in this group [163]. However, if a patient is taking another medication that can cause hyperkalemia, such as an angiotensin-converting enzyme inhibitor, monitoring should be done. Long-term studies in rats receiving high doses of spironolactone demonstrated an increased incidence of adenomas on endocrine organs and the liver, resulting in a black box warning by the FDA (www.drugs.com/pro/aldactone). The potential for spironolactone to induce estrogen-dependent malignancies in women remains controversial. However, the available data suggests there is no association between breast carcinoma and spironolactone ingestion, with more than 30 years of data [164, 165]. Patients should be counseled regarding this potential risk, but note that the risk is low. Still, patients with strong family history of breast cancer should likely not be prescribed spironolactone.

Cyproterone acetate is also a competitive inhibitor of the androgen receptor with a similar chemical structure to spironolactone, but with progestational activity and weak glucocorticoid activity [158, 161]. Outside of the USA, it is used at low doses (2 mg) in conjunction with ethinyl estradiol in oral contraception. At higher doses (300 mg daily), it is used in men for palliative treatment of prostate cancer and

has been associated with hepatotoxicity [166]. In FPHL, doses of 100 mg daily for the first 10 days of the menstrual cycle in premenopausal women and 50 mg daily in postmenopausal women have been associated with stabilization or improvement of hair loss and have been tolerated well. The response rate to cyproterone acetate is similar to spironolactone [161]. Hormonal adverse effects are also similar to spironolactone. There is a slightly increased risk of venous thromboembolism with combined oral contraceptive pills with cyproterone acetate as the progestin as compared to other progestins, but similar to those with desogestrel, drospirenone, or gestodene [166].

Flutamide, a nonsteroidal antiandrogen, is a more potent competitive inhibitor of the androgen receptor that is FDA approved to treat prostate cancer [167]. It has been used successfully at doses of 62.5–250 mg daily in combination with or without oral contraceptives for treatment of FPHL [167–169]. Liver function tests should be monitored as cases of fatal hepatitis have been reported, but hepatotoxicity is dose dependent [170]. Like the other antiandrogens, pregnancy and blood donation should be avoided. The use of flutamide in the treatment of FPHL may be limited by its high rate of side effects, which include abdominal pain, nausea, vomiting, diarrhea, dry skin, headache, transaminitis, and dyslipidemia [171].

Alopecia Areata

Alopecia areata (AA) is a T-cell-mediated autoimmune condition that causes non-scarring hair loss typically in smooth, well-demarcated patches on the scalp or other parts of the body. It is typically asymptomatic, though some patients may experience tenderness or pruritus of the scalp. It is unpredictably relapsing and remitting with a high rate of spontaneous regrowth, especially in the first year after onset, which makes it difficult to conduct meaningful studies. The more severe subtypes, ophiasis (band-like involvement along the temporal and occipital hairlines), totalis (AT;100% scalp hair loss), and universalis (AU;100% scalp and body hair loss), are less likely to have spontaneous regrowth, but it is possible.

Due to potential adverse effects of many of the systemic treatments used for AA, unclear benefit, and high rate of relapse, systemic therapy is typically reserved for those patients with extensive hair loss, defined as 50% or more scalp involvement, or for those that appear to be rapidly progressing toward 50% or more scalp hair loss [172, 173]. Still, there may be instances in which systemic therapy may be indicated for patients with less extensive AA, and discussing all therapeutic options along with their potential risks and benefits is recommended in order to create the best treatment plan for a particular patient.

Table 43.4 Dosing regimens for systemic corticosteroids in alopecia areata

Route	Medication	Dose	Interval[a]
Intravenous	Prednisolone	2 g	1 day per month
		100 mg	3 days per month
	Methyl. prednisolone	500 mg[b], 1 g	3 days per month
		5–25 mg/kg	3 days per month
	Dexamethasone	32–100 mg	3 days per month
		60 mg	1 day per month
Intramuscular	Triamcinolone	40 mg	Once monthly
Oral	Prednisone	500 mg	5 days per month
		5 mg/kg	1 day per month
	Prednisolone	300 mg	1 day per month
		5 mg/kg	1 day per month
		80 mg	3 days per month
	Methylprednisolone	15 mg/kg	3 days every 2–3 weeks
	Dexamethasone	2.5–5 mg	2 days per week
	Betamethasone	1–5 mg	2 days per week
		0.1 mg/kg	2 days per week
	Prednisolone	200 mg	1 day per week
		30 mg	3 days per week
	Prednisolone or prednisone	40 mg with slow tapering	Daily over 6 weeks or more

[a]Aside from a continuous tapering dose, the duration of a regimen can range from 3 months to 12 months
[b]The most common intravenous regimen is methylprednisolone 500 mg, 3 days per month

Systemic corticosteroids have been used for decades in the treatment of extensive AA. Many regimens have been published including oral, intramuscular, and intravenous routes and standard or pulsed dosing (weekly or monthly), which is favored by some due to reduced adverse effects associated with long-term corticosteroid use [174, 175]. See Table 43.4 for some dosing regimens. One randomized controlled trial was done using 200 mg prednisolone orally once weekly for 3 months followed by 3 months of observation [176]. Forty percent of patients (n = 8) had regrowth, but only two of those patients had complete regrowth and two of the patients relapsed. None of the patients on placebo had regrowth. A systematic review of all published studies using pulsed dosing of systemic corticosteroids for AA showed an overall 43% rate of complete response, defined as >75% hair regrowth and 51% complete response in pediatric-only studies [175]. The duration of follow-up varies greatly between studies, but the reported relapse rate was relatively low at 17% overall, but higher in the pediatric-only studies at 60%. Adverse effects were reported in 21% of patients, including epigastric pain, fatigue, headache, acneiform rash, and palpitations, and were considered of minor severity. Those more likely to respond had patchy alopecia, disease duration 6–24 months, and were in their first episode of AA [175]. Other reported side effects of systemic glucocorticoids are general weakness, acneiform eruption, weight gain, gastrointestinal upset, facial mooning, oligomenorrhea, osteoporosis, diabetes, and suppression of adrenocorticotropic axes [176].

Alternatively, if standard daily dosing is done, the systemic corticosteroids should be tapered gradually to avoid a rebound effect and to reduce the risk of adrenal suppression. Tapering regimens can vary greatly, but one proposed regimen starts with prednisone 40–60 mg daily (for adults) gradually tapered by 5–10 mg per week through 20 mg. Then tapering by 2.5–5 mg per week until 5 mg daily, after which it could be tapered by 1–2.5 mg per week until off [177]. Transitioning to monthly intralesional corticosteroid injections and/or topical corticosteroids, depending on the response, may also reduce the risk of relapse or flare. Topical minoxidil has also been helpful to reduce relapse [178]. These can be added when the dose is at 20 mg daily. At any point in the taper, if flare is suspected or adrenal suppression is suspected (see symptoms below), the taper should be temporarily halted, and hydrocortisone or an increased dose of the glucocorticoid should be given until the patient stabilizes. AM cortisol levels and a corticotropin stimulation test may be warranted at this time. Resumption of the taper at a slower rate can take place 2–4 weeks after stabilization of symptoms. Signs and symptoms of adrenal suppression include weakness, fatigue, nausea, vomiting, diarrhea, abdominal pain, fever, weight loss, myalgias, arthralgias, and malaise [177].

Intramuscular injections of triamcinolone (IM TAC) at 40 mg monthly can also have some benefit [179, 180]. Successful regimens, leading to more than 40% scalp hair regrowth, include monthly treatments for 3–6 months, with some cases followed by treatment every 1.5 months for 1 year. Compared to a pulsed regimen of 80 mg for 3 days every 3 months, 40 mg IM TAC every 1–2 months for one and a half years resulted in slightly higher response rate, relapse rate, and rate of adverse effects [179]. IM TAC also was associated with a higher rate of adrenal suppression measured by lab monitoring (AM cortisol, adrenocorticotropic hormone (ACTH), urine cortisol), but the lab tests normalized within 2 months without treatment. It is not clear, however, that these treatment regimens are equivalent, so this data cannot be extrapolated to other pulsed regimens.

Ultimately, systemic corticosteroid therapy does appear to be effective at least temporarily through a number of different regimens, including intramuscular, intravenous, and oral, pulsed and continuous. Evidence does not suggest that one regimen is consistently safer or more effective than another, except that low-dose continuous or pulsed regimens may not be as effective [179, 181]. It is also not clear that systemic corticosteroid therapy alters the overall course of the disease, but it does appear that there can be benefit in some cases. However, care must be taken in regard to monitoring for adverse effects. Annual DEXA scans may be indicated for long-term use in addition to supplementing calcium and vitamin D; gastrointestinal prophylaxis could be considered with a proton pump inhibitor; regular lab monitoring could be considered for electrolytes and renal function and glucose levels. Screening for cataracts or glaucoma history, checking blood pressure at each visit, checking fasting lipids, and monitoring psychiatric symptoms are also recommended [177].

Other traditional immunosuppressants have mixed evidence to support their use. These include methotrexate, cyclosporine, sulfasalazine, and azathioprine. These are sometimes used in conjunction with systemic corticosteroids. Mycophenolate mofetil showed no benefit in a small series, and oral tacrolimus was beneficial in one case [182, 183]. While they may be effective in some cases, overall, their side effect profile and high rate of relapse mean the risk to benefit ratio is high and their use in regular clinical practice is limited.

Cyclosporine (2–6 mg/kg/day) is a potent inhibitor of interleukin 2 (IL-2), which stimulates the proliferation and activation of T lymphocytes and plays an important role in AA. Published series often use it in conjunction with or without systemic corticosteroids with a response rate (>50% regrowth) of 25–76.7% [173, 181, 184–186]. Addition of corticosteroids, however, does not appear to improve its effectiveness, nor does it reduce the risk of relapse [185, 186]. Some series suggest that adverse effects are fewer with cyclosporine than systemic corticosteroids [186]. Cyclosporine use is typically limited to 1 year due to risks including nephrotoxicity, immune suppression, hypertension, and hypertrichosis of body hair.

Methotrexate (15–25 mg weekly) offers a safer long-term option than systemic corticosteroids or cyclosporine, but should not be used in women of childbearing age as it is an abortifacient. Its effectiveness both with and without oral corticosteroids ranges from 38 to 63% complete response in patients with AT/AU [187–189]. Response was seen as early as 3 months into treatment, but it may take 1 year or more [190]. Relapse rate is high. Hepatotoxicity is possible with liver fibrosis and cirrhosis reported with high cumulative doses. There are varying guidelines for liver biopsy, and monitoring of procollagen III peptide has been suggested [191, 192]. Leukopenia, nausea, and telogen effluvium can also be seen, and many medications can interact with methotrexate.

Azathioprine and sulfasalazine have also been used for AA. These also offer a longer-term option than systemic corticosteroids or cyclosporine, but still commonly cause adverse effects and have a high rate of relapse upon discontinuation. Azathioprine (2 mg/kg/day) resulted in a mean regrowth percentage of 52.3% out of 20 patients studied over the course of 6 months, with at least one patient having complete regrowth only after 10 months of continued treatment [193]. Another case series used a dose of 2.5 mg/kg/day and found a complete response rate of 43% in their patients after approximately 5 months [194]. Baseline TPMT (thiopurinemethyltransferase) levels are required, and close laboratory monitoring for myelosuppression must be done.

Sulfasalazine is an immunomodulatory drug more often used for inflammatory bowel disease and rheumatoid arthritis. It has been used in limited studies for AA with more than 60% regrowth in approximately 25% of patients and more than 10% regrowth in 68–79% of patients [195–199]. Dosing begins at 500 mg twice daily, then gradually increased up to a total of 3–4 g per day in split doses. Patients with response were treated for up to 4 years with doses reduced or increased as needed [197]. Initial laboratory abnormalities, if mild, may resolve without changing the dose. Unfortunately, sulfasalazine use is often limited by gastrointestinal distress and headaches.

Anecdotally, some practitioners use hydroxychloroquine (HCQ) for AA. Few case reports exist in the literature with mixed results [200, 201]. At a dose of 200 mg twice daily, those who did experience regrowth responded within 2–5 months. Several relapsed despite staying on therapy, and long-term data is unavailable for those who did not. However, its safety profile makes it an attractive choice, particularly in children and patients who have other autoimmune diseases.

Simvastatin/ezetimibe is a combination drug used to treat hyperlipidemia. Two case reports were published in which patients took the medication for their hyperlipidemia and had marked improvement of their AA, but notably did not have response to simvastatin alone [202, 203]. This led to a pilot study of 29 patients with AA with 40–70% scalp hair loss [204]. The dose was 40 mg simvastatin/10 mg ezetimibe, and the response rate (>20% regrowth) was 73% in patients with 40–70% scalp hair loss. Relapse occurred in those who discontinued the drug. Another study of 20 patients with more extensive AA showed mild response in only one patient [205]. Headaches and muscle cramps were reported, but mild; reported risks of simvastatin/ezetimibe also include diarrhea, muscle weakness, and rhabdomyolysis. There is also interaction with CYP3A4 inhibitors and risk of transaminitis. The mechanism of action is unclear, but statins are known to modulate lymphocyte activity, and ezetimibe appears to have an antioxidant effect and perhaps a role in autophagy [206]. Simvastatin has been shown to have an effect of janus kinase (JAK) inhibition as well [207].

As in other inflammatory skin disorders, targeted therapies have become attractive options for AA as they may be more effective and have a better safety profile. These include JAK inhibitors, for which studies and case reports are available. There is less data available for the following, but studies suggest they may be effective. These are abatacept (CTLA4 agonist), ustekinumab (IL-12/23p40 inhibitor), and apremilast (PDE4 inhibitor). Secukinumab (IL-17 inhibitor), dupilumab (IL-4 inhibitor), and tralokinumab (IL-13 inhibitor) have also been suggested based on their mechanisms of action. However, one must consider these carefully as they may not necessarily be effective. Past treatments thought to be promising have sometimes been disappointing. For example, TNF-alpha inhibitors have largely been deemed ineffective and have been associated with onset of AA [208, 209]. Alafacept, a soluble LFA-3-Ig fusion protein, prevents T-cell activation, but was also found to be ineffective in AA [210].

At this time, JAK inhibitors are the most promising emerging therapy for AA. Studies have shown that AA is mediated by interferon gamma producing NKG2D-expressing CD8+ T cells. They are recruited and activated by IL-2, IL-15, NKG2, and MHC ligands. Blockade of IL-2, IL-15, and interferon (IFN) gamma has been shown to prevent the development of AA in mouse models [211]. Janus kinases are downstream effectors of IFN-gamma and mediate IL-15 activation of T cells. The discovery of NKG2D polymorphisms in AA led to the understanding that this pathway was involved and that JAK inhibitors may be an effective treatment.

Current FDA-approved drugs in this class are ruxolitinib (JAK 1/2 inhibition primarily) and tofacitinib (pan-JAK inhibition). Ruxolitinib is approved for use in myelofibrosis and polycythemia vera, whereas tofacitinib is approved for use in rheumatoid arthritis. While JAK 1, 2, and TYK2 receptors are ubiquitous, JAK 3 receptors are found in hematopoietic, myeloid, and lymphoid cells [212]. Adverse effects include diarrhea and other GI side effects, headaches, liver function abnormalities, hyperlipidemia, infection, including herpes zoster, possible malignancy, and bowel perforation. Reduced response to vaccination is also possible [213]. Overall, the adverse effects due to immunosuppression are not significantly different from other targeted immunosuppressive therapies. Long-term risk, however, remains unknown.

Both ruxolitinib and tofacitinib have been studied with good results, but like other systemic treatments have a high relapse rate. One open-label clinical trial has been done with ruxolitinib (20 mg twice daily) in 12 patients with a baseline mean SALT score of 65%, 9 (75%) of whom had >50% regrowth within 3–6 months [214]. Within 3 months after discontinuation, all had increased shedding, but none reached their baseline. Minor infections, mild gastrointestinal symptoms, and low hemoglobin level were reported. Gene expression profiling showed that patients with low baseline IFN and cytotoxic lymphocyte signatures on scalp biopsies were less likely to respond to treatment.

More studies have been done with tofacitinib. In one two-center open-label clinical trial at 5 mg twice daily, 32% of patients had >50% regrowth after 3 months of treatment [215]. An additional 32% of patients had >5% but <50% regrowth. Those with AT/AU were less likely to respond during this time frame, but an additional retrospective analysis found that 58% of 65 patients had >50% response after 4–18 months of treatment, although some of the patients in the latter study were treated with prednisone (300 mg monthly for 3 doses) and/or were treated at higher doses of tofacitinib (up to 10 mg twice daily) [216]. It was also shown to be highly effective in 10 of 14 adolescent patients between the ages of 12 and 17 over the course of 2–16 months with mild adverse effects including headaches, upper respiratory infections, and mild liver transaminase elevation that resolved despite continuing therapy [217]. Caution is advised as the JAK/STAT pathway is ubiquitous and involved in many regulatory processes including growth hormone, which is known to regulate body growth via JAK 2 [212].

Abatacept is a soluble fusion protein that functions as a cytotoxic T-lymphocyte-associated antigen 4 (CTLA4) agonist that binds to CD80 and CD86 on antigen-presenting cells [218]. It thereby inhibits optimal T-cell activation by blocking the co-stimulatory pathway. In vitro, abatacept decreases T-cell proliferation and inhibits production of TNF-alpha, IFN-gamma, and IL-2. It is approved for use in rheumatoid arthritis. Polymorphisms in genes involved in the co-stimulatory pathway were found in genome-wide association studies, suggesting that abatacept may be an effective therapy [211]. An open-label, proof-of-concept, clinical trial was done with 15 patients given subcutaneous abatacept 125 mg once weekly for 6 months [219]. Patients had 30–100% scalp hair loss at baseline, and one patient had 98% regrowth and two others had up to 23% regrowth. Abatacept may be helpful for a subset of patients, but this study does not support its use.

Ustekinumab, a human monoclonal IgG1 antibody that inhibits the p40 subunit of IL-12 and IL-23, showed improvement of hair growth in three patients, with one showing complete regrowth after about 1 year [220]. The dose used was 90 mg subcutaneously every 12 weeks. The rationale of its usage was based on gene expression studies showing a significantly increased level of mRNA of IL-12/23p40 in scalp biopsies from patients with AA as compared to those of healthy controls [221]. However, there have been some case reports of patients developing AA while on 45 mg of ustekinumab q12 weeks [222, 223]. Ustekinumab is approved for use in psoriasis. Along the same lines, secukinumab, an IL-17 inhibitor approved for use in psoriasis is also of interest in AA, and a clinical trial is ongoing [224].

Apremilast, a phosphodiesterase 4 (PDE4) inhibitor, is also approved for use in psoriasis. PDE4 was also found to be upregulated in gene expression studies in AA [221], and one study showed that it prevented onset of AA in human skin grafts on mice [225]. No human studies or case reports are available at this time.

Interleukin-2 is known to be a mediator of disease activity in AA, but treatment with low-dose IL-2 has been associated with an increase in T regulatory cells, which may help to modulate the abnormal immune response in AA and other autoimmune diseases [226]. In the USA, IL-2 is commercially available under the name of aldesleukin and FDA approved for use in metastatic renal cell carcinoma and metastatic melanoma, in which they are used at high doses. One study showed that in four of five patients with extensive AA, subcutaneous IL-2, 1.5 MIU/d for 5 days, followed by three 5-day courses of 3 MIU/d at weeks 3, 6, and 9 was associated with at least partial response at 6 months after treatment [227]. Response was seen 2 months after the end of the treatment and improved at 6 months as well. Treatment adverse events were mild to moderate with asthenia, arthralgia, urticaria, and local reactions at injection sites. High-dose IL-2 is associated with exacerbation or onset of autoimmune disease and inflammatory disorders, but the low-dose regimen does not appear to do the same [226].

In summary, systemic therapy for AA consists of traditional and newer immunomodulators and immunosuppressants. The evidence is generally of poor quality, with small series, with variable disease severity and different endpoints. Duration of treatment and follow-up off of treatment as well as combination therapy make it very difficult to compare the medications and determine which are more effective than others. Nearly all the medications discussed carry risks associated with immunosuppression, but most are tolerated well by patients who are otherwise healthy. Overall, the effectiveness rate of systemic therapies appears to be comparable, 25–70% for >50% regrowth, with high rates of relapse upon discontinuation of treatment. Longer duration of disease and more extensive disease predict worse response to any treatment. Therapy still should be individualized based on the individual patient's health and preferences, including cost. Including topical or intralesional therapy with corticosteroids or minoxidil may help reduce the risk for relapse.

Case Report: Scarring Alopecia

A 19-year-old man presented with a history of ulcerative colitis and dissecting cellulitis of the scalp. He has previously been treated with doxycycline, dapsone, and topical antibiotics with minimal improvement. He presented to clinic after excision of an inactive scar on the posterior scalp with a flare of his overall condition with tenderness and drainage.

Past Medical/Surgical History

Ulcerative colitis *s/p* total colectomy with ileostomy

Social History

He is a student; he has never smoked, drinks alcohol, and does not use illicit drugs

Allergies

Penicillin

Previous Therapies

Doxycycline, dapsone, topical antibiotics, excision

Physical Exam

Several fluctuant nodules and sinus tracts with purulent drainage and exquisite tenderness on scalp, predominantly crown and vertex scalp

Acneiform erythematous nodules and atrophic scars on the face

Bacterial culture: Rare coagulase-negative staphylococcus

Management and Course

Due to the patient's history of inflammatory bowel disease, isotretinoin was deferred. Doxycycline 100 mg twice daily was started along with zinc 30 mg daily. After 2 months, his condition was uncontrolled. Intralesional injections of triamcinolone were added, and minocycline 100 mg twice daily replaced doxycycline. Chlorhexidine wash was started as well. He was maintained on this regimen, but could not discontinue without flare for 1 year. Therefore, adalimumab was initiated with 80 mg SC at day 0, followed by 40 mg SC at week 1 and every 2 weeks thereafter. Improvement was seen, but active disease continued, so he was started on clindamycin 300 mg twice daily and rifampin 300 mg twice daily for 6 weeks without improvement. Trimethoprim-sulfamethoxazole 1 DS tab twice daily was initiated with improvement seen in the first month. He stayed on this regimen with intralesional triamcinolone injections every 3–6 weeks for 3–4 years with periodic flares with any interruption, until he self-discontinued the systemic medications. He was clear for 2 months, then experienced a mild flare of both his acne conglobata and dissecting cellulitis. He resumed trimethoprim-sulfamethoxazole and has been maintained with this and topical and intralesional corticosteroids for 1 year to date. As he has had a total colectomy, he has been cleared for isotretinoin. He has declined resuming adalimumab, although he had experienced no adverse effects.

Case Report: Alopecia Areata

A 32 year-old woman presented with a 6-month history of alopecia areata and 4 months of alopecia universalis. She had been started on topical clobetasol cream twice daily without improvement. Of note, she had a history of ankylosing spondylitis, for which she had previously failed methotrexate and systemic corticosteroids. She was most recently on etanercept with mild control of her rheumatologic symptoms.

Past Medical History

Ankylosing spondylitis, mild plaque psoriasis, hypothyroidism

Medications

Levothyroxine, etanercept

Social History

Has three children, not planning to have more children
Has a copper intrauterine device
No smoking, no alcohol, no illicit drugs

Physical Examination

100% scalp and body alopecia, non-scarring

Management

Per patient, her rheumatologist and primary care provider believed that oral tofacitinib may be helpful for her ankylosing spondylitis and her alopecia universalis. Etanercept was discontinued. She was subsequently started on 5 mg twice daily. She was sometimes inconsistent and was on varying doses of 5-15 mg daily, and after 6 months, very minimal regrowth was seen along the frontal hairline. Thus, monthly intralesional triamcinolone injections were initiated. She also tried to be more consistent with her dosing. Regrowth was seen at 75% after 6 months of monthly injections, with continued growth to at least 95% without additional injections. She has continued on tofacitinib 11 mg extended release once daily. Of note, her ankylosing spondylitis has been very well-controlled.

References

1. Jimenez JJ, et al. Efficacy and safety of a low-level laser device in the treatment of male and female pattern hair loss: a multicenter, randomized, sham device-controlled, double-blind study. Am J Clin Dermatol. 2014;15(2):115–27.

2. El Taieb MA, et al. Platelets rich plasma versus minoxidil 5% in treatment of alopecia areata: a trichoscopic evaluation. Dermatol Ther. 2017;30(1).

3. Puig CJ, et al. Double-blind, placebo-controlled pilot study on the use of platelet-rich plasma in women with female androgenetic alopecia. Dermatol Surg. 2016;42(11):1243–7.

4. Bolduc C, et al. Primary cicatricial alopecia: other lymphocytic primary cicatricial alopecias and neutrophilic and mixed primary cicatricial alopecias. J Am Acad Dermatol. 2016;75:1101–17.

5. Fabbri P, et al. Scarring alopecia in discoid lupus erythematosus: a clinical, histopathologic and immunopathologic study. Lupus. 2004;13(6):455–62.

6. Patel P, Werth V. Cutaneous lupus erythematosus: a review. Derm Clinics. 2002;20(3):373–85.

7. Tebbe B, Orfanos CE. Epidemiology and socioeconomic impact of skin disease in lupus erythematosus. Lupus. 1997;6:96–104.

8. James JA, et al. Hydroxychloroquine sulfate treatment is associated with later onset of systemic lupus erythematosus. Lupus. 2007;16:401–9.

9. Pons-Estel GJ, et al. Possible protective effect of hydroxychloroquine on delaying the occurrence of integument damage in lupus: LXXI, data from a multiethnic cohort. Arthritis Care Res. 2010;62(3):393–400.

10. Callen JP, Camisa C. Antimalarial agents. In: Wolverton SE, editor. Comprehensive dermatologic drug therapy. New York: Elsevier Saunders; 2013. p. 241.

11. Marmor MF, et al. Recommendations on screening for chloroquine and hydroxychloroquine retinopathy (2016 revision). Ophthalmology. 2016;123(6):1386–94.

12. Braslow RA, et al. Adherence to hydroxychloroquine dosing guidelines by rheumatologists: an electronic medical record-based study in an integrated health care system. Ophthalmology. 2017;124(5):604–8.

13. Wahie S, Meggitt SJ. Long-term response to hydroxychloroquine in patients with discoid lupus erythematosus. Br J Dermatol. 2013;169:653–9.

14. Jessop S, et al. Drugs for discoid lupus erythematosus. Cochrane Database Syst Rev. 2009;(4):CD002954.

15. Dahl C, et al. Ustekinumab in the treatment of refractory chronic cutaneous lupus erythematosus: a case report. Acta Derm Venereol. 2013;93:368–9.

16. De Souza A, et al. Apremilast for discoid lupus erythematosus: results of a phase 2, open-label, single-arm, pilot study. J Drugs Dermatol. 2012;11:1224–6.

17. Winchester D, et al. Response to ustekinumab in a patient with both severe psoriasis and hypertrophic cutaneous lupus. Lupus. 2012;21(9):1007–10.

18. Cevasco NC, et al. A case-series of 29 patients with lichen planopilaris: the Cleveland Clinic Foundation experience on evaluation, diagnosis, and treatment. J Am Acad Dermatol. 2007;57(1):47–53.

19. Spencer LA, et al. Lichen planopilaris: retrospective study and stepwise therapeutic approach. Arch Dermatol. 2009;145:333–4.

20. Mehregan DA, et al. Lichen planopilaris: clinical and pathologic study of forty-five patients. J Am Acad Dermatol. 1992;27:935–42.

21. Assouly P, Reygagne P. Lichen planopilaris: update on diagnosis and treatment. Semin Cutan Med Surg. 2009;28:3–10.

22. Chieregato C, et al. Lichen planopilaris: report of 30 cases and review of the literature. Int J Dermatol. 2003;42:342–5.

23. Donati A, et al. Clinical and photographic assessment of lichen planopilaris treatment efficacy. J Am Acad Dermatol. 2011;64:597–8.

24. Racz E, et al. Treatment of frontal fibrosing alopecia and lichen planopilaris: a systematic review. J Eur Acad Dermatol Venereol. 2013;27:1461–70.

25. Garrido-Mesa N, et al. Minocycline: far beyond an antibiotic. Br J Pharmacol. 2013;169(2):337–52.

26. Griffin MO, et al. Tetracycline compounds with non-antimicrobial organ protective properties: possible mechanisms of action. Pharmacol Res. 2011;63(2):102–7.

27. Barbieri JS, et al. Duration of oral tetracycline-class antibiotic therapy and use of topical retinoids for the treatment of acne among general practitioners (GP): a retrospective cohort study. J Am Acad Dermatol. 2016;75(6):1142–50. e1141

28. Chiang C, et al. Hydroxychloroquine and lichen planopilaris: efficacy and introduction of lichen planopilaris activity index scoring system. J Am Acad Dermatol. 2010;62:387–92.

29. Mirmirani P, et al. Short course of oral cyclosporine in lichen planopilaris. J Am Acad Dermatol. 2003;49:667–71.

30. Karnik P, et al. Hair follicle stem cell-specific PPARgamma deletion causes scarring alopecia. J Investig Dermatol. 2009;129(5):1243–57.

31. Baibergenova A, Walsh S. Use of pioglitazone in patients with lichen planopilaris. J Cutan Med Surg. 2012;16:97–100.

32. Mesinkovska NA, et al. The use of oral pioglitazone in the treatment of lichen planopilaris. J Am Acad Dermatol. 2015;72(2):355–6.

33. Mirmirani P, Karnik P. Lichen planopilaris treated with a peroxisome proliferator-activated receptor gamma agonist. Arch Dermatol. 2009;145:1363–6.

34. Spring P, et al. Lichen planopilaris treated by the peroxisome proliferator activated receptor-gamma agonist pioglitazone: lack of lasting improvement or cure in the majority of patients. J Am Acad Dermatol. 2013;69:830–2.

35. Cho BK, et al. Efficacy and safety of mycophenolate mofetil for lichen planopilaris. J Am Acad Dermatol. 2010;62:393–7.

36. George SJ, Hsu S. Lichen planopilaris treated with thalidomide. J Am Acad Dermatol. 2001;45(6):965–6.

37. Joanique C, et al. Thalidomide is ineffective in the treatment of lichen planopilaris. J Am Acad Dermatol. 2004;51(3):480–1.

38. Erras S, et al. Rapid and complete resolution of lichen planopilaris in juvenile chronic arthritis treated with rituximab. Eur J Dermatol. 2011;21:116–7.

39. Jayasekera PS, et al. Case report of lichen planopilaris occurring in a pediatric patient receiving a tumor necrosis factor α inhibitor and a review of the literature. Pediatr Dermatol. 2016;33(2):e143–6.

40. Kreutzer K, Effendy I. Therapy-resistant folliculitis decalvans and lichen planopilaris successfully treated with adalimumab. J Dtsch Dermatol Ges. 2014;12(1):74–6.

41. McCarty M, et al. Lichenoid reactions in association with tumor necrosis factor alpha inhibitors: a review of the literature and addition of a fourth lichenoid reaction. J Clin Aesthet Dermatol. 2015;8(6):45–9.

42. Webster G. Failure of lichen planopilaris to respond to ustekinumab. Dermatol Online J. 2015;21(11).

43. Kossard S, et al. Postmenopausal frontal fibrosing alopecia: a frontal variant of lichen planopilaris. J Am Acad Dermatol. 1997;36:59–66.

44. Naz E, et al. Postmenopausal frontal fibrosing alopecia. Clin Exp Dermatol. 2003;28(1):25–7.

45. Samrao A, et al. Frontal fibrosing alopecia: a clinical review of 36 patients. Br J Dermatol. 2010;163:1296–300.

46. Tosti A, et al. Frontal fibrosing alopecia in postmenopausal women. J Am Acad Dermatol. 2005;52:55–60.

47. Banka N, et al. Frontal fibrosing alopecia: a retrospective clinical review of 62 patients with treatment outcome and long-term follow-up. Int J Dermatol. 2014;53(11):1324–30.

48. Ladizinski B, et al. Frontal fibrosing alopecia: a retrospective review of 19 patients seen at Duke University. J Am Acad Dermatol. 2013;68(5):749–55.

49. Tan KT, Messenger AG. Frontal fibrosing alopecia: clinical presentations and prognosis. Br J Dermatol. 2009;160:75–9.

50. Vanos-Galvan S, et al. Frontal fibrosing alopecia: a multicenter review of 355 patients. J Am Acad Dermatol. 2014;70(4):670–8.

51. Hirshburg JM, et al. Adverse effects and safety of 5-alpha reductase inhibitors (finasteride, dutasteride): a systematic review. J Clin Aesthet Dermatol. 2016;9(7):56–62.

52. Seale LR, et al. Side effects related to 5 α-reductase inhibitor treatment of hair loss in women: a review. J Drugs Dermatol. 2016;15(4):414–9.

53. Wiebe JP, et al. Progesterone-induced stimulation of mammary tumorigenesis is due to the progesterone metabolite, 5alpha-dihydroprogesterone (5alphaP) and can be suppressed by the 5alpha-reductase inhibitor, finasteride. J Steroid Biochem Mol Biol. 2015;149:27–34.

54. Bird ST, et al. Male breast cancer and 5α-reductase inhibitors finasteride and dutasteride. J Urol. 2013;190:1811–4.

55. Duijnhoven RG, et al. Long-term use of 5alpha-reductase inhibitors and the risk of male breast cancer. Cancer Causes Control. 2014;25(11):1577–82.

56. Vashi N, et al. Graham-Little-Piccardi-Lassueur syndrome. Dermatol Online J. 2011;17(10):30.

57. Yorulmaz A, et al. A case of Graham-Little-Piccardi-Lasseur syndrome. Dermatol Online J. 2015;21(6).

58. Bianchi L, et al. Graham Little-Piccardi-Lassueur syndrome: effective treatment with cyclosporin A. Clin Exp Dermatol. 2001;26(8):510–20.

59. Zegarska B, et al. Graham-little syndrome. Acta Dermatovenerol Alp Pannonica Adriat. 2010;19:39–42.

60. Alzolibani AA, et al. Pseudopelade of Brocq. Dermatol Ther. 2008;21(4):257–63.

61. Khumalo NP, Gumedze F. Traction: risk factor or coincidence in central centrifugal cicatricial alopecia? Br J Dermatol. 2012;167(5):1191–3.

62. Khumalo NP, et al. Hairdressing and the prevalence of scalp disease in African adults. Br J Dermatol. 2007;157(5):981–8.

63. Olsen EA, et al. Central hair loss in African American women: incidence and potential risk factors. J Am Acad Dermatol. 2011;64(2):245–52.

64. Callender VD, Onwudiwe O. Prevalence and etiology of central centrifugal cicatricial alopecia. Arch Dermatol. 2011;147(8):972–4.

65. Kyei A, et al. Medical and environmental risk factors for the development of central centrifugal cicatricial alopecia: a population study. Arch Dermatol. 2011;147:909–14.

66. Summers P, et al. Central centrifugal cicatricial alopecia—an approach to diagnosis and management. Int J Dermatol. 2011;50:1457–64.

67. Lewars M, et al. Follicular mucinosis. Indian Dermatol Online J. 2013;4(4):333–5.

68. Parker SR, Murad E. Follicular mucinosis: clinical, histologic, and molecular remission with minocycline. J Am Acad Dermatol. 2010;62(1):139–41.

69. Otberg N, et al. Folliculitis decalvans. Dermatol Ther. 2008;21:238–44.

70. Tietze JK, et al. Oral isotretinoin as the most effective treatment in folliculitis decalvans: a retrospective comparison of different treatment regimens in 28 patients. J Eur Acad Dermatol Venereol. 2015;29:1816–21.

71. Bunagan MJK, et al. Retrospective review of folliculitis decalvans in 23 patients with course and treatment analysis of long-standing cases. J Cutan Med Surg. 2015;19(1):45–9.

72. Brozena SJ, et al. Folliculitis decalvans—response to rifampin. Cutis. 1988;42(6):512–5.

73. Powell J, Dawber RP. Successful treatment regime for folliculitis decalvans despite uncertainty of all aetiological factors. Br J Dermatol. 2001;144:428–9.

74. Forrest GN, Tamura K. Rifampin combination therapy for nonmycobacterial infections. Clin Microbiol Rev. 2010;23(1):14–34.

75. Powell JJ, et al. Folliculitis decalvans including tufted folliculitis: clinical, histological, and therapeutic findings. Br J Dermatol. 1999;140(2):328–33.

76. Lyons RW. Orange contact lenses from rifampin. N Engl J Med. 1979;300(7):372–3.

77. Wozel G, Blasum C. Dapsone in dermatology and beyond. Arch Dermatol Res. 2014;306(2):103–24.

78. Lorenz M, et al. Hypersensitivity reactions to dapsone: a systematic review. Acta Derm Venereol. 2012;92:194–9.

79. Abeck D, et al. Folliculitis decalvans. Long-lasting response to combined therapy with fusidic acid and zinc. Acta Derm Venereol. 1992;72:143–5.

80. Brocard A, Dreno B. Innate immunity: a crucial target for zinc in the treatment of inflammatory dermatosis. J Eur Acad Dermatol Venereol. 2011;25:1146–52.

81. Fernandes P. Fusidic acid: a bacterial elongation factor inhibitor for the oral treatment of acute and chronic staphylococcal infections. Cold Spring Harb Perspect Med. 2016;6(1):a025437.

82. Sand FL, Thomsen SF. Off-label use of TNF-alpha inhibitors in a dermatological university department: retrospective evaluation of 118 patients. Dermatol Ther. 2015;28:158–65.

83. Navarini AA, Trueb RM. 3 cases of dissecting cellulitis of the scalp treated with adalimumab. Arch Dermatol. 2010;146(5):517–20.

84. Lim DT, et al. Spondyloarthritis associated with acne conglobata, hidradenitis suppurativa and dissecting cellulitis of the scalp: a review with illustrative cases. Curr Rheumatol Rep. 2013;15(8):346.

85. Salim A, et al. Dissecting cellulitis of the scalp with associated spondyloarthropathy: case report and review. J Eur Acad Dermatol Venereol. 2003;17(6):689–91.

86. Miletta NR, et al. Tinea capitis mimicking dissecting cellulitis of the scalp: a histopathologic pitfall when evaluating alopecia in the post-pubertal patient. J Cutan Pathol. 2014;41(1):2–4.

87. Badaoui A, et al. Dissecting cellulitis of the scalp: a retrospective study of 51 patients and review of the literature. Br J Dermatol. 2016;174:421–3.

88. Greenblatt DT, et al. Dissecting cellulitis of the scalp responding to oral quinolones. Clin Exp Dermatol. 2008;33(1):99–100.

89. Onderdijk AJ, Boer J. Successful treatment of dissecting cellulitis with ciprofloxacin. Clin Exp Dermatol. 2010;35(4):440.

90. Arabyat RM, et al. Fluoroquinolone-associated tendon-rupture: a summary of reports in the Food and Drug Administration's adverse event reporting system. Expert Opin Drug Saf. 2015;14(11):1653–60.

91. Scheinfeld N. Dissecting cellulitis (perifolliculitis capitis abscedens et suffodiens): a comprehensive review focusing on new treatments and findings of the last decade with commentary comparing the therapies and causes of dissecting cellulitis to hidradenitis suppurativa. Dermatol Online J. 2014;20(5):22692.

92. Bolz S, et al. Successful treatment of perifolliculitis capitis abscedens and suffodiens with combined isotretinoin and dapsone. J Dtsch Dermatol Ges. 2008;6(1):44–7.

93. Georgala S, et al. Dissecting cellulitis of the scalp treated with rifampicin and isotretinoin: case reports. Cutis. 2008;82(3):195–8.

94. Prasad SC, Bygum A. Successful treatment with alitretinoin of dissecting cellulitis of the scalp in keratitis-ichthyosis-deafness syndrome. Acta Derm Venereol. 2013;93:473–4.

95. Brandt HR, et al. Perifolliculitis capitis abscedens et suffodiens successflly controlled with infliximab. Br J Dermatol. 2008;159:506–7.

96. Wollina U, et al. Dissecting cellulitis of the scalp responding to intravenous tumor necrosis factor-alpha antagonist. J Clin Aesthet Dermatol. 2012;5(4):36–9.

97. Kobayashi H, et al. Successful treatment of dissecting cellulitis and acne conglobata with oral zinc. Br J Dermatol. 1999;141:1137–8.

98. Berne B, et al. Perifolliculitis capitis abscedens et suffodiens (Hoffman): complete healing associated with oral zinc therapy. Arch Dermatol. 1985;121(8):1028–30.

99. Health, N. I. O. Zinc: fact sheet for health professionals. 2016. https://ods.od.nih.gov/factsheets/Zinc-HealthProfessional/. Accessed 11 Feb 2017.

100. Maranda EL, et al. Treatment of acne keloidalis nuchae: a systematic review of the literature. Dermatol Ther (Heidelb). 2016;6(3):363–78.

101. Quarles FN, et al. Acne keloidalis nuchae. Dermatol Ther. 2007;20:128–32.

102. Broussard KC, et al. Erosive pustular dermatosis of the scalp: a review with a focus on dapsone therapy. J Am Acad Dermatol. 2012;66(4):680–6.

103. Patton D, et al. Chronic atrophic erosive dermatosis of the scalp and extremities: a recharacterization of erosive pustular dermatosis. J Am Acad Dermatol. 2007;57:421–7.

104. Tardio NB, Daly TJ. Erosive pustular dermatosis and associated alopecia succesfully treated with topical tacrolimus. J Am Acad Dermatol. 2011;65(3):e93–4.

105. Dall'Olio E, et al. Erosive pustular dermatosis of the leg: long-term control with topical tacrolimus. Australas J Dermatol. 2011;52(1):e15–7.

106. Feramisco JD, et al. Disseminated erosive pustular dermatosis also involving the mucosa: successful treatment with oral dapsone. Acta Derm Venereol. 2012;92(1):91–2.

107. Darwich E. Erosive pustular dermatosis of the scalp responding to acitretin. Arch Dermatol. 2011;147(2):252–3.

108. Di Lernia V, Ricci C. Familial erosive pustular dermatosis of the scalp and legs successfully treated with ciclosporin. Clin Exp Dermatol. 2016;41(3):334–5.

109. Ikeda M, et al. Erosive pustular dermatosis of the scalp successfully treated with oral zinc sulphate. Br J Dermatol. 1982;106(6):742–3.

110. Mastroianni A, et al. Erosive pustular dermatosis of the scalp: a case report and review of the literature. Dermatology. 2005;211(3):273–6.

111. Petersen BO, Bygum A. Erosive pustular dermatosis of the scalp: a case treated successfully with isotretinoin. Acta Derm Venereol. 2008;88(3):300–1.

112. Sperling LC, et al. Alopecias. In: Bolognia JL, Jorizzo JL, Schaffer JV, editors. Dermatology. London: Elsevier; 2012. p. 1.

113. Bansal M, et al. Atrichia with papular lesions. Int J Trichol. 2011;3(2):112–4.

114. Fernandez-Crehuet P, et al. Clinical and trichoscopic characteristics of temporal triangular alopecia: a multicenter study. J Am Acad Dermatol. 2016;75(3):634–7.

115. Ozcan D, Seckin D. N-Acetylcysteine in the treatment of trichotillomania: remarkable results in two patients. J Eur Acad Dermatol Venereol. 2016;30(9):1606–8.

116. Al-Kehnaizan S, Vitale P. Vitamin D-dependent rickets type II with alopecia: two case reports and review of the literature. Int J Dermatol. 2003;42(9):682–5.

117. Kumar V, et al. Alopecia in vitamin D-dependent rickets type II responding to 1alpha-hydroxycholecalciferol. Ann Trop Paediatr. 2010;30(4):329–33.

118. Yang X, Thai KE. Treatment of permanent chemotherapy-induced alopecia with low dose oral minoxidil. Australas J Dermatol. 2015. [Epub ahead of print].

119. Fiedler-Weiss VC, et al. Evaluation of oral minoxidil in the treatment of alopecia areata. Arch Dermatol. 1987;123(11):1488–90.

120. Gan DC, Sinclair RD. Prevalence of male and female pattern hair loss in Maryborough. J Investig Dermatol Symp Proc. 2005;10:184–9.

121. Hamilton JB. Patterned loss of hair in man: types and incidence. Ann N Y Acad Sci. 1951;53:708–28.

122. Yip L, et al. Role of genetics and sex steroid hormones in male androgenetic alopecia and female pattern hair loss: an update of what we now know. Australas J Dermatol. 2011;52:81–8.

123. Sinclair RD. Winding the clock back on female androgenetic alopecia. Br J Dermatol. 2012;166(6):1157–8.

124. Mella JM, et al. Efficacy and safety of finasteride therapy for androgenetic alopecia: a systematic review. Arch Dermatol. 2010;146(10):1141–50.

125. Kaufman KD, et al. Finasteride in the treatment of men with androgenetic alopecia. Finasteride male pattern hair loss study group. J Am Acad Dermatol. 1998;39(4 Pt 1):578–89.

126. Leyden J, et al. Finasteride in the treatment of men with frontal male pattern hair loss. J Am Acad Dermatol. 1999;40(6 Pt 1):930–7.

127. Olsen EA, et al. Global photographic assessment of men aged 18 to 60 years with male pattern hair loss receiving finasteride 1 mg or placebo. J Am Acad Dermatol. 2012;67(3):379–86.

128. Kelly Y, et al. Androgenetic alopecia: an update of treatment options. Drugs. 2016;76:1349–64.

129. Gonzalez ME, et al. Androgenetic alopecia in the paediatric population: a retrospective review of 57 patients. Br J Dermatol. 2010;163(2):378–85.

130. Whiting DA, et al. Efficacy and tolerability of finasteride 1 mg in men aged 41 to 60 years with male pattern hair loss. Eur J Dermatol. 2003;13(2):150–60.

131. Ramot Y, et al. Finasteride induced gynecomastia: a case report and review of the literature. Int J Trichol. 2009;1(1):27–9.

132. Amory JK, et al. The effect of 5alpha-reductase inhibition with dutasteride and finasteride on semen parameters and serum hormones in healthy men. J Clin Endocrinol Metab. 2007;92(5):1659–65.

133. Overstreet JW, et al. Chronic treatment with finasteride daily does not affect spermatogenesis or semen production in young men. J Urol. 1999;162(4):1295–300.

134. Samplaski MK, et al. Finasteride use in the male infertility population: effects on semen and hormone parameters. Fertil Steril. 2013;100(6):1542–6.

135. Steiner JF. Clinical pharmacokinetics and pharmacodynamics of finasteride. Clin Pharmacokinet. 1996;30(1):16–27.

136. Pole M, Koren G. Finasteride. Does it affect spermatogenesis and pregnancy? Can Fam Physician. 2001;47:2469–70.

137. Irwig MS, Kolukula S. Persistent sexual side effects of finasteride for male pattern hair loss. J Sex Med. 2011;8:1747–53.

138. Irwig MS. Androgen levels and semen parameters among former users of finasteride with persistent sexual adverse effects. JAMA Dermatol. 2014;150(12):1361–3.

139. Redman MW, et al. Finasteride does not increase the risk of high-grade prostate cancer: a bias-adjusted modeling approach. Cancer Prev Res. 2008;1(3):174–81.

140. Thompson IM, et al. The influence of finasteride on the development of prostate cancer. N Engl J Med. 2003;349(3):215–24.

141. Unger JM, et al. Long-term consequences of finasteride vs placebo in the prostate cancer prevention trial. J Natl Cancer Inst. 2016;108(12).

142. Iorizzo M, et al. Finasteride treatment of female pattern hair loss. Arch Dermatol. 2006;142(3):298–302.

143. Oliveira-Soares R, et al. Finasteride 5 mg/day treatment of patterned hair loss in normo-androgenetic postmenopausal women. Int J Trichol. 2013;5(1):22–5.

144. Price VH, et al. Lack of efficacy of finasteride in postmenopausal women with androgenetic alopecia. J Am Acad Dermatol. 2000;43(5 Pt 1):768–76.

145. Whiting DA, et al. Measuring reversal of hair miniaturization in androgenetic alopecia by follicular counts in horizontal section of serial scalp biopsies: results of finasteride 1 mg treatment of men and postmenopausal women. J Investig Dermatol Symp Proc. 1999;4:282–4.

146. Yeon JH, et al. 5 mg/day finasteride treatment for normoandrogenic Asian women with female pattern hair loss. J Eur Acad Dermatol Venereol. 2011;25(2):211–4.

147. Bowman CJ, et al. Effects of in utero exposure to finasteride on androgen-dependent reproductive development in the male rat. Toxicol Sci. 2003;74:393–406.

148. Clark RV, et al. Marked suppression of dihydrotestosterone in men with benign prostatic hyperplasia by dutasteride, a dual 5alpha-reductase inhibitor. J Clin Endocrinol Metab. 2004;89(5):2179–84.

149. Eun HC, et al. Efficacy, safety, and tolerability of dutasteride 0.5 mg once daily in male patients with male pattern hair loss: a randomized, double-blind, placebo-controlled, phase III study. J Am Acad Dermatol. 2010;63(2):252–8.

150. Gubelin Harcha W, et al. A randomized, active- and placebo-controlled study of the efficacy and safety of different doses of dutasteride versus placebo and finasteride in the treatment of male subjects with androgenetic alopecia. J Am Acad Dermatol. 2014;70(3):489–98.

151. Olsen EA, et al. The importance of dual 5alpha-reductase inhibition in the treatment of male pattern hair loss: results of a randomized placebo-controlled study of dutasteride versus finasteride. J Am Acad Dermatol. 2006;55(6):1014–23.

152. Boyapati A, Sinclair R. Combination therapy with finasteride and low-dose dutasteride in the treatment of androgenetic alopecia. Australas J Dermatol. 2013;54(1):49–51.

153. Jung JY, et al. Effect of dutasteride 0.5 mg/d in men with androgenetic alopecia recalcitrant to finasteride. Int J Dermatol. 2014;53(11):1351–7.

154. Boersma IH, et al. The effectiveness of finasteride and dutasteride used for 3 years in women with androgenetic alopecia. Indian J Dermatol Venereol Leprol. 2014;80(6):521–5.

155. Olszewska M, Rudnicka L. Effective treatment of female androgenic aloepcia with dutasteride. J Drugs Dermatol. 2005;4:637–40.

156. Bettoli V, et al. Is hormonal treatment still an option in acne today? Br J Dermatol. 2015;172(Suppl 1):37–46.

157. Marcondes JA, et al. The effects of spironolactone on testosterone fractions and sex-hormone binding globulin binding capacity in hirsute women. J Endocrinol Investig. 1995;18(6):431–5.

158. Sinclair R, et al. Hair loss in women: medical and cosmetic approaches to increase scalp hair fullness. Br J Dermatol. 2011;165(Suppl 3):12–8.

159. Young RL, et al. The endocrine effects of spironolactone used as an antiandrogen. Fertil Steril. 1987;48(2):223–8.

160. Famenini S, et al. Demographics of women with female pattern hair loss and the effectiveness of spironolactone therapy. J Am Acad Dermatol. 2015;73(4):705–6.

161. Sinclair R, et al. Treatment of female pattern hair loss with oral antiandrogens. Br J Dermatol. 2005;152(3):466–73.

162. Krunic A, et al. Efficacy and tolerance of acne treatment using both spironolactone and a combined contraceptive containing drospirenone. J Am Acad Dermatol. 2008;58(1):60–2.

163. Plovanich M, et al. Low usefulness of potassium monitoring among healthy young women taking spironolactone for acne. JAMA Dermatol. 2015;151(9):941–4.

164. Kim GK, Del Rosso JQ. Oral spironolactone in post-teenage female patients with acne vulgaris: practical considerations for the clinician based on current data and clinical experience. J Clin Aesthet Dermatol. 2012;5(3):37–50.

165. Mackenzie IS, et al. Spironolactone use and risk of incident cancers: a retrospective, matched cohort study. Br J Clin Pharmacol. 2017;83(3):653–63.

166. Martindale. Cyproterone acetate. Martindale: The Complete Drug Reference. Micromedex Healthcare Series [database online], The Royal Pharmaceutical Society of Great Britain; 2016.

167. Yazdabadi A, Sinclair R. Treatment of female pattern hair loss with the androgen receptor antagonist flutamide. Australas J Dermatol. 2011;52(2):132–4.

168. Carmina E, Lobo RA. Treatment of hyperandrogenic alopecia in women. Fertil Steril. 2003;79(1):91–5.

169. Paradisi R, et al. Prospective cohort study on the effects and tolerability of flutamide in patients with female pattern hair loss. Ann Pharmacother. 2011;45(4):469–75.

170. Wysowski DK, et al. Fatal and nonfatal hepatotoxicity associated with flutamide. Ann Intern Med. 1993;118(11):860–4.

171. Castelo-Branco C, et al. Long-term safety and tolerability of flutamide for the treatment of hirsutism. Fertil Steril. 2009;91(4):1183–8.

172. Olsen EA, et al. Alopecia areata investigational assessment guidelines—Part II. National Alopecia Areata Foundation. J Am Acad Dermatol. 2004;51(3):440–7.

173. Shapiro J. Current treatment of alopecia areata. J Investig Dermatol Symp Proc. 2013;16(1):S42–4.

174. Hordinsky M, Donati A. Alopecia areata: an evidence-based treatment update. Am J Clin Dermatol. 2014;15(3):231–46.

175. Shreberk-Hassidim R, et al. A systematic review of pulse steroid therapy for alopecia areata. J Am Acad Dermatol. 2016;74(2):372–4.

176. Kar BR, et al. Placebo-controlled oral pulse prednisoone therapy in alopecia areata. J Am Acad Dermatol. 2005;52(2):287–90.

177. Caplan A, et al. Prevention and management of glucocorticoid-induced side effects: a comprehensive review—gastrointestinal and endocrinologic side effects. J Am Acad Dermatol. 2017;76:11–6.

178. Olsen EA, et al. Systemic steroids with or without 2% topical minoxidil in the treatment of alopecia areata. Arch Dermatol. 1992;128(11):1467–73.

179. Kurosawa M, et al. A comparison of the efficacy, relapse rate and side effects among three modalities of systemic corticosteroid therapy for alopecia areata. Dermatology. 2006;212(4):361–5.

180. Seo J, et al. Intramuscular triamcinolone acetonide: an undervalued option for refractory alopecia areata. J Dermatol. 2017;44(2):173–9.

181. Jang YH, et al. A comparative study of oral cyclosporine and betamethasone minipulse therapy in the treatment of alopecia areata. Ann Dermatol. 2016;28(5):569–74.

182. Kanameishi S, et al. Successful hair regrowth in an acute diffuse form of alopecia areata during oral tacrolimus treatment in a patient with rheumatoid arthritis. J Eur Acad Dermatol Venereol. 2017;31(3):e137–8.

183. Köse O, et al. Mycophenolate mofetil in extensive Alopecia areata: no effect in seven patients. Dermatology. 2004;209(1):69–70.

184. Acikgoz G, et al. The effect of oral cyclosporine in the treatment of severe alopecia areata. Cutan Ocul Toxicol. 2014;33(3):247–52.

185. Shapiro J, et al. Systemic cyclosporine and low-dose prednisone in the treatment of chronic severe alopecia areata: a clinical and immunopathologic evaluation. J Am Acad Dermatol. 1997;36(1):114–7.

186. Yeo IK, et al. Comparison of high-dose corticosteroid pulse therapy and combination therapy using oral cyclosporine with low-dose corticosteroid in severe alopecia areata. Ann Dermatol. 2015;27(6):676–81.

187. Anuset D, et al. Efficacy and safety of methotrexate combined with low- to moderate-dose corticosteroids for severe alopecia areata. Dermatology. 2016;232(2):242–8.

188. Joly P. The use of methotrexate alone or in combination with low doses of oral corticosteroids in the treatment of alopecia totalis or universalis. J Am Acad Dermatol. 2006;55:632–6.

189. Lucas P, et al. Methotrexate in severe childhood alopecia areata: long-term follow-up. Acta Derm Venereol. 2016;96(1):102–3.

190. Hammerschmidt M, Mulinari Brenner F. Efficacy and safety of methotrexate in alopecia areata. An Bras Dermatol. 2014;89(5):729–34.

191. Bath RK, et al. A review of methotrexate-associated hepatotoxicity. J Dig Dis. 2014;15(10):517–24.

192. Kalb RE, et al. Methotrexate and psoriasis: 2009 National Psoriasis Foundation Consensus Conference. J Am Acad Dermatol. 2009;60(5):824–37.

193. Farshi S, et al. Could azathioprine be considered as a therapeutic alternative in the treatment of alopecia areata? A pilot study. Int J Dermatol. 2010;49(10):1188–93.

194. Vañó-Galván S, et al. Treatment of recalcitrant adult alopecia areata universalis with oral azathioprine. J Am Acad Dermatol. 2016;74(5):1007–8.

195. Aghaei S. An uncontrolled, open label study of sulfasalazine in severe alopecia areata. Indian J Dermatol Venereol Leprol. 2008;74(6):611–3.

196. Bakar O, Gurbuz O. Is there a role for sulfasalazine in the treatment of alopecia areata? J Am Acad Dermatol. 2007;57(4):703–6.

197. Ellis CN, et al. Sulfasalazine for alopecia areata. J Am Acad Dermatol. 2002;46(4):541–4.

198. Misery L, et al. Treatment of alopecia areata with sulfasalazine. J Eur Acad Dermatol Venereol. 2007;21(4):547–8.

199. Rashidi T, Mahd AA. Treatment of persistent alopecia areata with sulfasalazine. Int J Dermatol. 2008;47(8):850–2.

200. Nissen CV, Wulf HC. Hydroxychloroquine is ineffective in treatment of alopecia totalis and extensive alopecia areata: a case series of 8 patients. JAAD Case Rep. 2016;2(2):117–8.

201. Stephan F, et al. Successful treatment of alopecia totalis with hydroxychloroquine: report of 2 cases. J Am Acad Dermatol. 2013;68(6):1048–9.

202. Ali A, Martin JMIV. Hair growth in patients alopecia areata totalis after treatment with simvastatin and ezetimibe. J Drugs Dermatol. 2010;9:62–4.

203. Robins DN. Case reports: alopecia universalis: hair growth following initiation of simvastatin and ezetimibe therapy. J Drugs Dermatol. 2007;6:946–7.

204. Lattouf C, et al. Treatment of alopecia areata with simvastatin/ezetimibe. J Am Acad Dermatol. 2015;72(2):359–61.

205. Loi C, et al. Alopecia areata (AA) and treatment with simvastatin/ezetimibe: experience of 20 patients. J Am Acad Dermatol. 2016;74(5):e99–e100.

206. Kim KY, et al. SREBP-2/PNPLA8 axis improves non-alcoholic fatty liver disease through activation of autophagy. Sci Rep. 2016;6:35732.

207. Sandoval-Usme MC, et al. Simvastatin impairs growth hormone-activated signal transducer and activator of transcription (STAT) signaling pathway in UMR-106 osteosarcoma cells. PLoS One. 2014;9(1):e87769.

208. Strober BE, et al. Etanercept does not effectively treat moderate to severe alopecia areata: an open-label study. J Am Acad Dermatol. 2005;52:1082–4.

209. Tauber M, et al. Alopecia areata occurring during anti-TNF therapy: a national multicenter prospective study. J Am Acad Dermatol. 2014;70(6):1146–9.

210. Strober BE, et al. Alefacept for severe alopecia areata: a randomized, double-blind, placebo-controlled study. Arch Dermatol. 2009;145(11):1262–6.

211. Xing L, et al. Alopecia areata is driven by cytotoxic T lymphocytes and is reversed by JAK inhibition. Nat Med. 2014;20(9):1043–9.

212. Roskoski RJ. Janus kinase (JAK) inhibitors in the treatment of inflammatory and neoplastic diseases. Pharmacol Res. 2016;111:784–803.
213. Damsky W, King BA. JAK inhibitors in dermatology: the promise of a new drug class. J Am Acad Dermatol. 2017;76(4):736–44.
214. Mackay-Wiggan J, et al. Oral ruxolitinib induces hair regrowth in patients with moderate-to-severe alopecia areata. JCI Insight. 2016;1(15):e89790.
215. Kennedy Crispin M, et al. Safety and efficacy of the JAK inhibitor tofacitinib citrate in patients with alopecia areata. JCI Insight. 2016;1(15):e89776.
216. Liu LY, et al. Tofacitinib for the treatment of severe alopecia areata and variants: a study of 90 patients. J Am Acad Dermatol. 2017;76(1):22–8.
217. Craiglow BG, et al. Tofacitinib for the treatment of alopecia areata and variants in adolescents. J Am Acad Dermatol. 2017;76(1):29–32.
218. Moreland L, et al. Abatacept. Nat Rev Drug Discov. 2006;5(3):185–6.
219. Mackay-Wiggan J, et al. Subcutaneous abatacept in the treatment of moderate to severe alopecia areata. J Investig Dermatol. 2015;135:S41.
220. Guttman-Yassky E, et al. Extensive alopecia areata is reversed by IL-12/IL-23p40 cytokine antagonism. J Allergy Clin Immunol. 2016;137(1):301–4.
221. Suárez-Fariñas M, et al. Alopecia areata profiling shows TH1, TH2, and IL-23 cytokine activation without parallel TH17/TH22 skewing. J Allergy Clin Immunol. 2015;136(5):1277–87.
222. Tauber M, et al. Alopecia areata developing during ustekinumab therapy: report of two cases. Eur J Dermatol. 2013;23(6):912–3.
223. Verros C, et al. Letter: alopecia areata during ustekinumab administration: co-existence or an adverse reaction? Dermatol Online J. 2012;18(7):14.
224. Renert-Yuval Y, Guttman-Yassky E. A novel therapeutic paradigm for patients with extensive alopecia areata. Expert Opin Biol Ther. 2016;16(8):1005–14.
225. Keren A, et al. The PDE4 inhibitor, apremilast, suppresses experimentally induced alopecia areata in human skin in vivo. J Dermatol Sci. 2015;77(1):74–6.
226. Hordinsky M, Kaplan DH. Low-dose interleukin 2 to reverse alopecia areata. JAMA Dermatol. 2014;150(7):696–7.
227. Castela E, et al. Effects of low-dose recombinant interleukin 2 to promote T-regulatory cells in alopecia areata. JAMA Dermatol. 2014;150(7):748–51.

Dapsone in Dermatology

44

William Abramovits

Introduction

Dapsone is a nonsteroidal, antibacterial agent used in the treatment of several serious diseases. In dermatology, it is used to treat chronic conditions to avoid the concern for steroid associated side effects [1]. Examples include autoimmune bullous diseases like dermatitis herpetiformis or infectious diseases like leprosy [2]. Dapsone remains the primary drug treatment option for these and other dermatoses although it requires the monitoring of side effects that can potentially cause death [2, 3]. Dapsone is used topically (and has been used systemically) for acne due to its anti-inflammatory effects. Combined with pyrimethamine, it is used to treat malaria and an option after first-line medications (systemic corticosteroids) and second-line therapies (methotrexate, retinoids) failed [4]. Dapsone is effective with or without antimalarial in more than 50% of patients with cutaneous lupus erythematosus [5].

Dapsone belongs to the class of drugs known as sulfones that work by decreasing inflammation and stopping bacterial growth. Emil Fromm was the first to synthesize the compound in 1908 while researching azo dyes; its medical benefits were first discovered in the 1930s [6]. Later in the century, its anti-inflammatory properties would be applied to a vast array of dermatological diseases [6].

We review the chemistry, pharmacokinetics, mechanisms of action, indications, contraindications, and adverse events that may occur in the clinical use of dapsone.

Chemistry/Pharmacokinetics

The molecular structure of diaminodiphenyl sulfone (DDS) or dapsone (not a brand name) consists of a sulfur atom linking two aromatic amine rings (Fig. 44.1). Dapsone is

W. Abramovits, MD, FAAD
Baylor University Medical Center, The University of Texas
Southwestern Medical School, Dallas, Texas, USA
e-mail: dra@dermcenter.us

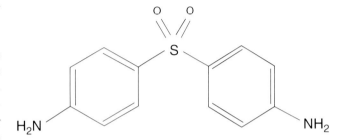

Fig. 44.1 Dapsone (diaminodiphenyl sulfone) $C_{12}H_{12}N_2O_2S$

manufactured as tablets (50 and 100 mg), oral suspension (2 mg/mL), and topical gel (5 and 7.5%). Due to the two aromatic rings, DDS is lipid soluble and water insoluble. High lipophilicity allows it to cross the lipid bilayer of cells efficiently. This may explain why obesity significantly reduces its plasma levels [7]. In tablet form, 70–80% of the DDS is absorbed by the gastrointestinal tract, enters the enterohepatic circulation, and becomes mostly bound to proteins. Its lipophilicity allows it to cross the placental barrier and pass into breast milk. The half-life of dapsone is about 30 h. The liver enzymes, N-acetyltransferase and N-hydroxylase acetylate dapsone form the by-products monoacetyl and diacetyl dapsone that are further metabolized and excreted in the urine and bile [8].

Mechanism of Action

Dapsone exerts its antibacterial properties through competitive antagonism with para-aminobenzoic acid (PABA) and functional inhibition of PABA to produce folic acid [9]. DDS competes with PABA for the active site of the bacterial enzyme dihydropteroate synthase. By inhibiting this enzyme, dapsone disrupts protein synthesis by preventing amino acid synthesis.

The anti-inflammatory properties of dapsone are exerted via the inhibition of the enzyme myeloperoxidase [9]. Neutrophils kill bacteria and use myeloperoxidase to convert

© Springer International Publishing AG 2018
P.S. Yamauchi (ed.), *Biologic and Systemic Agents in Dermatology*, https://doi.org/10.1007/978-3-319-66884-0_44

hydrogen peroxide into hypochlorous acid which can oxidize and damage local tissue via inflammation. Myeloperoxidase is inactivated at its intermediate form, and this prevents the accumulation of hypochlorous acid [9].

In diseases such as erythema elevatum diutinum and dermatitis herpetiformis, dapsone acts via inhibition of neutrophil chemotaxis and function. Dapsone may restore the chemotactic factors that inhibit accumulation of neutrophils [10].

Clinical Uses

The following are therapeutic uses of systemically and topically prescribed dapsone obtained from a PubMed® search starting in 2010 and ending at the time MEDLINE® was accessed for this chapter: acne vulgaris [topical and systemic], dermatitis herpetiformis [topical but mostly systemic], leprosy, erythema elevatum diutinum, hidradenitis suppurativa, delayed pressure urticaria, chronic idiopathic/spontaneous urticaria, neutrophilic urticarial dermatosis, polyarteritis nodosa, idiopathic thrombocytopenic purpura, lupus miliaris disseminatus faciei, autoimmune bullous diseases (including pemphigus vulgaris, pemphigus foliaceus, bullous pemphigoid, pemphigoid gestationis, linear IgA bullous dermatosis, epidermolysis bullosa, bullous systemic lupus erythematosus (BSLE), and ocular cicatricial pemphigoid), cutaneous lupus erythematosus (CLE), relapsing polychondritis, Henoch-Schönlein vasculitis, erosive pustular dermatosis of the scalp [topical], Behçet disease, familial Mediterranean fever, pyoderma gangrenosum, Sweet's syndrome, periodic fever, pyoderma gangrenosum-acnehidradenitis suppurativa (PASH) syndrome, granulomatous rosacea, lichen planus pemphigoides, lichen planus pigmentosus, oral lichen planus, circinate balanitis, cutaneous small-vessel vasculitis, erythema nodosum, panniculitis, dissecting cellulitis (perifolliculitis capitis abscedens et suffodiens), eosinophilic cellulitis (Wells' syndrome), amyopathic dermatomyositis, granuloma annulare [topical], annular elastolytic giant cell granuloma, granular C3 dermatosis, pustular psoriasis[topical and systemic], subcorneal pustular dermatosis, eosinophilic pustular folliculitis (Ofuji's disease), giant cell arteritis, and erythema multiforme.

Acne

Acne vulgaris affects millions of children and adults; it is an inflammatory disease characterized by comedones, papules, nodules, cysts, and scars [11]. Dapsone can be used as a topically applied gel at 5 and 7.5%. These concentrations are effective while safe for treating acne, and the 5% is reportedly gentle enough to use on sensitive skin [12, 13]. In one study the 5% gel produced a significantly greater reduction in acne lesions in female patients, which may be due to the

difference in hormones and skin textures or because women may be more likely to comply with twice a day regimens [14]. The 5% gel may be particularly effective in early stages of comedonal and non-comedonal acne particularly when used in combination with a retinoid [15]. The 7.5% gel is effective when applied once a day, making it easier for the 30–40% of patients who do not comply with twice-daily regimens [16–18]. The 7.5% formulation is well tolerated with improvement by 12 weeks [19]. Due to possible side effects, the oral form has been reserved for severe nodulocystic acne or acne resistant to other treatments. [20]

Dermatitis Herpetiformis

Dermatitis herpetiformis (DH) is an autoimmune blistering disease associated with gluten-sensitive enteropathy. Patients with autoimmune diseases such as thyroiditis, pernicious anemia, and type 1 diabetes show a higher prevalence [21]. The current standard of care for DH consists of a strict gluten-free diet and oral dapsone [22]. Similar to celiac disease, the pathology of DH is likely mediated by IgA class autoantibodies against one of the transglutaminases [2]. Although DH is essentially a bullous skin disease, it is classified as a cutaneous intestinal disorder caused by hypersensitivity to gluten [3]. A gluten-free diet can alleviate the cutaneous and intestinal symptoms, while dapsone can target skin eruptions [23, 24]. The dose commonly used is 100 mg per day (tapering with signs/symptoms control), with an average maintenance dose of 1 mg/kg/day [3]. Lesions may recur when dapsone is discontinued in the absence of a gluten-free diet [3].

Leprosy

Leprosy results from an infection caused by *Mycobacterium leprae*. Chronic leprosy is characterized by granulomas of the skin and mucous membranes and by peripheral nerve involvement. Leprosy can be exacerbated by pregnancy. Untreated, it can cause permanent damage to the skin, nerves, limbs, and eyes [25]. Treatment typically involves antimicrobials including dapsone [26, 27]. The type of leprosy dictates the time it will take for treatment to work. Paucibacillary leprosy can be successfully treated with 6 months of rifampicin and dapsone, while multibacillary leprosy may require dapsone and clofazimine for 2 years [28, 29]. Other options include moxifloxacin, ofloxacin, minocycline, and clarithromycin [30].

Erythema Elevatum Diutinum

Erythema elevatum diutinum (EED) is a rare skin disease characterized by persistent brown or red-purplish papules, nodules, or plaques [31]. Treatment of dapsone has been proven effective [31]. Side effects such as hypersensitivity syndrome may lead to discontinuation. In some patients EED relapses after stopping DDS [32]. Improvement may be obtained with the topical application of the gel. Orally administered dapsone may be needed for complete resolution [33].

Hidradenitis Suppurativa

Hidradenitis suppurativa (HS) is a chronic inflammatory cutaneous disease commonly involving intertriginous areas, such as the axilla, inner thighs, groin, buttocks, and pendulous breasts, but it may appear on any follicular skin [34]. Topical dapsone coupled with clindamycin may be sufficient to treat mild HS [34]. Doxycycline and minocycline have been the first-line systemic option in more widespread or severe cases [35]. Severe HS may require antibiotics per culture; ampicillin, clindamycin, rifampicin, fluoroquinolones, and metronidazole are often used, so are zinc, acitretin, hormone blockers, and oral prednisone [34, 36]. In one study DDS oral doses of 50–200 mg/day for 1–48 months led to improvement in 38% of cases, with adverse events occurring in 8%. Relapse was seen in patients that discontinued dapsone [37]. Adalimumab is the first drug approved by the FDA for HS and may currently be first line of therapy for moderate to severe HS.

Delayed Pressure Urticaria

Delayed pressure urticaria is characterized by hives at areas of pressure over the skin, like around the waist from tight belts; it can be managed with oral dapsone with a good therapeutic benefit lasting beyond the end of therapy. There are no significant effects related to age, gender, duration of therapy, or methemoglobinemia [38]. A retrospective study showed that 74% of patients ($n = 31$) with persistent symptoms obtained good or very good outcomes after receiving dapsone [38].

Chronic Idiopathic/Spontaneous Urticaria

Chronic idiopathic urticaria (CIU) is characterized by wheals for more than 6 weeks [39, 40]. It affects 0.5–1% of the population [41]. Dapsone appears to reduce the neutrophil adherence function mediated by integrins, thus inhibiting neutrophil migration to extravascular sites [39]. Primary treatment includes corticosteroids, cyclosporine, and omalizumab [40]. At the 4th International Consensus Meeting on CIU in 2012, dapsone was removed from the standard guidelines of care [41]. In refractory patients, dapsone may be used along with other treatments such as intravenous immunoglobulin, rituximab, and anticoagulants [42].

Neutrophilic Urticaria

Neutrophilic infiltrates are seen in a subset of patients with urticarial-like lesions that tend to be less responsive to therapy [43]. In a patient treated with an antihistamine, colchicine, and dapsone, only colchicine provided moderate benefit; anakinra achieved 100% control [43].

Polyarteritis Nodosa

Polyarteritis nodosa (PAN) is a type of systemic vasculitis characterized by necrotizing inflammatory lesions resulting from the affectation of medium-sized and small muscular arteries. The term PAN most likely stems from the classification changes and the modification of the epidemiology [44]. The first-line therapy includes a combination of glucocorticoids and cyclophosphamide or glucocorticoids alone, depending on the severity [44]. Many experts have recommended a less aggressive treatment regime for PAN such as colchicine or dapsone [44].

Thrombocytopenic Purpura

Idiopathic thrombocytopenic purpura (ITP) is thrombocytopenia with normal bone marrow in the absence of other etiologies. ITP is characterized by premature platelet destruction in the reticuloendothelial system due to autoantibodies that attach to platelet membrane proteins [45]. Dapsone at 100 mg/day for a minimum of 30 days results in a maximum of 20% long-term complete response rate and may be used before resorting to splenectomy [45].

Lupus Miliaris Disseminatus Faciei

Lupus miliaris disseminatus faciei (LMDF) is characterized as a chronic facial dermatosis with spontaneous regression in 2–4 years that leaves pock-like scars [46]. In one study, oral dapsone at 100 mg/day led to improvement after the first month, but cupuliform scars still developed [46].

Autoimmune Bullous Diseases

Autoimmune bullous disease (AIBD) encompasses a group of disorders that result from autoimmunity directed against basement membrane and/or intercellular adhesion molecules on cutaneous and mucosal surfaces [47]. AIBD includes linear IgA bullous dermatosis, DH, epidermolysis bullosa acquisita, bullous lupus erythematosus, bullous pemphigoid, mucous membrane pemphigoid (MMP), pemphigus vulgaris (PV), and pemphigus foliaceus (PF). Most studies conducted with dapsone have been on MMP and PV [47]. The maximum recommended dose for dapsone is 200 mg/day although there are reports of 300 mg/day being required [47].

Henoch-Schönlein Vasculitis

Henoch-Schönlein vasculitis (H-SV) is an acute IgA-mediated disorder. It is a systemic vasculitis disease that affects the skin, mucous membranes, and other organs. In one study, patients treated with dapsone 100 mg/day experienced fast and complete healing of the skin lesions [48].

Familial Mediterranean Fever

Familial Mediterranean fever (FMF) is a hereditary autoinflammatory disease that presents with fever and recurrent painful attacks involving polyserositis [49]. Dapsone given as a single dose of 2 mg/kg controlled the episodes in 50% of the cases and may be considered an alternative therapy in patients unresponsive to colchicine [49].

Sweet's Syndrome

Sweet's syndrome (SS) is an autoinflammatory disorder that typically presents with erythematous plaques. It is characterized by the abrupt onset of fever, peripheral neutrophilia, erythematous skin lesions, and diffuse neutrophilic dermal infiltrate. SS is associated with inflammatory bowel disease, infections, and hematologic entities [50]. Dapsone is a second-line agent after the first-line treatments such as corticosteroids and cyclosporine [50].

Granulomatous Rosacea

Granulomatous rosacea is a rosacea variant characterized by disseminated, red-brown papules and nodules located primarily in periocular and centrofacial areas. One case report showed remission and long-term stabilization in a patient treated with systemic dapsone [51].

Circinate Balanitis

Circinate balanitis is a manifestation of reactive arthritis that can occur independently [52]. Typically treated with topical corticosteroids, resistant cases may be successfully treated with a combination of dapsone and topical 0.1% tacrolimus ointment [52]. In a case report, circinate balanitis persisted after treatment with clobetasol propionate 0.005% cream but was cured by the tacrolimus/dapsone combination [52].

Cutaneous Small-Vessel Vasculitis

Cutaneous small-vessel vasculitis (CSVV) is characterized by neutrophilic inflammation that is mostly limited to the superficial cutaneous postcapillary venules. It typically manifests as symmetrically distributed palpable purpura of the lower extremities. Primary treatment for chronic CSVV includes dapsone at 50–200 mg/day singly or in combination with colchicine [53].

Eosinophilic Cellulitis (Well's Syndrome)

Eosinophilic cellulitis is a rare inflammatory skin disease characterized by tender, granulomatous eosinophilic infiltrates in the dermis with possible vesicles and urticarial plaques [54]. A patient treated with long-term therapy of dapsone at a dose of 50 mg/day was relapse-free at 1 year [55].

Subcorneal Pustular Dermatosis (Sneddon-Wilkinson Disease)

Subcorneal pustular dermatosis (SPD) is a rare, benign, pustular dermatosis [56]. Although dapsone-resistant cases have been increasingly reported, dapsone remains the first-line treatment [56].

Cutaneous Lupus Erythematosus

Cutaneous lupus erythematosus (CLE) is an inflammatory autoimmune disease with heterogeneous subtypes [4]. Antimalarials and systemic corticosteroids are typically recommended as first-line and long-term systemic treatment [4]. Dapsone is used as a second-line systemic treatment; it is effective with or without antimalarials [4].

Erosive Pustular Dermatosis of the Scalp

Erosive pustular dermatosis of the scalp (EPDS) is an idiopathic inflammatory disorder characterized by pustules, erosions, and crusting in alopecic areas that are atrophic, actinically damaged, or both [57]. Dapsone 5% gel is an effective treatment for EPDS [57].

Behçet Disease

Behçet disease (BD) is an autoinflammatory disease prevalent in Central and East Asia and the Eastern Mediterranean basin [58]. It is characterized by the "triple symptom complex" consisting of recurrent oral aphthosis, genital ulcers, and chronic relapsing bilateral uveitis [59]. In one study, dapsone was used as treatment 8.3% of the time, while drugs such as colchicine were used at a frequency of 78.3% [58]. These treatments were used for mucocutaneous manifestations [58].

Oral Lichen Planus

Oral lichen planus (LP) is an inflammatory disease that affects the mucous membranes of the mouth. Oral dapsone, tacrolimus, and retinoids are as efficacious as steroidal drugs for treating oral lichen planus [1]. Patients taking oral dapsone 100 mg/day for 3 months can avoid the associated side effects of chronic steroid use [1].

Eosinophilic Pustular Folliculitis (Ofuji's Disease)

Eosinophilic pustular folliculitis (EPF) is an idiopathic pruritic papulopustular dermatosis usually presenting with itchy papules and pustules in a circinate configuration. EPF affects the upper body while sparing the abdomen and lower extremities [60]. Indomethacin is the first-line oral medication for EPF, but dapsone has been shown to be efficacious [60]. Dapsone works by inhibiting eosinophil peroxidase activity and chemoattractant-induced signal transduction [60].

Pustular Psoriasis

Pustular psoriasis is a psoriasis variant characterized as small sterile pustules on an erythematous base, typically found on the knees and elbows [61]. A study tested dapsone in five patients that previously failed multiple topical and systemic treatments; four responded to oral dapsone and one to topical dapsone therapy [61]. The study found dapsone to be much safer than other systemic drugs and should be considered in the treatment of pustular psoriasis [61].

Neutrophilic Panniculitis

Neutrophilic panniculitis (NP) is an autoinflammatory disorder characterized by painful recurrent ulcerating subcutaneous nodules and by dense infiltrates of neutrophils in the deep dermis and septa [62]. Oral dapsone at 50–100 mg/day is the treatment of choice.

Linear Immunoglobulin A (IgA) Bullous Dermatosis

Linear immunoglobulin A (IgA) bullous dermatosis (LABD) is an autoimmune disorder that is characterized by subepidermal blistering elicited by IgA antibodies. The pathology takes place in the basal membranous zone of the skin and mucosal tissue [63]. Patients with LABD may benefit from dapsone but with a few side effects such as hemolytic anemia and alopecia [63].

Adverse Effects

The following side effects were listed in the same PubMed® review of dapsone over the past decade:

Dapsone is well tolerated at the normal doses given for dermatologic diseases, but some side effects may emerge at higher doses. Dapsone may lead to dose-related hemolytic anemia and methemoglobinemia. Patients that suffer from other disorders such as celiac disease may be predisposed to acute dapsone-induced methemoglobinemia [64].

Some patients experience adverse cardiovascular events when given higher dapsone doses; these include myocardial injury, shock, ventricular dysrhythmia, or cardiac arrest (occurring within the first 48 h of treatment) [64, 65].

Dapsone may lead to a hypersensitivity syndrome in about 0.3–3.6% of patients [66]. This typically occurs in the first 3–5 weeks after initiation of therapy. Its main signs are fever, generalized rash, lymphadenopathy, and hepatitis [66]. The syndrome can involve multiple organs and lead to life-threatening fulminant hepatitis [67].

Agranulocytosis is a serious and unpredictable manifestation of intolerance to dapsone typically presenting after 4–12 weeks of treatment [68]. In a case report, a patient with chronic urticaria developed livedo reticularis, a vascular pattern caused by swelling of the venules [69].

Pregnancy and Lactation

The use of dapsone as a therapeutic agent has been tested in the pregnant population. Adverse effects are less likely with intermittent use, but most adverse effects occur with long-term use of dapsone [70]. One study reported that dapsone therapy during pregnancy is thought to be safe, although there have only been 19 reported cases of exposure in the first trimester [71]. In pregnant women with leprosy, dapsone did not show an increase in the rate of abnormal outcomes [72]. Dapsone is excreted in the breast milk in quantities potentially toxic for newborns [72]. Patients should be informed about the lack of secured data.

Contraindications

Dapsone is contraindicated in patients who are allergic to the drug. A relative contraindication for dapsone therapy is glucose-6-phosphate dehydrogenase (G6PD) deficiency, an X-linked disorder affecting males [73]. Dapsone is contraindicated in patients with hypersensitivity to dapsone and related drugs (sulfonamides, para-aminobenzoic acid) or in patients with acute porphyrias and severe anemia [74]. DDS interferes with A1c monitoring leading to falsely low HgbA1c results in diabetic patients [75]. This may be due to it acting as an inhibitor of folic acid and reducing the life span of hemoglobin via oxidative stress on red blood cells [75]. Adverse reactions are reported with pyrimethamine-dapsone use; the rate for serious adverse reactions was 1:9100 prescriptions for malaria prophylaxis patients [76]. Dapsone must be used with caution in patients with G6PD deficiency, methemoglobin (Hb) reductase deficiency, cardiac insufficiency/heart failure, severe hepatopathy, pulmonary diseases, and co-medication with metHb-inducing drugs [77].

Laboratory Monitoring

Since adverse gastrointestinal effects including anorexia, abdominal pain, nausea, and vomiting can occur in patients receiving dapsone, periodic history and physical exams should be conducted during treatment [77]. Laboratory evaluation includes glucose-6-phosphate dehydrogenase (G6PD) and metHb reductase measurements; a complete blood count (CBC); a chemistry panel including bilirubin, alanine aminotransferase, aspartate aminotransferase, gamma-glutamyltransferase, and creatinine; and a urinalysis [77]. Follow-up evaluations should include a careful history and physical exam and a CBC every 2 weeks for the first 3–6 months and every 2–4 months thereafter with periodic chemistry panels [77, 78].

Conclusions

Dapsone is an old drug that found its way into a vast variety of treatment regimens and continues to do so. It may be a first- or second-line drug, safe when properly monitored and administered at the relatively low yet effective dose of 50–100 mg/day. At greater dosages, 200–300 mg/day, the risk of adverse effects such as methemoglobinemia increases significantly.

Many diseases benefit from dapsone, but more trials are needed to explore its full benefits as single agent or synergistic drug. This chapter reviewed the most recent literature and only presents a few of the many diseases resolved or alleviated by dapsone and provides insights into its use in untested conditions.

Case Report

A 61-year-old male presents for a routine follow-up of his dermatitis herpetiformis. He has been essentially free of lesions on a strict gluten-free diet and dapsone for 20 years. His initial dose of 100 mg/day has been lowered to 50 mg/day over the last 5 years, but attempts to lower it further result in vesicles around the elbows. Monitoring has consisted of complete blood counts and chemistries yearly, never showing abnormalities of significance. On a follow-up visit, the patient presented with an unusual facial erythema and slight edema and a perianal rash resembling intertrigo.

Past Medical History
- Hypertension
- Hyperlipidemia

Social History
- Nonsmoker and nondrinker
- Married
- Retired

Prior Therapies
- Topical steroids before the diagnosis of dermatitis herpetiformis

Physical Exam
- Mild erythematous, non-scaly patches on mid-face and perianally

Management
After questioning the patient, he recalled taking a new medication around the same time period the rash developed. Analysis of the medication showed that it contained gluten and the current flare was attributed to the medication. Subsequent discontinuation of the medication resolved the flare.

Medications that contain gluten:
(Data retrieved from a comprehensive list on Glutenfreedrugs.com)

The following medications contain gluten: Advil Liqui-Gels, Advil Migraine, Doryx 75 mg, Doryx 100 mg, Sanctura 20 mg, Tekturna HCT 150/12.5 mg, Tekturna HCT 150/25 mg, Tekturna HCT 300/12.5 mg, and Tekturna HCT 300/25 mg [79].

The following medications contain maltodextrin which occasionally is derived from a wheat source: Femcon Fe, Gabazolpidem-5 capsule kit, Junel Fe 1/20, Junel 1.5/30, Junel 1/20, Loestrin 1.5/30, Loestrin 1/20, Loestrin Fe 1.5/50, Loestrin Fe 1/20, Montelukast Chewable Tablets, Sentrazolpidem PM-5 capsule kit, Zenchent Fe Chewable, and Zeosa [79].

References

1. Singh AR, et al. Efficacy of steroidal vs non-steroidal agents in oral lichen planus: a randomized, open-label study. J Larngol Otol. 2017;131(1):69–76.
2. Yost JM, et al. Dermatitis herpetiformis. Dermatol Online J. 2014;20(12).
3. Clarindo MV, et al. Dermatitis herpetiformis: pathophysiology, clinical presentation, diagnosis and treatment. An Bras Dermatol. 2014;89(6):865–75.
4. Kuhn A, et al. S2k guideline for treatment of cutaneous lupus erythematosus. J Eur Acad Dermatol Venereol. 2017;31(3):389–404.
5. Klebes M, et al. Dapsone as second-line treatment for cutaneous lupus erythematosus? A retrospective analysis of 34 patients and a review of the literature. Dermatology. 2016;232(1):91–6.
6. Theirs BH, et al.. Dermatologic clinics. Philadelphia: Elsevier Saunders.
7. Moura FM, et al. Dapsone and body mass index in subjects with multibacillary leprosy. Ther Drug Monit. 2014;36(2):261–3.
8. van Zyl JM, et al. Mechanisms by which clofazimine and dapsone inhibit the myeloperoxidase system: a possible correlation with their anti-inflammatory properties. Biochem Pharmacol. 1991;42(3):599–608.
9. Kosseifi SG, et al. The dapsone hypersensitivity syndrome revisited: a potentially fatal multisystem disorder with prominent hepatopulmonary manifestations. J Occup Med Toxicol. 2006;1:9.
10. Staub J, et al. Successful treatment of PASH syndrome with infliximab, cyclosporine and dapsone. J Eur Acad Dermatol Venereol. 2015;29(11):2243–7.
11. Faghihi G, et al. The efficacy of 5% dapsone gel plus oral isotretinoin versus oral isotretinoin alone in acne vulgaris: A randomized double-blind study. Adv Biomed Res. 2014;3:177.
12. Thiboutot DM, et al. Efficacy, safety, and dermal tolerability of dapsone gel, 7.5% in patients with moderate acne vulgaris: a pooled analysis of two phase 3 trials. J Clin Aesthet Dermatol. 2016;9(10):18–27.
13. Lnde CW, et al. Cohort study on the treatment with dapsone 5% gel of mid to moderate inflammatory acne of the face in women. Skinmed. 2014;12(1):15–21.
14. Tanghetti E, Harper JC, Oefelein MG. The efficacy and tolerability of dapsone 5% gel in female vs male patients with facial acne vulgaris: gender as a clinically relevant outcome variable. J Drugs Dermatol. 2012;11(12):1417–21.
15. Tanghetti E, et al. Clinical evidence for the role of a topical anti-inflammatory agent in comedonal acne: findings from a randomized study of dapsone gel 5% in combination with tazarotene cream 0.1% in patients with acne vulgaris. J Drugs Dermatol. 2011;10(7):783–92.
16. Stein Gold LF, et al. Efficacy and safety of once-daily dapsone gel 7.5% for treatment of adolescents and adults with acne vulgaris: first of two identically designed, large, multicenter, randomized, vehicle-controlled trials. J Drugs Dermatol. 2016;15(5):553–61.
17. Jarratt MT, et al. Safety and pharmacokinetics of once-daily dapsone gel, 7.5% in patients with moderate acne vulgaris. J Drugs Dermatol. 2016;15(10):125–1259.
18. Bartless KB, et al. Tolerability of topical antimicrobials in treatment of acne vulgaris. J Drugs Dermatol. 2014;13(6):658–62.
19. Eichenfield LF, et al. Efficacy and safety of once-daily dapsone gel, 7.5% for treatment of adolescents and adults with acne vulgaris: second of two identically designed, large, multicenter, randomized, vehicle-controlled trials. J Drugs Dermatol. 2016;15(8):962–9.
20. Farrah G, Tan E. The use of oral antibiotics in treating acne vulgaris: a new approach. Dermatol Ther. 2016;29(5):377–84.
21. Mendes FB, et al. Review: dermatitis herpetiformis. An Bras Dermatol. 2013;88(4):594–9.
22. Burbidge T, et al. Topical Dapsone 5% gel as an effective therapy in dermatitis Herpetiformis. J Cutan Med Surg. 2016;20(6):600–1.
23. Plotnikova N, et al. Dermatitis herpetiformis. Skin Therapy Lett. 2013;18(3):1–3.
24. Cardones AR, et al. Management of dermatitis herpetiformis. Dermatol Clin. 2011;29(4):631–5.
25. Ozturk Z, et al. Leprosy treatment during pregnancy and breastfeeding: a case report and brief review of literature. Dermatol Ther. 2017;30(1).
26. Sung SM, et al. Diagnosis and treatment of leprosy type 1 (reversal) reaction. Cutis. 2015;95(4):222–6.
27. Mofin-Maciel BM, et al. Immunological evaluation during treatment of a case of borderline lepromatous leprosy. Rey Alerg Mex. 2016;63(4):413–9.
28. Goto M, et al. Guidelines for the treatment of Hansen's disease in Japan (third edition). Nihon Hansenbyo Gakkai Zasshi. 2013;82(3):143–84.
29. Eichelmann K. Leprosy, an update: definition, pathogenesis, classification, diagnosis, and treatment. Actas Dermosifiliogr. 2013;104(7):554–63.
30. Legendre DP. Hansen's disease (Leprosy): current and future pharmacotherapy and treatment of disease-related immunologic reactions. Pharmacoherapy. 2012;32(1):27–37.
31. Ortonne N. Cutaneous neutrophils infiltrates, Case 2. Erythema elevatum diutinum, late stage. Ann Pathol. 2011;31(3):173–7.
32. Seneschal J. Alternative procedure to allow continuation of dapsone therapy despite serious adverse reaction in a case of dapsone-sensitive erythema elevatum diutinum. Dermatology. 2012;224(2):115–9.
33. Frieling GW. Novel use of topical dapsone 5% gel for erythema elevatum diutinum: safer and effective. J Drugs Dermatol. 2013;12(4):481–4.
34. Scheinfeld N. Hidradenitis suppurativa: a practical review of possible medical treatments based on over 350 hidradenitis patients. Dermatol Online J. 2013;19(4):1.
35. Deckers IE, Prens EP. A update on medical treatment options for hidradenitis suppurativa. Drugs. 2016;76(2):215–29.
36. Yazdanyar S, et al. Dapsone therapy for hidradenitis suppurativa: a series of 24 patients. Dermatology. 2011;222(4):342–6.
37. Van der Zee HH, et al. Medical treatments of hidradenitis suppurativa: more options, less evidence. Dermatol Clin. 2016;34(1):91–6.
38. Grundmann SA, et al. Delayed pressure urticaria- dapsone heading for first-line therapy? J Dtsch Dermatol Ges. 2011;9(11):908–12.
39. Noda S, et al. Long-term complete resolution of severe chronic idiopathic urticaria after dapsone treatment. J Dermatol. 2012;39(5):496–7.
40. Kaplan AP. Treatment of chronic spontaneous urticaria. Allergy Asthma Immunol Res. 2012;4(6):326–31.
41. Maurer M. Revisions to the international guidelines on the diagnosis and therapy of chronic urticaria. J Dtsch Dermatol Ges. 2013;11(10):971–7.
42. Asero R. Current challenges and controversies in the management of chronic spontaneous urticaria. Expert Rev Clin Immunol. 2015;11(10):1073–82.
43. Belani H. Neutrophilic urticaria with systemic inflammation: a case series. JAMA Dermatol. 2013;149(4):453–8.
44. de Menthon M. Treating polyarteritis nodosa: current state of art. Clin Exp Rheumatol. 2011;29(1 Suppl 64):S110–6.
45. Kundu R. Age old dapsone in the treatment of idiopathic thrombocytopenic purpura—a case report with review. Am J Ther. 2013;20(6):e723–5.

46. El Benaye J. Dapsone efficacy in lupus miliaris disseminates faciei: two cases. Ann Dermatol Venereol. 2011;138(8–9):597–600.

47. Piette EW. Dapsone in the management of autoimmune bullous diseases. Dermatol Clin. 2011;29(4):561–4.

48. Mazille N. Dapsone for chronic skin lesions in 3 children suffering from Henoch-Schonlein vasculitis. Arch Pediatr. 2011;18(11):1201–4.

49. Salehzadeh F. Dapsone as an alternative therapy in children with familial Mediterranean fever. Iran J Pediatr. 2012;22(1):23–7.

50. Marzano AV. Autoinflammatory skin disorders in inflammatory bowel diseases, pyoderma gangrenosum and Sweet's syndrome: a comprehensive review and disease classification criteria. Clin Rev Allergy Immunol. 2013;45(2):202–10.

51. Ehmann LM. Successful treatment of granulomatous rosacea with dapsone. Hautarzt. 2013;64(4):226–8.

52. Bakkour W. Successful use of dapsone for the management of circinate balanitis. Clin Exp Dermatol. 2014;39(3):333–5.

53. Goeser MR, et al. A practical approach to the diagnosis, evaluation, and management of cutaneous small-vessel vasculitis. Am J Clin Dermatol. 2014;15(4):299–306.

54. Rabler F, et al. Treatment of eosinophilic cellulitis (wells syndrome)- a systematic review. J Eur Acad Dermatol Venereol. 2016;30(9):1465–79.

55. Coelho de Sousa V, et al. Successful treatment of eosinophilic cellulitis with dapsone. Dermatol Online J. 2016;22(7).

56. Watts PJ, et al. Subcorneal pustular dermatosis: a review of 30 years of progress. Am J Clin Dermatol. 2016;17(6):653–71.

57. Broussard KC, et al. Erosive pustular dermatosis of the scalp: a review with a focus on dapsone therapy. J Am Acad Dermatol. 2012;66(4):680–6.

58. Oliveira AC, et al. Behcet disease: clinical features and management in a Brazilian tertiary hospital. J Clin Rheumatol. 2011;17(8):416–20.

59. Rotondo C, et al. Mucocutaneous involvement in Behcet's disease: how systemic treatment has changed in the last decades and future perspectives. Mediators Inflamm. 2015;2015:451675.

60. Anjaneyan G, et al. Ofuji's disease in an immunocompetent patient successfully treated with dapsone. Indian Dermatol Online J. 2016;7(5):399–401.

61. Sheu JS, et al. Dapsone therapy for pustular psoriasis: case series and review of the literature. Dermatology. 2016;232(1):97–101.

62. Blanco I, et al. Neutrophilic panniculitis associated with alpha-1-antitrypsin deficiency: an update. Dr J Dermatol. 2016;174(4):753–62.

63. Akasaka E, et al. Diaminodiphenyl sulfone-induced hemolytic anemia and alopecia in a case of linear IgA bullous dermatosis. Case Rep Dermatol. 2015;7(2):183–6.

64. Swartzentruber GS. Metheoglobinemia as a complication of topical dapsone. N Engl J Med. 2015;372(5):491–2.

65. Kang KS, et al. Clinical outcomes of adverse cardiovascular events in patients with acute dapsone poisoning. Elin Exp Emerg Med. 2016;3(1):41–5.

66. Momen SE, et al. Erythema elevatum diutinum: a review of presentation and treatment. J Eur Acad Dermatol Venereol. 2014;28(12):1594–602.

67. Garcia A, et al. Fulminant hepatitis linked to dapsone hypersensitivity syndrome requiring urgent living donor liver transplantation: a case report. Pediatr Transplan. 2014;18(7):E240–5.

68. Milkova L, et al. Asymptomatic dapsone-induced agranulocytosis in a patient with chronic spontaneous urticaria. J Dtsch Dermatol Ges. 2014;12(8):717–9.

69. Semira, et al. Livedo reticularis associated with dapsone therapy in a patient with chronic urticaria. Indian J Pharmacol. 2014;46(4):438–40.

70. Brabin B, et al. Dapsone therapy for malaria during pregnancy. Drug Saf. 2004;27:633–48.

71. Ward S, et al. Antimalarial drugs and pregnancy: safety, pharmacokinetics, and pharmacovigilance. Lancet Infect Dis. 2007;7:136–44.

72. Nosten F, et al. Antimalaria drugs in pregnancy: a review. Curr Drug Saf. 2006;1(1):1–15.

73. Raj AC, et al. Dapsone in the treatment of resistant oral erosive lichen planus: a clinical study. J Indian Aca Oral Med Radiol. 2012;24(1):20–3.

74. Herrero-Gonzalez JE. Clinical guidelines for the diagnosis and treatment of dermatitis herpetiformis. Actas Dermosifiliogr. 2010;101(10):820–6.

75. Alison R, Rupali J. Dapsone interferes with hemoglobin A1c monitoring of diabetes in an HIV-infected patient. AIDS. 2013;27:299–301.

76. Phillips-Howard PA, et al. Serious adverse drug reactions to pyrimethamine-sulphadoxine, pyrimethamine-dapsone and to amodiaquine in Britain. J R Soc Med. 1990;83:82–5.

77. Gottfried W, Christian B. Dapsone in dermatology and beyond. Arch Dermatol Res. 2014;306(2):103–24.

78. Cohen PR, et al. Sweet's syndrome: a review of current treatment options. Am J Clin Dermatol. 2002;3(2):177–31.

79. http://www.glutenfreedrugs.com/newlist.htm. Accessed 23 March 2017.

Systemic Nonantibiotic Therapy in Acne and Rosacea

Guy Webster

Hormonal Therapy

Since acne is tied inextricably to androgen stimulation of the sebaceous gland it makes sense that hormonal manipulation is of value in acne treatment. To date, all systemic drugs that treat acne hormonally are feminizing so this approach is only useful in women. It is often assumed that only hyperandrogenic women will benefit from hormonal therapy but this is not the case. Women with normal androgens and regular menses will also respond to hormonal manipulation, although no study adequately addresses the issue.

In my opinion, spironolactone is the most effective commonly used anti-androgen in acne. The drug was introduced as a diuretic in 1959, was found to be feminizing and its use as an anti-androgen evolved without obtaining regulatory approval for these indications. It has a long history of safe use in the minds of dermatologists, but there is limited data in support of its safety. Shaw and White [1] studied 91 women comprising 200 person years of drug exposure and found menstrual irregularity and diuretic effect to be the most commonly reported adverse events. No serious events occurred.

Goodfellow et al. [2] reported on sebum secretion rates during 3 months of spironolactone therapy for severe acne. They found a dose dependent reduction in sebum secretion that was independent of androgen level. Shaw [3] reported a retrospective study of 85 women who received spironolactone 50–100 mg/day as monotherapy or adjunctive therapy for acne. 33% cleared and 33% had marked improvement.

There is generally positive evidence in the literature that spironolactone is effective in acne, but it is all in relatively small studies that fail to satisfy current standards for high grade evidence. Layton and coworkers [4] performed a hybrid systematic review of the literature and found that all trials were considered "at high risk for bias" and the quality of evidence was either low or very low and that the drug has yet to be proven to be effective in acne. Similarly, a Cochrane review of spironolactone use in hirsutism and acne failed to show evidence for effectiveness in acne [5]. Given the generic status of the drug and the cost of properly done trials it is unlikely that this lack of rigorous evidence will be remedied in the near future. Fortunately, the collective anecdotal evidence gives good support for the usefulness of this drug in acne.

Spironolactone appears to be a safe drug for treatment of acne. Although it is a potassium sparing diuretic it has been found that women treated for acne are not at risk of hyperkalemia [6]. Because of its hormonal activity a risk of breast cancer has been suggested to exist with spironolactone. A recent retrospective study [7] in over two million Danish women who received the drug revealed no statistically significant increase in breast or gynecologic cancers.

Spironolactone regimens have not been standardized and vary among expert practitioners. In general, higher doses (e.g., >100 mg/day) have more frequent side effects of breast tenderness or menstrual irregularity. Some physicians prescribe the drug along with OCP and others use it as monotherapy or maintenance monotherapy. In my practice I typically prescribe it at 100 mg/day and may decrease to 50/day after a good response, typically after 2 months. The response of acne is not quick; it's a matter of months not weeks, and I will usually start it with a more quick-acting drug, e.g., doxycycline, that is taken for the first 2 months or so. Patients are instructed that this is an off-label use, that a warning is given by the FDA about its use, and that if they become pregnant the drug should be discontinued.

Cyproterone acetate is an androgen blocker that is available in Europe as a combination contraceptive along with ethinyl estradiol and has been shown to be useful in acne therapy [8]. Other oral contraceptives (OCP) are also of use in treating acne. Drospirinone is a chemical relative of spironolactone and is available in several OCP preparations that have been shown to be effective in acne [9]. All combination

G. Webster, MD, PhD
Department of Dermatology, Sidney Kimmel Medical College of Thomas Jefferson University, Philadelphia, PA 19107, USA
e-mail: guywebster@yahoo.com

© Springer International Publishing AG 2018
P.S. Yamauchi (ed.), *Biologic and Systemic Agents in Dermatology*, https://doi.org/10.1007/978-3-319-66884-0_45

contraceptives that inhibit ovulation suppress androgen production and may be of use in acne therapy. Firm conclusions about the relative benefits of different OCP are hampered by a lack of comparative studies [10]. A recent meta-analysis compared the response of acne to antibiotic or OCP therapy [11] finding that antibiotics were superior at 3 months but equivalent to OCP at 6 months. Given the valid concerns regarding antibiotic overuse it may be that OCP are a better choice for long-term acne treatment. It must also be considered that OCP carry a very slight risk of thromboembolic disease. This risk if far lower than the clotting risk of pregnancy, so when used as contraception there is a favorable risk:benefit ratio to OCPs regarding clots. This cannot be said for acne which has no risk of thromboembolism. Certainly women desiring both treatment for acne and contraception can benefit from OCP for both indications.

Oral Retinoids

Isotretinoin is the retinoid useful in acne. Other oral retinoids, e.g., acetretin and etretinate have minimal effect on the sebaceous gland which is the main target of the drug in acne. Nelson and colleagues [12] have shown that isotretinoin effects are not a consequence of binding to nuclear retinoic acid receptors, but rather to a cytosolic ligand that induces apoptosis in sebocytes. Additionally, Dispenza et al. [13] demonstrated that isotretinoin can normalize an exaggerated innate immune response via TLR-2 bearing monocytes and dampen the response to *P. acnes*.

Isotretinoin Dosing and Relapse

In 1980 Farrell, Strauss and Stranieri [14] reported a small (14 patient) blinded 12 week study of 13-cis-retinoic acid treatment of severe acne where a dose dependent suppression of sebum production was observed along with marked improvement in the acne. At the highest dosage sebum was reduced to 10% or pretreatment levels. Side effects of desquamation, cheilitis, and dryness were noted. Laboratory abnormalities were minimal and did not require cessation of therapy. Later work [15] showed that prolonged remissions in acne were possible and that sebum production could remain suppressed long after cessation of therapy; up to 80 weeks in some individuals. A subsequent larger study in 150 patients compared 0.1, 0.5, and 1 mg/kg/day [16]. The drug was effective in all doses and no significant differences in acne improvement were seen between the groups. It was noted that 42% of those treated at the lowest dose required retreatment with the drug.

Dosing of isotretinoin has remained a matter of some controversy. Prescribers must weigh the benefits of minimizing side effects vs. the clinical response of the acne. Even low doses of isotretinoin are quite effective while the patient is taking them, it's clear that relapse is more frequent at lower dosages. In 1997 a group of acne experts reviewed the cases of 1000 acne patients who were treated with isotretinoin [17]. Fifty-five percent of the patients had severe acne and the rest mild or moderate acne. The panel concluded that most of the physicians aimed to achieve a target dose of 100–120 mg/kg.

More recently, a single center reported the use of 1.6 mg/kg/day for a cumulative dose around 290 mg/kg in 80 patients [18]. No adverse events lead to discontinuation of treatment. During the 3 years of the study 12.5% of the patients relapsed and required retreatment. All patients were acne-free at the end of the trial. A second study reported 180 patients treated with isotretinoin in varying dosages [19]. They were divided into two groups for analysis, those that received <220 mg/kg and those that received greater. The relapse rate at 1 year was 47.4% in the lower dose group and 26.9% in the higher dose group.

There are obvious difficulties in comparing the relapse rates among different studies using different regimens and different patients of differing severity. The authors of the high dosage papers note greater improvement over the generally accepted (but not rigorously proven) relapse rate of 15–20% at 100 mg/kg total dosage. But the differences were not huge in the first paper and actually much greater relapse occurred in the second. At issue is whether a few percentage points lesser relapse can be justified by the presumed risks of higher dosages. In these two papers at most 260 patients were treated with extra high dosages. This is far too small a number to prove equal safety with normal dosed isotretinoin and, for me, is not enough evidence to treat all acne patients at high dosage. To be sure there will be a few individuals who need the high dosage, and these publications give reassurance that it can be done safely.

What factors determine the likelihood of relapse following isotretinoin treatment? Dosage is clearly a factor and absorption of the drug is as important a variable as the size of the pill administered. Colburn and colleagues [20] showed in 1983 that the absorption of isotretinoin was decreased by 60% if taken on an empty stomach. Moreover the food needs to be quite fatty to get maximal absorption from the GI tract. The exact amount of fat is not well studied, but it appears (from FDA phase 3 submissions) to be substantial ....in other words a glass of milk or a spoon of peanut butter isn't enough to maximize absorption. This high variability can make it hard for a clinician to know how much drug his patient is actually getting and may account for great variability even within well-controlled studies. In addition the requirement of a fatty meal can run opposed to our instructions on how to control elevated triglycerides and with our patient's desires to remain slim. There is a newer formulation of isotretinoin, isotretinoin lidose, that minimizes the food effect and gets substantial absorption if taken on an empty stomach [21, 22].

Other factors that appear to promote post-isotretinoin relapse include early age of onset of the acne and need for the drug while still younger. Although the mechanism for this is not worked out, I assume it reflects a tendency to either an overactive sebaceous gland or excessive hypersensitivity to *P. acnes* that allows acne to recur. Likewise virilized women who have elevated androgens seem to more readily recover sebaceous activity post-isotretinoin and may need repeat treatment. More study in both of these areas is clearly needed.

Teratogenicity

The major issue with isotretinoin that prevents treating all acne patients with it is the risk of birth defects. Isotretinoin causes birth defects in at least 25% of babies exposed during the first trimester [23]. Isotretinoin embryopathy includes ear malformations, CNS defects, and cardiovascular defects. Pregnancy prevention programs have been instituted and are reasonably but far from completely effective in preventing fetal exposure. In the United States a more stringent iPLEDGE program supplanted its predecessor, SMART and seems to be somewhat better at limiting fetal exposure. One study reported that fetal exposure in SMART was 3.11 cases per 1000 courses and that iPLEDGE reduced that rate to 2.67 per 1000 [24]. A Canadian pregnancy prevention program identified 186 pregnancies out of 102, 308 courses of isotretinoin in females between 1996 and 2011 [25]. Of these 118 resulted in a live birth; with 11 cases of malformation.

In theory, proper use of two means of contraception should all but eliminate pregnancy on isotretinoin. Compliance with contraceptive requirements may be limited by a patient's circumstances, their understanding of the issues and their willingness to take risks and the influence of alcohol. It may be that injectable/implantable contraception should receive greater use going forward.

Other adverse events are far less problematic. Isotretinoin is a 35 year old drug and there should be no new problems that arise with it. Adverse events (Table 45.1) of dry skin, lips, elevated triglycerides are well known and are usually dose-dependent [26]. Less common problems are also listed in Table 45.1.

Table 45.1 Adverse events associated with isotretinoin therapy

Common
Dry skin and lips
Hypertriglyceridemia
Myalgia
Uncommon
Dry eye
Decreased night vision
Acne fulminans
Psychiatric disturbance
Hepatic irritation

Inflammatory Bowel Disease

Over the years scattered case reports and small retrospective studies have suggested a link between isotretinoin therapy and inflammatory bowel disease (IBD). Until relatively recently there have been no large studies that addressed the issue. In the past several years very large studies have reported on the incidence of IBD as a consequence of isotretinoin treatment [27, 28]. Invariably, they find no connection between the drug and the IBD. One study noted that there may be a protective effect in Crohn's disease [29], another found a link with antibiotic use and Crohn's [30], and another identified a link to acne but not to isotretinoin [27]. Interestingly, much of the support for a causal connection between the drug and IBD came from the US FDA drug adverse event reporting system that identified 2214 cases resulting from isotretinoin usage. Stobaugh and colleagues [31] analyzed the source of each of the case reports and found that 5.15% came from consumers, 6.0% from physicians, and 87.2% from lawyers.

Laboratory Abnormalities

Laboratory monitoring during isotretinoin treatment currently lacks a clear standard of performance [33]. The tests typically ordered are AST, ALT, CBC, Lipid panel, and HCG. Many physicians order tests monthly other less frequently. A meta-analysis by Lee et al. [32] found that significant abnormalities are rare in the published literature and that there was little rationale for monthly testing of all patients. Hansen and coworkers [34] similarly found that among their patients significant abnormalities were rare and that baseline and 2 month testing seemed sufficient. Webster and colleagues [35] reviewed the laboratory findings in 246 consecutive patients treated with isotretinoin. AST, ALT, GGT, CK, CBC, and lipids were measured. No significant CBC abnormalities occurred. AST and ALT elevations were mild and were not accompanied by a GGT elevation, indicating that their elevation was not from a hepatic source. Most AST and ALT elevations were accompanied by a CK elevation, indicating a muscular source. CK elevations were quite common and mostly in young men, and some were quite high, e.g., 4 × normal or greater. Invariably, these patients were engaging in strenuous physical activity and most were asymptomatic. Since this study was completed I have had one patient require hospitalization for rhabdomyolysis. These findings indicate that we may be missing significant problems by failing to measure CK in isotretinoin patients and that physically active young men must be treated carefully and probably advised to moderate their exercise. It is important to note that these patients were not matched to a control group so a definitive statement that isotretinoin causes CK elevation or damages muscle cannot be made. Indeed there are numerous papers documenting CK elevation and rhabdomyolysis in athletes taking no medication whatsoever.

Acne Fulminans

Acne fulminans is an explosive eruption that is classically accompanied by fever, arthralgia, leukocytosis, and ulcerative acne lesions. Over the past 30 years it has been observed that isotretinoin can trigger a skin-limited form of acne fulminans [35]. It typically occurs early in therapy of a patient with nodular trunk acne. High starting doses of isotretinoin seem to favor its development. The appropriate response is to lower or discontinue the isotretinoin and begin oral corticosteroids after which isotretinoin can be reintroduced. It is my practice to start most patients with severe trunk acne on both prednisone and isotretinoin both at 20 mg/day and taper away the prednisone after a few weeks.

Pseudotumor Cerebri

Pseudotumor cerebri is a rare complication of isotretinoin therapy. Its etiology and relation to the drug is uncertain. A recent case series has documented the safe use of isotretinoin in three acne patients who had previously had an episode of psuedotumor cerebri [36].

Bone Density

Changes in bone mineralization have been reported to result from isotretinoin therapy is a few small studies. A recent study of the safety of two formulations of isotretinoin looked at BMD in 476 patients before and after a course of 20 weeks [22]. Only one patient had a small decrease for which a drug-related effect could not be excluded.

Psychiatric Disorders

Since its approval, isotretinoin has had reports of psychiatric disturbances associated with therapy. Most were small case series or single patient reports and it was impossible to determine if there was really a risk. In 2008 a case control series of patients hospitalized for depression in Quebec were found to have a relative risk of 2.68 (CI 1.0–6.5) for isotretinoin exposure. In a safety study of 476 patients receiving isotretinoin that included psychologic evaluation of every patient, there were 56 adverse psychiatric events that included insomnia, anxiety, depression, ADD, mood swings, sleep disorder and panic attacks [22] no link to isotretinoin was established. Most recently, Huang and Cheng [37] performed a systemic review and meta-analysis of the literature concerning isotretinoin and depression. They found no difference in depression scores of patients treated with isotretinoin vs. an alternative therapy. The prevalence of depression after isotretinoin declined significantly and mean depression scores decreased over therapy. Thus the weight of the data indicates that isotretinoin does not induce affective disorders in the vast majority of patients. It must be borne in mind however that there is a possibility that a very small minority of outliers might exist for whom isotretinoin could trigger psychiatric problems.

References

1. Shaw JC, White LE. Long term safety of spironolactone in acne:results of an 8 year follow-up study. J Cutan Med Surg. 2002;6:541–5.
2. Goodfellow A, Alaghband-Zadeh J, Carter G, Cream JJ, Holland S, Scully J, Wise P. Oral spironolactone improves acne vulgaris and reduces sebum excretion. Br J Dermatol. 1984;111:209–14.
3. Shaw JC. Low dose adjunctive spironolactone in the treatment of acne in women: a retrospective analysis of 85 consecutively treated patients. J Am Acad Dermatol. 2000;43:498–502.
4. Layton AM, Eady EA, Whitehouse H, Delrosso JQ, Fedorowicz Z, van Zuuren EJ. Oral spironolactone for acne vulgaris in adult females:a hybrid systematic review. Am J Clin Dermatol. 2017;18(2):169–91. https://doi.org/10.1007/s40257-016-0245x.
5. Brown J, Farquhar C, Lee O, Toomath R, Jepson RG. Spironolactone vs placebo or in combination with steroids for hirsutism and/or acne. Cochrane Database Syst Rev. 2009;(2):CD000194. https://doi.org/10.1002/14651858.CD000194.pub2.
6. Plovanich M, Weng QY, Mostaghimi A. Low usefulness og potassium monitoring among healthy young women taking spironolactone for acne. JAMA Dermatol. 2015;151:941–4.
7. Lortscher D, Admani S, Satur N, Eichenfield LF. Hormonal contraceptives and acne: a retrospective analysis of 2147 patients. J Drugs Dermatol. 2016;15(6):670–4.
8. Van Waygen RG, van den Ende A. Experience in the long term treatment of patients with hirsutism and or acne with cyproterone acetate containing preparations. Exp Clin Endo Diabetes. 1995;103:214–51.
9. Barros B, Thiboutot D. Hormonal therapies for acne. Clin Dermatol. 2017;35:168–72.
10. Arowojolu AO, Gallo MF, Lopez LM, Grimes DA. Combined oral contraceptive pills for the treatment of acne. Cochrane Database

Syst Rev. 2012;(6):CD004425. https://doi.org/10.1002/14651858.cd004425.pub5.

11. Koo EB, Petersen TD, Kimball AB. Meta-analysis comparing efficacy of antibiotics versus oral contraceptives in acne vulgaris. J Am Acad Dermatol. 2014;71(3):450–9.

12. Nelson AM, Cong Z, Gilliland KL, Thiboutot DM. TRAIL contributes to the apoptotic effect of 13-cis retinoic acid in human sebaceous gland cells. Br J Dermatol. 2011;165(3):526–33.

13. Dispenza MC, Wolpert EB, Gilliland KL, Dai JP, Cong Z, Nelson AM, Thiboutot DM. Systemic isotretinoin therapy normalizes exaggerated TLR-2-mediated innate immune responses in acne patients. J Invest Dermatol. 2012;132(9):2198–205.

14. Farrell LN, Strauss JS, Stranieri AM. The treatment of severe cystic acne with cis-13-retinoic acid. Evaluation of sebum response and clinical response. J Am Acad Dermatol. 1980;3:602–11.

15. Strauss JS, Stranieri AM. Changes in long term sebum production from isotretinoin. J Am Acad Dermatol. 1982;6:751–6.

16. Stewart ME, Benoit AM, Stranieri AM, Rapini RP, Strauss JS, Downing DT. Effect of oral cis-13-retinoic acid at thjree dose levels on sustainable rates of sebum secretion and on acne. J Am Acad Dermatol. 1983;8:532–8.

17. Strauss JS, Rapini RP, Shalita AR, Konecky E, Pochi PE, Comite H, Exner JH. Isotretinoin therapy for acne: results of a multicenter dose-response study. J Am Acad Dermatol. 1984;10:490–6.

18. Cunliffe WJ, van de Kerkhof PC, et al. Roaccutane treatment guidelines: results of an international survey. Dermatology. 1997;194:351–7.

19. Cyrulnik AA, Viola KV, Gewertzman AJ, Choen SR. High dose isotretinoin in axcne vulgaris:improved treatment outcomes and quality of life. Int J Dermatol. 2012;51:1123–30.

20. Blasiak RC, Stamey CR, Burkhart CN, Lugo-Somolinos A, Morrell DS. High dose isotretinoin treatment and the rate of retrial relapse and adverse events in patients with acne vulgaris. JAMA Dermatol. 2013;149:1392–8.

21. Colburn WA, Gibson DM, Wiens RE, Hanigan JJ. Food increases the bioavailability of isotretinoin. J Clin Pharmacol. 1983;23:534–9.

22. Webster GF, Leyden JJ, Gross JA. Comparative pharmacokinetic profiles of a novel isotretinoin (isotretinoin-lidose). J Am Acad Dermatol. 2013;69:762–7.

23. Webster GF, Leyden JJ, Gross JA. Results of a phase III, double blind, parallel group noninferiority study evaluating the safety and efficacy of isotretinoin lidose in paruients with severe recalcitrant nodular acne. J Drugs Dermatol. 2014;13:665–70.

24. Lynberg MC, Khoury MJ, Lammer EJ, Waller KO, et al. Sensitivity, specificity and positive predictive value of multiple malformations in isotretinoin embryopathy surveillance. Teratology. 1990;42:513–9.

25. Shin J, Cheetham TC, Wong L, Niu F, et al. The impact of the iPledge program on isotretinoin fetal exposure in an integrated healthcare system. J Am Acad Dermatol. 2011;65:1117–25.

26. Henry D, Domuth C, Winquist B, Carney G, et al. Occurrence of preganacy and pregnancy outcomes during isotretinoin therapy. Can Med J. 2016;188:723–30.

27. Webster GF. Isotretinoin:mechanism of action and patient selection. Sem Cutan Med Surg. 2015;34:s86–8.

28. Alhusayen RO, Juurlink DN, Mamdani MM, et al. Isotretinoin use and the risk of inflammatory bowel disease. J Invest Dermatol. 2013;133:907–12.

29. Rashtak S, Khaleghi S, Pittlekow MR, Larson JJ, Lahr BD, Murray JA. Isotretinoin exposure and risk of inflammatory bowel disease. JAMA Dermatol. 2014;150:1322–6.

30. Racine A, Cuerg A, Bijon A, Ricordeau P, et al. Isotretinoin and risk of inflammatory bowel disease: a French nationwide study. Am J Gastroenterol. 2014;109:563–9.

31. Ungaro R, Bernstein CN, Gearry R, Hviid A, et al. Antibiotics associated with increased risk of new onset Crohn's disease but not ulcerative colitis. Am J Gastroenterol. 2014;109:1728–38.

32. Stobaugh DJ, Deepak P, Ehrenpreis ED. Alleged isotretinoin associated inflammatory bowel disease: disproportionate reporting by attorneys to the FDA. J Am Acad Dermatol. 2013;69:393–8.

33. Lee YH, Scharnitz TP, Muscat J, Chen A, Gupta-Elera G, Kirby JS. Laboratory monitoring during isotretinoin therapy for acne. JAMA Dermatol. 2016;152:25–44.

34. Hansen TJ, Lucking S, Miller JJ, Kirby JS, Thiboutot DM, Zaenglein AL. Standardized laboratory monitoring with use of isotretinoin for acne. J Am Acad Dermatol. 2016;75:323–8.

35. Dermatol Online J. 2017 May 15;23(5). pii: 13030/qt7rv7j80p. Laboratory tests in patients treated with isotretinoin: occurrence of liver and muscle abnormalities and failure of AST and ALT to predict liver abnormality.Webster GF1, Webster TG, Grimes LR.

36. Tintle SJ, Harper JC, Webster GF, Kim GK, Thiboutot DM. Safe use of therapeutic dose oral isotretinoin in patients with a history of pseudotumor cerebri. JAMA Dermatol. 2016;152:582–4.

37. Huang YC, Cheng YC. Isotretinoin treatment for acne and risk of depression: a systematic review and metaanalysis. J Am Acad Dermato. 2017;76(6):1068–76.e9. https://doi.org/10.1016/j.jaad.2016.

Oral Antibiotics in Dermatology: A Practical Overview with Clinically Relevant Correlations and Management Suggestions

James Q. Del Rosso and Suzanne M. Sachsman

Introduction

Oral antibiotics are frequently prescribed in dermatology practice, with their use related to treatment of both cutaneous infections and noninfectious inflammatory dermatologic disorders [1, 2]. Representing approximately 20% of all prescriptions written within the dermatology specialty, dermatologists prescribe more oral antibiotics per type of practitioner than any other medical specialty, including primary care; the majority of these oral antibiotic prescriptions are for treatment of noninfectious inflammatory dermatoses, such as acne and rosacea [1, 3, 4]. It is important to note that unlike treatment of most bacterial infections which usually respond to appropriate antibiotic therapy within a few to several days, antibiotic treatment of inflammatory skin disorders (such as acne and rosacea) is usually prolonged over a few to several months [1, 3–6]. Consistent with the common use of oral antibiotic agents to treat inflammatory skin disorders, oral tetracyclines comprise approximately three-fourths of all oral antibiotics prescribed by dermatologists, especially doxycycline and minocycline [1].

The goal of this chapter is not to serve as an encyclopedic review of all oral antibiotics that may be used for treatment of dermatologic conditions as a very thorough and recent review is already available [3]. Rather, the objectives of this chapter are to discuss specific oral antibiotic therapies that are commonly used in dermatology and to provide a practical overview on optimal antibiotic use for uncomplicated superficial cutaneous infections and noninfectious inflammatory dermatoses. *Emphasis is placed on the more frequently used antibiotic treatments* of *more commonly encountered cutaneous disorders*, such as superficial staphylococcal and streptococcal infections and facial inflammatory dermatoses (e.g., acne, rosacea, perioral dermatitis). Summary statements are provided for oral antibiotics that are used less frequently in outpatient dermatology, such as rifampin, clindamycin, linezolid, tedizolid, and dapsone.

Oral Penicillin Derivatives and Oral Cephalosporins

Dermatologic Applications of Oral Penicillins

The beta-lactamase-resistant oral penicillins and oral cephalosporins are adaptable for treatment of many uncomplicated bacterial skin infections caused by susceptible organisms. These agents are not generally recommended for treatment of common inflammatory facial dermatoses such as acne and rosacea, primarily due to concerns related to antibiotic resistance [1, 3, 7–9]. Of the oral beta-lactamase-resistant penicillins, dicloxacillin exhibits the most favorable pharmacologic and pharmacokinetic properties, with therapeutic activity against methicillin-sensitive *Staphylococcus aureus* (MSSA); these agents are not recommended for treatment of methicillin-resistant *S. aureus* (MRSA) [3]. The same is true for amoxicillin-clavulanate, which incorporates a beta-lactamase inhibitor (clavulanic acid) in combination with amoxicillin. Amoxicillin offers superiority over ampicillin, a structurally similar oral aminopenicillin antibiotic, demonstrating greater gastrointestinal (GI) absorption, lower incidence of diarrhea, adaptability to co-administration with food, and resistance to beta-lactamase when combined in the same tablet/capsule with clavulanic acid [3]. Isoxazolyl penicillins offer good coverage against both *Streptococcus pyogenes* and MSSA, which are associated with a variety of

J.Q. Del Rosso, DO, FAOCD, FAAD (✉)
Touro University Nevada, Henderson, NV, USA

JDR Dermatology Research, LLC,
9080 West Post Road, Suite 100, Las Vegas, NV 89148, USA

Private Dermatology Practice,
Thomas Dermatology, Las Vegas, NV, USA
e-mail: jqdelrosso@yahoo.com

S.M. Sachsman, MD
Division of Dermatology, David Geffen School
of Medicine at UCLA, Los Angeles, CA, USA
e-mail: SSachsman@mednet.ucla.edu

© Springer International Publishing AG 2018
P.S. Yamauchi (ed.), *Biologic and Systemic Agents in Dermatology*, https://doi.org/10.1007/978-3-319-66884-0_46

Table 46.1 Clinically relevant information with selected oral antibiotics used in dermatology

Drug	Usual dose	Comments
CEPHALEXIN	250–500 MG QID	Pharmacokinetic profile for skin not as favorable as cefdinir due to very short half-life and rapid renal clearance
		Not active against MRSA
CEFDINIR	300 MG BID	More prolonged tissue levels within skin than cephalexin
	600 MG DAILY	Not active against MRSA
AZITHROMYCIN	500 MG DAILY on first day followed by 250 MG DAILY on days 2 through 5	Dosage to left recommended for uncomplicated skin infections caused by susceptible bacteria
		Selective use for acne or rosacea; after initial loading dose may use 250 mg two to three times per week
DOXYCYCLINE	150–200 MG DAILY (infection)	Lower doses may be equally effective in rosacea
	150–200 MG DAILY (acne)	Enteric-coated and small tablet (scored) formulations reduce GI side effects
	20 MG BID or 40 MG DAILY with modified-release capsule (rosacea)	Administer with food to reduce GI upset
	50–200 MG DAILY (rosacea)	Avoid lying down flat after ingestion
		Photoprotection recommended
		Severe intractable cephalgia/visual disturbances/nausea and vomiting warrant evaluation for presence of papilledema
		Take doxycycline at least 1–2 h before oral ingestion of iron
MINOCYCLINE	100–200 MG DAILY (infection)	Caution about vestibular side effects; most likely to occur within first few days
	100–200 MG DAILY (acne)	Acute vestibular side effects reduced with weight-based dosing (using ER tablet) for acne
	1 MG/KG DAILY using extended-release (ER) tablet formulation (acne)	Drug hypersensitivity syndrome (DHS) most often occurs within the first 2–8 weeks after starting therapy; flu-like symptoms, facial edema, hepatotoxicity common; systemically may present with interstitial pneumonitis as predominant finding; watch for delayed development of autoimmune thyroiditis weeks to months after resolution of lupus-like syndrome that develops most often after months to years of use, usually without any skin changes, with polyarthralgias/arthritis of small peripheral joints (fingers/hands) most common; ANA* positive with several other autoantibodies potentially positive on serologic testing
		Monitor patients with cutaneous and/or mucosal dyspigmentation; may present as blue scars, blue lunula, gray or blue color of skin and/or mucosa (oral, ocular), brown macular discoloration often on legs
		Severe intractable cephalgia/visual disturbances/nausea and vomiting warrant evaluation for presence of papilledema
		Take minocycline at least 1–2 h before oral ingestion of iron
TRIMETHOPRIM-SULFACETAMIDE	160 MG/800MG BID (infection) (double-strength [DS] tablet)	Use for MRSA suggested if patient has failed or is unable to use doxycycline or minocycline
		Use for acne in selected cases that have failed other therapies and patient not a candidate for or refusing oral isotretinoin
		Lower dose may be effective in selected cases of acne; may use BID or DAILY
		Watch for potential signs of emerging DHS, Stevens-Johnson syndrome, and toxic epidermal necrolysis especially in the first few months after starting therapy
		Consider baseline and periodic monitoring of complete blood cell counts if to be administered for prolonged duration (acne)
CIPROFLOXACIN	500–750 MG BID	Take ciprofloxacin/fluoroquinolone agent at least 1 h before and not within 4 h after ingestion of dairy foods (i.e., milk, yogurt), fortified cereals, antacids, and/or vitamin/mineral supplements as failure to do so results in reduced GI absorption of the drug; this predisposes to antibiotic treatment failure

cutaneous bacterial infections encountered in the outpatient setting; the natural penicillins (penicillin G, penicillin V) are not active against MSSA or MRSA [3]. All oral penicillins primarily undergo renal elimination, with the exception of oxacillin [3]. Dosing of selected major oral penicillins used in outpatient dermatology is depicted in Table 46.1.

Adverse Effects Associated with Oral Penicillins

Hypersensitivity reactions, such as anaphylaxis/anaphylactoid reactions, are probably the major adverse effects (AEs) encountered clinically when prescribing oral penicillin derivatives. The diverse range of severity encompasses morbilliform skin eruptions to urticarial reactions to fatal or near-fatal anaphylaxis [3]. From a clinical perspective, it should be considered that all penicillins may cross-react. Therefore, if a patient is truly allergic to a penicillin (or cephalosporin) antibiotic, especially with a severe allergic reaction, avoidance of other penicillin and cephalosporin agents is recommended [3]. Other AEs associated with oral penicillins are antibiotic-associated diarrhea and *C. difficile*-associated colitis (much less common than the former); more serious AEs such as hemolysis, blood dyscrasias, and seizures are most commonly associated with high-dose parenteral administration of specific penicillin derivatives [3]. Assuming the clinical benefit is felt to outweigh the potential risks of therapy during pregnancy, the oral penicillins are generally rated as pregnancy category B [3, 10].

Dermatologic Applications of Oral Cephalosporins

Cephalosporins are beta-lactamase-resistant agents that have been divided into "generations" depending primarily on their spectrum of antibiotic activity; the first-generation cephalosporins, cephalexin and cefadroxil, and the third-generation cephalosporin, cefdinir, exhibit the most favorable antibacterial activity among oral cephalosporin agents against MSSA and non-enterococcal streptococci, with some activity against certain Gram-negative organisms [3, 11]. With the exception of cefdinir, which exhibits favorable antibacterial activity against MSSA and non-enterococcal streptococcal pathogens, it is generally accepted that second-, third-, fourth-, and fifth-generation cephalosporins exhibit increased activity against Gram-negative pathogens and lesser activity against Gram-positive pathogens, with many agents available for parenteral use only. Notably, individual differences in antibacterial coverages exist among specific agents in all generations [3, 11].

From a practical perspective, two oral cephalosporins that are commonly used in dermatology to treat uncomplicated cutaneous bacterial infections caused by susceptible pathogens are cephalexin and cefdinir. As with other cephalosporins, these agents are inactive against *Pseudomonas* spp. including *P. aeruginosa*, and unlike cefaclor (a second-generation agent), they are not active against *Haemophilus influenzae* [3, 11]. Cephalexin is best absorbed from an empty stomach, rapidly undergoes renal excretion, and warrants oral administration three to four times daily due primarily to its short serum half-life [3]. Unlike oral cephalexin, cefdinir exhibits a longer serum half-life and more prolonged persistence in the skin after oral administration, with favorable antibiotic activity against MSSA and *S. pyogenes* with twice daily or once daily administration [3, 11, 12].

Oral cephalosporins are often used in dermatology practice to treat uncomplicated superficial cutaneous infections caused by MSSA or non-enterococcal streptococci, such as folliculitis, cellulitis, and furunculosis [3, 11]. Other selected uses of oral cephalosporins that may be helpful in certain clinical situations include treatment of *H. influenzae* cellulitis with cefaclor and treatment of selected cases of gonorrhea or Lyme borreliosis with cefuroxime axetil [3].

Dosing of selected major oral cephalosporins used in outpatient dermatology is depicted in Table 46.1.

Adverse Effects Associated with Oral Cephalosporins

Hypersensitivity and urticarial skin reactions are reported to occur in 1–3% of patients treated with cephalosporin antibiotics, inclusive of both oral and parenteral administration [11]. Potential cross-reactivity/cross allergenicity between penicillins and cephalosporins has been noted to occur in anywhere from 1 to 10% of patients [3]. Overall, oral cephalosporin antibiotics are very well tolerated; GI toxicity such as nausea, vomiting, or diarrhea may occur, with antibiotic-associated colitis noted to be rare with oral formulations [3]. Vaginal candidiasis may occur in some cephalosporin-treated patients [3, 11]. Serum sickness-like reaction has been occasionally reported in association with oral cefaclor use, especially in children [13]. More serious AEs, such as hematologic toxicities, are infrequent and are usually seen in association with parenteral cephalosporin use [3].

Oral Macrolides and Azalide Agents

Dermatologic Applications of Macrolide and Azalide Agents

Macrolides and azalides are compounds that are structurally very similar; the major oral macrolide antibiotics used in dermatology are erythromycin and clarithromycin, with azithromycin being the major azalide agent [3, 14]. Oral erythromycin use for the treatment of acne, and also for treatment of commonly encountered superficial cutaneous staphylococcal bacterial infections, has been limited due to the prominent emergence of erythromycin-resistant causative organisms (i.e., *P. acnes* in acne; *S. aureus* in superficial cutaneous infections) [1, 4, 8, 14–17]. Clarithromycin is equally absorbed from the GI tract when administered with or without food, while azithromycin is absorbed better in the absence of food (1–2 h before food ingestion) [3]. Azithromycin elimination is predominantly via hepatic metabolism, while clarithromycin is primarily eliminated by renal excretion [3].

Oral macrolide/azalide agents *have* demonstrated efficacy for a variety of uncomplicated superficial cutaneous infections caused by susceptible bacteria, including folliculitis, infected wounds/skin ulcers, and cellulitis; MRSA is not responsive to macrolide or azalide therapy [3, 17, 18]. Other mucocutaneous infections that may be treated with macrolide/azalide agents include Lyme disease, erythrasma, erysipeloid, and several sexually transmitted diseases (STDs; non-gonococcal urethritis, syphilis, chancroid, lymphogranuloma venereum) [3, 19–21]. Azithromycin has demonstrated efficacy in the treatment of cat scratch disease, donovanosis, human and animal bites caused by *Pasteurella* spp. and *Eikenella* spp., and urethritis or cervicitis caused by *N. gonorrhea* or *C. trachomatis* [3, 19, 20]. Clarithromycin has demonstrated efficacy in the treatment of leprosy and atypical mycobacterial skin infections caused by a variety of *Mycobacterium* spp. [3, 19–22]. Both azithromycin and clarithromycin are active against *H. influenzae*, *Treponema pallidum*, *Toxoplasma gondii*, and *Borrelia burgdorferi* [3].

Although not considered a first-line agent, oral azithromycin has been used in selected cases to treat both acne and rosacea [1, 3, 7, 9, 14, 23–28]. Due to its prolonged persistence in cutaneous tissue, a variety of intermittent regimens have been suggested with oral azithromycin for acne and rosacea [3, 7–10, 14, 24–28]. Due to the marked global prevalence of *P. acnes* strains resistant to erythromycin, the use of this agent for the treatment of acne has diminished; oral erythromycin is also associated with a higher potential for GI upset than azithromycin and clarithromycin and is associated with some potentially significant drug-drug interactions with an enhanced risk of systemic toxicity when co-administered with certain other drugs (i.e., cyclosporine, carbamazepine) [1, 3–5, 7–9, 15, 29]. Dosing of selected major oral macrolide/azalide agents used in outpatient dermatology is depicted in Table 46.1.

Adverse Effects Associated with Oral Macrolide and Azalide Agents

The most predominant AEs associated with oral macrolide/azalide use are GI disturbances associated with erythromycin and metallic taste associated with clarithromycin [3, 14, 19]. Cardiac conduction abnormalities, including QT prolongation and torsades de pointes, have been associated primarily with systemic erythromycin use, with risk factors including higher age, high dosage, rapid administration, and history of cardiac disease [3]. Animal data support that macrolides/azalides can induce reactive oxygen species formation, mitochondrial membrane permeabilization, mitochondrial swelling, and cytochrome C release in cardiomyocyte mitochondria providing some

plausible scientific explanation for cardiac conduction changes and arrhythmias, including QT prolongation and torsades de pointes [30]. Sporadically reported AEs potentially associated with these agents have been fixed drug eruption, leukocytoclastic vasculitis, and hypersensitivity reactions with clarithromycin and hearing loss, angioedema, and hypersensitivity syndrome with azithromycin [3, 14, 19].

Oral Tetracyclines

Dermatologic Applications of Tetracycline Agents

Tetracycline agents are the most frequently utilized antibiotics in dermatology, representing approximately 75% of all oral antibiotics prescribed by dermatologists in the ambulatory practice setting; they are used to treat a broad range of cutaneous infections and even more commonly for noninfectious inflammatory dermatoses such as acne, rosacea, and perioral dermatitis [1, 3, 7, 8, 14]. Currently, doxycycline and minocycline are the most commonly prescribed tetracycline agents in the USA, with the majority of their use for facial inflammatory dermatoses (acne, rosacea, perioral dermatitis); these two agents offer advantages over tetracycline, including greater GI absorption, greater activity against *P. acnes*, lower prevalence of *P. acnes* resistance, reduced frequency of administration, and less binding within the GI tract by co-ingested metal ions found in dairy products, vitamin/mineral supplements, and antacids [1, 3, 4, 8, 9, 14, 29, 31].

Because of their broad range of antibiotic activity against MRSA and a diverse array of bacterial pathogens and spirochetes, doxycycline and minocycline are commonly used to treat a wide variety of cutaneous infections, including uncomplicated MRSA infections, several STDs, and Lyme disease [1, 3, 17, 21]. The biologic properties of tetracyclines which include anti-inflammatory effects unrelated to antibiotic activity appear to contribute therapeutically to their established efficacy for treatment of acne, rosacea, perioral dermatitis, and other noninfectious inflammatory and bullous skin disorders [2, 3, 14, 32, 35]. These biologic/anti-inflammatory properties unrelated to antibiotic effects include inhibition on neutrophil migration, diminished production of neutrophil chemoattractants by *P. acnes*, inhibition of matrix metalloproteinases associated with derma matrix degradation and modulation involving collagen and elastic tissue (e.g., collagenase, gelatinase), scavenger effect on reactive oxygen species, downregulation cytokines involved innate immune response, and inhibition of protein kinase C-associated granuloma formation [2, 3, 14, 32–35]. Sub-antibiotic dosing of doxycycline is achieved with the use of doxycycline 20 mg twice daily or with once daily administration of a specific modified-release 40 mg capsule formulation (doxycycline-MR) which is approved in the USA for treatment of papulopustular rosacea [34, 35].

The high lipophilicity of minocycline and doxycycline allows for concentrations in the skin, including the sebum-rich pilosebaceous unit [3, 4, 14, 31]. Co-ingestion of minocycline or doxycycline with iron may markedly reduce GI absorption; however, intake with food or with other metal ions has a more modest effect on impairing GI absorption [3, 29]. Doxycycline is primarily excreted via the GI tract; however, renal impairment prolongs the serum half-life of other tetracycline agents [3]. An extended-release (ER) tablet formulation of minocycline is available, specifically indicated only for treatment of acne and not for cutaneous infections, which allows for a slower drug accumulation, lower maximum drug concentration, and decrease in systemic drug exposure over time; minocycline-ER is dosed based on weight, with a target dose of 1 mg/kg/day [36]. Weight-based dosing of minocycline-ER has been shown to reduce the potential for acute vestibular side effects associated with minocycline use, such as vertigo [37].

For the purpose of clarification, the words doxycycline and minocycline refer to dosing and formulations that provide both the antibiotic and biologic properties and can be used to treat cutaneous infections; minocycline-ER and doxycycline-MR refer to formulations that are used to treat inflammatory acne and papulopustular rosacea, respectively, and not for cutaneous infections. Dosing of selected major oral tetracycline agents used in outpatient dermatology is depicted in Table 46.1.

Doxycycline and minocycline are the predominant tetracycline agents currently used by dermatologists in the USA [1, 2, 8, 14]. The predominant use of these agents in dermatology is for acne and rosacea, including primarily papulopustular rosacea, but also for ocular rosacea and granulomatous rosacea [1, 3, 4, 8, 14]. For acne and papulopustular rosacea, their use is continued usually over at least a few months in order to gain adequate control of the eruption, allowing for transition to topical therapy alone to sustain control of the disorder and reduce continued risk of antibiotic resistance [1, 3, 4, 7–9, 14, 23]. Sub-antibiotic dose doxycycline is amenable for more prolonged treatment of papulopustular rosacea, including as monotherapy, due to lack of antibiotic selection pressure and avoidance of emergence of antibiotic-resistant bacterial strains; data for use in acne are limited but may be beneficial in some cases of mild to moderate acne severity, especially with more prolonged use over at least 6 months [1, 5, 32, 34, 38–40].

Importantly, doxycycline and minocycline are frequently used to treat uncomplicated cutaneous MRSA infections and are commonly utilized as first-line therapy, with incision and drainage incorporated when cutaneous abscess is present [3, 17, 18, 41, 42]. Doxycycline is considered the treatment of choice for rickettsial infections such as Rocky Mountain spotted fever and African tick bite fever, and for lymphogranuloma venereum, and is also used for spirochete infections, including primary syphilis (second line), early Lyme disease, yaws, and pinta [3, 21]. Tetracyclines are no longer considered to be a therapeutic option for uncomplicated or disseminated gonorrhea, and use of any tetracycline agent for granuloma inguinale, despite initial improvement or clearance, has been associated with a high risk of therapeutic failure [3, 21]. Minocycline or doxycycline have been used successfully for treatment of cutaneous *M. marinum* infections (e.g., fish tank granuloma), used preferably at maximum dose (200 mg/day) and ideally for durations of at least 12–16 weeks [3, 22]. Management of other atypical mycobacterial infections is dependent on type of organism, severity/extent of disease, and immunologic status of the patient, with many cases involving combination therapy with other agents; further details on management have been reviewed elsewhere [3, 22].

Tetracyclines have been sporadically reported in small studies and case reports to be effective, alone and/or in combination with other agents, in the treatment on several noninfectious dermatologic disorders, including immunobullous disorders (e.g., bullous pemphigoid; combination with niacinamide), sarcoidosis (minocycline, doxycycline), pityriasis lichenoides et varioliformis acuta (tetracycline), pityriasis lichenoides chronica (tetracycline, minocycline), pyoderma gangrenosum (minocycline), oral lichen planus (doxycycline, minocycline), cetuximab-related acneiform eruption (minocycline and topical tazarotene), and hidradenitis suppurativa [2, 3, 32, 43, 44]. Minocycline is considered to be first-line therapy for confluent and reticulate papillomatosis [2, 3].

Adverse Effects Associated with Oral Tetracycline Agents

Tetracycline is no longer commonly used in dermatology due to need for greater frequency of administration, higher prevalence of *P. acnes*-resistant strains than doxycycline and minocycline, less predictable GI absorption with higher chelation by co-administered metal ions in foods (e.g., milk, yogurt, fortified cereals) and vitamin/mineral supplements, and intermittent problems with supply and manufacturing [3–5, 7–9, 14, 29, 31].

The most common AEs associated with doxycycline use are dose-related phototoxicity and GI side effects ("pill esophagitis") [3, 8, 9, 14]. The former may be obviated by ultraviolet light (i.e., sun) avoidance and broad-spectrum sunscreen use, and the latter mitigated by administration with food and use of an enteric-coated formulation or the small tablet formulation of doxycycline [3, 14, 45].

Minocycline is associated with acute vestibular side effects (vertigo, dizziness, tinnitus) in some patients, which develops early on after starting therapy, and may be obviated by use of minocycline-ER weight-based therapy if treating acne [3, 9, 14, 37]. Cutaneous and mucosal hyperpigmentation may also occur with use of minocycline, especially with more prolonged durations of use [3]. Multiple cases of drug hypersensitivity syndrome (DHS; drug reaction with eosinophilia and systemic symptoms [DRESS]) have been reported in association with minocycline use; patients commonly present within 2–6 weeks after initiation of therapy with flu-like symptoms, diffuse erythema, pharyngitis, facial swelling, and systemic effects such as hepatitis and/or pneumonitis and/or delayed autoimmune thyroiditis [3, 8, 9, 14, 46, 47]. Systemic lupus-like syndrome and autoimmune hepatitis have also been associated with minocycline use, usually occurring after chronic administration over months to years, although some cases may occur earlier [3, 9, 46].

Sporadic reports of benign intracranial hypertension (BIH; pseudotumor cerebri) have been reported with use of tetracycline agents, including tetracycline, minocycline, and doxycycline [3, 7–9, 14]. Affected patients may present with intractable cephalgia, diplopia, photophobia, nausea, and/or vomiting. If BIH is suspected, the suspected agent should be discontinued, and ophthalmologic evaluation is recommended to evaluate for presence of papilledema.

Oral Trimethoprim-Sulfamethoxazole

Dermatologic Applications of Trimethoprim-Sulfamethoxazole

Trimethoprim-sulfamethoxazole (TMP-Sulfa) is well absorbed after oral administration with biotransformation of both components partially by hepatic metabolism and the remainder dependent on renal excretion (20–60% of parent compounds excreted unchanged) [3]. The antibacterial activity of TMP-Sulfa includes MRSA, MSSA, several streptococcal stains, and some *Pseudomonas* spp. other than *P. aeruginosa* [3]. In dermatology, TMP-Sulfa is used selectively as an alternative agent for refractory inflammatory acne and for treatment of uncomplicated cutaneous MRSA infections [3, 7–9, 14, 25, 41, 42, 48]. Use of TMP-Sulfa in combination with incision and drainage proved to be superior in achieving clearance of uncomplicated MRSA-induced skin abscesses than incision and drainage alone [49]. Dosing of oral trimethoprim-sulfamethoxazole used in outpatient dermatology is depicted in Table 46.1.

Adverse Effects Associated with Oral Trimethoprim-Sulfamethoxazole

Due to the potential for TMP-Sulfa to induce rare yet severe AEs that are often associated with significant morbidity or mortality, use of this agent warrants careful consideration of the anticipated therapeutic benefits versus possible risks along with dedicated patient education. Less severe cutaneous reactions which often occur within the first few weeks of use in up to 5% of immunocompetent patients include morbilliform eruptions, urticaria, fixed drug eruption, and pruritus [3]. The most concerning AEs associated with use of TMP-Sulfa are cutaneous reactions and hematologic effects [3, 46, 48]. TMP-Sulfa may induce DHS (DRESS), Stevens-Johnson syndrome (SJS), or toxic epidermal necrolysis (TEN), usually manifesting within 2–6 weeks after starting therapy; approximately 30% of cases of SJS/TEN are induced by sulfonamide antibiotics, most often TMP-Sulfa [46, 48]. The risk of TEN associated with the use of TMP-Sulfa in adults is estimated overall to be 2.6/100,000 exposures, increasing to 8.4/100,000 exposures in HIV-infected individuals [3, 46, 48]. The development of flu-like symptoms, "hives," painful skin, "sore throat," or mouth "sores" reported by the patient warrants discontinuation of therapy and clinical assessment as these findings may suggest the onset of DRESS or SJS/TEN. Onset of a very severe "sore throat" may suggest the presence of agranulocytosis.

A diverse array of hematologic reactions can occur at any point during therapy with TMP-Sulfa, including thrombocytopenia, neutropenia, agranulocytosis, aplastic anemia, and pure red cell aplasia [3, 48]. TMP-Sulfa should be used cautiously in patients with folate deficiency or in those with megaloblastosis [3]. If long-term treatment with TMP-sulfa is anticipated, baseline and periodic monitoring of complete blood cell counts may be prudent; however, there are no specific monitoring recommendations [3].

Oral Fluoroquinolones

Dermatologic Applications of Oral Fluoroquinolones

There are several oral fluoroquinolones available in the marketplace, with ciprofloxacin and levofloxacin the most commonly prescribed [3]. Fluoroquinolones are concentration-dependent antibiotics, are well absorbed from the GI tract with or without food (with the exception of norfloxacin), and are predominantly eliminated via renal excretion (with the exception of moxifloxacin) [3, 50–52]. Importantly, administration within 1 h before or 4 h after ingestion of metal ions found in dairy products (e.g., milk), fortified cereals, antacids, and vitamin/mineral supplements markedly reduce the GI absorption of most fluoroquinolones, including ciprofloxacin [3, 29, 50–52].

The antibacterial spectrum of fluoroquinolones is primarily against Gram-negative organisms including *P. aeruginosa*, with variable activity against Gram-positive bacteria; in vitro and clinical activity against *S. aureus* (including MRSA) and *S. pyogenes* has been reported with some fluoroquinolones; however, emergence of resistance is often rapid, especially with *S. aureus* (including MRSA) [3, 17, 18, 41, 42]. Ciprofloxacin exhibits antibacterial activity against *Bacillus anthracis*; ciprofloxacin and levofloxacin demonstrate activity against *Mycobacterium* spp., including *M. fortuitum*, *M. kansasii*, and *M. tuberculosis* [3].

The ability of fluoroquinolone agents to achieve high concentrations in the skin supports their use for treatment of uncomplicated cutaneous infections caused by Gram-negative bacterial pathogens, such as infected ulcers, folliculitis (including hot tub folliculitis caused by *P. aeruginosa*), cellulitis, toe web space infections, lower extremity ulcers in diabetic patients, and abscesses [3, 50, 51]. Ciprofloxacin has the greatest activity against *P. aeruginosa* compared to other fluoroquinolones, is a treatment of choice for cutaneous anthrax, and may be used as a second-line agent for treatment of chancroid and granuloma inguinale [3, 21]. Dosing of oral fluoroquinolones used in outpatient dermatology is depicted in Table 46.1.

Adverse Effects Associated with Oral Fluoroquinolones

The most common AEs associated with use of fluoroquinolones are GI related, including nausea, vomiting, and diarrhea [3, 51, 52]. A diverse array of CNS side effects have also been reported with these agents, including cephalgia, dizziness, sleep disturbance, seizures, hallucinations, and depression [3, 52]. Avoidance of fluoroquinolones in children is recommended due to concerns about impairment in cartilage formation [3]. Multiple cases of tendonitis and tendon rupture have been reported associated with fluoroquinolone use, may be delayed in onset, and appear to be associated with risk factors such as corticosteroid use, increased age, sports-related physical activity, renal failure, diabetes, rheumatologic disease, and history of tendinopathy [3, 53]. Hypersensitivity reactions, including anaphylaxis/anaphylactoid reactions, and photosensitivity, have been reported with fluoroquinolones, including ciprofloxacin [3, 51, 52].

Summary Points with Selected Oral Antibiotics

- Oral clindamycin is sometimes utilized to treat cutaneous MRSA infections; however, resistance to this agent may be prevalent in some communities [3, 17, 41, 42]. The D zone test should be utilized by laboratories to confirm that inducible resistance to clindamycin is not present as cross-resistance may occur when *S. aureus* strains are erythromycin-resistant [3, 42].
- Rifampin is sometimes used in combination with other oral antibiotics, such as clindamycin or TMP-Sulfa for treatment of MRSA infections. Monotherapy with rifampin is avoided due to rapid emergence of resistance [3, 41, 42].
- Rifampin is potent enzyme inducer resulting in increased metabolism of several other drugs. This can result in reduced therapeutic effects of the drugs undergoing enhanced metabolic clearance. An illustrative example is decreased efficacy of oral contraceptives resulting in breakthrough bleeding and/or unintended pregnancy [3, 29].
- Oral linezolid, an oxazolidinone antibiotic, exhibits complete oral bioavailability and has activity against multidrug-resistant MRSA, vancomycin-resistant staphylococci, penicillin-resistant streptococci, and vancomycin-resistant enterococci; with regard to MRSA therapy, its use should be reserved for cases that have failed other agents including doxycycline, minocycline, TMP-Sulfa, clindamycin/rifampin, and/or vancomycin [3].
- Oral tedizolid is a newer oxazolidinone antibiotic that exhibits properties similar to those of linezolid; however, some in vitro microbiologic evaluations have suggested that tedizolid may be active against some staphylococcal and enterococcal strains that are resistant to linezolid and/or vancomycin [54–56]. Tedizolid, administered 200 mg once a day for 6 days, has been shown to be equivalent in efficacy to linezolid, given 600 mg every 12 h for 10 days [54–56]. Tedizolid is recommended for the treatment of adult patients with cutaneous infections caused by susceptible Gram-positive bacteria, including MSSA, MRSA, several streptococcal bacterial strains including *S. pyogenes*, and *Enterococcus faecalis* [54, 56]. As with linezolid, this agent is reserved for cases that have failed other agents

General Management Considerations with Oral Antibiotic Therapy

- Although product labeling with some oral antibiotics includes general and non-specific statements suggesting periodic laboratory monitoring, there are no specific published laboratory monitoring guidelines with penicillins, cephalosporins, macrolides/azalides, tetracyclines, and fluoroquinolones [3, 8, 9, 14, 52].
- Other than with rifamycin antibiotics, such as rifampin, there is no definitive evidence that oral antibiotics (including penicillins, cephalosporins, macrolides, tetracyclines, fluoroquinolones) reduce the efficacy of combination oral contraceptives [3, 29]. Population-based data suggest that such interactions do not appear to occur; however, it is not possible to totally exclude the potential for such interactions if the potential risk is low. Physicians

are encouraged to suggest to patients to utilize additional precautions to prevent pregnancy.

- Dermatologic conditions where oral antibiotic use is not usually needed are inflamed epidermal cysts and chronic venous leg ulcers; oral antibiotic therapy has not been shown to accelerate healing of noninfected venous ulcers; however, colonization with drug-resistant bacteria is promoted [17].
- More recent published guidelines on perioperative antibiotic prophylaxis and studies evaluating the risk of post-surgical infection after dermatologic surgical procedures have resulted in a definite shift away from routine perioperative administration of prophylactic antibiotics [17]. The reader is encouraged to refer to published guidelines in order to review recommendations in detail as several clinical scenarios may need to be considered [57–60].
- The use of oral antibiotics is discussed in guidelines and "consensus" publications that address the management of both acne and rosacea [1, 7, 23, 61, 62]. These are suggested as further reading to those clinicians who regularly treat patients with these common dermatologic disorders.
- Treatment of moderate and severe acne with oral antibiotic therapy should always be coupled with a rational topical regimen; the goal is to discontinue oral antibiotic therapy once adequate suppression of new acne lesion development is achieved, with topical therapy continued to sustain the therapeutic benefit [1, 3–5, 7–9, 14–16, 23].
- As the pathophysiology of rosacea has not been associated with the presence of causative bacteria, an antibiotic effect is not believed to be needed in order to achieve improvement of papulopustular rosacea [62, 63]. It is suggested that when oral therapy for papulopustular rosacea is felt to be warranted, that sub-antibiotic dose doxycycline be on azelaic acid, ivermectin, in order to avoid antibiotic selection pressure and emergence of antibiotic-resistant bacterial organisms [1, 3, 5, 62, 64].

References

1. Del Rosso JQ, Webster GF, Rosen T, Thiboutot D, Leyden JJ, et al. Status report from the scientific panel on antibiotic use in dermatology of the American acne and rosacea society part 1: antibiotic prescribing patterns, sources of antibiotic exposure, antibiotic consumption and emergence of antibiotic resistance, impact of alterations in antibiotic prescribing, and clinical sequelae of antibiotic use. J Clin Aesthet Dermatol. 2016;9(4):18–24.
2. Bhatia N. Use of antibiotics for noninfectious dermatologic disorders. Dermatol Clin. 2009;27(1):85–9.
3. Kim S, Michaels BD, Kim GK, Del Rosso JQ. Systemic antibacterial agents. In: Wolverton SE, editor. Comprehensive dermatologic drug therapy. 3rd ed. Philadelphia, PA: Elsevier-Saunders; 2013. p. 61–97.
4. Leyden JJ, Del Rosso JQ, Webster GF. Clinical considerations in the treatment of acne vulgaris and other inflammatory skin disorders: a status report. Dermatol Clin. 2009;27(1):1–15.
5. Del Rosso JQ, Zeichner JA. The clinical relevance of antibiotic resistance: thirteen principles that every dermatologist needs to consider when prescribing antibiotic therapy. Dermatol Clin. 2016;34(2):167–73.
6. Nagler AR, Milam EC, Orlow SJ. The use of oral antibiotics before isotretinoin therapy in patients with acne. J Am Acad Dermatol. 2016;74:273–9.
7. Gollnick H, Cunliffe W, Berson D, Dreno B, Finlay A, et al. Management of acne: a report from the global alliance to improve outcomes in acne. J Am Acad Dermatol. 2003;49(suppl 1):S1–S38.
8. Del Rosso JQ. Topical and oral antibiotics for acne vulgaris. Semin Cutan Med Surg. 2016;35(2):57–61.
9. Del Rosso JQ, Kim G. Optimizing use of oral antibiotics in acne vulgaris. Dermatol Clin. 2009;27(1):33–42.
10. Leachman SA, Reed BR. The use of dermatologic drugs in pregnancy and lactation. Dermatol Clin. 2006;24(2):167–97.
11. Del Rosso JQ. Cephalosporins in dermatology. Clin Dermatol. 2003;21(1):24–32.
12. Package insert, cefdinir (Omnicef), Medicis Pharmaceuticals.
13. Hebert AA, Sigman ES, Levy ML. Serum sickness-like reactions from cefaclor in children. J Am Acad Dermatol. 1991;25(5 Pt 1):805–8.
14. Del Rosso JQ. Oral antibiotics. In: Shalita AR, Del Rosso JQ, Webster GF, editors. Informa healthcare. London: Informa Healthcare; 2011. p. 113–24.
15. Leyden JJ. The evolving role of Propionibacterium acnes in acne. Semin Cutan Med Surg. 2001;20:139–43.
16. Bowe WP, Leyden JJ. Clinical implications of antibiotic resistance: risk of systemic infection from Staphylococcus and Streptococcus. In: Shalita AR, Del Rosso JQ, Webster GF, editors. Informa healthcare. London: Informa Healthcare; 2011. p. 125–33.
17. Del Rosso JQ, Rosen T, Thiboutot D, Webster GF, Gallo RL, et al. Status report from the scientific panel on antibiotic use in dermatology of the American acne and rosacea society part 3: current perspectives on skin and soft tissue infections with emphasis on methicillin-resistant Staphylococcus aureus, commonly encountered scenarios when antibiotic use may not be needed, and concluding remarks on rational use of antibiotics in dermatology. J Clin Aesthet Dermatol. 2016;9(6):17–24.
18. Stevens DL, Bisno AL, Chambers HF, et al. Practice guidelines for the diagnosis and management of skin and soft tissue infections. Clin Infect Dis. 2005;41:1373–406.
19. Scheinfeld N, Tutrone WD, Torres O, et al. Macrolides in dermatology. Clin Dermatol. 2003;21(1):40–9.
20. Parsad D, Pandhi R, Dogra S. A guide to selection and appropriate use of macrolides in skin infections. Am J Clin Dermatol. 2003;4(6):389–97.
21. Rosen T, Vandergriff T, Harting M. Antibiotic use in sexually transmitted diseases. Dermatol Clin. 2009;27(1):49–61.
22. Bhambri S, Bhambri A, Del Rosso JQ. Atypical mycobacterial cutaneous infections. Dermatol Clin. 2009;27(1):63–73.
23. Zaenglein AL, Pathy AL, Schlosser BJ, Alikhan A, Baldwin HE, et al. Guidelines of care for the management of acne vulgaris. J Am Acad Dermatol. 2016;74(5):945–73.
24. Sandoval LF, Hartel JK, Feldman SR. Current and future evidence-based acne treatment: a review. Expert Opin Pharmacother. 2014;15(2):173–92.
25. Amin K, Riddle CC, Aires DJ, Schweiger ES. Common and alternate oral antibiotic therapies for acne vulgaris: a review. J Drugs Dermatol. 2007;6(9):873–80.
26. Modi S, Harting M, Rosen T. Azithromycin as an alternative rosacea therapy when tetracyclines prove problematic. J Drugs Dermatol. 2008;7(9):898–9.

27. Fernandez-Obregon A. Oral use of azithromycin for the treatment of acne rosacea. Arch Dermatol. 2004;140(4):489–90.

28. Dereli T, Inanir I, Kilinç I, Gençoğlan G. Azithromycin in the treatment of papulopustular rosacea. J Dermatol. 2005;32(11):926–8.

29. Del Rosso JQ. Oral antibiotic drug interactions of clinical significance to dermatologists. Dermatol Clin. 2009;27(1):91–4.

30. Salimi A, Eybagi S, Seydi E, Naserzadeh P, Kazerouni NP, Jalal PJ. Toxicity of macrolide antibiotics on isolated heart mitochondria: a justification for their cardiotoxic adverse effect. Xenobiotica. 2016;46(1):82–93.

31. Leyden JJ, Del Rosso JQ. Oral antibiotic therapy for acne vulgaris: pharmacokinetic and pharmacodynamic perspectives. J Clin Aesthet Dermatol. 2011;4(2):40–7.

32. Webster G, Del Rosso JQ. Anti-inflammatory activity of tetracyclines. Dermatol Clin. 2007;25(2):133–5.

33. Golub LM, Ramamurthy NS, Menamara TF, et al. Tetracyclines inhibit tissue collagenase activity: a new mechanism in treatment of periodontal disease. J Periodontal Res. 1984;19:651–5.

34. Del Rosso JQ. Anti-inflammatory dose doxycycline in the treatment of rosacea. J Drugs Dermatol. 2009;8(7):664–8.

35. Del Rosso JQ. A status report on the use of subantimicrobial-dose doxycycline: a review of the biologic and antimicrobial effects of the tetracyclines. Cutis. 2004;74(2):118–22.

36. Plott RT, Wortzman MS. Key bioavailability features of a new extended-release formulation of minocycline hydrochloride tablets. Cutis. 2006;78(4 Suppl):6–10.

37. Fleischer AB, Dinehart S, Stough D, Plott RT. Safety and efficacy of a new extended-release formulation of minocycline. Cutis. 2006;78(4 Suppl):21–31.

38. Skidmore R, Kovach R, Walker C, Thomas J, Bradshaw M, et al. Effects of subantimicrobial-dose doxycycline in the treatment of moderate acne. Arch Dermatol. 2003;139(4):459–64.

39. Walker C, Preshaw PM, Novak J, Hefti AF, Bradshaw M, et al. Long-term treatment with sub-antimicrobial dose doxycycline has no antibacterial effect on intestinal flora. J Clin Periodontol. 2005;32(11):1163–9.

40. Thomas J, Walker C, Bradshaw M. Long-term use of subantimicrobial dose doxycycline does not lead to changes in antimicrobial susceptibility. J Periodontol. 2000;71(9):1472–83.

41. Cohen PR, Grossman ME. Management of cutaneous lesions associated with an emerging epidemic: community-acquired methicillin-resistant Staphylococcus aureus skin infections. J Am Acad Dermatol. 2004;51(1):132–5.

42. Elston DM. Methicillin-sensitive and methicillin-resistant Staphylococcus aureus: management principles and selection of antibiotic therapy. Dermatol Clin. 2007;25(1):157–64.

43. Alhusayen R, Shear NH. Scientific evidence for the use of current traditional systemic therapies in patients with hidradenitis suppurativa. J Am Acad Dermatol. 2015;73:S42–6.

44. Abdulmajeed A. Pityriasis Lichenoides chronica responds to minocycline in three patients. Int J Dermatol. 2016;55:1027–9.

45. Del Rosso JQ. Oral doxycycline in the management of acne vulgaris: current perspectives on clinical use and recent findings with a new double-scored small tablet formulation. J Clin Aesthet Dermatol. 2015;8(5):19–26.

46. Knowles SR, Shear NH. Cutaneous drug reactions with systemic features. In: Wolverton SE, editor. Comprehensive dermatologic

47. Wu PA, Anadkat MJ. Fever, eosinophilia, and death: a case of minocycline hypersensitivity. Cutis. 2014;93:107–10.

48. Bhambri S, Del Rosso JQ, Desai A. Oral trimethoprim/sulfamethoxazole in the treatment of acne vulgaris. Cutis. 2007;79(6):430–4.

49. Talan DA, Mower WR, Krishnadasan A, Abrahamian FM, Lovecchio F, et al. Trimethoprim–sulfamethoxazole versus placebo for uncomplicated skin abscess. NEJM. 2016;374(9):823–32.

50. Hooper DC, Wolfson JS. The fluoroquinolones: pharmacology, clinical uses, and toxicities in humans. Antimicrob Agents Chemother. 1985;28(5):716–21.

51. Walker RC, Wright AJ. Symposium on antimicrobial agents: the quinolones. Mayo Clin Proc. 1987;62(11):1007–12.

52. Liu HH. Safety profile of oral quinolones: focus on levofloxacin. Drug Saf. 2010;33(5):353–69.

53. Kim GK, Del Rosso JQ. The risk of fluoroquinolone-induced tendinopathy and tendon rupture: what does the clinician need to know? J Clin Aesthet Dermatol. 2010;3(4):49–54.

54. Hussar DA, Nguyen A. Dalbavancin, tedizolid phosphate, oritavancin diphosphate, and vedolizumab. JAPhA. 2014;54(6):658–62.

55. Crotty MP, Krekel T, Burnham CA, Ritchie DJ. New gram-positive agents: the next generation of oxazolidinones and lipoglycopeptides. J Clin Microbiol. 2016;54(9):2225–32.

56. Zhanel GG, Love R, Adam H, Golden A, Zelenitsky S, et al. Tedizolid: a novel oxazolidinone with potent activity against multidrug-resistant gram-positive pathogens. Drugs. 2015;75(3):253–70.

57. Wright TI, Baddour LM, Berbari EF, et al. Antibiotic prophylaxis in dermatologic surgery: advisory statement 2008. J Am Acad Dermatol. 2008;59(3):464–73.

58. Rosengren H, Dixon A. Antibacterial prophylaxis in dermatologic surgery: an evidence-based review. Am J Clin Dermatol. 2010;11(1):35–44.

59. Bae-Harboe YS, Liang CA. Perioperative antibiotic use of dermatologic surgeons in 2012. Dermatol Surg. 2013;39(11):1592–601.

60. Rossi AM, Mariwalla K. Prophylactic and empiric use of antibiotics in dermatologic surgery: a review of the literature and practical considerations. Dermatol Surg. 2012;38(12):1898–921.

61. Del Rosso JQ, Harper JC, Graber EM, Thiboutot D, Silverberg NB, et al. Status report from the American Acne & Rosacea Society on medical management of acne in adult women, part 3: oral therapies. Cutis. 2015;96(6):376–82.

62. Del Rosso JQ, Thiboutot D, Gallo R, Webster G, Tanghetti E, et al. Consensus recommendations from the American Acne & Rosacea Society on the management of rosacea, part 3: a status report on systemic therapies. Cutis. 2014;93(1):18–28.

63. Del Rosso JQ, Gallo RL, Tanghetti E, Webster G, Thiboutot D. An evaluation of potential correlations between pathophysiologic mechanisms, clinical manifestations, and management of rosacea. Cutis. 2013;91(3 Suppl):1–8.

64. Del Rosso JQ, Baldwin H, Webster G. American Acne & Rosacea Society rosacea medical management guidelines. J Drugs Dermatol. 2008;7(6):531–3.

drug therapy. 3rd ed. Philadelphia, PA: Elsevier-Saunders; 2013. p. 747–56.

Sonic Hedgehog Pathway Inhibition in the Treatment of Advanced Basal Cell Carcinoma

Patrick Armstrong, Stephanie Martin, and Gary Lask

Introduction

Basal cell carcinoma (BCC) is the most common type of skin cancer, comprising about 80% of non-melanoma skin cancer. In the United States, there are over 2.8 million new cases diagnosed each year [1]. Incidence is highest in those who have fair skin and thus less pigmentary protection and a tendency to burn with sun exposure. Men are more commonly affected than women, at a ratio of 1.5–2:1. The incidence of BCC is increasing over time, up to 20–80% over the last 30 years in the USA, with similar increasing rates reported in other areas of the world [2]. Speculation for this increase includes an aging population, changes in sun protective habits, changes in the environment, and increased prevalence of immunosuppression.

Despite the high incidence of BCC, mortality from BCC remains low. The significant majority of BCCs remain localized to the skin and are most commonly treated with surgical procedures such as standard excision, curettage and electrodessication, or Mohs micrographic surgery. Radiation therapy can also be utilized as primary treatment when surgery is either contraindicated or the patient is not amenable to surgery. Radiation can also be used as adjuvant treatment in certain high-risk patients. Additional superficial treatments have utility in select situations and include photodynamic therapy (PDT), intralesional injections (5-fluorouracil or bleomycin), and topical therapies (such as imiquimod or 5-fluorouracil). However, approximately 1% of patients with BCC develop advanced disease and may have little efficacy or significant morbidity from standard therapies [3].

Pathogenesis of Basal Cell Carcinoma

Most cancers in humans arise from epithelial cells and are thought to result from genotoxic insults causing mutations responsible for abnormal growth and proliferation. The most frequent insult that contributes to the development of non-melanoma skin cancer is ultraviolet (UV) radiation, which is known to produce genetic mutations through the formation of dipyrimidine dimers in cell DNA. Episodes of intense sun exposure and resulting sunburns appear to be the primary environmental risk factor for development of BCC, as opposed to cumulative UV exposure that has been demonstrated a major risk factor for squamous cell carcinoma (SCC) [4].

Basal cell carcinoma has unique growth requirements as it is reliant on a specific connective tissue stroma to promote growth. Such a relationship is analogous to the interdependent relationship between the epithelium of a developing hair follicle and its surrounding stroma. It has been hypothesized that the characteristic indolent nature and low rate of transformation to a metastasizing tumor is likely due to an unconditional dependence on growth factors produced by mesenchymal fibroblasts. Since malignant epithelial cells are unable to travel in the body en masse with their stroma, metastatic growth is inhibited. This concept is supported by experimental data in which autotransplantation of BCC without supporting stroma resulted in development of keratinaceous cysts, rather than proliferating tumors [5].

The Role of the Hedgehog Pathway in Basal Cell Carcinoma

Research into the genetics of nevoid basal cell carcinoma (NBCC) syndrome (Gorlin-Goltz syndrome) has shed significant light into the molecular and signaling processes in

P. Armstrong, MD
Division of Dermatology, UCLA Medicine, Los Angeles, CA, USA
e-mail: phatpat86@gmail.com

S. Martin, MD (✉)
UCLA/WLA VA Derm Surgery Fellowship Program,
Dermatologic Surgery and Mohs Micrographic Surgery,
Department of Dermatology, VA Greater Los Angeles Healthcare
System, Los Angeles, CA, USA
e-mail: stephanie.jeanne.martin@gmail.com

G. Lask, MD
Dermatology Laser Center, David Geffen School of Medicine
at UCLA, Los Angeles, CA, USA
e-mail: glask@mednet.ucla.edu

© Springer International Publishing AG 2018
P.S. Yamauchi (ed.), *Biologic and Systemic Agents in Dermatology*, https://doi.org/10.1007/978-3-319-66884-0_47

BCC, most importantly the critical involvement of hedgehog (Hh) signaling pathway in driving tumorigenesis. The *Hedgehog (HH)* and *patched* genes were initially discovered from genetic analysis of the fruit fly *Drosophila melanogaster*. The genes were found to be involved in embryogenesis and normal tissue development. The human hedgehog pathway is complex, with three identified *hedgehog* genes (*Sonic hedgehog (SHH)*, *Desert hedgehog (DHH)*, and *Indian hedgehog (IHH)*) and two *patched* genes (*PTCH1* and *PTCH2*). The effects of the Hh pathway are primarily exerted by proteins encoded by the *glioblastoma (GLI)* family of genes through altering nuclear gene expression with resultant increase in proliferation, inhibition of apoptosis, and stem cell self-renewal. Specifically in human skin, the SHH signaling plays an integral role in the differentiation and proliferation of hair follicles and sebaceous glands, as well as the maintenance of stem cell populations [6]. A constant supply of cutaneous stem cells is crucial for skin homeostasis through continual tissue turnover and wound healing.

Family-based linkage analysis of individuals affected with NBCC syndrome led to the identification of mutations of human homolog *Patched 1 (Ptch1)* gene on chromosome 9 [7]. PTCH1 is a highly conserved 12-pass transmembrane protein that regulates the hedgehog signaling pathway through its inhibitory effect on the 7-pass transmembrane G-protein-coupled receptor smoothened (SMO) through constitutive binding. When PTCH1 is bound in the extracellular domain by the human homolog hedgehog protein ligands (SHH, DHH, IHH), the inhibitory effect on SMO is released, allowing SMO migration to the tip of the primary cilium resulting in downstream activation of the hedgehog pathway through GLI transcriptional activity (Fig. 47.1).

NBCC syndrome is a rare autosomal dominant condition in which a nonfunctional single copy of Ptch1 is either inherited or acquired through a germline mutation. It is associated with characteristic developmental defects including odontogenic keratocysts, calcification of the falx cerebri, palmoplantar pits, neurologic defects (agenesis of the corpus callosum, developmental delay), and skeletal abnormalities (bifid ribs, syndactyly, craniofacial malformations) [8]. *Ptch1* is thought to act as a tumor suppressor gene, following Knudson's two-hit model for neoplasia. Given that there is only one functional *Ptch1* gene expressing allele in NBCC syndrome, an inactivating "second-hit" mutation of the functional copy leads to complete loss of *Ptch1* expression and thus constitutively active signaling through the Hh pathway. This explains the significant propensity for neoplasia in NBCC syndrome, with patients developing numerous basal cell carcinomas, predomi-

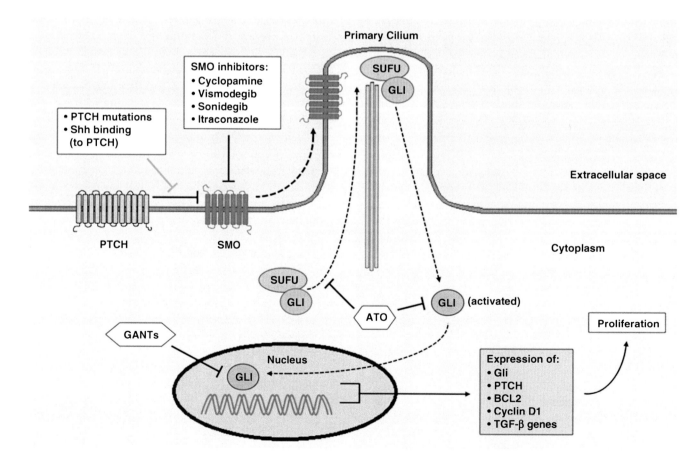

Fig. 47.1 *ATO* arsenic trioxide, *GANTs* GLI antagonists, *PTCH* patched protein, *SMO* smoothened protein, *SUFU* suppressor of fused

nantly in sun-exposed areas. Additionally, there is an increased risk of developing other neoplasms, including medulloblastoma, ovarian fibromas, and cardiac fibromas. Murine mutant models of *Ptch* [+/−] knockout mice, analogous to humans with NBCC syndrome, have been shown to develop only a few BCCs over their life span, similar to sporadic human BCCs. Exposure to ultraviolet B (UVB) or X-rays in these mice produces growth of numerous BCCs, further supporting the role of Ptch1 as a tumor suppressor and the role of UV and ionizing radiation in BCC development [9].

The vast majority of human BCCs are sporadic and, like NBCC syndrome, are similarly driven by hedgehog pathway signaling. Genetic analysis has shown *Ptch1* to be the most frequently mutated gene in sporadic BCCs, with up to 80% demonstrating loss of function in at least one allele and the remainder having activating downstream gain-in-function mutations in the *SMO* gene [10]. These mutations, which upregulate Hh signaling and increase GLI expression, appear to be necessary and possibly sufficient for sporadic BCC formation. The second most commonly found mutation in sporadic BCCs is seen in the p53 tumor suppressor gene. Point mutations with UV signatures have been observed in over 50% of cases of BCC [11]. Interestingly, those with inherited mutations in p53 (Li-Fraumeni syndrome) have a significantly increased risk of multiple malignancies, but do not have an increased propensity to develop BCCs, suggesting that p53 mutations may be a secondary event and not necessary for tumorigenesis [12].

Despite common molecular signaling pathways, a wide variation in clinical and histological features of BCC subtypes exists. There has been significant controversy over the cell of origin. Recently, mouse models have provided evidence that BCCs can arise from both the bulge of the follicle, as well as the interfollicular epidermis [13, 14].

Advanced Basal Cell Carcinoma

Advanced BCCs fall into two categories, locally advanced BCC (laBCC) and metastatic BCC (mBCC). LaBCC includes primary tumors that invade surrounding structures (i.e., cartilage, bone, muscle, or local lymph nodes). Metastatic BCC is defined as spread to distant sites from the primary tumor, including the skeletal system, other organ systems, and non-regional lymph nodes. Management of laBCC can be challenging, as surgery may be appear to be a feasible treatment but can have a high risk of recurrence or result in significant morbidity from functional impairment or disfigurement. The utility of radiation therapy for laBCC is often limited due to high risk of recurrence, prior failure of radiation, sensitivity to radiation (i.e., radiation-sensitive diseases such as xeroderma pigmentosa or NBCC), or limited access to treatment.

The incidence of metastatic BCC is exceedingly rare (0.0028–0.5%) and typically evolves from large, ulcerated, locally invasive cases subjected to prolonged neglect or avoidance of medical care [15]. Metastasis most commonly spreads to the lymph nodes, lungs, and bones. The natural history of metastatic BCC has a poor prognosis with reported median survival time of approximately 8 months when sign of nodal metastases are present [16].

Until recently, there were few options for patients with laBCC and mBCC. New BCC-targeted treatments acting through inhibition of the Shh pathway have demonstrated significant efficacy in the treatment of advanced BCC.

Sonic Hedgehog Inhibition in the Treatment of Basal Cell Carcinoma

Smoothened Inhibitors

SMO has been the primary target in the development of Shh-inhibitive treatments. Cyclopamine, a naturally occurring alkaloid derived from the corn lily, *Veratrum californicum*, was the first compound discovered to inhibit SMO [17]. It was found that sheep who consumed the plant during pregnancy gave birth to offspring with birth defects including holoprosencephaly and cyclopia. The mechanism of action of cyclopamine involves binding to SMO, preventing active configuration of the protein and antagonizing downstream Hh signal transduction [18]. This observation led to testing cyclopamine as an anticancer drug in light of the recent implications of Shh signaling in BCC tumorigenesis. A small, clinical, proof-of-concept study demonstrated efficacy of topical cyclopamine to cause regression of BCCs in humans prior to surgical excision, but was not a practical for therapy given the need for reapplication every few hours [19]. Murine studies demonstrated BCC growth inhibition in vivo with systemic cyclopamine; however, the medication had many limitations for human use secondary to significant toxicity, poor oral bioavailability, and suboptimal pharmacokinetic/pharmacodynamic profiles [20]. The shortcomings of cyclopamine lead to the development of additional SMO inhibitors in the treatment of cancer.

Vismodegib

Vismodegib is an orally dosed, second-generation cyclopamine derivative that acts by binding directly to SMO, inhibiting its function in downstream Shh signal transduction. It was approved by the FDA in January 2012 as the first-in-class Shh pathway inhibitor for the treatment of laBCC and mBCC [21]. Approval was based on the pivotal Phase II study ERIVANCE, a multicenter study of 104 patients with two treatment cohorts: unresectable laBCC and mBCC [22]. A control group was not assigned given the small sample size. Based on Phase I safety data, all patients received vismodegib 150 mg daily. The primary endpoint was the objective response rate (RR). A response in laBCC was defined as ≥30% tumor size reduction or complete resolution of tumor ulceration (if present at baseline). A response in mBCC was defined as ≥30% decrease in sum of the longest diameter of target lesions. Efficacy analysis by independent review of the laBCC group ($n = 63$) revealed an RR of 43% (95% CI, 31–56) and in the mBCC group ($n = 33$) an RR of 30% (95% CI, 16–48). A complete response (absence of residual BCC on analysis of a biopsy specimen) was observed in 21% of the laBCC.

Side effects with vismodegib are frequent and can be significant. The side effect profile is often the limiting factor in continued treatment and should be weighed with the drug's potential benefits. In the initial ERIVANCE study, all patients reported a treatment-related adverse event, although the majority of these were low grade (ranked mild-to-moderate) in severity. The most frequently encountered side effects were muscle spasms (68%), alopecia (63%), dysgeusia (51%), weight loss (46%), fatigue (36%), nausea (29%), anorexia (23%), and diarrhea (22%). There was a moderate rate of serious adverse events during the study (25%), including seven deaths. These deaths were seen in patients with underlying comorbidities, and there was no consistent pattern of adverse events or evidence for causality by vismodegib. Of note, the high observed rate of alopecia and dysgeusia are considered to be on-target effects due to inhibition of normally active Shh signaling in hair follicles and taste buds.

Since the approval of vismodegib, multiple additional clinical trials have been performed providing additional efficacy and safety data. A recent systematic review and pooled analysis of 704 patients demonstrated higher efficacy than the independent review analysis from the ERIVANCE study [23]. Objective RR in laBCC had a weighted average of 64.7% (95% CI: 63.7–65.6) and average complete response rate of 31.1% (95% CI: 30.4–31.8); mBCC had an objective RR average of 33.6% (95% CI: 33.1–34.2) and complete response average of 3.9% (95% CI: 3.3–4.4). Additionally, one randomized, double-blinded, placebo-controlled study examined the use of vismodegib in the treatment of 41 patients with NBCC syndrome and found that the annual incidence of new BCCs per group decreased significantly (2 vs. 29, $p < 0.001$), and the size of pre-existing BCCs decreased as well (−65% vs. 11%, $P = 0.003$) [24]. Side effects in the NBCC patients were significant, resulting in 54% of patients discontinuing treatment. Upon cessation of vismodegib, nearly all of the BCCs that regressed while on therapy subsequently recurred. Although the medication demonstrated efficacy in prevention and treatment of BCCs in NBCC syndrome, there are no clear guidelines for the use of vismodegib for long-term prevention of BCC given patients have a relatively normal life span and the side effect profile may not be tolerable for lifelong treatment if started at a younger age.

Analysis of long-term treatment data has also suggested seemingly paradoxical increased risk for developing non-BCC malignancies in patients treated with vismodegib. A case-control study of 55 patients and 125 controls demonstrated a hazard ratio of 6.37 (95% CI: 3.39–11.96), indicating increased risk of developing non-BCC malignancies [25]. The most common malignancy observed in the study was cutaneous SCC, with a hazard ratio of 8.12 (95% CI: 3.89–16.97). The majority of SCCs developed within 1 year of starting treatment. A possible explanation observed in SMO inhibitor-treated medulloblastoma cells is the selection for cancer cells with upregulation in alternative signaling pathways, such as RAS/MAPK [25, 26]. Such upregulation permits these cells to escape dependence on upstream signaling from the hedgehog pathway. Increased RAS signaling has been associated with many cancers and could increase risk of developing other malignancies. A notable weakness of the case-control study was the inability to control for UV exposure. The vismodegib group was noted to have a statistically significant earlier onset of their first BCC (mean age difference of 7 years) and may have a higher amount of UV exposure, predisposing them to develop other cutaneous malignancies. Until future prospective studies fully evaluate this potential risk, it may be prudent for patients on SMO inhibitors to be monitored at frequent intervals for development of non-BCC cutaneous malignancies.

Sonidegib

Sonidegib is an orally dosed SMO inhibitor that acts by binding to SMO. It is not derived from cyclopamine and is structurally distinct from vismodegib. It was approved by the FDA in June 2015 for treatment of locally advanced basal cell carcinoma that has either recurred following surgery or radiation therapy or in patients who are not candidates for surgery or radiation therapy [27]. Approval was based on results from the multicenter Phase II BOLT trial on patients with mBCC or laBCC not amenable to surgery or radiation [28]. Patients were randomized in a 1:2 ratio to receive either 200 mg (lowest active dose; $n = 79$) or 800 mg (maximum tolerable dose; $n = 151$) daily. The primary endpoint was an objective RR in both treatment arms. An objective RR in the 200 mg group was 43% for laBCC and 15% for mBCC, and in the 800 mg group was 38% for laBCC and 17% for mBCC. Although the 800 mg dose was anticipated to have higher antitumor activity, no additional efficacy was found over the 200 mg dose. The 200 mg dose also exhibited a more benign side effect profile, with a lower rate of serious adverse events (14% vs. 30%).

The side effect profile for sonidegib is similar to that of vismodegib, presumably due to on-target effects from SMO inhibition. The most frequently reported adverse events with sonidegib 200 mg daily were muscle spasms (49%), alopecia (43%), dysgeusia (38%), nausea (33%), elevated creatinine kinase (29%), fatigue (29%), weight loss (27%), diarrhea (24%), and myalgia (19%). An increased frequency of these adverse events was observed in the 800 mg dose group. Differences from vismodegib's side effect profile were elevated creatine kinase and increased lipase levels (8%), which were also the most common of the severe adverse effects reported. Of note, one case of rhabdomyolysis was reported by investigators in the 200 mg dose group. Due to these musculoskeletal adverse reactions, a baseline CPK prior to initiation is recommended, as well as regular interval monitoring as clinically indicated [27]. Furthermore, clinicians should monitor patients closely if they are taking additional medications with known myotoxic side effect profiles, such as statins.

The advent of a second commercially available SMO inhibitor offers additional options in the treatment of advanced BCC. Vismodegib appears to be the treatment of choice for mBCC, as it has explicit FDA approval for this indication and seems to have a superior efficacy to sonidegib in treating mBCC based on indirect comparison of response rates. However, some have suggested that sonidegib may have similar efficacy to vismodegib in treatment of laBCC based on indirect comparison after adjusting for the more stringent response rate criteria used in the BOLT study [29]. At this time, the true comparative efficacy between sonidegib and vismodegib are not known and will require head-to-head randomized controlled trials to elucidate. Additionally, given that sonidegib is a relatively novel drug, additional safety data is needed to assess its use in long-term treatment of BCC.

Neoadjuvant Use of SMO Inhibitors for Locally Advanced BCC

The role of SMO (and other hedgehog pathway) inhibitors as a neoadjuvant treatment to surgery has possible utility in treatment of laBCC, but evidence for its use is not yet well established. Advantages of neoadjuvant SMO inhibition followed by definitive surgical treatment include transient exposure to poorly tolerated SMO inhibitor side effects and potential decreased postsurgical defect size. A small, open-label study evaluated the use of vismodegib 150 mg daily for 3–6 months to decrease tumor size in high-risk BCCs prior to surgery [30]. There was a dropout rate of 29% due to side effects of vismodegib. Of patients who completed adjuvant treatment (average 4-month treatment duration), there was a reduction of surgical defect size by 27% (95% CI, −45.7 to −7.9%, $P = 0.006$). After a mean follow-up of 11.5 months, recurrence was observed in one patient who was being treated for a previously recurrent infiltrative BCC and did not complete a full course of vismodegib. The findings of this study provide some support for the role of SMO inhibitor use to decrease defect size in laBCCs where surgery could be curative but might otherwise be avoided due to risk of excessive disfigurement and morbidity.

Resistance to SMO Inhibitors

Despite the significant clinical response of many advanced BCCs to SMO inhibitors, approximately 5–10% of patients demonstrate primary resistance with progression and no response. In patients who do respond, long-term efficacy is often mitigated by the development of tumor-acquired resistance to these medications with regrowth of tumors despite continued therapy. This phenomenon was first described in the treatment of BCCs with vismodegib in a case series that demonstrated regrowth of at least one tumor in 21% of patients with advanced BCC after a mean of 56 weeks [31]. Several potential mechanisms have been proposed that have been demonstrated in mouse models of medulloblastoma, a malignancy known to be dependent on increased Shh pathway signaling similar to BCC.

Multiple point mutations in SMO have been described that appear to confer resistance to SMO inhibitors. The first documented mutation associated with resistance was in a vismodegib Phase I trial for medulloblastoma. A patient with a *PTCH1* mutation initially responded but then progressed after 1 month of treatment and was found to have acquired a new mutation in *SMO* (D473H) [32]. A subsequent study analyzed protein configuration in resistant BCC tumors using computer simulation of SMO in a similar D473Y mutation, as well as a new SMO mutation identified in a case of primary resistance (G497W). Both mutations were found to interfere with the vismodegib binding site, conferring a mechanism for SMO inhibitor resistance [33]. Interestingly, distinct point mutations have been described in tumors resistant to sonidegib in mice, suggesting that different SMO inhibitors may select for different mutations [34]. The degree of cross-resistance to different SMO inhibitors conferred by these point mutations is not known.

Another mechanism of SMO inhibitor resistance is seen through amplification (duplication) of genes. One study demonstrated amplification of *GLI* genes in medulloblastoma tumors resistant to sonidegib that was mutually exclusive from resistance conferred through point mutations [34]. These *GLI*-amplified resistant tumors were found to have a 2–20-fold higher expression of *GLI* mRNA. Not all of the resistant tumors analyzed in the study were found to have amplification of *GLI* genes, leading to investigation of possible upregulation of GLI signaling through compensatory pathways. An increase in PI3K signaling was found in many of the resistant tumors, occurring in those both with and without concurrent amplification of *GLI* genes. These findings provide evidence for mechanisms allowing GLI signaling in tumors to escape SMO inhibition. Based on these findings, the investigators found combined treatment with sonidegib and PI3K/mTOR inhibitors in a mouse model appeared to delay development of tumor resistance and produce a greater number of complete responses compared to sonidegib alone.

Additional Hedgehog Pathway Inhibitors

Currently, vismodegib and sonidegib are the only Shh inhibitors approved in the treatment of BCC in humans. Several medications with other FDA-approved treatment indications have also been demonstrated to inhibit parts of the Shh pathway. Additionally, there are multiple molecules that are known to inhibit the Shh pathway that are in preliminary stages of research. This section reviews additional select Shh inhibitors with some prospect for treatment of BCC (summarized in Table 47.1).

Alternate SMO Inhibitors

Itraconazole, an FDA-approved antifungal, has been shown to inhibit the Shh pathway in a mechanism distinct from vismodegib and sonidegib. It appears to block SMO migration to the tip of the primary cilium [35]. Itraconazole has been demonstrated to effectively inhibit *GLI* expression in vitro cells with the vismodegib-resistant mutation, SMO^{D477G} [36]. These investigators also exhibited that in vitro treatment with both itraconazole and arsenic trioxide, which target different loci in the Shh pathway, cumulatively inhibited all other known SMO mutants and *GLI2* overexpression. These findings suggest combination therapies targeting more than one component of the Shh pathway may be more effective in combating resistance. A small, open-label, Phase II clinical study treating BCC patients with itraconazole alone was performed and found a reduction in GLI mRNA by 65% and a reduced tumor area of 24%; patients previously treated with vismodegib did not show significant changes in tumor size or proliferation [37]. Another small clinical study of patients with mBCC resistant to typical SMO inhibitors found that combination treatment with itraconazole and arsenic trioxide decreased *GLI* mRNA expression by 75% [38]. The best clinical responses observed were

stable disease; no regression of tumors occurred. The authors concluded that the scheduling and dosing in the study may not have been frequent or high enough to obtain maximal inhibition of the Shh pathway. Further studies are needed to better evaluate ideal dosing and the efficacy of itraconazole in the treatment of BCCs in humans.

GLI Inhibitors

GLI transcription factors are the terminal effectors in Shh pathway signaling that promote proliferation and survival of BCCs. Although inhibition of upstream Shh signaling has shown to be effective in decreasing GLI function, upregulation of GLI activity by Shh and SMO independent pathways can occur, as seen in SMO inhibitor-resistant tumors. Direct targeting of GLI makes for an ideal target in the treatment of advanced BCCs, especially in the context of SMO inhibitor resistance.

Arsenic trioxide (ATO) is a chemotherapeutic agent that is FDA approved for the treatment of promyelocytic leukemia [39]. Its mechanisms appear to be multiple and are not completely understood. Relevant to the inhibition of the Shh pathway, ATO has been demonstrated to have inhibitive properties through binding directly to GLI1 and GLI2 [40]. It has also been found to prevent the accumulation of GLI in the primary cilium, a necessary step for downstream Shh signaling [41]. There have been some studies exploring ATO in combination with itraconazole for the inhibition of GLI and treatment of BCC, as described above.

GLI antagonists, or GANTs, are small molecules that were discovered to inhibit GLI-mediated gene transcription within the nucleus of cells [42]. Two molecules have been described: GANT-58 and GANT-61. Both compounds have been shown to have in vitro and in vivo activity against GLI function. GANT-61 was found to inhibit GLI binding to DNA in the nucleus and is speculated to have the most

Table 47.1 Signaling Pathway Driving Tumorigenesis in BCCs

Shh inhibitor	Mechanism of action	Notable side effects	Status[a]
Vismodegib	SMO inhibition via direct binding	Muscle spasms, alopecia, dysgeusia, weight loss, fatigue, nausea, vomiting	FDA approved
Sonidegib	SMO inhibition via direct binding	Elevated CPK, elevated lipase; otherwise similar profile to vismodegib	FDA approved
Itraconazole	Prevents translocation of SMO to primary cilium	Nausea, diarrhea, rash, headache	Research[b]
Arsenic trioxide	GLI inhibition via (1) direct binding and (2) prevention of GLI migration to primary cilium	Numerous toxicities of multiple organ systems, metabolic dysregulation	Research[b]
GANT 58	Blocks GLI function within the nucleus by unclear mechanism	Under investigation	Research
GANT 61	Interferes with GLI binding to DNA	Under investigation	Research
Forskolin (topical)	GLI degradation in proteasomes mediated by increased cAMP and phosphorylation by PKA	Under investigation	Research

[a]Status in clinical treatment of basal cell carcinoma
[b]FDA approved for clinical indications other than treatment of BCC
SMO smoothened protein, *GANT* GLI antagonist, *PKA* protein kinase A

potential as a GLI inhibitor. GANTs have not yet been evaluated for Shh pathway inhibition in BCC and have yet to be tested in clinical trials for cancer.

Activation of the PKA pathway has also been demonstrated to nonselectively decrease GLI activity, apparently through phosphorylation and subsequent degradation of GLI proteins by proteasomes [43, 44]. A mouse model of SMO inhibitor-resistant mice showed significant *GLI* mRNA reduction and inhibition of BCC growth via PKA activation with the topical application of cyclic-AMP agonist forskolin [45].

Future Directions

The discovery of the Shh pathway and its role in the pathogenesis of basal cell carcinoma has led to the development of novel therapies. SMO inhibitors are a significant milestone in the targeted treatment of malignancy, offering major improvements in morbidity and mortality in many cases of advanced BCC. Further evaluation of these medications as neoadjuvant therapies to surgery to decrease morbidity and disfigurement in laBCC is warranted. Although the multiple mechanisms of SMO inhibitor resistance convey challenges to treatment, continued research and further understanding will assist in improving systemic therapies in advanced BCC. Development of newer Shh pathway inhibitors, such as those targeting GLI further downstream in the Shh pathway, may exhibit more efficacy than the current SMO inhibitors. Furthermore, combinations of drugs that act on different loci of the Shh pathway, as well as concurrent targeting of other pathways implicated in upregulation of GLI activity, may prove more efficacious than monotherapy alone. Combination therapies may become especially relevant in the context of managing drug resistance in advanced BCC.

Case Report

A 68-year-old Caucasian male presented with a large, non-healing tumor of the scalp that had been progressively enlarging for many years. A punch biopsy demonstrated infiltrative basal cell carcinoma. The lesion had not been treated previously. A total body computed tomography scan demonstrated evidence of local invasion of the underlying temporal bone but no distant metastases, consistent with a tumor stage of T3.

Past Medical History
- Hypertension

Social History
- Smokes cigarettes, 1 pack per day
- Drinks 6 beers daily
- Divorced
- Retired, formerly worked in construction

Previous Therapies
- None

Physical Exam
- 6 × 9 cm friable tumor with 1.5 cm central ulceration located on the left frontotemporal scalp
- Significant male-pattern alopecia involving the vertex, frontal scalp, and temples

Management
The patient's basal cell carcinoma was classified as locally advanced; due to the involvement of underlying bone structures, he was not an ideal surgical candidate. He was sent for a radiation-oncology consultation for possible radiation therapy. However, the patient had limited transportation and lived a far distance from the radiation treatment center. The patient instead opted for treatment with vismodegib. He was started on the standard vismodegib dose of 150 mg daily. On follow-up 2 months later, the patient was noted to have a significant decrease in tumor size and resolution of central ulceration. He experienced grade 1 adverse effects from treatment with muscle spasms, dysgeusia, and worsening of scalp alopecia. The patient found these side effects tolerable and has remained on vismodegib for a total of 8 months with clinical remission of his tumor and no disease progression.

References

1. Mohan S, Chang A. Advanced basal cell carcinoma: epidemiology and therapeutic innovations. Curr Dermatol Rep. 2014;3:40–5.
2. Bolognia JL, Jorizzo JL, Schaffer JV. Dermatology. London: Saunders; 2012.
3. Walling HW, Fosko SW, Geraminejad PA, Whitaker DC, Arpey CJ. Aggressive basal cell carcinoma: presentation, pathogenesis, and management. Cancer Metastasis Rev. 2004;23(3-4):389–402.
4. Armstrong BK, Kricker A. The epidemiology of UV induced skin cancer. J Photochem Photobiol B. 2001;63(1-3):8–18.
5. Van Scott EJ, Reinertson RP. The modulating influence of stromal environment on epithelial cells studied in human autotransplants. J Invest Dermatol. 1961;36:109–31.
6. Blanpain C, Fuchs E. Epidermal homeostasis: a balancing act of stem cells in the skin. Nat Rev Mol Cell Biol. 2009;10(3):207–17.
7. Gailani MR, Bale SJ, Leffell DJ, DiGiovanna JJ, Peck GL, Poliak S, et al. Developmental defects in Gorlin syndrome related to a putative tumor suppressor gene on chromosome 9. Cell. 1992;69(1):111–7.
8. Gorlin RJ. Nevoid basal cell carcinoma (Gorlin) syndrome. Genet Med. 2004;6(6):530–9.
9. Aszterbaum M, Epstein J, Oro A, Douglas V, LeBoit PE, Scott MP, et al. Ultraviolet and ionizing radiation enhance the growth of BCCs and trichoblastomas in patched heterozygous knockout mice. Nat Med. 1999;5(11):1285–91.
10. Athar M, Li C, Kim AL, Spiegelman VS, Bickers DR. Sonic hedgehog signaling in basal cell nevus syndrome. Cancer Res. 2014;74(18):4967–75.
11. Rady P, Scinicariello F, Wagner RF Jr, Tyring SK. p53 mutations in basal cell carcinomas. Cancer Res. 1992;52(13):3804–6.
12. de Zwaan SE, Haass NK. Genetics of basal cell carcinoma. Australas J Dermatol. 2010;51(2):81–92. quiz 3-4

13. Youssef KK, Lapouge G, Bouvree K, Rorive S, Brohee S, Appelstein O, et al. Adult interfollicular tumour-initiating cells are reprogrammed into an embryonic hair follicle progenitor-like fate during basal cell carcinoma initiation. Nat Cell Biol. 2012;14(12):1282–94.

14. Wang GY, Wang J, Mancianti ML, Epstein EH Jr. Basal cell carcinomas arise from hair follicle stem cells in Ptch1(+/−) mice. Cancer Cell. 2011;19(1):114–24.

15. Lo JS, Snow SN, Reizner GT, Mohs FE, Larson PO, Hruza GJ. Metastatic basal cell carcinoma: report of twelve cases with a review of the literature. J Am Acad Dermatol. 1991;24(5 Pt 1):715–9.

16. von Domarus H, Stevens PJ. Metastatic basal cell carcinoma. Report of five cases and review of 170 cases in the literature. J Am Acad Dermatol. 1984;10(6):1043–60.

17. Incardona JP, Gaffield W, Kapur RP, Roelink H. The teratogenic Veratrum alkaloid cyclopamine inhibits sonic hedgehog signal transduction. Development. 1998;125(18):3553–62.

18. Taipale J, Chen JK, Cooper MK, Wang B, Mann RK, Milenkovic L, et al. Effects of oncogenic mutations in smoothened and patched can be reversed by cyclopamine. Nature. 2000;406(6799):1005–9.

19. Tabs S, Avci O. Induction of the differentiation and apoptosis of tumor cells in vivo with efficiency and selectivity. Eur J Dermatol. 2004;14(2):96–102.

20. Lipinski RJ, Hutson PR, Hannam PW, Nydza RJ, Washington IM, Moore RW, et al. Dose- and route-dependent teratogenicity, toxicity, and pharmacokinetic profiles of the hedgehog signaling antagonist cyclopamine in the mouse. Toxicol Sci. 2008;104(1):189–97.

21. Prescribing information: ERIVEDGE (vismodegib) capsule for oral use 2015. http://www.accessdata.fda.gov/drugsatfda_docs/label/2015/203388s005s006s007s008lbl.pdf.

22. Sekulic A, Migden MR, Oro AE, Dirix L, Lewis KD, Hainsworth JD, et al. Efficacy and safety of vismodegib in advanced basal-cell carcinoma. N Engl J Med. 2012;366(23):2171–9.

23. Jacobsen AA, Aldahan AS, Hughes OB, Shah VV, Strasswimmer J. Hedgehog pathway inhibitor therapy for locally advanced and metastatic basal cell carcinoma: a systematic review and pooled analysis of interventional studies. JAMA Dermatol. 2016;152(7):816–24.

24. Tang JY, Mackay-Wiggan JM, Aszterbaum M, Yauch RL, Lindgren J, Chang K, et al. Inhibiting the hedgehog pathway in patients with the basal-cell nevus syndrome. N Engl J Med. 2012;366(23):2180–8.

25. Mohan SV, Chang J, Li S, Henry AS, Wood DJ, Chang AL. Increased risk of cutaneous squamous cell carcinoma after vismodegib therapy for basal cell carcinoma. JAMA Dermatol. 2016;152(5):527–32.

26. Zhao X, Ponomaryov T, Ornell KJ, Zhou P, Dabral SK, Pak E, et al. RAS/MAPK activation drives resistance to Smo inhibition, metastasis, and tumor evolution in Shh pathway-dependent tumors. Cancer Res. 2015;75(17):3623–35.

27. ODOMZO (sonidegib) capsules, for oral use 2015. http://www.accessdata.fda.gov/drugsatfda_docs/label/2015/205266s000lbl.pdf.

28. Migden MR, Guminski A, Gutzmer R, Dirix L, Lewis KD, Combemale P, et al. Treatment with two different doses of sonidegib in patients with locally advanced or metastatic basal cell carcinoma (BOLT): a multicentre, randomised, double-blind phase 2 trial. Lancet Oncol. 2015;16(6):716–28.

29. Burness CB, Scott LJ. Sonidegib: a review in locally advanced basal cell carcinoma. Target Oncol. 2016;11(2):239–46.

30. Ally MS, Aasi S, Wysong A, Teng C, Anderson E, Bailey-Healy I, et al. An investigator-initiated open-label clinical trial of vismodegib as a neoadjuvant to surgery for high-risk basal cell carcinoma. J Am Acad Dermatol. 2014;71(5):904–11.e1.

31. Chang AL, Oro AE. Initial assessment of tumor regrowth after vismodegib in advanced basal cell carcinoma. Arch Dermatol. 2012;148(11):1324–5.

32. Rudin CM, Hann CL, Laterra J, Yauch RL, Callahan CA, Fu L, et al. Treatment of medulloblastoma with hedgehog pathway inhibitor GDC-0449. N Engl J Med. 2009;361(12):1173–8.

33. Pricl S, Cortelazzi B, Dal Col V, Marson D, Laurini E, Fermeglia M, et al. Smoothened (SMO) receptor mutations dictate resistance to vismodegib in basal cell carcinoma. Mol Oncol. 2015;9(2):389–97.

34. Buonamici S, Williams J, Morrissey M, Wang A, Guo R, Vattay A, et al. Interfering with resistance to smoothened antagonists by inhibition of the PI3K pathway in medulloblastoma. Sci Transl Med. 2010;2(51):51ra70.

35. Kim J, Tang JY, Gong R, Lee JJ, Clemons KV, Chong CR, et al. Itraconazole, a commonly used antifungal that inhibits hedgehog pathway activity and cancer growth. Cancer Cell. 2010;17(4):388–99.

36. Kim J, Aftab BT, Tang JY, Kim D, Lee AH, Rezaee M, et al. Itraconazole and arsenic trioxide inhibit hedgehog pathway activation and tumor growth associated with acquired resistance to smoothened antagonists. Cancer Cell. 2013;23(1):23–34.

37. Kim DJ, Kim J, Spaunhurst K, Montoya J, Khodosh R, Chandra K, et al. Open-label, exploratory phase II trial of oral itraconazole for the treatment of basal cell carcinoma. J Clin Oncol. 2014;32(8):745–51.

38. Ally MS, Ransohoff K, Sarin K, Atwood SX, Rezaee M, Bailey-Healy I, et al. Effects of combined treatment with arsenic trioxide and Itraconazole in patients with refractory metastatic basal cell carcinoma. JAMA Dermatol. 2016;152(4):452–6.

39. List A, Beran M, DiPersio J, Slack J, Vey N, Rosenfeld CS, et al. Opportunities for Trisenox (arsenic trioxide) in the treatment of myelodysplastic syndromes. Leukemia. 2003;17(8):1499–507.

40. Beauchamp EM, Ringer L, Bulut G, Sajwan KP, Hall MD, Lee YC, et al. Arsenic trioxide inhibits human cancer cell growth and tumor development in mice by blocking hedgehog/GLI pathway. J Clin Invest. 2011;121(1):148–60.

41. Kim J, Lee JJ, Gardner D, Beachy PA. Arsenic antagonizes the hedgehog pathway by preventing ciliary accumulation and reducing stability of the Gli2 transcriptional effector. Proc Natl Acad Sci U S A. 2010;107(30):13432–7.

42. Lauth M, Bergstrom A, Shimokawa T, Toftgard R. Inhibition of GLI-mediated transcription and tumor cell growth by small-molecule antagonists. Proc Natl Acad Sci U S A. 2007;104(20):8455–60.

43. Huntzicker EG, Estay IS, Zhen H, Lokteva LA, Jackson PK, Oro AE. Dual degradation signals control Gli protein stability and tumor formation. Genes Dev. 2006;20(3):276–81.

44. Pan Y, Bai CB, Joyner AL, Wang B. Sonic hedgehog signaling regulates Gli2 transcriptional activity by suppressing its processing and degradation. Mol Cell Biol. 2006;26(9):3365–77.

45. Makinodan E, Marneros AG. Protein kinase a activation inhibits oncogenic sonic hedgehog signalling and suppresses basal cell carcinoma of the skin. Exp Dermatol. 2012;21(11):847–52.

Update in Immunotherapies for Melanoma

Sabrina Martin and Roger Lo

Introduction

The initial treatment of many melanoma cases is surgical, as most thin melanomas can be cured with wide local excision. However, once a patient develops disseminated disease, systemic medications are warranted. In the past, traditional chemotherapy agents did little to improve survival. Among those, dacarbazine was the most effective. In recent years, a deeper understanding of the pathogenesis of melanoma has led to an expansion in the treatment options. These new medications can be organized into two categories: those that target pathway alterations caused by gene mutations ("targeted therapy") or those that augment the immune system to fight off the cancer ("immunotherapy").

Targeted Therapy

The key to targeted melanoma therapy revolves around the mitogen-activated protein (MAP) kinase pathway (Fig. 48.1). As a regulator of cell proliferation, constitutive activation of the MAP kinase pathway can lead to the progression of melanoma [1]. Around 40–60% of melanomas contain an activating mutation in BRAF. A majority of those are activating mutations that cause a change at codon 600 from valine to glutamic acid (BRAF V600E) [2, 3].

Vemurafenib and dabrafenib are inhibitors of mutated BRAF and therefore used to treat melanoma. In a phase III trial, vemurafenib was compared to dacarbazine in 675 patients with either untreated stage IIIc or stage IV disease. Overall survival was calculated at 6 months and found to be 84% for vemurafenib and 64% for dacarbazine. Overall survival and progression-free survival were 13.6 and 9.7 months

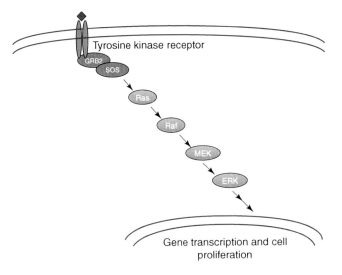

Fig. 48.1 MAP kinase pathway. Activation of the tyrosine kinase receptor initiates a cascade that results in cell proliferation

for vemurafenib versus 5.3 and 1.6 months for dacarbazine. The most common side effects were grade 1–2 adverse events such as arthralgia (50%), fatigue (43%), photosensitivity (37%), and rash (32%). The more severe, grade 3–4 adverse events included squamous cell skin cancer (SCC) (19%), keratoacanthomas (KA) (10%), rash (9%), and abnormal liver function tests (11%) [3]. Although rare, it should be noted that vemurafenib may cause QT prolongation [4].

In a phase III trial, dabrafenib was compared to dacarbazine in 250 patients with either untreated stage III or stage IV disease. Overall survival favored dabrafenib but was not statically significant. Progression-free survival was 5.1 months for dabrafenib versus 2.7 months for dacarbazine. The most common grade 2 adverse events were hyperkeratosis (12%), palmar-plantar erythrodysesthesia (6%), pyrexia (8%), and fatigue (5%). More severe grade 3 or 4 events were uncommon. SCCs or KAs occurred at 2% or 4% for grade 2 and 3, respectively.

Common to both BRAF inhibitors was the development of SCCs and KAs in patients. These cancers usually developed

S. Martin, MD • R. Lo, MD, PhD (✉)
Division of Dermatology, Department of Medicine,
University of California, Los Angeles, 200 Med Plaza,
Suite 450, Los Angeles, CA 90095, USA
e-mail: SLMartin@mednet.ucla.edu; RLO@mednet.ucla.edu

© Springer International Publishing AG 2018
P.S. Yamauchi (ed.), *Biologic and Systemic Agents in Dermatology*, https://doi.org/10.1007/978-3-319-66884-0_48

shortly after initiation of the medication and were treated surgically. Further studies demonstrated that these patients had pre-existing RAS mutations in their skin. When subjected to BRAF inhibition, these RAS mutations paradoxically increased signaling in the pathway, causing development of SCCs and KAs [5].

While the development of BRAF inhibitors was a considerable breakthrough, it was not effective as monotherapy, as acquired resistance to the medication limited progression-free survival. The MAP kinase pathway was reactivated, usually facilitated through a secondary mutation in genes such as RAS, BRAF, and MEK [6–10]. MEK inhibitors, such as trametinib and cobimetinib, block the same MAP kinase pathway, but further downstream. These are used in combination with BRAF inhibitors for BRAF-positive melanomas [11].

In a phase III trial, trametinib was compared to dacarbazine or paclitaxel in 322 melanoma patients that had not received prior BRAF inhibitor treatment. Overall survival rate at 6 months was 81% versus 67%. Progression-free survival was 4.8 months for dabrafenib versus 1.5 months for dacarbazine [11]. The most common side effects were rash, diarrhea, fatigue, and edema. Other notable side effects included cardiac issues such as a decreased ejection fraction or ventricular dysfunction and ophthalmologic issues such as vision changes and reversible chorioretinopathy. No SCCs or KAs were seen.

The combination of BRAF and MEK inhibitors results in improved outcomes. Cobimetinib plus vemurafenib versus vemurafenib alone has shown to increase mean survival to 22.3 months from 17.4 months. Progression-free survival is also increased to 12.3 months from 7.2 months. Combination groups had higher rates of adverse events, including elevations in gamma-glutamyl transferase, creatine phosphokinase, and alanine transaminase as well as serious side effects of fever and dehydration [12]. Trametinib in combination with dabrafenib compared to monotherapy with BRAF inhibitors (either dabrafenib or vemurafenib) has also shown increased mean survival and progression-free survival. Combination of trametinib with dabrafenib was more likely to cause diarrhea, chills, or fever [13]. Of note, combination therapy showed significantly less instances of SCC or KAs than BRAF monotherapy [14].

Immunotherapy

Another strategy is to encourage the immune system to recognize and eradicate the melanoma. When an antigen-presenting cell (APC) displays intracellular proteins to the T cell, there needs to be a co-stimulatory signal for the T cell to become activated. This occurs when a B7 molecule binds to CD28 on the T cell. If an inhibitory signal is sent instead (creating a "checkpoint"), the T cell is not activated. This can occur when a B7 molecule on the APC binds to the cytotoxic T-lymphocyte antigen 4 (CTLA-4) receptor on the T cell or when a programmed cell death ligand (PD-L1) from a tumor cell binds to the programmed cell death 1 receptor (PD-1) on a T cell. The basis of immunotherapy is to bypass this immune system checkpoint so that the T cells recognize and target the cancer cells [15].

Ipilimumab is a monoclonal antibody that binds CTLA-4 and approved for treatment of metastatic melanoma and as adjuvant therapy in high-risk cases. One phase III trial comparing ipilimumab plus dacarbazine versus dacarbazine alone found a 5-year survival rate of 18% versus 9%. A phase III trial examining ipilimumab to glycoprotein 100 vaccine showed a 2-year survival rate of 24% versus 14% [16]. A larger 1861 patient pooled analysis found that median overall survival was 11.4 months and that the survival curve plateaued around 21% after 3 years regardless of prior therapy [17]. The side effects of ipilimumab are immune related and very common, with up to 85% affected. Common grade 3 or higher side effects include diarrhea, liver toxicity, and rash. Most cases can be treated with immunosuppression, either with corticosteroids or a TNF alpha inhibitor. Of importance, side effect treatment does not affect tumor response to ipilimumab [18].

Pembrolizumab and nivolumab are monoclonal antibodies that bind PD-1. A study comparing two different doses of pembrolizumab (2 mg/kg or 10 mg/kg) versus chemotherapy found an overall 2-year survival rate of 36, 38, and 30% [19]. More impressively, the progression-free survival rate at 2 years was 16, 22, and less than 1% [20]. Nivolumab has been compared to chemotherapy in a few phase 3 trials and has shown improved overall survival (73% vs. 42% in one study) as well as longer progression-free survival [21, 22]. Notably, tumors that expressed more PD-L1 did respond better, but even some tumors without PD-LI expression showed a response [20]. The side effects are also immune related and occur in 71% of patients. Most common were fatigue, diarrhea, rash, and itching. Only 10% had grade 3 or higher reactions [23].

PD-1 inhibitors are currently the most effective checkpoint inhibitors for melanoma compared with CTLA-4 inhibitors. Nivolumab has a better overall 2-year survival rate of 55% versus 43% with less adverse events than ipilimumab [24]. Combination of pembrolizumab or nivolumab with ipilimumab has also shown better response rates, but with more frequent and more severe adverse events [25]. More research is examining the option of combination or sequential treatment with both types of checkpoint inhibitors. Some tumors are resistant to PD-1 inhibitors, such that no response or relapse is seen with treatment. Studies have shown that the resistant rate can be innate (60%) or acquired (25%) [26–28]. As this area is further explored, new medications and combined treatment regimens will likely develop.

Current Treatment Recommendations and Doses

Systemic medications are used in the setting of metastatic melanoma. Dosing regimens are listed in Table 48.1. Immunotherapy is central to treatment. Most patients are started on a PD-1 inhibitor, possibly in combination with ipilimumab. Treatment is administered until disease progression, intolerable side effects, or maximum clinical benefit is derived. If a tumor has a BRAF mutation, treatment course may be switched to a BRAF and MEK inhibitor, or the two may be added to immunotherapy. Radiation for brain metastasis or palliative surgery may also be done. Studies are ongoing to determine the preferred sequence and combinations of systemic treatments. Tumor sequencing information may help individualize treatment regimens in the future [29].

Surgery has long been the mainstay of treatment for earlier stage melanoma. However, a renewed focus on adjuvant and neoadjuvant therapy has occurred as the target and immunotherapy options have expanded. For stage III disease, adjuvant therapy with ipilimumab or interferon alpha is approved but not commonly done. Interferon alpha is often poorly tolerated, and subsequent clinical trials have shown less consistent results with treatment. High dose ipilimumab can be given at 10 mg/kg every 3 weeks for four doses and then every 12 weeks for up to 3 years but also has significant side effects. Given this, one should consider enrollment in a trial for expanded systemic options. Several phase III trials are examining the use of nivolumab or pembrolizumab as well as low-dose ipilimumab, vemurafenib, or dabrafenib plus trametinib. Neoadjuvant therapy for high-risk melanoma is not approved, but phase I and II trials are underway for nivolumab with or without ipilimumab and dabrafenib plus trametinib [30].

Numerous clinical trials are ongoing and available to patients, especially in the setting of standard treatment failure. These trials are examining new medications, different dosing schedules, and different combinations of pre-existing medications. Given the impressive progression in the past few years, melanoma treatment is likely to change rapidly with the hope of improving patient outcomes.

Case

A 77-year-old Hispanic female developed a mole on her left ankle. It was initially small and dark in color, but, over the course of 4 years, grew in size and became more raised. Her podiatrist performed a biopsy that showed malignant melanoma. She underwent an excision with clear margins. Histological examination revealed a 6.2 mm nodular melanoma with positive lymphovascular involvement. Genetic testing was positive for the BRAF V600E mutation. She then underwent sentinel lymph node biopsy, which showed no evidence of disease. Brain MRI and whole-body PET showed no evidence of disease. However, 2 months later, two skin nodules on her left leg grew and biopsies revealed in transit melanoma metastases.

Past Medical History
Diabetes
Hypertension

Social History
No past or current smoking
No alcohol use

Physical exam
Large linear hypopigmented scar, left ankle
Two smaller linear scars, left thigh, left shin

Management
Patient was started on PD-1 therapy. She received nivolumab 240 mg IV infusions every 2 weeks. Unfortunately, the patient developed multiple small and large interval nodules on her shin after 4 cycles, so treatment was discontinued. No other definitive metastases were found in scans of the chest, abdomen, or pelvis. She was enrolled in a clinical trial and started on a combination of pembrolizumab plus a TLR9 agonist injected into the metastatic leg lesions. After 1 month consisting of two pembrolizumab infusions and 4 weekly TLR9 agonist injections, patient wished to discontinue the trial. All medications were stopped and discussions regarding a dabrafenib plus trametinib trial were considered. However, in the interim, the patient noted a delayed response of her leg nodules to the prior trial injections. She was instead restarted on the original trial and will continue to be monitored.

Table 48.1 Frequently used metastatic melanoma medications

Medication	Dosage and frequency
Vemurafenib	960 mg PO BID
Dabrafenib	150 mg PO BID
Cobimetinib	60 mg once per day on days 1 to 21 of each 28-day cycle
Trametinib	2 mg orally once daily
Ipilimumab	3 mg/kg every 3 weeks for four doses (metastatic disease)
	10 mg/kg every 3 weeks for four doses, then every 12 weeks for up to 3 years (adjuvant setting)
Nivolumab	240 mg IV every 2 weeks
Pembrolizumab	2 mg/kg IV every 3 weeks

References

1. Beeram M, Patnaik A, Rowinsky EK. Raf: a strategic target for therapeutic development against cancer. J Clin Oncol. 2005;23:6771–90.
2. Curtin JA, Fridlyand J, Kageshita T, Patel HN, Busam KJ, Kutzner H, et al. Distinct sets of genetic alterations in melanoma. N Engl J Med. 2005;353:2135–47.

3. McArthur GA, Chapman PB, Robert C, Larkin J, Haanen JB, Dummer R, Ribas A, et al. Safety and efficacy of vemurafenib in BRAF(V600E) and BRAF(V600K) mutation-positive melanoma (BRIM-3): extended follow-up of a phase 3, randomised, open-label study. Lancet Oncol. 2014;15:323–32.

4. Flaherty L, Hamid O, Linette G, Schuchter L, Hallmeyer S, Gonzalez R, et al. A single-arm, open-label, expanded access study of vemurafenib in patients with metastatic melanoma in the United States. Cancer J. 2014;20:18–24.

5. Su F, Viros A, Milagre C, Trunzer K, Bollag G, Spleiss O, et al. RAS mutations in cutaneous squamous-cell carcinomas in patients treated with BRAF inhibitors. N Engl J Med. 2012;366:207.

6. Poulikakos PI, Persaud Y, Janakiraman M, Kong X, Ng C, Moriceau G, et al. RAF inhibitor resistance is mediated by dimerization of aberrantly spliced BRAF(V600E). Nature. 2011;480:387–90.

7. Nazarian R, Shi H, Wang Q, Kong X, Koya RC, Lee H, et al. Melanomas acquire resistance to B-RAF(V600E) inhibition by RTK or N-RAS upregulation. Nature. 2010;468:973–7.

8. Shi H, Moriceau G, Kong X, Lee MK, Lee H, Koya RC, et al. Melanoma whole-exome sequencing identifies (V600E)B-RAF amplification-mediated acquired B-RAF inhibitor resistance. Nat Commun. 2012;6:724.

9. Shi H, Hugo W, Kong X, Hong A, Koya RC, Moriceau G, et al. Acquired resistance and clonal evolution in melanoma during BRAF inhibitor therapy. Cancer Discov. 2014;4:80–93.

10. Hugo W, Shi H, Sun L, Piva M, Song C, Kong X, et al. Non-genomic and immune evolution of melanoma acquiring MAPKi resistance. Cell. 2015;162(6):1271–85.

11. Flaherty KT, Robert C, Hersey P, Nathan P, Garbe C, Milhem M, et al. Improved survival with MEK inhibition in BRAF-mutated melanoma. N Engl J Med. 2012;367:107–14.

12. Ascierto PA, McArthur GA, Dréno B, Atkinson V, Liszkay G, Di Giacomo AM, et al. Cobimetinib combined with vemurafenib in advanced BRAF(V600)-mutant melanoma (coBRIM): updated efficacy results from a randomised, double-blind, phase 3 trial. Lancet Oncol. 2016;17:1248–60.

13. Long GV, Stroyakovskiy D, Gogas H, Levchenko E, de Braud F, Larkin J, Ascierto PA, McArthur GA, Dréno B, Atkinson V, Liszkay G, Di Giacomo AM, et al. Combined BRAF and MEK inhibition versus BRAF inhibition alone in melanoma. N Engl J Med. 2014;371:1877–88. https://doi.org/10.1056/NEJMoa1406037.

14. Robert C, Karaszewska B, Schachter J, Rutkowski P, Mackiewicz A, Stroiakovski D, et al. Improved overall survival in melanoma with combined dabrafenib and trametinib. N Engl J Med. 2015;372:30.

15. Koller KM, Wang W, Schell TD, Cozza EM, Kokolus KM, Neves RI, et al. Malignant melanoma—the cradle of anti-neoplastic immunotherapy. Crit Rev Oncol Hematol. 2016;106:25–54. https://doi.org/10.1016/j.critrevonc.2016.04.010.

16. Hodi FS, O'Day SJ, McDermott DF, Weber RW, Sosman JA, Haanen JB, et al. Improved survival with ipilimumab in patients with metastatic melanoma. N Engl J Med. 2010;363:711.

17. Schadendorf D, Hodi FS, Robert C, Weber JS, Margolin K, Hamid O, et al. Pooled analysis of long-term survival data from phase II and phase III trials of ipilimumab in unresectable or metastatic melanoma. J Clin Oncol. 2015;33:1889.

18. Horvat TZ, Adel NG, Dang TO, Momtaz P, Postow MA, Callahan MK, et al. Immune related adverse events, need for systemic immunosuppression, and effects on survival and time to treatment failure in patients with melanoma treated with ipilimumab at Memorial Sloan Kettering Cancer Center. J Clin Oncol. 2015;33:3193–8. https://doi.org/10.1200/JCO.2015.60.8448.

19. Hamid O, Puzanov I, Dummer R, Schachter J, Daud A, Schadendorf D, et al. Final overall survival for KEYNOTE-002: pembrolizumab versus investigator-choice chemotherapy for ipilimumab-refractory melanoma. Abstract 11070, presented at the 2016 European Society for Medical Oncology meeting.

20. Ribas A, Hamid O, Daud A, Hodi FS, Wolchok JD, Kefford R, et al. Association of pembrolizumab with tumor response and survival among patients with advanced melanoma. JAMA. 2016;315:1600.

21. Weber JS, D'Angelo SP, Minor D, Hodi FS, Gutzmer R, Neyns B, et al. Nivolumab versus chemotherapy in patients with advanced melanoma who progressed after anti-CTLA-4 treatment (CheckMate 037): a randomised, controlled, open-label, phase 3 trial. Lancet Oncol. 2015;16:375–84. https://doi.org/10.1016/S1470-2045(15)70076-8.

22. Robert C, Long GV, Brady B, Dutriaux C, Maio M, Mortier L, et al. Nivolumab in previously untreated melanoma without BRAF mutation. N Engl J Med. 2015;372:320.

23. Weber JS, Hodi FS, Wolchok JD, Topalian SL, Schadendorf D, Larkin J, et al. Safety profile of nivolumab monotherapy: a pooled analysis of patients with advanced melanoma. J Clin Oncol. 2017;35:785–92. https://doi.org/10.1200/JCO.2015.66.1389.

24. Schacter J, Ribas A, Ling GV, Arance A, Grob JJ, Mortier L, et al. Pembrolizumab versus ipilimumab for advanced melanoma: Final overall survival analysis of KEYNOTE-006. Abstract 9504, American Society of Clinical Oncology 2016 annual meeting.

25. Wolchok JD, Chiarion-Sileni V, Gonzalez R, Piotr Rutkowski P, Grob JJ, Cowey CL, et al. Updated results from a phase III trial of nivolumab (NIVO) combined with ipilimumab (IPI) in treatment-naive patients (pts) with advanced melanoma (MEL) (CheckMate 067). Abstract 9505, American Society of Clinical Oncology 2016 annual meeting.

26. Hugo W, Zaretsky JM, Sun L, Song C, Moreno BH, Hu-Lieskovan S, et al. Genomic and transcriptomic features of response to anti-PD-1 therapy in metastatic melanoma. Cell. 2016;165:35–44.

27. Shin DS, Zaretsky JM, Escuin-Ordinas H, Garcia-Diaz A, Hu-Lieskovan S, Kalbasi A, et al. Primary resistance to PD-1 blockade mediated by JAK1/2 mutations. Cancer Discov. 2017;7:188–201.

28. Zaretsky JM, Garcia-Diaz A, Shin DS, Escuin-Ordinas H, Hugo W, Hu-Lieskovan S, et al. Mutations Associated with Acquired Resistance to PD-1 Blockade in Melanoma. N Engl J Med. 2016;375:819–29.

29. Coit DG, Thompson JA, Algazi A, Andtbacka R, Bichakjian CK, Carson WE 3rd, et al. Melanoma, version 2.2016, NCCN clinical practice guidelines in oncology. J Natl Compr Cancer Netw. 2016;14:450–73.

30. van Zeijl MC, van den Eertwegh AJ, Haanen JB, Wouters MW. (Neo)adjuvant systemic therapy for melanoma. Eur J Surg Oncol. 2017;43:534–43.

Patient Advocacy Organizations

49

Catie Coman

Overview of a Patient Advocacy Organization

A patient advocacy organization is a type of nonprofit, charitable entity that focuses on improving the health and well-being of individuals who share a particular chronic disease or disability or a set of diseases or disabilities. Also known as a voluntary health agency, patient advocacy organizations typically work in one or more of the following service areas: disease education, patient support, government relations, public health communications, and access to care and research.

The work of patient advocacy organizations should not be confused with the work of a patient advocate. While there is some crossover in function, patient advocates largely focus on helping individuals navigate the health-care system using a case-management approach. Patient advocacy organizations work on systemic issues affecting the health of their patient population as well as provide "mass" education available to a wide audience. Rarely do patient advocacy organizations offer direct service support such as access to community programs, counseling, transportation, or other types of services typically associated with social work.

There are about 20 organizations in the USA concerned with the range of dermatological diseases [1]. These include common, immune-mediated conditions such as atopic dermatitis, psoriasis, and vitiligo to rare skin diseases like pemphigus and pemphigoid. These organizations are governed by a lay board of directors often comprised of patients and/or caregivers, and most have a separate medical or scientific advisory board of health-care providers and/or research scientists.

49

C. Coman, MA
Health Advocacy Partners,
Portland, OR, USA
e-mail: ccoman@healthadvocacypartners.com

Core Programs

All of the services provided by patient advocacy organizations in dermatology can be grouped into three central programmatic areas: education, advocacy, and research.

Education

All dermatology patient advocacy organizations provide some level of basic disease education to their patient and caregiver audiences. This education takes the form of print booklets and pamphlets, disease-specific websites, support groups, Webinars, live health events, print magazines and newsletters, and e-newsletters.

Larger and more well-funded patient advocacy organizations offer expanded disease education through apps, videos, social media, and call centers. These services as well as those mentioned earlier are usually offered free of charge to patients and their families.

Advocacy

Organization advocacy activities fall into two broad areas. The first focuses on advocating at a federal level for increased funding for disease-specific research at the National Institutes of Health (NIH), Centers for Disease Control (CDC), and other government agencies. Larger dermatology patient advocacy organizations may also work to advocate for better health policies at the federal level for their patient communities.

The second area of advocacy activity is in ensuring patients have access to care. This includes access to safe, effective and affordable treatments, and access to health-care specialists able to treat the symptoms of the disease affecting their community and/or related comorbid conditions of that disease. These activities are undergirded by the philosophy that the decision for type and methods of care is one that belongs to the patient and their doctor only.

© Springer International Publishing AG 2018
P.S. Yamauchi (ed.), *Biologic and Systemic Agents in Dermatology*, https://doi.org/10.1007/978-3-319-66884-0_49

Access to care advocacy is conducted in several different arenas. Patient advocacy organizations work directly with payors to articulate burden of disease and need for access to treatment without oppressive bureaucracy. These organizations also work with state and federal lawmakers to curb onerous health insurance practices such as step therapy, prior authorization, cost transference to patients in the form of higher co-payments and coinsurance for branded drugs, and outright denial to cover needed medications. Additionally, patient advocacy organizations work with drug manufacturers to reduce costs of drugs and provide patients with financial support for prescription costs.

Research

The motivation to accelerate the discovery of better treatments and a cure is a key driver for research activities by patient advocacy organizations.

Many of the organizations serving patients with skin disease provide seed grants to researchers with innovative ideas in order that these researchers may get a body of data that supports an NIH or other large research grant applications. These grants fund basic science, translational research, and other research areas supporting understanding in population health such as burden of disease and health-related quality of life impacts.

Dermatology advocacy organizations also actively support and promote clinical trial participation among their patient community. Increasingly, these organizations are involving patients—at the request of industry researchers—to provide input on clinical trial protocol with the goal of making the trial more patient centric. Some organizations create and populate tissue or biobanks and related clinical data in their specific disease areas for use by researchers.

Larger and more established advocacy organizations collect, analyze, and publish patient-reported data with the goal of quantifying impacts of the disease on quality of life. This data also serves to identify other issues in the patient community such as mis- and underdiagnosis, symptom impact, side effects, disease complications, access to care issues, etc. As well, this data informs organization public health messaging and program development and implementation.

Benefits of Partnering with Patient Advocacy Organizations

Patient advocacy organizations can serve as an important adjunct to clinical care. At the most fundamental level, advocacy organizations offer health-care providers medically reviewed, patient education materials for use in office. These materials range from disease overview pamphlets to specifics on using topical, oral, and biological medications. Beyond

patient literature, advocacy organizations offer patients ongoing education and peer support with the goal of creating activated patients, which in turn, lead to improved health outcomes [2].

Another key area of collaboration between the physician office and a patient advocacy organization is in the area of access to care. In addition to working at the state and federal level to influence policies and laws that ease barriers to patient access to treatments and medical specialists, advocacy organizations also assist individuals in accessing care. These services include providing tools, templated letters, information and assistance on appealing insurance denials, and other insurer methods of controlling cost at the expense of patient access.

National Eczema Association

National Eczema Association (NEA) is the sole patient advocacy organization serving people with eczema in the USA. NEA provides people with eczema and their families the information and services they need to best manage their condition while funding research to better understand and treat the disease.

NEA is dedicated to improving the health and quality of life for individuals with eczema through research, education, peer support, and advocacy initiatives.

Research

The NEA research agenda focuses on high-value/high-yield projects that provide clues to eczema pathogenesis, symptom evolution, its impact on quality of life, and new approaches to treatment. Each year, the organization awards grants to qualified researchers with small but innovative projects that add to the canon of understanding eczema and its bearing on patients. In recent years, NEA has funded research exploring novel treatments for pruritus, atopic dermatitis comorbidities, and skin barrier function in atopic dermatitis [3].

The National Eczema Association also collects and analyzes patient-reported data from its community and publishes on the findings with the goal of elucidating the true impact of eczema symptoms on patient and family quality of life, treatment satisfaction, access to care issues, symptom progression, and patient preference.

Education

The National Eczema Association provides approximately six million people a year with disease management and wellness education. The organization manages a large website that includes basic information on eczema, how it is treated, potential triggers, etc. NEA provides additional digital patient education in the form of monthly e-newsletters, frequent Webinars, live question and answer sessions on social media, and downloadable fact sheets.

Printed patient education materials include booklets and brochures on the range of disease topics and a biannual patient magazine. Patients receive these materials by requesting them directly from NEA or through their physicians' office.

All NEA's educational materials are written by health education experts and reviewed by members of their medical editorial board for accuracy.

Lastly, the organization hosts live health education events in the form of patient and physician conferences and forums in cities around the USA.

With regard to physician education, National Eczema Association leads a coalition of patients and physician thought leaders tasked with developing programs that prepare health-care providers to effectively treat eczema patients. The coalition is spearheading the development of national medical education programs focused on the latest research and best practices in eczema care.

Peer Support

NEA sponsors a growing online support group, Eczema Wise (www.inspire.com/groups/national-eczema-association), where patients exchange information, get answers to their questions about eczema, and provide each other with encouragement. The organization also hosts live support groups in 11 states and facilitates telephone- and email-based support services staffed by volunteer peer mentors.

Advocacy

NEA works with a network of patient leaders who advocate at the state and federal level, as well as in the private sector, on issues critical to the eczema community. The organization has a threefold advocacy strategy that includes, raising awareness among lawmakers on the impact of eczema; pressing for laws that ensure access to affordable, effective treatments; and increasing the amount of federal money for eczema research.

For more information on how the National Eczema Association supports health-care providers and their patients, go to www.nationaleczema.org or call, 415-499-3474.

References

1. CSD Members and Affiliates—Coalition of Skin Diseases. CSD Members and Affiliates—Coalition of Skin Diseases. Coalition of Skin Diseases. 2017. http://coalitionofskindiseases.org/members/. Accessed 29 Apr 2017.
2. Hibbard J, Greene J. What the evidence shows about patient activation: better health outcomes and care experiences; fewer data on costs. Health Affairs. 2013;32(2):207–14. https://doi.org/10.1377/hlthaff.2012.1061.
3. NEA Funded Research. National Eczema Association. 2013. https://nationaleczema.org/research/nea-funded-research/. Accessed 30 Apr 2017.

Index

© Springer International Publishing AG 2018
P.S. Yamauchi (ed.), *Biologic and Systemic Agents in Dermatology*, https://doi.org/10.1007/978-3-319-66884-0